Fundamentals of

COMPLEMENTARY
AND ALTERNATIVE
MEDICINE

Fourth Edition

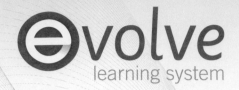
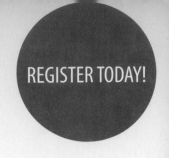
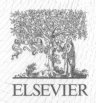

Fundamentals of
COMPLEMENTARY
AND ALTERNATIVE
MEDICINE

Fourth Edition

MARC S. MICOZZI, MD, PhD
Adjunct Professor
Department of Physiology & Biophysics
Georgetown University School of Medicine
Washington, DC;
Former Director
Center for Integrative Medicine
Thomas Jefferson University Hospital
Philadelphia, Pennsylvania

With forewords by

C. EVERETT KOOP, MD, ScD
Former Surgeon General of the United States;

AVIAD HARAMATI, PhD
Professor, Departments of Physiology & Biophysics and Medicine
Georgetown University School of Medicine
Washington, DC

and

GEORGE D. LUNDBERG, MD
Former Editor-in-Chief, Journal of the American Medical Association, 1982-1999; and
Medscape, The Medscape Journal of Medicine and eMedicine from WebMD, 1999-2009
Consulting Professor, Stanford University
President and Chair, The Lundberg Institute

SAUNDERS

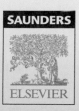

ELSEVIER

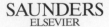

SAUNDERS
ELSEVIER

3251 Riverport Lane
St. Louis, Missouri 63043

Notices

Knowledge and best practice in this field are constantly changing. As new research and experience
broaden our understanding, changes in research methods, professional practices, or medical treatment
may become necessary.

Practitioners and researchers must always rely on their own experience and knowledge in evaluating
and using any information, methods, compounds, or experiments described herein. In using such
information or methods they should be mindful of their own safety and the safety of others, including
parties for whom they have a professional responsibility.

With respect to any drug or pharmaceutical products identified, readers are advised to check the
most current information provided (i) on procedures featured or (ii) by the manufacturer of each
product to be administered, to verify the recommended dose or formula, the method and duration of
administration, and contraindications. It is the responsibility of practitioners, relying on their own
experience and knowledge of their patients, to make diagnoses, to determine dosages and the best
treatment for each individual patient, and to take all appropriate safety precautions.

To the fullest extent of the law, neither the Publisher nor the authors, contributors, or editors,
assume any liability for any injury and/or damage to persons or property as a matter of products
liability, negligence or otherwise, or from any use or operation of any methods, products, instructions,
or ideas contained in the material herein.

Library of Congress Cataloging-in-Publication Data

Fundamentals of complementary and alternative medicine / [edited by] Marc S. Micozzi ; with forewords
by C. Everett Koop, Aviad Haramati, and George Lundberg. 4th ed.
    p. ; cm.
  Rev. ed. of: Fundamentals of complementary and integrative medicine. c2006.
  Includes bibliographical references and index.
  ISBN 978-1-4377-0577-5 (hardcover : alk. paper) 1. Alternative medicine. I. Micozzi, Marc S.,
1953- II. Fundamentals of complementary and integrative medicine.
  [DNLM: 1. Complementary Therapies. WB 890 F981 2011]
  R733.F86 2011
  615.5 dc22

              2009043446

Vice President and Publisher: Linda Duncan
Senior Editor: Kellie White
Senior Developmental Editor: Jennifer Watrous
Publishing Services Manager: Catherine Jackson
Senior Project Manager: David Stein
Design Direction: Amy Buxton

Printed in the United States

Last digit is the print number: 9 8 7 6 5 4 3 2

Dedicated to Edio D. Micozzi (1927-2007)
To my departed father Edio
Who taught me the Latin I needed to know
In modern medicine, question the *status quo*
And of it, remember to always ask, *cui bono*

Acknowledgment to the team at University of
Texas Medical Branch—Galveston who worked
by hurricane lamp during Hurricane Ike to
complete their chapters on time.

And new philosophy calls all in doubt
The element of fire is quite put out
The sun is lost, and the earth, and no man's wit
Can well direct him where to look for it

And freely men confess that this world's spent
When in the Planets, and the Firmament
They seek so many new; they see that this
Is crumbled out againe to his Atomies

'Tis all in pieces, all cohaerence gone;
All just supply, and all relation

John Donne (1572-1631),
Physician and Metaphysician,
Written in 1611

Contributors

Mones S. Abu-Asab, Ph.D.
Senior Research Biologist
Laboratory of Pathology
National Cancer Institute
National Institutes of Health
Bethesda, Maryland

Hunter "Patch" Adams, MD
Executive Director of Gesundheit Institute
Arlington, Virginia

Amy L. Ai, PhD
Professor, University of Pittsburgh
Pittsburgh, Pennsylvania

Hakima Amri, PhD
Director, CAM Master of Science Program in Physiology
Department of Physiology & Biophysics
Georgetown University Medical Center
Washington, DC

Donald A. Bisson, RRPr
Ontario College of Reflexology
New Liskeard, Ontario, Canada

Gerard C. Bodeker, EdD
Nuffield Department of Medicine
Division of Medical Sciences
University of Oxford;
Department of Epidemiology
Mailman School of Public Health
Columbia University
New York, New York

Emma Bragdon, PhD
Director of the Foundation for Energy Therapies, Inc.
Director of Spiritual Alliances, LLC
Woodstock, Vermont

Michael Carlston, MD
Editorial Advisory Board,
HOMEOPATHY: The Journal of the Faculty of Homeopathy
Private Practice
Santa Rosa, California

Claire Monod Cassidy, PhD, Dipl Ac, LAc
Director, Windpath Healing Works, LLC
Bethesda, Maryland

Patrick Coughlin, PhD
Professor, Department of Anatomy
Philadelphia College of Osteopathic Medicine
Philadelphia, Pennsylvania

Judith DeLany, LMT
Director, Neuromuscular Therapy Center
St. Petersburg, Florida

Kevin V. Ergil, MA, MS, LAc
Associate Professor, Finger Lakes School of Acupuncture
   and Oriental Medicine of New York Chiropractic
   College
Seneca Falls, New York

Marnae C. Ergil, MA, MS, LAc
Professor, Finger Lakes School of Acupuncture
   and Oriental Medicine of New York Chiropractic
   College
Seneca Falls, New York

Susan M. Gerik, MD
Associate Professor of Pediatrics and Family Medicine
University of Texas Medical Branch
Galveston, Texas

Sherry W. Goodill, PhD, BC-DMT, NCC, LPC
Clinical Professor and Chairperson
Department of Creative Arts Therapies
Drexel University
Philadelphia, Pennsylvania

Howard Hall, PhD, PsyD, BCB
Associate Professor
Division of Developmental/Behavioral Pediatrics
   and Psychology
Rainbow Babies and Children's Hospital
Case Medical Center
Cleveland, Ohio

Rhiannon Harris, FIFPA
Editor-in-Chief, International Journal of Clinical
   Aromatherapy
Provence, France

Mariana G. Hewson, PhD
Synthesis Consulting in Healthcare and Education
Madison, Wisconsin

John A. Ives, PhD
Director, Brain, Mind, and Healing
Samueli Institute
Alexandria, Virginia

Wayne B. Jonas, MD
President and CEO
Samueli Institute
Alexandria, Virginia

John M. Jones, DO, MEd
Professor of Family Medicine
Chair, Department of Osteopathic Principles
   and Practice
William Carey University College of Osteopathic
   Medicine
Hattiesburg, Mississippi

Joseph Katzinger, ND
Salugenecists, Inc.
Shoreline, Washington

Richard A. Lippin, MD
Founder, International Arts-Medicine Association
Southampton, Pennsylvania

David F. Mayor, MA, BAc, MBAcC
Research Associate, Department of Physiotherapy
University of Hertfordshire
Hatfield, United Kingdom
Undergraduate and MSc Supervisor
London College of Traditional Acupuncture
   and Oriental Medicine
London, United Kingdom

Donald McCown, MAMS, MSS, LSW
The Mindfulness Institute
Jefferson-Myrna Brind Center of Integrative Medicine
Philadelphia, Pennsylvania

Radheshyam Miryala, MD
Assistant Professor of Surgery, Division of Emergency
   Medicine
Assistant Professor of Family Medicine, University
   of Texas Medical Branch
Galveston, Texas

Daniel E. Moerman, PhD
William E. Stirton Professor Emeritus of Anthropology
University of Michigan-Dearborn
Dearborn, Michigan

Paul Nolan, MCAT, MT-BC, LPC
Director of Music Therapy Programs
Department of Creative Arts Therapies
Drexel University
Philadelphia, Pennsylvania

Kerry Palanjian, MBA
Principal, Shiatsu On-Site
Corporate Massage Services
Hatboro, Pennsylvania

Joseph E. Pizzorno, Jr, ND
Editor-in-Chief, *Integrative Medicine, A Clinician's Journal*
Seattle, Washington;
President Emeritus
Bastyr University
Kenmore, Washington

Daniel Redwood, DC
Associate Professor, Cleveland Chiropractic College,
   Kansas City
Overland Park, Missouri

Denise Rodgers MDiv
Association for Development of Mind/Body Potential
Bastrop, Texas

**Hari M. Sharma, MD, DABP, FCAP, FRCPC,
   DABHM**
Professor Emeritus
Former Director, Division of Cancer Prevention
   and Natural Products Research
Department of Pathology, College of Medicine
Provider for Ayurveda, Center for Integrative
   Medicine
The Ohio State University
Columbus, Ohio;
Chair, Integrated Medicine Committee, American
   Association of Physicians of Indian Origin
Fellow, National Academy of Ayurveda, Ministry
   of Health and Family Welfare, Government
   of India

Victor S. Sierpina, MD
WD and Laura Nell Nicholson Family Professor of
   Integrative Medicine Professor, Family Medicine
University of Texas Distinguished Teaching
   Professor
University of Texas Medical Branch
Galveston, Texas

Devna Singh, MD
Family Medicine and Integrative Medicine Practitioner
Optimal Health Dimensions
Fairfax, Virginia

Pamela Snider, ND
Executive and Senior Editor
Foundations of Naturopathic Medicine Project
Associate Professor, National College of Natural
    Medicine
Portland, Oregon

Kevin Spelman, PhD, MCPP
Bioanalytical Chemistry and Drug Discovery Section
National Institute on Aging
Baltimore, Maryland

Robert T. Trotter II, PhD
Arizona Regent's Professor
Department of Anthropology
Northern Arizona University
Flagstaff, Arizona

Christine Vlahos, MSPT
Sloane Stecker Physical Therapy
New York, New York

Richard W. Voss, DPC, MSW, MTS
Professor of Social Work
West Chester University
West Chester, Pennsylvania

Michael I. Weintraub MD, FACP, FAAN, FAHA
Clinical Professor of Neurology and Internal Medicine
New York Medical College
Valhalla, New York;
Adjunct Clinical Professor of Neurology
Mt. Sinai School of Medicine
New York, New York

Kenneth G. Zysk, PhD, DPhil
Department of Cross-Cultural and Regional Studies
University of Copenhagen
Copenhagen, Denmark

Reviewers

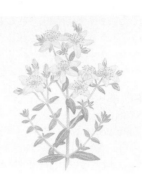

Maryalyse Adams Mercado, MD
First Choice Community Healthcare
Department of Family Medicine
Albuquerque, New Mexico

David A. Bray, CMD, DAc, Dipl. CH (NCCAOM)
Guangzhou University of Traditional Chinese Medicine
Hunan University of Traditional Chinese Medicine
Toronto, Ontario

Todd Caldecott, ClH, RH(AHG)
Vancouver, British Columbia

Lisa Ann Conboy, MA, MS, ScD
Instructor
Osher Research Center
Harvard Medical School
Boston, Massachusetts

Gautam Desai, DO, FACOFP
Kansas City University of Medicine and Biosciences
Associate Professor of Family Medicine, Executive
    Director, Kesselheim Center for Clinical Competence/
    Family Medicine
Kansas City, Missouri

Joan Engebretson, DrPH, AHN-BC, RN
University of Texas Health Science Center—Houston
Professor/School of Nursing, Department of Integrated
    Nursing Care
Houston, Texas

Tyson Gibbs, PhD
Associate Professor
Department of Anthropology
University of North Texas
Dallas, Texas

Earlene Gleisner, Reiki Master, RN
Laytonville, California

Richard Gold, PhD, LAc
Pacific College of Oriental Medicine
Professor/Asian Body Therapy
San Diego, California

**Yoon-Hang (John) Kim, MD, MPH, DABMA
    (MD MPH FAAMA)**
Georgia Integrative Medicine
Tyrone, Georgia

Mitchell Kossak, PhD
Lesley University
Division Director/Expressive Therapies
Cambridge, Massachusetts

Margaret Krassy, EdD, MPH, RN,C
Holistic Impressions
Alternative Medicine Consultant and Educator
Great Falls, Virginia

Ruth Levy, MA Expressive Therapies, MSW, LICSW
Lesley University
Assistant Professor, Assistant Director/Expressive
    Therapies Division
Cambridge, Massachusetts

Anne McCaffrey, MD, MPH
Medical Director
Marino Center for Integrative Health
Cambridge, Massachusetts

Anthony A. Miller, MEd, PA-C
Professor & Director
Division of Physician Assistant Studies
Winchester, Virginia

Susan Salvo, BEd, LMT, NTS, CI, NCTMB
Louisiana Institute of Massage Therapy
Practitioner, Instructor, Author
Lake Charles, Louisiana

Robert Schwartz, ND, LAc
Physician, Gorge Family Health and Aesthetic
    Medical Center
The Dalles, Oregon

Elaine Stillerman, LMT
Mother Massage
New York, New York

Catherine Ulbricht, PharmD, MBA
Natural Standard Research Collaboration
Adjunct Assistant Professor/School of Pharmacy
Somerville, Massachusetts

Lisa Upledger, DC, FIAMA, CST-D
Upledger Institute
Palm Beach Gardens, Florida

Joy Weydert, MD
Children's Mercy Hospital and Clinics
Kansas City, Missouri

Beth Wolfgram, MS, RD, CSSD, CD, CSCS
Adjunct Faculty Member & Sports Dietitian/Nutrition
    Department and Athletic Department
University of Utah
Salt Lake City, Utah

Foreword

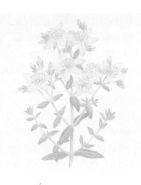

For more than 50 years I have tried to identify the mix of personal attributes and technical skills that make one an outstanding doctor. I am sure that most physicians in the United States have pondered the same question. Now, through the work of the C. Everett Koop Institute at Dartmouth I have an opportunity to influence the way medical students are trained. The Institute, working in partnership with the Dartmouth Medical School and the Dartmouth-Hitchcock Medical Center, is actively engaged in training physicians for the new century.

Because doctors must remain abreast of a growing volume of new information, our medical schools help both their graduates and society by producing physicians who are computer literate and comfortable with telemedicine. As a scientific pursuit, medicine should take advantage of the technologic innovations that allow us to better serve the lifetime learning needs of physicians as well as the health education needs of patients. Nonetheless, because medicine is also an art, doctors still need to listen to their patients. This aspect of medical practice has not changed.

As I travel across the country many of the people I meet are eager to share their ideas for improving the nation's health care system. The most common complaint I hear focuses on poor communication in the doctor-patient relationship. Too many patients feel that their physician does not really listen to them. When the patient attempts to explain his or her problem, the doctor interrupts. Subsequently, when the doctor tries to explain what conditions the patient has and attempts to outline a treatment regimen, the patient is confused because the physician does not communicate to the level of the patient's understanding.

From my perspective, medical students need to master the art of listening to and communicating with their patients just as much as they need to learn the fundamentals of human biology. We have found at the Koop Institute that a student's communication skills are greatly improved by having to explain the first principles of health promotion and disease prevention to second graders. Medical students who choose to participate in programs sponsored by the Koop Institute work in and with local communities from their very first year. Some choose to advise junior high and high school students on the

risks associated with alcohol, tobacco, and sexually transmitted diseases; others help rural physicians take better advantage of the computer revolution.

Just as a physician should be sensitive to the feelings of a patient and the needs of the community, he or she must be conversant with major trends and developments in society. I would like to tell you about one current trend that is of interest to me. Studies conducted at Harvard Medical School and reported in the *New England Journal of Medicine* focused on attitudes toward complementary and alternative medicine in the United States. They indicate that one-third of adult Americans regularly use some kind of complementary or alternative treatment even though it was not covered by insurance and they had to pay for it themselves. This is an opportune time for us to take a second look at such alternative treatment approaches as acupuncture, botanical medicine, homeopathy, and others; not to offer these treatment modalities blindly but to expose them to the scientific method. Physicians have to depend on facts—on empirical data—when they determine treatment strategy for a particular patient. Today we do not have enough data on the potential of alternative approaches to help or harm human health. It is time to discover the value of these treatment regimens. We can conduct the necessary studies and assemble the data that doctors and health policy makers need, a type of biomedical research that would be a prudent long-term investment.

In my lifetime we have achieved great successes in the fight against infectious diseases. We have more work to do in our effort to improve the quality of life and make people more comfortable as they endure chronic health problems such as cancer, heart disease, and arthritis. Drugs and surgery can be useful tools in the effort to treat these diseases, but when possible I would like to see us increase the range of approaches that can be used. My experience as a doctor has taught me that often a mix of different approaches is necessary to achieve success. We need to be flexible and adaptable because the diseases that challenge us certainly are not static.

A recent trend that concerns me is the growth of drug-resistant bacteria. Today it is easy to forget that prior to the development of antibiotics in the 1940s a child's ear infection could be a frightening and fatal experience. I well remember patients with serious complications and death caused by the lack of antibiotics. If drugs we have depended on for decades are compromised, we may return to a time when even routine infections could be dangerous. As both a grandfather and a physician, I would hate to see that happen.

There is an element of good news in this picture. If some of the synthetic drugs we have developed are no longer as dependable as they once were, studies have shown that the botanical substances these drugs are based on are still effective in treating disease. I have never claimed to be an expert on botany or ecology, but current trends suggest that we need to do more. We need to conserve the plants that may contain the medicines of the future and, more important, we need to learn what local experts seem to understand about the pharmacologic properties and uses of these medicines.

Reduced health care costs are an important by-product of the work we are doing at the Koop Institute. Our students know that the physician of the future must be a health educator first and foremost. Today, the challenge is to treat the patient once he or she has gone to the hospital. Tomorrow, the challenge will be to keep the patient out of the hospital in the beginning.

Preventive medicine means education, empowerment, and personal responsibility. Many patients want alternatives to invasive medical procedures and long stays in the hospital. Physicians can conserve time and resources by teaching patients how to reduce their risk of cancer, heart disease, and other life-threatening diseases. As our students know, the most inexpensive treatment is to keep the patient from becoming sick in the first place. Demand reduction in the health care system is the most immediate cost-saving effort.

I think that alternative/complementary therapies may potentially be an important part of this overall educational process. One must have an open mind about complementary therapies and understand belief systems that emphasize the mind-body connection. At a time when many Americans complain of stress, make poor nutritional choices, and are increasingly concerned about environmentally induced illnesses these messages could not be more timely.

Many people are confused about alternative medicine, and I do not blame them. For many Americans alternative therapies represent a *new* discovery, but in truth, many of these traditions are hundreds or thousands of years old and have been used by millions of people worldwide. To ease the uncomfortableness of the word *alternative* one must realize that while treatments may look like alternatives to us, they have long been part of the medical mainstream in their cultures of origin.

When I worked in Washington as Surgeon General for 8 years, President Reagan had an important credo in his approach to foreign policy: "Trust but verify!" So it is with complementary and alternative medicine. So many people have relied on these approaches for so long that they may have something of value to offer. Let us begin the necessary research so that we could have substantive answers in the near future.

One reason such research is worth doing is that 80% of the world's people depend on these alternative approaches as their primary medical care. For years, we have attempted to export Western medicine to the developing world. The sad truth is that the people we are attempting to help simply cannot afford it. I have doubts about how much longer we can afford some of it ourselves. It is possible that in this new millennium, we may be more ready to ask the peoples of the developing world to share their wisdom with us.

During the nineteenth century, American medicine was an eclectic pursuit where a number of competing ideas and approaches thrived. Doctors were able to draw on elements from different traditions in attempting to make people well. Perhaps there is more to this older model of American medicine than we in the twentieth century had been willing to examine. My experience with physicians has convinced me that they are healers first. As such, they are willing to use any ethical approach or treatment that has been proven to work. However, in the opinion of many doctors, there is not yet a definitive answer on the value of complementary and alternative medicine. I would like us to undertake the study and research that will provide definitive answers to prudent questions about the usefulness of complementary and alternative medicine for society at large.

C. Everett Koop, MD, ScD
Former Surgeon General of the United States
Senior Scholar, The Koop Institute at Dartmouth,
Hanover, New Hampshire

Foreword

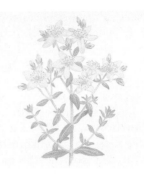

As I write these words in early February 2010, I am returning from my first trip to India. The purpose of my visit was to lead a delegation of six prominent leaders in Complementary and Integrative Medicine from prestigious academic medical centers in the United States at the invitation of the Ministry of Health in India, Department of AYUSH (Ayurveda, Yoga, Unani, Siddah, and Homeopathy). The expressed goal of the Indian Government was to inform our delegation about the evidence-base for Ayurvedic Medicine, and to give us first-hand exposure to the use of traditional Indian medicine in clinical practice and in education, and to explore potential research projects in this area. My own specific objective was to determine whether anything we saw or heard about Traditional Indian Medicine should eventually be included in the curriculum for physicians and other health professionals in the United States.

What struck me during this intense 7-day visit, was the chasm that exists, even in India, between those trained in traditional medical practices and those trained in Western allopathic medicine. Many of the traditionalists feel that centuries of continued practice provides sufficient rationale for the use of various medical approaches (what in Europe constitutes "historic use" in terms of regulatory approval), irrespective of whether these therapies have been "proven" by modern scientific means, whereas most of those conventionally trained express a healthy skepticism and demand clear and unambiguous data to support the use of any therapy or medicinal plant.

This tension is very familiar to me. A decade ago, I helped launch a public lecture series on complementary and alternative medicine (CAM) at Georgetown University School of Medicine. At that time, a fellow colleague and I established a "mini-medical school" series at Georgetown University aimed at informing the public about the advances in medical science and health. For several years, over 200 men, women, and young adults, ranging in age from 16 to 83 years, would come to the medical center on 8 Tuesday nights in the Fall and Spring semesters to hear some of our finest faculty teachers lecture on a myriad of medical issues. In response to our surveys inviting suggestions for future topics, many participants kept requesting lectures on CAM. Initially, we did not know what to make of these requests, but eventually we invited our fellow faculty member, Dr. Hakima Amri, to develop an eight-lecture series on CAM.

Thus began my education into this field, and I quickly realized that the public was eager to learn more about these treatment approaches and ancient medical systems. In contrast, the academic medical community was, in general, wary of venturing into areas many deemed unproven and unscientific. Our purpose in offering the public lecture series on CAM was to provide the best evidence available for what was harmful, what was safe and beneficial, and what aspects of CAM were simply unknown or untested.

This initial foray into a rather controversial field bore fruit. In December 1999, in an effort that demonstrated considerable courage, the leadership at the National Center for Complementary and Alternative Medicine at the National Institutes of Health issued a call for grant proposals from allopathic schools (conventional medicine and nursing) to develop curricular modules that would integrate CAM into the conventional training of physicians and other health professionals. The initiative led to important interactions between like-minded academic leaders of Integrative Medicine who were interested in determining, in an objective fashion, what aspects of CAM ought to be part of a medical curriculum. Those initial efforts led to a landmark series of articles that were published in the October 2007 issue of *Academic Medicine*, which addressed such topics as *rationale for CAM education in health professions training programs, what should students learn about CAM, and instructional strategies for integrating CAM into the medical curriculum.*

At Georgetown University School of Medicine, in addition to introducing CAM-relevant material into the medical and nursing curricula, our faculty in the Department of Physiology and Biophysics created an innovative graduate degree program of study in CAM. The mission of the program is to provide advanced study in the science and philosophy of predominant CAM therapies and disciplines and to train students to objectively assess the safety and efficacy of various CAM modalities. The program seeks to understand the mechanistic basis for CAM therapies such as acupuncture, massage, herbs and supplements, and mind-body interactions. By embedding CAM principles and paradigms firmly into a conventional basic/clinical sciences context, our intent is to prepare a new generation of health care providers, educators, and researchers for the challenging task of delivering the health care of the future; namely, a multidisciplinary approach to improved wellness emphasizing health maintenance and disease prevention.

However, literacy in CAM, for students and faculty in our program, as well as for others around the nation, depends on an authoritative, comprehensive textbook that can provide the basic information regarding the philosophy and science for many of the CAM therapies. Fortunately, Dr. Marc Micozzi has done the field a great service by producing an outstanding text, entitled, *Fundamentals of Complementary and Alternative Medicine*. Joined by a list of distinguished experts in the field of complementary and integrative medicine, Dr. Micozzi introduces the reader to the foundations of CAM, the contexts for the use of CAM, and thorough, evidence-based descriptions of the predominant CAM therapies and traditional medical systems. The writing is easy to understand and the focus is sharp. Each chapter is referenced appropriately, and the reader is directed to several suggested additional readings. For the past few years, my colleagues at Georgetown have relied on this excellent work and have made it required reading for our program. In the new fourth edition, Dr. Micozzi has made significant additions to the scope of the textbook, including a new and important section on mind-body-spirit.

It is essential that the health care practitioner of the future, either in the United States or elsewhere in the world, be able to bridge the current chasm between conventional and traditional medicine. Recently, the Consortium of Academic Health Centers for Integrative Medicine (www.imconsortium.org) defined Integrative Medicine as *"the practice of medicine that reaffirms the importance of the relationship between practitioner and patient, focuses on the whole person, is informed by evidence, and makes use of all appropriate therapeutic approaches, healthcare professionals and disciplines to achieve optimal health and healing."* If we are to produce practitioners who can truly address the needs of their patients, they must be knowledgeable about all therapeutic approaches, both conventional and those from other traditions, and be willing and interested to develop working relationships with practitioners from various disciplines. This textbook by Dr. Micozzi goes a long way in providing the reader with a fundamental understanding of complementary and integrative medicine. It is a journey worth taking and on which we at Georgetown University have seriously embarked.

Aviad Haramati, PhD
February 2010

Your "Good Medicine" Guide to CAM

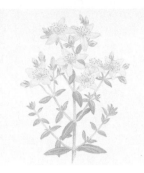

There is no complementary or alternative medicine (CAM). There is only medicine; medicine that has been tested and found to be safe and effective—use it; pay for it. Medicine that has been tested and found not to be safe and effective—don't use it; don't pay for it. And medicine that is plausible but has not been tested—test it; and then place it into one of the two prime categories. If safe and effective, integrate it into mainstream medicine. Strange as it may seem to some readers, this prescription for action applies equally to medical practices taught in standard "Western" medical schools and practiced by licensed U.S. MDs and also to all those practices taught in those "other" health education institutions and practiced by so-called "alternative" practitioners. Sadly, there are many diagnostic and therapeutic practices in both camps yet to be properly tested and acted on.

The landmark theme issue of JAMA published in late 1998 demonstrated that it was possible, and responsible, to apply well-established scientific methods to the study of many CAM practices and begin that great parsing into "safe and effective" or "not safe or effective." That JAMA also convincingly illustrated that it was respectable for U.S. MDs to talk seriously with their patients about CAM. The science of CAM (yes or no) is much clearer now; some CAM works, much does not.

Americans, and people of all countries, use the methods and products called CAM, for better or worse. They deserve such medical treatments to be informed by "best evidence." Doctors of many types and the public observe patients improving, even recovering, after an encounter with a "healer," regardless of the modality that healer applied. Such anecdotal experiences lead patients and practitioners to believe, even fervently, that the modality applied caused the therapeutic success, when actually only time and biology produced the success.

There is a vast historical, cultural, experiential, and increasingly clinical and evidentiary literature about that body of practice termed "CAM." I know of no other one place where the interested reader can find a better collection of accurate and objective information about such CAM as the Micozzi text, *Fundamentals of Complementary and Alternative Medicine,* now into its fourth edition (first edition, 1996). Those persons who are biased (and there are still many) both for and against CAM in general and with specific CAM modalities may or may not be swayed by the voluminous content in this 624-page tome. But the editor Marc Micozzi, MD, PhD, and his 50 assembled authors deserve our thanks and praise for bringing us this detailed and compelling updated product to clarify this field of increasing importance as it becomes more and more integrated into the mainstream.

George Lundberg, MD
January 2010

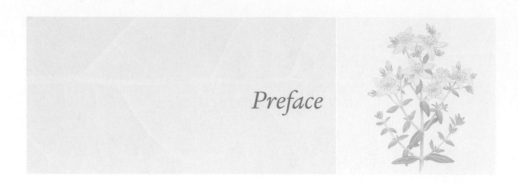

Preface

BACKGROUND

During the U.S. Bicentennial Year of 1976/77 I had the opportunity to live, study, and work in East and Southeast Asia, during which I was exposed to a much broader perspective on health and healing than what I had theretofore been able to observe in western premedical and medical education. My scholarship was awarded by the Henry Luce Foundation, New York, NY, which has sent 35 consecutive groups of 15 graduate students each year to work in Asia. The Luce Scholars are comprised of graduate students in law, journalism, architecture, fine arts, philosophy, and other topics, and my exposure to students outside medicine was just as enlightening to developing a broader perspective on medicine as a social institution as well as a science.

Pointedly, while I was in my room in New York (at the old St. Regis Hotel) where the final interviews were being held to select the Luce Scholars for 1976, Ivan Illich, MD, had appeared on *Good Morning America* to discuss his new book *Medical Nemesis*. His arguments helped bring home the **need** to find alternatives to the invasive, high-cost, high-tech medicine of the late twentieth century, even while Asian and indigenous medical systems provided me the **opportunity** to observe real choices in healing, providing a balance to the excesses of western biomedicine.

These experiences have profoundly influenced my work, and especially the creation of these texts, over the past 30 years. Today, students are able to learn about these healing traditions without traveling to Asia or studying traditional societies, in light of new curricula being offered such as that at Georgetown University School of Medicine.

This book is now being used in programs such as the Master's Degree in Physiology, CAM Track at Georgetown University School of Medicine, now graduating its sixth consecutive class. This program and others are an example of how the medical curriculum is being supplemented to give health professions students the tools to understand a broader perspective in medicine and to be prepared to work in a post-biomedical paradigm. Students take science-based courses, acquire CAM-related knowledge, and learn the skills to critically analyze the available

evidence of CAM studies. I wish to here acknowledge the inspiration that comes from teaching these students each year and the creativity of the faculty members working together under the directorship of Dr. Hakima Amri (who is a contributor to this text and my co-author on our chapter in the "Mind Body" section, and in an upcoming Elsevier publication) as well as all those who have supported and nourished this program.

BENEFIT OF THIS BOOK TO THE HEALTH PROFESSIONS

The need for more *science* is often identified as an issue in understanding alternative/complementary therapies. In this textbook we address that issue, and also answer the need for more *sciences* in the study of CAM. For example, the social sciences are also critical for an understanding of the foundations of human knowledge and experience that underlay and support the practice of ancient healing traditions, which we call here complementary/alternative medicine and which social scientists, such as medical anthropologists, call ethnomedicine. For those many readers of this textbook, now entering its fourth edition, it is important to realize that among other things, this work is a complete textbook of medical approaches to healing. New chapters on Siddha and Unani Medicine and South American ethnomedical healing traditions enhance and round out our coverage of the world's great healing traditions. This text brings forward the best scholarship on ancient healing traditions in application to our understanding of CAM. Some of the earliest translations of classical medical texts were not very sophisticated in terms of the medical terminology used for translation into English. With contemporary scholarship and translations we now see that it was not the ancient healing traditions that appeared unsophisticated but the old English translations.

For those with an orientation to understanding from where this knowledge originates and how it has been promulgated as part of our global cultural patrimony, we must move beyond the standard basic science curriculum of modern medical education and the clinical trials, protocols, and "cookbook recipes" of "integrative medicine."

CONTENTS AND ORGANIZATION

The format of the book has been expanded into six sections instead of four for this edition. The first section serves as an introduction to the field of complementary and alternative medicine, discussing the history, characteristics, translation, and issues in alternative and integrative medicine. The sections next move into the subjects of ecology, vitalism, psychoneuroimmunology, mind-body approaches, and biophysical devices. Given this foundation, the book then moves the reader into thorough descriptions of the development and key concepts of the most prevalent complementary and alternative therapies being used in the United States. Topics covered include homeopathy, massage and manual therapies, chiropractic, osteopathy (new chapter), herbal medicine, aromatherapy, naturopathic medicine, and nutrition and hydration. There are also two unique appendices on herbal medicine, located on the Evolve site to accompany this book: common herbs in clinical practice, and Native American herbs.

The section on Mind-Body Medicine provides an overview of all mind-body medical modalities, including background on neurohumoral physiology and psychoneuroimmunology (PNI), energy healing (new chapter), biophysical modalities and devices (new chapter), creative arts and movement therapies (new chapter), and humor. The final two sections introduce and provide comprehensive overviews of the traditional medical systems of Chinese medicine: acupuncture, (new chapter) Qi Gong, shiatsu, Tibetan medicine (located on the Evolve website) and Ayurveda, the traditional medicines of India, and Yoga, as well as Siddha, Sufism, and Unani Medicine. The sixth and final section continues the global perspective with discussions of healing systems from Africa and the Americas.

In addition to providing background from the biological sciences, this book takes a broader approach compared with other texts on complementary, alternative, and integrative medicine. The social sciences, including social history and medical anthropology, provide the origins of the underlying science that informs one unique approach of this text to the study of CAM. In this edition, the Preface and the introductory section is meant to serve as a primer for those students and faculty who wish to use this work as a foundational text in the "basic sciences" of health and healing.

The behavioral and social sciences generally, and medical anthropology in particular, provide a disciplined approach (literally, as academic disciplines and as fields of practice) to understanding human biology and culture, and human nature in the context of nature, as particularly relevant to the naturalistic approaches of

alternative/complementary medicine, and what is, in fact, often called "natural medicine." These approaches have tremendous value in understanding the aspects of medical practice and healthcare that are compelled, or chosen, and those that represent true alternatives on a global basis. Although biomedical science and clinical trials provide many answers to human medicine, we here offer an approach whereby other kinds of knowledge about health and healing may additionally be brought to bear in a serious and disciplined manner. Thus this expanded fourth edition of *Fundamentals of Complementary and Alternative Medicine* presents the world's healing traditions, including those from the western world, that continue to offer real alternatives and choices for health and healing to both practitioners and patients in the twenty-first century.

EVOLVE WEBSITE

New to this edition is a companion website, located at http://www.evolve.elsevier.com/Micozzi/complementary. Follow the directions to sign up for these free resources:
* References for all chapters in the book
* Image collection
* Tibetan Medicine chapter
* Native American and common herb appendices
* Discussion questions for each chapter

As you read, this Evolve icon ⊜ indicates there is additional material on the website that will enhance the book's content.

NOTE TO THE READER

While recovering and re-interpreting the ancient and traditional knowledge and wisdom about health and healing as now proven by contemporary scientific investigations, it is also important to take what we have learned about medicine in the twentieth century and form a new synthesis that represents a whole, or truly "holistic" approach, for the twenty-first century. We must be prepared to live in a post-biomedical paradigm. Consumers described by social scientists as "cultural creatives" (numbering some 50 million people) are already there. This text provides the fundamentals to the health professions to be prepared to meet them, and help lead them, to a better, more optimistic, more complete kind of healthcare that recognizes the limits of biomedical technology as well as the limitless possibilities of human capabilities and the boundless human spirit.

FINIS
Marc S. Micozzi
February 2010

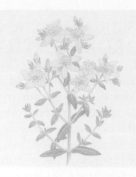

Introduction

THE ROLE OF SCIENCES IN MEDICINE

In addition to the biological sciences, the social sciences, including social history and medical anthropology, provide the origins of the underlying disciplines that inform the approach of this text to the study of CAM. In this edition, the Preface and Introduction are meant to serve as a primer for those students and faculty who wish to use this work as a foundational text in all the "basic sciences" of health and healing.

HOW TRADITIONAL MEDICAL SYSTEMS CAN BE UNDERSTOOD

Anthropology is a relatively recent discipline that studies traditional beliefs and behaviors in human societies. Taking the perspective of George Stocking, an anthropologist and historian, we can see how anthropology evolved in the academic arena to study peoples, times, and places that had not already been "claimed" by other established academic disciplines in the early twentieth century. From a contemporary standpoint, most scholars that we think of as "historians" consider themselves *social historians,* while they think of anthropologists as *cultural historians.* The whole concept of culture itself can be seen as a uniquely American contribution to the field of anthropology and more broadly social sciences. This feature (culture) also distinguished American anthropology from British-European social anthropology during the early twentieth century until British anthropologist A. Radcliffe-Brown taught at the University of Chicago and began building a bridge between the two.

With the appearance of anthropology on the scene as an academic discipline, it emerged where historians had long been studying the past through their analysis of documentary records (documentary history) and where early archaeologists were unearthing cultural materials from the past. Thus one domain of early anthropology became the study literally of "pre-historic man," that is, the study of the biology and, where possible, culture of humans who existed before written languages (prehistory). Human societies that predate written languages and records thus became a domain of anthropology. Recovery of early fossils of hominids provided the basis for studying biology, and the recruitment of archaeology for recovering artifacts (such as stone tools, and so forth) became the basis for studying prehistoric technology and culture. Anthropology found a niche among the prior academic disciplines of History, Oriental Studies, Classics, and other pillars of academia.

Since anthropology was able to study human biology and culture from "pre-historic" humans, a logical extension was to "pre-literate" or "primitive peoples" in the contemporary world of the late nineteenth century where there were likewise no documents or written records available. Therefore the spoken language (vs. written records) became another route to understanding through the development of anthropological linguistics. The colonial experiences of this era provided ample opportunity for European anthropologists to study "primitive" peoples where there were no written records.

The United States at the end of the nineteenth century presented a different picture than that of Europe and its colonies in Africa and Asia. In the United States, Native Americans were fast disappearing peoples who also did not have written records, thus lending themselves to study by the new field of anthropology. Franz Boas was an immigrant to the United States from Europe and become known as the "Founder" of American Anthropology. He studied both **biology and culture** (a useful alliance for medical anthropology). In contrast to European social anthropology, which sought *generalizable rules* for the **structure and function** of human societies, because Boas and American anthropologists encountered peoples and societies that were fast disappearing from the earth, they became interested in the *unique features* of each group or tribe—thus the concept of **culture.** The early methods of American anthropology relied on the "informant interview" reflected as early as the publications of the *Bureau of American Ethnology* in the 1880s. In describing interviews with the Lakota Sioux, for example, there is a repeating footnote: "But *Two Crows* denied this," in distinction to what other members of his tribe generally answered to questions regarding their customs. While building a consensual view of what constituted culture as *shared, learned knowledge and behavior,* it was recognized even at the dawn of ethnography that there are variations within the *culture*. This insight opened the door to the eventual anthropological study of *personality* within culture (famously by Ruth Benedict during WWII, a student of Alfred Kroeber at the University of California—Berkeley, who in turn had been a student of Boas).

The once centrality of the **informant interview** methodology is illustrated by Boas himself at turn of the twentieth century. He was studying the Native Americans of the Northwest Coast of North America (who are unique in representing a culture that practiced sedentism—living in permanent settlements vs. nomadic encampments—but without engaging in agriculture). His field notes have an entry: "Today was wasted. I could not talk to anyone because they all went to *potlatch*." In the later development of the methodology of **participant observation,** watching the potlatch itself would become central in understanding the social functioning of these peoples in addition to simply asking them about their beliefs and behaviors.

Through the evolution of anthropology it thus came to have these attributes:

a. Theory: humans have biology and culture (and both have been and are evolving)
b. Methodology: informant interview, participant observation
c. Principles: through biology and culture humans interact with, and adapt to, their environments
d. Practices: understanding human biology and culture, and their interplay, in ways that enhance human success at sustenance, subsistence, reproduction, and health (and the counter-argument that some human behavior is not adaptive, or maladaptive, for the species—but in fact may be protective for other species on earth, as per the Gaia Hypothesis of Chapter 4)

These academic approaches can be applied specifically to the study of health and disease. Taking the approach of physical anthropology to human biology and evolutionary biology, biological attributes can be seen as adaptations to the environment in [what is now called] *Health Ecology*. A particular emphasis on human biology, understanding biological evolution, is known as *Evolutionary Biology* or *Darwinian Biology*. These academic orientations add to our understanding of human health, complementing the essentially typological approach of modern, reductionist biomedical science.

At a meeting of the American Anthropological Association in Denver in 1986, the ethnographer George Foster (who had written the seminal ethnography, *The Image of Limited Good* (1965), to explain agrarian, peasant societies) stated: *"Medical anthropology does best when it contributes to anthropological theory and method."* At this end of the spectrum, medical anthropology is another domain for extension of classical anthropology into human health and medical practices. At the other end of the spectrum is the application of medical anthropology to help improve the health of the world's peoples. Medical anthropology as *applied anthropology* involves those with the academic training in anthropological theory and methods, and principles, studying the health of specific populations, and using those studies to improve access to health care, and health and nutritional status, of affected populations. Medical anthropologists also work as part of health care teams in *clinical anthropology* to help deliver care with *cultural competence* to those from other cultural traditions. In a general sense, medical anthropologists through their studies of population health can help formulate national health policies, and bilateral and multilateral international health assistance programs.

CAM AS ETHNOMEDICINE

The development of ethnoscience and ethnomedicine in the 1960's provided a basis for seeing indigenous health traditions as part of culture and empirical systems of knowledge that are rational and adaptive. Thus early western perceptions moved away from ethnomedicine as "superstition, myth and magic," in, for example, Sir James Frazier's *The Golden Bough,* in the late nineteenth century. WHR Rivers, the British anthropologist and physician (a common combination at that time), established as early as the 1920's that what we call ethnomedicine today represents an internally ordered, rational system of beliefs about health and disease that is generally adaptive to a given environment and provides a society as part of its culture with tools to cope with illness and disease. These tools almost always include the use of *materia medica,* primarily plants, from the local environment that are biologically active and have medicinal properties. A premise of *ethnobotany* is: just as it is adaptive for peoples to learn to harvest or grow plants for foods, [thus] they learn as part of culture to harvest or grow plants for medicines. Ethnomedicine includes the capability both to *diagnose* and to *treat* illnesses. Ethnomedical theories of disease and illness include the development of classification typologies based on the causation of diseases. In the mind-body continuum of ethnomedicine, disease causation systems may be based on naturalistic causes (as we would find analogies in western biomedicine) and/or personalistic (or supernatural) causes. Ideas about disease originating from curses, voodoo deaths (which have actually been documented in western medicine, see my book with Michael Jawer, *The Spiritual Anatomy of Emotion*, Rochester VT: Park Street Press, 2007), and envy as a source of illness, are personalistic causes. Foster's *Image of Limited Good* (1965) describes how curses arise from envy; the admiring eye is the "Evil Eye," so that "good" must be either hidden or shared. A heavy emphasis on the ethos of sharing in a culture may underlie a deep-seated image of limited good. Disorders in the division of good lead to illness; a disorder in the community leads to a disorder in the human body.

There are also diseases that literally blow into the body, such as *hangin*, or "wind sickness" of Southeast Asia, and *susto*, or startle response. These causations may straddle the personalistic and the natural. The paper on "Classification of Skin Diseases Among the Subanum," in an early anthology of medical anthropology, compiled by David Landy in 1977, illustrates several features. While the Subanum generally agreed among themselves as to the categories of skin diseases, there was frequently disagreement as to how to categorize a specific example of skin diseases. Therefore knowledge of the categories was part of the culture-learned behavior that is passed down and shared, but the ability to apply the knowledge varied based on the abilities and experiences of members of the cultural group. Having a disease classification system based on causation of disease—either natural or supernatural (personalistic) causes—does not make a health care system in itself. The "diagnostic" system of disease classification may confer a benefit to a culture in understanding in its own terms disease as a result of disorder within the cosmos or within the community. As shared knowledge, passed down, disease classification forms part of culture. The development of a health care system (see below) is based on **cultural** ideas about health and healing but represents part of the **social** structure.

Body-Mind Singularity vs. Dualism

In ethnomedical systems, furthermore, there is no distinction between the mind and the body (dating back in western philosophy to the "Cartesian" duality splitting the study of mind from body). Therefore, for example, what we call a psychological problem may literally be manifest as a somatic pain, or "somatization," in indigenous societies. The mind-body unity of ethnomedicine sometimes contributes to its perception by western biomedicine as being "spiritual" or "magico-religious." Whereas the practice of western biomedicine has divided both diagnoses and treatments of mental vs. physical diseases into the professional practices of psychology/psychiatry and internal medicine, respectively, ethnomedicine engenders healing for mental disorders through physical interventions, and for physical disorders through "spiritual" interventions. It is now being recognized in western science that the mind and the body are connected through neurological, endocrinological and immunological pathways documented by science (so-called, "psychoneuroimmunology," or PNI).

Social Evolutionary Perspectives on Ethnomedical Classification of Illness and Healthcare Systems

Social Type	Subsistence	Illness Causation	Healers
Nomadic	Hunter-gatherer, foraging	Self, ancestors, deity, "outsiders"	Shamans, diviners
Village	Simple horticulture	Community members, simple ethnopathology	Shamans, magico-religious healers, spiritual mediums, herbalists
Nomadic Pastoralists	Herding, animal domestication	Imbalances in hot and cold	Healers, spiritual mediums, exorcists
Chiefdoms	Sedentary agriculture	Imbalances in "humors"	Healers, spiritual mediums, herbalists, shamans
Early states	Complex agriculture	Imbalances	Same as above, plus priests
Civilizations	Irrigation agriculture	Individual behavior, moral failings, imbalances, elaborate ethnopathology	Priests, physicians, folk and religious healers
Modern, Industrial	Mechanized	Germs, genes, lifestyles, elaborate pathologies	Physicians, folk healers, alternative practitioners
Postmodern	Information	Mind-body, imbalances "humors"	Integration

Adapted from Fabrega H Jr: *Evolution of healing and sickness*, Berkeley, 1997, University of California Press.

FINAL WORDS

Medical anthropology provides a disciplined approach (literally, as an academic discipline and as a field of practice) to understanding human biology and culture, and human nature in the context of nature. These approaches have tremendous value in understanding those aspects of medical practice and health care that are compelled, or chosen, and those that represent true alternatives on a global basis. Although biomedical science and clinical trials may not hold all the answers to human medicine, anthropology provides an approach whereby other kinds of knowledge about health and medicine may be brought to bear in a serious and disciplined manner. Thus this expanded fourth edition of *Fundamentals of Complementary and Alternative Medicine* presents the world's healing traditions, including those from the Western world, that continue to offer real alternatives and choices for health and healing to both practitioners and patients in the twenty-first century.

Marc S. Micozzi, MD, PhD
Bethesda, MD, and Rockport, MA

About the Author

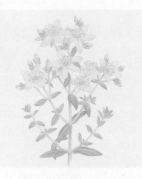

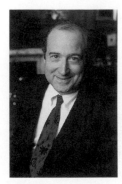

Marc Micozzi is a physician-anthropologist who has worked to create science-based tools for the health professions to be better informed and productively engaged in the fields of complementary and alternative (CAM) and integrative medicine. He was the founding editor-in-chief of the first U.S. journal in CAM, *Journal of Complementary and Alternative Medicine: Research on Paradigm, Practice and Policy* (1994) and the first review journal in CAM, *Seminars in Integrative Medicine* (2002). In addition to editing this textbook through four editions, he served as series editor for Elsevier's Medical Guides to Complementary and Alternative Medicine with 18 titles in print on a broad range of CAM therapies and therapeutic systems. In 1999, he edited *Current Complementary Therapies* for Current Science Press, focusing on contemporary innovations and controversies, and *Physician's Guide to Complementary and Alternative Medicine,* for American Health Consultants. With Springer Publishers he has just published the texts *CIM in Cancer Care & Prevention,* and *The Practice of Integrative Medicine: A Legal and Operational Guide.* He organized and chaired continuing education conferences on the theory, science, and practice of CAM in 1991, 1993, 1995, 1996, 1998, and 2001.

Prior to this work, Dr. Micozzi published original research on diet, nutrition, and chronic disease as a Senior Investigator in the intramural Cancer Prevention Studies program of the National Cancer Institute from 1984-1986. He continued this line of research when he was appointed Associate Director of the Armed Forces Institute of Pathology and Director of the National Museum of Health and Medicine in 1986. His early work on carotenoids (including lycopene), iron and cancer (collaborating with Nobel laureate Baruch Blumberg), anthropometric methods for time-related assessment of nutritional status, and other research made important contributions to this field. He was recognized for his work as the recipient of the John Hill Brinton Young Investigator Award at Walter Reed Army Medical Center in 1992, at which time he was jointly appointed as a Distinguished Scientist in the American Registry of Pathology, an affiliated, congressionally

chartered research and educational organization. He edited and co-edited two comprehensive technical volumes on application of clinical trials methods to new investigations of the role of micronutrients and macronutrients in cancer. He has published 275 articles in the medical, scientific, and technical literature.

In 1995, he returned to Philadelphia to serve as Executive Director of the College of Physicians. He managed all aspects of the college's professional and public educational programs, operations, and physical revitalization of the organization, including creation of the C. Everett Koop Community Health Information Center, which provided state-of-the-art information to consumers on health, wellness, and CAM. The White House Commission on CAM recognized this work on behalf of consumer health information in 2001.

Dr. Micozzi also actively collaborated with Former U.S. Surgeon General C. Everett Koop for over 25 years with the National Museum of Health and Medicine and as a medical and scientific advisor to Dr. Koop Life Care Corporation, where he worked on new developments with the FDA regarding review of dietary supplements. Over the past several years Dr. Micozzi has developed his own formulations for dietary, herbal, and nutritional supplements for a variety of applications and has reviewed thousands of publications on hundreds of nutritional supplements and herbal remedies, including bringing to light little known herbal remedies from the Southern African continent.

In 2002, he became Founding Director of the Policy Institute for Integrative Medicine in Bethesda, MD, working to educate the U.S. Congress, policymakers, the health professions, and the general public about needs and opportunities for CAM and integrative medicine. From 2003-2005, he accepted an additional interim appointment as Executive Director of the Center for Integrative Medicine at Thomas Jefferson University in Philadelphia. He is an Adjunct Professor in the Department of Medicine at the University of Pennsylvania and in the Department of Physiology & Biophysics at Georgetown University, and a faculty member for the new CAM curricula at Drexel University in Philadelphia and at University of California School of Business at Irvine. He lectures widely in continuing medical education courses that use his basic texts. Contact e-mail: marcsmicozzi@aol.com.

Contents

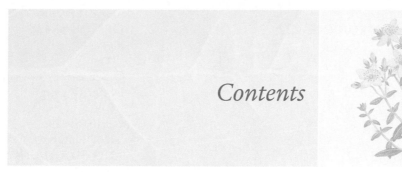

CHAPTER

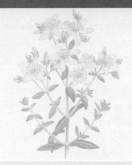

1

CHARACTERISTICS OF COMPLEMENTARY AND ALTERNATIVE MEDICINE

MARC S. MICOZZI

This section provides an introduction to the whole topic of complementary and alternative medicine (CAM), its themes and terminology, and the various contexts relative to its proper interpretation. In addition, this section addresses issues in so-called "integrative medicine," which represents the attempt to bring legitimate CAM therapies into the continuum of mainstream healthcare. The chapters provide a social and cultural recontextualization of CAM. The ubiquitous use of plants and natural products among alternatives is introduced through underlying themes from both the social and the biological sciences.

As introduction to complementary and alternative medicine (CAM), these chapters discuss social and cultural factors, an integrative medical model, and global dimensions of CAM practice. Also, the social history of the use of CAM is introduced through the concept of "vitalism" in intellectual and medical discourse, which is important to the understanding of the common themes of bioenergy and self-healing in the following Section Two. ∾

The different medical systems subsumed under the category *complementary and alternative* are many and diverse, but these systems have some common ground in their views of health and healing. Their common philosophy can be called *a new ecology of health,* sustainable medicine, or "medicine for a small planet."

ROLE OF SCIENCE

Allopathic medicine is considered the "scientific" healing art, whereas the alternative forms of medicine have been considered "nonscientific." However, perhaps what is needed is not *less science* but *more sciences* in the study of complementary and alternative medicine (CAM). Some of the central ideas of biomedicine are very powerful but may be intellectually static. The study of dead tissue cells, components, and chemicals to understand life processes and the quest for "magic bullets" to combat disease are based on a reductionist, materialist view of health and healing. Tremendous advances have been made over the past 100 years by applying

1

these concepts to medicine. However, the resulting biomedical system is not always able to account for and use many observations in the realms of clinical and personal experience, natural law, and human spirituality.

Contemporary biomedicine conceptually uses Newtonian physics and preevolutionary biology. Newtonian physics explains and can reproduce many observations on the mechanics of everyday experience. Contemporary quantum physics (quantum mechanics) recognizes aspects of reality beyond Newtonian mechanics, such as matter-energy duality, "unified fields" of energy and matter, and wave functions (see Chapters 10 and 11). Quantum physics and contemporary biology-ecology may be needed to understand alternative systems. Nuclear medicine uses the technology of contemporary physics, but biomedicine does not yet incorporate the concepts of quantum physics in its fundamental approach to human health and healing. Contemporary biomedicine measures the body's energy using electrocardiography, electroencephalography, and electromyography for diagnostic purposes, but it does not explicitly enlist the body's energy for the purpose of healing.

The biomedical model relies on a projection of Newtonian mechanics into the microscopic and molecular realms.

As a model for everything, Newtonian mechanics has limitations. It works within the narrow limits of everyday experience. It does not always work at a *macro* (cosmic) level, as shown by Einstein's theory of relativity, or at a *micro* (fundamental) level, as illustrated by quantum physics. However useful Newton's physics has been in solving mechanical problems, it does not explain the vast preponderance of nature: the motion of currents; the growth of plants and animals; or the rise, functioning, and fall of civilizations. Per Bak once stated that mechanics could explain why the apple fell but not why the apple existed or why Newton was thinking about it in the first place.

Mechanics works in explaining machines. But no matter how popular this metaphor has become (with acknowledgment of *National Geographic*'s popular "incredible machine" imagery), the body is not a machine and it cannot be entirely explained by mechanics. It is becoming increasingly clear that an understanding of energetics is required. This duality between the mechanical and the energetic has been accepted in physics for most of the past century. This duality is famously illustrated by the fact that J. J. Thomson won the Nobel Prize for demonstrating that the electron is a particle. His son, George P. Thomson, won the Nobel Prize a generation later for demonstrating that the electron is a wave.

"Hard scientists," such as physicists and molecular biologists, accept the duality of the electron but sometimes have difficulty accepting the duality of the human body. The "soft sciences," which attempt to be inclusive in their study of the phenomena of life and nature, are often looked on with disdain according to the folklore of the self-styled "real" scientists. However, real science must account for all of what is observed in nature, not just the conveniently reductionistic part.

The biological science of contemporary medicine is essentially preevolutionary in that it emphasizes typology rather than individuality and variation. Each patient is defined as a clinical entity by a diagnosis, with treatment prescribed accordingly. The modern understanding of the human genome does not make this approach to biomedical science less preevolutionary. Both the fundamentals of inheritance (Mendel) and those of natural selection (Darwin and Alfred Russel Wallace) were explained long before the discovery of the structure of the gene itself. Although modern biology-ecology continues to explore the phenomena of how living systems interact at the level of the whole—which cannot be seen under a microscope or in a test tube—molecular genetics continues to dissect the human genome.

It may seem outrageously complex to construct a medical system based on the concepts of modern physics and biology-ecology while maintaining a unique diagnostic and therapeutic approach to each individual. This would indeed be complex if not for the fact that the body is its own entity, a part of nature, and each body has an innate ability to heal itself.

One way of studying and understanding alternative medicine is to view it in light of contemporary physics and biology-ecology and to focus not just on the subtle manipulations of alternative practitioners, but also on the physiological responses of the human body. When homeopathy or acupuncture is observed to result in a physiological or clinical response that cannot be explained by the biomedical model, it is not the role of the scientist to deny this reality, but rather to modify our explanatory models to account for it. In this way, science itself progresses. In the end there is only one reality. Integrative (or alternative) medical systems, which are relatively "old" in terms of human intellectual history, always have been trying to describe, understand, and work with the same reality of health and healing as biomedicine. Whereas contemporary biomedicine uses new technologies in the service of relatively old ideas about health and healing, alternative methods use old technologies whose fundamental character may reflect new scientific ideas on physical and biological nature (Boxes 1-1 and 1-2).

> If biomedicine cannot explain scientific observations of alternative medicine, the biomedical paradigm will be revised.

Science must account for *all* of what is observed, not just part of it. That is why physics has moved beyond Newtonian mechanics—biology beyond typology. Is it possible for a biomedical model to be constructed for which its validity includes observations from CAM? Although it may be necessary to wait for new insights from physics and biology to understand CAM in terms of biomedicine, clinical pragmatism dictates that successful

BOX 1-1

A Note about Nomenclature

Although the term *complementary and integrative medicine (CIM)* was used in the third edition, *complementary and alternative medicine* was used in the title of the first two editions of this text to which we now return, no longer a victim of fashion. The word *alternative,* or the term *complementary and alternative medicine,* now seems to be culturally encoded in the English language.

Alternative medicine has been used to refer to those practices explicitly used for the purpose of medical intervention, health promotion or disease prevention which are not routinely taught at U.S. medical schools nor routinely underwritten by third-party payers within the existing U.S. health care system.

Such a definition seems to be a diagnosis of exclusion, meaning that alternative medicine is everything not presently being promoted in mainstream medicine. This definition may remind us of a popular song from the 1960s called "The Element Song," which offers a complete listing of the different elements of the periodic table (set to the tune of "I Am the Very Model of a Modern Major General" from Gilbert and Sullivan's *The Pirates of Penzance*). It ends with words to this effect: "These are the many elements we've heard about at Harvard. And if we haven't heard of them, they haven't been discovered." I have likened the recent "discovery" of alternative medicine to Columbus's discovery of the Americas. Although his voyage was a great feat that expanded the intellectual frontiers of Europe, Columbus could not really discover a world already known to millions of indigenous peoples who had complex systems of social organization and subsistence activities. Likewise, the definitional statement that alternative forms of medicine are not "within the existing U.S. health care system" is a curious observation for the tens of millions of Americans who routinely use them today.

therapeutic methods should not be withheld while mechanisms are being explained—or debated. We live in a world filled with opportunities to observe the practice of integrative medicine; all that remains is to apply scientific standards to its study. In the meantime, patients are now waiting for mainstream physicians to understand the mechanisms of CAM. Also, we can come to understand the underlying intellectual content and history of alternative forms as complete systems of thought and practice.

WELLNESS

The CAM systems generally emphasize what might be called "wellness" by the mainstream medical system. The goal of preventing disease is shared by integrative and mainstream medicine alike. In the mainstream medical model this involves using drugs and surgery to prevent disease in those who are only at risk, rather than reserving these powerful methods for the treatment of disease. I have called this trend the *medicalization* of prevention. In this approach, one can continue to engage in risky lifestyle behaviors while medicine provides "magic bullets" to prevent diseases that it cannot treat. Wellness in the context of complementary medicine is more than the prevention of disease. It is a focus on engaging the inner resources of each individual as an active and conscious participant in the maintenance of his or her own health. By the same token, the property of being healthy is not conferred on an individual solely by an outside agency or entity, but rather results from the balance of internal resources with the external natural and social environment. This latter point relates to the alternative approach that relies on the abilities of the individual to get well and stay healthy (Box 1-3).

BOX 1-2

Complementary and Alternative Medicine on the American Frontier, 1492-1942

Among the early exchanges to occur between European explorers (then settlers) and Native Americans were diseases and medical treatments. In the New World, Europeans were not surprised to find Native American remedies effective in light of the sixteenth-century "law of correspondences," which held that remedies could be found in the same locales where diseases occur. In the New World most Europeans, and thence Americans, found themselves for most of history from 1492 until as late as 1942 on the frontier where there was often no doctor. And often that was not such a bad thing.

Native Americans also readily adopted "big medicine" from European "physick" and early surgical practices as well, from the early Spanish conquistador Cabeza de Vaca (1530), eventually taking the French word for physician (*médecin*) and incorporating it into their own languages to express something previously unknown.

Europeans were in turn impressed by Native American resort to the healing power of nature and to spiritual healing. Nature in the New World provided a bounty of new medicinal plants and foods (whereas in Europe there had been only 16 cultivars—before chocolate, corn, squash, tomatoes, peppers, potatoes, and other foods of the Americas). In the English colonies beginning at Jamestown (1607) herbs, such as sassafras, were readily adopted. In Pennsylvania, William Penn (1680) himself became well acquainted with native herbs and other healing-spiritual practices such as the sweat lodge of the Delaware Indians (see Chapter 35).

Continued

BOX 1-2

Complementary and Alternative Medicine on the American Frontier, 1492-1942—cont'd

Many of the earliest books to come out of the English colonies were natural histories, serving as "herbals," that documented the occurrence of medicinal plants in various parts of the colonies: John Josselyn (1671) on New England, and John Lederer (1670), Robert Beverley (1705), John Lawson (1709), and John Brickell (1737) on Virginia and the Carolinas. John Wesley, later founder of the Methodist Church in England, wrote a similar book on Georgia (1737) during his two-year service as chaplain in Savannah. These regions are very biodiverse with many plant species because they represent the southern edge of the most recent geologic glaciations (see Chapter 4).

Later the best known of such herbal chronicles was *Travels through North and South Carolina, Georgia, East and West Florida, the Cherokee Country, etc.* by William Bartram, professor of botany at the College of Philadelphia (later, the University of Pennsylvania) who was consulted by Lewis and Clark prior to their own travels. (Bartram's *Travels* is the one book carried by the fictional Civil War character Inman—not only for its practical value but because "it made him happy"—in his journey to Cold Mountain in the 1997 landmark novel of the same name by Charles Frazier).

Physicians were rare on the expanding frontier, which prevented "regular medicine" (such as bleeding by lancet, leeches, and cupping; and blistering, puking, and purging—of which Francis Bacon had said, "The remedy is worse than the disease") from taking root where there were effective natural and home remedies. The American "self-help" book first took hold on the frontier with the publication in 1734 of *Every Man His Own Doctor, Or, The Poor Planter's Physician* by John Tennent of rural Spotsylvania County, Virginia, describing many native American herbal remedies. The potent American ginseng of Appalachia quickly became an international commodity with exportation to China. Frontiersman Daniel Boone for a time earned a living as a "sanger," gathering the herb in the wild.

Perhaps the most popular self-help book of all was *Gunn's Domestic Medicine, or Poor Man's Friend,* by Dr. John C. Gunn of Knoxville, Tennessee, continuously in print from 1830 to 1920. It is mentioned, for example, in Mark Twain's *Huckleberry Finn* (1885) and in John Steinbeck's *East of Eden* (1952).

In 1774, the leading American physician, Benjamin Rush (see Chapter 22), published a treatise on the importance of Native American remedies, and he later advised Lewis and Clark in 1803. Amazingly only one man died on the expedition, which implied that nature was a healthier place than Civilization. Charles Dickens described the unhealthy conditions of "civilized" areas in grim detail in his *American Notes* (1842). The "west cure, rest cure, and nature cures" became recommended means of recuperating from the illnesses of nineteenth-century civilization. This cure was used to good effect by future President Theodore Roosevelt, for example.

Other journeys of exploration expanded the frontier and the reach of frontier medicine, including those of Zebulon Pike (1806; before Lewis and Clark had even returned), Hugh Campbell (1833; with Dr. John Scott Harrison, who was son of President William Henry Harrison and father of President Benjamin Harrison and who died of alcoholism just prior to his father's election in 1840), John C. Frémont (1836-1848), and John Wesley Powell (named for the aforementioned Methodist minister), sometimes accompanied by colorful "mountain men" like Jedediah Smith, Jim Bridger, and Kit Carson.

Andrew Jackson's election in 1828 had provided a second American revolution with the ascendency of the common man along with his medicines. A backlash against the regular medicine of the elites was accompanied by the formal organization of natural healing by Samuel Hahnemann (see Chapter 24), Samuel Thomson (see Chapter 21), Franz Joseph Gall, and later John Harvey Kellogg (see Chapter 21). By the middle of the nineteenth century, the natural remedies of frontier medicine represented a well established and widely available form of health care in America.

During the Civil War, after the Union naval blockade of the South began working in 1862, the Confederacy found it difficult to obtain manufactured medicines and turned to natural remedies, publishing a pamphlet listing native herbs that could be used for treatment: snakeroot, sassafras, partridgeberry, lavender, dogwood, tulip tree, and red and white oak. Confederate Medical Corps kits contained many of these remedies toward the end of the war. After the Civil War came the heyday of patent (herbal) remedies, including Dr. Pepper, Dr. John Pemberton's Coca-Cola, and Dr. Hire's Root Beer, still enormously popular today as "soda," "pop," "tonic," and "root beer."

The term *quacks* (from the German *quacksalver* "quicksilver" or "mercury," which was actually a toxic regular medical treatment of the time) began to be applied to the practitioners of natural remedies (considered useful on the American frontier from the 1500s to the 1850s) suddenly at about the time the American Medical Association was organized in 1847—in reaction to the formation of the American Homeopathic Association in 1842.

Physicians and scientists who made real health advances with the use of natural healing in the mid- to late-nineteenth century (Thomson; Vincent Priessnitz [the water cure]; Russell Trall [the nature cure]; Nikola Tesla, pioneer of electromagnetism) were rounded up in the judgment of twentieth-century history together with true charlatans like Thomas Alva Edison, Jr. (son of the inventor, who did his best to put Tesla, the true genius of electricity and bioenergy, out of business), John Romulus Brinkley, Dr. C. Everett Field, and Norman Baker. This label came to include hypnotists and "magnetic" healers (e.g., Franz Anton Mesmer) and the emerging manual therapists (e.g., Andrew Taylor Still, Daniel David Palmer) of the nineteenth century who originated in and were also initially a phenomenon of the rural frontier. In retrospect, the exploits of nineteenth-century and early-twentieth-century charlatans seem quaint in comparison with the organized havoc wreaked on the public health during the last quarter century by the drug and insurance industries.

BOX 1-2

Complementary and Alternative Medicine on the American Frontier, 1492-1942—cont'd

The great unexamined assumption for today's reader is that natural healing in the later nineteenth century became "quackery." This attitude betrays something of a triumphalist approach to the wonders of twentieth-century medicine, whereas twenty-first-century American medicine in many ways has become nothing to celebrate. The vast majority of Americans were once able to leave "frontier medicine," for two or three generations, and enjoy medical practice and health care marked by well-trained physicians they knew and trusted, and the widespread availability of compassionate health services in hospitals that were accountable to their own communities. In the twenty-first century Americans now subsidize and sustain with hundreds of billions of dollars each year (16% of gross domestic product—the largest share in the world, but resulting in only the fortieth best health status among nations) a largely ineffective, inequitable, unsustainable health care system for the benefit of an unaccountable corporate-government-research complex of vested interests—marked by the arrogance and intransigence of mainstream biomedical research elites, excessive corporate profiteering through "blockbuster" drugs and direct-to-consumer marketing (rather than true therapeutic breakthroughs), and the mirage of "biotech" cures, as well as the substitution of hard-won medical knowledge and clinical judgment by insurance company bureaucracies that results in withholding of care and health care rationing (ironically, that which had been the greatest fear under the "socialized medicine" of a single-payer system). For several decades many have awaited the next "miracle" drug, biotech breakthrough, and, now, medical information technology for solutions to our health care crisis. This book illustrates that often it is ancient knowledge and wisdom about healing that, when adapted to new circumstances, provide truly innovative approaches to health problems.

In today's economy, the health care *crisis* is rapidly moving toward *collapse*. Many Americans may find themselves back on the medical frontier, where fortunately the natural healing and remedies once spurned (including some in this book) are still abiding in the contemporary consumer movement labeled as "complementary/alternative medicine."

BOX 1-3

Prevention versus Acute versus Chronic Disease

In Western allopathic medicine careful distinctions are made between modalities for preventing disease, for treating acute disease, and for treating chronic disease.

Because complementary and alternative medicine (CAM) modalities generally address the causes rather than the symptoms of disease, CAM strategies for prevention, for treatment of acute disorders, and for treatment of chronic disorders may often be the same or similar.

Ambulatory CAM Care Versus Residential CAM Care
CAM modalities are now widely available in the United States in both health care and non–health care settings. However, they are generally offered only as ambulatory care. Although there is much that can be accomplished by a CAM practitioner in a clinical setting, ambulatory care clients often experience a "reduced" form of the full potential benefits. Traditional Chinese, Ayurvedic, naturopathic, and other CAM "cures" involve the client's being "admitted" for residential care in a healthful environment over prolonged periods where all aspects of the client's experience are directed toward a healing response. Here, for example, diet is part of therapy and not something assigned to institutional food services as in modern hospitals. Although CAM modalities are generally gentler and less potent than modern biomedical technology, the potency of a full residential CAM cure can be remarkable.

SELF-HEALING ENERGY

The body heals itself. This might seem to be an obvious statement, because we are well aware that wounds heal and cells routinely replace themselves. Nonetheless, this is a profound concept among CAM systems, because self-healing is the basis of *all* healing. External manipulations simply mobilize the body's inner healing resources. Instead of wondering why the body's cells are sick, alternative systems ask why the body is not replacing its sick cells with healthy cells. The body's ability to be well or ill is largely tied to inner resources, and the external environment—social and physical—has an impact on this ability.

What is the evidence for self-healing? The long and common history of clinical observations of the "placebo effect," the "laying on of hands," or "spontaneous remissions" may be included in this category. To paraphrase Carl Jung: Summoned or unsummoned, self-healing will be there. Self-healing is so powerful that biomedical methodology mainly designs double-blind, controlled clinical trials to see what percentage of benefit powerful drugs can add to the healing encounter.

A related concept is that the body has energy (see Chapters 10 and 11). Accordingly, as a living entity, the body is an energetic system. Disruptions in the balance and flow of energy cause illness, and the body's response to energetic imbalance leads to perceptible disease. Because the body heals itself, the body can also make itself sick. Restoring or facilitating the body to restore its own balance restores health. The symptoms of a cold, flu, or allergy are caused by the body's efforts to rid itself of the offending agent. For example, by raising the body's temperature, a fever reduces bacterial reproduction (like an antibiotic, fever is literally bacteriostatic), and sneezing physically expels offending agents (see Figure 1-1 and Chapter 24).

Pathologists know that there are only so many ways that cells can look sick, because cellular reactions have a defined repertoire for manifesting malfunction. We have also learned a great deal over the past 100 years by correlating the appearance of dead tissue cells under the microscope with clinical diagnosis and prognosis. However, studying dead tissue cells for clinical significance does not allow direct observation of the dynamic energy of living cells, systems, organisms, and communities. Although correlation of the appearance of stained tissue cells under a microscope to clinical conditions is a powerful concept in medicine, alternative forms of medicine appear to provide a path to study the energy of living systems for health and healing, perhaps before the development of overt disease, as so often encountered among the many "functional complaints" in modern medicine (see Chapter 2).

NUTRITION AND NATURAL PRODUCTS

The reliance on nutrition and natural products is fundamental to CAM and does not play merely a supportive or adjunctive role. Nutrients and plant products are taken into the body and incorporated in the most literal sense. They provide the body with energy in the form of calories and with the material resources to stay healthy and get well.

Because the basic plan of the body, as a physical entity and as an energy system, evolves and exists in an ecological context, what the body needs it obtains from the environment in which it grew. Lao Tzu said that "what is deeply rooted in nature cannot be uprooted." The human organism is designed to obtain nutrients from natural food sources present in the natural environment, and the body is often best suited to obtain nutrients in their natural forms (see Chapters 22 and 25).

PLANTS

Plants are an important part of nature relative to health and a dominant part of the nature in which humans evolved. In addition to producing the oxygen that we breathe, plants are seen as sources of nutrients, medicines (e.g., phytochemicals), and essential oils (e.g., volatiles for inhalation and transdermal absorption); some systems also view plants as sources of vibrational energy. Many systems see the use of plants as sources of nutrients in continuity with their use as sources of medicine, paralleling contemporary biomedical guidelines for nutrition as disease prevention. As in Chinese medicine, foods exist in continuity with medicines among plant sources (Boxes 1-4 and 1-5).

INDIVIDUALITY

The emphasis of CAM is on the whole person as a unique individual with his or her own inner resources. Therefore the concepts of normalization, standardization, and generalization may be more difficult to apply to research and clinical practice compared with the allopathic method. Some believe that alternative forms of medicine restore the role of the individual patient and practitioner to the practice of medicine; the biomedical emphasis on standardization of training and practice to ensure quality may leave something lost in translation back to restoring the health of the individual (see Chapter 24).

> The focus on the whole person as a unique individual provides new challenges to the scientific measurement of the healing encounter. Mobilizing the resources of each individual to stay healthy and get well also provides new opportunities to move health care toward a model of wellness and toward new models for helping solve our current health care crisis, which is largely driven by costs. ∾

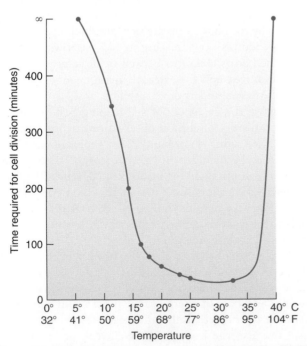

Figure 1-1 Relation between rate of cell division for *Bacillus mycoides* and temperature. (Data from *Encyclopaedia Britannica*, 1954 ed, s.v. "Bacteriology.")

If the body heals itself, has its own energy, and is uniquely individual, then the focus is not on the healer

BOX 1-4

Garlic: Food or Drug?

Garlic (*Allium sativum*) has been widely promoted as a remedy for colds, coughs, flu, chronic bronchitis, whooping cough, ringworm, asthma, intestinal worms, fever, and digestive, gallbladder, and liver disorders. Investigators have explored its use as a treatment for mild hypertension and hyperlipidemia, Heavy consumption may lead to lengthened clotting times, perioperative bleeding, and spontaneous hemorrhage. Numerous studies over a long period have documented garlic's irreversible inhibitory effect on platelet aggregation and fibrinolytic activity in humans.

Unlike many other herbs, garlic is also a biologically active *food* with presumed medicinal properties, including possible anticancer effects. Clinical studies of garlic in humans address three areas: (1) effect on cardiovascular system–related disease and risk factors such as lipid levels, blood pressure, glucose level, atherosclerosis, and thrombosis; (2) protective associations with cancer; and (3) clinical adverse effects. There are multiple clinical studies with promising but conflicting results. There is high consumer usage of garlic as a health supplement.

Scant data, primarily from case-control studies, suggest that dietary garlic consumption is associated with decreased risk of laryngeal, gastric, colorectal, and endometrial cancer and adenomatous colorectal polyps. Single case-control studies suggest that dietary garlic consumption is not associated with breast or prostate cancer.

Cholesterol levels have been related to use of garlic as well. Thirty-seven randomized trials, all but one in adults, consistently showed that, compared with use of a placebo, use of various garlic preparations led to small, statistically significant reduction in total cholesterol at 1 month (range of average pooled reductions, 1.2 to 17.3 mg/dL). Garlic preparations studied included standardized dehydrated tablets, "aged garlic extract," oil macerates, distillates, raw garlic, and combination tablets. Statistically significant reduction in low-density lipoprotein (LDL) levels (range, 0 to 13.5 mg/dL) and in triglyceride levels (range, 7.6 to 34.0 mg/dL) also were found. One multicenter trial involving 100 adults with hyperlipidemia found no difference in lipid outcomes at 3 months between persons who were given an antilipidemic agent and persons who were given a standardized dehydrated garlic preparation.

Garlic has a range of biological activities. Twenty-seven small, randomized, placebo-controlled trials, all but one in adults and of short duration, reported mixed but never large effects of various garlic preparations on blood pressure outcomes. Most studies did not find significant differences between persons randomly assigned to take garlic and those randomly assigned to take a placebo.

Adverse effects of oral ingestion of garlic are "smelly" breath and body odor. Other possible, but not proven, adverse effects include flatulence, esophageal and abdominal pain, small intestinal obstruction, contact dermatitis, rhinitis, asthma, bleeding, and heart attack. How frequently adverse effects occur with oral ingestion of garlic as a food and whether they vary for particular garlic preparations are not established. Adverse effects of inhaled garlic dust include allergic reactions such as asthma, rhinitis, urticaria, angioedema, and anaphylaxis. Adverse effects of topical exposure to raw garlic include contact dermatitis, skin blisters, and ulcerative lesions. Frequency of reactions to inhaled garlic dust or topical exposure to garlic is not established. Whether adverse effects are specific to particular preparations, constituents, or dosages should be elucidated. In particular, adverse effects related to bleeding and interactions with other drugs such as aspirin and anticoagulants warrant further study.

Research Questions on Garlic
- Whether oral ingestion of garlic (fresh, cooked, or as supplements) compared with no garlic, other oral supplements, or drugs lowers lipid levels, blood pressure, glucose levels, and cardiovascular morbidity and mortality
- Whether garlic increases insulin sensitivity and antithrombotic activity
- Associations between garlic use and the occurrence of precancerous lesions, cancer, and cancer-related morbidity and mortality
- Types and frequency of adverse effects of oral garlic, topical garlic, and inhaled garlic dust
- Interactions between garlic and commonly used medications

BOX 1-5

Ginger: Food or Drug?

Like garlic, ginger can be considered as both a popular ingredient in prepared foods and an effective medicinal plant remedy. Ginger has long been known and used for its antinausea effects and calming properties on the stomach—thus, the traditional popular beverages ginger ale and ginger beer. It is particularly useful for nausea associated with pregnancy and with chemotherapy, for which acupuncture is also a useful alternative therapy.

but on the healed. Although this concept is humbling to the role of practitioner as heroic healer, it is liberating to realize that in the end, each person heals himself or herself. If the healer is not the sole source of health and healing, there is room for humility and room for both patient and practitioner to participate in the interaction.

For the purposes of this book, a functional definition of CAM is offered, limited here to what may be called *complementary medical systems*. Complementary medical systems are characterized by a developed body of intellectual work that (1) underlies the conceptualization of health and its precepts; (2) has been sustained over many generations by many practitioners in many communities; (3) represents an orderly, rational, conscious system of knowledge and thought about health and medicine; (4) relates more broadly to a way of life (or lifestyle); and (5) has been widely observed to have definable results as practiced.

Although the term *holistic* has been applied to the approach to the "body as person" among CAM systems, I apply holism to the medical system itself as a complete system of thought and practice (what I have called "health beliefs and behaviors," Chapter 2). This system of knowledge is therefore shared by patients and practitioners—the active, conscious engagement of "patients" is relative to the focus on *self-healing* and *individuality* that are among the common characteristics of these systems.

In this regard it might be considered that we are trying to document here the "classic" practice of CAM systems. In trying to build a bridge between a well-developed system of allopathic medicine and complementary medical systems, it is necessary to have strong foundations on both sides of this bridge. It is not possible to apply these criteria to the work of individual alternative practitioners who have unilaterally developed their own unique techniques over one or two generations (what might be called "unconventional"), just as it is not possible to build a bridge to nowhere. This definition is meant to apply to systems of *thought* and not just techniques of practice. Often an underlying philosophy of individual practitioners surrounds new techniques they have developed, or new techniques may be subsumed under existing systems of practice.

Eclecticism is itself a historical form of alternative medicine that drew from among different traditions and was popular in the United States in the nineteenth century. In such a system, treatment is determined by the needs of each individual patient, not limited to what one given system has to offer. At present a chiropractor may practice in an Ayurveda clinic; osteopaths may practice in allopathic clinics; and chiropractors, osteopaths, or allopaths may use acupuncture. *Naturopathy,* in some ways the most recent of homegrown alternatives from the Euro-American tradition, consciously uses a variety of traditions ranging from acupuncture to herbal medicine. I have termed naturopathy *neoeclecticism,* with the underlying philosophy that the body heals itself using resources found in nature (see Chapter 21).

In the end a given system develops in answer to human needs. Alternatives vary widely, but their characteristics cluster around the self-healing capabilities of the human organism and the human organism's ability to use (and reliance on) resources present in nature. What is constant and at the center of such CAM systems is the individual human. Therefore, if the focus is not on the medical system itself but on the person at the center, there is really only one system.

FUNDAMENTALS

Contemporary biomedicine is a scientific paradigm with a particular history, as much influenced by social history as by scientific laws. In the laudable effort to make medicine scientific, we have emphasized that knowledge about the world, including nature and human nature, must be pursued using the following criteria: (1) *objectivism*—the observer is separate from the observed; (2) *reductionism*—complex phenomena are explainable in terms of simpler, component phenomena; (3) *positivism*—all information can be derived from physically measurable data; and (4) *determinism*—phenomena can be predicted from a knowledge of scientific law and initial conditions. We all know that this is not the only way of "knowing" things, but it became the twentieth-century test to determine whether knowledge is "scientific."

In fact, science simply requires *empiricism*—making and testing models of reality by what can be observed, guided by certain values, and based on certain metaphysical assumptions. Science itself is a system of human knowledge. Scientists often detect differences between metaphysical reality and the scientific models constructed through human intellectual activity. These new thoughts about the nature of medicine do not represent a new science so much as they represent a new philosophy.

Therefore the four criteria just listed are not always applicable. In the science of physics, objectivism is ultimately not possible at the fundamental level because of the *Heisenberg uncertainty principle,* which states that the act of observing phenomena necessarily influences the behavior of the phenomena being observed. Contemporary biological and ecological science has produced a wealth of observations about interactions among living organisms and their environments in transactional, multidirectional, and synergic ways that are not ultimately subject to reductionist explanations. For positivism and determinism to provide a complete explanation, we must assume that science has all the physical and intellectual tools to ask the right questions. However, the questions we ask are based on the history of science itself as part of the history of human intellectual inquiry.

A final point about alternative systems: In a way that is perhaps particular to the United States, complementary and alternative medicine systems imply the importance of individuality and choice. In an era in which the active engagement of the individual in his or her own health is a paramount goal, the importance of individuality and choice could not be greater.

CHAPTER

2

TRANSLATION FROM CONVENTIONAL MEDICINE

MARC S. MICOZZI

What has been labeled "alternative medicine" in the United States is, first of all, a social phenomenon and consumer movement of significant dimensions. The term *complementary medicine* has been used interchangeably with *alternative medicine* and is a more accurate functional description of this social phenomenon, because patients in the United States generally use "alternative medicine" as an *adjunct* to (not a replacement for) conventional medical care. Much of what we call "complementary and alternative medicine" in the United States, in fact, represents time-honored traditions of medical practice originating in other countries and other cultures or during earlier periods of European and American society.

One of the most important distinctions we can make in studying and understanding CAM is to note the differences between two types of practices: (1) practices that are many years or centuries old and have a large body of practitioners and patients and a well-developed fund of clinical "wisdom" that is encoded into the belief system of a particular society or subgroup of people, and (2) practices that have been developed recently by one or a few

practitioners in isolation from peers and without benefit of scientific testing and clinical studies (what may be called "unconventional therapy"). Practices in this second category often fit conceptually within the biomedical model but simply have not been tested using the standards of biomedical research and practice.

For example, with regard to the topics in this volume, CAM systems (alternatives) in the first category of time-tested traditions include the traditional medicine of China (with heterogeneous practice styles), manual therapies (osteopathy, chiropractic, massage), and homeopathy. Many time-tested traditions have in common, to a greater or lesser extent, aspects of mind-body medicine, a focus on nutrition and natural products, hands-on interaction between practitioner and patient, and an emphasis on listening to the patient. The five common characteristics of complementary and alternative medicine described in this book are (1) a wellness orientation, (2) a reliance on self-healing, (3) an inference that bioenergetic mechanisms play a role, (4) the use of nutrition and natural products in a fundamental role, and (5) an emphasis on individuality.

Because homeopathy, for example, stresses the importance of eliciting detailed symptoms and symptom complexes from the patient (and is not a system for placing patients into disease-based diagnostic categories), the practitioner must spend a great deal of time listening to the patient. The therapeutic benefits (and diagnostic value) of listening to the patient continue to be actively recognized among the "talk therapies" of contemporary mainstream medical practice in psychiatry and psychology, as well as general clinical practice (Adler, 1997).

Because CAM therapies do not necessarily stress the assignment of patients to disease-based diagnostic categories, they are routinely prepared to deal with "functional" disorders and complaints (e.g., headache, pain, gastrointestinal dysfunction, menstrual dysfunction, other "subjective" symptoms) that do not carry a pathological diagnosis. Many CAM systems see these functional disorders as precursors of disease (rather than, for example, results of disease) and approach the clinical intervention on that basis.

HOLISM AND VITALISM

Various CAM systems also refer to the importance of "energy" in the development of disorders and diseases and in their treatment and cure. Energy has a dynamic quality and is not measured in the usual ways that conventional medicine is accustomed to describing things, on the basis of materialist, reductionist biomedical mechanisms. The idea that whole, living systems and organisms have a "vital energy" that may not be present in nonliving entities or in parts or portions of an organism is an ancient concept among human cultures that is also reflected in European and U.S. intellectual traditions (Figure 2-1).

CAM medical systems are sometimes considered vitalistic and holistic compared with allopathic medicine, which is considered materialistic and reductionistic (Table 2-1). Vitalism contends that there is an "energy" to living organisms that is nonmaterial. *Vitalism* is a nonecological concept historically and posits nonnaturalistic explanations for life. *Holism* is an ecological concept that the totality of biological phenomena in a living organism or system cannot be reduced, observed, or measured at a level below that of the whole organism or system (Smuts, 1926). Holism as an ecological concept is not consistent with the vitalist idea that living systems are independent of nature. Holism was meant to be both antimechanistic and antivitalist.

It is generally interpreted that vitalism and holism go together in studying the characteristics of CAM. However, some interpretations of homeopathy, for example, rely on a vitalist mechanism while basing therapy on an essentially reductionist approach; that is, a whole organism's energetic mechanism is postulated to explain the effect elicited by minute doses of specific materia medica in pills. Likewise, in Chinese medicine the post-1949 traditional

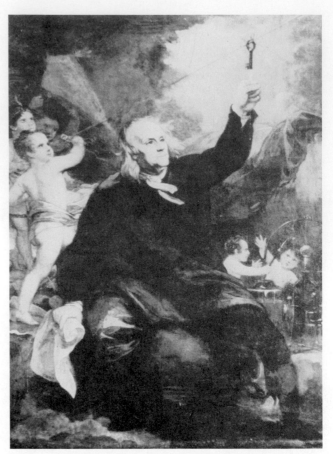

Figure 2-1 Poets, philosophers, and scientists of the late eighteenth and early nineteenth centuries were all interested in vitalism—finding the energy that animated life and the universe. Here Benjamin Franklin is shown in a heroic pose by Benjamin West figuratively "taming lightning." In fact, Franklin, like his contemporaries, was searching for insights into nature and human nature, not just exploring electricity in a contemporary utilitarian sense. Later, scientists thought that reductionist, materialist explanations substituted for the need for vitalist interpretations.

TABLE 2-1

Vitalism and Holism in Complementary Medicine

Biomedicine	Complementary medicine
Reductionist	Holistic
Materialist	Vitalist

Chinese medicine style of practice veers toward a reductionist model while maintaining an essentially vitalist mechanism. Since 1978 the World Health Organization (WHO) has referred to traditional (cultural) medical systems as holistic, meaning "viewing humans in totality within a wide ecological spectrum, and emphasizing the view that ill health or disease is brought about by imbalance or disequilibrium of humans in the total ecological system and not only by the causative agent and pathogenic mechanism" (WHO, 1998).

Historically, we might say that premodern medical systems could understand medicine only on the basis of observations of the whole organism, whose components were not well known or understood. Modern reductionist biomedical science has allowed knowledge to be built on the basis of studying dead parts and pieces of the whole organism (e.g., tissue cells, DNA). A postmodern medicine might permit translation of the biomedical model back to the realm of the whole, vital organism. For example, new imaging technologies that permit observation of living cells for diagnostic and therapeutic purposes may provide one mechanism.

This view might consider that biomedicine has new technologies generally in the service of old ideas about health and healing, whereas CAM systems represent old technologies that may be interpreted in light of new ideas about health and healing.

Outcomes-based research has begun to be helpful in demonstrating the therapeutic benefit (or lack of benefit) of alternative (integrative) practices that are unexplainable on the basis of postulated mechanisms of action foreign to the biomedical model. In this way, some regard such ideas as nonsense, or perhaps more precisely, "unsense." However, some sense may be made of these ideas by considering a medical ecological or adaptational model.

MEDICAL ECOLOGY AND THE ADAPTATION MODEL

For medical traditions that have been encoded and carried as knowledge in different cultures for many years, it is possible to study the adaptiveness and adaptive value of these practices. What benefits do these traditions confer on members of a society who follow certain health-related beliefs and practices?

Human physiology allows adaptation to occur in response to environmental pressures in the short term in the individual. Evolution allows adaptation to occur over the long term in the population. Human culture is learned behavior that also has adaptive value.

At the end of the nineteenth century, European interpretations regarded traditional medical practices as myth, superstition, or magic (and sometimes madness), as illustrated in Sir James Frazer's *The Golden Bough* (1890). During the twentieth century, social scientists searched for the functional meanings and purposes of medically related traditions. European and North American social scientists began describing the meanings of traditional medical practices in the 1920s. For example, if traditional societies, through plant domestication and agriculture, learn to obtain nutrients (foods) from the environment in which they live, they may also learn to obtain medicines from their environments and to develop therapeutic techniques to provide medical care.

As previously stated, many contemporary CAM paradigms and practices derive from complex and sophisticated ancient health systems and from indigenous cultures closely in touch with their natural and social environments. These health systems form part of the adaptation of these societies and cultures to their respective environments, representing integral components of traditional societies (Micozzi, 1983). Health-related beliefs and behaviors that are widespread and persistent merit study to determine their adaptive value (Table 2-2).

To accept the validity of the premise for scientific investigation of integrative (alternative) medical systems, one need only accept the possibility (or probability) of the adaptiveness of human belief and behavior systems that are persistent and widespread. The adaptiveness of human behavior is an important concept to both social and biological scientists. Whether human behavior is adaptive represents a persistent question in intellectual discourse. Some point to cultural practices that are widespread and

TABLE 2-2

Representation of Traditional Health Systems

Conceptual paradigm	Health system component	Methodology	Representation
"Social reality"	Health beliefs Health behaviors • Health practices, wellness maintenance • Care seeking, illness perceived —Structural-functional access —Cultural access	Informant interview/survey Participant observation	Cognitive Observational
"Scientific reality"	Health outcomes, disease defined	Technical evaluation: health and nutrition status indicators	Analytical

that persist over generations as evidence of the adaptiveness of such practices.

Although many hold out the symbolic power of beliefs and the transcendental value of ideas regardless of "adaptive" value, belief and behavior systems can often be demonstrated in a scientific sense to have associated outcomes relative to human health and disease. The British anthropologist-physician W.H.R. Rivers (1924) showed that traditional health systems are not magic or superstition but represent rational, ordered systems of knowledge and useful ways of understanding and interacting with the environment.

Bringing together social science and biomedical science in a more effective and integrated way requires rigorous application of the social sciences to the study of health and medicine. Social scientists often study health belief systems without adequately measuring health outcomes in a scientific sense, whereas biomedicine measures outcomes scientifically without being able to study the underlying belief systems. Social and cultural factors are amenable to study by techniques extrinsic to biomedical science. A conceptual paradigm may be considered to have reached the limits of explanation or inquiry when dependent variables can be measured but independent variables are unknown or immeasurable in the system of study (Kuhn, 1973). If health outcomes are considered *dependent* variables, the explanatory limits of biomedical science are exceeded, because relevant *independent* variables are not made an explicit component of the explanatory model.

For example, there are different ways of explaining how manual therapies work. Although their clinical applications and associated health outcomes have been accepted on the basis of biomechanical mechanisms, many manual therapy traditions invoke the manipulation of bioenergy as the mechanism.

BIOENERGETIC EXPLANATIONS FOR MANUAL THERAPIES

First, all manual therapies imply that touching the patient in a particular manner is a primary means of therapy. The traditional view of the "laying on of hands" is to focus the attention of both practitioner and patient on the intention to heal and on the practitioner undertaking to treat the patient.

Manual therapies as CAM combine several approaches to healing traditions. Manual therapies can be seen to include North American historic traditions such as osteopathy and chiropractic and, more recently, "body work" (e.g., massage therapy, rolfing, Trager method, applied kinesiology, Feldenkrais method). Asian manual systems include Chinese tui na and Japanese shiatsu. Techniques that are often viewed as manual therapy but more explicitly relate to manipulation of bioenergy are the Asian systems of qigong (qi gong) and reiki and the North American technique of therapeutic touch.

The founder of *chiropractic*, Daniel David Palmer, was originally an "energy healer" or "magnetic healer," as was the founder of traditional *osteopathy*, Andrew Taylor Still. Both traditions were established within a few years and a few hundred miles of each other in the American Midwest of the 1890s. In addition to embracing the concept of "vital energy," both Palmer and Still also rejected the use of drugs, which were especially toxic during that period of history (Palmer, 1910; Still, 1902). In this regard, Still and Palmer were joined by such mainstream medical figures as Sir William Osler and Oliver Wendell Holmes. In a famous statement to the Massachusetts Medical Society (publisher of the *New England Journal of Medicine*) in 1860, Holmes opined that if the entire materia medica of contemporary medicine were sunk to the bottom of the sea, it would be all the better for humankind and all the worse for the fishes. However, chiropractic and traditional osteopathy went further by specifically identifying themselves as "drugless healing," which found many adherents, in reaction to the therapeutic excesses in mainstream medicine. After World War II, osteopathy was largely mainstreamed into modern medicine, which was partially driven by the chronic shortage of medical personnel in the U.S. military (who recruited DOs to supplement MDs), as well as the desire of osteopaths to participate in the full benefits of medical mainstream training and practice.

Therapeutic touch and *healing touch* are more recent developments, largely promulgated initially by two nurses in the United States, Dolores Krieger and Dora Kunz. Healing "touch" is notable in that the patient is not actually physically touched. The technique therefore may be explained as a form of "energy healing" (perhaps the form most in practice in clinical settings in the United States) rather than manual therapy. The hands of the practitioner are thought to manipulate the flow of energy around the patient's body (Krieger, 1979; Kunz, 1991).

Other forms of hand-mediated healing include polarity therapy, Tibetan-Japanese reiki, Japanese jin shin jyutsu, external qigong, touch for health, reflexology, acupressure, and shiatsu massage.

Bioenergetic mechanisms are invoked to explain clinical observations of the efficacy of therapeutic touch. These concepts are difficult to translate into clinical medicine, which at the same time recognizes that there is experimental reality beyond the realm of the contemporary biomedical paradigm.

AYURVEDA

Bioenergetic mechanisms have also been invoked in attempting to understand some aspects of Ayurveda, or the traditional medicine of India (see Chapters 29 to 32). Traditionally, Ayurveda is not simply a medical system; rather, it is described as the science of *longevity* and relates more to what we would think of as a way of life or "lifestyle." A contemporary form of Ayurveda as provided by Maharishi Ayurveda represents a revival of Ayurvedic traditions lost through centuries of foreign rule (Moslem/ Mogul and European/ British) in India, blended with "bioenergetic" interpretations of mechanism.

Empirically, Ayurveda makes use of correspondences among five cosmic elements of earth, air, fire, water, and space (similar to ancient Greek concepts and "humoral" Western medical systems extending into the nineteenth century). There are three constitutional body types based on the balance of three *doshas,* which represent these five elements as they occur in the human body (Table 2-3). The three primary body types *(prakriti)* represent an empirical system for describing predisposition to illness, proscribing against unhealthy behavior, and prescribing for treatment of disease. The three primary body types of vata, pitta, and kapha may be roughly translated to the Sheldon somatotypes of twentieth-century Western science describing body

constitution as ectomorph, mesomorph, and endomorph. Ayurveda also demonstrates systematic correspondences among a number of cosmic elements, seasons, constitutions, personalities, diseases, and treatments.

The idea that body constitution predisposes to certain diseases is an old one, and in biomedicine this idea now finds expression in the association of genetic factors with disease, a current preoccupation of contemporary biomedical science.

CHINESE MEDICINE

As with Ayurveda, we can also think of Chinese medicine as an empirical tradition of systematic correspondences making reference to five cosmic elements ("five phases") that dates back to about 3000 BC (Table 2-4). Although for

TABLE 2-3

Characteristics of Three Constitutional Types in Ayurveda

	Dosha		
	Vata	Pitta	Kapha
Somatotype (Sheldon)	Ectomorph	Mesomorph	Endomorph
Body type	Light, thin	Moderate	Solid, heavy
Skin type	Dry	Reddish	Oily, smooth
Personality	Anxious	Irritable	Tranquil, steady
Digestion	Irregular, constipation	Sharp	Slow
Activity	Quick	Medium	Slow, methodical
Season	Winter	Fall	Spring
Diseases	Hypertension	Inflammation	Sinusitis
	Arthritis	Inflammatory bowel disease	Respiratory diseases
	Rheumatism	Skin diseases	Asthma
	Cardiac arrhythmia	Heartburn	Obesity
	Insomnia	Peptic ulcer	Depression

TABLE 2-4

Correspondences of the Five Phases in Chinese Medicine

Category	Wood	Fire	Earth	Metal	Water
Organ	Liver	Heart	Spleen	Lungs	Kidney
Bowel	Gallbladder	Small intestine	Stomach	Large intestine	Urinary bladder
Season	Spring	Summer	Late summer	Autumn	Winter
Time of day	Before sunrise	Forenoon	Afternoon	Late afternoon	Midnight
Climate	Wind	Heat	Damp	Dryness	Cold
Direction	East	South	Center	West	North
Development	Birth	Growth	Maturity	Withdrawal	Dormancy
Color	Cyan	Red	Yellow	White	Black
Taste	Sour	Bitter	Sweet	Pungent	Salty
Sense organ	Eyes	Tongue	Mouth	Nose	Ears
Odor	Goatish	Scorched	Fragrant	Raw fish	Putrid
Vocalization	Shouting	Laughing	Singing	Weeping	Sighing
Tissue	Sinews	Vessels	Flesh	Body hair	Bones

comparative purposes Chinese medicine is often treated as a homogeneous monolithic structure, this view neglects the changing interpretations of basic paradigms offered by Chinese medicine through the ages and the synchronic plurality of differing opinions and ideas over thousands of years (Unschuld, 1985).

Likewise, I prefer to use the term *China's traditional medicine* or *traditional medicine of China*. The popular term "traditional Chinese medicine" is a twentieth-century invention, concoction, or perhaps convention that blends certain aspects of Chinese medicine with a scientific underpinning put into place by the Communist government of Mao Tse-Tung to provide basic health care to the Chinese population.

Much of what the Chinese medical practitioner does is thought to influence the flow or balance of the body's energy, called "qi." In my view, the Chinese concept of qi, which is translated as "energy," "bioenergy," or "vital energy," has a metabolic quality, because the Chinese character for qi may be described as vapor or steam rising over rice (Figure 2-2). The term *rice* has a specific quality that we associate with a specific food, but it also has a generic meaning, "food" or "foodstuff." For example, the character "rice hall" is used to describe a restaurant in Chinese. The elusive meaning of qi may therefore be likened more to living metabolism than to the energy that we associate with electromagnetic radiation.

Energy or qi also has the dynamic qualities of "flow" and "balance." Because flow and balance are dynamic, they may be described in changing terms from one patient to the next or in the same patient from one day to the next (again, without the use of static, fixed pathological diagnostic categories). Such concepts present great challenges in translation to the biomedical model.

Acupuncture is a major modality for the manipulation of qi. Clinical observations of efficacy are increasing, and some biomedical explanations focus on the physiological effects of skin puncture and modulation of neurotransmitter substances. Some experiments indicate that the acupuncture needle has the same effect when it is merely held in place over the appropriate point (without puncturing the skin). If acupuncture needles operate by influencing the flow of energy, which is not limited by internal or external barriers, then puncturing the skin is not a necessary part of the mechanism of action. Perhaps practical Chinese acupuncturists simply found a way to hold the needles in place by puncturing the skin when they were trying to influence more than two acupuncture points simultaneously (and had only two hands to hold the needles in place).

HOMEOPATHY

Homeopathy challenges certain assumptions of allopathic medicine with the concept that "like cures like." A symptom may be seen as an attempt on the part of the body to correct itself, to fight disease, and to restore balance (homeostasis). For example, in the case of fever this may be seen as an adaptation to bacterial infection. Increased temperatures (above the normal body temperature) are seen to slow the rate of bacterial reproduction significantly (Figure 2-3). In this way, raising body temperature above normal is bacteriostatic and, as with many antibiotics, may slow bacterial growth, which gives the immune system a chance to clear the infection.

Homeopathy originally gave the name "allopathic" medicine to the "regular" medical mainstream approaches

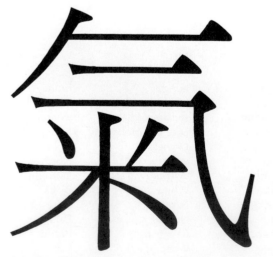

Figure 2-2 The Chinese character *qi*, described as vapor or steam rising over rice.

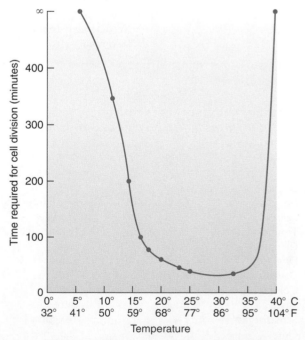

Figure 2-3 Relation between rate of cell division for *Bacillus mycoides* and temperature. (Data from *Encyclopaedia Britannica*, 1954 ed, s.v. "Bacteriology.")

of the time (early nineteenth century) because the medical focus is on the elimination or control of symptoms. In homeopathy, symptoms are everything, and describing them is the primary goal and guide to therapy. In classic homeopathy an empirical approach is taken by administering "provings" of substances (largely materia medica) in minute doses and observing whether the patient shows clinical improvement. This practice may also be considered reductionistic. Because many symptoms tend to improve over time, these provings cannot be considered controlled experiments, but the same observation may be applied to the administration of "cures" in other traditions as well.

NATUROPATHIC MEDICINE AND HERBALISM

Naturopathy is the most recent of alternative approaches to have developed as a complete system in North America (see Chapter 21). It emphasizes the healing power of nature and can also be understood in terms of the adaptational model. In practice, contemporary naturopathy is eclectic, consciously drawing on a number of models and systems (e.g., Chinese medicine, Ayurveda, homeopathy, manual therapies, Islamic healing) in an effort to fit the patient profile and the clinical problem with appropriate medical systems and techniques. Naturopathy is well organized in a few western states (notably Oregon, Washington, and Montana) and in Connecticut and northern New England but may be practiced in a less formal fashion in other parts of the United States.

The use of nutrition, herbs, natural remedies, and other natural products is an important component of naturopathic medicine. Medical traditions around the world, from the most basic shamanistic approaches to healing to the highly complex and sophisticated systems of Chinese and Ayurvedic medicine, make use of medicinal plants in relation to their biological activity. Homeopathy (often included in the range of practice of naturopathic medicine) is also based largely on minute doses of materia medica.

From the standpoint of evolutionary biology, it is not surprising that plants develop biologically active constituents as an adaptation to compete in nature with each other and with animal species. Because plants form a primary feature of the terrestrial environment in which humans evolved, it is also not surprising that human physiology and metabolism are adapted to obtaining nutrients and medicines from plants in their environments. Societies learn over time which plants have value, and how to obtain, harvest, and prepare them, and encode this knowledge and behavior into their cultures. In addition to the traditional medical settings for the use of medicinal plants, an eclectic system of herbal medicine has historically developed in the West, which can be referred to as "Western herbalism." Biologically active constituents of plants include carbohydrates,

glycosides, tannins, lipids, volatile oils, resins, steroids, alkaloids, peptides, and enzymes.

Volatile oils form the primary basis of the practice of aromatherapy. The active constituents have various physiological effects throughout the body (Table 2-5 and Box 2-1). Because biologically active constituents are present in combination in medicinal plants, they are often observed to have synergistic effects. These synergistic effects have been useful, for example, in the application of crude extracts of medicinal plants to antibiotic-resistant bacterial infections and to chloroquine-resistant malaria. However, it is difficult to translate this approach to the active ingredient model of reductionist biomedical research, as described in Chapter 4.

TABLE 2-5

Medicinal Plant Constituent Actions

Respiratory	Gastrointestinal	Neural
Expectorant	Emetic	Sedative
Antitussive	Antiemetic	Stimulant
Immunomodulative	Laxative	Cardiotonic
	Spasmolytic	Antidepressant

BOX 2-1

Medicinal Plants as Adaptogens: Ginseng

Another concept that is difficult to translate to biomedicine, and another category of medical plant constituent action, is that of *adaptogen*. An adaptogen has the interesting and nonpharmacological property of helping the body to adapt to whatever changes in environment may occur and to maintain homeostasis. Thus, it helps keep you warm if it is cold, or stay cool if it is hot; stay awake when you need to be up, or sleep when it is time to retire; be alert when that is called for, or relax when it is time to restore your energy. This "tonic" property is not accounted for in Western pharmacology but is consistent with physiology, in which essentially the same metabolic mechanisms must adapt to constantly changing circumstances.

Ginseng is the prototype medicinal plant among adaptogens. There are Chinese Ginseng, Siberian Ginseng, and American Ginseng. In a good illustration of the diffusion of Western herbalism, American ginseng was rapidly brought into the modern Chinese pharmacopeia when Chinese emigrants to the United States "discovered" it (there is that word again) and rapidly brought it into common use. American ginseng is highly prized, and it is "wild-crafted" today by American "sangers" in the Appalachian Mountains who closely guard the secret of where and how to locate ginseng for gathering.

GLOBAL PERSPECTIVES

Understanding complementary medical systems described here as "traditional" or "cultural" medicine in an ecological model, we can compare and contrast how they fit into their indigenous settings with how they are interpreted in the contemporary United States. In the U.S. health care system, we assume traditional herbal medicines to be of value only when their active principal or ingredient is known and can be purified for mass production. However, this "active ingredient" approach to medicinal plants and traditional medicine reflects a particular conceptual paradigm rather than a particular truth about how natural medicines may work. On the basis of findings from U.S. biomedical plant-screening programs, therapeutic benefits are often observed to be limited. However, methodologies used in biomedicine often overlook the effects by which traditional medicines produce results because of a fixed and defined view of what constitutes therapeutic action. Although traditional health systems have acknowledged use in management of chronic, low-level conditions, they are assumed to be of no value in providing acute or emergency care. In some countries (China, Vietnam, Nicaragua), however, traditional medicine is mandated and used effectively for trauma and major acute diseases; historically, this resulted from political and economic exclusion from other health care technologies. Much research already exists in other countries (often in languages other than English).

Traditional medicines are now seen as valuable because they serve as sources of leads for new pharmaceuticals (so-called biodiversity prospecting), and the potential medical value of tropical rainforest species provides a basis for support to preserve and conserve regional biodiversity. However,

TABLE 2-6

Old Assumptions and New Perspectives on Complementary Medical Systems

Old assumptions	New perspectives
"Primitive"	Holistic
Ineffective	Cost effective
Marginalized	Locally available
Extinct	Renewed
Should be regulated	Should be studied
Provides prospects for biomedicine	Valid in own right
Active ingredient model	Synergistic activity

this biodiversity prospecting assumption overlooks the role of traditional medical systems in addressing the needs of the people from whence come the medicinal plants and the knowledge about their appropriate use. Whereas old views assume the marginalization of traditional medical systems, a new perspective looks to them to provide complementary therapies and, in some cases, new solutions to our contemporary "health care crisis" (Table 2-6).

Much of what is called complementary or integrative (alternative) medicine in the United States represents primary care for 80% of the world's people (WHO, 1998). In this way, CAM may be considered to represent appropriate technology and affordable, sustainable medicine both for indigenous people traditionally and now for industrialized societies as well, on a global basis.

☉ Chapter References can be found on the Evolve website at http://evolve.elsevier.com/Micozzi/complementary/

CHAPTER 3

ISSUES IN INTEGRATIVE MEDICINE

MARC S. MICOZZI

As discussed in Chapters 1 and 2, one of the major popular health movements of the twenty-first century is widespread interest in, and utilization of, what has been called "alternative," "complementary," or, now, "integrative medicine." Following recognition by the medical and scientific community during the 1990s, there has been a corresponding movement among medical practitioners, administrators, academicians, and scientists to incorporate these modalities into their existing spheres of research, practice, and teaching. These movements are now leading the private sector, through health systems and insurers, and the public sectors of state and federal governments to invest more deeply and broadly in integrative medicine from the standpoint of public health and health care practice.

In recent years, estimates indicated that the American public made more visits to alternative practitioners than to primary care physicians. Utilization of herbal remedies and dietary supplements is now supported by an estimated $30 billion industry in the United States. The 2004 report on complementary and alternative medicine (CAM) utilization by the U.S. National Center for Health Statistics,

the largest and most methodologically sophisticated survey to date, indicated that almost three quarters of Americans had used CAM at some point in their lives and almost two thirds had used CAM sometime in the prior year. These statistics seem to indicate "once a user, always a user" (Barnes et al, 2004).

Significantly, American consumers have paid for most of these products and services as out-of-pocket costs, receiving only limited if any insurance or tax benefits until recently (see later discussion). It is also estimated that the out-of-pocket amount spent by consumers for alternative care exceeds the out-of-pocket copayments and deductibles consumers make for health care covered by insurance. These observations are important when making assumptions or debating the roles of third-party payers in the provision of health care. A reality for health care professionals is that one last bastion of traditional fee-for-service medicine resides among alternative and many integrative practitioners. Furthermore, the workforce supplying alternative, complementary, and integrative care is strikingly small compared with the current workforce of approximately 600,000 practicing physicians (see Availability of Services).

NOMENCLATURE AND PHILOSOPHIES OF CARE

In trying to develop a nomenclature for these modalities for descriptive purposes in the 1990s, the medical and scientific professions advanced various labels, such as "nontraditional," "unconventional," "unorthodox," "holistic," and "wholistic" (the latter a revival from the 1960s). In the midst of the call for greater scientific evidence and objectivity, these labels had the characteristic of betraying cultural values, prejudices, and judgments about the validity and appropriateness of such modalities. The more properly descriptive terminology of "alternative and complementary medicine" became generally accepted at the time. "Alternative" came to imply a mutual exclusivity with regard to the regular practice of medicine, whereas "complementary" was more accurate in describing a compatibility between the utilization and acceptance of these modalities as an adjunct to, and not a replacement for, regular medicine. As feared by many, "integration" has generally meant dominance by the mainstream biomedical complex in terms of practice, economic, and professional constraints.

"Integrative medicine," at its best, implies an active, conscious effort by the health professions and medical science to seek and sort out the evidence for and application of various complementary modalities for appropriate incorporation into the continuum of health care within the current parameters of the health care system. A potentially irresolvable philosophical question relates to the intangible costs and benefits of integration within one system versus the continued existence of pluralism among healing choices for consumers. "Integration" is interpreted to mean improved standards of evidence, quality, appropriateness, and availability of care within the mainstream health care system. "Alternatives" imply greater choices to consumers for those (perhaps relatively few) willing and able to create their own menu of healing modalities.

One view pivots on the present workforce situation (Micozzi, 1998), which may dictate that more appropriate care will be provided to more Americans through continued integration than with an uncoordinated landscape of different practices, each vying for primacy within as-yet incompletely defined, articulated, and accepted evidence-based scopes of practice. These considerations regarding "integration" may be overriden by current concerns about the economic crisis in health care (which is really a social crisis brought about by pursuing nineteenth-century ideas about healing using expensive, invasive twenty-first-century technologies). The existing health care infrastructure of clinics and hospitals may simply be unsustainable, which leads to serious consideration about providing health services outside of health care facilities (Box 3-1).

BOX 3-1

The Nature Cure as a Remedy for Health Care

- The U.S. health care system is in crisis and does not appear to be sustainable. Fortunately, alternative approaches to much of health and wellness are available.
- Presently, three quarters of Americans use health services now labeled as "complementary and alternative medicine" (CAM) for health and wellness.
- Americans now pay for CAM services primarily out of pocket. These payments now exceed total out-of-pocket charges for all outpatient mainstream health services.
- CAM services in the United States are usually available only in an outpatient (ambulatory care) setting in private offices or health care facilities. This setting provides only limited potential for the full therapeutic benefits of CAM.
- Many people would benefit from the application of CAM therapies and protocols ("a cure") over successive days of treatment (residential care) outside of health care facilities in more healthful environments.
- CAM care can be provided in more healthful environments and at lower costs than in health care facilities while providing vastly enhanced levels of hospitality.*
- Resorts, natural springs, spas, and campgrounds are ideal settings for providing many CAM health and wellness services together with the benefits of a restful, stress-free, relaxing, and healthy environment.
- Historically in the United States, and in much of Europe and Asia today, CAM may be thought of as natural medicine, or "nature cures." There is a great deal of now largely forgotten historical evidence regarding the benefits of "nature cure" obtained during the late 1700s, 1800s, and early 1900s in the United States.
- The hidden or forgotten history of American medicine is highly relevant to fully understanding the potential benefits of CAM and natural healing today.

There is a tremendous opportunity to integrate the historically proven benefits of "nature cure" with contemporary CAM therapies in natural settings.*

*See Claire Cassidy, Chapter 5, "modern biomedicine can barely function in the absence of carefully controlled environments and perfectly sterile conditions."

MODALITIES OF CARE

Many of the different physical modalities variously described as alternative, complementary, and integrative medicine can be seen to exist on a continuum with regular medicine and are believed and increasingly proved to have a measurable, physiological effect on the body. In this textbook, we have found it useful and instructive to arrange these techniques from "least invasive" to "most invasive" (see Figure 5-4). Such an array also provides the beginnings of an approach to cost-effectiveness analyses in light of the general correlation between degree of invasiveness and costs, both the cost of providing the care and the cost of managing the known and accepted complications of that care.

One such array is provided by meditation, talk therapies, bioenergetic manipulation, massage, physical manipulation, insertion, ingestion, injection, and surgery. Alternative/complementary systems of practice are then organized around the use of one or more of these techniques. For example, Chinese medicine uses bioenergy (qi), manipulation (tui na, qigong), insertion (acupuncture needles), and ingestion (herbs and foods) for medicinal purposes, approximating a more "complete" system of care. Chiropractic is traditionally limited to manipulative therapy, although many chiropractors incorporate acupuncture, herbal medicine, and nutrition into their individual practices.

Thus, individual practitioners within one system of care may incorporate other healing modalities that are traditionally outside that system of care (e.g., physician or chiropractor who incorporates acupuncture). Finally, individual techniques, when practiced in a manner that is removed from the traditional system of care (what may be called "formulary approaches"), are increasingly proved to be effective. For example, in the traditional practice of Chinese medicine (as may be found in China or in the urban United States in Chinatowns) the client generally seeks the services of a seventh-generation Chinese practitioner who may also want to incorporate herbs, manipulation, and other remedies for the treatment of a medical condition, despite historic debates among various Chinese practitioners over the use of herbs versus acupuncture. Meanwhile, in the United States, a licensed physician may attend a 6-week course in acupuncture in California and become a licensed acupuncturist. Research shows that acupuncture provided by the physician on a "formulary" basis is effective and may meet cultural expectations better for the average American when delivered by a practitioner in a white coat in an antiseptic clinic than with delivery of care in Chinatown (Cohen et al, 2007).

AVAILABILITY OF SERVICES

The availability of these modalities is determined by (1) the existence, number, and location of practitioners trained (and licensed, where applicable) to provide these services and (2) access to these practitioners through, in increasing order of complexity, clinics, hospitals, academic medical centers, health care systems, and networks. Individual practices have often thrived independent of the mainstream health care system. Given the dimensions of the movement, it is often striking how few "alternative" providers presently exist relative to the mainstream medical workforce. Manual and manipulative therapies are relatively well represented,

with approximately 300,000 massage therapists and more than 50,000 licensed chiropractors. There are approximately half that number of osteopaths, with perhaps fewer than one quarter of them maintaining any practice in manipulative therapy. Manipulative therapy is also relatively well regulated, with licensure for chiropractic in all 50 states and the District of Columbia and accreditation of graduate schools of chiropractic, whereas osteopathy has been fully subsumed under the credentialing processes of mainstream medicine.

In contrast, other fields of complementary medicine are sparsely represented. There are approximately 10,000 licensed acupuncturists in the United States, with licensure available in most states and the District of Columbia. Approximately 3000 are MD-acupuncturists, and the remainder in this category include a number of traditional Chinese practitioners. There are approximately 3000 homeopaths, most of them licensed physicians. There are approximately 4000 naturopaths, with licensure available only in a dozen states, primarily in the northwestern United States and New England, and five accredited graduate schools, primarily in the northwest and southwest. Naturopathy represents the practice of an eclectic style of medicine and Western herbalism, drawing from the herbal traditions of other cultures worldwide. Hundreds of Ayurvedic practitioners may exist, with many following highly individuated practices and others ascribing to a tightly controlled Maharishi Ayurveda school of practice in North America. In another tradition from India, thousands of yoga masters offer somewhat attenuated training in a variety of yoga, primarily designed as a meditative practice, intended to influence the physical body (Hatha Yoga). Energy healers now come from several organized schools of energy healing nationwide. The practice of energy healing is widespread among members of the U.S. nursing professions through healing touch and therapeutic touch and among a number of physical therapists, who may also include such modalities as craniosacral therapy.

MODELS OF INTEGRATION

To provide integrated care, the health care system requires access to licensed health care providers and training of existing providers in one or more modalities of complementary care. The health care system may provide credibility, appropriate practice environments, and access to new clients for practitioners. Often the health care system has opportunities to make capital investments in facilities required to provide care that are not available to individual practitioners. Sometimes the success of the integrated care clinic is based on attracting the individual practitioner's existing client base, whereas the individual practitioner comes to the health care system looking for new referrals. An important area for expansion of services is represented by appropriate referrals from within the health system hosts to their integrated clinics and inpatient services.

When complementary medical services are added onto existing services (instead of selectively replacing them), they become a cost center rather than a cost-effective source of savings. In response to consumer demand, some managed care systems have offered access to a network of complementary care providers who have agreed to accept reduced rates. For example, an innovative approach is to create a network of licensed "holistic" health providers, which offers an insurance rider to employers, unions, and associations for access to members at negotiated rates. These networks may be developed as part of corporate wellness programs, so that access to alternative providers becomes another employee benefit and factor for retention and recruitment of employees who seek these kinds of services.

Academic medical centers offer a further opportunity to develop the integration of clinical research and training with the practice of integrative medicine. Many academic medical centers adopt an "arms-length" relationship with CAM with internally isolated efforts at research or teaching or practice that are not at all functionally integrated.

Integrated care has been taken to imply the provision of various medical modalities under the supervision of a physician. To the extent that such physician-supervised centers function as full-service (or even fuller-service) primary care facilities, the concern is that if primary care "gatekeepers" refer patients for complementary care, they may never come back. Within a health care system, an integrative medical practice may be successfully managed as part of a primary care referral system for general hospital services. The national American Whole Health Network, based on a successful clinic in Chicago and intended to provide integrated medical services under physician supervision, was unable to receive adequate physician patient referrals nationally and had to embark on costly direct-to-consumer marketing. One response to the concern about physician referrals, developed by the late William Fair, Sr., a leader in integrated care, was a facility for complementary care not supervised by a physician. This concept, initially developed as Synergy Health, opened in New York City in the late 1990s under the name Haelth.

Another important direction in integrated medicine takes the provision of complementary care beyond the primary care provider and gatekeeper to the integration of appropriate complementary medical modalities into a medical specialty practice for the management of chronic diseases. The initial primary care focus of integrated medicine is being supplemented by information on integrative medicine targeted to medical specialists.

EFFECTIVENESS AND COST EFFECTIVENESS

The establishment and expansion of the CAM research program at the National Institutes of Health (NIH) by leaders in the U.S. Congress has increasingly emphasized clinical trials research to create the research database for evidence on the efficacy or lack of efficacy of available alternative medical modalities. Therefore the health care system has access to increasingly available, abundant, and credible data on effectiveness. Understanding the appropriateness and cost effectiveness of care requires health care utilization research to better understand (1) patient motivation and satisfaction, (2) willingness to pay for care, (3) preference for one effective modality of care over another, (4) willingness to substitute care, (5) multidisciplinary guidelines for best practices in disease management, and (6) related types of analyses that can better inform health care decision makers, whether policy makers, administrators, or consumers. The Agency for Healthcare Research and Quality has worked within a limited budget to provide important analyses on the effectiveness and cost effectiveness of various modalities in the management of low back pain, the most common cause of disability in working Americans; pharmaceuticals, surgery, spinal manual therapy, acupuncture, massage, and other therapies are all available at various levels of accessibility, cost, and effectiveness.

The U.S. Health Resources and Services Administration is currently sponsoring projects for development and dissemination of best practices for the treatment of lower back pain, for example, as well as an Internet-based distance learning network for applied aspects of the management and administration of integrative medical practice. Under the Health Insurance Portability and Accountability Act (HIPAA, originally the Kennedy-Kassebaum bill, developed by the Congressional Energy and Commerce Committee), the Center for Medicare and Medicaid Services is mandated to develop current practice terminology (CPT) codes for every therapy "in commerce," which implies that codes will exist for CAM therapies currently in practice and for which consumers are paying. These codes will provide a basis for expanded reimbursement of CAM by Medicare and Medicaid and serve as a precedent for other third-party payers. For improved effectiveness and cost savings to be realized by consumers, the health care system, and third-party payers, it is necessary to determine which therapeutic options can be appropriately and specifically provided to which patients in what order for cost-effective medical management.

PRODUCTS FOR THE PRACTICE OF INTEGRATIVE MEDICINE

Reliance on the appropriate use of nutrients and herbs is a critical and fundamental component of many integrative medical practices (see Figure 5-4). Presently in the United States, these natural products are widely available and are classified and regulated as dietary supplements. As such, they are regulated by the U.S. Food and Drug Administration (FDA) for identity, purity, and safety, but not for efficacy. However, unlike with pharmaceuticals, information about the health effects may not be provided on the product label or with the product. Credible third-party research is increasingly available on the efficacy of herbal and nutritional ingredients. In addition, the medical profession is increasingly recognizing the importance of dietary supplementation for optimal health and for the prevention and management of many medical conditions (Fairfield et al, 2002). Practitioners of integrative medicine are able to maintain a medical standard of information and practice about herbal and nutritional ingredients. One requirement is to develop and maintain an appropriate clinic- or hospital-based formulary of high-quality sources of herbs and nutrients, available in appropriate forms, doses, and combinations.

Not only is the regulatory environment chaotic, but much of the natural products industry does not operate to medical and scientific standards, many irresponsible marketing claims are made, and many medical and scientific professionals are not knowledgeable about the science behind herbal and nutritional medicine. This volatile mix produces much confusion and misinformation on both sides, even promulgated periodically by such well-intentioned sources as the *New England Journal of Medicine.* Most medical professionals are presently on their own in trying to understand the proper indications, ingredients, and dosages for the appropriate scientific use of herbal and nutritional remedies. Consumers can only look to health professionals for guidance. New information technologies are being brought online to provide distributors, consumers, and practitioners fair and accurate information about the appropriate use of dietary supplements (see Chapter 22).

REGULATION

The practice of integrative medicine is based on incorporating various nonconventional modalities in a more conventional medical setting—for example, MDs may include Chinese or Ayurvedic protocols in their practices. The other, equally important, half of integrative medical care is the prescription of dietary supplements.

In this regard, it is essential that practitioners have accurate and appropriate information about dietary supplements and that the supplements themselves be of the highest quality—or at least of a quality high enough to ensure that they will benefit health in the way intended. In the medical community, both of these issues fall under the category of pharmacy practice and hospital formulary.

The current regulatory environment is based on some of the same criteria that are made to apply to pharmaceuticals, but at the same time (1) much of the natural products industry does not operate to the same medical and scientific standards, (2) many irresponsible marketing claims are made, and (3) many medical and scientific professionals are still not knowledgeable about the science

behind herbal and nutritional medicine. This volatile mix produces much confusion and misinformation on both sides, documented periodically by such august sources as the *New England Journal of Medicine.* Medical professionals are largely on their own in trying to understand the proper indications, ingredients, and dosages for the appropriate scientific use of herbal and nutritional remedies. And consumers can only look to practitioners for guidance.

This situation can be improved only with the active participation of the health professions, pharmacists, integrative medical physicians, naturopathic medical physicians, and others who recommend natural supplements as part of the practice of health care.

PHARMACY FOR INTEGRATIVE MEDICAL PRACTICES: LEGISLATIVE AND REGULATORY ENVIRONMENT

Before 1994, the FDA regulated dietary supplements as foods in most circumstances. Then, under the Dietary Supplement Health and Education Act (DSHEA) of 1994 (amended in 1998) dietary supplements and dietary ingredients were regulated as a category unto themselves—neither foods nor, as some wished, drugs. Under DSHEA, the FDA has the power to regulate all dietary supplements in several ways (Box 3-2).

Lack of FDA regulatory authority is frequently misrepresented—sometimes by the FDA commissioner

---

BOX 3-2

FDA Power of Regulation Under DSHEA

In regard to accurate information:
- To obtain injunctions against the sale of products making false claims
- To sue any company making claims that a product cures or treats disease

In regard to safety and quality:
- To require good manufacturing practices (GMPs), including ensuring ingredient identity and product potency, cleanliness, and stability (although it was not until 2003, some 9 years after the passage of DSHEA, that the government published proposed rules for dietary ingredient and supplement GMPs, and were finalized in 2007.)
- To refer those engaging in the sale of toxic or unsanitary products for criminal action
- To seize products that pose an unreasonable risk of illness and injury
- To stop sales of entire classes of products if they pose an imminent health hazard
- To stop products from being marketed if the FDA does not receive sufficient safety data in advance under "generally recognized as safe" (GRAS) provisions

DSHEA, Dietary Supplement Health and Education Act; *FDA,* Food and Drug Administration.

herself or himself—according to a report released by the House Committee on Government Reform in July 2001.

According to testimony recorded before Congress, the FDA does not always appear to understand or implement the authority Congress had already given it to regulate dietary supplements.

The FDA was also given responsibility to carry out educational efforts regarding dietary supplements under DSHEA in 1994 but has often acted as if it has not educated itself, let alone the health professions. The FDA took 15 years to develop new good manufacturing practices for dietary supplements, which were finally disseminated by 2008.

Nonetheless, even with sufficient regulation, the safety and quality of dietary supplements still depends to an extent on medical vigilance and voluntary industry compliance—especially since, after the 2004 congressional elections, further changes to DSHEA were not legislated. This situation may not be as dire as it sounds, however. In his memoirs, Senator Orrin Hatch (R-Utah; 2002), co-chair of the Congressional Caucus on Complementary and Alternative Medicine and Dietary Supplements, documents the unprecedented involvement of citizens and commercial groups in successfully getting DSHEA passed. With such strong consumer and commercial interest, it is likely that what is somewhat sketchily covered by regulation still may be achieved by better information and the education of consumers and health professionals, as, for example, was indicated by this author to the hearings of the U.S. House of Representatives Committee on Government Reform, Subcommittee on Health and Human Rights, on the topic "Dietary Supplement Health and Education Act of 1994: Ten Years After," in March 2004.

The best way to bring about improvements under the current legislation is to work with the active and growing U.S. natural products and dietary supplements industry. Some responsible natural products suppliers, manufacturers, and distributors are beginning to recognize that the integration of herbal and nutritional medicine into integrative and naturopathic medical practice mandates higher standards of product ingredients and information about their appropriate use.

QUESTIONS ON THE PROPER USE OF HERBAL MEDICINES

It is important to keep in mind that as integrative medicine goes mainstream, there can be misdirection of supplement use (Box 3-3). St. John's wort (SJW, *Hypericum perforatum*), *Gingko biloba*, kava kava (*Piper methysticum*), and ephedra (*Ephedra sinensis*) have all come under public attack in recent years based on misuse of the herb in question. Each case, explained in the following sections, illustrates a different aspect of misinformation about, and/or misuse of, herbal remedies.

BOX 3-3

General Guidelines for the Use of Herbal Medicines

- The clinician should take a careful history of the patient's use of herbs and other supplements
- An accurate medical diagnosis must be made before the use of herbs for symptomatic treatment
- *Natural* is not necessarily *safe*: attention should be paid to product quality, dosage, and potential adverse effects, including herb-drug and herb-herb interactions.
- Many herbal treatments should be avoided in pregnancy (and contemplated pregnancy, because fertility is not a perfect science) and lactation.
- Herbal medicines should be given to children with care, and the appropriate dosage based on weight should be used.
- Adverse effects should be recorded, and the dosage reduced or the product discontinued. It can be carefully restarted to ascertain whether or not it is the source of the problem.

ST. JOHN'S WORT

SJW is considered an effective treatment for mild to moderate depression. One recent study tested SJW in patients with depression severe enough to warrant hospitalization. The problem is that there has been no practical experience on what the appropriate SJW dosage or regimen might be in such severely depressed patients. The study found SJW to be ineffective (the conventional antidepressant was also ineffective in this study), and patients were deprived of needed mainstream psychotherapy when there was initially no plausible reason to believe that SJW might be appropriately used in this population. This circumstance raised questions about the ethicality of such an experiment in the first place.

It is important not to ignore "historic use" and to assume that herbs can be "prescribed" just like drugs, when these substances are moved into the mainstream. Another study reported in spring 2002 showed no difference between placebo and conventional medication in the treatment of severely depressed patients who were also given 14 to 16 hours of intensive personal care from highly trained mental health professionals. Perhaps the real message regarding severe depression is that neither herbs nor drugs can be expected to completely substitute for "hands-on" therapeutic care.

GINGKO

Gingko is well established as an effective treatment for mild dementia and has been demonstrated to improve memory in those with documented memory impairment. However, it has been marketed irresponsibly as a generic memory enhancer, which led to a misguided study of gingko showing no effects when standard tests of memory were used in those without cognitive impairment. The subsequent promotion of the study findings has led to great confusion and the claim that gingko does not help memory in anyone, when in fact an inappropriate study population was chosen, either accidently due to ignorance or deliberately due to malice. Again, historic use is ignored at the potential peril of both researchers and study participants.

KAVA KAVA

Kava kava is well accepted under historic use for its actions as a muscle relaxant and sleep inducer. However, among the anecdotal experiences of approximately 70 million users, kava kava was claimed in a report titled "In-Depth Investigation into [European Union] Members States Market Restrictions on Kava Products" to cause rare serious liver toxicity. Liver toxicity is not uncommon with many prescription and over-the-counter drugs, and there are hundreds of deaths due to liver failure each year from the routine use of over-the-counter acetaminophen, for example. Joerg Gruenwald, MD, demonstrated that the assignment of liver toxicity to the use of kava kava in the cases cited by the European Union study was high questionable. This leads to the issue of whether kava kava, which is an effective treatment for anxiety, should be banned or whether, instead, a responsible approach to risk-benefit should be developed, as with many other treatments potentially manifesting side effects. The case-by-case analysis by Gruenwald and colleagues at the Phytopharm Consulting Group in Berlin, Germany, found several alternative explanations for liver toxicity in those taking kava kava. Nonetheless, many retailers have voluntarily taken kava kava off the shelves in response to these claims. This demonstrates the loss to the public of a potentially valuable product for reasons that are not scientifically sound.

EPHEDRA

Ephedra has been used by millions for weight loss, but it was also inappropriately used as a performance enhancer—in this latter case, leading it to be listed on a number of autopsy reports as contributing to fatalities among otherwise healthy individuals. An FDA-commissioned report in 2003 stated in its final ruling that five deaths could be attributed directly to ephedra. To put this number in perspective, the American Herbal Products Association reports that about 12 to 17 million people took ephedra in 1999, their latest numbers. The *Nutrition Business Journal* estimated that 2002 ephedra sales were $1.25 billion. Regardless, these fatality reports led to ephedra's being taken off the market in 2004, although the ban did not affect sales of over-the-counter cold medications such as decongestants, which often contain ephedrine in synthetic form. (There has subsequently been regulation to place synthetic ephedrine–containing remedies behind the pharmacy counter.)

It was only in 2005 that a Utah-based Nutraceutical Corporation successfully challenged the ephedra ban, which led a judge to rule that, in accordance with DSHEA, the FDA could not place the burden to prove safety on dietary supplement manufacturers as it does on drug and device makers. The court allowed the sale of ephedra products containing less than 10 mg of ephedra.

Because the federal government has also recognized obesity as a major risk factor for many diseases, and because effective weight loss regimens elude many overweight individuals, does ephedra have a role? Is it possible to have safe, medically supervised application of appropriate ephedra formulations for weight loss, or does ephedra have no place whatsoever in contemporary use?

Abuse of herbal products adulterated with therapeutic drugs and contaminants (a particular problem with imports from overseas, particularly China) is also a serious safety issue. Consumers, health professionals and responsible elements of the U.S. natural products industry all suffer when irresponsibly adulterated products are imported from abroad. A much heralded clinical trial conducted by the National Center for Complementary and Alternative Medicine (NCCAM) at the NIH on use of the Chinese herbal formulation PC-SPES to treat prostate cancer was undermined by the unwitting use of adulterated herbs. A further dilemma was created when NCCAM stopped the trial after it discovered the adulteration, but study participants demanded to continue because they had found relief from the treatment. Some natural products from China have even been contaminated with the dangerous antibiotic chloramphenicol, which may cause bone marrow aplasia, as recently as 2002.

Thus, some voluntary improvements in manufacturing and marketing standards in the natural products industry will be required for effective integration into medical practice (Box 3-4).

INTEGRATIVE PRACTICE: SOME SOLUTIONS

Reliance on the appropriate and safe use of diet, nutrients, and herbs is a critical and fundamental component of integrative medical practices. To properly address this area, attention needs to be focused on medical education and public policy issues.

MEDICAL EDUCATION

The issues considered thus far point to the clear need for improved education on dietary supplements and integrative medicine in medical schools, postgraduate medical training programs, and continuing medical education (CME) courses. CME programs are met with the challenge

BOX 3-4

Problems with "Integrative" Medical Research

Part of the development of integrative medicine involves mainstream biomedical research on the effects of herbal medicines in established use. When mainstream biomedical scientists are turned loose to conduct clinical research on complementary and alternative medicine (CAM), especially herbal medicines, they have access to unprecedented levels of funding, state-of-the-art technologies, and new patient populations, but they often lack the rudimentary knowledge about historical use that would be known to any reader of this text. These new studies in new populations, outside the regular practice of CAM, often cause controversy.

Certain herbal remedies, regulated as dietary supplements, are now commonplace in the United States, with their application often supported by historic use. Two aforementioned examples of well-established herbal remedies are *Gingko biloba* for improvement of memory in those with medically documented memory impairment and St. John's wort (SJW) for improvement of mood in ambulatory patients with mild to moderate depression. Well-publicized, controversial studies of each of these herbs have been conducted recently that illustrate some of the challenges faced in conducting contemporary research on historically established herbal remedies.

Gingko has been a well-established treatment for cognitive impairment and dementia. As of 10 years ago, over 40 studies had already been performed showing these benefits, which were documented in a meta-analysis. Since then there have been several clinical trials that substantiated the use of gingko for this purpose. Gingko has other uses as well. From year to year it has been the most popular herbal remedy in Europe and the United States.

Although prior evidence, and responsible use of gingko, shows benefits for the treatment of cognitive impairment and dementia, a well-publicized study involving healthy volunteers without cognitive impairment was published in the *Journal of the American Medical Association (JAMA)* in August 2002. The 6-week psychological study predictably showed that gingko did not improve memory in elderly adults without cognitive impairment. The study was conducted at an undergraduate college by psychologists and their undergraduate students. Although the results did not emanate from clinical researchers at an academic medical center and were not surprising given the existing body of clinical research on the appropriate use of gingko, the results were treated as a major news event by the public media. Experts contended that the study, which tested one brand of gingko of unknown potency, has flaws.

By the spring of 2003, this study and the publicity surrounding it was raising many questions. A high-level conference for the functional foods and nutraceuticals industry, sponsored by Hoffmann-La Roche, Pfizer, and others, addressed the topic on March 6, 2003. A question was posed: the federal government is presently supporting research on dietary supplements, but what is the reward for that investment and are these studies asking the right questions about traditional herbal medicines?

As interest in research on traditional remedies grows, researchers will have access to new populations and powerful research capabilities and methodologies. Knowledge of the traditional and appropriate use of herbal remedies, and their applications in integrative medicine, is an important part of the equation.

Other recent studies conducted on St. John's wort illustrate the difficulties of studying traditional herbal remedies in new populations. In April 2001, Shelton et al published a study in *JAMA* entitled a "Randomized Controlled Trial of St. John's Wort in Major Depression." The many (over 30) studies performed on SJW before that had generally showed it to be effective in treating mild to moderate depression but not major depression.

The new study selected 200 patients with severe depression, whereas SJW is not used or recommended for treatment of severe depression or for hospitalized patients or patients undergoing active psychiatric treatment. This study confirmed the findings of prior studies that adverse side effects of SJW were low, especially compared with those of antidepressants.

Shortly after the Shelton et al study was published, several physicians, researchers, and leading authorities in the psychiatric community responded. The most common theme of the rebuttals centered on the actual foundation of the study. Whereas Shelton et al openly refuted many of the landmark studies based on mild to moderate depression, the Shelton study enrolled only patients with severe depression.

As noted earlier, the study was published in *JAMA* in April 2001. The following month, May 13 to 18, it was disclosed at the Annual Meeting of the American Psychiatric Association held in Chicago that 43 of the 200 participants of the study dropped out of the study early. In the published study, however, Shelton et al had reported that only 28 individuals dropped out. After being called to question by his peers, Shelton disclosed (2 months later, in July 2001, in his response to rebuttal letters) that the dropout rate had again been adjusted to 33. How accurate was record keeping? Was it 28, 33, or 43? In addition, in his response letter, Shelton stated, "We did note the possibility of a sampling bias in our article."

Two physicians at the Council for Responsible Nutrition in Washington, D.C., found additional flaws in the Shelton et al study and went so far as to say that the authors may have acted unethically according to the World Medical Association Declaration of Helsinki by exposing 200 patients known to be suffering from severe depression both to a placebo and to an herbal extract that the researchers themselves did not believe worked even for mild forms of depression. This clearly fails to comply with item 19 of the Helsinki Declaration, which states, "Medical research is only justified if there is a reasonable likelihood that the populations in which the research is carried out stand to benefit form the results of the research."

As evidenced by Shelton's clear and express repudiation of preceding studies on the effects of SJW, he clearly held no belief that there was a reasonable likelihood that the study group would benefit in any way from the study. Yet he subjected these patients to the study.

BOX 3-4

Problems with "Integrative" Medical Research—cont'd

Two physicians in the Department of Epidemiology and Social Medicine at the Albert Einstein College of Medicine in New York called the authors' math into question. Although Shelton et al claim an 80% power to detect their response rate, Dr. Cohen and Dr. Marantz state that "Shelton and associates only had a power of 46% to find a statistically significant difference."

Another group of physicians in similar positions at leading psychiatric institutions ran Shelton's numbers and found similar discrepancies. They offered two notable rebuttals that would have put Shelton et al back on the ethical side of the fence:

To remove the discrepancies between placebo and St. John's Wort why didn't they add a third arm to their research ... an antidepressant drug ... to see its affects on severe depression. At least this way, they would have been able to maintain some level of belief that the study would benefit the patients they were experimenting on—thus staying within the Helsinki Declaration of medical research ethics.

We suggest a proper conclusion ... might read ... "The efficacy of St. John's Wort in patients with mild to moderate depression WAS NOT EVALUATED" ... much clearer and more concise than, ... "St. John's Wort was not effective for treatment of major depression."

Writing about this study in *Advances in Therapy* in February 2002, Behnke et al noted that the *JAMA* study selected patients from psychiatric institutions who had suffered from major depression for more than 10 years and whose current depressive disorder had lasted for 2.5 years before they entered the study, and that the severity of disease and the study population were not appropriately selected for the SJW treatment. Behnke et al also showed SJW to be 80% as effective as drug therapy for mild to moderate depression and to be safe.

Another study reported in *JAMA* in April 2002 found that neither SJW nor drug therapy produced effects that were significantly different from those for the placebo control. This study enrolled patients with "moderately severe major depression." The dosages of both SJW and the drug varied for different patients. The authors' review identified several studies performed before 1996 that reported positive effects for SJW. They also cited five studies that showed SJW treatment to be comparable to drug therapy and four studies showing SJW to be superior to placebo conducted since 1996. The historically established use for SJW has been in the management of mild to moderate depression, not of severe depression, the treatment of which is likely to be in the hands of a psychotherapist.

Integrative medical research is problematic in many ways and is not likely to be able to supplant knowledge of historical use, which is the foundation for the practice of CAM.

---

that current practitioners generally have had little to no exposure to these topic areas.

According to surveys conducted by the Center for Research in Medical Education and Health Care at Thomas Jefferson University, Philadelphia (http://www.jefferson.edu), the majority of today's medical students in all graduation years and in all current classes want more education in integrative medicine. The proportion is increasing with each graduating year. Among medical school classes, the proportion is relatively high in the first year (when entering students carry the culture of the general population), declines somewhat in the second and third years (as students become professionalized and generally witness little reinforcement for the teaching of integrative medicine), and rises again in the fourth year (after students have been exposed to the problems and questions of patients).

The literature of integrative medicine is in the process of creation, with a need for both "basic science" and clinical texts, and journals in integrative medicine. Elsevier Health Sciences (subsuming the former C.V. Mosby of St. Louis, W.B. Saunders of Philadelphia, and Churchill-Livingstone of Edinburgh and London) has developed many titles in complementary medicine, including a series Medical Guides to Complementary and

Alternative Medicine for which this text served as the foundation (http://www.elsevierhealth.com). Much curriculum and faculty development remains to be done in this area, and the traditional support of state and federal governments for medical education and training could help provide medical schools with the needed resources and incentives. In the interim, it is incumbent upon providers of health care services to help stimulate appropriate CME and in-service training for health professions staffs so that practitioners can be knowledgeable and helpful to their patients seeking guidance on the use of dietary supplements and integrative medicine.

PUBLIC POLICY ISSUES

Unlike with pharmaceuticals, and at the risk of repeating these critical points, DSHEA mandates that information about health effects can *not* be provided on the product label or with the product as a product insert. Due to the increasing availability of credible third-party research on the efficacy of herbal and nutritional ingredients, as well as increasing recognition by the medical profession of the importance of dietary supplementation for optimal health, it is incumbent upon practitioners of integrative medicine to maintain a medical standard of information and practice about herbal and nutritional ingredients. One approach to this requirement is to develop and maintain the capability for a clinic- or hospital-based formulary of appropriate, effective, and high-quality sources of herbs and nutrients.

It also bears repeating that new information technologies are being brought online to provide distributors, consumers, and practitioners fair and accurate information about the appropriate use of dietary supplements. The Tai Sophia Institute in Columbia, Maryland (http://www.tai.edu/maryland-chi.html), the University of Exeter in the United Kingdom (http://www.ex.ac.uk), and other sources are committed to developing accessible databases on dietary supplements for professional reference in the practice of integrative medicine.

State governments have developed a traditional role in regulating medical practice and in supporting medical education. The federal government maintains a unique and critical role in stimulating and supporting medical research, regulating medical products and devices, protecting the public health, and helping build health care infrastructure, and is now paying approximately one third of the costs of health care in America. Policy makers at the state and federal levels should become more knowledgeable about the needs and opportunities relative to integrative medicine.

As mentioned earlier, a bipartisan Congressional Caucus on Complementary and Alternative Medicine and Dietary Supplements was organized to help serve this purpose, co-chaired in the Senate by Tom Harkin (D-Iowa) and Orrin Hatch (R-Utah) and in the House of Representatives by Dennis Kucinich (D-Ohio) and Dan Burton (R-Indiana), who has also chaired the Committee on Government Reform and its Subcommittee on Health and Human Rights. In 2006, a new House Caucus on Dietary Supplements was formed with Representatives Chris Cannon (R-Utah) and Frank Pallone (D-NJ), as well as a Caucus on Complementary and Alternative Medicine continuing with Rep. Burton. Some professional groups are beginning to work with members of these caucuses and other elected representatives to broaden and deepen federal support for appropriate analyses and applied programs on dietary supplements and integrative medicine. However, the effort to work with public policy leaders is poorly organized and undermined by the desire of most "integrative medicine" programs, within their mainstream biomedical institutions, to maintain the status quo and not to rock the boat for federal funding for biomedical education and research.

Although funding for NCCAM has increased each year since its creation was mandated by Congress in 1992, it is critical that other federal agencies charged with administering programs related to health resources and services, primary care, health professions training and workforce development, consumer education, health services research, and other areas direct their efforts to address the important challenge and opportunity of integrative medicine. Integrative medicine has an important role that requires further articulation in current congressional actions on medical liability insurance reform and the national patient safety and quality assurance initiative, not to mention the chimera of authentic healthcare reform. Public support together with private innovation, and respect for the art and science of the traditions of medical practice, has been the hallmark of medical advancement, and this should continue to be the case for integrative medicine.

Chapter References can be found on the Evolve website at http://evolve.elsevier.com/Micozzi/complementary/

ECOLOGICAL PHARMACY: FROM GAIA TO PHARMACOLOGY

KEVIN SPELMAN

First, the world of life, taken as a whole, forms a single system bound to the surface of the earth; a system whose elements, in whatever order of association they may be considered, are not simply thrown together and moulded upon one another like grains of sand, but are organically interdependent like . . . molecules caught in a capillary surface.
—PIERRE TEILHARD DE CHARDIN, 1943

THE GAIA HYPOTHESIS: STARTING WITH THE WHOLE, THE INTERDEPENDENCE OF ORGANISM AND ENVIRONMENT

Pierre Teilhard de Chardin, a visionary French Jesuit, paleontologist, biologist, and philosopher who was fascinated with evolution and its connection with spirituality, seems to have recognized the limitations of reductionism. He insisted that life must be studied in its totality on a large scale as a single system. As he contemplated the Earth and its life forms in the 1940s, he suggested the term *geobiology* to embrace all life systems and their environment as a self-organizing whole (Galleni, 1995).

Within two decades of de Chardin's writing, a significant paradigm shift took place from the quantitative clockworks view to an exploration of the qualitative emergent view of self-organizing systems and even life itself. A system's approach was starting to be supported in other sciences. For example, in Germany Hermann Haken developed his nonlinear laser theory and Manfred Eigen experimented on catalytic cycles (Capra, 1996); in the United States Heinz von Foerster focused his interdisciplinary team on self-organization; in Belgium Ilya Prigogine grasped the now understood connection between nonequilibrium systems and nonlinearity; meanwhile in Chile Humberto Maturana was postulating autopoiesis and life.

These paradigms that all converged on systems as a whole, coupled with Teilhard de Chardin's insistence that the Earth must be studied as a unity, with both geological and biological points of view (Galleni, 1995), perhaps led the British atmospheric chemist James Lovelock to one of the biggest revolutions in viewing our planet that possibly we will ever know (Lovelock et al, 1974).

Lovelock worked as a consultant to the U.S. National Aeronautics and Space Administration (NASA) in the early 1960s. NASA contracted Lovelock to aid in the quest to detect life on Mars. Lovelock, contemplating the chemistry of the atmosphere, found that an atmosphere out of chemical equilibrium was the signature of life on a planet. An atmosphere rich in oxygen and methane, for instance, indicates the presence of organisms that are responsible for the uneven mix. Earth has just such an atmosphere (Lovelock, 1979). Through this investigation Lovelock had a flash of insight one day: the planet Earth as a whole is a self-organizing system. He saw the unity of the biosphere—a global organism (Turney, 2005).

Just a few years later, the further study of these features of the Earth resulted in the idea that life vigorously regulated terrestrial conditions, a sort of planetary homeostasis (Turney, 2005). By observing the geological evidence and paleoclimatic evidence, Lovelock, influenced by ecology, physiology, cybernetics, and systems analysis, hypothesized that the ocean's salinity, the gaseous atmospheric concentration, and the surface temperatures were maintained within narrow ranges by feedback loops of organisms responding to variations in their environment (Lovelock, 1979).

Lovelock postulated that the climate and chemical composition of the Earth's surface are kept in homeostasis at an optimum by and for the biosphere (Lovelock et al, 1982). The notion was that the biosphere adaptively regulated the Earth (Lovelock et al, 1974). In time, Lovelock (1995) viewed self-organization as emerging from the ensemble of biota and environment. He saw the flow of sunlight on the planet and feedback systems from living organisms to automatically generate comfortable life conditions that synchronistically evolved with the needs of the organisms on the planet. He called this idea of a living planet the *Gaia hypothesis.*

A model as whole and beautiful as Gaia was predictable. Chemists and physicists probing matter were finding that nature did not consist of isolated components, but rather appeared as a complex web of relations between the various parts of a unified whole. As Heisenberg expressed decades before the Gaia hypothesis was formulated, "the world thus appears as a complicated tissue of events, in which connections of different kinds alternate or overlap or combine and thereby determine the texture of the whole" (Capra, 1982).

Life has existed on Earth for over 3.8 billion years (Lenton, 2002). During this time, the Earth's surface has been subject to increasing solar luminosity and declining volcanic and tectonic activity, and to such perturbations as massive asteroid impacts (Lenton, 2002; Lovelock et al, 1974; Watson et al, 1978). For example, despite the fact that the heat of the sun has increased by 25% over the last 4 billion years, the Earth's surface temperature has remained constant, which creates an agreeable environment for life (Lovelock, 1987). The Gaia hypothesis suggests that practically all metabolisms are intimately connected to the flow of chemical compounds (Lovelock, 1989). For instance, the greenhouse gases of carbon dioxide, methane, and sulphur compounds can produce highly reflective clouds, thus affecting the temperature of the Earth's surface and, in turn, influencing the metabolism of life on the planet (due to temperature change), which again changes the flow of chemical compounds to the surface and atmosphere (Kleidon, 2004).

It seems that life affects the Earth's surface environment at a planetary level, significantly increasing the cycling of free energy, essential elements, and water; inducing extreme thermodynamic disequilibrium of the atmosphere; and altering the chemistry of the atmosphere, oceans, land surface, and crust (Lovelock, 1987). In turn, the state of the environment influences life, creating feedback loops between life and its environment (Lenton, 2002). These circular processes are organized through feedback loops that are found in every living system. The unusual aspect of the Earth's hypothesized feedback loops is that they link together living and nonliving systems. For instance, the Gaia theory weaves together plants, microorganisms, and animals with rocks, oceans, and the atmosphere (Capra, 1996).

In this construct, life and the environment evolve together as one system, so that not only does the species that leaves the most progeny inherit the environment, but the environment that favors the most progeny is itself sustained (Kirchner, 2003). This life-enhancing dance of environment and organism can be understood as an emergent property of evolution, because life-enhancing effects would be favored by natural selection (Lenton, 1998). This relationship also requires a radical rethinking of the neo-Darwinist view of evolution. Lovelock deduced the following principles from his observations of the planet (Lovelock, 1989):

1. Life is a global phenomenon. There cannot be sparse life on a planet. It would be as unstable as half of a buffalo. Living organisms must regulate their planet; otherwise, the inevitable forces of physical and chemical evolution would render it uninhabitable.

2. Gaia theory supplements Darwin's great vision. The evolution of the species needs to be considered hand in hand with the evolution of their environment. The two processes are closely linked as a single indivisible process. To say that the organism that leaves the most progeny succeeds is not enough. Success also depends on coherent coupling between the evolution of the organism and the evolution of its material environment.

3. Finally, Gaia theory requires a mathematical model that accepts the nonlinearity of nature without being overwhelmed by the limitations imposed by the chaos of complex dynamics. The theory makes the seemingly irrelevant observations of ecological oscillations relevant (Lotka, 1925).

At its simplest, the idea that the entire ensemble of living organisms in its interaction with the environment—the biosphere—can be considered a single system has become the basis for a whole series of unfolding programs of research (Turney, 2005).

Now, some 40 years after Lovelock's realization, a statement issued from a joint meeting in 2001 of the International Geosphere-Biosphere Programme, the International Human Dimensions Programme on Global Environmental Change, the World Climate Research Programme, and the International Biodiversity Programme in a meeting in Amsterdam to study our planet begins, "The Earth System behaves as a single, self-regulating system comprised of physical, chemical, biological and human components." It seems the science of Gaia has become conventional wisdom (Turney, 2005).

Even some scientists who do not agree with the Gaia hypothesis acknowledge what Lovelock's vision has added to the study of earth sciences (Turney, 2005; Volk, 2002). The very term *earth science* exists because of Lovelock's work. Volk (2002), who does not embrace the implications of the Gaia hypothesis, says, "I was inspired by Lovelock's early writings to move into issues about the effects of life on a global scale that led to technical work I would not otherwise have accomplished. . . . Gaia became a way of thinking, a mantra to be mindful of the biggest scale." Many critics accept that it is essential to understand the Earth system as a unity, rather than as a set of disconnected components (Kirchner, 2003).

One of the issues is the defining feature of a complex system like Gaia that makes it extremely difficult to analyze, namely, that the planet is not a well-designed machine, but a complex ensemble of life that constantly rebuilds itself within a range of variable parameters, like all living organisms. This creates a model impossible to analyze from a reductionist perspective (Kirchner, 2003).

Yet a deeper reservation is that a living planet has all the hallmarks of scientific communities coming to grips with a major paradigm shift, a revolution in science (Kuhn, 1962). Whether or not one agrees with the enchanted vision of a biotic Earth, the issue is more than academic. Given the havoc created by our own species, it is vital to comprehend how our planet functions and how it is likely to respond to immature fostership (Lenton, 2002).

Capra (1996) points out that the conception of the universe as an interconnected web of relations is one of the major themes that recur throughout modern physics. The elucidation of the patterns and relationships between a system's components may yield models that provide a more accurate depiction of reality. He goes on to suggest that Gaia is a mere realization of this line of reasoning. Moreover, such a systems approach may provide a wider perspective for understanding the process of evolution, inviting us to recognize that humans belong to a process that is much more grand than the human species.

COHERENT COUPLING, EXPANDING THE COEVOLUTION CONSTRUCT: ADAPTATION TO THE ENVIRONMENT

Isolating the organism from its environment has been a fundamental tenet of the study of biological processes. In many laboratories around the world this practice is still followed in hopes of gaining further insight into life processes. However, this may lead to incomplete conclusions. Maturana and Varela (1987) proposed that, because organisms are inexorably interwoven with their environments, it is impossible to speak of environment and organism as separate entities. They presented this interrelationship as *structural coupling* (later called "coherent coupling") in their landmark book the *Tree of Knowledge*. They define coherent coupling as a history of recurrent interactions leading to the structural congruence between two (or more) systems (Maturana et al, 1987).

In other words, autopoietic (self-organizing) unities, such as organisms and environment, can undergo coupled histories of structural change due to their consistent and constant interactions. Coherent coupling recognizes the congruence between autopoietic systems. This congruence can include the system and its environment or systems affecting systems. In this paradigm, the environment is seen as a medium, which illustrates the interwoven nature of organism and environment. Development of the autopoietic systems involved thereby arises from transformations that each invokes in the other. This very much challenges the neo-Darwinist evolutionary theory, which in some authors' opinions drastically underestimate the effects and inseparability of the environment and organism (Cairns, 1996; Scapini, 2001; Thaler, 1994). Such an interdependent relationship is considered unique and diachronic and is a defining principle of an organism and the environment (Scapini, 2001).

The construct of coherent coupling dictates that organism and environment are mutually enfolded in multiple ways, and what constitutes the world of a given organism is enabled by that organism's history of coupling with its environment (Varela et al, 1991). Indeed, on a human level it is well accepted at this juncture that our intertwining with our environment provides constant perturbation requiring a systemic reorganization of physiological function (Schulkin, 2003).

Although some researchers are realizing the profound effect the environment has on physiological function, especially in regard to health and disease, other researchers have taken it a step further. Cairns' group (Cairns et al, 1988) published an extremely controversial paper some years ago stating that mutations can be environmentally directed. Following up on Cairns' work a few years later, Thaler (1994) came to the same conclusion, declaring that the environment can invoke genotypic change and postulating that both the environment and the organism's *perception* of the environment can induce genetic engineering genes to rewrite themselves and thus rewrite sections of DNA code. Cairns and Thaler were suggesting a complex engagement of organism and environment. What they perhaps did not know was that they had just provided Maturana and Varela with molecular evidence for their coherent coupling construct. This greatly challenged the prevalent neo-Darwinists' perspective that views mutations as random events, not specifically adaptive as suggested by Cairns and Thaler. Such a non-Darwinian response, well beyond haphazard natural selection, infers a primary form of intelligence that had developed billions of years ago (Pechere, 2004).

The construct of coherent coupling provides the understanding of an autopoietic system's ability to be extensively shaped by interactions with its environment over time, and vice versa. Many may see this as the fitting of a system to its environment, but this is not what is meant by coherent coupling. Rather, this construct denotes congruence between an autopoietic system and environment due to changes prompted by each one. It is also important not to confuse this construct with the concept of coevolution, a subset of evolution that includes population genetics and theoretical ecology. Although coevolution accounts for species-species or species-environment interaction, it differs from the coherent coupling paradigm in that the species are still seen separately from their environment and surrounding species. Coevolution still follows the central dogma of biology: Information flows from DNA to RNA to protein and, by extension, to the cell and on to multicellular systems. Crick (1970) originally formulated this dogma as a negative hypothesis stating that information cannot flow from protein to DNA. What this central dogma of biology implies is that a cell's experience has no effect on DNA sequence (Figure 4-1).

Maturana and Varela (1987) challenged the central dogma by implying that experience can have an effect on DNA. They pointed out that the confusion is in viewing DNA as "uniquely responsible" instead of as having an "essential participation." Although the organisms and environment are recognized as autonomous in the coherent coupling model, they are also recognized as inseparably engaged in mutually affecting relationships. The result is ontogenic adaptation of the organism to its medium: the changes of state of the organism correspond to the change of state of the medium (Maturana, 1975). Thus organisms are seen as shaped due to historical recurrent interactions with their environment, just as the environment has been shaped by its interactions with the organism.

On a microcosmic scale, for instance, cellular membranes have coherently coupled with the abundance of sodium and calcium ions. This is seen through the specialization of proteins in the membrane to allow for active transport and the inclusion of metabolic processes that include sodium and calcium. This implies that the genome adapted to the reoccurring experience of the membrane with sodium and/or calcium. On a macrocosmic scale, the paradigm of coherent coupling leads to an easy realization of the Gaia hypothesis whereby the planetary environment (e.g., temperature, ocean salinity, and atmospheric gases) is modified by various species and, in turn, these species phenotypically and genotypically morph to the environment. It can be stated that all "evolution is coevolution" and that all "development is codevelopment." Could it be that all evolution and all development are environmental coupling?

Ultimately interpreting Maturana and Varela's work results in the idea that the coupling of organisms with a high capacity for adaptation goes beyond response to the physicochemical dimension; the morphological, physiological, and psychological plasticity of an organism firmly embeds that organism in its surroundings, creating a dynamic response to recursive perturbations. Put simply, the phenotype depends to a significant degree on the environment, and this is a necessary condition for integrating the developing organism into its particular habitat (Gilbert, 2002).

COUPLING OF HUMANS WITH PHYTOCHEMISTRY: PLANT-HUMAN COALITIONS

The constant interwoven nature of organism and environment requires some sort of exchange of information to account for species plasticity. Markos (1995) defines this exchange that allows species to read their environment, thus integrating into Gaia, as "informational flow." The informational flow relevant to the discussion between plants and humans is, in its most basic form, chemistry—molecular messaging—although there are likely many other cues that are important to plant-human coalitions.

The secondary metabolites of plants are well known to modulate the interrelations—both positive (i.e., attractant) and negative (i.e. repellent)—among plants and their consumers. The presence of secondary compounds in plants provides information to other species, and due to a reiterative history of interactions, generates a mutual enfolding between plants and humans: plants have always provided oxygen, shelter, clothing, food, and medicine for humans. In turn, we transport, seed, cultivate, and, with our metabolic waste, fertilize plants and provide carbon dioxide.

Higher primates have been evolving and have been exposed to plant chemistry for about 88 million years. The higher primates, considered to be omnivores, are nevertheless primarily herbivores. Over such an evolutionary

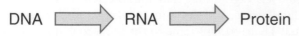

Figure 4-1 The central dogma of biology.

time scale, all higher primates relied on the predictability of vegetative parts of plants as food sources (Johns, 1996). This includes *Homo sapiens,* with 5 to 7 million years of exposure to phytochemistry. Of course, this contact with various plant parts exposed the consumer to thousands of secondary metabolites. Estimates of the number of plants in the early human diet range from 80 to 220. Clearly if *Homo sapiens* regularly consumed such a number and volume of plant foods, its members were exposed to a very high number of phytochemicals. A very conservative estimate would be in the range of 80,000 to 220,000, and the number is quite likely much higher. Ames et al (1990) makes an estimate of the number of secondary metabolites in the current human diet taking into account only those secondary metabolites that are also known to function as pesticides. He observes that even with the great reduction in variety in the human diet compared to our hunter-gatherer ancestors, the modern number of secondary metabolites in the diet is about 10,000 compounds. Thus, even now we are exposed to a great amount of "information" from plants.

If we have coherently coupled with plants, then by default this means that plants have shaped us through informational molecular exchange—and vice versa, we have shaped plants. This shaping, if the hypothesis is solid, should range from DNA to protein. It is easy to see that humans have shaped plants by looking at the cultivation of crops; the original species of any of the crop plants has changed drastically due to human intervention. It is not quite as easy to recognize that plants have shaped us, though one obvious, well-known example is the "shaping" of the cytochrome P-450 (CYP 450) genes. This ancient superfamily of enzymes consists mostly of microsomal and mitochondrial proteins and in humans represents about 75 different CYP 450 genes (Danielson, 2002) (Figure 4-2).

Danielson (2002) points out that CYP 450 genes allow animals to generate a metabolic resistance to plant compounds designed to dissuade grazers and also allow plants to generate new compounds to deter herbivory. He goes on to point out that these CYP 450 genes in plants and animals have been engaged in a cyclical process, generating novel compounds in plants and generating resistance in animals. Jackson (1991) discusses the observation that

particular plant compounds, such as alkaloids, glycosides, phenolics, uncommon proteins, unusual free amino acids, steroids, essential oils, terpenes, and resins, are capable of altering the metabolism and potentially changing the biological fitness of humans as well as their domesticated animals, and even the obligate parasites of each species. She points out that detoxification of plant compounds represents an avenue of potentiating individual and group shifts in gastrointestinal function, structure, and endocrine metabolism. But this influence on physiology does not just stop with transient functional effects.

CYP 450 genes have an unusual ability to evolve rapidly, following a quick-paced, nonlinear time course (Danielson, 2002; Nelson et al, 1993). A large-scale expansion of the CYP 450 gene family is thought to have provided a cache of proteins from among which novel isoforms provided adaptive strategies for metabolizing plant compounds. The resulting diversity in these genes is believed to be due to the recurring exchange of molecular information between the secondary metabolites of plants and mammals needing new enzymes to detoxify these plant compounds (Gonzalez et al, 1990). Therefore, the rich exposure of humans to phytochemistry ultimately promoted human biological variability affecting our genes (Gonzalez et al, 1990; Jackson, 1991; Nelson et al, 1993). Was it haphazard mutations that led to such abilities? Or were genotypic changes environmentally directed, as Cairns' and Thaler's work suggest?

Another example of coherent coupling between plants and humans is the steroid receptors. Specifically, the estrogen receptor is the earliest member of the steroid receptor family (Hawkins et al, 2000; Wu et al, 2003). The gene structure and ligand-binding properties of the classical estrogen receptor (ER-α) are known to be highly conserved for 300 million years of vertebrate evolution. Thus, the binding of an estrogenic chemical to ER-α in fish, amphibians, reptiles, birds, and mammals (including humans) shows relatively little difference (Katzenellenbogen et al, 1979; Pakdel et al, 1989; Welshons et al, 2003; White et al, 1994). The orthodox view that this protein occurs only in vertebrates needs revision: The microbial organisms known as mycorrhiza, living on the roots of plants, have a receptor called "NodD," which has a high amount of genetic homology with the human estrogen receptor. Plants also express a protein identical to the human 5α-reductase enzyme (Fox, 2004; Li et al, 1997). Steroids and flavonoids, produced by plants, bind these proteins (Baker, 1992; Gyorgypal et al, 1991). Thus, molecules that have a shape and electronegativity similar to that of the estrogens are used as a communication strategy between plants and fungi (Gyorgypal et al, 1991).

An evolutionary perspective suggests that the communication strategy of plants pertains to us as well. Phytochemical messenger molecules used by symbiotic soil fungi can be sequestered by humans, bind to estrogen receptors, and thereby influence gene expression. Fox (2004) attempts to explain the fact that the NodD and

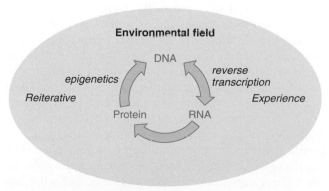

Figure 4-2 The central dogma of biology revised.

estrogen receptor share no common evolutionary ancestry by invoking the construct of convergent evolution—that is, these different species have responded to similar environmental signals, via natural selection, with the same adaptive traits. However, this leaves the homology between these proteins to mere chance. If we view this through the lens of the coherent coupling paradigm, it offers an example of interspecies plasticity in response to environmental context.

Through this lens, humans and plants would be seen to shape themselves to mutual signals. Wynne-Edwards (2001) postulates that plants chosen for domestication may have a higher occurrence of phytoestrogens. This could potentially enhance the ovulatory cyclicity in women, which might mean more humans to cultivate more crops, an arguable benefit for the particular plant species. Wynne-Edwards goes on to point out that humans have receptors in the nose and cheeks that bind native steroids and plant compounds, which in turn signal the brain. Studies have demonstrated that mammals will consume steroids in foods at some times and reject them at other times, depending on physiological and reproductive conditions (e.g., in pregnancy, rats will reject foods with steroids in them). Thus, true to the coherent coupling paradigm, there is a plasticity of response between animals and plants (Figure 4-3).

Of significance, the effects of flavonoids, nonsteroidal secondary metabolites of plants, share key similarities in mycorrhiza and mammals. Flavonoids can regulate gene transcription in both groups. Moreover, some of these flavonoids can modulate the endocrine system and regulate mammalian physiology through activity on steroid receptors and prostaglandin-synthesizing enzymes (Baker, 1995). In addition, humans express a protein, the 5α-reductase enzyme, that is homologous in sequence and identical in function (the reduction of steroid substrates) to a plant protein (Fox, 2004; Li et al, 1997). Hence, it should come as no surprise that plants have a long history of utilization in treating endocrine ailments; currently, phytochemistry is being explored for the regulation of human fertility. This leads Baker (1992) to suggest that flavonoids may have an evolutionary role in steroid hormone activity. More importantly, this is an obvious example of informational exchange between plants and humans.

That flavonoids are considered conditionally essential nutrients (Challem, 1999) adds to the intrigue. In other words, humans have "coupled" with these particular flavonoid "signals" to such a degree that they enhance our long-term health (Manthey et al, 1998; Martinez-Valverde et al, 2000). One wonders how many other plant compounds, with regular consumption, enhance human health. As research on plant metabolites continues, it is increasingly obvious that many phytochemicals are at least favorable to, if not necessary for, human health. Considering only the vitamins and minerals of plant origin makes it obvious that human physiological processes are dependent on the phytochemistry of plants. Moreover, the evolutionary history of humans' ingesting plants with a multitude of phytochemicals suggests that the interface of myriad phytochemicals with animal systems may be informative about pharmacology.

HORMESIS AND XENOHORMESIS—ADAPTATION TO THE PHYTOCHEMICAL ENVIRONMENT

There are a number of reasons that the complex chemistry that is inherent in the ingestion of a plant produces different effects than does an isolated chemical. Of these reasons, pharmacokinetic potentiation, pharmacodynamic convergence, and hormesis and xenohormesis are the best known and the easiest to discuss in the existing framework of pharmacology. Pharmacokinetic potentiation involves processes related to absorption, distribution, metabolism, and excretion, whereas pharmacodynamic convergence involves modulation of multiple biochemical pathways, membrane dynamics, receptor binding cooperativity, and shifts in the degrees of freedom of proteins (enzymes and receptors). Although both of these modes of activity are unique to the ingestion of chemical mixtures, they are commonly put under the rubric of synergy, even though they would ideally be discussed separately. The last mode, hormesis, has been well established by the field of toxicology, and the concept is slowly encroaching into physiology and pharmacology. Regardless of the scientific discipline of origin, it is a useful construct for understanding how plant chemistry interfaces with living systems. Xenohormesis provides an overarching construct to encompass much of what has been previously discussed.

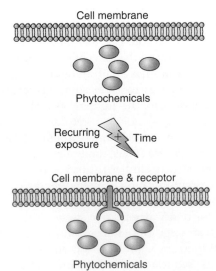

Figure 4-3 Coherent coupling between phytochemistry and eukaryotic cells.

HORMESIS DEFINED

The term *hormesis* is derived from the greek word *hormon* meaning "to excite." In other words, on ingestion of a hormetin, physiological processes are stimulated into activity. Simply put, hormesis is a paradoxical effect of a toxic chemical or radiation at low dose (Trewavas et al, 2003). Stebbing (1982) defined hormesis as low-dose stimulation followed by higher-dose inhibition. A more complete definition by Calabrese, who has spent the last 15 years bringing hormesis back to the attention of physiologists and pharmacologists, is "an adaptive response characterized by biphasic dose responses of generally similar quantitative features with respect to amplitude and range of the stimulatory response that are either directly induced or the result of compensatory biological processes following an initial disruption in homeostasis" (Calabrese et al, 2002). The idea behind hormesis is a dose-response relationship, a beneficial physiological upregulation induced by small doses of a toxin. Many terms have been used to describe this effect (Table 4-1), including the common *biphasic dose response.*

Calabrese and Baldwin (2002) point out that not only have the hormesis dose-response phenomena been labeled with diverse terminology but there are also several biological "laws" referring to hormesis (see Table 4-1). Although this suggests that the phenomenon has repeatedly been "discovered" by different research groups, it is also a comment on the unfortunate lack of conceptual integration across scientific disciplines.

What the hormesis dose-response data suggest is that there is a common regulatory strategy for biological resource allocation and a plasticity of regulatory processes dependent on environmental perturbations due to a long history of coherent coupling (Spelman, 2006) or coevolution with phytochemistry.

TABLE 4-1

Previous Terms Applied to the Hormesis Dose Response

Compensatory response	Bell shaped
Facilitation-inhibition	β curve
Intermediate disturbance hypothesis	Bidirectional
Paradoxical dose responses	Biphasic
Reverse response	J shaped
Stimulatory-inhibitory	U shaped
Subsidy-stress gradient	

Previous Laws Referring to Hormesis
Hebb law
Yerkes-Dobson law
Arndt-Schulz law

From Calabrese EJ, Baldwin LA: Defining hormesis, *Hum Exp Toxicol* 21(2):91, 2002.

HISTORY OF HORMESIS: POLITICALLY SUSPECT BUT SCIENTIFICALLY SOLID

As mentioned, the hormetic response is oriented toward dose-response effects of substance. Although Calabrese and coworkers have brought this construct back into acceptance in the sciences, it had long been recognized in ancient systems of pharmacology.

For example, in the 5000-year-old Ayurvedic system there is a tenet that *everything*, even poisons, can be used as medicine if properly utilized. Thus, very small amounts of heavy metals were used to rejuvenate the system in the weak, convalescing, and aging. In the sixteenth century Paracelsus (Philippus Aureolus Theophrastus Bombast von Hohenheim), a Swiss chemist, was known to use toxic substances, with particular attention to dose (Gurib-Fakim, 2006; Wood, 1992). Although there is much skepticism about this therapy, it is written that his results were particularly positive (Wood, 1992). Nonetheless, Paracelsus's therapies included the use of heavy metals, and centuries later this led to use of the well-known term *quack* derived from the German word *quacksalver* or "quicksilver," an old term for mercury. By the late 1800s published research had demonstrated that chemicals that were toxic to yeast could stimulate growth and respiration if used in lower dosages (Calabrese et al, 1999).

By the 1920s a researcher committed a blunder in the politics of science by associating the phenomena of hormesis with homeopathy (Calabrese, 2006). Considering that this was only a few years after issuance of the Flexner Report, an association with homeopathy was a death sentence to any scientific hypothesis, irregardless of the existence of reproducible evidence. Although the Flexner Report had resulted in the needed elimination of many of the illegitimate schools of medicine of the early twentieth century, it also, apparently by design, put on its hit list any school teaching a system of medicine other than allopathy. It did not help matters that there was also a paucity of explanations based on the biochemical understanding of hormesis at that time (Stebbing, 1982). However, laboratory observations of the hormesis phenomenon continued unbiased in other parts of the world, and a German journal, *Zell-Stimulations Forschungen*, was established to report hormetic effects (Calabrese et al, 1999). By 1943 the scientific method cut through the politics in the United States. Researchers at the University of Idaho reproducibly observed the phenomenon, calling it "hormesis," unaware of its previous labels (Calabrese et al, 1999).

About 50 years later a newsletter of original research, *Stimulation Newsletter*, which lasted just over a decade, reported the enhancement of plant growth and yield by exposure to low-dose radiation (Calabrese et al, 1999). Upon the arrival of the 1980s, despite lingering skepticism about the hormesis phenomenon, a book providing a lengthy review of the research on radiation hormesis was published in the United States

(Luckey, 1980). By the end of the twentieth century, through the work of the Calabrese group, a substantial database of dose-response studies demonstrating hormesis to be common and reproducible had caught the attention of physiologists and pharmacologists (Calabrese, 2006). Hormesis as a scientific principle is solid. But is it here to stay?

UTILITY OF HORMESIS: UNDERSTANDING HUMANS AND THEIR RELATIONS TO THE ENVIRONMENT

Hormesis is not just relevant to poisons such as heavy metals, synthetic pesticides, radiation, and pollutants (Calabrese et al, 1999). Needed substances such as vitamins, minerals, and oxygen are also toxic at excessive doses (Calabrese et al, 1999). Nor is this principle only observed with natural compounds. This principle applies to endogenous compounds as well. Biosynthetic compounds moving through the human system, such as the adrenalines, adenosine, androgens, estrogens, nitric oxide, opioids, many peptides, and prostaglandins, all may have beneficial effects at low concentrations but detrimental effects at high concentrations (Calabrese, 2006). Some pharmaceuticals are also known to conform to this principle. For example, low doses of antibiotics may actually enhance reproduction of pathogenic bacteria, whereas higher doses are toxic to these microbes (Calabrese et al, 1999). Probably the best known and most commonly consumed hormetin is alcohol. Alcohol, a solvent, can clearly be toxic. However, at low doses alcohol is known to be beneficial to health and protective against cardiovascular diseases and some cancers.

Calabrese and Baldwin (2002) suggest that the hormesis response provides a biological buffering response to protect against environmental and endogenous insults. The observation of this response in so many different organisms and cell types against such diverse chemical groups (and radiation) suggests a systemwide feedback response resulting in upregulation of many regulatory processes (Calabrese et al, 1999) and an evolution-wide biological strategy (Calabrese et al, 2002). By overcompensating to an initial disruption caused by an environmental stressor, an organism is protected against the possibility of further exposures (Calabrese et al, 1999).

The hormetic dose-response effects seen for so many phytochemicals also suggests that the mode of activity for health enhancement by fruits, vegetables, and spices may be due, at least partially, to the evolutionary protective response previously mentioned. Furthermore, it argues against a strictly antioxidant mode for plant-based foods, which has become a common assumption among many clinicians and researchers. Like exercise and caloric restriction, many phytochemicals may act as mild stressors to induce an adaptive response via upregulation of multiple genes producing a protective effect (Calabrese, 2005; Mattson et al, 2006) (Box 4-1).

BOX 4-1

Well-Researched Plant Compounds That Are Beneficial at Low Doses but Detrimental at High Doses

Allyl isothiocyanate
Caffeic acid
Catechins
Curcuminoids
Hypericin
Limonene
Perillyl alcohol
Quercetin
Resveratrol
Sulforaphane

From Trewavas A, Stewart D: Paradoxical effects of chemicals in the diet on health, *Curr Opin Plant Biol* 6(2):185, 2003; Mattson MP, Cheng AW: Neurohormetic phytochemicals: low-dose toxins that induce adaptive neuronal stress responses, *Trends Neurosci* 29(11):632, 2006.

At this juncture, some researchers thinking outside the box are applying the hormesis construct to grasp the relationship between the natural pesticides occurring in plants and human health. Many of the secondary compounds plants produce are antifeedants, antimicrobials, and insecticides for the plants' protection (Poitrineau at al, 2003). The well-respected researcher Bruce Ames points out that of all the pesticides in the diet, both those that are naturally produced by the plant itself and synthetic pesticides applied to the plant by farmers, 99.9% are naturally occurring (Ames et al, 1990). This becomes particularly relevant to human health in that many of these natural "pesticides," such as flavonoids (Baker, 1998) and coumarins (Zangerl et al, 2004), are known to be beneficial to human health in multiple ways, including through anticancer activity and beneficial cardiovascular effects (Baba et al, 2002; Hamer et al, 2006; Hollman et al, 1997; Hoult et al, 1994; Knekt et al, 1996; Lin et al, 2001; Nijveldt et al, 2001). At low doses these compounds appear to activate adaptive cellular stress-response pathways (Mattson et al, 2006). At high doses, however, many of these compounds can become carcinogenic (Trewavas et al, 2003).

What this also suggests is that diets high in animal-based foods and processed foods may lack the protective effect of diets high in phytochemicals (Johns, 1996). Ames and Gold (2000) point out that about 80% of U.S. and 75% of U.K. citizens eat insufficient fruit and vegetables to provide minimal protection against cancer. After summarizing 200 epidemiological studies, Block et al (1992) reported that consumption of a diet rich in phytochemicals from fruits and vegetables reduced cancer risks by about 50%. Knoops et al (2004) found that in individuals aged 70 to 90 years, adherence to a phytochemical-rich diet was associated with a more than 50% lower rate of all-cause and cause-specific mortality. Norris et al (2003) showed that good health habits, one of which includes consumption of a phytochemical-rich diet, are associated with a 10- to 20-year delayed progression of morbidity. What might seem paradoxical to the casual observer is that many phytochemicals, evolutionarily derived to protect plants from predators, are detrimental to health at high doses (Figure 4-4).

Xenohormesis

The majority of life forms on the planet either feed on, or live in, close proximity to photosynthesizing organisms (photoautotrophs). Thus there is a long-term evolutionary relationship between photoautotrophs and heterotrophs (fungi and animals). Much of this relationship is based on the secondary metabolites from plants. Plants are known to synthesize secondary metabolites in response to environmental conditions. These phytochemicals, in turn, may be utilized by their surrounding heterotrophic neighbors as cues to impending environmental changes. Thus, when ingested or absorbed by coexisting life forms, such as bacteria, fungi, animals, or humans, certain phytochemicals may provide a chemical signature of the state of the environment (Howitz et al, 2008).

The polyphenols are one example of phytochemical compounds carrying information about environmental conditions. This class of compounds includes the anthocyanidins, catechins, chalcones, flavanones, flavones, isoflavones, and tannins. Spelman et al (2006) suggested that the metabolic expense of generating such molecules would generate a "chemical economy," an efficient and multiple use of one molecule. Indeed, these molecules are known to be multifunctional in that they are antioxidants, antibiotics and fungicides, herbivory deterrents, and ultraviolet radiation protectants. However, they are also known to play a role as signaling molecules, carrying environmental information to heterotrophs. Stafford (1991) proposed that the original role of the polyphenols was as signaling molecules and that their other properties evolved later. Flavonoids do provide cues to plant development (Taylor et al, 2005), and it has also been proposed that flavonoids were the original steroid signaling molecules (Baker, 1992).

Accumulating evidence does suggest that mammals sense stress-signaling molecules. The mammal that could respond to molecules such as the polyphenols would have an advantage over those competitors that could not interpret these environmental cues. A possible explanation for this phenomenon is based in evolutionary biology. Kushiro et al (2003) proposed that the biosynthetic pathways for signaling compounds originated in a common ancestor of plants and animals. As the phyla diverged, the heterotrophs eventually lost their ability to synthesize polyphenols, but retained the ability to respond to these messenger molecules. The retention of the ability to respond to these molecular cues likely allowed for an anticipatory adaptation to environmental changes (Howitz et al, 2008).

At the least, recurring interactions between phytochemicals and heterotrophic proteins on an evolutionary time scale may have generated conditional requirements for some phytochemicals (Spelman et al, 2006). The consumers of these molecules have been shown to respond by inducing cellular defenses and resource conservation (Howitz et al, 2003). For example, it is well known that the polyphenols butein, fisetin, and the well-publicized resveratrol extend life in fungi, nematodes, flies, fish, and mice (Westphal et al, 2007). In addition, concentrations of polyphenols required to extend life span in the laboratory (approximately 10 μM) are detectable in the leaves and fruits of stressed plants (Howitz et al, 2008). This interspecies hormesis, a mode of interpreting stress signals from surrounding organisms to improve survival potential, has been termed *xenohormesis* (Howitz et al, 2003).

The xenohormesis hypothesis varies from the hormesis model in that the stress occurs in one organism and the coexisting species, which have evolved to sense the surrounding chemical ecology, are the beneficiaries (Howitz et al, 2008). In regard to the age-old game of adaptation to the environment, it is sensible to propose that absorbed phytochemicals carry information about the status of the environment and imminent changes in an animal's food supply. Moreover, considering the evidence that stress-induced plant compounds upregulate pathways that provide stress resistance in animals and humans and an evolutionary imperative for anticipatory adaptation, plant consumers would sensibly have modes to perceive these chemical cues and react to them in ways that are beneficial.

An illustration of the relationship between human health and plant chemistry

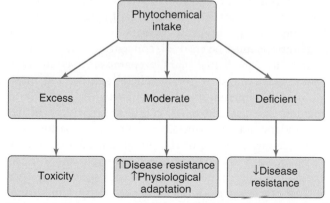

Figure 4-4 Exposure to secondary plant metabolites, many of which were selected to protect plants against bacteria, insects, and herbivores, can be protective to human health. In excess doses, however, many of these natural microbicides and insecticides are toxic. In insufficient doses, human health may be compromised. At ideal doses human health may be enhanced due to the hormesis principle, and the individual may therefore be more resistant to disease processes and better able to respond to changing environmental circumstances. (Adapted from Johns T: *The origins of human diet and medicine: chemical ecology*, Tucson, 1996, University of Arizona Press, p 213.)

The hormesis and the xenohormesis hypotheses are not mutually exclusive. Responses to absorbed toxins (hormesis) and the ability to respond to molecules of environmental origin as molecular signals (xenohormesis) were likely concurrent developments in evolution. Howitz and Sinclair (2008) point out that in an animal's response to complex mixtures of phytochemicals both responses are likely at play.

This environmental coupling may have resulted in a conditional dependence on phytochemicals for the modulation of particular proteins. For example, the nucleotide-binding sites of protein kinases appear to bind the polyphenolic flavonoids and stilbenes with reasonable affinity. The evidence indicates that these polyphenols do not compete with the enzyme's nucleotide substrates; rather they bind elsewhere (Gledhill et al, 2007; Howitz et al, 2003). Molecules such as resveratrol and quercetin have been found to bind not to conserved domains but to hydrophobic pockets (Gledhill et al, 2007). This may partially explain their ability to modulate multiple proteins. Howitz and Sinclair (2008) suggested that this is consistent with the driving of these polyphenol-protein interactions by selective pressures rather than by coincidental binding. This also suggests that these interactions are likely potentiating with one another and with endogenous regulators.

There are also data demonstrating that many of these compounds bind to the same binding pockets as endogenous regulators (Baker, 1992). Both types of interactions open the door to the claims of synergy so often cited for multicomponent extracts from medicinal plants (Spelman et al, 2006). At the least, the ingestion of phytochemical cocktails likely involved multiple interactions that go well beyond ligand binding and involve subtler molecular dynamics (Spelman, 2005) (see Molecular Modes of Activity later in the chapter).

The xenohormesis hypothesis makes a number of predictions that rest squarely on organisms' relationship of coupling with their environment (Lamming et al, 2004). First, there is likely a substantial cache of medicinal molecules that are upregulated in stressed plants that can benefit the user. Second, xenohormetic phytochemicals serve as messenger molecules by interacting with a variety of enzymes involved in regulating stress responses and survival. Third, these molecules should be relatively safe for human consumption. Fourth, there may be conserved domains in enzymes and receptors that do not interact with endogenous molecules (Howitz et al, 2008). Last, many phytochemicals, due to a history of recurrent interactions with heterotrophic proteins, may have developed a structural congruence that potentiates the effects of endogenous regulatory molecules. If the aforementioned predictions hold true, then xenohormesis may provide the philosophical underpinnings explaining why many phytochemicals have been documented to enhance health.

The xenohormesis hypothesis, when fully recognized, has implications for the foundations of pharmacology.

Although classical pharmacology is based on high affinity and selectivity, many physiologically active phytochemicals are known to function with broad specificity and low affinity (Ágoston et al, 2005). This creates a quandary for the pharmacological paradigm, because many phytochemicals are known to affect multiple proteins. Although polyvalent binding (binding of a small molecule to multiple proteins) is considered an inferior pharmacological strategy by pharmaceutical standards, it may have been the original mode of upregulation of defensive physiological responses and provide distinct evolutionary and pharmacological advantages.

DANGER OF A SECOND REJECTION FROM THE POLITICAL HALLS OF SCIENCE

Although the argument just described is based on solid science, a logical extension of this argument is the use of food and medicinal plants for enhancement of health. Many opponents of the view that plants have therapeutic value claim that there is not enough of any one chemical in plants to make them therapeutically useful (Spinella, 2002), Although this argument explains why medicinal plants are sometimes called "crude drugs," it also demonstrates a gross misunderstanding of the pharmacology of complex mixtures. Furthermore, it completely misses the hormesis phenomenon.

Thus the argument that food and medicinal plants are not effective for inducing physiological change because they are too dilute to have activity contradicts the entire database of hormesis studies demonstrating that minute doses of substance do induce a general and reproducible biological response. At the same time, the hormesis principle should call into question the practice of concentrating an active constituent from a plant by standardization. Although the quality and identity of medicinal plant preparations must be ensured, concentration of one constituent in a medicinal plant preparation may, in some cases, breach the dose for beneficial activity and move toward a detrimental dose, particularly if the compound operates through a hormetic mode of activity. Nonetheless, understanding hormesis can help the allopathic community appreciate one of the possible modes of activity for medicinal plants. The hormesis principle was dropped like a hot potato in the early part of the twentieth century because of the association with homeopathy. Will hormesis again be shunned because it is invoked as an explanation to understand the action of medicinal plants? One would hope that science would cut through petty politics in the interest of human health.

When hormesis is viewed in an ecosystem context, hormetic responses as measured by the effects on growth can turn out to be a result of altered competition between species. If a competitor, parasite, or disease of a species is more susceptible to a certain chemical than the species itself, then the species will experience a relief from a resource-demanding stress factor and hence increase growth at low concentrations of that chemical. This is the basic principle behind the beneficial effect of pharmaceuticals such as penicillin on vertebrates and leads to the xenohormesis hypothesis.

ECOLOGICAL PHARMACY: THE UNDERPINNINGS OF PHARMACOLOGY

The aforementioned evidence logically leads to the end point of a discussion on pharmacology; that is, how has adaptation to phytochemical exchange influenced the physiological processes of organisms consuming plants? A key point is that ingestion of plants, a process that has been going on for 300 million years for vertebrates, 88 million years for higher primates, and 7 to 10 million years for humans, leads to exposure to an array of plant compounds in every swallowed bolus. Never has the consumption of edible foodstuffs involved a single, isolated compound. This is of pharmacological significance: our current model in pharmacology attempts to induce physiological change through the ingestion of one chemical at a time.

In an unspoken oversight of the medical sciences, the rationale for the approach of isolation and purification of active constituents from "crude drugs" has never been made explicit. The general conclusion drawn from a century of research on isolation of active constituents from medicinal plants is that medicinal plants typically contain numerous active compounds (Gilbert et al, 2003; Singer et al, 1962; Spelman, 2005; Spelman et al, 2006; Williamson, 2001). A key point regarding the politics surrounding the use of food and medicinal plants to promote human health is that multiconstituent plant medicines were not forsaken because of research that demonstrated harmful or ineffective activity, but because they were too complex to study in their multiconstituent form (Vickers, 2002). Nevertheless, pharmacological modeling has used isolation as a fundamental tenet of inducing physiological shifts in humans. Unfortunately, this methodology is deficient in revealing the mode of activity of the bulk of food and medicinal plants because it neglects the possibility of synergic, additive, or antagonist activity of multiconstituent remedies (Cech, 2003). Moreover, it grossly simplifies human health to only those parameters observed in reductionist models.

According to a pharmacological paradigm supported by a foundation of human adaptation to the informational input from plants, our physiological processes, down to the level of our genes, have undergone a history of recurring biochemical interactions with complex phytochemistry that has lead to the structural congruence of humans and plants. The previously discussed shifts in DNA, the homology of proteins, and the ligand-receptor relationship between humans and plants are examples of structural congruence. Humans have integrated with plants so that multiple concurrent biochemical perturbations are ordinary. Reiterative exposure to minute doses of numerous plant metabolites provides constant stimuli for biological adaptation (Jackson, 1991). In turn, this adaptation has had profound effects on human health.

Jackson (1991) aptly calls attention to system stability, writing that system diversity is proportional to system stability. Another way of expressing this in regard to human health is that the stability of health may be seen as a function of exposure to phytochemical diversity. Keith and Zimmermann (2004) suggest that many genes might need complementary action to modify disease processes. In other words, therapy could be more effective if pharmacological agents engaged with more than one biochemical site. Quite likely, the majority of the multitude of plant constituents that ancient humans regularly consumed throughout their evolution had a positive affect on many of the health-modifying genes because of the millions of years of history of recurring exposure to multicomponent phytochemical mixtures. Observations do indicate that people who consume a phytochemical-rich diet have a significantly better health status than those who have a diet low in phytochemicals (McCarty, 2004). It is quite likely that phytochemicals interface with a large percentage of the estimated 10,000 health-modifying genes (Keith et al, 2004). Unfortunately the current number of pharmacological targets, approximately 300 to 400, is anemic compared with the phytochemical-gene interface that occurs in diets rich in plant-based foods.

A pharmacological model that accounts for millions of years of exposure to arrays of phytochemicals provides not only a recognition of plants as sources of medicines but also a multitarget approach that single-chemical, stand-alone interventions cannot offer (Keith et al, 2004). And it returns us to the origins of pharmacology, in which what humans regularly ingested, somewhere between 80 and 220 plants with an estimated 80,000 to 220,000 secondary metabolites, modified multiple physiological processes in a concerted manner. The understanding of the translational response of numerous proteins to multiple perturbations, such as provided through phytochemistry, holds promise for the fields of medicine and biology not because it is a new insight, but because it is an ancient process that shaped human physiology. Such a paradigm shift would also advance the understanding of biological molecular networks and open up further therapeutic strategies.

MOLECULAR MODES OF ACTIVITY

CELLULAR MEMBRANE AND SIGNAL TRANSDUCTION

Cellular morphology is the result of a nonlinear and dynamic molecular flux, especially related to the cell membrane. Although the membrane has been described as a system driven by thermodynamic equilibrium (Aon et al, 1996), it is more accurately seen as an emergent structure consisting of highly asymmetrical structures and phase transitions (Perillo, 2002).

Typically, mammalian cellular plasma membranes consist of about eight major classes of lipids (Simons et al, 2004) and includes embedded proteins in its bilipid structure. Because signal transduction and the complex behavior of chemical reactions is coupled to the dynamics of membranes, the membrane has been closely scrutinized in hopes of further understanding the cell's ability to receive, process, and respond to information. Unfortunately there has been (and still is) an epistemological divide between the analysis of the complex behavior involved in biochemical events and the structural aspects of the membrane involved in signaling phenomena, especially in relation to signal transduction involving exogenous molecules (Perillo, 2002).

Until very recently, explanations of signal transduction were based on a linear model that defined successive steps in the decoding process and focused on compounds with high affinity and selectivity. However, the membrane, key in its interactions with the ensemble of phytochemicals to which early humans were consistently and constantly exposed, may also respond to compounds that do not exhibit high affinity and high selectivity for a particular receptor species. Ignoring these interactions may lead to erroneous conclusions in the basic sciences.

Significantly, systems properties of heterogenous molecular ensembles could induce minute difference in the strength of attractive forces among molecules and increased degrees of freedom within a pharmacological system (Buehler, 2003). Just as phase separations and self-assembly processes are systems properties of molecular ensembles, a pharmacological systems approach is required to understanding a phytochemical matrix interacting with another biological system (Spelman, 2005). The author proposes three modes of activity based on recently elucidated behaviors of the cell membrane, two that involve the bilipid membrane and one that is based on concerted activity.

1. Cooperative Binding by Receptors: Receptor Mosaics

The discovery of direct receptor-receptor interactions rigorously challenges the historical belief that the receptor is the minimal unit for drug recognition and activity and therefore that high-affinity, high-specificity compounds are superior ligands (Kenakin, 2004). The existence of various types of receptor mosaics, clusters of receptors functioning as a unit that demonstrate cooperative binding, suggests a plasticity of the steric conformation of receptors (Agnati et al, 2005). In the receptor mosaic model each receptor is seen as a subunit of a multimeric protein.

Recall the cooperative binding of oxygen to hemoglobin. After one oxygen molecule binds to hemoglobin, the affinity of the other binding pockets for oxygen increases. Thus, the likelihood of subsequent binding of oxygen molecules is increased.

Cooperativity is considered a mode of self-regulation by multimeric proteins (Koshland et al, 2002) and is hypothesized to be so for receptor systems as well (Agnati et al, 2005). In receptor mosaics the conformational change caused by the binding of the first ligand is transmitted to adjacent receptors with reciprocal contact to change the affinity for subsequent ligand binding. The change in affinity is due to the conformational change induced by the first bound ligand, which induces sequential changes of the multimeric protein's neighboring subunits. This change in protein conformation may make subsequent binding easier (positive cooperativity) or more difficult (negative cooperativity).

Because a phytochemical matrix consists of hundreds of compounds, including groups of constituents that vary slightly in their structure but are based on a common backbone (Yong et al, 2004), there may be both high-affinity ligands and low-affinity ligands for a given receptor. Once the high-affinity ligand binds to a species of receptor, other receptors, because of intramolecular transfer of the conformational change to the adjacent peptides, may be able to bind the lower-affinity ligands and play a role in cellular messaging. Accordingly, the search for only high-affinity compounds within such a matrix may miss lower-affinity compounds that could bind within receptor mosaics due to cooperative binding. This suggests one possible molecular explanation of the synergistic effects so often invoked by phytotherapists to suggest that plant medicines and foods cannot be reduced to an "active" constituent. The receptor mosaic model also suggests the need for an expansion of the traditional pharmacological methodology of searching for only high-affinity ligands within plant chemistry (Figure 4-5).

2. Shifts in Membrane Electronics and/or Shape: Nonspecific Membrane Interactions by Exogenous Molecules

Many components of signal transduction, such as receptors, are anchored in the plasma membrane and therefore are subject to the biochemical milieu of the plasma membrane. Of the four basic receptor signaling modes—gated ion channels, metabotropic receptors, receptor enzymes, and the steroid receptor—three are directly linked to plasma membrane processes. This lipid-rich two-dimensional environment allows for hydrophobic interactions that lead to alterations in component access, orientation, and effective concentration (Weng et al, 1999). Hence, modulation of the molecular organization of the membrane may have an effect on signal transduction.

Many drugs are amphiphilic or hydrophobic molecules, and a common site of action for these compounds is the plasma membrane (Perillo, 2002). Among the amphiphilic compounds, many of the central nervous system depressants (Goodman et al, 2001) will, because of

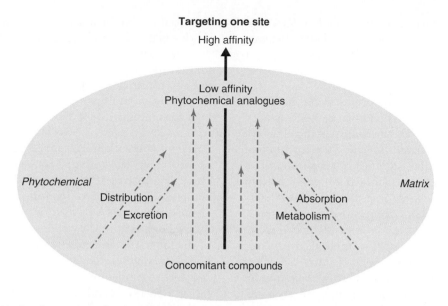

Figure 4-5 Under the current pharmacological model, only high-affinity and high-selectivity compounds are sought, and compounds with lower affinity for receptor (and enzyme) binding are overlooked. In contrast, the receptor mosaic model holds that the low-affinity compounds typically accompanying high-affinity compounds in plant extracts may cooperatively bind, affecting signal transduction. In addition, the concomitant compounds commonly improve the pharmacokinetics (absorption, distribution, metabolism, and excretion) of the low-high affinity compounds.

their molecular properties, self-aggregate into micelles (Perillo, 2002). Despite significant molecular investigation into modes of activity for some of the hydrophobic drugs (e.g., the local anesthetics) no specific receptors for them have been revealed (Franks et al, 1984; Schreier et al, 2000). Rather, these compounds demonstrate activity at the plasma membrane surface (Perillo, 2002).

Hydrophobic and amphiphilic compounds, and the resulting micelles, may induce shape changes, membrane disruption, vesiculation, and solubilization (Schreier et al, 2000). Consequently, exogenous molecules may generate membrane asymmetries that result in membrane tensions (Garcia et al, 2000; Perillo et al, 2001). As expected given the thermodynamics of open systems far from equilibrium, the membrane perturbations caused by curvature tensions and the flux of molecular movements from one monolayer to the other shift the resting state of the membrane and reorganize cellular shape (Perillo, 2002). Changes in the curvature of the membrane, as well as its composition, lead to demonstrated changes in the function of the membrane when it interfaces with an exogenous molecule (Farge et al, 1993; Garcia et al, 2002; Mui et al, 1993). Given that protein conformation is dependent on molecular interactions, structural change may also induce alterations in protein conformation (Simons et al, 2004). This could result in signal transduction.

Notably, many of the secondary compounds of plants are amphiphilic or hydrophobic (e.g., hyperforin in St. John's wort, the curcuminoids in *Curcuma longa* [turmeric], alkylamides in *Echinacea* species) and would accordingly likely display similar behavior. Given the evolutionary history of plant ingestion by humans, membrane interactions with "nonactive" compounds in plants were likely routine. Consumption of a plant led to ingestion of active constituents *and* other phytochemicals that influenced membrane dynamics. Consequently, with recognition of evolutionary precedent, the combination of compounds affecting the membrane with active compounds binding to receptors was part of routine physiology. This may be a partial explanation of why many isolated plant constituents do not appear to function in the same way as they do when given in a whole-plant extract.

3. Polyvalent Activity: Biochemical Convergence

The last two modes of activity were discussed in relation to the realm of an isolated cell. However, signal transduction involves networks of cells, tissues, and organs. Following the science of physics, molecular biology is slowly moving from study of the components of signaling to investigation of the context in which the signaling occurs. Study at the molecular level of components alone will not advance the understanding of when and why cells interact in their typically nonlinear, nonlocal, multiple feedback loops (Maini, 2002).

Physiology does not run in linear, sequential processes involving one chemical at a time. Robust systems, like living organisms, are likely quite responsive to numerous but subtle chemical perturbations (Ágoston et al, 2005). Thus multisystem analysis will probably be found to be essential to understanding signaling networks (Plavec et al, 2004). Allowing for models that include multitarget and multipathway assaying could clearly elucidate the informational connectivity of networks. Aon et al (1996) refer to the network of interactions established between dynamic subsystems through common intermediates or effectors (hormones and second messengers) as *dynamic coupling*.

It is well established that the overall combination of nonnutritive phytochemicals appears to be key to plants' positive effects on health, that the health-giving effects of plants are *not* always related to the nutrient content (McCarty, 2004), and that significant consumption of secondary compounds from plants plays an important role in the prevention of chronic diseases (Liu, 2003). Although some constituents are interfacing with receptors and membranes, others are influencing pharmacokinetics. For example, concomitant compounds, frequently considered excipient nonactive constituents, can affect absorption, distribution, metabolism, or excretion of other constituents, enhancing (or antagonizing) their bioavailability (Eder et al, 2000). Moreover, as the xenohormesis hypothesis suggests, many of the excipients removed from our foodstuffs and medicinal preparations may upregulate beneficial physiological processes.

Recognition of such subtle perturbation would eventually allow the understanding of a disease-modifying molecular network and further pharmacological target potential. Monitoring of targets tripped by polyvalent groups of compounds will almost certainly lead to the recognition of yet further biochemical connectivity. Moreover, as our knowledge of the range of perturbable sites improves, proteins expressed by what are now considered mere "housekeeping" genes will likely be recognized as disease modifying. The outcome could be an expansion of the understanding of the disease-modifying gene network and further therapeutic targets (Keith et al, 2004). Such a perspective will likely lead to the acknowledgement that a multitarget perturbation, as happens with the consumption of any plant product, holds the potential for significantly more therapeutic activity than single-chemical, stand-alone interventions.

The ingestion of plants leads not only to the potential for multiple compounds to interface with multiple targets, but also for single compounds, due to their broad specificity, to engage multiple targets. Generally, the pharmacological sciences consider these molecules "dirty" because of their lack of selectivity. Such molecules are thought to have more potential for producing adverse events because of "off-target" effects than does a highly selective chemical. However, dozens, if not hundreds, of multifunctional compounds have been identified in natural products chemistry that are known to be quite safe (Corson et al, 2007). For example, the well-known phytochemical group of the salicylates are known to interact with multiple proteins. The ubiquitous catechins, such as epigallocatechin-3-gallate, have demonstrated considerable chemopreventative activity via induction of apoptosis, inhibition of multidrug resistance pumps, promotion of cell cycle arrest, and inhibition of cyclooxygenase-2 (Khan et al, 2006). The curcuminoids are documented to engage over 60 molecular targets to protect against cancer and regulate the expression of inflammatory enzymes, cytokines, adhesion molecules. and cell survival proteins (Goel et al, 2008). The not uncommon resveratrol modulates the function of over two dozen enzymes and receptors, leading to protection against cancer, atherosclerosis, and diabetes while promoting endurance (Howitz et al, 2008).

Csermely et al (2005) have found using network models of pharmacology that the partial inhibition of multiple targets offered by a mixture of chemicals is often more efficient than the complete inhibition of a single target. For example, Wald and Law (2003) suggest that a combination of six drugs at subclinical doses—a baby aspirin, three blood pressure drugs (at half the standard dose), a statin, and 800 mcg of folic acid—could extend life by 11 years (Figure 4-6).

Targeting multiple sites

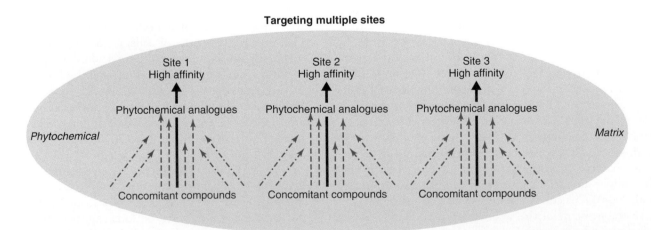

Figure 4-6 Physiology is a complex process that operates in a symphonic manner with multiple receptors, enzymes, and genes being affected at any given moment. When a plant extract or food is ingested, the phytochemicals triggers many sites concurrently, which can then converge on a positive outcome.

In addition, in a meta-analysis encompassing 56,000 patients with hypertension, Law et al (2003) concluded that combinations of two or three drugs at half the standard dose delivered therapeutic effects comparable to those of one or two full-dose antihypertensive medications. Not surprisingly, the multiple low-dose drug combination was preferable because of the reduction in side effects. Clinicians have historically overcome single-target insufficiency by using combination drug therapy such as seen in today's clinical protocols for treatment of human immunodeficiency virus infection, tuberculosis, and cancer. Csermely et al (2005) propose that partial drug inhibition by multiple drugs could prove to be a superior pharmacological strategy to strong inhibition by one drug at a single target. This is likely due to the need for complementary action on multiple targets to modify disease processes (Keith et al, 2004).

When combinations of various pharmacological compounds are screened, the natural outcome will almost certainly necessitate further exploration of the connectivity of physiological pathways. Borisy et al (2003) discuss the unexpected but beneficial interactions that a systematic screening of combinations of small molecules reveals. They report, for example, that an antipsychotic agent coupled with an antiprotozoal drug demonstrates antineoplastic activity and that a fungistatic agent coupled with an analgesic produces antifungal activity against resistant strains of *Candida albicans*. In these instances, however, these ensemble properties never would have been realized if the effects had been broken apart and studied in isolation.

If the ensemble properties of a chemical matrix are necessary for physiological and pharmacological effects, and it appears that they are, then the purification process from whole plant to isolated compound is inadequate for the elucidation of pharmacological activity (Wagner, 1999; Wang et al, 2004). Moreover, the phytochemical matrix, rather than the phytochemical isolate, offers an opportunity for an enhanced perspective. The study of phytochemical matrices interfacing with mammalian systems, with the addition of improved technology, will almost certainly elucidate biochemical pathway connectivity that has been unattainable with previous methodology. The medical sciences would do well to heed Etxeberria (2004), who suggests that the properties of a unity cannot be accounted for by accounting for the properties of its components. Here again it remains true that the whole is greater than the sum of the parts.

⊖ Chapter References can be found on the Evolve website at http://evolve.elsevier.com/Micozzi/complementary/

SOCIAL AND CULTURAL FACTORS IN MEDICINE

CLAIRE MONOD CASSIDY

There are a great many health care systems in the world. All share the goals of alleviating the suffering of the sick, promoting health, and protecting the wider society from illness.

Despite this universality, systems differ profoundly. They differ in degree of expansion into the world, so that some systems are practiced only locally, as among a single rainforest tribe, whereas others have spread to every corner of the globe. They differ in degree of technology, from systems that require virtually none to others that can barely function in the absence of electricity and perfect sanitation. Most importantly, these systems differ in their perceptions of the sick and well human body and in the ways in which they deliver health care.

These similarities and differences have been systematically studied for more than 100 years. As a result, we can now discuss both why so many systems exist and how differences among them matter. Basically, health care systems arise and persist because each one serves a need. Moreover, patients report satisfaction with care—no matter what kind—if that care is delivered in a manner that meshes with their cultural expectations. The form health

care takes is first and fundamentally a matter of sociocultural interpretation. In other words, the "truth" that guides any health care system is relative and is learned.

This point, although implied by the very existence of numerous health care systems, surprises North Americans because, almost alone in the world, we have encouraged the belief that there is only one "best" health care approach. This belief is couched in language that argues for the primacy of scientific medicine, including the claim that only one medicine—biomedicine or allopathy—is scientific. As the voices of other types of practitioners gain strength, however, and as the world's cultural diversity increasingly bears in on Americans, it becomes clear that most of what we know, even scientific fact, is culturally modeled. We remain unaware of this situation most of the time because our cultural assumptions are learned at an early age and are embedded within us to the point that we take them for granted. Only when these assumptions are challenged, as they will be by the material in this book, do we become aware of them. Once aware, we can choose either to expand our thinking or to defend the status quo.

This chapter offers an opportunity to expand thinking through a series of conceptual models that contextualize the variety of health care systems. It considers three questions:

1. What are the many health care realities?
2. How do they resemble each other?
3. What are the implications of the differences?

REALITY, INTERPRETATION, AND RELATIVITY

A psychiatrist told me about a Mormon woman who came to him deeply distressed because 20 years and four children into her second marriage, she realized that she would be spending eternity with her first husband, a man who had died 6 months after their wedding. Mormon couples can be married both for this life and for "eternity," and she and her first husband had chosen to be linked in both ways. Now her first husband was a stranger to her, and she desperately wanted to spend the afterlife with her present husband and children. To his credit the psychiatrist realized that he could not help this patient. He called a Mormon colleague who quickly linked the patient with a bishop of the Mormon Church. In a single visit the bishop helped the woman straighten out her fears about the afterlife.

Why could the first psychiatrist not help the patient himself? Because he did not share her reality model. He could have denied her suffering and told her "not to be so silly." Instead, he took a logical and compassionate step and linked the sick woman with health care workers who did share her reality model.

Consider another example. On a chilly wet day, a young woman laughingly pointed out her red tights and red boots to me, saying, "I always wear red on my feet on days like this, to keep me cooking from below up." Was this an amusing poesy shared on an elevator? A sign of psychosis? Certainly, this remark did not make sense from within the biomedical model. But an acupuncturist would understand that the cold element, water, is chased by the hot element, fire, and the symbolic color of fire is red. A similar behavior pattern would be recognized by practitioners of Ayurveda, the traditional medicine of India, or curanderismo, the folk medicine tradition of Mexico, Central America, and many Hispanic people in the United States. It also survives in mainstream America when a mother boots up her kids on rainy days to keep them warm and to prevent colds.*

These stories provide small illustrations of the statement that the form health care takes is first and fundamentally a matter of interpretation. The wide variety of lifeways shows that humans have found many different ways to answer the same life questions. We can enjoy these differences much as we enjoy a good conversation, or we can grapple with their meanings and implications. Those involved in delivering health care must grapple with these differences.

Unfortunately, the same derisive tone that labels the interpretation of personal experience as merely superstition is also found in comparisons of medical belief systems. If one is modern then others are, by inference, outmoded; if one is based on fact then others must be laced with superstition. In this way, biomedicine is seen as somehow more true than any alternative system could possibly be.... Such a view ... fails to consider the internal logic of other explanatory models. But most health systems are logical and rational systems of thought if the underlying assumptions are known; this does not necessarily mean that these assumptions are correct, only that they can be viewed as having been reached by the coherent use of reason. (Snow, 1993)

Grappling with issues of meaning can be difficult if we do not even know why we are reacting with laughter, anger, or defensiveness. The process of socialization—into our culture as children and into our profession as adults—provides us with truths and logical structures that answer life's questions well. We even learn to deal with the ambiguities and inconsistencies within what we have learned, and we may not notice that we believe two mutually incompatible things until someone with a different perspective points it out to us. Even then, why should we question our own truths or pay other truths heed? Strange answers make no sense and provide little guidance or comfort. It is tempting to think that others are irrational or ignorant. In the following quotation, a biomedical practitioner rejects user models of health care while insisting on the truth of his own reality, but would he be likely to convince mothers with this tone of voice?

Mothers may not believe this, but colds are not caused by standing in drafts, going without a hat, or getting feet wet. They occur when one sneezing, coughing child shares germs with another. (Sears, 1991)

That there are numerous cogent *models* of reality is often disturbing to people. In the West, battles have been fought and lives lost in defense of the ideal of a singular reality (Ames, 1993). Earlier in our history the search for this reality was mainly expressed in religious terms, but for more than 150 years, many have believed that science provides that singular reality. By this logic, health care practices that are not considered scientific are not trustworthy, and the path to acceptance demands "scientific research."

This situation helps explain why the preceding psychiatric example might be shrugged off. Lay people are known to have beliefs, and clinicians must deal with them. But the point of this discussion is that *everyone*

---

*That the remark makes sense within the logic of humoral models does not mean that practitioners would say that red boots "work," that is, that the boots themselves, or their color specifically, prevented the young woman from being invaded by cold damp. To determine whether an action is instrumental requires an entirely different level of analysis.

has beliefs, and *all* realities are constructed; the facts of science are as culturally contextualized as those of law, theology, or social manners. Scientific fact is only as stable as the logic that produced it and the systems that apply it. Thus, science also experiences paradigm shifts. Plasma physics operates by a different logic and perceives reality differently from Newtonian physics; population biology is quite a different kettle of fish from Linnaean systematics; and an ecological or holistic approach to gathering scientific knowledge is very different from a reductionistic one.

The curious thing about modular reality is that you are likely to find exactly what you expect. The observer is not separate from the observed (see discussion of the Heisenberg uncertainty principle in Chapter 1). Expectations are based on assumptions and the application of logic. When the assumptive base changes, so does the logic and, as a result, the appropriate response. Consider, for example, streptococcal pharyngitis. According to biomedicine the *Streptococcus* bacterium causes the sore throat. Logically, one could treat with antibiotics to destroy that bacterium. However, approximately 20% of the population carries this germ in their throats without developing an illness (Greenwood et al, 1994). Only a minority of people who are exposed to the bacterium contract a sore throat. Thus, other factors must be involved; the presence of the bacterium, although necessary, is not sufficient. Most "holistic" health care systems, such as homeopathy, Ayurveda, and Chinese medicine, understand this concept and focus more attention on the other factors—the reacting body, the person—than on infectious microorganisms. Care is aimed at strengthening the person rather than destroying bacteria.

But surely, you might ask, people use universal definitions for such material body parts as the heart or blood? Not necessarily. For example, although everyone might agree that the heart is a pulsating organ located in the center of the chest, its energetic and spiritual capabilities are debated. Biomedical thinkers describe the heart as a pump, using a material and mechanical metaphor. Even biomedical physicians, however, once thought of the heart as the "seat of the soul," a memory our society revisits in many romantic songs. This idea still is active in Chinese medical thought, in which the physical heart beats while the energetic "Heart" fills the role of sovereign ruler: "Sovereign of being and pivot of life, the heart is the guarantor of the unity of a person's existence" (Larre et al, 1995, p. 174). In Chinese anatomy the heart even has a special "Protector," an organ unknown in biomedical anatomy.

Again, in biomedicine, blood is a living red substance that contains red and white cells and carries food, enzymes, hormones, and oxygen; it is complex and constantly renews itself. In popular Jamaican thought, however, blood does not renew itself. Its purity (a social rather than medical concept) determines one's success in life (Sobo, 1993). Following this logic, many Jamaicans are loath to give or receive blood for transfusions. Resistance to donating blood (e.g., among Jehovah's Witnesses; Ontario Consultants on Religious Tolerance, n.d.) or to receiving organ transplants (O'Connor, 1995) is common wherever people believe the soul imbues all body parts.

CULTURAL RELATIVITY

For each of the preceding examples a reader might ask, "Who's right?" This is not a useful question, however, because answers are judged "right" from within the logic of the model in use. "Rightness" also is modular or relative.

A truly useful question is, "How does this model serve its users?" To be able to ask this question, one must stand back from one's own beliefs and models and recognize them as constructed and not exclusively correct. To ask this question is to practice *cultural relativity*.

Cultural relativity is a technique for dealing with the many ways in which people explain themselves. It tells practitioners and researchers to remain in a fairly neutral, nonjudgmental stance, *knowing the values of people without adopting or rejecting them* (Kaplan, 1984). From this position, clinicians, researchers, or students can observe their own perceptions and those of others and understand how these interpretations serve users' lives. They can avoid becoming mired in determining which method is true, because nothing is exclusively true when all realities are constructed.

On the other hand, ideas can be true in certain contexts or situations; that is, they make sense to their users. Therefore the observer must learn to synthesize his or her position with those of others, so as to design an effective response strategy. For example, if people think of penicillin as a cooling drug and therefore hesitate to use it to treat a "cold" illness such as pneumonia, the practitioner can neutralize the cold of penicillin by suggesting that the patient take the medicine along with a food perceived as "hot" (Harwood, 1977). Alternatively, as in the previous example of the Mormon woman, the clinician can refer a patient to a practitioner whose reality model more closely resembles that of the patient.

The practice of cultural relativity is pivotal to the study of medicine, because each system of medicine provides a different set of ideas about the body, disease, and medical reality. Readers will find it much easier to absorb and use this material if they can willingly—even playfully—step aside from their current beliefs and appreciations to let in new ones.

THE BEHAVIORAL FIELD OF HEALTH CARE

What belongs under the rubric of health care? Once we know, we can examine which components are addressed by which particular health care system, because no single system addresses the whole.

FIELD OF HEALTH CARE FROM EGO'S POINT OF VIEW

Imagine that each person is immersed in a potential field of health care that instructs how to prevent illness, treat illness, and, more positively, enhance wellness. Figure 5-1 depicts this idea as three triangles (shown as nonoverlapping, although in reality they do overlap, at least partially). The three triangles are embedded in a semicircle labeled "historical, cultural, and social environment," which reminds us that all health care is delivered within a context of experience, belief, and expectation that is not always obvious to us.

The central triangle deals with health care as it is delivered to groups of people, and the right and left triangles deal with health care that is received primarily by individuals or families. The small circle in the center represents a person, Ego,* to whom all the contents of the field are available. Lines at the bottom of the drawing mark the health condition, from increasing health (left) to decreasing health (right). The central triangle covers prevention, that is, the avoidance of sickness without seeking high-level wellness.

Each triangle is divided into three sections. Section 1 represents the forms of health care that Ego can seek and

---

*"Ego" is used in the anthropological or genealogical sense, that is, the person from whose point of view the figure is to be understood. It is not used in the common psychiatric sense, that is, the "I" that deals with reality.

---

deliver without the intervention of a specialist. Examples include praying, exercising, brushing teeth, bathing, eating fruit, cleaning house, paying utility bills for receipt of electricity and pure water, taking dietary supplements, washing and bandaging minor wounds, and taking an analgesic or sleeping to treat a headache.

Section 2 represents a degree of complexity or severity that requires specialist intervention. Most health care needs fall at this level, and most health care systems deliver most care at this level. At this level of wellness, we might find Ego seeking help with finding appropriate work, consulting a dietary specialist, taking a parenting class, or learning meditation techniques. Under treatment, we would find Ego seeking help for traumas, discomforts, or malfunctions that have not responded to home remedies or that Ego believes require the attention of a specialist. This section also includes ongoing care and control of chronic conditions and handicaps. Prevention at this level involves preventive dental care, screening tests, vaccinations, and community prevention activities, such as pure food and drug controls and pollution prevention—activities of which Ego is generally unaware and over which he or she has little control.

Section 3 represents a high degree of complexity and intensity that few specialists emphasize and that Ego calls on rarely. This level of treatment deals with extreme illnesses, malformations, and trauma, including care that is delivered in emergency departments, operating rooms, and intensive care units. This level in the prevention triangle deals with responses to major catastrophes such as

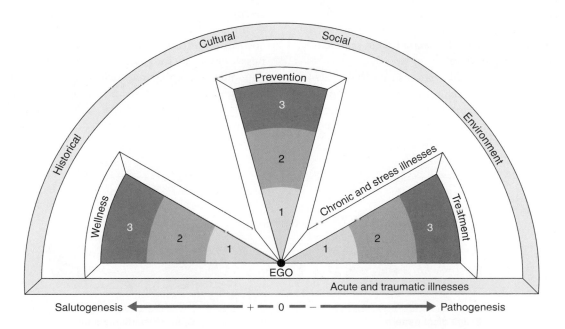

1	Self-care
2	Lower intensity specialist care
3	Higher intensity specialist care

Figure 5-1 The behavioral field of health care from the perspective of an individual.

epidemics and earthquakes. In the wellness triangle this level deals with an issue that is not easily expressed in English and is generally described in terms with psychological and spiritual overtones, such as *self-actualization, enlightenment,* or *awakening.*

Note that the cost of health care rises from level 1 to 3, attaining the highest cost in the prevention and treatment triangles at level 3 but, paradoxically, potentially the lowest cost at wellness level 3.

Now having drawn and laid out this concept in a linear form, I must critique it. The alert reader already will be asking questions such as, What if Ego has diabetes and is taking all kinds of proactive steps to increase wellness despite his or her condition? What about healing communities that increase wellness for terminally ill patients? Where do healthy pregnant women belong on this figure? These are appropriate criticisms: distinctions among the sections are not as precise in real life. A healthy woman who seeks a midwife's care during delivery might belong in wellness section 2, whereas one who delivers in a hospital with biomedical intervention belongs in treatment section 2—not because she is sick, but because her pregnancy is being treated as if it were an illness, as it has been for most North American women since the middle of the twentieth century.

FIELD OF HEALTH CARE FROM THE POINT OF VIEW OF VARIANT PRACTICES OR SYSTEMS

Activities included in the wellness triangle in Figure 5-1 range from those that are widely accepted in our society, such as diet and exercise, to behaviors such as praying that many do not classify as health related (but see Dossey, 1997). Why include them here?

The dominant biomedical system's materialist effort to segregate medicine from religion grew out of the secularist urge to embrace science late in the nineteenth century; this concept is artificial and is not shared by most of the world's health care systems. Indeed, most systems argue that the nonmaterial aspects of the body-person are as real and cogent as the material aspects and, further, that there is no true separation of these aspects.

> Sister Erma Allen once told me of having healed a small boy who had cut his head; she had silently said the [blood-stopping] verse over and over while at the same time applying ice to the wound. I asked how she knew that it was not the *ice* that had stopped the bleeding. After a pause she reprimanded me gently, "God sewed it with *His* needle, darlin'." (Snow, 1993)

The fact that biomedicine prefers materialist explanations also implies that it does not deliver care in all parts of the triangles. This is equally true for other systems. Each emphasizes a distinctive viewpoint (explanatory model) and develops expertise in only some of the potential areas of health care. For example, biomedicine has had great success in treating acute illness and trauma. Its control of technology allows for remarkable success in extending life and in producing pharmaceuticals and technology to address the physical and physiological components of disease. Simultaneously, however, biomedicine is criticized for its relatively ineffective care of many chronic conditions and for repeated inefficiencies in human kindness and humane care, areas that easily escape its materialist model.

Other systems, notably the so-called holistic systems, *integrate* human development into their usual care patterns. These systems also control technologies and techniques that address physical and physiological functioning. Patients praise these systems for their care of chronic conditions and for their efforts to enhance wellness, which include weaning patients from excessive dependence on pharmaceuticals and even on health care specialists.

Figure 5-2 portrays these different approaches. Note that neither the biomedical system nor the Chinese medical

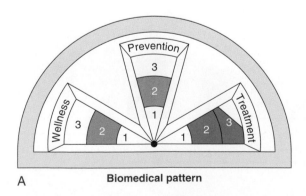

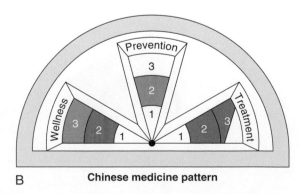

A   **Biomedical pattern**

B   **Chinese medicine pattern**

■ Strong emphasis
■ Moderate emphasis

Figure 5-2 The behavioral field of health care, highlighting the components addressed by two particular health care systems. **A,** Biomedicine. **B,** Chinese medicine.

system deals much with prevention on a mass scale. That is the prerogative of different specialists, especially of public health specialists.

Two vital points emerge from the field discussion and recur throughout this chapter, as follows:

1. No one health care system addresses the whole field.
2. All health care systems address a considerable part of the field.

The logical corollaries are (1) no one system is best for everything, and (2) existing systems overlap considerably in what they offer. There is a temptation to argue that societies ought to achieve economies of scale by making sure that only the best survive. However, considering our discussion of cultural relativity, it is impossible to define "best" in a manner that satisfies everyone. Logic demands that we determine who will be served well by which system and why. We will return to this issue after discussing some of the important ways in which health care systems differ.

CULTURAL CONCEPT OF THE HEALTH CARE SYSTEM

A cultural medical system is a complex of beliefs, models, and linked activities that providers and users consider useful in bettering health or well-being and in relieving stress and disease (Box 5-1).

This definition makes it clear that a health care *system* is complex and multilayered. Even simple systems, such as

---

BOX 5-1

Components of a Health Care System

1. A developed theory of the body-person, known as the explanatory model (Kleinman, 1980). This theory includes the causes of malfunction, as well as appropriate ways to address this malfunction.
2. Plans to educate and train new practitioners through apprenticeship, schooling, or both.
3. A health care subsystem that delivers care to needy persons.
4. Associated means of producing substances or technologies necessary to delivery systems and educational subsystems.
5. Professional organizations of practitioners who monitor each other's practices and promote the system to potential users.
6. A legal mandate that provides for the official recognition of practitioners and maintains a minimum standard of quality.
7. A social mandate that informally reveals levels of community acceptance, as by frequency of use, willingness to pay, and stereotypes about practitioners, among other markers.

---

those limited in scope to one ethnic group, are difficult for one person to master or describe. Larger systems are correspondingly more complex, encompassing a wide range of viewpoints, numerous subspecialties, and distinctive styles of practice. Biomedicine includes specialties ranging from the intensely material practice of surgery to the much more relational specialties of family medicine and psychiatry. Biomedical complexity is compounded by the fact that it is practiced rather differently in different countries.

Even the best simultaneous translator is going to have trouble dealing with the fact that *peptic ulcer* and *bronchitis* do not mean the same things in Britain that they do in the United States; that the U.S. *appendectomy* becomes the British *appendicectomy;* that the French tendency to exaggerate means there are never headaches in France, only migraines, and that the French often refer to real migraines as "liver crises"; that the German language has no word for chest pain, forcing the German patient to talk of heart pain, and that when a German doctor says "cardiac insufficiency" he may simply mean that the patient is tired. . . . How can [bio]medicine, which is commonly supposed to be a science, . . . be so different in four countries whose peoples are so similar genetically? The answer is that while [bio]medicine benefits from a certain amount of scientific input, culture intervenes at every step of the way. (Payer, 1988)

This complexity is equally true of Chinese medicine, which embraces many *styles,* including traditional Chinese medicine (TCM), Worsley five element style, French energetic, and numerous Japanese, Korean, and other styles. Even community-based or folk systems may have different specialties. Lakota (Sioux) people distinguish medicine men and women who emphasize herbal treatment from holy men and women who practice shamanically (Hultkrantz, 1985). The Dineh (Navajo) recognize three types of diagnosticians and singers who work with ritual, herbs, and the psychosocial body to deliver health care (Morgan, 1977). Biomedicine is famous for its numerous *specialties,* and other health care systems also offer specializations.

On a much smaller scale than the system or the style is the *technique* (Figure 5-3). A technique is comparatively simple; it might be a single therapy and often can be practiced without being linked to an explanatory model, detailed training, or professional oversight. Some practitioners specialize in offering single therapies, such as bee-sting injections, colonic irrigations, biofeedback, specific dietary supplements, or Swedish massage.

Single-therapy practitioners can provide *symptomatic relief* to their patients, but they cannot provide *systematic care,* that is, care guided by a well-developed model of how the body-person works, how the malfunction arose, and how intervention can help. The expansive power and persistence of health care systems correlate with the effectiveness of their explanatory models and linked therapeutic modalities.

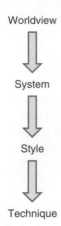

Figure 5-3 Scale of complexity in understanding health care.

SYSTEMS EMBEDDED IN LARGER CONSTRUCTS

But where do explanatory models come from? As noted earlier, health care systems are embedded in the sociocultural system surrounding them. This provides access not only to natural resources but also to ideas, assumptions, and patterns of logic. All these are reflected in explanatory models and health care delivery formats. In formal terms, health care systems are guided by the worldview principles of their society. The larger and more heterogeneous the surrounding society, the wider the range of health care ideas that society can encompass.

Nevertheless, certain worldviews tend to predominate. In the United States and Europe the *hierarchical* or *reductionistic* worldview dominates. This worldview model emphasizes hierarchies of value, a tendency to be judgmental, and appreciation for competition, forcefulness, "modernity," and materialism (Cassidy, 1994; Kenner, 2002). Biomedicine reflects these patterns in (1) its concern for the expertise of the practitioner over that of the layperson or patient; (2) its tendency to magnify the importance of some specialties or diseases over others (cardiology over pediatrics, cancer over asthma); (3) its preference for specialist-delivered technological treatment modalities that cause obvious reactions in the physical body (surgery, pharmaceuticals); and (4) its focus on end-stage physical malfunction while generally ignoring less-developed conditions and rejecting nonmaterial explanations of cause.

> [Cartesian] assumptions permeate Western society and form the modus operandi of conventional medicine. They have led to our belief in rationalism, causality, objectivity, and the separation of [bio]medicine and psychiatry. The assumptions work very well in acute emergency situations, but are limited when illness becomes chronic. . . . Cartesian thinking can be classified broadly as yang, and its inferred opposite as yin. Chinese philosophic thought can therefore be seen to be inclusive of Western thought, while Western thought has no way of incorporating Chinese holistic thinking. (Greenwood et al, 1994)

Other Western health care systems literally originated in reaction to biomedicine (allopathy), including homeopathy, osteopathy, naturopathy, chiropractic, and Christian Science. Others have been imported from Asia, such as Chinese medicine and Ayurveda. All argue (not always convincingly) that their approaches to care are more egalitarian, less judgmental, and gentler than biomedicine. Several offer nonmaterialist explanations of cause and care. In making such arguments, these systems are calling on another worldview currently held in the United States, namely, the *relational* (ecological or holistic) worldview. This worldview sees all things as connected in a network of relationships and considers how people, things, and energy interact and how these interactions can better the whole. Reflected into health care, this idea means that practitioners model health in terms of achieving balance (homeostasis), and patients are seen to have expertise different from that of the practitioner but expertise nonetheless. Thus, practitioner and patient form a partnership, and patients take some responsibility for their own care and development.

PROFESSIONALIZED AND COMMUNITY-BASED SYSTEMS

The terms *professionalized systems* and *community-based* systems distinguish between systems that serve large, heterogeneous patient populations and those smaller, more localized systems that serve culturally homogeneous populations.

A professionalized system tends to be found in urban settings, is taught in schools with the aid of written texts, and demands formal, usually legal, criteria for practice (Foster et al, 1978; Shahjahan, 2004). Students enter the system by choice and are approved by entrance examinations. They become practitioners on completing a designated plan of study, passing more examinations, and often being licensed by the state or nation. Health care typically is delivered on a one practitioner–to–one patient basis in locales that have been set aside for this purpose, such as offices, clinics, and hospitals. Practitioners form membership organizations dedicated to policing their respective specialties and presenting them in a positive light to outsiders. The dominant health care systems of modern nations always are professionalized systems. Examples include Ayurveda, biomedicine, Chinese medicine, chiropractic, homeopathy, osteopathy, and Unani (the traditional system of Pakistan and neighboring Muslim nations).

Community-based systems, also known as *folk* or *tribal* systems, are less expanded than professionalized systems, although they may have equally complex explanatory models and equally lengthy histories. These systems are found in both urban and rural settings, and training is often by apprenticeship. People enter training sometimes by inheritance but most often by receiving a call from the unseen world, indicating that he or she has the special capacity necessary to become a healer. Training ends when the teacher considers the student ready to practice. Rather than taking written examinations, students are tested by practicing medicine under guidance; essentially the community itself determines whether a student is "good enough." Care is often offered in people's homes, and community-based healers often practice on a part-time basis. Some folk healers form professional associations, with the same goals as professionalized doctors. Examples of community-based systems include Alcoholics Anonymous and similar urban self-help groups, curanderismo (among the most expanded of folk systems), rootwork (an African-derived system used by some African Americans), and traditional health care in Native American and Euro-American rural groups.

Box 5-2 provides sources for details about community-based systems in North America.

A third type of system is often called "popular" health care. Popular health care is not organized systematically; rather, it consists of simple techniques associated with the care of particular conditions. Examples include using cranberry juice for bladder infections, chicken soup for

colds, and hot toddies for sore throats. Much of what is published in general-reader magazines or discussed on talk shows is popular medicine. It is typically presented using biomedical terminology and is often simplified biomedicine.

Distinctions of complexity among health care systems are not absolute. For example, most professionalized systems continue to insist on considerable hands-on training, similar to apprenticeships. Some folk systems, especially urbanized ones, train practitioners in schools and do not expect students to have received a call to practice; these practitioners often earn their living through full-time health care work.

LANGUAGE ISSUES

Distinctions made in this section deal with differences of *scale* (Cassidy, 2008). A *system* is remarkably more complex than a *technique* or a single *therapy;* a professionalized system is expanded further than a community-based system. Failure to understand this point can lead to confusion and can also result in invalid "data." For example, researchers attempting to describe attitudes toward those in nonbiomedical practices often offer respondents lists of "alternative therapies" of completely different scale, from garlic supplementation (a small-scale, single therapy a layperson can select from reading a popular magazine) to Ayurvedic medical care (a large-scale, professionalized urban health care system). Creating a list of such wildly different scalars cannot yield meaningful data; it is as pointless as comparing a baseball bat to the entire Olympics, or an orange to a grocery chain.

This problem is common in commentary about alternative and complementary medicine, because one system (biomedicine) has been set up as "standard" while everything else, of whatever scale of complexity, has been set aside into the "other" category. This "contrast habit," itself, is invalid, and it is hoped that a wider view of medical care will soon result in all medical systems being seen as alternatives to one another. Meanwhile, one must be careful of terms that lend themselves to scalar confusion. The single term *acupuncture* can refer to a system, a modality, or simply a needling technique. Which does a given writer or speaker mean? *Massage* can mean a single technique, or it can refer to a rapidly professionalizing and systematizing practice. Some people use the term *medicine* to refer exclusively to biomedicine; for most, however, *medicine* is a term that encompasses all the ways in which people deliver health care.

Another confusing term is *traditional* (a good one not to use). Biomedical publications often refer to their own practice as "traditional medicine," categorizing all other practices by a term such as "alternative." However, when biomedicine is referred to as "modern" medicine, its worldwide nature is being contrasted with the indigenous systems of non-Western societies, which are then called "traditional." Systems other than biomedicine are used

---

BOX 5-2

Sources Describing Community-Based Systems in North America

American Folk Medicine (Hand, 1976)

Black Elk: The Sacred Ways of a Lakota (Black Elk et al, 1990)

Cry of the Eagle: Encounters with a Cree Healer (Young et al, 1989)

Curanderismo: Mexican-American Folk Healing (Trotter et al, 1997)

Ethnic Medicine in the Southwest (Spicer, 1979)

Feeling the Qi: Emergent Bodies and Disclosive Fields in American Appropriations of Acupuncture (Emad, 1998 [dissertation])

Healing by Hand: A Cross-Cultural Primer for Manual Therapies (Oths, 2004)

Healing Traditions, Alternative Medicine and the Health Professions (O'Connor, 1995)

Herbal and Magical Medicine: Traditional Healing Today (Kirkland et al, 1992)

Masters of the Ordinary: Integrating Personal Experience and Vernacular Knowledge in Alcoholic Anonymous (Scott, 1993 [dissertation])

Powwowing in Union Country: A Study of Pennsylvania German Folk Medicine in Context (Reimansnyder, 1989)

Ritual Healing in Suburban America (McGuire, 1994)

Susto: A Folk Illness (Rubel et al, 1984)

The Hands Feel It: Healing and Spiritual Presence Among a Northern Alaskan People (Turner, 1996)

This Other Kind of Doctors: Traditional Medical Systems in Black Neighborhoods in Austin, TX (Terrell, 1990)

Walkin' over Medicine (Snow, 1993)

worldwide, so the expanded systems are sometimes classified as the "Great Tradition" systems and others, in contrast, as "little tradition" or "folk" systems.

In summary, it is most effective to refer to health care systems by their specific names and to distinguish clearly the scale at which one wants to speak or write.

MODALITIES OF HEALTH CARE

Whatever the other aspects of their character, all health care practices care for people. To do so, these practices use a variety of interventions, such as surgery, injection or ingestion of pharmaceuticals, use of biologicals or botanicals, needling, dietary management, manipulation, bodywork, meditative exercises, dancing, music therapy, art therapy, water and heat treatments, bioenergetic manipulation, talk therapy, shamanic journeying, sitting meditation, and prayer.

Figure 5-4 sorts selected modalities along a line from intensely to lightly physically invasive. This correlates roughly with a movement from materialist to nonmaterialist views of the body-person. The more invasive modalities enter the physical body by cutting, pricking, insertion, or ingestion. Less invasive techniques involve touching the surface of the body. Even softer modalities access energetic or spiritual levels of the body without touching the skin. Even techniques that break into the body have differing degrees of intensity: replacing a hip is more intrusive than removing a cataract. Pharmaceutical drugs generally are more toxic than phytomedicines (semipurified plant medicines), which are in turn more forceful

than herbs. However, forcefulness does not connote effectiveness. Mild and gentle modalities can be as effective as intrusive ones.

Actual health care systems employ several of these modalities and can be roughly mapped with regions of the line in the figure, which provides further evidence that each system emphasizes certain parts, but not the entire spectrum, of health care options.

For example, a community-based system such as curanderismo uses bodywork, dietary manipulation, herbs, first-aid techniques, and shamanic techniques to treat a wide range of physical, psychosocial, and spiritual malfunctions (Rubel et al, 1984; Spicer, 1979; Trotter et al, 1997). Ayurveda offers surgery, a variety of water treatments from purges to baths, numerous biological and herbal remedies, bodywork, dietary management, and both sitting and moving forms of meditation (Krishan, 2003; Morrison, 1995). Biomedicine is unusual in focusing at the left of the line in Figure 5-4, the most invasive region, but associated practitioners such as physical therapists, nurses, and psychotherapists use modalities farther to the right along the line.

EXPLANATORY MODELS

We have discussed intervention modalities, but we have yet to understand the "madness" behind each method. Each system has its own explanatory model that summarizes the perceptions, assumptions, beliefs, theories, and facts that guide the logic of health care delivery. To develop the idea of the explanatory model, we explore how different

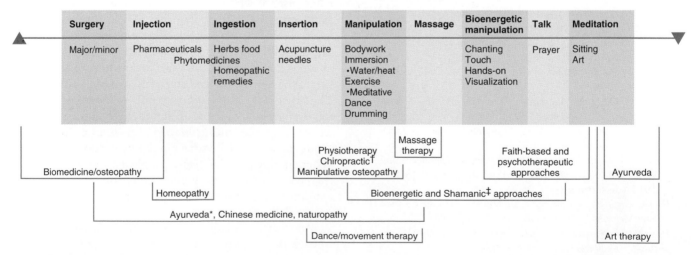

Techniques favored by selected health care systems

Surgery	Injection	Ingestion	Insertion	Manipulation	Massage	Bioenergetic manipulation	Talk	Meditation
Major/minor	Pharmaceuticals Phytomedicines	Herbs food Homeopathic remedies	Acupuncture needles	Bodywork Immersion •Water/heat Exercise •Meditative Dance Drumming		Chanting Touch Hands-on Visualization	Prayer	Sitting Art

Biomedicine/osteopathy

Homeopathy

Ayurveda*, Chinese medicine, naturopathy

Physiotherapy Chiropractic† Manipulative osteopathy

Massage therapy

Dance/movement therapy

Faith-based and psychotherapeutic approaches

Bioenergetic and Shamanic‡ approaches

Ayurveda

Art therapy

* Ayurveda also provides minor surgery.
† Some chiropractors offer dietary management, acupuncture needling, etc.
‡ Many Shamanic practitioners also provide herbs.

Figure 5-4 Relative physical invasiveness of selected therapeutic techniques, from most invasive *(left)* to least invasive *(right)*.

systems perceive the body-person and sickness and disease, their preferred causal explanations, and the preferred relationship between patients and practitioner.

CONCEPTS OF THE BODY-PERSON

There is not one human body, not one anatomy, not one physiology, but many. To understand any system, we must understand its concept of the body. Figure 5-5 depicts the body-person as four intersecting circles. The figure is simplified, because even within each of the circles, there are many ways in which systems can phrase their material, energetic, spiritual, or social perceptions of the body-person.

The biomedical model of the body-person focuses on the physical body, specifically the structure of its tissues and the movement and transformation of chemicals within cells. Classic chiropractic and osteopathic* models of the body are also materialistic, emphasizing connections and communications between bones, nerves, and muscles and the rest of the physical body, although newer versions increasingly employ an "energy" model to help explain changes. Note that such primarily materialist systems "enter" the body through the physical route and view this aspect as the goal of treatment, only hesitantly accepting that the psychosocial being may also be affected.

Other medical systems focus initial care on other aspects of the body-person and characteristically assume that care will redound on all parts. Several systems begin with "energy," and much current research aims to develop this concept (Jobst, 2004; Oschman, 2003; Stux et al, 2001). Existing systems use traditional language; for example, homeopathy views the physical body as having three significant layers and the body-person as having three distinct aspects (Vithoulkas, 1980), each imbued with *vital spirit* or *vital energy*. Acupuncture analyzes the physical body in terms of the flow of energy through

---
*Osteopathy originated as a manipulative system. Currently, only a minority of practitioners maintain this tradition; the remainder practice biomedicine (allopathy) or a combination.

pathways, or *meridians,* that do not directly correlate with known anatomical entities. The energy that flows through and animates the material body is called *qi* (*ch'i, ki*) and closely resembles the homeopathic concept of vital spirit or the Ayurvedic concept of *prana.*

Biofield or bioenergetic therapies intervene in aspects sometimes referred to as energy "whorls," "emanations," or "auras," and specialists identify them somewhat differently. Wirkus (1993), using bioscience terminology, refers to the thermal, electromagnetic, and acoustic fields. Brennan (1988), using esoteric science terminology, labels these three as the etheric, astral, and mental bodies. Bruyere (1989) focuses on chakras.

Spiritual and shamanic healers also work with nonmaterial and normally invisible bodies. Most believe that these spiritual forces imbue the physical body, although some say they extend beyond it, and some say that parts can travel (as during sleep), be removed (by exorcism), or get lost (Eliade, 1964; Ingerman, 1991, 1994; Targ et al, 1999).

Psychotherapists typically begin work with the psycho-social body, that is, the "person" who lives within the other bodies and interacts with the world outside. Terms for this aspect include *mind* and *emotions,* as well as technical terms that each subspecialty uses to showcase its particular explanatory model.

The several bodies are not separate: only one body-person stands before the practitioner seeking help. But who can say where the physical body, with its ongoing chemical and electrical changes, merges into the energetic body and where the latter extends into the spiritual body? All are immersed in the psychosocial body. For what a person believes greatly affects how he or she will respond to illness and to treatment or what he or she will deliver in the way of health care.

With the exception of heavily materialist models that perceive themselves as treating the physical body and only reluctantly acknowledge the psychosocial body, all health care systems argue that there are both material and nonmaterial aspects to the body (Figure 5-5) and that intervention in one area will affect all others. Thus, when a professional acupuncturist needles a patient who is having

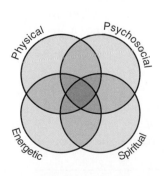
The four bodies

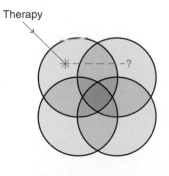
Therapeutic goal assumption of materialist systems

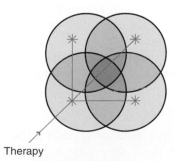
Therapeutic goal assumption of nonmaterialist systems

Figure 5-5 The four bodies addressed by health care.

an asthma attack, he or she enters the energetic body and moves energy. The acupuncturist expects the physical, psychosocial, and spiritual bodies to respond as well: the bronchial tubes will dilate, and pain, anxiety, and fear will dissipate. These changes are not thought to be coincidental; according to this system's explanatory model, all the aspects of the body can work at ease when energy flows smoothly. Similarly, a shamanic practitioner offers healing first through the spiritual body, but assumes that harmoniousness will result in improved function in all bodily aspects. Gathering scientific evidence for bodily interrelatedness is the subject of the field of psychoneuroimmunology (Martin, 1999; Moss et al, 2002).

CONCEPTS OF SICKNESS, DISEASE, AND IMBALANCE

Although often used generically, the terms *sickness* and *illness* formally refer to an experience of discomfort or malfunction. Disease and imbalance, however, are abstracted concepts. Thus a person has an illness or sickness, and a practitioner assigns meaning to this experience by diagnosing and explaining what has happened. The answers provided by the practitioner are guided by the explanatory model of his or her health care system. Cultural learning also guides the expression of the patient's illness and the practitioner's diagnostic values, so much so that even the pain people feel and report is related to such learned aspects of being as gender and ethnicity (Bachiocco et al, 2002; Bates, 1996; Bates et al, 1995; Emad, 1994).

A system's preferred malfunction concept is closely linked to its perception of the body-person, particularly whether a system tends to perceive cause as primarily *external* or *internal* (Cassidy, 1982, 1995; Fabrega, 1974; Foster et al, 1978; Helman, 2000; Kleinman, 1980; Lindenbaum et al, 1993; Mattingly et al, 2000; Murdock, 1980). Most health care systems accept that both occur, although most also prefer to emphasize either the invader or the responding organism. External models argue that malfunctions attack from outside the body-person, invading and destroying. Internal models argue that something must first go wrong internally, which allows outer influences to penetrate where they previously could not. These conceptual differences affect each system's view of patient and practitioner. External theorists see the patient as passive and the practitioner as authority, whereas internal ideology interprets the patient as responsible and the practitioner as partner to that responsibility.

DISEASE

The concept of *disease* is preferred by external models. In this view the body-person is relatively passive, whereas the surrounding environment teams with danger. Body-persons are thought to respond similarly to invaders; that is, one person with mumps, leukemia, or pneumonia

experiences it much as others do. If people are similar and the environment is dangerous, it is logical to emphasize the actions of the invader, and to find that every different type of invader creates a different disease. These assumptive patterns lead to the naming of many different diseases, and a major function of practitioners is to distinguish among them (diagnose *disease*). Their second job is to remove, destroy, or immobilize invaders, and thereby cure the patient.

This model has long been preferred by biomedicine and has yielded familiar metaphors (Sontag, 1977). Tumor cells and microorganisms that have been awaiting their chance in "reservoirs" invade human "victims." The body "wages war," and surgeons and physicians are "warriors in white," battling the invaders.* Diseases that fit this classic model have distinctive symptoms and signs, have single causes, and respond to specific therapies. Treatment results in cure. To emphasize the separation between ailments and patients, the former often are called *disease entities*.

Only a minority of the disease entities defined by biomedicine fit the invasion model. Chronic, degenerative, and stress-related disorders frustrate the system because they do not have specifiable boundaries, single causes, or predictable outcomes. These disorders force biomedicine to consider explanations that fall outside the usual framework: (1) the body-person is not passive but plays some part in the genesis of disease; (2) many (often unspecifiable) factors must interact before disease arises; (3) some of these factors might be psychosocial; and (4) the practitioner's role is less to prescribe than to educate. The area of biomedicine that best reflects this opening state of mind is that of "lifestyle" diseases, or conditions that arise from and can be ameliorated by changes in how people behave and believe. Interestingly, even this door has not opened too widely; most lifestyle discussions still focus on ameliorative factors that address the physical body, such as diet and exercise. Biomedical practitioners who recommend visualization or meditation are likely to consider themselves "avant-garde."

As noted, chiropractic and osteopathy share biomedicine's primarily material and mechanistic view of disease, although these systems focus on the spine and nerves rather than cells and chemicals. Patient instructions also tend to take a physical form, such as a change in diet or more exercise.

IMBALANCE

Many health care systems stress internal models of disorder and emphasize *imbalance* rather than disease. Their therapeutic goal is to return the person to a state of

---

*Similar metaphors are used to describe the need for exorcism: invasion by an evil entity demands a spiritual battle to defeat it. Faith-based systems that use exorcism therapeutically also use external models of disease causation.

balance. These systems often name conditions according to their process within the person. For example, in Chinese medicine, *rising Liver fire* describes a person's condition momentarily or repeatedly, but it is not a free-standing and categorical concept such as the biomedical disease entity *hepatitis*.

Balance can be perturbed by external invaders or by interruptions in the smooth working of the internal milieu. External causes, however, rarely harm a body-person who is in balance. Health care therefore tends to the self-protective abilities of the body-person, maintaining and strengthening them. This is not curing but healing; the practitioner's goal is not to battle the invader or fix the patient but rather to prune, weed, and plant within the patient, enabling the person to grow a vibrant internal garden in which all aspects of his or her body-person function harmoniously despite the vagaries of the external environment.

Treatment within internal-cause systems is individualistic, because the logic of this model is such that each person is considered to have a unique history and constitution that affect how he or she will respond to the myriad circumstances of life. The practitioner examines the current condition of the patient, relates it to the patient's social and medical history, and then selects therapy on the basis of the entire assessment.

Although diet, exercise, rest, and other physical interventions are prescribed, these are usually offered in formats that also address the spiritual and energetic bodies. For example, exercises such as yoga, t'ai chi, or qigong offer movement, energy balancing and storage, and meditation simultaneously. A patient might be advised to develop his or her spiritual and emotional body through creative activities such as art, dance, and chanting, or may be encouraged to minimize vulnerability to psychic attack by meditation, shamanic journeying, or prayer. Diet counseling may include attention not only to nutrient content but also to seasonal, constitutional, and essential (as opposed to literal) temperature appropriateness.

CONSTITUTIONAL TYPES

The disease entity and imbalance models represent ideals. Practitioners know that neither model works all the time. Thus, biomedicine recognizes as *syndromes* those conditions with multiple linked causes, not all of which can be specified. Similarly, internal-cause systems know that individuality is not absolute, because people do present commonalities or patterned responses to similar challenges.

Many health care systems have developed sophisticated models to link certain constitutional types with the probability of the development of particular illnesses. In the European and Middle Eastern system that preceded biomedicine, persons were categorized as melancholic, phlegmatic, sanguine, or choleric. Although current biomedical practitioners may view these concepts with an indulgent smile, the underlying idea is by no means absent in modern biomedicine. In the mid-twentieth century, bioscientists attempted to link physical and psychosocial diseases with the endomorphic, mesomorphic, and ectomorphic types (Sheldon et al, 1949). At present there is much interest in type A personalities, which are said to be linked to heart disease, and type C, linked to cancer. A popular diet links blood type to diet (Adamo, 1996). Constitutional typologies are well developed in the Ayurvedic system (the *doshas* of pitta, vata, and kapha) and in some styles of Chinese medicine (the five elements of wood, fire, earth, metal, water). The old European categories survive in the hot-cold systems of Latin America and the Philippines.

Figure 5-6 summarizes the data of this section in a linear model. The "categorical disease entities" model forms one extreme on a continuum, with the "process-related imbalance" model at the other end. At the midpoint are patterned responses, including constitutional types. At the end featuring diseases, the individual person essentially has been deleted from the argument ("One person suffers much like others, so focus on identifying the disease"), whereas at the other extreme the person is

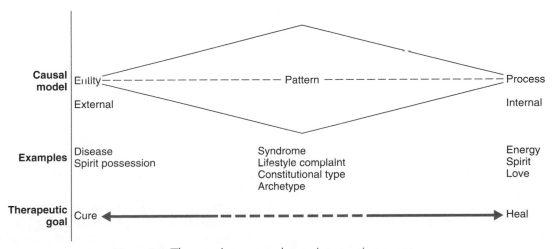

Figure 5-6 Three major approaches to interpreting symptoms.

the final focus and arbiter of interpretation ("In this individual these symptoms mean *x*, which I know from experience of him/her . . . They may mean *y* in another individual"). In the middle are positions that share both interpretive energies ("Certain characteristics make it more likely that he or she will experience these symptoms, so perhaps I can reduce my diagnostic chore").

LANGUAGE ISSUES

Biomedical disease entity names have become standard vocabulary, but these diseases (not the symptoms) are "real" only to people who use the biomedical model. Practitioners of other systems may use these terms out of familiarity to communicate with patients or granting agencies or to complete insurance claim forms, but within their own systems of health care, these labels have little cogency. Acupuncturists, for example, treat what their patients and referring physicians call "depression," but the concept does not exist in Chinese medicine. Research has shown that in samples of people with the biomedical diagnosis of depression, Chinese medical practitioners can recognize at least five distinct energetic imbalance conditions (Schnyer, 2002; Schnyer et al, 2001). The significant point is that two patients with the same biomedical diagnosis might appropriately receive different diagnoses and therapies from a Chinese medicine practitioner.

Practitioners and scientists therefore must be careful in their use of biomedical terminology, not assuming that it is sufficient to describe what is understood by other systems. Specialists should describe the symptoms and then, if they wish, affix a biomedical label while clearly stating that the biomedical label may not reflect the way of knowing of another system. This can serve its purpose, because symptoms are recognized everywhere; it is the interpretations that differ. By focusing on symptoms, the malfunction labels of the other systems would begin to take on the kind of reality that now is owned only by the biomedical labels. The medical conversation would become more accurate and broader.

CONCEPTS OF DEEP CAUSE

External and internal causative factors mentioned so far can be understood as proximate causes of malfunction. With the issue of deep cause, we contemplate why *this* person at *this* time or in *this* place has become ill in *this* way. We want to consider sociocultural answers, not epidemiological ones. We explore the issue first by returning to our discussion of the body-person and considering the developmental nature of sickness, and second by considering the intentional component of sickness.

Developmental Nature of Sickness
An ancient chicken-and-egg philosophical argument questions whether the physical body comes first, giving rise to nonmaterial constructs such as emotions and mind, or whether mind (spirit, soul) comes first and animates the physical body. Materialist models prefer the first argument, whereas nonmaterialist models favor the second.

This choice affects both the theory and the politics of health care. If one accepts as real only what one can see, hear, or measure with machines, delivering care to the nonmaterial bodies is, at the least, puzzling and more likely ridiculous. Efforts to test nonmaterialist systems include designing machinery to "prove" that the claimed bodies exist, such as using electrical point locators to find acupuncture points and meridians or Kirlian photography to find auras. Materialists suspect nonmaterialist practitioners of misleading their patients or achieving effects primarily by activating the placebo response. Cynics also argue that nonmaterialist practitioners have their greatest successes in the care of functional, or psychosomatic, diseases. Such diseases are disvalued in materialist systems precisely because they lack specific material signs such as germs, malfunctioning genes, tumor cells, abnormal metabolic values, or broken bones. Materialists suspect that those who have functional conditions are not really sick.

Nonmaterialist thinkers consider malfunction in the nonmaterial aspects of the body to be as real as physical malfunction. All patient complaints signal true distress; the diagnostic concern is not with triaging between the real and the imaginary, but with identifying what aspect of the person will respond most efficaciously to treatment.

Many such systems use a developmental model of malfunction, in which sickness starts in the nonmaterial bodies and is expressed in the physical body only later. They fault materialist systems for paying attention only to end-stage (i.e., physical) malfunction and failing to treat conditions before they become entrenched. They further argue that a focus on the material level alone provides only symptomatic relief and ignores deep cause, allowing underlying malfunctions to remain unaddressed. Nonmaterialist systems assume that care can modify all parts of the body-person. Some also claim that as persons heal, they cycle backward through layers of long-buried symptoms until finally they express the oldest symptoms, release them, and are well. This pattern is called the "law of cure."

For example, a child might experience a spiritual trauma such as loss of intimacy (Jarrett, 1998). Afterward this child has eczema. Later still the child has allergies and asthma. Untreated, the original spiritual wound or deep cause has been magnified and becomes overt and disabling. Appropriate treatment of the asthma not only will relieve wheezing but also might instigate a recrudescence of eczema and grief until the spiritual wound is healed.

Thus, by the logic of internal-cause systems, it is advantageous to treat complaints before malfunction is manifested physically. Nonmaterial complaints are real because any suffering affects the whole body-person.

Systems that use only nonmaterial therapies, such as bioenergetic healing, psychotherapy, and shamanism, focus care on the nonmaterial aspects of the person but expect that the physical body will respond. However, many systems use a combination of material and nonmaterial therapeutic modalities. The techniques themselves often have a layered character. For example, acupuncture points have multiple functions and in combination have predictable and specific physical, spiritual, and emotional effects (Ross, 1995). The same is true of herbal remedies and some forms of bodywork. Nonmaterialist models also view the person as having an active role in creating and treating his or her own condition. The role of practitioner is reformulated from authority to facilitator, from the one who does the curing to the one who helps persons heal themselves. As treatment is administered, such practitioners encourage patients to consider what attitudes of mind or spirit may have played a part in their illness and to explore new, life-enhancing ways of believing and behaving—wellness training. The goals of nonmaterialist health care are to care for the nonsomatic aspects of the patient so completely that the somatic aspect rarely suffers.

Unfortunately, in the hands of some practitioners the focus on patient responsibility becomes excessive, and patients feel guilt about their sickness. The materialist emphasis on the patient as the victim of disease can be equally harmful, resulting in patients who feel helpless to change themselves or learn health-enhancing behaviors.

Intentional Component of Sickness

Whereas practitioners discuss proximate and deep causes of sickness, medical social scientists recognize another cross-cutting domain of causality and contrast, called the "naturalistic" and "personalistic" explanatory approaches. According to the *naturalistic* approach, the causes of sickness are found in the natural world and lack intention; they cause malfunction by unintentionally ending up in the wrong place or by causing damage as they go about their own lifeways. Sickness is considered a normal experience of life, natural and inevitable. The *personalistic* approach, in contrast, maintains that some form of intention is present, and sickness is an unnatural result of one's own misbehavior or of attracting the attention of the wrong entities (Foster et al, 1978).

When a person says he or she has lung cancer and attributes it to 30 years of smoking, the person speaks in a naturalistic mode. However, if the person complains of having been inveigled into smoking or declares that this habit is an expression of weak character, the person is moving in a personalistic direction. If people attribute their cancer to the corrective or punitive actions of a spiritual entity such as God, they speak fully in the personalistic mode.

These tendencies coexist in most health care systems, although one or the other usually is emphasized. Professionalized health care systems generally prefer naturalistic explanations such as microorganisms, malformations, toxins, age-related degeneration, winds, hot and cold, or damp and dry. Within these systems, however, some practitioners recognize, even specialize in, the personalistic approach. In biomedicine, psychiatry and psychology emphasize this structure, usually attributing malfunction to troubles in the psychosocial body rather than in the spiritual or energetic bodies. In other major systems, practitioners deal with expressions of self-distrust or the results of psychic attacks in much the same way as they deal with physical conditions.

Faith-based systems are primarily personalistic in approach. They ask patients to confess ways in which they have angered God, who may have retaliated by sending disease. Some also recognize invasion by evil spiritual entities and offer exorcism as a treatment. Prayer is offered to alleviate pain and prevent sickness. Some faith-based systems also practice the "laying on of hands."

> "But she seems to be an intelligent woman," one family practitioner kept repeating as he told me of the woman who had refused the surgical removal of uterine fibroids. What he viewed as a completely medical (and secular) situation his patient took to be a tangible sign of divine displeasure. . . . God would heal her if it would be his will; no scalpels necessary. (Snow, 1993)

Shamanic systems combine naturalistic and personalistic approaches. Natural events, such as experiencing a severe emotional or physical shock, may cause parts of the soul to be lost. The shaman recognizes the situation from the symptoms and takes a spiritual journey to retrieve the soul parts. Again, a person with an insufficient degree of psychic protection may be psychically attacked by someone else, either purposefully, during an argument, or even by being looked at with envious eyes. The shaman's task is to heal the psychospiritual wound and then help the patient to develop stronger personal protective skills. Shamans also serve communities by mediating arguments, changing weather, and treating physical illness with herbs and psychospiritual support.

Notice that the naturalistic-personalistic frame cuts across the materialist-nonmaterialist frame. Naturalistic explanations often deal with causes that are nonmaterial, such as temperature changes or wind invasions. Similarly, personalistic explanations can be materialist; some people see, hear, or feel entities such as ghosts and spirits, and material objects such as hair and fingernails store aspects of soul and thus can be used to heal or harm. Most importantly, however, even when the system and practitioner prefer naturalistic explanations, patients regularly demand to know, "Why me, Lord?" and offer answers couched in the personalistic framework.

CONCEPTS OF THE PRACTITIONER-PATIENT RELATIONSHIP

Systems that prefer external causative models characteristically view the body-person as passive, a victim, and, logically enough, interpret the practitioner as active, the one who cures. By contrast, systems that prefer internal causative models view the body-person as active and as already capable of healing. The practitioner's task is to facilitate the discovery of this capacity and develop it. The patient in this model has life expertise, and the practitioner must use medical expertise in partnership with the patient.

Some patients are passive regardless of what is asked of them, and others always demand a say in their care. The biomedical literature discusses this issue under the rubrics of external locus and internal locus of control. However, this chapter makes the point that not only practitioners or patients but entire systems are modeled to emphasize one style of caregiving. Systems that want patients to be passive find active patients frustrating, irritating, and intrusive. Systems that want patients to be active find passive patients unresponsive, helpless, and in denial.

A lucid practitioner might be able to match his or her style to the patient's needs, providing either authoritarian or relational (patient-centered) care to fit the situation. However, practitioners also have preferences and personal styles that cannot be modified easily. Students are likely to select health care practices that fit their personal styles.

MAKING SENSE OF ALL THE VARIABILITY

The chapter began with the claim that health care systems vary in many ways and that the variety can be analyzed with the help of conceptual models. Now we must ask, "How can this information be applied in a world in which patients use many health care modalities and practitioners are advised to understand and sympathize?"

This section explores this question by discussing an example that compares biomedicine and Chinese medicine. I have developed a conceptual map that allows any system to be rapidly compared with another (Figure 5-7). I end by summarizing what makes biomedicine unusual, yet convinced that it is normative.

COMPARISON OF CARE IN TWO MEDICAL SYSTEMS

As discussed, biomedicine prefers reductionistic, categorical explanatory models, whereas Chinese medicine prefers relational, process-oriented explanatory models (Beinfield et al, 1991; Cassidy, 2002; Kaptchuk, 1983; Lock et al, 1988; Stein, 1990). Both are heterogeneous

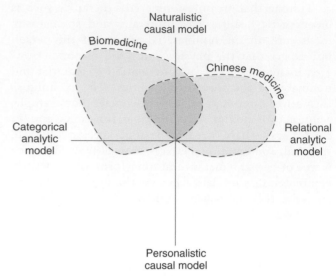

Figure 5-7 A cognitive map for health care systems.

systems, so relational tendencies can be found in biomedicine, and categorical tendencies exist in Chinese medicine. How different do these preferences really make these two systems?

Similarities Between Biomedicine and Chinese Medicine

1. Both aim to provide comprehensive health care, which includes health-enhancing, preventive, reproductive, acute and chronic illness, and trauma care.
2. Both prefer to deliver care in specific locales such as clinics or hospitals and in practitioner-to-patient dyads; group-based and home- or community-based practices are viewed as possible but nonmodal.
3. Both prefer naturalistic explanations of malfunction, arguing that impersonal forces are the main sources of ill health. However, if sometimes reluctantly, both also recognize that personalistic explanations sometimes make sense.
4. Both subsume a wide range of practices or specialties. Although specialties within internal medicine represent the intensively reductionistic naturalistic components of biomedicine, psychiatry veers toward personalistic explanatory models, and immunotherapy, clinical ecology, and approaches emphasizing lifestyle intervention have a relational flavor. Again, although some styles of acupuncture practice aim to be primarily relational and holistic in outlook, the post-1949 TCM style veers toward the reductionistic model and borrows many ideas from biomedicine.

Differences Between Biomedicine and Chinese Medicine

1. Biomedicine focuses on trauma, acute illness, and end-stage chronic disease intervention. Although prevention is discussed as part of biomedical care,

wellness is not a core concept. Chinese medicine emphasizes wellness and preventive care, and treats chronic and acute illness conditions, but avoids surgery (see Figure 5-2).

2. Biomedicine emphasizes materialist explanations, whereas Chinese medicine emphasizes nonmaterialist explanations based on a distinctive concept of qi (ch'i, vital energy). Their views of anatomy and physiology and their favored bodily metaphors (machinery and warring vs. gardening) are distinctly different.

3. Biomedicine emphasizes the physical body as the locus for intervention, recognizes but remains uncomfortable with the concept of the psychosocial body, and largely denies the existence of the energetic and spiritual bodies. By contrast, Chinese medicine uses the energetic body as the locus for intervention and assumes that interventions at that level will redound on all the other bodies.

4. Biomedicine sees humans as biologically similar; therefore, diseases will present similarly and can be treated similarly. Chinese medicine sees each human as unique and assumes that even if symptoms appear to be similar, the deep cause might be dissimilar; thus, care should be delivered individualistically.

5. Biomedicine has defined an immense universe of distinct disease entities, assumes they will present similarly in most people, focuses much energy on disease diagnosis, and defines success as cure. Controlling or palliating symptoms is considered a lesser success, and death is commonly thought of as a failure. Chinese medicine focuses on the flow of energy within the body and between the patient and the cosmos. Ill health arises when this flow is disrupted or impeded or when there is insufficient energy. Because this can happen in many ways, the practitioner also spends much time diagnosing by assessing the character of the flow, hearing the patient's story, and listening in on the energetic body (e.g., by taking the pulses). Imbalance is viewed as commonplace and natural, and there is little to cure; instead the practitioner hopes to maintain or improve the coherence of the body-person, that is, heal the person. Death is also deemed natural; the dying patient can use acupuncture to ease pain and to achieve a final energetic balance.

CONCEPTUAL MAPPING OF HEALTH CARE SYSTEMS

It is possible to map differences among health care systems to allow these similarities and differences to be rapidly grasped and applied. Figure 5-2 maps the systems in terms of individual needs; Figure 5-7 redraws Figure 5-2 in terms of the conceptual models explored in this chapter.

Figure 5-7 shows a matrix with the categorical (reductionistic) versus relational (process-related) worldview represented on the horizontal axis and the naturalistic to personalistic causal model on the vertical axis. Using this map, we can—hypothetically—locate virtually any system of health care in such a way as to compare it rapidly with any other system. Knowing more about the terrain of systematic health care differences makes it easier to understand and use the insights from other systems of health care. Practitioners can use such information to design research, to make themselves and their patients aware of their own prejudices, and to listen more openly to the users of different health care systems.

Figure 5-7 maps only the two systems cited in our example; readers are encouraged to map others as they learn about them in this text. Note, however, that each of the two systems mapped covers a wide area. Biomedicine, although clearly within the realm of categorical naturalistic thinking, spills over the horizontal line into personalistic models (psychology, psychiatry) and over the vertical line into relational territory (family practice, psychoneuroimmunology, lifestyle arguments). In fact, biomedical practice overlaps the Chinese medicine outline at the center of the figure.

The map also shows that in terms of preferred worldview, Chinese medicine is opposite that of biomedicine. On the other hand, it is similar to biomedicine in its general preference for naturalistic causal explanations. These twin characteristics map Chinese medicine into the upper right quadrant. Note again, however, the wide range of practice under the umbrella of Chinese medicine. The more symptomatic and categorical styles of practice map left toward the reductionistic quadrant, and the traditional shamanistic components of Chinese medicine map below the horizontal line.

This map reminds us that no single health care system serves the whole field, and that systems differ but also share similarities.

WHY BIOMEDICINE FINDS OTHER SYSTEMS UNCONVENTIONAL

Although not drawn onto the map, the other health care systems tend to cluster more centrally or to the right of the center on both sides of the horizontal axis. Thus the mapping exercise also provides a visual clue as to why biomedicine, from its perch in the upper left quadrant, might find the other systems unconventional. They are nonmodal when judged from biomedicine's position. Biomedicine is equally unconventional when viewed from the position of most systems. From a worldwide viewpoint, biomedicine is unusual in the following ways:

1. Its intense attachment to materialist interpretive models
2. Its focus on the physical body, almost to the exclusion of other possibilities
3. Its focus on the disease, often to the virtual exclusion of the person
4. Its vast development of disease types
5. Its highly technological delivery system

6. The invasiveness of its care modalities
7. Its emphasis on acute disease, trauma, and end-stage malfunction, with relatively little focus on prevention or wellness
8. Its high cost

Despite these oddities, biomedicine considers itself conventional and other systems "alternative." How did this situation come about, and why is it not surprising to most Western urban people? Furthermore, why is it difficult for people to consider biomedicine as just one more alternative?

Health care is not free of culture or politics. In the United States, we are accustomed to thinking of biomedicine as the best system because it is the most expanded, being practiced in every country in the world, although Chinese medicine and homeopathy are close seconds. Biomedicine also has the largest educational, legal, and economic mandate. Finally, its explanatory model closely fits the dominant European and North American worldview paradigm: categorical or reductionistic.

As part of the expression of this worldview, many state that biomedicine is the most scientific system. This argument is controversial and must be examined carefully.

Science is a particular method for gathering information and constructing knowledge. In contrast to other systems—such as theology, which allows for revelation, and law, which allows for precedence—science demands that information be sought in the natural world and that interpretations be tested for accuracy. This is extremely unusual; it means that a person's opinion or mere observation and consequent certitude are not enough to make the person's position acceptable to scientists. Instead, the person must show that he or she has gathered data systematically and accounted for potential biases, then must submit his or her interpretations to others for examination and retesting. Furthermore, the researcher is enjoined to be a relativist; that is, not to become enamored with his or her interpretations but to hold them always as *models* of reality or approximations. This provides remarkable training in humbleness, and to be frank, not many researchers achieve it.

ROLE OF SCIENCE

Euro-American society in particular has developed science to be *the* believable knowledge method, the knowledge orthodoxy since the late nineteenth century. The determination with which Westerners cling to their cultural preference concerning the power of science approaches a religious fervor. Biomedicine gradually took on the cloak of scientism with the rise of clinical medicine in the early nineteenth century, moving toward a laboratory-based experimental model by the late nineteenth century. Although the experiment is only one way to gather valid data by use of the scientific method, this became accepted as the "scientific" approach. By the early twentieth century,

American biomedicine already contrasted itself to other systems by claiming to be experimental and thus uniquely scientific. Given that the other major systems are generally not experimental—they depend on well-developed clinical observation skills and experience guided by their explanatory models—it becomes clear why a system that perceives itself as scientific can consider nonscientific systems as inferior *in our cultural milieu*.

> The biomedical model assumes diseases to be fully accounted for by deviations from the norm of measurable biologic (somatic) variables. It leaves no room within its framework for the social, psychological, and behavioral dimensions of illness. . . . The biomedical model has thus become a cultural imperative, its limitations easily overlooked. In brief, it has now acquired the status of dogma. In science, a model is revised or abandoned when it fails to account adequately for all the data. A dogma, on the other hand, requires that discrepant data be forced to fit the model or be excluded. (Engel, 1977)

But is biomedicine really scientific if judged from the perspective of science rather than cultural preference? Recent studies suggest that only 30% of what biomedicine achieves has been tested adequately (Altman, 1994; American Iatrogenic Association, n.d.; Andersen, 1990). A full 70% of practice uses the same well-developed clinical observation skills and experience guided by the explanatory model that powers the other health care systems.

Those who can stand back dispassionately—that is, those who really do think like scientists—understand that a great deal of the argument over which systems are modal or alternative is really an argument over cultural turf. As such, victory in this argument serves the usual political purpose of maintaining power by insisting on the virtue of one's own values, often by attacking the perceptions of one's rivals, but these are political, not scientific, acts.

IMPORTANCE OF VIEWING HEALTH CARE AS A MATTER OF CULTURAL MODELING

That health care is a matter of cultural modeling rather than scientific truth is important to practitioners whose goals are to relieve suffering. It also is important to those who want to be scientific in their thoughts and choices. Differences must be addressed. So, pragmatically, we end by asking, "Who do the differences serve?" and "How do the differences serve?"

USERS OF ALTERNATIVE MEDICINE

Demand for nonbiomedical health care in Europe and North America is at a peak that has not been seen for about 150 years. Surveys of users of alternative or integrative medicine tell similar stories. People want to feel cared for, and biomedicine's emphasis on laboratory medicine, factoring of the person out of the diagnostic and treatment equation, invasive treatments associated with high levels of painful side effects,* rushed delivery of care, and immensely high cost all connote an uncaring system and are making biomedicine unattractive to increasing numbers of people.

Who are these people? Early surveys indicated that the users of the major nonbiomedical systems were mainly urban, female, and well educated, with middle to high incomes (Cassidy, 1998a; Cassileth et al, 1984; Eisenberg et al, 1993, 1998; McGuire, 1994); today CAM is used by all demographic groups. Original users—"early adopters"— were in excellent positions to judge the quality of the care they received from the variety of practitioners that they consulted, and they passed on their success stories. This point matters, because mainstream practitioners and researchers often attacked nonbiomedical health care by saying that the users are being misled, either purposefully by the practitioners or by their own desires, distress, and ignorance.

Such defensive, politically motivated arguments are increasingly weakened by the following:

1. Studies show that where health care is obviously pluralistic, lay people are astute at matching systems with complaints (Cassidy, 1998a; Young, 1981).
2. On the whole, patients report satisfaction with alternative health care (Cassidy, 1998b; Eisenberg et al, 1998; Emad, 1994; Gould et al, 2001; O'Connor, 1995; Paterson et al, 2004; Work-shop on Alternative Medicine, 1994).
3. Rapidly accumulating results of scientific research on alternative treatments show that they are often as effective or more effective, or safer, than biomedical treatments for identical conditions, or that they provide valuable complementary effects when biomedicine is in use (Benor, 1993; Byrd, 1988; Carlston, 2003; Cassidy, 2002; Church, 2007; Edzard et al, 2001; Jacobs et al, 1994; Jobst, 1995; McTaggart, 2007; O'Connor, 1995; Reilly et al, 1994; see also articles in *Journal of Alternative and Complementary Medicine, Alternative Therapies,* and other journals; access MEDLINE; and see reports of the National Institutes of Health Center for Complementary and Alternative Medicine).
4. Methodological skills for analyzing systems that differ deeply from biomedicine are developing rapidly (Cassidy and Thomas 2007; Cassidy, 1995; Edzard et al, 2001; Grimes, 2003; Jonas et al, 2003; MacPherson et al 2007; Paterson and Schnyer 2007; Wisnesky et al, 2005).

*Approximately 20% of illnesses that lead to hospitalization are iatrogenic, that is, caused by the biomedical care itself (Greenwood et al, 1994).

CONSTITUENCY FOR ALTERNATIVE MEDICINE

Current biomedical discussion on the best use of nonbiomedical alternatives focuses either on annexing particular techniques (in the process, jettisoning the systemic embedding of the techniques in their native explanatory models) or on using the alternatives adjunctively (e.g., recommending acupuncture as adjunctive therapy to minimize the side effects of chemotherapy). Readers are now prepared to interpret these proposals as expressions of a biomedical perspective that claims its health care reality is superior to all others.

Of course, the situation looks a little different from the viewpoints of alternative practitioners, as well as from the perspective of potential patients, many of whom are glad that modern health care provides a menu of alternatives from which to choose. At times, for example, Chinese medical practitioners might want to use biomedicine adjunctively, and some biomedical diagnostic techniques are well integrated into nonbiomedical systems of health care.

Many would benefit if the U.S. health care system were organized so that several alternatives were widely available and people learned about them from childhood (Box 5-3).

Note that this discussion assumes that there is space for all forms of health care. This should be true in a democratic society, and it is true in the sense that all the systems already exist and serve people. The drive behind current research is to discover what services each system can provide and to compare their effectiveness in providing these services. Interestingly, this drive will fail if it is expressed solely in terms of conditions or complaints, which is only half the equation. The other half consists of the people who are to receive the

BOX 5-3

Beneficiaries of Widely Available Alternative (or Integrative) Health Care Systems in the United States

- Those who have a high need for affiliation and who therefore want a relational style of health care
- Those who want to alleviate symptoms gently or with fewer side effects
- Those who will not take "hopeless" for an answer
- Those who want to prevent disease or enhance wellness
- Those who interpret the body-person as having more than a physical aspect and who want to be able to address the energetic, psychosocial, and spiritual bodies when receiving or delivering health care
- Those who are concerned with the end-stage focus and invasiveness of typical biomedical care

care. There always will be a range of desires and needs; some patients will always prefer care that is technological and has rapid overt effects, whereas others will always prefer care that is relational, gentle, and virtually contemplative.

It is hoped that the world's people will become more skilled at using all our health care resources and options, to make it possible for everyone—practitioners and patients—to know enough about their options to triage care successfully in a manner that maximizes patient satisfaction and health while minimizing suffering, iatrogenic disease, and cost.

It remains for you to consider your own goals for practice. Where do you fall on the various continua discussed in this chapter? Are you satisfied with the care that you deliver, or would you like to modify some rough spots? How can the existing range of medical options help you do so? How can developing your skill and referral base in alternatives to your own medicine aid your current or future patients?

SUMMARY

This chapter introduces concepts that are fundamental to understanding values and issues in the practice of health care and provides a sociocultural context and models that will be useful in understanding the practices described in subsequent chapters.

Health care is fundamentally a matter of sociocultural interpretation. It should now be clear that health care systems differ in important ways and that no one system provides all the answers, or even the best answers, for all users or circumstances. Differences among systems are not random but are driven and logically organized by underlying assumptive patterns that are revealed in explanatory models, therapeutic modalities, and styles of practice.

These differences are *not* unbridgeable; the concepts developed in this chapter should allow most practitioners and researchers to approach even strange ideas with new appreciation, as well as provide them with tools that allow for better communication and understanding. After all, the deepest and most common goal of all health care systems is to relieve pain and prevent suffering.

ACKNOWLEDGMENTS

Special thanks to Haig Ignatius, MD, MAc, and Marc Micozzi, MD, PhD, for their generous reading of the original chapter in its draft stages. More thanks to Jean Edelen for bibliographic help with the newer version. Continuing thanks to many colleagues whose deep thinking about medical philosophical and practice issues guides and sustains my own explorations. And to my husband and daughter, always, your love and support are most precious.

🄮 Chapter References can be found on the Evolve website at http://evolve.elsevier.com/Micozzi/complementary/

CHAPTER

6

VITALISM: FLOW, CONNECTION, AND THE AWARENESS OF BEING ALIVE

DAVID F. MAYOR

Life is nothing but a word which means ignorance, and when we characterize a phenomenon as vital, it amounts to saying that we do not know its immediate cause or its condition.

—CLAUDE BERNARD (1813-1878)

Physical events can be looked at in two ways: from the mechanistic and from the energic standpoint.

—CARL GUSTAV JUNG (1875-1961)

Vitalism has been defined as "the doctrine that the origin and phenomenon of life are due to or produced by a vital principle, as distinct from a purely chemical or physical force" (Onions, 1933, p. 2364). In some form or other, this belief occurs throughout what is now labelled as complementary and alternative medicine (CAM). To understand its enduring power, it is helpful to consider how we experience being alive and the ways we think about this. This chapter then traces the historical development of vitalism. A selection of healing practices is described in terms of their fundamental propositions and the ontological status that they confer on the vital principle. The chapter concludes with a discussion of the vitalist dialectics of

CAM and an attempt to delineate the most significant characteristics of vitalism in the context of twenty-first-century medicine.

TIME AND LIFE—THE BASIC QUESTIONS

What is life? How do we even know that we ourselves are alive, or that others are? What connects us to the living, and what differentiates the living from the dead? How much of our world is alive? Why do some of us appear more vital than others? Are we born with a certain amount of vitality that we can dissipate and that runs out when we die, or does it fluctuate so that we feel more alive at some times than others? Are there ways we can enhance our aliveness, situations that injure it (such as drug abuse, illness, many childbirths, too much sex, or, as in Chinese Medicine, "taxation fatigue" of *qi*, the vital energy)?

If we are fortunate enough to have time for reflection and self-awareness, such questions may arise for all of us—perhaps in wonderment as children, or more existentially as

61

adolescents before the business of life sweeps us along, or during illness, or as oldsters with leisure time or increasing levels of pain, or finally as lovers standing temporarily outside of time. It is not really surprising, given our shared humanity, that the answers we have come up with over the centuries are based on and expressed with only a few basic metaphors (Boers, 1999; Johnson, 2007), from wherever we hail. Whether our sense of being alive comes from inner awareness or outer attention, we appear to recognize life in similar ways (Kuriyama, 1995). But we do need to set aside time for this consideration. Thomas Hobbes (1588-1679), his birth precipitated by his mother's terror of the Spanish Armada (of which he wrote, "My mother dear / Did bring forth twins at once, both me and fear"), described the natural state of humankind as "solitary, poore, nasty, brutish, and short" (Hobbes, 1651). In his version of prehistory based on struggle and competition, time for anything but staying alive would be available only for a favored few. A more Romantic view (as expressed the following century in France by Jean-Jacques Rousseau and others) might be that the prehistoric world was some kind of primitive harmonious paradise in which awareness of life could flourish, before being spoiled by civilization and its conventions and limitations. In reality, significant leisure time to explore the deeper questions of life may not have ever been available, even among a favored few, until the "axial age" of classical antiquity (ca. 800 to 200 BC) (Kuriyama, 1995).

PRECURSORS I: THE LIFE-BREATH

A scientist may say that the study of life is the study of organisms, and so it is necessarily about how these maintain their organization and structure. However, the lived body as experienced in feeling is very different from the "structural corpus" (Ots, 1994), the body as conceived in thought (Hall, 1975b; Lowen, 1976; Sandner, 1986). On a very simple level, we sense, we move. Life is sensation and movement, as well as organization, even at the cellular level (Lipton, 2005). We need both to live in this world.

If we take our attention within the body, we may sense many movements—flows, pulsations, vibrations, expansions and contractions, changing balances of heat and cold. In particular, we breathe, and we soon become aware that to cease breathing is threatening to life. The entering breath brings life; breath leaving may even signal its end.

We also need food and drink to live, of course, in particular to fuel the visible, tangible, physical body. But the breath remains somehow more mysterious, less graspable, and so has been taken as a key to life in many cultures ("an *almost* visual, tangible image of the fluidly conceived life flowing through the body"; Hultkrantz, 1953, p. 180 [my italics]). It connects us with the world, the inner and outer, what is above and what is below. But what happens to it inside us, or outside us? Are there purely inner breaths, "breath-souls"? Is breath indeed a

form of the winds we can feel outside of ourselves in nature (Kuriyama, 1995), or is our understanding of such outer winds derived from our experience of breath (Rank, 1968)? Is there indeed one all-embracing wind of nature, a "life-breath" that connects all things? For many North American peoples, for example, there is but one word to denote life, breath, and wind (Reichard, 1974). For many indigenous peoples around the world, illness is carried literally on the wind, such as the *angin* or wind sickness of the Malaysian Archipelago (Laderman C, 1991).

CLASSICAL ANTIQUITY

In ancient Egypt, the *ka* was the vital force, housing the more subtle soul (*ba*) and distinguishing the living from the dead (Budge, 1899). Breathed into us by the goddess of childbirth when (or possibly even before) we are born, leaving the body at death but remaining earthbound, it required sustenance through incense as well as food and drink in the afterlife. The ka, one of several immaterial aspects of a person, was both symbol and source of the transmission of life from the gods to men and was depicted as two arms extended in embrace, indicating the imparting of vital essence. The flow of this essence from the divine could be hindered by wrongdoing (Clark, 1978). By the axial age, described by Karl Jaspers (1883-1969) as "a pause for liberty" between ages of empire, "a deep breath bringing the most lucid consciousness" (Jaspers, 1953), similar breath-souls were of fundamental importance in the philosophies of the three great civilizations of India, China, and Greece, present both in the world about us and in our inner worlds.

In India, the cosmic breath-soul was, and still is, known as *prana*. The *Atharvaveda,* one of the earliest Vedic hymns dating back even to before 800 BC, is entirely devoted to *prana* and its subcategories *apana*, *udana*, *samana*, and *vyana*. In the somewhat later literature of *Ayurveda,* the traditional medicine of India (see Chapter 29), the physiology of prana as breath is emphasized (Zysk, 1995), while one of the main limbs of postclassical *yoga* (see Chapter 31) is *pranayama*, or "breath control" (Feuerstein, 1990). More than this, though, "*pranayama* . . . is an attention directed on one's organic life . . . a calm and lucid entrance into the very essence of life" (Eliade, 1958, p. 58). In both Ayurveda and yoga, prana (particularly vyana) moves, or is moved, through fine channels in the body known as *nadi* (Zysk, 1995). Vyana is also responsible for the circulation of the blood (Singh, 2004). The three principle nadi of yoga—*susumna, ida,* and *pingala*—are sometimes seen as corresponding to the three great mythological rivers of India, the Sarasvati, the Ganga (Ganges), and the Yamuna (Jumna) (White, 1996).

In traditional Chinese thought, there is a close relationship between wind (*feng*, 风) and what is termed *qi* (氣, or 气 in modern, simplified characters) (Kuriyama, 1995). At times qi "means the spirit or breath of life in living creatures, at other times the air or ether filling the sky and surrounding the universe, while in some contexts it denotes the basic substance of all creation" (de Bary et al, 1960, p. 193n). In a broad sense qi pervades and sustains the universe (Kuen, 2000), moving and flowing in all directions (de Bary et al, 1960) and is very much a multi-dimensional concept (Matsumoto et al, 1988), referring to anything that cannot be observed directly (Birch et al, 1999) or that is perceptible (in its effects) but intangible (Wiseman, 1990). "It is both a principle of unity and coherence that connects all things and a potential, an immanent life force in the world that is knowable only in the various changing aspects it assumes" (Robinet, 1997, p. 8). In a narrower sense, qi can be considered as a breath-soul, like prana in Ayurveda (although as Chinese medicine became more formalized, the nutritive-materialist aspect of *gu qi, 谷气*, was emphasized rather than the respiratory-shamanic; Hayashi, 1995). Qi also "begets movement and heat" (Beinfield et al, 1991). As with pranayama in Indian yoga, working with the qi is fundamental to the self-cultivation practices of *qigong* (气功) (see Chapter 28): qi and the related *jing* (精, essence, sometimes translated as semen or "configurative potential"; Milburn, 2001; Robinet, 1997) should not be wasted, but conserved. One modern commentator has defined qi as "nothing else than my bodily awareness of being alive" (Ots, 2006). Such awareness may be heightened in illness or pain (Boers, 1999; He et al, 1996).

Corresponding to some extent to the Indian nadi are the *jingluo* (经络, channels) of Chinese medicine (see Chapter 26), along which some forms of qi travel. Indeed, it is quite possible that some of the ideas underpinning acupuncture (see Chapter 27) and qigong derived in part from earlier Indian developments (Filliozat, 1991; Miura, 1995), because the earliest references to qi occur only in the writings of Confucius (Kong Fuzi, 551-479 BC) (Kuriyama, 1995) and the first known descriptions of vessels (*mai, 脉*) in Chinese medicine are found in the *Zuo Zhan* of around 310 BC (Sivin, 1995). The mai (based more on a multidimensional subjective experience of the body than objective investigation; Lo, 2001) carry both qi and blood, and are still relatively undifferentiated compared to the later, more elaborated jingluo of the medical classics (Lo, 1998). As with the inner-outer correspondence of nadi and rivers, much has been made of that between the jingluo and the canals and roads of Han dynasty imperial China (Allan, 1997; Ots, 2006; Unschuld, 1985). And as with prana, qi can be divided into functional subcategories within the body (*zong qi* [宗气], *zhen qi* [真气], *ying qi* [营气], *wei qi* [卫气], and so forth; Maciocia, 1989). A shift toward such systematization of knowledge and away from patients' perceptions of pain, illness, and the movements of qi is already evident in the *Lingshu*, a classic text on acupuncture dating back to around 70 BC (Hsu, 2001).

In Greece as in Egypt, India, and China, the breath-soul, the *pneuma* (πνεῦμα), evolved over time and so has many overlapping meanings. For Homer, around 800 BC, the breath of life or *pnoie* (πνοή, cognate with pneuma)

vivified the body, inhaled with the air and passing to the blood and heart (French, 1969). The body of Homeric man was thus permeable to winds and drives, emotions were "breathed into him by a god" (Vernant, 1989). For Hippocrates (ca. 460-377 BC), pneuma was taken in from food and drink as well as air (Kuen, 2000). Around 440 BC Diogenes of Apollonia would write of life as pneuma moving like warm currents through the vessels (*phlebes, φλέβες*)of the body (Yoke, 2000). For Plato (420-340 BC) almost a century after, both blood (*aima, αἷμα*) and breath moved through the same channels (Mendelsohn, 1964). A little later Aristotle (384-322 BC) considered pneuma to act as intermediary between *psyche, ψυχή* (prime mover of the breath) and *soma, σῶμα* (Hall, 1975a). For Aristotle, matter was not inert, but "in a way all things are full of soul" (Solmsen, 1957).

Again in the fourth century BC, Diocles of Karystos distinguished between outer and inner (psychic) pneuma, the latter arising from the exhalations of the blood (Kuen, 2000); Praxagoras (b. ca. 340 BC) then differentiated pneuma from blood, the heart being the seat of pneuma, whence it was distributed throughout the body via the arteries and nerves, with blood being carried by the veins (Kuriyama, 1999). For the later Stoics, pneuma both was immanent in the universe (Lloyd et al, 2002) and pervaded the body (French, 1969), although Kuriyama has argued that for the Stoics pneuma was based on "the experience of an active life driven not by outer winds or divine influence, but by changes interior to and defining the self" (Kuriyama, 1995, p. 27). In late antiquity, for Galen (129 to ca. 201), the smooth coursing of pneuma throughout the body was essential to consciousness, perception, and action, and disruptions in its flow accounted for afflictions ranging from minor twitches and dizziness to epilepsy and paralysis (Kuriyama, 1995).

In Latin, the life-breath was known as *spiritus* or *anima*, the consciousness or rational soul as *animus* (Lewis, 1904). However, for the Epicurean Lucretius (ca. 99-55 BC) anima and animus were still part of the same breath (French, 1969). Epikouros (Epicurus) himself (341-270 BC) thought the breath-soul was distributed throughout the body, with a central animus in the chest (Konstan, 2005) governing a more widely distributed anima (Hall, 1975b).

There are long Indian and Chinese traditions of self-cultivation practice based upon awareness or direction of the prana or qi within the body, but despite the Delphic adage "know thyself" (γνωθι σεαυτόν, gnothi seauton), such methods were not apparently practiced in ancient Greece or Rome (Yamada, 1995). Despite this, and clear cultural differences, there are some striking basic similarities between prana, qi, and pneuma:

- They are neither completely immaterial nor material.
- They are similar to but differ from both wind and breath, and are in some sense more than either.
- They are considered to flow along ducts within the body.

- They act as a connecting medium between the body and the outer world, and between different parts of the body, or between body and mind.
- Illness or dysfunction will occur if flow is uneven or blocked, diverted or reversed (Fields, 2001; Hayashi, 1995; Kuriyama, 1999; Lo, 1998; Motoyama, 1981; Robinet, 1997; Rochat de la Vallée, 2006; Singh, 2004; Sivin, 1995; Unschuld, 1985).

OTHER CULTURES AND SOME GENERALIZATIONS

Throughout history there have been comparable, although not identical, concepts in many cultures. Some examples are listed in Table 6-1.

Soul is often multiple, usually dual, encompassing both free-soul(s) and body-soul(s) (Hultkrantz, 1953; VanStone, 1974). The free-soul, relatively immaterial, is experienced in trance states or associated with thoughts and memories. The body-soul, relatively material, arises from observation and inner sensation. Among the Netsilik Eskimo and Western Déné, for example, the "general life-soul . . . seems to flow through the entire body as a uniform energy." Different body-souls may also inhabit different organs (heart, kidney, liver) (Hultkrantz, 1953). This is the case in both Indian (Zysk, 1995) and Chinese medicine (Maciocia, 1989), for example. Both free- and body-souls may derive originally from the breath-soul, as with the *hun* ("cloud soul," 魂) and *po* ("bone soul," 魄) in Taiwanese Daoism (Schipper, 1993). There is often such a polarization of souls, with the free-soul considered "pure" or "good" and the body-soul "impure" or "bad" (Levy, 1998), or the free-soul "white" and the body-soul or flesh "black" (Shoko, 2007). In many cultures, including our own, there is also an intimate connection between blood and the breath of life. Blood-soul (Frazer, 1911) and breath-soul may not be distinguished, they may be complementary, or one may predominate over the other.

Shigehisa Kuriyama has proposed that the breath-soul developed as an internalization of the experience of external winds (Kuriyama, 1995). In this he is supported by the "experiential realism" of philosophers George Lakoff and Mark Johnson (1999), who consider that "the core of our conceptual systems is directly grounded in

TABLE 6-1

Some Examples of the "Life-Breath" or "Breath-Soul" and Its Channels (If Known)

Culture	Name	Flows Through	Source
Ancient Egypt	*ka*	*metw*	Clark, 1978
Judaism	*ruach*		Kuen, 2000
India	*prana*	*nadi*	Zysk, 1995
Tibet	*rlung*	*rtsa*	Janes, 2001
China	*qi* (氣, or 气)	*jingluo*	Maciocia, 1989
Japan	*ki*	*keiraku*	Birch et al, 1997
Korea	*gi*	*kyungrak*	Kim, 1964
Vietnam	*khí*	*kinh tuyên*	Ton, 2008
Cambodia	*khyal*		Hinton et al, 2005
Greece	*pneuma*	*phlebes*	Yoke, 2000
Rome	*spiritus*		Lewis, 1904
Cree (Canada/U.S.)	*ahtca'k*		Hultkrantz, 1953
Huna (Polynesia)	*ha*		King, n.d.
Warao (Venezuela)	*hina*		Briggs, 1996
Akan (Ghana)	*hónhōm*		Konadu, 2007
Karuk (California)	*imya*		Hultkrantz, 1953
Kung (Kalahari)	*n/om or num*		Biesele et al, 1996; Katz, 1982
Malay (Malaya)	*nyawa*		Antares et al, n.d.; Laderman, 2001
Maori (New Zealand)	*mauri*		Lévy-Bruhl, 1927; National Library of New Zealand, 2008
Juaneño (California)	*piuch*		Hultkrantz, 1953
Bella Coola (Canada)	*sxixmänoäs likt'*	"invisible lines"	McIlwraith, 1948
Dakota (Canada/U.S.)	*ni*		Walker, 1979
Navaho (U.S.)	*nílch'i*		McNeley, 1981
Inuit (Arctic)	*silla*		Wikipedia: Silap inua, n.d.

NOTE: Stefan Stenudd (b. 1954) has compiled a comprehensive, if unreferenced, listing of such terms (Stenudd, 2008). However, it should be noted that this life-soul, present in and connecting all things, is distinct from concepts of nonordinary (or supernatural) power such as *sekhem* (ancient Egypt), mana (Melanesia), *megbe* (Bambuti, Africa) or *orenda* (Iroquois) (Arbman, 1931; Budge, 1899; Codrington, 1891; Durkheim, 1912/1995; Eliade, 1971).

perception, body movement, and experience of a physical and social character" (Lakoff, 1987, p. xiv). In other words, the metaphors and metonymies in which we think are based on our sensory and motor interactions with the *outer* world: we transfer them from outside to inside (e.g., from wind to the breath within).

The inner world of the body is difficult to access, even experientially. It is hard to find words to describe inner sensations or movements, or even to localize them (Lewis et al, 1939). This is a world of process, of continuity and connection, of flow and streaming, wave and gurgle, rather than of isolated parts, concepts, bits and bytes, a "land of natural anarchy and inner harmony" as against "the exterior, fragmented view of things" (Schipper, 1993). Awareness here is at a more primitive, even preverbal, level, the level of anima rather than animus.

It is tempting to speculate on the profound effect of intrauterine life on our later ability to feel our way into our own bodies (as well as conceptualize the world about us). It may be no coincidence that some self-cultivation methods in qigong utilize what is called "embryonic breathing" (Huang et al, 1987). At some level, this intrauterine life with its sense of a *participation mystique* (Lévy-Bruhl, 1926) with our enfolding world continues within us as we develop, even if rapidly overlaid by an education that emphasizes consciousness, predominantly externally directed and visual, rather than intuition and imagination, inner-directed, tactile, and proprioceptive.

PRECURSORS II: THE FIRE OF LIFE

After the first breath we take, the warmth of the human embrace is our earliest experience in life (Lakoff et al, 2000). Even when *imagining* mental contact with another, the most common felt experience is one of warmth and touch (Reed, 1996). Throughout the world, and throughout history, vital processes have been associated with warmth, heat, fire, or flame (Hall, 1975b), whereas absence of heat is associated with death (Hufford, 1988). (Excess heat, as in fever, may be viewed as dangerous to life, or as healing in itself [Lohff, 2001].)

If life is movement, fire is the most active of the elements (fire, air, water, earth). World literature is full of references to the fire of life, and in particular to the felt fires of love, lust, feeling, and passion in general. Fire was also often a central metaphor for the divine in nature—"ever moving, self-moving, moving other things," in the words of Dionysius the Areopagite (Peter the Iberian, 452-491?) (Dionysius, 1894), although this sort of fire was considered *ethereal* or "pure" and so distinguished from *visible* or "vulgar" elemental fire (Pagel, 1958; Shaffer, 1978).

A cooking or furnace fire at the core of the body is a central metaphor in many forms of yoga and *tantra* (Child, 2007; Fields, 2001), as well as in Chinese medicine (Maciocia, 1989) and mystical practices (Robinet, 1997).

The association of fire with life was taken up by the Pythagoreans (Berkeley, 1744/1871) and Heraclitus (ca. 500-460 BC) (Hall, 1975a), was present in the writings of Hippocrates (Lloyd, 1966) and Democritus (ca. 480-370 BC), for whom body-soul or vital principle was composed of atoms of fire (French, 1969); in Plato (420-340 BC), for whom fire was the "animal spirit" of both microcosm and macrocosm (Mendelsohn, 1964); in Aristotle (Hall, 1975a), for whom "animal heat" connected soul and body (Fraser, 1871); and also in Epicurus and Lucretius (French, 1969), who embellished on Democritus in their understanding of soul as atomic fire. The Stoics went one further, identifying both pneuma and Aristotle's superlunary "ether" ($\alpha\iota\theta\acute{\eta}\rho$, *aither*) (Cantor et al, 1981b) with the vital heat of the world-soul (Fraser, 1871).

For Galen, too, there was "innate heat," a "vital flame" in living matter (Porter, 2003), and in this he was followed by Avicenna (ca. 979-1037) (Mendelsohn, 1964) and other Unani practitioners (see Chapter 30). Even for Paracelsus (Philippus Aureolus Theophrastus Bombast von Hohenheim, 1493-1541), despite his rejection of the Aristotelian elements (Pagel, 1958) and much of Galenic medicine, fire and life were fundamentally equivalent (Bachelard, 1949). "Vital heat" moved further toward center stage following publication of the *Physiologia* of Jean Fernel (1497-1558) (Sherrington, 1946), in which he distinguished it from elemental heat. Francis Bacon (1561-1626), for example, described the vital spirit of the body as flamelike (Pagel, 1935), "a mysterious combination of flammeous and aerial nature" (Bacon, 1623).

Bacon also stated "that the remedy is worse than the disease," which was later modified by dramatist John Fletcher to "the medicine is worse than the malady."

For Marcus Marci (1595-1667), too, the life principle was flamelike and distributed throughout the body (Pagel, 1935). In alchemy, such fire retained a central role (Jung, 1968). More matter of factly, the British surgeon-general John Hunter (1728-1793), who first elucidated the circulatory system, considered life as "animal fire" released from food as the result of respiration (French, 1969) and as being particularly active in the blood (Levere, 1981). "Natural heat" later played a pivotal part in Thomsonian herbalism (see later and Chapters 21 and 22).

PRECURSORS III: ANIMAL SPIRITS

With Saint Augustine (354-430), spiritus as breath-soul became completely disengaged from matter (Kuen, 2000), a "mind-soul" (animus) rather than a "body-mind-soul" (anima). This early division would have a profound influence on many developments throughout history in the West.

Until the Renaissance, however, Western medicine remained based on the teachings of Galen, for whom pneuma-like animal spirits ($\pi\nu\epsilon\acute{\upsilon}\mu\alpha$ $\varphi\upsilon\chi\iota\kappa\acute{o}\nu$, *pneuma physicon*) occupied brain and nerves, mediating between and connecting will and muscle (Duffin, 2000; French, 1981). Other spirits included the vital spirit or *pneuma zoticon* (πνεῦμα ζωτικόν) in the heart, and the natural spirit in the liver (University of Virginia Health System: Galen, n.d.). Galen based his animal spirits and vital spirit on those of the rationalist Eristratos of Chios (310-250 BC) (Wheeler, 1939). Virtually identical spirits were also described in the Greco-Arabic system of Unani medicine (see Chapter 30). Thus pneuma still served as a common denominator of all phenomena and allowed all forms of being—from human to minerals—to maintain their cohesiveness and growth and to transform into other forms of being. In Elizabethan times, Galen's three types of spirit continued to mediate between the vital heat generated from food and the body itself: natural spirits (vaporlike and carried in the veins), vital spirits (transmitting heat through the arteries), and animal spirits (still, as with Galen, acting through the nerves, and partaking of both body and soul) (Tillyard, 1963). Francis Bacon, for example, considered the latter as aspects of the irrational or sensible soul (as opposed to the animus). In mainland Europe, Paracelsus and Jan Baptist van Helmont (1577-1644) proposed a multiplicity of souls and *archaei* to fulfil a variety of functions (Hall, 1975a).

With René Descartes (1596-1650), soul and body were finally—and seemingly still irrevocably in Western biomedicine—torn asunder (Hall, 1975a), as were mind (*res cognitans*) and matter (*res extensa*). Animal spirits within the nerves became merely rapidly moving particles, flamelike yet of "a certain very fine air or wind" (Mendelsohn, 1964), without any inner activity of their own. His mechanical model of the workings of muscle has been compared with the hydraulic system of the French King Louis's garden with its water-driven machinery (Jackson, 1970) and the Cartesian ether was but the by-product of the mutual abrasion of particles (Hall, 1975a). Following Descartes, in the eighteenth century the body was seen by many as a form of clockwork (Bajollet, 1735; Borelli, 1680), with the living being differentiated from the nonliving just by the presence of more organized movement (Hall, 1975b).

The body as a machine was envisioned based upon human mechanical inventions, and this unfortunate metaphor remains in full force with, for example, the *National Geographic Society*'s breathless and popular descriptions of the human body as the "incredible human machine" (Rosten, 1975/2007). Animal spirits were reduced to an epiphenomenon of the blood for anatomists such as William Harvey (1578-1657) and Thomas Willis (1621-1675) (Hall, 1975a; Mendelsohn, 1964) although for their French colleague Raymond de Vieussens (1641-1715), blood remained the main seat of the "vital spirit" (Allen et al, 1984). Nature had ceased to be an organic being that matured through self-development. However, in alchemy—a relatively "hidden" (some might say "mystical") tradition in the West that emphasized the centrality of experiential

or sensed living reality—"the spirit of the world and of matter" still guaranteed that the world "is alive and full of life" (Amadou, 1953).

RISE AND FALL OF MAINSTREAM VITALISM

At the beginning of the eighteenth century there was a tension in the West between Cartesian mechanists like Joseph Addison (1672-1719), for whom the body was "a Bundle of Pipes and Strainers, fitted to one another after so wonderful a manner as to make a proper Engine for the Soul to work with" (Addison, 1711) and others such as George Berkeley (1685-1753), for whom the animal spirits of the nerves corresponded to the "net of fire, and rays of fire in the human body" in Plato's *Timaeus* (Berkeley, 1709), and the "vital spirit of the world" was identified with pure fire, ether, light, and even the Chinese *tian* (天, heaven) (Berkeley, 1744/1871). This was not as unusual as it may seem now: Immanuel Kant (1724-1804), the foremost thinker of the Enlightenment, as well as the philosopher Friedrich von Schelling (1775-1854), similarly identified fire or ether as the original "world-spirit" (Schaffer, 1978; Tatar, 1978). Earlier Isaac Newton (1642-1727) had speculated that the ether is in some sense the source of matter, and matter but a lower form of ether—both being permeated by Spirit (Grabo, 1930). Further, he surmised that an "electric spirit" allied to fire and "more subtile than common Air or Vapour" might maintain life and prevent decay (Home, 1993).

As investigations on electricity gathered momentum in the eighteenth century, there were those who moved beyond machinery and identified it with the *Anima Mundi* or *flamma vitalis* (Millburn, 1976) or, like John Wesley (1703-1791), with God's spirit of love made manifest (Wakefield, 1976) or with the ether (Heimann, 1973, 1981; Wikipedia: William Watson, n.d.; Wilson, 1746). Joseph Priestley (1733-1804), the first electrical-chemical polymath, considered electricity to be both a manifestation of the immortal soul (Bragg, 2004) and a form of "phlogiston" (PJH, 1968) (yet another hypothetical substance—without color, odor, taste, or weight, but supposedly liberated in burning; Wikipedia: Phlogiston theory, n.d.). Nineteenth-century Romantic scientists continued to describe electricity as itself the life force (Brandis, 1795; Oken, 1809-1811; Hall, 1975b), as its essence (the link between spirit and matter) (Segala, 2001), or as the agent of the vital principle (Prout, 1816).

Vitalism arose as a conservative, more measured response to mechanism and atomistic physicochemical reductionism (Lain Entralgo, 1948). A key figure here was the prominent chemist-cum-physician Georg Ernst Stahl (1660-1734) (also one of the originators of the phlogiston theory). He dispensed with (animal) spirits as intermediary between material and immaterial, and influenced by Paracelsus and van Helmont he suggested instead that the *immaterial* soul (anima) or "moving principle" acts directly upon inert matter by means of motion (not necessarily flow) (French, 1969). His soul gave life to matter, although not itself alive (Hall, 1975a). For Stahl, the "organizing energy" or order implicit in "organism" is what distinguishes living from dead bodies (Cheung, 2008). Thus in Germany, the "vital force" (*Lebenskraft*) developed as a quite abstract concept (Medicus, 1774), as a universal "formative drive" (*Bildungstrieb*) (Blumenbach, 1787), or as an "organizing principle" operating according to a "rational plan" (Müller, 1833-1834). The abstract nature of this concept did not prevent doctors such as Christoph Wilhelm Hufeland (1762-1836), in his influential 1797 book *Macrobiotics, or the Art of Prolonging Human Life,* from putting forward the view that medicine should be based on cultivation of the vital force rather than its depletion (Hufeland et al, 1958).

In France, Stahl's philosophy was reinterpreted at the influential medical faculty in Montpellier, first by the more mechanistic François Boissier Sauvages de la Croix (1706-1767), using the word *âme* ("soul") rather than anima, and then by his student Paul Joseph Barthez (1734-1806), later one of Napoleon's physicians, who preferred the more straightforward *principe vitale* or "vital principle" (Haigh, 1975; Wheeler, 1939). This principle was expressed in the collaboration of *"forces sensitives"* and *"forces motrices"* working together in the body, and was distinct from both rational soul and the body itself (Haigh, 1977), although Barthez held that it is single and on death becomes one with the animating *"principe universel"* of God's universe (Hall, 1975b). His student Jean Guillaume Grimaud (1750-1789) subdivided the holistic principe vitale once more, into external and internal motor forces (forces motrices) and an internal vital sense (*sens vital intérieur*), "lower" and centered in the stomach (Haigh, 1975; Williams, 2008). For Barthez's near-contemporary Xavier Bichat (1771-1802), creator of the modern science of histology, life was not one fundamental force, nor yet threefold, but the "collection of those functions which resist death" (Bichat, 1800). These *propriétés vitales* he considered as similar to gravity and other physical forces (Wheeler, 1939).

During the nineteenth century the mechanistic physicochemical view gained complete ascendancy in biology and medicine. Gradually the intimate connection that had held since Galen's time between pneumatic animal spirits that flow and particular structures within which they flow was superseded by (or amalgamated with) other models of flow, within nerves (Hillman, 1999). (Harvey's description of the circulation of the blood had long undermined traditional accounts of the vital and natural spirits [Wheeler, 1939].) The flow or obstruction of electricity in nerves, for example, was considered by many to uphold or undermine health (Wilson, 1750), and this understanding led in turn to the use of electrical stimulation to effect cure (Cloquet, 1826; Molenier, 1768; Philip, 1817). Oxygen was discovered in 1774 by Priestley, and although it was still considered as a universal "vital force" by the Romantic writer Novalis (Friedrich von Hardenberg, 1772-1801) (Tatar, 1978), the vivifying air also lost much of its mystique. In 1811, Gottlieb Sigismund (Konstantin Sigizmundovich) Kirchoff (1764-1833) presented his findings on the extraction of glucose from starch to the academy of sciences in St. Petersburg (Gillespie, 1973), furthering the demystification of the body's heat and energy.

Whereas in the early 1800s Jean-Baptiste Lamarck (1744-1829) still considered an elementary, ubiquitous, and ethereal "fire" as responsible for the movements of living organisms (French, 1981), from 1828, when Friedrich Wöhler (1800-1882) first synthesized organic material (such as urea), there was a gradual elimination of any need to believe in a vital principle or life force to explain the perceived inadequacies of physicochemical explanations (Needham, 2005). In mid-century, Justus von Liebig (1803-1873) demonstrated that body heat derives solely from the chemical processes of oxidation and combustion (Liebig, 1843), although in many ways he was also a vitalist (Benton, 1974; Lipman, 1967; Wheeler, 1939), while Eduard Pflüger (1829-1910) went on to reduce all life to the "intramolecular warmth" of oxidation (Hall, 1975b). William Benjamin Carpenter (1813-1885) (Carpenter, 1850) and Hermann von Helmholtz (1821-1894) (Hall, 1975b) again reduced "vital" "cell-force" to chemical and physical forces. And in 1897 Wilbur O. Atwater (1844-1907) and Edward B. Rosa (1873-1921) showed that the laws of thermodynamics apply to life as well as to inorganic matter (although the argument that life has some negentropic property has persisted; Wheeler, 1939). Even "neovitalist" Ernst Haeckel (1834-1919) defined life as "nothing but a connected chain of very complicated material phenomena of motion" (Haeckel, 1868) or "a physicochemical process" (Haeckel, 1899). "The entire internal process of feeling experience" was discounted (Conger, 1988).

Vitalism weakened and retreated before each new scientific discovery, and as Kaptchuk (2006) has argued, effectively migrated to an alternative medical worldview that was being created in the nineteenth century, where it was welcomed and eventually merged with other important forms of vitalism. This shift was accentuated in the twentieth century, with the emphasis in mainstream medicine on biomedical diagnosis of disease labels rather than the individual's state of illness.

MESMER'S *FLUIDUM*

In the eighteenth century, there were many attempts to group together different forms of energy (heat, light, electricity, magnetism) as forms or modifications of an underlying universal ether. In 1775, the Viennese physician Franz Anton Mesmer (1734-1815) announced the existence of what he called "animal magnetism," a universal fluid bringing together aspects of the "universal gravity" of his medical dissertation (Carlson, 1960), magnetism, light, and the Hippocratic *ignis subtilissimus* (Zweig, 1933), responsible for the properties of both organic and inorganic matter, and to be found within "the substance of the nerves" (Wyckoff, 1975). The previous year he had treated a certain Fraülein Österlin with magnets and an iron-based drink, whereupon she experienced the sensation of a stream flowing down through her body (and was then cured of her various—possibly hysterical—ailments) (Palfreman, 1977). Mesmer went on to develop a controversial therapy on the basis of this case, his own "rapture" when alone in nature, and his theory of animal magnetism (Benz, 1989). He taught that harmony with the cosmic fluid is health and that all disease is due to an unequal distribution of or "obstacles" to the flow of the *fluidum*. The fluidum can be manipulated by healers to restore equilibrium and therefore health (Mesmer, 1980).

In 1778 Mesmer relocated to Paris, where his methods became both popular and controversial (Darnton, 1968). Seven years later, "mesmerism" was investigated by a commission of the French Royal Académie des Sciences under Louis XVI, which included such prestigious figures as the new American ambassador Benjamin Franklin (1706-1790), the chemist Antoine-Laurent Lavoisier (1743-1794), the physician Joseph Guillotine (1738-1814), and the academy's president, Alphonse LeRoy. They ignored Mesmer's request for an investigation based on clinical outcomes and concluded that the fluidum, invisible and intangible, is inexplicable "on purely rationalistic terms" and so nonexistent, with the crises provoked in his patients due principally to "imagination" (Zweig, 1933). The French Société Royale de Médecine concurred in a separate report, advising prospective members against using mesmerism (Commissaires de la Société Royale de Médecine, 1784); however, one of its committee members, botanist Antoine-Laurent de Jussieu (1748-1836), did acknowledge that Mesmer's methods were effective (even curative) and agreed with him that some kind of subtle fluid ("animal heat") may play a significant role in maintaining health (Jussieu, 1784). Even before these investigations, Franklin had written of animal magnetism: "I . . . must doubt its Existence till I can see or feel some Effect of it" (Begelow, 1904). They were thus almost bound to fail and banished mesmerism to the fringes of the conventional medical world. Here, however, it flourished. Many of Mesmer's ideas were paralleled by developments in the "Romantic science" of the early nineteenth century (which, like alchemy, emphasized a self-investigational approach to gaining knowledge) and became a critical component of allied currents in medical thought (Fuller, 1982). In particular, the view that flow dissolves petrifaction has been considered the point of departure for all "Romantic medicine" ("flow is the counterpart to reification") (Asendorf, 1993).

Mesmer's followers were divided. The "fluidists" understood the fluidum as analogous to a physical electromagnetic vibration that resembled more recognized scientific energies. The "animists" interpreted the fluidum as ethereal, reducing it to an epiphenomenon of little consequence. Will or thought was more important. For the novelist Charles Dickens (1812-1870), for example, as well as many of his contemporary fellow mesmerists, the operator was no longer just a mediator for magnetic fluid, but harnessed, focused, and transmitted it using will power (Kaplan, 1975), whereas Honoré de Balzac (1799-1850) described thought or will as an "imponderable fluid" flowing like electricity through the body (Balzac, 1837). By the mid-nineteenth century, mesmerism had intermingled with several mystical and occult traditions and became allied to a range of unconventional therapies and practices, from phrenology to clairvoyant medical diagnosis, telepathy, and spiritualism (Darnton, 1968). Between the fluidist and animist poles were various intermediate versions, each spawning its complex lineage yet all sharing the distinctive mesmeric view that life's agency and healing potential can be found in something—whether a vital energy or in the mind—distinct from the ordinary physicochemical forces of Victorian science. Mesmerism thus became the inspiration for many unconventional therapies.

"FLUIDISM" MODERNIZED

Spiritualism, with its levitations, ectoplasmic emissions, table turning, spirit rapping, and spirit photographs, became a mass phenomenon in the nineteenth century (Braude, 1989; Goldsmith, 1999; Moore, 1977; Oppenheim, 1988). In keeping with the times, and perhaps to avoid the stigma of association with what was now excommunicated from official science, attempts were made to explain these manifestations in terms of force (rather than fluidum), with one spiritualist and magnetic healer (mesmerist), John Murray Spear (1804-1887), even constructing a spirit-designed mechanical messiah designed to be powered by the life force (Moore, 1977). In 1844 Karl Ludwig von Reichenbach (1788-1869), retired discoverer of creosote and paraffin, published his findings on what he called "odic force" (allied to electricity, magnetism, and heat), to which he found certain people were particularly sensitive (Reichenbach, 1977). In 1853 Robert Hare (1781-1858), inventor of the oxyhydrogen blowpipe at the age of 20 and then a professor of chemistry at the University of Pennsylvania for over 30 years, felt it his duty during retirement "to stem the tide of popular madness which, in defiance of reason and science, was fast setting in favor of the gross delusion called spiritualism," but the following year became a convert himself, later even acting as a medium (Answers.com: Robert Hare, n.d.; Hare, 1855). He coined the scientific-sounding term *psychic force*, developing a spirit-scope to measure mesmeric and spiritual presences (McClenon, 1984; Moore, 1977). The prominent physicist William Crookes (1832-1919) used the same term slightly later (Kottler, 1974). "Astral force" was one of several related terms used by theosophists such as Charles W. Leadbeater (1847-1934) to describe the "super-physical forces" involved in spiritualist *seances* (Leadbeater, 1900). Electricity, only recently tamed by science, was co-opted by Helena Petrovna Blavatsky (1831-1891), cofounder of the Theosophical Society, for whom "electric vital fluid" or "soul-electricity" was produced by the cerebral pile of man (Blavatsky, 1888). Mysterious forces have also featured prominently in science fiction, from the "Vril" of Edward Bulwer-Lytton (1803-1873) in 1871 (Bulwer, 1871) to "the force" of Star Wars.

The ether too, respectably mechanized and then described in mathematical terms by Victorian science (Cantor et al, 1981a), was often referred to. Crookes, for example, wrote that "ether vibrations" might be responsible for telepathy (Wilson, 1971), physicists Balfour Stewart (1828-1887) and Peter Guthrie Tait (1831-1901) described a hierarchy of ever more energetic ethers between gross matter and God (Stewart et al, 1875), and even as late as the 1930s physicist Oliver Lodge (1851-1940) believed that an "ethereal body" might mediate between body and mind (Lodge, 1933). "Etheric force" and "etheric currents" in the body were claimed as the basis of the induction resonance motion devices of John Worrell Keely (1827-1898) (Paijmans, 1998). However, with the publication by Albert Einstein (1879-1955) of the special theory of relativity in 1905, the ether fell out of scientific fashion, although variants are still alive and well in twenty-first-century quantum physics (Duffy, n.d.). Since the 1980s—perhaps partly in reaction to the notoriety of Einstein's $e = mc^2$—many writers have favored the phrase *subtle energy.*

Such name substitutions indicate a concern for keeping the vital fluidum on a par with the currently accepted terms of science. In 1975 Fritjof Capra (b. 1939) published his influential book *The Tao of Physics,* comparing qi with the quantum field of modern physics. Partly as a result, in addition to "subtle energy," a particularly tenacious label in recent decades has been the term *quantum,* popularized by Deepak Chopra (b. 1946) (Chopra, 1989), although already in the mid-1980s considered overused or employed so vaguely as to be meaningless ("quantum silliness") by those critical of CAM (Stalker et al, 1985). Quantum fields have been evoked since to explain healing (Rein, 1998), particularly nonlocal healing (Schwartz et al, 2007), or "paraphysical" phenomena (King, 1990), and writers such as Mae-Wan Ho and James Oschman continue to explore the place of quantum physics as an explanatory model for CAM practices (Ho, 1993; Oschman, 2000, 2003).

HEALING ENERGY

Many "new" methods of healing appeared in the twentieth century, the best-known early survivor being *reiki* (霊気), developed in 1922 by Mikao Usui (1865-1926) (Miles, 2006). Mokichi Okada (1882-1955) created his *johrei* (浄霊) method shortly after. These were followed by the "polarity therapy"

of Randolph Stone (Rudolph Bautsch, 1890-1981) in the late 1940s (Sills, 1989), unorthodox or "paranormal" healing in the 1950s (Rose, 1954), and "therapeutic touch," devised by Dolores Krieger (b. 1935) in the early 1970s. Krieger's method is aimed at restoring the free flow of prana within the patient (Krieger et al, 1979). It was further developed as "healing touch" by Janet Mentgen (b. 1938) and "quantum-touch" by polarity therapist Richard Gordon (b. 1948) (Gordon, 1999). More recent methods include the syncretist "pranic healing" of Choa Kok Sui (b. 1952) (Sui, 2004), *seichim* (a reiki add-on devised by Patrick Zeigler after spending a night in the Great Pyramid) (Shewmaker, 2000), and countless other idiosyncratic variants.

Although sometimes unaware of their heritage, methods of "spiritual healing" bear the characteristic mesmeric style of manipulating unseen and refined vital forces that evade biomedical detection, and some explicitly speak of "an electromagnetic dimension which can become depleted or unbalanced . . . [causing] the blockage of energy flow, requiring physical or spiritual cleaning in order for healing to occur" (Glik, 1988, p. 1201). There may be a moralizing dimension to this (as in ancient Egypt, mentioned earlier, or in "New Thought," later). Thus healers Ambrose and Olga Worrall (1899-1972 and 1906-1985, respectively) believed that we can "insulate ourselves by wrong thinking or wrong living" from the supply of life energy around us. In this situation, "we are like batteries that need recharging," and the healer acts "as a conductor between the source of supply and the patient" (Worrall et al, 1969). (Ambrose Worrall coined the term *paraelectricity* for the energy of healing [Beltzer, n.d.].) Others query whether the energy manipulated is "channelled" through the healer, originates in the healer, or originates within the patient (Benor, 2001; McClean, 2006). Whatever the model adopted, successful healing is considered to provide "proof" of the force or energy involved, with secondary evidence in the sensations of heat, tingling, or vibration frequently reported by healees (Fuller, 1989; Krieger, 1979). Despite the suspicions—and even hostility—of colleagues, more and more researchers from conventional science hover on the edge of this type of healing and continue to investigate the phenomenon (Benor, 2001; Beutler et al, 1988; Schwartz et al, 2007).

OSTEOPATHY, CHIROPRACTIC, AND MASSAGE

Osteopathy (see Chapter 17) was founded by Andrew Taylor Still (1828-1917), who in 1874 abandoned his career as a self-taught physician to become a magnetic (mesmeric) healer and a few years later a bone setter (Gevitz, 1988b). In addition to experiencing episodes of clairvoyance and channelling, Still had connections to metaphysical, Mind Cure, and spiritualist groups (Gevitz, 1988c). In 1874 he discovered that misaligned bones impede the flow of fluids and blood, and so developed the system of osteopathy. He wrote that "all diseases are mere effects, the cause being a partial or complete failure of the nerves to properly conduct the fluids of life," more generally that "it is necessary that there be liberty of blood, nerves, and arteries from the generating-point to its destination." For Still, health depended on the uncongested free play of "life-giving current" through the system (Still, 1897). In the United States, the mesmeric influence has since been bred out of osteopathy, which renders it practically indistinguishable from mainstream medicine (Baer, 1987; Gevitz, 2004).

The system of *cranial* osteopathy, however, created by Still's student the osteopathic physician William Garner Sutherland (1873-1954) (Sutherland, 1990), is still controversial, as are its offspring, the "light-touch therapies" of osteopath John E. Upledger (b. 1932). Foremost of these is craniosacral therapy, developed between 1975 and 1983 very much in accordance with Still's original ideas (albeit to release restrictions in the craniosacral system and so improve the functioning of the *central* nervous system), and often used by nonosteopaths (Upledger, 2008). In 1977 to 1980, Upledger, with Zvi Karni, also developed the methods of somatoemotional release, focusing on the release of trauma-induced holding patterns (somatic and emotional) and "energy cysts" within the tissue (Upledger, 2002). The biodynamic craniosacral therapy of Franklyn Sills (b. 1947) has grown in a slightly different direction, bringing together the "implicate order" of quantum physicist David Bohm (1917-1992) (Bohm, 1980) with Sutherland's concepts of "creative intelligence" and the "breath of life" in an ordering or "biodynamic" principle or life force (Sills, 2001-2004).

A quite different gentle, noninvasive, osteopathically based form of body therapy is Ortho-Bionomy or "the correct application of the laws of life," developed in the 1970s by Arthur Lincoln Pauls (1929-1997). Pauls frequently quoted Still's "rule of the artery," believing that blockages in blood flow should be corrected (Patel, 2007). As with craniosacral methods, Ortho-Bionomy fosters inner awareness in both patient and practitioner (Overmyer, 2008). Another innovator who originally called himself an osteopath (although he never trained as such officially) was Tom Bowen (1916-1982) (Baker, 2001). He began his practice of the Bowen technique in the 1950s (Albrecht et al, 2000). Some Bowen practitioners write about the method as a "method of moving blocked energy" (Olafimihan et al, 2002), and this is something he apparently talked about informally with his students (Burgess, 2008).

Mesmeric vital energy took a somatic and even mechanical twist in the creation of chiropractic (see Chapter 18), currently the third largest doctoral-level health care profession, after medicine and dentistry, in North America (Wardwell, 1992). Discovered in 1895 by Daniel David Palmer (1845-1913), chiropractic's origin is another marriage of the indigenous healing craft of bone setting (Cooter, 1987) and the American tradition of mesmeric healing (Beck, 1991). For 10 years before his discovery of chiropractic, Palmer worked (like Still) as a magnetic healer, occasionally using hand passes and magnetic rubbings of the spine (Fuller, 1982). In an intuitive flash (or, some say, clairvoyant communication; Beck, 1991), he realized that "putting down your hands" (mechanical adjustment) worked better than an esoteric "laying on of hands" (magnetic activity administered from a distance). Others have suggested that Palmer probably borrowed some of his ideas from Still (Baer, 1987; Fuller, 1989).

As with Still, even 20 years after Palmer abandoned his magnetic clinical work, Palmer's mesmeric heritage is readily evident in his writings: "Disease is a manifestation of too much or not enough energy. Energy is liberated force; in the living being it is known as vital force. . . . It is an intelligent force, which I saw fit to name Innate, usually known as spirit" (Beck, 1991). Disease is a disruption in this "Innate" or "intelligent force," for which the nervous system is the conduit. Through alignment of the spine, the nerves are freed so that the force can move without interference and produce healing. Vital energy is guided and shaped by the structure of the body, and the noncorporeal agency of life is housed in the nerves and guarded by the spinal vertebrae. D.D. Palmer's son Bartlett Joshua Palmer (1882-1961) at first marketed his father's emphasis on the Innate, or Universal Intelligence, inherent in all, and on the single cause of "dis-ease" as "interference with the supply of mental impulse": "The Chiropractor removes the obstruction, adjusts the cause, and there are going to be effects" (Palmer, 1911). Many later chiropractors have tended (at least outwardly) to distance themselves from such potentially contentious statements (Fuller, 1989). Naprapathy, for example, developed by chiropractor Oakley Smith in 1907, emphasizes work on the spine and its connective tissue rather than anything more subtle (National College of Naprapathic Medicine, 2008).

Massage (see Chapter 15) is one of the earliest and most pervasive varieties of healing (Sigerist, 1961). In the West, "Swedish massage" has been the best-known approach for nearly 200 years, developed originally by Per Henrik Ling (1776-1839) and based on the techniques used in the Chinese method of *tuina* (although without any acknowledgement of the role of qi) (Maanum et al, 1985). Over the last century many unconventional massage therapies practiced in the West have increasingly found their rationale in vital energy theory. Examples of methods derived in part from the yoga model include Ayurvedic massage (Douillard, 2004), *breema* (Frey, 2001), Narendra Mehta's *champissage* (Indian head massage) (McGuinness, 2007), Thai massage (Gold, 2007), and rolfing (Rolf, 1977), with its own offshoots such as Aston-Patterning (Aston, 1998) and Hellerwork (Heller et al, 2004). More numerous are those that hold some concepts in common with the acupuncture model: acupressure (Kolster, 2007), *chi nei tsang* (*qi nei zang*, 气内臟) (Chia, 2007; Marin, 1999), *do-in* (導引) (Rofidal, 1983), *tuina* (推拿) (Xu, 2003), and *zhiya* (指壓); *amatsu* (Amatsu

Therapy Association, n.d.) and *anma* (按摩, or *amma*) (Mochizuki, 1995), including various forms of *shiatsu* (指圧) (Beresford-Cooke, 2003; Namikoshi, 1969; see Chapter 20), the very subtle *seiki soho* of Akinobu Kishi (b. 1945) (Davies, 1998), *watsu* (Dull, 1993), *jin shin jyutsu* (Burmeister, 1997), and *jin shin do* (仁神导) (Teeguarden, 2002); and even Balinese traditional massage (Segarra, n.d.). Others with a partial energy focus include Esalen massage, based among other sources on Swedish massage and the sensory awareness methods of Charlotte Selver (1901-2003); reflexology (Carter, 1969; Keet, 2008; Norman et al, 1989; see Chapter 19); and its offshoot metamorphic technique (Saint-Pierre et al, 1989). Methods such as the Trager approach (or "Trager psychophysical integration") of Milton Trager (1908-1997) may not explicitly refer to energy, but (like Ortho-Bionomy) emphasize the freeing of "blocks" within the body and the enhanced sensitivity of both client and therapist in their shared experience (Liskin, 1996).

ACUPUNCTURE AND ITS OFFSHOOTS

The first detailed accounts of acupuncture reached Europe in the 1680s, although it was not actually practiced there for nearly another 140 years, in France. Stripped of any references to qi or the jingluo, it was medically fashionable from 1825 until 1832, before being replaced by mesmerism as the latest fad (Mayor, 2007). In the United States, in the 1820s acupuncture was brought to the attention of the Philadelphia medical community with the publication of a translation by Benjamin Franklin Bache (1792-1864), grandson of the great inventor and printer, of a French textbook on the subject (Morand, 1825). For the remainder of the nineteenth century, acupuncture was reduced to a technique for local pain relief, often confused with simple puncture for anasarca or dropsy (Churchill, 1828; Dantu, 1825; Elliotson, 1827; Munro, 1874; Tweedale, 1823). As late as the tenth edition of the influential *Textbook of Medicine* by Sir William Osler (1849-1919), acupuncture was referenced as an effective treatment for lumbago, or low back pain (Osler, 1919, p. 101), before being removed in subsequent editions after Osler's death by those who thought they knew better than him.

In the late 1920s, acupuncture resurfaced, again in France, when George Soulié de Morant (1878-1955) translated qi as "energy," "for want of anything better" (Soulié de Morant, 1985), influenced by the *élan vital* propounded by philosopher Henri Bergson (1859-1941) (Bergson, 1914), and despite the qualms of his colleagues (Needham et al, 1956).

Since the 1960s, acupuncture has enjoyed increasing success in Europe and North America, so providing an important ideological boost and infusion of credibility for CAM in general. It is now one of the most rapidly growing health care professions, supported by a considerable research effort (Han, 1987; MacPherson et al, 2007).

This success has come at a price, however. As with their nineteenth-century predecessors, many acupuncturists with conventional medical training use acupuncture as a purely physical technique (e.g., "dry needling" of "myofascial trigger points"; Seem, 1993) based on physiological principles (Sato et al, 2002), with little regard for traditional notions or methods such as qi and the jingluo or pulse taking. Some have equated the jingluo with blood vessels (Kendall, 2002; Schnorrenberger, 2006). Others have made some connection between qi and electricity, and—sometimes in line with the electrodynamic field theory of Harold Saxton Burr (1889-1973) (Burr, 1973; Crane, 1950) or the direct current perineural transmission conjectures of Robert O. Becker (b. 1923) (Becker et al, 1985)—use electronic equipment to measure bioelectrical activity at acupuncture points and/or to stimulate them, for instance with electrical, electromagnetic, or laser devices (Mayor, 2007).

At the other end of the spectrum, the complex and multidimensional concept of qi has been hijacked by Western concepts of "vital energy." It is overly simplistic to equate qi and "energy" (Porkert, 1983), just as it is to discard it altogether or equate it with bioelectricity, but such attitudes have even percolated back to China (Kendall, 2002; Kuen, 2000). In the words of one standard Chinese textbook, "Qi is energy that moves" (Shuai, 1992).

Although Stahl used the term *energia*, "energy" only came into general use in science in the mid-nineteenth century, as a more precise substitute for the ambiguous term *force* (Martin, 1981; Tait, 1876). Many contemporary acupuncturists glibly use the word *energy* and talk of "vital energy" (Motoyama, 1981) and of "energy circulating" through meridians (Motoyama et al, 1978). However, qi is neither "substance" nor "energy" (Wiseman et al, 1995). "Qi = energy is an equation that does not compute" (Birch et al, 1999). The translation of qi as "matter-energy" is also inexact (Sivin, 1987), except for a handful of texts written since the eleventh century (Robinet, 1997).

This is not to deny the value of a model of acupuncture based on the bodily experience and mental concepts of flow. Patients do indeed frequently report sensations of movement in the body (along the channels) during acupuncture treatment (Buck, 1986). We must, however, tread cautiously whenever we are tempted to reduce the statements of one medical system to those of another, even (or perhaps especially) if we find notions derived from fluid anatomy or the physics of energy attractive because of our unconscious cultural bias. Both "subtle" and gross anatomy have their place in acupuncture.

As with osteopathy, chiropractic, and massage, there is a spectrum of acupuncture needling methods, from the vigorous intramuscular stimulation method discovered by Chan Gunn in 1973 (Gunn, 1996) to the palpatory subtleties of *toyohari*, developed by Kodo Fukushima (1910-2007?) and others in the 1950s (Fukushima, 1991). In general, it is probably fair to say that practitioners of the gentler approaches have more sympathy with the concept of qi. Both "touchy-feely" traditional acupuncturists and those who practice medical acupuncture and do not want to stray outside the bounds of conventional science are slowly learning to accept that each point of view has its merits and that there is plenty of room for different types and traditions of acupuncture.

Methods derived from acupuncture but not using needles divide into those in which there is direct contact between patient and practitioner and those in which some technical device comes between them.

ACUPUNCTURE-DERIVED METHODS INVOLVING PATIENT CONTACT

"Zero balancing" is a gentle system of bodywork developed in the early 1970s by Fritz Smith (b. 1929), a doctor, osteopath, and acupuncturist, on the basis of his studies of rolfing, yoga, and meditation, among other methods. Smith considers qi as "energy," its main characteristic being movement, whether in currents or as an undefined field. Zero balancing treatment aims to restore a smooth flow of energy throughout the body, but in the context of body structure. During treatment, there may be involuntary responses (as in other body-centered therapies), "caused by resistance to the passage of energy through a dense or congested area of the body" (Smith, 1986, 2005).

In 1964, chiropractor George Goodheart (1918-2008) invented the system of "applied kinesiology" (AK) based on muscle-strength testing (Kendall et al, 1949). Goodheart found that many factors can positively or negatively affect muscle strength, and his system evolved rapidly. He soon claimed to be able to evaluate the activity (overenergy or underenergy) of the acupuncture channels with AK (Walther, 1976). A simplified version was popularized as "touch for health" by John F. Thie (1933-2005) in the 1970s (Thie et al, 1973), and a description of another simple muscle-testing procedure, the Bi-Digital O-Ring Test (BDORT), was published by Yoshiaki Omura (b. 1934) in 1981 (Yamamoto, 2008). Both AK and the BDORT have been used to test many different aspects of body (and mind) function.

John Diamond (b. 1934) was the first to attempt an integration of AK with psychotherapy (Diamond, 1979). In 1979, Roger Callahan (b. 1925), a clinical psychologist, studied with Diamond and found that simple stimulation (tapping) at an acupuncture point on the Stomach channel was able to release a patient from severe, lifelong phobia. On the basis of this experience he developed "thought field therapy"—so called because thoughts held in the mind appeared to have an informational expression in the energy field of the body (Callahan et al, 2001). In 1995, one of those he had trained, Gary Craig, launched "emotional freedom techniques," a simplified version of thought field therapy that eliminates muscle testing, substituting instead a standard algorithm of tapping on all

the meridians. In 2000 Fred Gallo published a textbook on his own energy diagnostic and treatment methods (Gallo, 2000). More recently Phil Mollon has designed "psychoanalytic energy psychotherapy" for practitioners whose background is in more traditional psychotherapies (Mollon, 2008). All these approaches now make up the field of "energy psychology" (Gallo, 2005).

"Quantum mysticism" (Wikipedia: Quantum mysticism, n.d.) has raised its head here too, with authors such as Johnjoe McFadden and Arnold Mindell exploring in depth the quantum nature of the mind (McFadden, 2000, 2002; Mindell, 2000) and others such as Peter Fraser, Bruce Lipton, Lynne McTaggart, and Dean Radin describing how fields or flow of information or intention may be involved in healing or other "paranormal" phenomena (Fraser et al, 2008; Jonas et al, 2003; Lipton, 2005; McTaggart, 2003, 2007; Radin, 2006).

ACUPUNCTURE-DERIVED METHODS— THE MACHINE AS INTERMEDIARY

Apart from devices that stimulate acupuncture points with measurable, physical energy, there are many types of equipment that purport in some way to detect, harness, amplify, balance, or otherwise alter the energies of the jingluo or related systems of the body to improve health. Most of these are based on methods created in the 1950s: *ryodoraku* (Yoshio Nakatani), electroacupuncture according to Voll or EAV (Reinhold Voll, 1909-1989), and auriculotherapy/auricular medicine (Paul Nogier, 1908-1996). Related methods from the 1970s include the "apparatus for measuring the function of the meridians and the corresponding internal organs," or AMI (1972; Hiroshi Motoyama, b. 1925), MORA therapy (created in 1975 by Franz Morell and Erich Rasche), and the VEGAtest (developed in 1978 by Helmut W. Schimmel, 1928-2003, and known originally as the "vegetative reflex test"). Most of these and their derivatives have now become complex computerized systems that bear little resemblance to the traditional practice of acupuncture (Mayor, 2007).

OTHER "ENERGY" TECHNOLOGY

Methods such as AK, the BDORT, Nogier's "vascular autonomic signal" and their numerous progeny, as well as EAV and the VEGAtest, have much in common with the earlier technologies of dowsing (Weaver, 1978), radiesthesia (Mermet, 1959), and radionics (Tansley, 1975). There have been attempts to explain these precursors in terms of conventional science (Tromp, 1949), whereas the VEGAtest and other EAV-related devices have sometimes been described as methods of biofeedback to encourage acceptability (Mayor, 2007). However, they are still caught in the mesmeric trap: they either involve some kind of nonphysical energy (with considerable self-training required to become proficient, or perhaps sensitive to the body states or energy involved), or they are dependent on intention or the mental state of the operator-practitioner and/or patient (certainly they also require at least a "suspension of disbelief" to be used effectively). In either case their results are difficult to replicate, so that they remain controversial, if intriguing.

There are other technologies that are claimed to reveal life energy dysfunctions within the body but remain controversial. Examples are Kirlian photography (a serendipitous discovery in 1939 by Semyon Davidovich Kirlian, 1900-1980 and Valentina Khrisanthovna Kirlian, d. 1971) (Krippner et al, 1973), with its echoes of spirit photography, and electrocrystal therapy (developed in 1988 by Harry Oldfield) (Niblock et al, 2000), whose antecedents include shamanic practices (Eliade, 1964) and Reichenbach's investigations into the odic force (Reichenbach, 1851). Crystals on their own have been used both to detect and to treat energetic imbalances within the body, and may be associated with methods using color or sound (McClean, 2006).

T'AI CHI CH'UAN, QIGONG, AND YOGA

Acupuncture, Oriental massage, and healing methods were not the only significant imports to the West in the second half of the twentieth century. Yoga, with its emphasis on prana was long established (see Chapter 31), with a proliferation of approaches under the influence of Theosophy earlier in the century. A number of "soft" martial arts (using the opponent's force, rather than meeting force with force) soon became popular as well, in particular *t'ai chi* (*taiji*, 太极) (Frantzis, 2006) and *ki aikido* (氣合氣道) (Tohei, 1976), both qi-based arts. These, together with yoga and the Pilates method ("contrology") of Joseph Pilates (1880-1967), based in part on yoga postures and breathing (Robinson et al, 2000), have contributed to a ready acceptance of qigong (see Chapter 28), as well as various spinoffs such as Jun Konno's *ai chi* (Adami, 2002), and countless "new" forms of meditation (often formulated in nineteenth-century vitalist terms; Miura, 1989) (see Chapter 7).

Although the physical aspects of yoga have become readily established in the West, the traditional theories of the nadi and prana that underpin both *hatha yoga* and *tantra yoga* are less accepted (Dazey, 2005). There are those, however, who have explored the byways of tantra and related practices (such as the "interior alchemy" of Daoism, as distinct from qigong; Robinet, 1997), and in particular *kundalini*, the (usually) unconscious or instinctive corporeal energy envisaged as a sleeping serpent coiled at the base of the spine (susumna channel) (Flood, 1996). Rousing the kundalini, whether wittingly or unwittingly, can lead to dramatic experiences of "energy-sensation" or "currents" when "blocks" in the susumna or other nadi are encountered, and these may be accompanied by psychological disturbance (Krishna, 1971; Sannella, 1976).

Such explorations are best undertaken under the guidance of an experienced teacher (see, e.g., Tweedie, 1979).

LIFE AND GRAVITY

Whereas Mesmer considered gravity to be an aspect of the vital fluidum, for other eighteenth-century physicians such as Herman Boerhaave (1668-1738) (Schaffer, 1978) and François Boissier Sauvages de la Croix (de la Croix, 1763), life is what overcomes the deadening force of gravity. Thus, although movement and the interplay with gravity is an essential attribute of life, and a sense of kinesthetic flow is at the very core of dance, it is surprising that apart from the 5Rhythms movement meditation practice first devised by Gabrielle Roth in the 1960s (Roth, 1998, 1999), other CAM movement, dance, and posture therapies rarely mention any sort of life force or energy. Rolando Toro Mario Araneda (b. 1924), for example, founder of the Biodanza system ("dance with life" or "dance of life"—originally called "Psicodanza"), writes about a relearning of life's primordial functions based on instinct to counter the repressive structures fostered by consumer society and totalitarian ideologies, but not about the life energy as such (Araneda, 2008). However, most movement, dance, and posture approaches certainly do emphasize self-awareness as a key. This is true of the Feldenkrais method of Moshé Feldenkrais (1904-1984) (Feldenkrais, 1990) and the Alexander technique of F. Matthias Alexander (1869-1955) (Jones, 1997), for instance.

THE MIND, TRANCE, AND CHANNELLING

The animist position that the mind, rather than any subtle force or energy, is the primary arbiter of health, was taken up by many of Mesmer's followers. One in particular was very influential in America. Phineas P. Quimby (1802-1866) first worked as a magnetizer or magnetic healer (reconstituted names for a mesmerist) in Portland, Maine, but soon came to believe that disease follows from "a wrong direction given to the mind" and healing correspondingly from changes in mental state (Dresser, 1969). His student Warren F. Evans (1817-1889) published the first book on "Mind Cure" or "New Thought," in which he advocated cultivating deep meditative states to contact the divine healing energy within (Evans, 1869), "a battery and reservoir of magnetic life and vital force" (Evans, 1874).

Quimby's other notable student was Mary Baker Eddy (1821-1919), a former patient who went on to found the system of Christian Science. More radical and doctrinaire than Evans, she declared that all disease, pain, misfortune, and evil are illusion, Divine (rather than individual) Mind being the only reality. The illusion of illness thus can be overcome through prayer, which leads to healing. Eddy denied any relationship with Mind Cure, mesmerism, or other methods of healing, but her venomous denunciations of Quimby, forbidding of "laying on of hands," and descriptions of animal magnetism as "malicious" (Tatar, 1978) reveal her origins only too clearly, assuring Christian Science a place in the history of vital energy (Feldman, 1963; Schoepflin, 1988).

By the late 1890s, New Thought authors such as Ralph Waldo Trine (1866-1958) had also replaced the fluidum with a dematerialized "Divine inflow [of] Infinite Intelligence and Power," with the healer's *mind* as "channel" (Trine, 1897). "Channeling spiritual power through your thoughts" was also central to the method later popularized by Norman Vincent Peale (1898-1993) as the "power of positive thinking," which he claimed would lead to "peace of mind, improved health, and a never-ceasing flow of energy" (Peale, 1952). Norman Cousins (1915-1990), well-known for his personal battles against illness, was another who emphasized the capacity of the human mind and body to regenerate: "The life-force may be the least understood force on earth" (Cousins, 1979).

New and updated forms of mind-based approaches to healing are particularly prevalent in the United States, examples being "a course in miracles" (Schucman, 1975), "prosperity consciousness" (Chopra, 1993; Cole-Whittaker, 1983), and "living love" (Keyes, 1989). Beyond any organization, the notion of "what you think is what is real" and a focus on love infuse important sectors of the modern CAM community, resonating through history in surprising ways. Quimby's 1859 declaration that "Love or True Mind heals all" (Dresser, 1969) could almost have been taken from Bernie S. Siegel's best-seller *Love, Medicine and Miracles* (Siegel, 1986), or even perhaps vice versa.

Over a century ago, William James (1842-1910) wrote of the "verbiage" of Mind Cure, and how the "Gospel of Relaxation" of the "Don't Worry Movement" was becoming pervasive (James, 1902). The meditation, relaxation, and breathing techniques involved partially derived from somnambulistic or mesmeric trance states (see, e.g., Davis, 1885) but also, James considered, from New England transcendentalism and Hinduism. They certainly prepared the way for the adoption of the many Asian-style and other meditation and relaxation methods that for many are associated with CAM.

In spiritualism, the trance states of animist mesmerism were used to contact noncorporeal realities and beings. Healing dispensations, medical diagnosis, and medical advice were common products of "tuning-in," as much as clairvoyance or clairaudience. This movement was later reincarnated in the New Age scene of the 1970s and 1980s (Melton, 1988). As with some forms of "past lives therapy" (Netherton et al, 1978), phenomena such as "experiencing the healing powers of interplanetary Brotherhoods and curing their medical ailments by soul travel to different planes of reality" (Levin et al, 1986, p. 890) are frequently direct descendants of animist mesmerism. Associations such as the Spiritual Frontiers Fellowship founded by Arthur Ford, Edgar Cayce's Association for Research and Enlightenment (Carter, 1972), and the Great White Brotherhood (Prophet, 1976) involve a panoply of spiritual beings contactable during mesmeric trances (in today's parlance, during altered states of consciousness, channelling, higher states of awareness, or transmissions from spiritually evolved beings). Such associations are rarely organized as professional healing bodies, and indeed their methods routinely exceed the limits of healing practice, categorizable instead as alternative or emergent religions.

PSYCHOLOGICAL ENERGIES

Of all the mesmeric forces, the most complex, prolific, and hidden ones lie concealed in psychology. Significant aspects of clinical psychology's origins are connected with attempts to legitimize, mainstream, or find the real source of mesmerism and vital energy. In 1843 the Scottish physician James Braid (1795-1860) sought to clean up mesmerism's tainted reputation by changing its name to *hypnosis*, after Hypnos (Υπνος), the Greek god for sleep. He postulated that mesmeric manifestations were "entirely attributable to the mechanical pressure on an excited state of the nervous system" and that the effects were due to a mental force, not magnetism, and certainly not some mysterious fluid (Braid, 1899).

Hypnosis became a major concern in psychology and retains its importance in some areas of conventional medicine (Heap et al, 2002). Together with such forms of passive volitional intention as guided imagery (Hall et al, 2006) and the autogenic training of Johannes Schultz (1884-1970) (Linden, 1990), derived in part from post-mesmeric methods of autosuggestion and with parallels in yoga (Bird et al, 2002), it has contributed to the formation of such modern cognitive-behavioral mind-body interventions as biofeedback (Schwartz et al, 2000), the relaxation response (Benson et al, 2001), and the reexamination of older self-control practices such as meditation (West, 1987). These mind-body interventions shift between conventional and nonconventional. Beginning as academic pursuits, they have become valuable intellectual and clinical resources for CAM, lending it significant credibility and allowing the vital force to be conceptualized in psychosomatic terms or within the current mind-body framework. They are the "lowest," most scientific aspects of the mesmeric legacy, a kind of legitimate mesmerism, and have generated much research (e.g., Eccleston et al, 2003; Izquierdo de Santiago et al, 2007; Ostelo et al, 2005). "Behaviorism" itself, created by John B. Watson (1878-1958), emphasized external behavior and reactions rather than internal mental states. It has been described by one opponent as "soulless psychology," the "Newtonian psychology par excellence" (Graham, 2001).

Like Watson's original behaviorism as well as much hypnotherapy, "cognitive-behavioral therapy" (CBT), which started life as "rational therapy" in the hands of Albert Ellis (1913-2007) during the 1950s (Ellis, 1975), is a psychotherapeutic method with a goal-oriented approach, which makes it particularly amenable to research. A more direct spinoff of hypnosis is "neurolinguistic programming" (NLP), created by Richard W. Bandler (b. 1950) and John Grinder (b. 1940) in the 1970s from "modelling" therapists such as the psychiatrist and medical hypnotherapist Milton Erickson (1901-1980). Here again, the approach is goal oriented, one key to success being for the therapist to know in advance the desired outcome of the intervention (Bandler et al, 1979). Both CBT and NLP encourage brief rather than prolonged therapy, but they differ in that CBT pays no or little attention to the unconscious mind, whereas NLP makes use of unconscious behaviors and communication, although without the need to translate this into conscious form. No mysterious forces here—just the mind and its reasons.

Rather different was the method of psychoanalysis originally developed by Sigmund Freud (1856-1939) in the 1890s on the basis of his studies in hypnosis with Josef Breuer (1842-1925). They initially proposed that disorders of the mind might result from "a block that interferes with the normal current of feeling in such a way as to cause stagnation and overflow" (Breuer et al, 1974). Both used hydraulic and electrical language to describe their new way of working (e.g., flows, dams, charges, discharges, excitation, cathexis, currents of energy, resistance, tension) (Zweig, 1933). To the horror of most of his contemporaries, Freud considered the will and force of life not as a form of *higher* intelligence, but as *instinctual,* defining "libido," the energy of instinct, as a drive toward sexual gratification (Stafford-Clark, 1967). In his later writings, he redefined it as a drive toward *any* form of pleasurable bodily sensation (Wolff et al, 1990) or even as the energy of all the life instincts (Hall, 1954). James Hillman has pointed out that the linguistic roots of the term *libido* encompass notions of pleasure, pouring (flow), and freedom, as well as sexuality (Hillman, 1999).

For Carl Gustav Jung (1875-1961), unlike Freud, libido was once more not so much instinctual as *intentional,* a neutral "psychic energy" in some ways like water, "canalized" (Jung, 1928/1969), flowing down gradients, associated with light and creative heat (Jung, 1967). He distinguished libido from "vital energy" (Jung, 1969), comparing it instead with Melanesian *mana,* which he interpreted as a qualitative, not quantitative, power or influence, present in the atmosphere of life, although in a way supernatural rather than physical (contrast p. 64, earlier). He also explained it as a drive rather than a force, akin to the "Will" of Schopenhauer, Aristotle's *horme* (Ορμή), Plato's *eros* (Ερως), or Bergson's *élan vital* (Jung, 1969). It could also be compared with the "nonenergetical" psychoid "entelechy" of Hans Driesch (1867-1941) (Driesch, 1914, 1929), a concept that in turn contributed to the morphogenetic field theory of Rupert Sheldrake

(b. 1942) (Sheldrake, 1981). Closing the loop, Sheldrake's "morphic resonance" has been compared with Jung's concept of synchronicity as an acausal connecting principle (Piirto, 1999).

Wilhelm Reich (1897-1957) developed Freud's concept of libido in a rather different way, concentrating on its physical expression and simultaneous psychological content (Kelley, n.d.). Libido here is a real energy ("orgone" or "bioenergy"), discharged during emotional expression and sexual orgasm (DeMeo, 1998) and manifesting physically as static (but not galvanic) electricity (Trettin, 1997). Reich considered the flow of life and its block in the frozen patterns of our personal histories ("character armor") as both ultimately derived from the same *energetic* source ("orgonotic streaming") (Reich, 1972). It is noteworthy that in 1921, even before Reich published his major work, the novelist D.H. Lawrence (1885-1930) was writing that illness can arise from the blocking of flow within the body, suppressing the sensual will. For Lawrence, as for Reich, this could also lead to *psychological stunting of whole generations,* not just individuals (Lawrence, 1971). Reich's orgone has been uncritically equated with Keely's "etheric force" and the "scalar electromagnetics" of Thomas Bearden (Davidson, 1987).

Alexander Lowen (1910-2008), one of Reich's foremost pupils, focused on the release of the chronic muscular holding patterns of the character armor, tensions associated with reduced vitality (Lowen, 1973) and emotional conflict, unresolved and probably repressed (Lowen, 1975). He expunged Reich's provocatively named "orgone" in favor of a blander "bioenergy" and posited that all living processes can be reduced to its manifestations (Lowen, 1958). For Lowen, although nerves may mediate our inner perceptions and coordinate responses, "the underlying impulses and movements are inherent in the body's energetic charge, in its natural rhythms and pulsations," blood in particular being "the energetically charged fluid of the body" (Lowen, 1976, pp. 51, 52). Inevitably, it has been suggested that orgone is identical to qi (Senf, 1979).

John Pierrakos (1921-2001), who codeveloped "bioenergetic analysis" with Lowen, went on to found the Institute of Core Energetics in 1980, integrating this work with insights from his study of Eastern traditions and the psychic explorations of his wife, Eva Pierrakos (1915-1979). Like Lowen, he understood that "pain results when the energy flow is blocked," but also emphasized that a free flow of energy both from and into the "core" of the person is necessary for spiritual development (quoted in Chubbuck, 2006).

There are many other neo-Reichian therapies, such as the Kelley-Radix work of Charles R. Kelley (1922-2005) (Kelley-Radix, 2009), the "biosynthesis" approach of David Boadella (b. 1931), and the "biodynamic psychology" of Gerda Boyesen (1922-2005) (Boyesen, 1994). Stanley Keleman has combined his experience with chiropractic, bioenergetic analysis and other therapeutic approaches in what he calls "formative psychology" ("your body is your energy"; Keleman, 1975). More information on these therapies, all of which owe considerable debt to Reich and his concept of orgone energy, can be found in the specialist journal *Energy and Character* founded by Boadella in 1970 (International Institute for Biosynthesis, 2008). A useful review of the web of connections between these various forms of bodywork and the world of dance has been written by Helen Payne (Payne, 2006).

Reichian therapy is of course not the only bodywork method to focus on muscle relaxation. The Rosen method (Marion Rosen, b. 1914) is also intended to release chronic muscular tension. Rosen's teacher Lucy Heyer had found that treating patients with breathwork, movement, and massage enabled them to contact their emotions more freely in subsequent sessions of Jungian analysis. As Reich intuited, working with breathing and body awareness enables contact with the unconscious (Rosen et al, 2003); in a sense, in an overrationalized life, the body becomes the unconscious "shadow" (Conger, 1988).

Holotropic Breathwork, created in the mid-1970s by Stanislav Grof (b. 1931) and his wife Christina, involves both intensified breathing and bodywork in a group setting, and is believed to facilitate access to nonordinary states of consciousness. Although Grof does not theorize about the role of vital energy in this work, participants commonly report greater awareness of somatic processes and bodily impulses, in particular feeling where energy is blocked or streaming within the body (Collinge, 2000; Taylor, 2003).

Another author who emphasizes the importance of inner focus and of feelings within the body is Eugene T. Gendlin (b. 1926). The method of "Focusing" developed by him and his colleagues involves awareness of the "physical sense of meaning," the "felt sense"—not just body sensation, not just feelings or thoughts, but body-mind awareness of a total situation (Gendlin, 1981) or of "our ongoing life process" (Wikipedia: Eugene Gendlin, n.d.).

A very different approach to "flow" is that of Mihaly Csikszentmihalyi. Although he writes of "a loss of the feeling of self-consciousness" and "the merging of action and awareness" in flow, he also repeatedly emphasizes the importance of a clear purpose, concentration, and sense of control (Wikipedia: Flow, n.d.). In other words, he explicitly intends his method to "fortify the self" rather than enable a letting go into deep contact with the inner flows of the body. As with CBT and NLP (and to an extent the "what you think is what is real" positive thinkers), his aim is to foster better outward goal-directed behavior ("higher, faster, stronger") (Csikszentmihalyi, 1992). To the ego, the animus, or rational mind, the interior of the body remains a shadowy unknown world (Becker, 1997; Conger, 1988). The body itself is in danger of being disowned (Young, 2006), "felt more as one object among other objects in the world than as the core of the individual's own being" (Laing, 1969).

HOMEOPATHY AND THE "SPIRIT-LIKE VITAL FORCE"

For much of the nineteenth century, homeopathy was the most serious challenge to conventional Western medicine, particularly in the United States (Rothstein, 1992). Created by Samuel Christian Hahnemann (1755-1843), classical homeopathy espouses the belief that whatever symptom complex a substance can cause in a healthy person, infinitesimally small amounts of the same substance can cure diseases with the same symptom configuration. The small dosage has the capacity to evoke the spirit-like vital force (*dynamis*), everywhere present in the organism and maintaining both the sensations and activities of all its parts in harmony. Hahnemann described the rationale of his approach in *The Organon of Rational Healing*, first published in 1810 and in its sixth edition by 1842 (Hahnemann, 1983). The book begins with his account of how "pathologically untuned vital force," the "inner essence of disease," may lead to the "disagreeable sensations" of disease, emphasizing that the influence of medicines is dynamic, not material. Progressive dilution in the form of "potentization" or "dynamization" of homeopathic remedies using a method he called "succussion" renders them even more effective.

Hahnemann several times likens the "dynamic, virtual action" of medicines to the invisible force of magnetism, their effects "perceived by the nervous sensitivity everywhere present in the organism." Moreover, "the dynamic forces of mineral magnetism, electricity, and galvanism act no less homeopathically and powerfully on our vital principle than medicines actually called homeopathic" (Hahnemann, 1983, pp. 16, 21, and 209). He further states that "it is impossible only through the efforts of the intellect to recognize the spirit-like force itself," although in contrast "it is possible to create a very grave disease by acting on the vital principle through the power of imagination and to cure it in the same way" (Hahnemann, 1983, pp. 21 and 23). Toward the end of the *Organon* he writes effusively of the healing force of Mesmer's animal magnetism as "a marvelous, priceless gift of God to man," emphasizing the role of the "strong and benevolent will" of the mesmerizer to "transmit human force" to the debilitated. In contrast, he abhors the "monstrous derangement of the entire being termed *clairvoyant trance*" (Hahnemann, 1983, pp. 210-212). Hans Burch Gram (1786-1840), an influential early American homeopath, also had a strong interest in mesmerism (Fuller, 1989).

The origins of Hahnemann's "spirit-like vital force" go back to Paracelsus and van Helmont, as well as the more recent vitalism of Stahl (Coulter, 1977). At its inception, homeopathy also shared some characteristics with animal magnetism. Today other parallels may be highlighted. Following Hahnemann's aside on the dynamic force of electricity, the prominent homeopath George Vithoulkas (b. 1932), for instance, has written on the equivalence of "electrodynamic energy" and the "vital force" (Vithoulkas, 1980), and the work of Jacques Benveniste (1935-2004) on electronic digitizing of signals from ultra-low dilutions (Jonas et al, 2006) has been used as the basis for various computerized therapeutic devices, including variants of the VEGAtest, as well as for justification of older technologies such as radionics (see earlier). (Interestingly, the original radionic device created by Albert Abrams [1863-1924] included a "dynamizer," although not for the purpose of potentization [Wilson, 1998].) Homeopathy suffered a serious decline in the first half of the twentieth century (Kaufman, 1971), but currently is enjoying a serious revival and has generated considerable conventional biomedical research and debate (Ernst et al, 1998) (see Chapter 24).

As with osteopathy, chiropractic, acupuncture, and psychology, there are of course different approaches to homeopathy, from the "classical," with its dependence on Hahnemann's spirit-like vital force, to the everyday use of low-potency remedies and "isopathy" (use of potentized disease agents), where such subtleties are less of a consideration.

Related methods include the anthroposophic medicine of Rudolf Steiner (1861-1925) and Ita Wegman (1876-1943), in which treatment aims to enhance the life force of the patient as an axis for improved health and deepened self-knowledge (Steiner et al, 1996), and the flower remedies of Edward Bach (1886-1936), who believed that health was a result of mental or emotional balance and that the unique energetic property of a plant could be used to rectify an imbalance and restore the awareness of "wholeness" (Bach, 1990). Such self-knowledge is one of the aims of treatment with the Bach remedies (Dr Edward Bach Centre, n.d.). Although not potentized using succussion, the Bach remedies are classified as homeopathic remedies in the United States. A number of other flower essence systems now exist.

Rather different is the 12 tissue salts system of Wilhelm Schüssler (1821-1898). Although his remedies are homeopathically potentized, Schüssler considered both disease and the effects of the tissue salts to be chemically based rather than involving any vital force (Boericke et al, 1986). As within homeopathy itself, a polarization between vitalist and materialist approaches is evident here.

HERBALISM, NATUROPATHY, AND THE *VIS MEDICATRIX NATURAE*

Hippocrates considered that the body contains within itself the power of self-healing, *physis* (φύσις (Garrison, 1929). Thomas Sydenham (1624-1689), the "English Hippocrates," wrote similarly of the *vis medicatrix naturae* (the healing power of nature) (Neuburger, 1926). Early in the eighteenth century, Richard Mead (1673-1754), another eminent physician whose ideas influenced Mesmer (Mesmer, 1980), identified "nature" itself with the immaterial principle of

life (Neuburger, 1926), and in the 1770s the influential professor of medicine at Edinburgh University William Cullen (1712-1790), reinstated the term *vis conservatrix et medicatrix naturae* (Neuburger, 1926), although in a different sense (Hiroshi, 1998). He considered that life consists "in the excitement of the nervous system, and especially of the brain, which unites the different parts, and forms them into a whole," and that "powers, which have a tendency to hurt and destroy the system, often excite such motions as are suited to obviate the effects of the noxious power," these "motions" being the vis medicatrix naturae (Cullen, 1777). Like Hufeland, Cullen preferred to assist the body's healing (with "tonics") rather than depleting it (with laxatives and purgatives) (University of Virginia Health System: William Cullen, n.d.).

The earliest American natural healing movement was Thomsonian herbalism. Samuel Thomson (1769-1843), a farmer burdened by the back-breaking nature of his work, came to realize that exposure to cold temperatures can be a key cause of illness. On the basis of Galen's humoral pathology (Berman, 1951), and borrowing from indigenous colonial-frontier and Indian treatments, he created a system based on restoring the body's "natural heat" using predominantly herbs and steam baths. The Thomsonian movement eventually developed into the profession of eclectic medicine, with a strong following in Europe (Griggs, 1981). Although Thomson himself did not use terms such as the vis medicatrix naturae or vital force (Fuller, 1989), later herbalists such as the break-away physicomedicalists (Haller, 1997) came to insist that treatment must be in harmony with nature and the vital force and must assist the latter instead of destroying it (Brown, 1985). As with homeopathy, herbalism as a profession suffered an eclipse in the United States in the early twentieth century (Rothstein, 1988) (probably less so in Europe), but more recently has once again begun to flourish (Brown, 1985; Hoffmann, 2003) (see Chapter 22). Other systems of herbal medicine are also much more in evidence in the West than even a few years ago. These include Chinese herbal medicine (see Chapter 26), Tibetan medicine (see Evolve Site), and Ayurveda (see Chapter 29)—all three of which have a vitalist core (*qi, rlung, prana*)—as well as traditional methods transplanted from other cultures (see, e.g., Chapters 34, 35, and 38).

Herbal medicine is in many respects closely allied to the ecological movement and the "Gaia hypothesis" of James Lovelock (b. 1919), in which the earth's biosphere, atmosphere, oceans, and soil form one single self-preserving system, virtually a living organism in itself (Lovelock, 1979, 2006). In this context, the vis medicatrix naturae begins to take on new meanings. In particular, "earth energies" have frequently been explored using dowsing or divining, the paths they take likened to the jingluo of acupuncture (Graves, 1978; Skinner, 1982). In the late 1940s, there were even attempts to amplify the vis medicatrix naturae electrically (Eeman, 1950).

Enhancing the vis medicatrix naturae was a key concept in the nineteenth-century health reform movement (Whorton, 1988) and the later eclectic approach known as "naturopathy," based on the *Naturheilkunde* of German practitioners such as Sebastian Kneipp (1821-1897) and Lorenz Gleich (1798-1865) (Lohff, 2001). Thus Sylvester Graham (1794-1851), founder of the influential "Grahamism" health movement, aware of the focus on the stomach by Grimaud and other Montpellier vitalists, stressed the need to support the "vital power" provided by digestion. A Presbyterian minister, he also inveighed against the excesses of "artificial" city life and the dangers of masturbation and alcohol, which could so easily deplete the body (Donegan, 1986; Fuller, 1989). The physicomedicalists warned not only against masturbation and excess venery, but even prolonged nursing of children, for the same reason (Haller, 1997). Other health reformers such as Russell T. Trall (1812-1877) and William A. Alcott (1798-1859) took a similar puritanical line, considering sexual intercourse more frequently than once a month as excessive, for example (Donegan, 1986). Trall also advocated contraception as a better alternative for women "compelled" to bear children that were a constant drain upon their life forces (Cayleff, 1988) and instructed fledgling hydropathic practitioners on the connections of their own methods with mesmerism (Fuller, 1989).

The Naturopathic Society of America and American School of Naturopathy were both founded in 1901 by Kneipp's follower, the water cure therapist Benedict Lust (1872-1945) (Cooksey, 2001). He defined naturopathy as "the art of natural healing and the science of physical and mental regeneration on the basis of self-reform, natural life, clean and normal diet," with the use of various CAM therapies but "to the exclusion of poisonous drugs and nonadjustable surgery" (Fishbein, 1932). John Harvey Kellogg (1852-1943), a prominent second-generation health reformer and Seventh Day Adventist, similarly promoted a no-drug philosophy, with "only such means employed as NATURE can best use in her recuperative work" (Fuller, 1989). Like many other naturopaths, he laid considerable emphasis on the avoidance of constipation, labelling it in a distant and very American echo of Mesmer as "the most destructive blockage that has ever opposed human progress" (Whorton, 1988). Another key figure was Chicago-based Henry Lindlahr, whose system of "Nature Cure" was based on the principle that "every acute disease is a healing effort of Nature" (Lindlahr, 1913). In Britain, Lindlahr's methods were popularized by practitioners such as James C Thomson (1887-1960) and Stanley Lief (1892-1963), and in 1945 the Nature Cure Association (founded in 1925) merged with the British Association of Naturopaths to form the British Naturopathic Association.

Although legal constraint may have prevented the widespread adoption of naturopathy as a unifying ideology for all natural therapies, its basic philosophy has spilled over into many fields. In the words of Jack Reginald

(J.R.) Worsley (1923-2003), founder of one particularly influential five-element acupuncture tradition, "Only Nature can cure disease. Practitioners only assist Nature, acting as instruments of Nature in putting the patient back on the path to health" (Worsley, 1985, p xi). Despite its virtual disappearance as an independent profession in North America by the 1970s (Gort et al, 1988), naturopathy is once more established today (see Chapter 21).

DIALECTICS OF COMPLEMENTARY AND ALTERNATIVE MEDICINE—THE RETURN OF VITALISM

Vitalism is, by definition, a movement in opposition to a purely physicochemical science, part of a recurring dialectic of the immaterial and the material that occurs throughout history.

Conventional science, including biomedicine, is inevitably reductionist, often perceived as needing to grind phenomena down into manageable, measurable particles. As a generalization, in contrast CAM therapies tend to look at the "big picture," the whole, the wave and flow of things. A result is that CAM practices in the 1970s frequently adopted the label "holism," and holistic methods were seen to share a common thread of belief in a "universal Life Energy" (Bauman et al, 1978), with the aim of opening "pathways or flows" within the body (Otto et al, 1979)—although the original definition of holism by the South African soldier, statesman, and scholar Jan Christiaan Smuts (1870-1950) as "the tendency in nature to form wholes that are greater than the sum of the parts through creative evolution" was antivitalist as well as antireductionist (Smuts, 1926). Other labels for holistic medicine such as "alternative" and "complementary" are, like "vitalism," oppositional terms, defined in relation to "orthodox" or "conventional" medicine.

Language and emphasis change over time, but a list of congruent polarities might look something like that in Table 6-2.

Polarization inevitably occurs within CAM as well, as mentioned earlier for mesmerism, osteopathy, chiropractic, acupuncture, psychotherapy, homeopathy, and related methods. And there is clearly quite a gulf between the abstract mind fields of the quantum theorists and the flows and feelings of the bodyworkers (although both concern *connection*).

The CAM label itself is a compromise, but at least allows rapprochement, although the risk of polarization and conflict remains (quackbusters vs. neohippies). Vitalism is often associated with liberalizing or democratic tendencies (Darnton, 1968; McClean, 2006; Moore, 1977), but stark reminders of misinterpretation can be seen in its elevation to a "gospel of energy" by the Italian Futurists and military in World War I (will, struggle, "dynamic

TABLE 6-2

Vitalism and Some Possible Congruent Polarities

Physicochemical	Vitalist
Mechanism	Spirit
Matter	Ether
Establishment	Counterculture (Roszak, 1969)
Neo-Darwinian/ competitive	Neo-Romantic/ cooperative (Amato, 2002)
Expert led	Democratic
Male dominated	Feminist
Particle	Wave (Cassidy, 2004)
Fragments, parts	Connections, field
Separation, alienation	Participation, enfoldment
Cool	Warm
Reductionism	Holism
Hard science	Touchy-feely
Quantitative	Qualitative
Evidence based	Unknowable
Technocratic medicine	Hands-on or interactional healing
Removal of symptoms	Nourishment and support of health
Intervention (linear, one-directional)	Self-regulation (cybernetic, feedback looping)
Outcome	Process
Objectively verifiable	Subjectively experienced
Factual knowledge	Self-awareness
Animus	Anima
Rational	Intuitive
Left-brained	Right-brained
Conscious	Unconscious
Ego	Id
Visual	Tactile, proprioceptive
Outer-directed observation	Inner sensing, interiority
Mind, disembodied	Body, embodied
Central nervous system	Autonomic nervous system (Wilhelm, 1962)
Structure/organization	Movement/change
Gross anatomy	Subtle energy
Tension	Relaxation
Block	Flow
Pain (Hankey, 2006)	Pleasure
Contraction	Expansion
Holding	Breathing

And so forth.

sensations," . . . violence) (Thompson, 2008) and in the fact that so many of the innovators mentioned earlier—Freud, Reich, Rosen, Feldenkrais, Gendlin, for example—were emigrés from a Europe under the authoritarian regime of the Nazis. Paradoxically, some forms of natural medicine actually flourished in Nazi Germany, homeopathy in particular (Abgrall, 2000), which was even tested on the inmates of the Dachau concentration camp (Hale, 2003).

Of course, life is not so schematically dualistic in practice. There are various forms of vitalism and mechanism, not a simple single spectrum with "extreme" vitalism at one end and "extreme" mechanism at the other (Benton, 1974). How we think and perceive depends on many different factors: "vitalistic or mechanistic judgements . . . are largely determined by nonscientific beliefs or prejudices" (Wheeler, 1939). Some of us will be more inclined to the Cartesian "I think, therefore I am" (Descartes, 1649/1988), others to "I feel, therefore I live." It is interesting, for example, that in most fields of CAM women practitioners tend to outnumber men (Cayleff, 1988; Donegan, 1986; Gevitz, 1988a; Kaufman, 1988; Schoepflin, 1988). On the other hand, mechanists may become vitalists in older age (Wheeler, 1939), although the contrary trend is also possible. In the past, new branches of medical science have been founded by insisting on theoretical concepts not reducible to those accepted at the time (Kaitaro, 2008). "Yesterday's liminal becomes today's stabilized, today's peripheral becomes tomorrow's centered" (Turner, 1974).

As the neo-Confucian Zhu Xi (1130-1200) wrote of the eternally oscillating relationship between *qi* and *li* (form, reason, principle of organization, 理), "Throughout the universe, there is no *qi* without *li*, nor *li* without *qi*" (Yoke, 2000). Both are necessary to life.

CONCLUSION—VITALISM IN TWENTY-FIRST-CENTURY COMPLEMENTARY AND ALTERNATIVE MEDICINE

Much of human reason is based on metaphor (Lakoff, 1987), and much of this is grounded in visceral, lived experience (Johnson, 2007). In particular, the basic metaphors of vitalism are present for all of us, usually unacknowledged. Whether they originate in our genes or in our inner, intrauterine, or early life experience; are intellectually molded later on by our sociocultural environments; or are part of our individual energy or thought fields, they are there whether we like it or not, whether we consider ourselves cool rationalists or hot-blooded intuitives. Even in *imagined* interaction with a partner, "it would seem as if images of energy patterns [are] one of the psyche's natural language or symbol systems" (Reed, 1996). As one writer on vitalism has put it, vitalist views are too "resilient and complex to be corroded by mere facts" (Brooke, 1971). The endless fascination throughout history with mysterious energies and forces—pneuma, electricity, animal magnetism, quantum fields, and so forth—attests to their significance for us as humans.

This is particularly clear in literature and popular culture, where vitalism remains a pervasive influence. Sustained in the writing of influential Romantic authors such as Percy Bysshe Shelley (1792-1822) (Grabo, 1930), his wife Mary Wollstonecraft Shelley (1797-1851) (Shelley, 1831), and Honoré de Balzac (Balzac, 1831) as well as by post-Romantics such as Gustav Meyrink (1868-1932) (Meyrink, 1915) and D.H. Lawrence (e.g., in *Women in Love*, with its ubiquitous flows of kundalini-like "fierce electric energy") (Lawrence, 1999), it is difficult even now to find a novel that, in some form or other, does not make use of the language of vitalism, whether consciously or unconsciously. What a society considers to be its "mainstream" views may actually be shared only by a numerical minority (Moore, 1977). Folk (medical) traditions from around the world lay stress on "the flow, transmission, and balance of life energies" (Hufford, 1988), as for instance in the positive or negative *vibraciones* of *curanderismo* (see Chapter 37).

As can be seen from the ubiquity of various forms of vitalism in the many CAM practices mentioned earlier, its multivalent possibilities have made it endlessly attractive. Its very imprecision allows for enormous flexibility and adaptibility, explanatory models morph and coalesce, and there are so many strands to its history that it is now probably impossible to disentangle them. However, some aspects of vitalism do appear consistently across the various modalities of CAM, more or less in the order shown in Figure 6-1.

In conventional medicine it is sometimes too easy for a person to become a thing, an irrelevant spectator, overwhelmed by a mechanical world of technology, tests, and

Flow Connection	Within the body, between people, or between the individual and something greater
Awareness	Increased; usually of bodily (or body-mind) processes; often of something flowing (pulsing, moving, tingling), or of breath
Breath	More underlying than overt in some CAM modalities

Figure 6-1 Vitalism aspects in complementary and alternative medicine.

surgery in which stress may adversely affect self-healing. The vitalist perspective, on the other hand, aligns itself with coherent, life-affirming principles. The vitalist universe is not random, detached, or mindless; it is benign, coherent, and hospitable. Instead of a medicine whose central issues can seem coldly mechanical and buried in inaccessible molecular biology, vitalism instinctively invites a person to experience a unifying, transcendent, and reassuring ontological presence. Whatever the outcome of scientific investigations of vitalist medical traditions, vitalism's attractiveness for practitioners and patients is likely to remain a growing presence in health care, provided we can give it the necessary time in our own new "axial age" (Lambert, 1999).

Acknowledgements

To Ted Kaptchuk, for giving me free rein in rewriting his original chapter on vitalism for this edition, to Ton Than Thy for her transliteration of Vietnamese terms, and to Rodger Watts of Donica Publishing for assistance with Chinese characters.

⊖ Chapter References can be found on the Evolve website at http://evolve.elsevier.com/Micozzi/complementary/

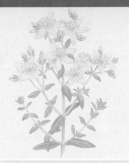

CHAPTER

7

MIND-BODY THOUGHT AND PRACTICE IN EARLY AND LATE AMERICA

DONALD McCOWN
MARC S. MICOZZI

Most forms of complementary and alternative medicine can be seen to draw on a "mind-body" connection. The complementary medical approaches described in this section explicitly make use of physiological mechanisms by which mental states are reflected in direct biological responses. Likewise, although "bioenergy" is invoked in many complementary modalities and alternative medicine therapies, energy medicine itself uses this energetic property as the sole means and primary mode of cure. Ultimately, mind and energy may be reflected in the "consciousness" approach of many complementary and alternative medicine forms of traditional healing. ∾

Thinking and practice regarding mind-body approaches dates to early American history and has continued until its resurgence in late, or "postmodern," American history. This thinking and practice did not originate from early physiological medical studies nor from the current recognition of psychoneuroimmunology in medical science (the topic of the next chapter in this section). Like complementary and alternative medicine in general, it arose in the popular consciousness from nonmedical cultural and spiritual

movements based on experiential and existential (not experimental) thinking, studies, and philosophies.

OVERSEAS BEGINNINGS

It is possible to date a European intellectual connection to Asian spiritual thought and practice to as early as the ancient Greek histories of Herodotus, Alexander the Great's Indian campaign in 327 to 325 BC (Hodder, 1993), or Petrarch's mention of Hindu ascetics in his *Life of Solitude*, written 1345 to 1347 (Versluis, 1993). A more substantive start, however, would be 1784, which marks the founding by British scholars and magistrates of the Asiatic Society of Bengal, from which quickly flowed first translations of Hindu scriptures directly from Sanskrit texts into English. Sir William Jones was the preeminent member of the group. His tireless work included translations of Kalidasa's *Sakuntala* (1789), Jayadeva's *Gitagovinda* (1792), and the influential *Institutes of Hindu Law* (1794). His early tutor in Sanskrit, Charles Wilkins, holds the distinction of making the first translation of the *Bhagavad*

Gita (1785). In 1788, the group founded a journal, *Asiatik Researches,* that was widely circulated among the intelligentsia, including the second U.S. president John Adams, an enthusiastic subscriber (Hodder, 1993; Versluis, 1993). The effect of this flow of scholarly and objective information about Indian culture and religion began a profound shift in Europe's view of the East—"from the earlier presupposition of the East as barbarous and despotic, to a vision of an exotic and highly civilized world in its own right" (Versluis, 1993, p. 18).

The new language, ideas, images, and narratives embedded in such texts immediately touched something in poets, philosophers, and artists, particularly in England and Germany—powerful influences on the development of American culture. In England, the Romantics embraced all things "Oriental" as a celebration of the irrational and exotic. Their use of the scriptures, stories, lyrics, and images becoming ever more available to them from Hinduism, Buddhism, Confucianism, and Islam was not discrete, but rather an amalgam. Their drive was not for a practical use of these new elements of discourse in expressing some tacit knowledge heretofore inexpressible; to the contrary, as Versluis (1993) notes, "their Orientalism was not serious but rather a matter of exotic settings for poems" (p. 29). The latter confounding of international relations by "Orientalism" (Said, 1978) was an unforeseen serious consequence. Johann Gottfried von Herder, Johann Wolfgang von Goethe, and the Romantics who followed them in Germany found "Oriental" thought a refreshing alternative to the stifling rationality (and then nationality) of their time. Yet, again, their usage of the new material available was not entirely pragmatic. Their philosophical and poetic insights could have been expressed in the preexisting discourse of Christian mysticism, Neo-Platonism, and Hermeticism and the charismatic movement. What the use of Oriental religious discourse by a poet of spiritual power such as Novalis (Freidrich von Hardenberg) did do was to suggest that the full range of Eastern and Western religious expression pointed to a Transcendent reality, and that all—*in essence*—offered truth (Versluis, 1993). It is this last point that brings us to America, to the Transcendentalists, and, at last, to the pragmatic use of the Eastern discourses to better understand and express a personal tacit knowledge.

AMERICAN BEGINNINGS

In writers such as Ralph Waldo Emerson and Henry David Thoreau, and in the utopian vision of the Transcendentalist Old Concord Farm and other communities, the influence of Eastern thought is evident (Brooks, 1936; Hodder, 1993; Versluis, 1993). Through the *Dial,* their journal that did much to shape American Transcendentalism, they brought out translations of Hindu, Buddhist, and Confucian texts, and of the Sufi poets, such as Hafiz, Rumi, and Saadi. In these "transcendentalations" a new, rich brew began to find ways to give voice to tacit experience.

It is possible to see both Emerson and Thoreau as natural (and learned) contemplatives whose entwined literary and spiritual lives reflect experiences that demanded a larger discourse than the West provided for more explicit understanding and more elaborated communication. Emerson's early (1836) essay "Nature," written before his deep engagement with Eastern thought, contains a description of such an experience:

> Crossing a bare common, in snow puddles, at twilight, under a clouded sky, without having in my thoughts any occurrence of special good fortune, I have enjoyed a perfect exhilaration. Almost I fear I think how glad I am. In the woods, too, a man casts off his years, as the snake his slough, and at what period so ever of life is always a child. In the woods, is perpetual youth. Within these plantations of God, a decorum and a sanctity reign, a perennial festival is dressed, and the guest sees not how he should tire of them in a thousand years. In the woods, we return to reason and faith. There I feel that nothing can befall me in life,—no disgrace, no calamity, (leaving me my eyes,) which nature cannot repair. Standing on the bare ground,—my head bathed by the blithe air, and uplifted into infinite space,—all mean egotism vanishes. I become a transparent eye-ball. I am nothing. I see all. The currents of the Universal Being circulate through me; I am part or particle of God.

As Emerson began reading the amalgam of Oriental writings in earnest, which consumed him for the rest of his life, his enterprise became the essentialization (distillation) and integration of the insights that supported his experience and vision on both a personal and a cultural scale. Versluis notes that, "For Emerson . . . the significance of Asian religions—of all human history—consists of assimilation into the present, into this individual here and now" (1993, p. 63). He was reading and feeling and thinking his way toward a universal, literally Unitarian religion. (Imagine if the early New England settlers had not thought to provide "commons" as the centerpieces of their settlements as spiritual practices evolved from Puritanism to Congregationalism to Unitarianism.)

It seems Thoreau had a different enterprise underway, using the same materials. Where Emerson was grappling with universals and theory to make sense of the world, Thoreau was intent that particulars and practice would make sense of his own world. Though he had only the translated texts to guide him, he did more than just *imagine* himself as an Eastern contemplative practitioner. He wrote to his friend, H.G.O. Blake, in 1849, "rude and careless as I am, I would fain practice the yoga faithfully. . . . To some extent, and at rare intervals, even I am a yogin" (quoted in Hodder, 1993, p. 412). Thoreau offers descriptions of his experience, such as this from the "Sounds" chapter of *Walden:*

> I did not read books that first summer; I hoed beans. Nay, I often did better than this. There were times when

I could not afford to sacrifice the bloom of the present moment to any work, whether of the head or hands. I love a broad margin to my life. Sometimes, in a summer morning, having taken my accustomed bath, I sat in my sunny doorway from sunrise till noon, rapt in a revery, amidst the pines and hickories and sumachs, in undisturbed solitude and stillness, while the birds sang around or flitted noiseless through the house, until by the sun falling in at my west window, or the noise of some traveller's wagon on the distant highway, I was reminded of the lapse of time. I grew in those seasons like corn in the night, and they were for me far better than any work of my hands would have been. They were not time subtracted from my life, but so much over and above my usual allowance. I realized what the Orientals mean by contemplation and the forsaking of works.

Like Emerson, Thoreau read the "Orientals" back into his own experiences, to help express that which was inexpressible without them. A journal entry from 1851 states, "Like some other preachers—I have added my texts—(derived) from the Chinese and Hindoo scriptures—long after my discourse was written" (quoted in Hodder, 1993, p. 434). That original inarticulate discourse of ecstasy in nature was capable of transformation with the insights he found in the translations of Jones and Wilkins. It was the here-and-now value of the new language, images, and stories that counted. An emphasis on the moment-to-moment particulars of nature and his own experience was the central concern of his later life. He became, in his own words, a "self-appointed inspector of snowstorms and rainstorms," which is, perhaps, as cogent a description of an alternative practitioner as any from the Eastern traditions.

Although India and, particularly, Hindu thought have taken the prime place in the discussion so far, America's engagement with the East by the middle of the nineteenth century also included East Asian culture, with Chinese, Korean, and Japanese arts, literature, and religion—including the Buddhism of these areas—shaping the intellectual direction of an emerging American modernism. For example, the work of Ernest Fenollosa, American scholar of East Asian art and literature, and convert to Tendai Buddhism, brought this spirit into wider intellectual discourse (Bevis, 1988; Brooks, 1962). Fenollosa represents a more specific, scholarly, but no less engaged, use of the East by an American. A few lines from Fenollossa's poem "East and West," his Phi Beta Kappa address at Harvard in 1892, reflect a growing need of Western thought for contemplative space. Addressing a Japanese mentor, Fenollossa says, "I've flown from my West / Like a desolate bird from a broken nest / To learn thy secret of joy and rest" (quoted in Brooks, 1962, p. 50).

At Fenollossa's death, his widow gave his unpublished studies of the Chinese written language and notebooks of translations from the classical Chinese poet Li Po to the American poet Ezra Pound, for whom a whole new world opened. Pound's Chinese translations drawn from Fenollossa's work radically transformed the art of the time. Indeed,

Pound had arguably the most powerful influence of any single poet in shaping the poetry, not only of his modernist contemporaries, but of the generation that would come to maturity in the middle of the twentieth century.

Although Pound's use of Eastern influences was mainly stylistic, a very different sort of poet, Wallace Stevens, used his own encounter with the East—studying Buddhist texts and translating Chinese poetry with his friend the scholar-poet Witter Bynner—to better understand and express his tacit experience (Bevis, 1988). Perhaps "The Snow Man," an early poem (written in 1908 and first published in 1921), suggests this (Stevens, 1971, p. 54).

The Snow Man, 1908; 1921
—Wallace Stevens

One must have a mind of winter
To regard the frost and the boughs
Of the pine-trees crusted with snow;

And have been cold a long time
To behold the junipers shagged with ice,
The spruces rough in the distant glitter

Of the January sun; and not to think
Of any misery in the sound of the wind,
In the sound of a few leaves,

Which is the sound of the land
Full of the same wind
That is blowing in the same bare place

For the listener, who listens in the snow,
And, nothing himself, beholds
Nothing that is not there and the nothing that is.

One can also cite a description of an alternative, meditative stance, using an image from the poet's Connecticut landscape, and rhetoric from his East Asian studies, perhaps. Yet it is possible that this is *also* an articulation of personal experience. Stevens did not study meditation formally, but, like Thoreau, he was a prodigious walker. In any season or weather, a perambulation of 15 miles or so—in a business suit—was a common prelude to writing (Bevis, 1988). This is neatly captured in a few lines from "Notes for a Supreme Fiction": "Perhaps / The truth depends on a walk around a lake, // A composing as the body tires, a stop / To see hepatica, a stop to watch / A definition growing certain and // A wait within that certainty, a rest / In the swags of pine trees bordering the lake" (Stevens, 1971, p. 212).

A transparent eyeball. An inspector of snowstorms. A mind of winter. These are powerful metaphors to describe experiences that sought and found elaboration through encounters with Eastern thought. For these individuals, there was a willingness to use whatever comes to hand—from whatever culture or tradition suggests itself or is available—to understand what is happening in the here and now. This stance reflects a perennial American pragmatism, which endures today in much of the discourse of complementary and alternative and "integrative" medicine: Hatha Yoga mixes with Buddhist meditation, whereas Sufi poetry and Native American stories illuminate teaching points, and the expressive language of the Christian and Jewish contemplative traditions hovers in the background.

In the same early time frame, a more specific connection to Buddhism began developing, as well. Of the major traditions in the Oriental amalgam, Buddhism appears to have been the least understood and the most scorned during the earlier part of the nineteenth century. Reasons include Christian defensiveness and hostile reporting from the mission field; a portrayal of Buddhist doctrines as atheistic, nihilistic, passive, and pessimistic; and even the contagious anti-Buddhist biases of the Hindu scholars themselves who taught Sanskrit to the English translators of the Asiatic Society of Bengal (Tweed, 1992; Versluis, 1993). The "opening" of Japan to the United States in the 1850s commencing with Commodore Matthew Perry's visit, and the subsequent travels, study, and writing of American artists, scholars, and sophisticates, including Ernest Fenollossa, Henry Adams (great-grandson of the aforementioned John Adams), John LaFarge, and Lafcadio Hearn (all had direct contact with Buddhism) did much to increase interest and sympathy for Buddhism. Then, the 1879 publication of *The Light of Asia,* Edwin Arnold's poetic retelling of the life of the Buddha, drawing parallels with the life of Jesus, turned interest into enthusiasm. Sales estimates of between 500,000 and a million copies put it at a level of popularity matching that of, say, *Huckleberry Finn* (Tweed, 1992) or the number one bestseller of that time, *Ben Hur,* by retired Civil War General and adventurer Lew Wallace.

Buddhism became a new possibility for those at the bare edge of the culture who intuited the tidal shift of Christian believing that Matthew Arnold had poignantly articulated in the final stanzas of "Dover Beach" in 1867.

On Dover Beach with Matthew Arnold, 1867

The Sea of Faith
Was once, too, at the full, and round earth's shore
Lay like the folds of a bright girdle furled.
But now I only hear
Its melancholy, long, withdrawing roar,
Retreating, to the breath
Of the night-wind, down the vast edges drear
And naked shingles of the world

Ah, love, let us be true
To one another! for the world, which seems

On Dover Beach with Matthew Arnold, 1867—cont'd

To lie before us like a land of dreams,
So various, so beautiful, so new,
Hath really neither joy, nor love, nor light,
Nor certitude, nor peace, nor help for pain;
And we are here as on a darkling plain
Swept with confused alarms of struggle and flight,
Where ignorant armies clash by night.

And for some, Buddhist belief became a formal identity. Madame Olga Blavatsky and Henry Steele Olcott, founders of the Theosophical Society (and the alternative practice of Theosophical medicine), were long engaged with Buddhism. In Ceylon in 1880, they made ritual vows in a Theravada temple to live by the five precepts and take refuge in the Buddha, the teachings, and the community. The most powerful event, however, was the face-to-face encounters with Buddhist masters afforded by the Parliament of World Religions, particularly the Theravadin Anagarika Dharmapala and the Rinzai Zen Master Soyen Shaku. Both of these teachers continued to raise interest in Buddhism through subsequent visits. In fact, Soyen Shaku bears significant responsibility for the popularization of Buddhism through the present day. The vision of Buddhism that he presented fit perfectly with the early modern scientific and moral outlooks. The themes he presented—"an embrace of science combined with the promise of something beyond it, and a universal reality in which different religions and individuals participate, but which Buddhism embodies most perfectly" (McMahan, 2002, p. 220)—still resonate. (These themes resonate with contemporary reconciliation of ancient, traditional Ayurvedic precepts with quantum mechanics and fundamental particle physics in the formulations of *Maharishi Ayurveda*.) He also had a "second-generation" impact through the 1950s and 1960s, as he encouraged his student and translator for the Parliament visit, the articulate Zen scholar D.T. Suzuki, to maintain a dialogue with the West through visits and writing (McMahan, 2002; Tweed, 1992).

It is important to note that the character of Buddhist "believing" during this period was an engagement with philosophy and doctrine, a search for a replacement for the Judeo-Christian belief system that some felt was no longer sustaining. Consider that two other Buddhist "bestsellers" beside Arnold's *Light of Asia* were Olcott's *Buddhist Catechism* and Paul Carus's *Gospel of Buddha,* whose titles even reflect a Christian, belief-oriented approach to Buddhism. In the best Evangelical Protestant tradition comes the story of the first "Buddhist conversion" in America. In Chicago in 1893, Dharmapala was speaking on Buddhism and Theosophy to an overflow crowd in a large auditorium. At the end of the talk, Charles Strauss, a Swiss-American businessman of Jewish background, stood up from his seat in the audience and walked deliberately to the front. One can imagine the hush and expectancy. As planned in advance, he then—to use an Evangelical Protestant phrase—"accepted" Buddhism, repeating the refuge vows for all to hear (Obadia, 2002; Tweed, 1992).

The connection of most of the 2000 or 3000 Euro-American Buddhists and the tens of thousands of sympathizers at this time (Tweed, 1992) was, with a few exceptions, intellectual. The popular appeal of Buddhism was as a form of *belief*, not as a form of spiritual *practice*. According to Tweed (1992), the fascination with Buddhist believing reached a high-water mark around 1907 and declined precipitously thereafter. A small nucleus of Euro-Americans interested in the academic or personal study of Buddhism maintained organizations and specialized publishing, but few Asian teachers stayed in the United States, and impetus for growth was lost. Dharmapala, in 1921, wrote in a letter to an American supporter, "At one time there was some kind of activity in certain parts of the U.S. where some people took interest in Buddhism, but I see none of that now" (In Tweed, 1992, p. 157). Charges by the status quo religious and cultural powers that Buddhism was passive and pessimistic—terrible sins in a culture fueling itself on action and optimism—drowned dissenting Buddhist voices (Box 7-1).

In the aftermath of World War II the applications of Eastern thought to Western experience developed a powerful momentum. Western soldiers, many drawn from professional life into active duty, were exposed in great numbers to Asian cultures, from India, Burma, and China. In Japan, physicians, scientists, and artists and intellectuals who held posts in the occupation forces were exposed to a culture that included the aesthetic, philosophical, and spiritual manifestations of Japanese Buddhism, particularly its Zen varieties.

Some stayed to study, and East-West dialogues that had been suspended were resumed, such as with D.T. Suzuki and Shinichi Hisamatsu. Most important for the discourse of mind-body medicine and psychotherapy, American military psychiatrists were exposed to Japanese psychotherapy, particularly that developed by Shoma Morita, which is based on a paradox that had enormous repercussions in Western practice. Instead of attacking symptoms as in Western approaches, Morita asked his patients to allow themselves to turn toward their symptoms and fully experience them, to know them as they are (Dryden et al, 2006; Morita, 1928/1998).

Morita therapy was of interest and intellectually available to those Westerners in Japan for two powerful reasons. First, it is a highly effective treatment for what Western practitioners would identify as anxiety-based disorders; reports of rates of cure or improvement of more than 90% are common (Morita, 1928/1998; Reynolds, 1993). Morita developed a diagnostic category of *shinkeishitsu* for the disorders he targeted, which he describes as anxiety disorders with hypochondriasis (Morita, 1928/1998). Second, Morita did not develop his work in cultural isolation. Working contemporaneously with Charcot, William James, Sigmund Freud, and Carl Gustav Jung, Morita read, referenced, and critiqued Western developments. He was particularly interested in the therapies that paralleled his own in certain ways, such as Freud's psychoanalysis, S. Weir Mitchell's nineteenth-century rest therapy (also rest cure, West cure, and nature cure), Otto Binswanger's life normalization therapy, and Paul DuBois's persuasion therapy (LeVine, 1998). It integrated East and West—from an *Eastern* perspective.

Although the entire regimen of Morita therapy, a four-stage, intensive, residential treatment has rarely been used in the United States—David Reynolds (1980, 1993) has adapted it and other Japanese therapies for the West—two of its basic insights had immediate and continuing effects. The first is the paradox of turning toward rather than away from symptoms for relief. The second is the insistence on the nondual nature of the body and mind. Although the influence of Zen is easily seen in his therapy, Morita did not wish to promote a direct religious association, fearing that the treatment might be seen as somehow less serious, exacting, and effective (LeVine, 1998). Paradoxically, perhaps the Zen connection actually drew the interest of the Westerners.

BOX 7-1

Three Buddhisms in America

It is important to note that the narrative that has shaped the discourse of alternative medical professionals today sidelines the story of ethnic Asian Buddhism in America. Religion scholar Richard Hughes Seager (2002) describes three Buddhisms in America:
1. Old-line Asian-American Buddhism, with institutions dating back into the nineteenth century
2. Euro-American or convert Buddhism, centered in the Westernized forms of Buddhism—often generically parsed as Zen, Tibetan, and Theravada (or Vipassana or Insight), which are centered on meditation practice; and Soka Gakkai International, an American branch of a Japanese group, which with a rich mix of Asian Americans, Euro-Americans, and substantial numbers of African Americans and Latino Americans is the most culturally diverse group and is centered on chanting practice rather than meditation
3. New immigrant or ethnic Buddhism, which is most easily parsed by country of origin

 Morita Therapy: Mushoju-shin and the Stages of Treatment.

In the nutshell version of Morita therapy, the Zen term *mushoju-shin* points to the end, or the beginning. It describes a healthy attention. In Morita's (1928/1998) metaphor, it is the attention you have when you are reading while standing on the train. You must balance,

(Continued)

Morita Therapy: Mushoju-shin and the Stages of Treatment.—cont'd

hold the book, read, remember the next station, and be aware of others. That is, you cannot focus on any one thing too tightly. You must be willing to be unstable, to be open to whatever happens, and to be able to respond and change freely. In short, you are not "self" focused; rather, mind-body-environment are one. "This is the place from where my special therapy begins" (p.31), says Morita. It is also the place that Morita therapists are required to inhabit as they work.

First Stage: Isolation and Rest. (5 to 7 Days)
Disposition: After careful assessment to ensure safety, patients are isolated and asked to remain in a lying down posture, except to use the bathroom.
Instructions: Experience the anxieties and illusions that arise; let them run their course, without trying to change or stop them.
Purpose: There is a Zen saying that if you try to eliminate a wave with another wave, all you get is more waves, more confusion. This becomes clear.

Second Stage: Light Occupational -Work. (5 to 7 Days)
Disposition: Isolation is maintained; there is no conversation or distractions. Sleep is restricted to 7 or 8 hours a night. Patients must be working during the day, and may not return to the room to rest.
Instructions: Move gently into mental and physical activity again, tidying the yard by picking up sticks and leaves, and moving into more effortful activities over time. Allow physical and mental discomfort to be just as it is.
Purpose: Break down the "feeling-centered attitude" by de-emphasizing judgments of comfort and discomfort and promoting spontaneous activity of mind and body.

Third Stage: Intensive Occupational Work. (5 to 7 days)
Disposition: Same as in stage two.
Instructions: Patients are assigned more strenuous labor, such as chopping wood and digging holes, and are encouraged to do art or craft projects that please them and to be spontaneous.
Purpose: Learn to be patient and to endure work, build self-confidence, and own their subjective experiences.

Fourth Stage: Preparation for Daily Living (5 to 7 days)
Disposition: Patients may interact purposefully with others but not to speak of their own experience, and may leave the hospital grounds for errands.
Instructions: The work and activities are not chosen by the patient.
Purpose: Learn to adjust to changes in circumstances; to not be attached to personal preferences. Prepare for return to the natural rhythms of living.

Zen had a double-barreled influence in America, particularly in the postwar "Zen boom" years of the 1950s and 1960s, touching both the intellectual community and the popular culture. With the first barrel, it had significant impact on the serious discourse of scholars, professionals, artists, and Western religious thinkers. One person was so profoundly influential in conveying the spirit of Zen that he epitomizes this impact: D.T. Suzuki. As a young man, you will remember, Suzuki had played a role in the Buddhist enthusiasm of the 1890s and 1900s as translator for Soyen Shaku. Suzuki had then lived for a time in the United States, working for Open Court, a publishing company specializing in Eastern thought, and had married an American woman. After the war, Suzuki returned to the West, where he continued to write books of both scholarly and popular interest on Zen and Pure Land Buddhism, traveled and lectured extensively in the United States and Europe, maintained a voluminous correspondence, and affected an incredibly varied range of thinkers. Three short examples involving Thomas Merton, John Cage, and Eric Fromm give a glimpse into the effects of Suzuki's Zen on intellectual discourse.

The Trappist monk Thomas Merton was greatly influenced by Suzuki's work—which he had first known in the 1930s before entering the monastery. An engagement with Eastern religious and aesthetic thought—particularly Zen, and particularly through Suzuki's work—shaped Merton's conception of and practice of contemplative prayer, which has had a powerful influence on Christian spiritual practice to the present day (e.g., Merton, 1968; Pennington, 1980). Merton began a correspondence with Suzuki in 1959, asking him to write a preface for a book of translations of the sayings of the "Desert Fathers." Merton's superiors felt such collaboration in print was "inappropriate," yet in practice, they encouraged Merton to continue the dialogue with Suzuki, one telling him, "Do it but don't preach it" (Mott, 1984, p. 326). This stance represented a reversal of the earlier Buddhist fusion of *belief* without *practice*. The dialogue did indeed continue, with each endeavoring to explore and understand Christianity and Zen from their own perspectives. The relationship meant so much to Merton that, although his vocation had kept him cloistered in the Monastery of Gethsemane in Kentucky from 1941, he sought and gained permission from his abbot to meet Suzuki in New York City in 1964, Merton's first travel in 23 years (Merton, 1968; Mott, 1984; Pennington, 1980). Suzuki summed up the burden of their two long talks this way: "The most important thing is Love" (Mott, 1984, p. 399).

The composer John Cage, who was deeply influenced by Hindu, Buddhist, and Daoist philosophy and practice, regularly attended Suzuki's lectures at Columbia University in the 1950s. His statement that in choosing to study with Suzuki he was choosing the elite—"I've always gone—insofar as I could—to the president of the company" (Duckworth, 1999, p. 21)—suggests the value of Suzuki's thought to him and to much of the avant garde. The Zen influence on Cage's work is captured in his conception of his compositions as "purposeless play" that is "not an attempt to bring order out of chaos, nor to suggest improvements in creation, but simply to wake up to the very life we are living, which is so excellent once one gets one's mind and desires out of the way and lets it act of its own accord" (Cage, 1966, p. 12). Suzuki's expansive sense of play is reported by Cage (1966) in an anecdote: "An American lady said, 'How is it, Dr. Suzuki? We spend the evening asking you questions and nothing is decided.' Dr. Suzuki smiled and said, 'That's why I love philosophy: no one wins'" (p. 40).

The psychoanalyst Erich Fromm (the author of *Escape from Freedom,* about the attraction of fascism before and during World War II) was one of many in the psychoanalytic community of the time to be drawn to Zen and Suzuki's exposition of it. At a conference held in Mexico in 1957 entitled "Zen Buddhism and Psychoanalysis" and attended by about 50 psychoanalytically inclined psychiatrists and psychologists, Suzuki was a featured speaker and engaged in dialogue particularly with Fromm and the religion scholar Richard DeMartino. A book of the lectures was published after the conference (Fromm et al, 1960). Fromm suggests that psychoanalysis and Zen both offer an answer to the suffering of contemporary people: "The alienation from oneself, from one's fellow man, and from nature; the awareness that life runs out of one's hand like sand, and that one will die without having lived; that one lives in the midst of plenty and yet is joyless" (p. 86). The answer, then, would not be a cure that removes symptoms, but rather "the presence of well being" (p. 86; Fromm's italics). Fromm defines well-being as "to be fully born, to become what one potentially is; it means to have the full capacity for joy and for sadness or, to put it still differently, to awake from the half-slumber the average man lives in, and to be fully awake. If it is all that, it means also to be creative; that is, to react and respond to myself, to others, to everything that exists" (p. 90). For Fromm, the work was not just to bring the unconscious into consciousness, as Freud suggested, but rather to heal the rift between the two. What was most intriguing for Fromm in the possibilities Zen offered for such a project was *koan* practice—the use of paradoxical or nonrational questions, statements, and stories to back the student's ego-bound intellect against a wall, until the only way out is through. This process of amplifying the root contradiction of ego-consciousness, leading to its overturning—*satori,* or enlightenment—was the subject of DeMartino's contribution to the conference and book. Fromm drew a parallel between this process and the work of the analyst, suggesting that the analyst should not so much interpret and explain, but rather should "take away one rationalization after another, one crutch after another, until the patient cannot escape any longer, and instead breaks through the fictions which fill his mind and experiences reality—that is, becomes conscious of something he was not conscious of *before*" (p. 126).

Love, play, and well-being: it was not just Suzuki's erudition that attracted so many, it was his embodiment of what he taught. Alan Watts, the scholar-entertainer to whom we shall turn next, who got to know Suzuki at the Buddhist Lodge in London in the 1920s, described him as "about the most gentle and enlightened person I have ever known; for he combined the most complex learning with utter simplicity. He was versed in Japanese, English, Chinese, Sanskrit, Tibetan, French, Pali, and German, but while attending a meeting at the Buddhist Lodge he would play with a kitten, looking right into its Buddha nature" (Watts, 1972). Suzuki should have the last word on his way of being, and what he wished to communicate to others:

> We cannot all be expected to be scientists, but we are so constituted by nature that we can all be artists—not, indeed, artists of special kinds, such as painters, sculptors, musicians, poets, etc., but artists of life. This profession, "artist of life" may sound new and quite odd, but in point of fact, we are all born artists of life and, not knowing it, most of us fail to be so and the result is that we make a mess of our lives, asking, "What is the meaning of life?" "Are we not facing blank nothingness?" "After living seventy-eight, or even ninety years, where do we go? Nobody knows," etc., etc. I am told that most modern men and women are neurotic on this account. But the Zen-man can tell them that they have all forgotten that they are born artists, creative artists of life, and that as soon as they realize this fact and truth they will all be cured of neurosis or psychosis or whatever name they have for their trouble. (Fromm et al, 1960, p. 15)

Certainly, such a vision of unfettered creativity and immediate relief from the pains of living would be resonant in postwar American culture.

It should be noted, however, that in the 1950s and 1960s, despite his tremendous stature, Suzuki was also criticized—accused by the *academic* Buddhist community of being a reductionist "popularizer" of Zen and dismissed by the *practice* community as one who did not sit in meditation with enough discipline and regularity. On the one hand, these may be valid charges, yet on the other, they may be significant reasons for Suzuki's influence. This was a time when Western intellectuals were in search of new rhetoric and new philosophy to help express and ground their shifting experiences and intuitions; for many, it was a time of wide-ranging dialogue, of exploring possibilities, of framing a debate, rather than a time of grounding, of digging in, of focus on details. Indeed, the charges might simply be moot, when Suzuki's enterprise is cast in the mode of his teacher Soyen Shaku, or even the mode of Ralph Waldo Emerson, of attempting to universalize spiritual experience. In his dialogue with Christian mysticism, for example, Suzuki (1957) found it possible that "Christian experiences are not after all different from those of the Buddhist" (p. 8).

Just as Suzuki epitomized the intellectual reach of the Zen boom, it may be possible to capture the more popular facets of the time and continue the story through the 1960s by focusing on a single character: the transplanted Englishman Alan Watts. Watts's eccentric career as a scholar-entertainer travels a ragged arc from the 1930s to the early 1970s, along the way touching most of the important figures and movements in the meeting of Eastern and Western religious thought and practice, particularly as they offered insights that could be used in psychotherapy. The arc described here is drawn with the help of his autobiography, *In My Own Way* (1972), whose punning title suggests the paradox of sustaining a powerful public self to earn a living while discussing the dissolution of the ego, and Monica Furlong's feet-of-clay biography, whose original title, *Genuine Fake* (1986), carries an ambiguous truth.

An intellectually precocious and sensitive religious seeker, Watts spent his early years at King's School, Canterbury, which is next to the ancient cathedral. There, the history-steeped atmosphere and rich liturgical expression cast a spell and created a love of ritual that never left him. In his adolescent years at the school, he developed an interest in Buddhism, which he was able to defend on a very high level in debates with faculty. He wrote to Christmas Humphries, the great promoter of Buddhism and Theosophy, and the founder of the Buddhist Lodge in London, who assumed the letters were from a faculty member. When they finally met, Humphries became a mentor, providing guidance for reading and practice, and connecting Watts to other Asian scholars, including D.T. Suzuki. By 1935, having foregone an Oxford University scholarship to study what appealed to him, Watts published his first book, written at age 19, *The Spirit of Zen,* which was almost a guidebook to the densities of Suzuki's *Essays on Zen.* Watts's studies expanded, he came to read and write Chinese at a scholarly level, and he read deeply in Daoism, as well as Vedanta, Christian mysticism, and Jung's psychology.

Through the Buddhist Lodge, he met a mother and adolescent daughter, Ruth Fuller Everett and Eleanor. Ruth had been a member of the ashram-cum-zoo, as Watts called it, of Pierre Bernard—known as "Oom the Magnificent"—who catered to the New York society ladies by teaching Hatha Yoga and Tantrism. Through that association, she learned of Zen Buddhism and, taking Eleanor as a traveling companion, set off for Japan. The two became the first Western women to sit in meditation in a Zen monastery. Years later, Ruth married a Zen teacher and eventually became a teacher herself. Watts and Eleanor courted, in a way, and attended meditation sessions together.

Watts's practice at the time was simply to be in the present moment, learned from the independent spiritual teachers J. Krishnamurti (who called it "choiceless awareness") and G.I. Gurdjieff (who called it "constant self-remembering"). He was becoming frustrated with his inability to concentrate on the present and discussed this with Eleanor on their walk home from a session at the Buddhist Lodge. Eleanor said, "Why try to concentrate on it? What else is there to be aware of? Your memories are all in the present, just as much as the trees over there. Your thoughts about the future are also in the present, and anyhow I just love to think about the future. The present is just a constant flow, like the Tao, and there's simply no way of getting out of it" (Watts, 1972, pp. 152-153). That was *it.* He came to think of this as his true

way of life and continued to practice in this way in various guises throughout his lifetime.

The couple married and moved to the United States, just ahead of the war in Europe. After all his resistance and protest, at this point in his development Watts felt drawn to try to fit himself into a vocation that made sense in the West. With his rich Anglican background, the logical choice was the priesthood of the Episcopal Church. Although he had no undergraduate degree, Watts proved the depth of his learning and entered Seabury-Western Seminary in Chicago for a 2-year course of study. In his second year, his standing was so far advanced that he was excused from classes and undertook expansive theological reading in personal tutorials. His researches resulted in the book *Behold the Spirit,* which brought insights from the Eastern religions into profound dialogue with a Christianity he painted as in need of refreshment. Reviewers in and outside the church greeted it warmly. Ordained, he was made chaplain of Northwestern University, where his feeling for ritual, his skills as a speaker, and his ability to throw a great party brought quick success. Yet tensions in his growing family and his own tendency for excess ended his career; the church in 1950 did not take affairs and divorce lightly.

With a new wife and no job, Watts's prospects were indeed uncertain as he began work on a new book, *The Wisdom of Insecurity* (1951). An influential friend, Joseph Campbell, managed to get Watts a grant from the Bollingen Foundation, funded by one of C.G. Jung's wealthy patients, to support research on myth, psychology, and Oriental philosophy. The book, fueled perhaps by the indigence and indignities of his situation, brought him to the directness and clarity of expression that characterize his work from here on. Here is a description of working with pain by trusting that the mind "has give and can absorb shocks like water or a cushion" (p. 96):

> How does the mind absorb suffering? It discovers that resistance and escape—the "I" process—is a false move. The pain is inescapable, and resistance as a defense only makes it worse; the whole system is jarred by the shock. Seeing the impossibility of this course, it must act according to its nature—remain stable and absorb.
>
> . . . Seeing that there is no escape from the pain, the mind yields to it, absorbs it, and becomes conscious of just pain without any "I" feeling it or resisting it. It experiences pain in the same complete, unselfconscious way in which it experiences pleasure. Pain is the nature of this present moment, and I can only live in this moment. . . .
>
> This, however, is not an experiment to be held in reserve, as a trick, for moments of crisis. . . . This is not a psychological or spiritual discipline for self-improvement. It is simply being aware of this present experience, and realizing that you can neither define it nor divide yourself from it. There is no rule but "Look!" (pp. 97-99)

In no time, Watts landed on his feet, invited into a position at the founding of the American Academy of Asian Studies in San Francisco, a precursor of today's California Institute of Integral Studies. He also landed in creative ferment. Instead of business people and diplomatic and government officials learning Asian languages and culture that were the anticipated students, the academy drew artists, poets, and religious and philosophical thinkers who were open to the kind of exploration for which Watts and his faculty colleagues had prepared their whole lives. Students included the Beat poet Gary Snyder, with whom Watts struck up a deep friendship; Michael Murphy and Richard Price, who would found *Esalen Institute;* and Locke McCorkle, who would become a force in *est* (Erhard Seminars Training). As Watts added administrative duties to his teaching, he brought in an amazing range of guest lecturers, old friends such as D.T. Suzuki; his ex-mother-in-law Ruth Fuller Sasaki, who spoke on Zen koan practice; Pali scholar G.P. Malalasekera and Theravada Buddhist monks Pannananda and Dharmawara; and the Zen master Asahina Sogen. As the academy found its place in the community, local connections were made with Chinese and Japanese Buddhists. Through the academy, the Zen Master Shunryu Suzuki came to understand the need for a Western Zen institution, later creating the San Francisco Zen Center. Watts himself spoke and gave workshops up and down the West Coast and began a relationship with the Berkeley radio station KPFA, the first community-funded station in the United States, broadcasting regularly and appearing as well on the educational television station KQED. He was stirring what was fermenting and that would soon distill itself as a kind of renaissance.

The core of the Beat writers coalesced for a moment in 1956 in San Francisco, and Jack Kerouac captured it in his novel *The Dharma Bums* (1958). Its central character is the poet and Zen student Japhy Ryder (Gary Snyder), whom the narrator Ray Smith (Kerouac) idolizes for his "Zen lunatic" lifestyle, combining Zen discipline and aesthetics with freewheeling sensuality. One scene in the novel recounts the Six Gallery poetry reading, at which Snyder, Philip Whalen, Michael McClure, and Philip Lamantia read, and Allen Ginsberg's incantation of *Howl* did, indeed, scream for a generation about the agonies of 1950s fear and conformity (and fear of conformity, and conformity as a form of dealing with fear). *The Dharma Bums,* coming fast on the heels of Kerouac's bestselling *On the Road* (1957), drew a huge readership of the young and aspiring hip, who saw in Ryder/Snyder a new template for living, a chance to go beyond the confines of suburban expectations. This fueled the Zen boom from the popular culture side, prompting complaints from the Western Zen community of practitioners and academics about the authenticity of the Beats' Buddhism. Both the popular and elite outlooks drew a chastening commentary from Watts in his essay "Beat Zen, Square Zen, and Zen" (1958/1960), as he showed that their differences arose from the same fundamental background and impulse:

> The Westerner who is attracted to Zen and who would understand it deeply must have one indispensable qualification: he must understand his own culture so thoroughly that he is no longer swayed by its premises unconsciously. He must really have come to terms with the Lord God Jehovah and with his Hebrew-Christian conscience so that he can take it or leave it without fear or rebellion. He must be free of the itch to justify himself. Lacking this, his Zen will be either "beat" or "square," either a revolt from the culture and social order or a new form of stuffiness and respectability. For Zen is above all the liberation of the mind from conventional thought, and this is something utterly different from rebellion against convention, on the one hand, or adapting to foreign conventions, on the other. (p. 90)

Watts, already a friend and admirer of Snyder, whom he exempted from his criticisms due to Snyder's level of Zen scholarship and practice, soon came to count the rest of the Beats as friends and accepted many of them as "serious artists and disciplined yogis" (Watts, 1972, p. 358). He had connections to many seemingly disparate worlds. There were old guard spiritual seekers, like expatriate friend Aldous Huxley; members of the highest circles of art, music, and literature; Asian meditation teachers from many different traditions and cultures; psychotherapists of every stripe; and the old guard bohemians, the Beats, and the students. All of whom, as the 1960s began, would come together to create a culture into which Watts was not fitted, but built.

A catalyst of the new culture in the revolutionary 1960s was the beginning of experimentation with lysergic acid diethylamide (LSD) and other psychedelic drugs in the 1950s, and the publicity surrounding it. Aldous Huxley's descriptions of his experiences in *The Doors of Perception* (1954) were illuminating, but for Watts, it was about embodiment—that his once ascetic and severe "Manichean" friend had been transformed into a more sensuous and warm man made the promise real. Watts's own controlled experiments, in which he found his learning and understanding of the world's mystical traditions and meditative practices extremely helpful, resulted in powerful experiences, followed (inevitably) by enthusiastic essays and broadcasts, as well as by a book, *Joyous Cosmology: Adventures in the Chemistry of Consciousness* (1962). His position as a proponent of the drugs for experienced, disciplined explorers of consciousness helped fan an interest—the more so when Watts coincidentally was given a 2-year fellowship at Harvard just as Timothy Leary and Richard Alpert (later Ram Das) were beginning their engagement with psychedelics. The spread of psychedelics beyond the specialists added a key facet to what Roszak (1969) dubbed the "counterculture": "It strikes me as obvious beyond dispute, that the interests of our college-age and adolescent young in the psychology of alienation, oriental mysticism, psychedelic drugs, and communitarian experiments comprise a cultural constellation that radically diverges from values and assumptions that have been in the mainstream of our society since at least the Scientific Revolution of the seventeenth century" (quoted in Furlong, 1986, p. 143).

Just as the 1950s Zen boom can be captured in the Fromm-Suzuki meeting in Mexico in 1957, the 1960s can, perhaps, be captured in a meeting—admittedly much larger—the "Human Be-In" at the polo field in Golden Gate Park, San Francisco, in 1967. A procession led by Snyder, Ginsberg, and Watts, among others, circumambulated the field as in a Hindu or Buddhist rite to open the day. Tens of thousands found their way there, dressed in colorful finery, raising banners, dropping acid, listening to the Grateful Dead, Jefferson Airplane, and Quicksilver Messenger Service, and digging the mix of the crowd—Timothy Leary and Richard Alpert, political radical Jerry Rubin, Zen Master Shunryu Suzuki, and activist-comedian Dick Gregory suggest the organizers' intention to unify "love and activism." The be-in became a model for gatherings around the United States and the world. The color, light, and promise of the day were captured by Paul Kantner of Jefferson Airplane in "Won't You Try/Saturday Afternoon" (Kantner, 1967). The soaring harmonies and instrumental arrangement convey a fuller experience; but if you cannot listen, try to visualize the following stanza:

> Saturday afternoon,
> Yellow clouds rising in the noon,
> acid, incense and balloons;
> Saturday afternoon,
> people dancing everywhere,
> Loudly shouting "I don't care!"
> It's a time for growing,
> and a time for knowing love . . .

And another shift had already begun. At the leading edge of cultural change, seekers had learned what was to be learned from psychedelic experience and were turning toward the practice of meditation. As Watts (1972) put it in his unique blend of the pontifical and the plain, "When one has received the message, one hangs up the phone" (p. 402). Where an infrastructure for teaching and practice of Zen Buddhism already existed, such as in San Francisco, seekers turned in that direction, following Watts and Snyder. Another infrastructure had also been building, since 1959, using a mass marketing model to encompass much of the Western world: the Maharishi Mahesh Yogi's Transcendental Meditation (TM). This was an adaptation of Hindu mantra meditation for Western practitioners, in which the meditator brought the mind to a single pointed focus by repeating a word or phrase—in TM, the mantra was secret, potently exotic, and specially chosen for the meditator (Johnston, 1988; Mahesh Yogi, 1963). The Beatles, among many other celebrities, discovered (or were "recruited" into) TM in 1967, which brought it to prominence on the world stage. (When the Beatles invited one of the Hindu yogis to visit London, he responded, "London? I am London.") The connection seemed direct. Perhaps the psychedelic experience linked more directly to Hindu meditation than to Zen, as well. Watts (1972) describes this from his own experience: "LSD had brought me into an undeniably mystical state of consciousness. But oddly, considering my absorption in Zen at the time, the flavor of these experiences was Hindu rather than Chinese. Somehow the atmosphere of Hindu mythology slid into them, suggesting at the same time that Hindu philosophy was a local form of a sort of undercover wisdom, inconceivably ancient, which everyone knows at the back of his mind but will not admit" (p. 399). TM was able aggressively to take advantage of the publicity available to it. In 1965, there were 350 TM meditators in the United States, and by 1968, there were 26,000; by 1972, there were 380,000; and by 1976, there were 826,000. (Later Deepak Chopra was able to vault onto the *New York Times* bestseller list with appropriated ancient Ayurvedic wisdom by asking each of the TM meditators to buy 10 copies of his first book.) The marketing strategy targeted specific populations, giving the practice and its benefits a spiritual spin, a political change spin, or a pragmatic self-help spin depending on the target. The pragmatic approach, designed to reach the middle class, middle-management heart of the market, was given impetus through scientific research into TM's physical and psychological outcomes (e.g., Seeman et al, 1972; Wallace, 1970), which subsequently captured the attention of the medical establishment. The result was development of and research on medicalized versions, such as the relaxation response (Benson, 1975) and clinical standardized meditation (Carrington, 1998). The factors at work here—translation into Western language and settings, popular recognition, adoption within scientific research in powerful institutions, and the use of sophisticated marketing and public relations techniques—represent a model for success in the building of new social movements (Johnston, 1988).

On both the substantive and popular levels, then, the market for Eastern and Eastern-inflected spiritual practices grew steadily. Looking from 1972 back to himself in 1960, Watts provides perspective on this growth:

> In my work of interpreting Oriental ways to the West I was pressing a button in expectation of a buzz, but instead there was an explosion. Others, of course, were pressing buttons on the same circuit, but I could not have believed—even in 1960—that [there would be] a national television program on yoga, that numerous colleges would be giving courses on meditation and Oriental philosophy for undergraduates, that this country would be supporting thriving Zen monasteries and Hindu *ashrams,* that the *I Ching* would be selling in hundreds of thousands, and that—wonder of wonders—sections of the Episcopal church would be consulting me about contemplative retreats and the use of mantras in liturgy. (1972, p. 359)

At the turn of the decade of the 1960s, through political dislocations, waves of immigration, and economic opportunism, new teachers from many of the Eastern traditions became available to offer instruction in the

West. At the same time, Westerners of the post–World War II cohort who studied in the East, or with Eastern teachers in the West, began to find their own approaches and voices for teaching as well.

The 1970s were a time of institution building on an unprecedented scale, a time in which, for example, Buddhism in America took its essential shape. Watts only flashed on this, only saw the promised land from afar. He died in 1973, at age 58, of a heart attack. His health had been in decline for some time, due to overwork and problems with alcohol. And in that, his example was again prophetic—foreshadowing the revelations in the 1980s of many spiritual teachers' feet of clay.

THE WEST WENT A LONG WAY TO FIND WHAT IT LEFT AT HOME

The injunctions to relieve suffering and to live a more integrated, creative life by paying attention to what is arising in the present moment and turning toward discomfort—mindfulness and acceptance—are easily located within the three Abrahamic religions, the ones closest to home. But the encrustation of tradition and the carelessness of familiarity hide them quite well.

In Judaism, there is the marvelous text from Ecclesiastes (3:1-8), given here in the King James Version, which may ring in your ears with the "To everything turn, turn, turn" motion of the chorus of the song by Pete Seeger.

> To every thing there is a season, and a time to every purpose under the heaven: a time to be born, and a time to die; a time to plant, and a time to pluck up that which is planted; a time to kill, and a time to heal; a time to break down, and a time to build up; a time to weep, and a time to laugh; a time to mourn, and a time to dance; a time to cast away stones, and a time to gather stones together; a time to embrace, and a time to refrain from embracing; a time to get, and a time to lose; a time to keep, and a time to cast away; a time to rend, and a time to sew; a time to keep silence, and a time to speak; a time to love, and a time to hate; a time of war, and a time of peace.

There is also the tradition that everything should be blessed. Indeed, when one hears good news the blessing traditionally said is, "Blessed are you G-d, Sovereign of the Universe (who is) good and does good." On hearing bad news such as the death of a friend or relative one says, "Blessed are you G-d, Sovereign of the Universe, true judge." Such blessings acknowledge G-d as the source of everything, good or bad (Kravitz, 2008). In Christianity, the natural mode for many is to do for others, to focus outward. This "Letter to a Christian Lady" from C.G. Jung (who had carved over the doorway of his home in Zurich, "summoned or unsummoned, G-d will be there"), which was made into a text for speaking by Jean Vanier (2005, pp. 63-64), is a refreshing corrective:

> I admire Christians,
>   because when you see someone who is hungry or thirsty,
>   You see Jesus.
>   When you welcome a stranger, someone who is "strange,"
>   you welcome Jesus.
>   When you clothe someone who is naked, you clothe Jesus.
>   What I do not understand, however,
>   is that Christians never seem to recognize Jesus
>   in their own poverty.
>   You always want to do good to the poor outside you
>   and at the same time you deny the poor person
>   living inside you.
>   Why can't you see Jesus in your own poverty,
>   in your own hunger and thirst?
>   In all that is "strange" inside you:
>   in the violence and the anguish that are beyond your control!
>   You are called to welcome all this, not to *deny* its existence,
>   but to accept that it is there and to met Jesus *there*.

The Christian contemplative teacher Richard Rohr (1999) suggests that, for him, Jesus' refusal of the drugged wine as he hung on the cross is a model of the radical acceptance of what is happening in the moment (Box 7-2).

Growth and definition of Buddhism in America occurred as a great variety of teaching and practice became available as the turn away from psychedelic culture to more disciplined and thoughtful practice began as the 1960's

---

BOX 7-2

Rumination by Sufi Poet Rumi

The Sufi poet Rumi makes the injunction for acceptance come alive in "The Guest House," a poem translated by Coleman Barks (1995, p. 109) that has become a very common teaching:

This being human is a guest house.
Every morning a new arrival.

A joy, a depression, a meanness,
some momentary awareness comes
as an unexpected visitor

Welcome and entertain them all!
Even if they are a crowd of sorrows,
who violently sweep your house
empty of its furniture,
still, treat each guest honorably.
He may be clearing you out
for some new delight.

The dark thought, the shame, the malice,
meet them at the door laughing and invite them in.

Be grateful for whatever comes,
because each has been sent
as a guide from beyond.

waned. There was a range of Eastern and Western teachers in Hindu, Buddhist, Sufi, and the independent and occult traditions. There were new takes on Western traditions such as the Jesus People or Jesus Freak manifestation of Christianity, and the resurgence of interest in the mysticism of Kabbalah in Judaism. Yet, in tracing the discourse of mindfulness, by far the most influential tradition was Buddhism. This turn-of-the-decade moment is a fruitful place to focus, as all of the elements at play today came into view.

This was a time of growth. For example, the San Francisco Zen Center, which had been started for Western students under the teaching of Shunryu Suzuki Roshi in 1961, expanded in 1967 to include a country retreat center at Tassajara Hot Springs, for which more than a thousand people had contributed money; and by 1969, the center had moved to larger quarters in the city and had established a series of satellite locations. The Zen presence in the United States was the most well established, whereas Tibetan and Theravada-derived teaching and practice infrastructures were in earlier developmental stages. It is these three traditions, generalized, that represent the shape that Buddhism in America has taken.

The task of characterizing and defining something that could be called *American Buddhism* is an enormous task, because it requires the parsing of, at a minimum, two phenomena under that title. Prebish (1999) suggests that identifying two divisions approximating "Asian immigrant Buddhism" and "American convert Buddhism" can be informative; it should be noted, however, that there is considerable disagreement among researchers about how and if such distinctions can be made. For our purposes it might reasonably be said that the former group is more interested in preserving religious and community traditions, whereas the latter is more interested in transforming religious traditions for an elite population.

That American convert Buddhism is the preserve of an elite is indisputable and is an extremely important factor in the development of the popularity of alternative medicine. The group is highly educated, economically advantaged, politically and socially liberal, and overwhelmingly of European descent. This was as true of the crowd at the World Parliament of Religions in 1893, as it was of the students and intellectuals who made the shift from psychedelic experience to meditative experience, and as it is now of the medical, mental health care, and other professionals exploring the roots of alternative medicine. Indeed, there is a continuity not just of types, but of persons (Coleman, 2001; Nattier, 1998).

The signal characteristic of the American converts is a focus on meditation, almost to the exclusion of other forms of Buddhist practice and expression (Prebish, 1999). It is not surprising, then, that the expressions of world Buddhism they have "imported" for their use (as Nattier, 1998, would characterize it) are the meditation-rich Zen, Tibetan, and Theravada-derived traditions. A quick overview of the development and essential practice of each in the United States may be of value.

Zen was the first wave and the "boom" of Buddhism in America. In keeping with the elite nature of American interest, the highly aristocratic Rinzai sect, represented by Soyen Shaku and D.T. Suzuki, was influential until the 1960s. Rinzai emphasizes *koan* practice leading to *satori* or *kensho*—concentrating on a paradoxical question or story to heighten intensity and anxiety until a breakthrough occurs. This is central in the dialogues of D.T. Suzuki, Fromm, and DeMartino, for example. In the 1960s, however, the more popular Soto Zen sect began to reach out of the Japanese American communities to American converts. Two of the most important figures in this shift and in the development of Buddhism in America, are from this community: Shunryu Suzuki and Taizan Maezumi. Maezumi Roshi founded the Zen Center of Los Angeles in 1967 to reach Western students. He was in the Harada-Yasutani lineage, which includes koan practice and significant intensity and push for enlightenment. Two Western teachers were also part of this lineage and began their teaching at this same period: Robert Aitken founded the Diamond Sangha in Hawaii in 1959, and Philip Kapleau founded the Rochester Zen Center in 1966. Shunryu Suzuki Roshi of the San Francisco Zen Center was of a more traditional Soto lineage and presented an approach that must have clashed with what most of his students would have read or known about Zen. His focus was not on enlightenment but on what he presented as the heart of the matter, just sitting. That is, "Our zazen is just to be ourselves. We should not expect anything—just be ourselves and continue this practice forever" (quoted in Coleman, 2001, p. 71). Zen in its original Chinese form, Chan, as well as Korean (Son) and Vietnamese (Thien) forms, arrived much later in the United States. Yet, teachers such as the Korean Seung Sahn, and the Vietnamese Thich Nhat Hahn have had significant influences on Buddhism in America—particularly the genuine witness of "engaged Buddhism" advocate Thich Nhat Hahn, who was nominated for the Nobel Peace Prize by Martin Luther King, Jr., for his peace work during the Vietnam War.

The foundational teachers mentioned here have authorized others to carry on their lineage of teaching. These others have often gone on to found their own centers. Some have hewn closely to their teachers' approaches, whereas others have continued to make adaptations to bring Zen to more Americans. To suggest the flavor of this process, in the Maezumi line, John Daido Loori founded Zen Mountain Monastery in Mount Tremper, New York, keeping more toward traditional monastic training, yet creating a highly advanced computer-based communications and marketing infrastructure. Bernard Glassman Roshi, Maezumi's heir, has extended not simply Zen training, but a deeply felt social engagement, from highly successful initiatives to bring education and employment opportunities to the homeless in Yonkers to the founding of the Zen Peacemaker Order (Prebish, 1999; Queen, 2002). In Kapleau's line, Toni Packer, who had been his successor in Rochester, became disillusioned by the traditional hierarchy and protocols and left that all behind to form an independent center with a Zen spirit all but devoid of the tradition—including that of lineage (Coleman, 2001; McMahan, 2002).

If it were possible to characterize "typical" Zen practice, one might see most of the following (Coleman, 2001; Prebish, 1999): protocols for meeting teachers and entering and leaving meditation halls, including bowing; chanting, often in the original Asian language; ceremonial marking of changes in status, anniversaries of events, and the like; and a meditative engagement with manual work around the center. Central to Zen is the sitting practice, *zazen*, in which the adherence to correct physical posture is considered extremely important. Initial instruction may be to count one's breaths—say, to 10—and, when the attention has wandered, just to notice that this has happened and begin the count again. When capacity for concentration has grown, one may begin *shikantaza*, "just sitting" with full awareness, without directing the mind (Coleman, 2001; Suzuki, 1970). Retreats, or *sesshins*, are intensely focused on sitting meditation, with short periods of walking meditation in between; retreats are rarely longer than 7 days.

Tibetan teachers began to leave Tibet in response to the Chinese repression in the 1950s that killed or drove more than a third of the population into exile. Buddhism's central role in the culture made teachers and monastics a major target. While a few scholars had come to the United States in the 1950s—notably Geshe Wangal, Robert Thurman's first teacher—it was not until 1969 that Tibetan teachers reached out seriously to American students. Tarthang Tulku established the Tibetan Nyingma Meditation Center in Berkeley. The basic approach was very traditional, with students asked to undertake hundreds of thousands of prostrations, vows, and visualizations before meditation instruction is given. Tarthang Tulku created the Human Development Training Program to teach Buddhist psychology and meditation techniques to a professional health care and mental health care audience, and created as well the Nyingma Institute to support Buddhist education and study. In 1971, Kalu Rinpoche, who had been asked by the Dalai Lama to teach in North America, came first to Vancouver to start a center and later created a center in Woodstock, New York (Coleman, 2001; Seager, 2002).

Chogyam Trungpa, who had escaped from Tibet to India in 1959, came to the West to study at Oxford University; during the years he spent in the United Kingdom, he moved away from the traditional monastic teaching role and eventually gave up his vows. In 1970, as a lay teacher, he came to the United States, where he had an instant effect. He had arrived after the "boom," after the Beats, but "Beat Zen" described him better than any type of Zen master. Allen Ginsberg became a student, and many of the original Beat contingent taught at the Naropa Institute (now Naropa University) in Boulder, Colorado, which Trungpa founded. The appeal to the counterculture was swift and far reaching. In a very short time, he created a thoroughgoing infrastructure, including a network of practice centers (now worldwide) and developed a "secular path" called "Shambhala Training," to make the benefits of meditation practice and Buddhist psychological insights more available. Trungpa's approach to teaching was not the traditional one, but an amalgam that included much that he had learned from his Oxford education in comparative religion as well as wide-ranging exposure to Western psychology, which flavor finds its way into the new translations offered by Shambhala Publications. He not only powerfully shaped Tibetan Buddhism in the West, he offered spiritual perceptions that had a much wider reach—particularly the idea of "spiritual materialism," which he defined in this way: "The problem is that ego can convert anything to its own use, even spirituality. Ego is constantly attempting to acquire and apply the teachings of spirituality for its own benefit" (Trungpa, 1973).

Tibetan Buddhist practice in America is richly varied; characterizing it in a paragraph is a hopeless challenge. It is the most exotic and sensual of the three traditions under consideration. The iconography and rituals are complex; the teachers are often Tibetan, rather than Westerners as is common in the other traditions. There is considerable emphasis on textual study. The ritual relationship of student to teachers is hierarchical and devotional. Many of the difficult issues of "belief" that are subdued in the other traditions are right at the surface in Tibetan doctrine and practice—karma, rebirth, realms of supernatural beings. And the practices themselves are guarded, only revealed by initiation, face to face with an authorized teacher. Vajryana or tantric practice, roughly conceived, includes visualization by the meditator of himself or herself with the attributes of a particular enlightened being. Less traditional teachers work differently. Trungpa began his students with sitting meditation much like that of his friend Shunryu Suzuki. The *dzogchen* teachers have an approach that seems easily accessible to Western students, a formless meditation akin to shikantaza in Zen. Within the tradition, this is considered a high teaching, available only after years of preparation. In the West, however, it is offered differently. Lama Surya Das, a Westerner, explains: "One surprise is that people are a lot more prepared than one thinks. Westerners are sophisticated psychologically, but illiterate nomads (as in Tibet) are not" (quoted in Coleman, 2001, p. 109). Retreats in the Tibetan tradition may be adapted for Americans as day long or weeks long, or as more traditional lengths such as 3 months or 3 years.

Vipassana meditation is the latest tradition to flower in North America. It is drawn from Theravada Buddhist practice, the tradition most directly connected to the historical Buddha, and perhaps the most conservative. Theravada was an early and profound influence on the development of Buddhism in the United Kingdom and Europe, dating back to the nineteenth century, through colonial connections. In the United States, the connection came much later, in the Buddhist Vihara Society of Washington, DC, founded in 1966, with teachers Dickwela Piyananda and Henepola Gunaratana, and also as young Americans in the Peace Corps or traveling in southern Asia in the 1960s came into contact with Theravada teachers, such as Mahasi Sayadaw, S.N. Goenka, and U Ba Khin. The influential Vipassana or Insight movement in the United States can be said to have begun when two of those young Americans, Joseph Goldstein and Jack Kornfield, came together to teach Vipassana at Chogyam Trungpa's request at Naropa Institute in 1974. Their connection, which also included Goldstein's friend Sharon Salzberg, another of the travelers to become a teacher, deepened. In 1975, under their leadership, the Insight Meditation Society (IMS) was founded, in rural Barre, Massachusetts. IMS grew quickly into a major retreat center, as the Insight approach found broad appeal. In 1984, Jack Kornfield left IMS for California to found Spirit Rock Meditation Center, which quickly became a second wing in American Vipassana practice (Coleman, 2001; Fronsdal, 2002; Prebish, 1999).

The Insight movement is the most egalitarian and least historically conditioned of the three traditions under consideration. Ritual, ceremony, and hierarchy are deemphasized, and meditation is of central importance. In contrast to Zen orderliness and Tibetan richness, there is ordinariness and a very American democratic, individualistic atmosphere. Students and teachers alike wear casual clothes and are known by first names. Teachers are less authority figures than "spiritual friends," and language is more psychological than specifically Buddhist. Vipassana is highly psychologized; in fact, many, if not a majority, of Vipassana teachers in the Insight movement are trained psychotherapists.

Meditation practice commonly includes two forms, concentration on the breath and open awareness (insight) of whatever is arising in the moment. Practices for cultivating loving kindness, as well as compassion, sympathetic joy, and equanimity, are also a part of training. Retreats are commonly 10 days in length, with long days of intense practice in silence. A typical schedule would find retreatants rising at 5:00 in the morning and moving through periods of sitting and walking (walking periods are as long as sitting periods, in contrast to the short breaks in Zen) with breaks for meals, until 10:00 in the evening (Coleman, 2001; Fronsdal, 2002; Prebish, 1999).

Perhaps most important for the discourse is not the differences in these three traditions, but rather the essential similarities. Stephen Batchelor (1994) neatly summarizes:

> The distinctive goal of any Buddhist contemplative tradition is a state in which inner calm (*samatha*) is *unified* with insight (*vipassana*). Over the centuries, each tradition has developed its own methods for actualizing this state. And it is in these methods that the traditions differ, *not* in their end objective of unified calm and insight.

If the 1960s and 1970s were the period of foundation and growth, the 1980s and 1990s could be seen as the painful passage to maturity. In the many Buddhist centers around the United States, large but intimate communities had grown up, often with charismatic leaders. In most instances, the sharp discipline of Asian monastic practice, with celibacy and renunciation at its core, had been replaced by more casual, worldly, "extended family" types of community. As Suzuki Roshi told the San Francisco Zen Center, and Downing (2001) construed as a warning, "You are not monks, and you are not lay people" (p. 70). There was no map, as communities sought ways forward. Perhaps the scandals around sexuality, alcohol, finances, and power that began to plague these institutions could not have been avoided and were necessary in catalyzing change. By 1988, Jack Kornfield could write, "Already upheavals over teacher behavior and abuse have occurred at dozens (if not the majority) of the major Buddhist and Hindu centers in America" (quoted in Bell, 2002). None of the three traditions was spared. A précis of a scandal from each will help illustrate the commonality of the problems and the importance of their aftermaths and resolutions.

At the San Francisco Zen Center, Suzuki Roshi appointed Richard Baker his successor, not just as abbot but as principal authority over the entire enterprise, which included associated meditation centers and successful businesses such as the Tassajara Bakery and Greens Restaurant. Following Suzuki's death in 1971, Baker held a tight rein over the institution, with little input from board members or other authorized teachers. In 1983, the board called a meeting, and the outcome was Baker's taking a leave of absence. This was precipitated by an incident in which it became obvious that Baker, married himself, was having a sexual relationship with a married female student—indeed, the wife of a friend and benefactor. This was not an unprecedented situation; Baker had a considerable history of infidelities with students. There was more: in a community in which the residents willingly worked long hours for low wages, Baker spent more than $200,000 in a year, drove a BMW, and had his personal spaces impeccably furnished with antiques and artwork. Further, Baker had surrounded himself with an inner circle of "courtiers" and failed to treat other senior members who had been ordained by Suzuki Roshi as valued peers. The most painful thing for the community was Baker's reaction: he did not comprehend that he had done anything wrong. More than 10 years after "the apocalypse," as it came to be known, he stated, "It is as hard to say what I have learned as it is to say what happened" (quoted in Bell, 2002, p. 236; Downing, 2001).

In Chogyam Trungpa Rinpoche's organization, excess was framed as "crazy wisdom" and accepted by many; in fact, failure to accept it was characterized as failure to understand the teaching. Trungpa's sexual liaisons with female students, his destructive meddling in students' lives and relationships, his drunkenness, and his aggressive, even violent outbursts were well known. He was both open and unapologetic about his behavior (Bell, 2002, Clark, 1980, Coleman, 2001). Trungpa chose a Westerner, Osel Tendzin, as his heir. When Trungpa died in 1987, Tendzin became what amounted to supreme ruler of the enterprise, holding untouchable spiritual and executive power. In 1988, it was revealed to members that Tendzin had tested positive for human immunodeficiency virus and that, although he was aware of his condition, he had continued to have unprotected sex with male and female members. Not only had Tendzin known of his condition, but board members had known as well and had kept silent (Bell, 2002, Coleman, 2001). Tendzin, at the urging of a senior Tibetan teacher, went into retreat and died soon after.

At the end of an IMS retreat taught by an Asian Theravada teacher, Anagarika Munindra, a woman came forward to say that she had had sex with the teacher during the retreat. The woman had been psychologically troubled, and this had traumatized her further. The IMS guiding teachers were divided as to how to handle the situation—how much to reveal publicly, and how to deal with Munindra, who had returned to India. Kornfield pushed for complete disclosure and an immediate confronting of Munindra. As he put it, "If parts of one's life are quite unexamined—which was true for all of us—and something like this comes up about a revered teacher, it throws everything you've been doing for years into doubt. It's threatening to the whole scene" (quoted in Schwartz, 1995, p. 334). Eventually, Kornfield was sent by the board to India to speak directly with Munindra, who agreed to apologize to the community.

In the aftermath and resolution of all of these incidents, American Buddhism lost its idealized self-image and came to the maturity it carries now. In this process common themes and practices arose. Leadership power moved away from the charismatic models and was rationalized and distributed more widely, with checks and balances, and boards accountable for oversight. Ethics were addressed formally with statements and policies. The model of teacher-student interaction was scrutinized, and methods for diluting intensity were developed and instituted, as possible. Of course, this remains the most difficult of all relationships to manage, because meditation training carries the teacher-student dyad into areas of intimacy and power differential analogous to those in psychotherapy.

A universalizing and secularizing discourse draws together four themes. The first theme is the need for an expanded vocabulary of words, images, and ideas with which to express tacit experience. As more experience comes into shared language—verbal or nonverbal—the possibilities for teaching expand. The second theme is the drive for universalizing of the experiences and language surrounding them. This may emerge as explicitly spiritual language, as with Emerson or D.T. Suzuki, or in more secular language, as in the mindfulness-based interventions. The third theme, more specific, is the discovery or rediscovery of the principle of turning *toward* suffering and taking on the attitude of acceptance. This is a universal insight that is both spiritual and psychological in nature, and suggests that such a distinction is of little expressive value. As the verbal and nonverbal discourse of mindfulness continues to expand, universalize, and secularize, the potentials for teaching expand as well. But this is only possible if the fourth theme is considered: the fact that this discourse is predominantly a product of an elite social group, with significant socioeconomic advantages and a level of education that is "right off the charts" (Coleman, 2001, p. 193). As professionals and members of an elite, we teach from our own experience and give voice to it in language that may reflect that elite position. Therefore, we must continually be sensitive to, and learn from, the language of our clients, patients, and students.

One window into the possibilities of expanding discourse is suggested in the work of the postmodern theologian Don Cupitt (1999), who undertook an exercise in "ordinary language" theology. He collected and analyzed more than 150 idiomatic expressions in English that use the term *life*. His hypothesis was that these idioms have arisen as the overall population's reaction to the shifts in religion or spirituality from the mid-nineteenth century onward—the era of the development of the East-West discourse under consideration. He suggests that for a great many people, *life* has become the privileged religious object. Consider, for example, the switch since the mid-twentieth century from funerals oriented toward the deceased's place in the hereafter to a "celebration of the life of" the deceased. It might be said of the deceased that "she loved life." Phrases like "the sanctity of life," "the value of life," "the quality of life" have become current since the 1950s; in fact, in health care, there are scales to measure "quality of life." And then there is the imperative phrase "Get a life!" that became so popular in the 1990s. What are its implications as a spiritual phrase?

The usual rhetoric about spirituality and religion in contemporary Western culture is that it has been *secularized*. Cupitt suggests just the reverse, that ordinary life has been *sacralized*. We can trace the roots of this shift back again to the mid-nineteenth century: Thoreau recorded this new attitude in *Walden*, as he went to the woods to "live deliberately," as he put it. Says Cupitt (1999),

> It is clear straightaway that Thoreau is not going to live in the wilderness for any of the Old World's traditional reasons. He's not going into the desert like Elijah or Muhammad to listen out for the voice of God; he's not going like Jesus or Anthony to be tempted of the devil; and he's not going, like Wittgenstein or Kerouac, in order to seek relief for his own troubled psychology. He's going to try to find out for himself what it is to be a human being with a life to live. (p. 21)

This attitude is of considerable importance. For example, a poem such as Mary Oliver's "The Summer Day," with the last lines "Tell me, what is it you plan to do/With your one wild and precious life?" dropped into the silence of a class creates a sacred space and a sacred pause for reflection. It is secular liturgy.

Another window into the further possibilities is suggested by the sociologist of religion Robert Wuthnow. In *After Heaven: Spirituality in America since the 1950s* (1998), he maps out three approaches to spirituality that may suggest language, images, metaphors, and assumptions that will promote connection of contemporary Americans to alternative practices. The approaches he names follow the arc of the narrative of this chapter: the traditional *spirituality of dwelling,* the contemporary *spirituality of seeking,* and the emerging *spirituality of practice.*

Dwelling spirituality dominates in settled times in history, when it is possible to create stable institutions and communities, when sacred spaces for worship can be *inhabited.* The metaphor of this spirituality is a *place.* In the narrative we've been following, the hundred years from mid-nineteenth to mid-twentieth century were dwelling times. In America, the overwhelming majority of the population identified with Jewish or Christian tradition. Towns were small, church buildings and synagogues were central, often " commons" occupied the center of town, and one—and one's entire family—simply *belonged.* Lives were spent from infancy to funeral within a community, a place. The few at the end of the nineteenth century who saw and felt the withdrawal of the tide of the sea of faith— the first Buddhists—were anomalous harbingers.

Seeking spirituality dominates in unsettled times, when meaning must be negotiated, and all that is on offer may be explored. Wuthnow notes that a major shift was beginning in the America of the 1950s, as the culture became more fluid, complex, and threatening to individual identities. The opening to new possibilities from the East, and from the culture of recovery and self-help, brought new products and perspectives into the spiritual marketplace. The seeking of the 1960s and 1970s was pervasive, and continues today, as the market becomes more fragmented and the culture more unstable.

The metaphor for seeking spirituality is a journey.

Practice spirituality is the new bright edge in the culture. In a profound way, it integrates both dwelling and seeking. It requires setting aside a sacred space-time for the practice, yet that space-time is potentially fluid. Further, practice spirituality begins to reconcile or mediate the split between dwelling and seeking. Practice encourages both discipline and wide-ranging exploration, and can be undertaken within the shelter of an organization and community or pursued independently. There is not a metaphor for practice, but rather an impulse and attitude to "live deliberately," as Thoreau and Cupitt suggest.

It is here, now, in this emerging moment, with a democratic and ethical view of spiritual teacher-student relations, a secular spirituality of life, and a drive for the paradoxical fluidity and stability of spiritual practice that alternative medical interventions are growing and evolving. With 150 years of evolving discourse behind and within alternative thought and practice we may finally be ready to reap the rewards by a radical reorganization of our ideas and approaches to health care in America.

🌐 Chapter References can be found on the Evolve website at http://evolve.elsevier.com/Micozzi/complementary/

CHAPTER 8

NEUROHUMORAL PHYSIOLOGY AND PSYCHONEUROIMMUNOLOGY

HAKIMA AMRI
MARC S. MICOZZI

NEUROHUMORAL MECHANISMS

The autonomic nervous system (ANS) maintains homeostasis by a series of humoral and nervous system interactions that continually occur on a subconscious, involuntary level. The ANS sends nervous impulses to all parts of the body as directed by the integration of several complex biofeedback mechanisms.

The information from these biofeedback loops is integrated in the central nervous system (CNS), and appropriate neural directives are passed along to the organs of respiration, circulation, digestion, excretion, and reproduction via the ANS.

Thus the body is maintained in a state of dynamic equilibrium, continually responsive to stimuli from internally monitored systems and environmental influences.

The functional anatomy of the ANS has important implications for therapeutics (Table 8-1). The division of the system into two major parts—sympathetic and parasympathetic—provides a series of checks and balances to regulate body functions. This division enables an ongoing dialogue between the two parts to maintain dynamic equilibrium. The opposition of two vital forces may be likened to the Asian concept of the yin and the yang, in which the interaction of these opposing forces maintains the balance and harmony of humans and the universe (see Chapters 1 and 2). Accordingly, each of the two forces may take on some characteristics of the other. An analogy lies in the sympathetic and parasympathetic divisions of the nervous system, which are antagonistic, with a few notable exceptions. Coronary and pulmonary blood vessels are dilated by both divisions of the ANS, whereas the vessels supplying blood to skeletal muscles may be dilated by the sympathetic system in exercise or by the postganglionic parasympathetic neurotransmitter at rest.

The unique short-term and long-term adaptability of the human organism to environmental stimuli is facilitated by the actions of the ANS. The so-called fight-flight or defense-alarm responses are promulgated by the *sympathetic nervous system*, which raises blood oxygenation and pressure, regulates blood flow to the musculoskeletal system for activity and to the skin for thermal regulation,

TABLE 8-1

Sympathetic and Parasympathetic Divisions of the Autonomic Nervous System

	Sympathetic	Parasympathetic
Synonym	Adrenergic	Cholinergic
Preganglionic fiber	Short	Long
Neurohumoral agent*	Acetylcholine	Acetylcholine
Ganglion location	Paravertebral	End organ
Postganglionic fiber	Long	Short
Neurohumoral agent*	Norepinephrine	Acetylcholine
Extraautonomic sites	Adrenal medulla	Neuromuscular junction
Evolutionary role	Fight-flight/defense-alarm	Relaxation response, vegetative functions
Activators	Multiple	Specific
Blockers	Diffuse, nonspecific	Selective, cholinesterase
Degradative enzymes	Monoamine oxidase, methyltransferase	

*These compounds are referred to as *neurohumoral* agents because they are present both in the general circulation and within nervous tissue. They are *neurotransmitters* because they manifest their activity across presynaptic or postsynaptic junctions during transmission of nerve impulses.

and causes retention of fluids and electrolytes in a state of arousal. These acute physiological responses are adaptive in the short term and allow long-term survival of the human organism.

The "relaxation response" is mediated by the dynamic opponent of the sympathetic system—the parasympathetic system. The *parasympathetic nervous system* directs the normative functions of the organism, allowing development of an ongoing state of well-being and physiological equilibrium. The maintenance of vegetative functions has facilitated human development and cultural evolution. The ability to relax has allowed humans to reserve some portion of physical and mental energy for the pursuit of activities peripheral to primary survival. This ability has given humans their unique cultural attributes, which enable each individual to express the inclination for creativity. The selective responsiveness of the ANS has enabled humans, both as individuals and as a species, to make the successful adaptation to the environment that has characterized human evolution.

The anatomical divisions corresponding to the functional autonomy of the sympathetic and parasympathetic nervous system can be traced along the length of the brain and spinal column (Figure 8-1). The ANS begins with cranial nerve X, the vagus, a single bundle of parasympathetic nerves that originates from the brainstem and courses throughout the body. Cranial nerves III, VII, and IX also send some parasympathetic fibers to the eyes, nose, and salivary glands. *Vagus* means "wanderer" in Latin, and no other nerve interfaces at so many diverse points along the functional anatomy. Passing down along the spinal cord, the cervical, thoracic, and lumbar divisions send sympathetic nerves throughout the body. Finally, the sacral divisions of the spinal cord send a few parasympathetic nerves to the lower regions of the body.

Each nerve of the ANS has two longitudinal divisions as it passes from the CNS to the end organs. The initial,

or *preganglionic,* nerve fiber originates in the CNS and terminates in a nerve ganglion. Here it synapses with a new continuation—the postganglionic nerve fiber. This *postganglionic* fiber originates in the ganglion and terminates at a site of action. Autonomic nerve impulses travel in a continuum along the preganglionic fiber, through the synapse, and onto the postganglionic fiber to the site of action. In the sympathetic division, the preganglionic fibers are short and end in nearby ganglia, which occur in chains along the thoracic and lumbar vertebrae. From there, the postganglionic fibers travel to the diverse sites of action. In the parasympathetic system the preganglionic fibers are long and travel into ganglia located near end organs. From there, postganglionic fibers traverse a short distance to the sites of action.

The occurrence of *synapses* in the ganglia, between the preganglionic and postganglionic fibers, is important to therapy. Local anesthetics affect nerve conduction in the nerve fiber. Otherwise, these nerve impulses may be influenced by activities at the synaptic junction site. The interactions that occur in the synapse are a microcosm of neurophysiology and serve to distinguish the sympathetic system functionally from the parasympathetic system. These distinctions are used extensively in therapy. Each of these systems makes use of characteristic neurohumoral agents for the unique transmission of nervous impulses throughout the body. The preganglionic fibers of both divisions use *acetylcholine* as the neurotransmitter across the synapse. The postganglionic parasympathetic transmitter is also acetylcholine, but the sympathetic transmitter is *norepinephrine*. The exclusive postganglionic use of acetylcholine as the parasympathetic and norepinephrine as the sympathetic neurotransmitter holds throughout the ANS, except in the case of sweating of the palms, soles, and axilla, where the autonomic innervation is adrenergic, but the neurotransmitter is acetylcholine. Because these neurohumoral compounds used in the transmission of impulses across the

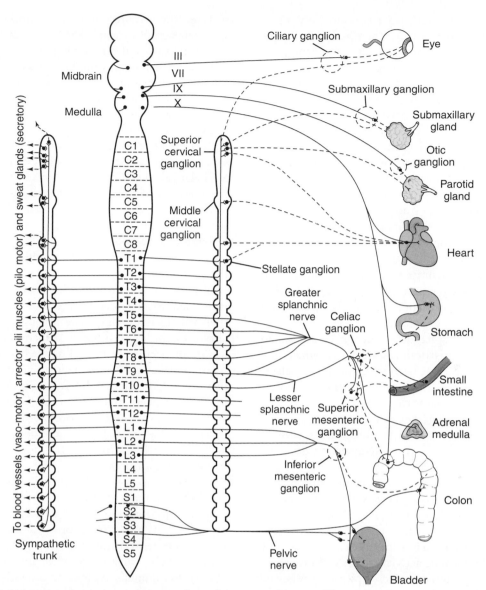

Figure 8-1 Autonomic nervous system and cranial nerves. (From Williams PL: *Gray's anatomy,* Edinburgh, 1995, Churchill Livingstone.)

synaptic junction are distinct chemical entities, they tend to accumulate at their sites of release. Such an occurrence would limit effectiveness of the ANS in providing sensitive, instantaneous regulation of body systems. Thus the synaptic sites maintain extensive and sophisticated mechanisms for the reuptake and degradation of released neurohumoral transmitters, and the synaptic junctions are kept clear of accumulated active compounds on an ongoing basis.

Specific enzymes degrade norepinephrine in the sympathetic postganglionic synapses, as well as their metabolic products. The concentration of these metabolites may be increased in certain pathological conditions and detected by analytical chemical techniques.

The enzyme responsible for the breakdown of acetylcholine in the postganglionic parasympathetic synapse is *acetylcholinesterase.* Although acetylcholine itself cannot practically be administered even when its properties are desired, a "functional dose" may be given through inhibition of its breakdown by cholinesterase. Thus, anticholinesterases form the basis for parasympathetic nervous stimulation in clinical therapeutics. A phenomenon known as *denervation hypersensitivity* greatly depends on this system of reuptake and degradation. When the autonomic innervation to an organ is anatomically interrupted (denervation), the postganglionic synaptic site loses its induced degradative enzymes, and the synaptic receptor becomes extremely sensitive (hypersensitive) to the neurohumoral agent. Thus any amount of the original neurohumoral agent introduced into the site by the circulation, through administration or otherwise, will have a magnified effect because the activity will not be mitigated by action of its appropriate degradative mechanism.

The functional divisions of the ANS have great pathophysiological and therapeutic significance. For example, the entire gastrointestinal (GI) tract is extensively inner-vated by nerve fibers from both the sympathetic and the parasympathetic divisions. As previously discussed, the parasympathetic ganglia, where preganglionic fibers synapse with postganglionic fibers, are located near the sites of action in end organs. In the case of the GI tract, the parasympathetic ganglia lie in two areas of the esophageal, gastric, intestinal, and colonic walls: the Auerbach myenteric plexus and Meissner submucous plexus. These ganglia may be congenitally absent, as in Hirschsprung disease, or destroyed by a number of pathogenic agents. The resultant disease depends on the location of the deficiency or insult along the GI tract.

With destruction of the parasympathetic ganglia, there is prolonged, unopposed sympathetic stimulation. The characteristic effect is for the diseased segment to become constricted, with impaired motility and loss of peristaltic action. The segment of the GI tract proximal to the constriction lesion becomes extensively dilated as a pathological response to the event.

Achalasia of the esophagus is such a condition, in which a local area of constriction leads to proximal dilation of the esophagus. It has been thought that achalasia is caused by degenerative disease of the parasympathetic vagus nerve, which innervates this area.

Pyloric stenosis of the gastric outlet is a similar condition. A ganglionic megacolon, or Hirschsprung disease, is caused by a congenital lack of parasympathetic ganglion cells in the intestinal tract.

Chagas disease, or South American trypanosomiasis, caused by the parasitic organism *Trypanosoma cruzi,* may be associated with both megaesophagus and megacolon resulting from the toxic degeneration of the intraluminal nerve plexus through *T. cruzi* infection. On the other hand, selective loss of sympathetic activity occurs in Horner syndrome, with the characteristic triad of ptosis, miosis, and anhydrosis (lid lag, pupillary constriction, and loss of sweating). Horner syndrome occurs with injury to the cervical sympathetic trunk and unopposed parasympathetic innervation.

Unfortunately, no autonomic therapeutic agents are available for the effective treatment of disorders such as Horner syndrome or irreversible disorders of the GI tract. However, autonomic agents to treat diseases of the circulatory and respiratory systems are common therapies in medicine. These same neurohumoral mechanisms involved in medical therapeutics may also be used in a nonspecific manner by many of the "mind-body" techniques of complementary, integrative, and alternative medicine.

PSYCHONEUROIMMUNOLOGY

The Romans' view of *mens sanum in corpore sano,* "a sound mind in a sound body," as well as the Greek physician Galen's observation that women suffering from depression had a predisposition toward developing breast cancer, reflected the early recognition of mind-body interactions and their significance in health and disease. Understanding the connection and functioning of the mind has been the subject of discussions from the ancient era and transcended the Renaissance and modern times. This is witnessed by the philosophical writings of Pythagoras that "the brain served as the organ of the mind and the temple of the soul," and Anaximander, another Greek philosopher, that "mind gives body a life force" (Cassano, 1996). The European Renaissance was marked by the work of Leonardo da Vinci and Michelangelo. Da Vinci was mostly interested in answering the question of how the brain processes sensory inputs; Michelangelo, an expert in anatomy, painted detailed structures of the human brain (Meshberger, 1990). René Descartes, a post-Renaissance philosopher, declared the connection between the body and the soul to be located in the pineal gland (Lokhorst et al, 2001). The development of electrochemistry in the eighteenth and nineteenth centuries led to the identification of different gases and their role in maintaining life through respiration, which also made the lungs the new indispensable organ to be seriously considered. It is basically what Hippocrates and Avicenna called the "air element" that distributes the spirits inside the body (Tercier, 2005). The importance of breathing started then to occupy the discussion about what animates living beings. The twentieth century was marked by remarkable technological developments, especially imaging, in which the functional brain is visualized and its metabolites measured.

Thus, it was not until studies in the 1950s and 1960s verified the impact of stress on overall health that mind-body connection research started to become a focus of attention. In 1964, Solomon and Moos described the interaction between mind and body as a result of stress exposure. The early work of Rasmussen et al showed (1957) that animals exposed to stress had increased susceptibility to infection. George Engel's view that genetics is not the only cause of poor health and that social and psychological factors have a direct impact on all biological processes further expanded this new, holistic medical model referred to as "psychoneuroimmunology," or PNI (Engel, 1977; Lutgendorf et al, 2003). Subsequent research strongly suggested that the higher cognitive and limbic emotional centers are capable of regulating virtually all aspects of the immune system and therefore play a significant role in health and disease (Ader R et al, 1991; Blalock, 1994; Reichlin, 1993). The pioneering work of Besedovsky et al (1975) revealed the role of hormones and cytokines in modulating the brain and immune functions (Besedovsky et al, 1975). The Institute of Medicine issued two reports titled *Health and Behavior* (1982, 2001) with a special focus on understanding the role and interactions of the biological, behavioral, and social factors in health and disease.

Autonomic and neuroendocrine processes constitute the mind-body pathways of communication. The ANS innervates the bone marrow, thymus, spleen, and mucosal surfaces, the areas where immune cells develop, mature, and encounter foreign proteins (Felten et al, 1992). This innervation involves sympathetic, parasympathetic, and nonadrenergic noncholinergic fibers. As discussed earlier, signal transduction occurs through epinephrine, norepinephrine, acetylcholine, and neuropeptides. These chemical messengers exert tissue-specific inflammatory or antiinflammatory effects on immune target tissues, and nerves and inflammatory cells mutually influence each other in a time-dependent manner (Watkins, 1995). Development and aging of the immune system and ANS appear to be closely related (Ackerman et al, 1989; Bellinger et al, 1988). Levels of natural killer (NK) cells, considered the first line of immune defense against viral infections, were found dramatically reduced in individuals exposed to chronic life stress as well as in those with major depression. The levels of NK cells were found to return to normal levels after the depression episodes subsided (Irwin and Miller, 2007). Studying 245 patients who had depression and were stratified by smoking habits, Jung and Irwin (1999) found that the combination of depression and smoking caused a more pronounced decline in levels of NK cells than depression or smoking alone. Several studies published in the past 25 years have clearly showed that behavior affects immunity and have deciphered neuroimmune pathways governing the observed effects. The neuroimmune system also affects behavior, functioning as a bidirectional highway of communications involving neuropeptides and cytokines. It has been hypothesized that altered cytokine profiles, including levels of interleukin-1 (IL-1), IL-6, and tumor necrosis factor, might contribute to symptoms of depression, such as insomnia and fatigue (Irwin and Miller, 2007).

The neuroendocrine pathway constitutes the second indirect communication channel involving the hormonal regulation of immune cell function. Immune cells have surface receptors for endorphins, enkephalins, and the various hormones, such as growth hormone, thyroid-stimulating hormone, sex hormone–releasing hormones, vasopressin, and prolactin (Blalock, 1994; Felten et al, 1992). The release of many of these hormones is intimately related to thoughts and emotions and has a profound effect on immune system function. The "molecules of emotion" therefore govern the immune response through the endocrine system, leading to either suppression or enhancement (Pert et al, 1998). The neuroendocrine peptide corticotropin-releasing hormone (CRH) received a special attention, especially after it was found that depressed patients had elevated central CRH levels as measured in the cerebrospinal fluid. Furthermore, acute administration of CRH centrally caused dramatic reduction in innate and cellular immune responses in animal models (Irwin et al, 1987, 1989; Strausbaugh et al, 1992). These studies showed that the central action of this neuropeptide could affect the peripheral immune response. CRH is considered as the major neuroimmunoendocrine integrator.

Because thoughts, feelings, emotions, and perceptions alter immunity (Watkins, 1995), complementary therapies targeted at these areas should affect health and elicit changes in pathological conditions (Watkins, 1994).

Epilepsy illustrates this point (i.e., the effect of the mind on the brain). Epileptic seizures can be triggered by stressful events (Fenwick, 1998), and negative emotions exacerbate the condition. A potential mechanism is the activation of the cytokine network (Hulkkonen et al, 2004), which corresponds to seizure activity, but whether it is cause or effect remains unclear.

The reverse scenario is reflected in a long-term study involving healthy World War II veterans who were asked to write about their war experiences and themselves. The essays were rated on a scale ranging from extreme optimism to extreme pessimism. When the study participants reached the age of 45, health status positively correlated with optimistic scoring at the beginning of the study (Peterson et al, 1993). Recently, a new approach using multiplex immunoassay was applied to assess the relationship of 11 T-cell cytokines and chemokines to behavior. Mommersteeg et al investigated whether cytokine and chemokine profiles correlated to hostility in 304 healthy Dutch military males before deployment. In addition to finding that hostility was related to various clusters of proinflammatory and antiinflammatory cytokines and chemokines and to potential risk factors including age, body mass index, smoking, drinking, previous deployment, early life trauma, and depression, the authors found that "hostility was significantly related to decreased interleukin 6/chemokine secretion and increased pro- and antiinflammatory cytokines" (Mommersteeg et al, 2008).

EVIDENCE FOR PSYCHONEUROIMMUNOLOGICAL MEDIATION OF THE EFFECTS OF COMPLEMENTARY AND ALTERNATIVE THERAPIES

The use of PNI-related techniques has dramatically increased in the United States. According to a recent survey, one in five adults reported using one or more mind-body therapies during the previous year (Wolsko et al, 2004). Relaxation techniques, guided imagery, hypnosis, and biofeedback are the most frequently used modalities. Patients sought these PNI-related techniques for treatment of chronic diseases such as anxiety (34%), depression (26.5%), headaches (18.5%), back or neck pain (18%), heart problems or chest pain (18%), arthritis (14.8%), digestive disorders (12.4%), and fatigue (12.1%). The authors estimated that the absolute numbers of patients using the modalities listed were as follows: for back and neck pain, 11.2 million; for anxiety, 6.3 million; and for fatigue, 6.8 million. Between 29% and 55% of patients found these therapies "very helpful" for their respective health condition. A recent study on the prevalence of complementary and alternative medicine (CAM) use in the military population showed that 37% of the 1305 individuals in a random sample of active duty and Reserve and National Guard members contacted between December 2000 and July 2002 had used at least one CAM modality in the previous year (Smith et al, 2007).

What is the evidence that complementary, integrative, and alternative therapies work through the previously outlined mind-body pathways? To date, few studies have actually investigated the *mechanism of action* of these therapies. Some data suggest that the activity of the ANS may be altered by chiropractic intervention (Beal, 1985; Bouhuys, 1963), hypnosis (DeBenedittis et al, 1994; Neild et al, 1985), conditioning (Hatch et al, 1990), and acupuncture (Han et al, 1980; Jian, 1985). Other studies have indicated that the benefit derived from acupuncture (Kasahara et al, 1992) and spinal manipulation (Vernon et al, 1986) might be mediated through endorphin release.

Several studies demonstrate that acupuncture-induced analgesia is blocked by naloxone, an opioid antagonist, which indicates that an opioidergic mechanism mediates the acupuncture analgesic response (Mayer et al, 1977; Sjolund et al, 1979). In electroacupuncture, electrical pulses are applied via acupuncture needles. Opioid and nonopioid pathways govern the antinociceptive effect induced by electroacupuncture. However, the PNI-mediated mechanism in electroacupuncture occurs at the level of neuronal nitric oxide synthase, nitric oxide expression and synthesis in the brain, and the therapeutic response induced by acupoint ST36 (Ma, 2004).

Recently, a new hypothesis on the mechanism of acupuncture involving neutrophins and cytokines has been postulated (Kavoussi et al, 2007). The beneficial effects of acupuncture on inflammatory pain, as well as neurodegenerative and psychiatric diseases, could indeed be mediated by nerve growth factor, brain-derived neurotrophic factor, neurotrophin 3, or neurotrophin 4/5, as well as by IL-1, IL-2, IL-6, tumor necrosis factor α, and transforming growth factor β. The dynamic crosstalk between the central and peripheral nervous systems could shed light on the mechanism of acupuncture (Du, 2008).

Acupuncture has also been used to relieve stress and anxiety, which are known to affect the immune response. In a study investigating the effects of acupuncture in women with anxiety, Arranz et al tested several immune functions: adherence, chemotaxis, phagocytosis, basal and stimulated superoxide anion levels, lymphocyte proliferation in response to phytohemagglutinin A, and NK activity of leukocytes (neutrophils and lymphocytes). Ten 30-minute sessions of manual acupuncture using 19 acupoints were administered to 34 women aged 34 to 60 with anxiety, as assessed by the Beck Anxiety Inventory, and 20 healthy controls. The investigators found that the most positive effects of acupuncture on the immune parameters appear 72 hours after a single session and persist for 1 month after the full treatment regimen. The abnormal immune profiles of women with anxiety were normalized and the immune functions significantly enhanced by acupuncture (Arranz et al, 2007).

Using state-of-the-art technology (e.g., two-dimensional electrophoresis-based proteomics) and an animal model for neuropathic pain, Sung et al (2004) detected 36 proteins that were differentially expressed in the brains of injured animals compared with controls. Most interestingly, normal levels of these proteins were restored after the injured animals were treated with electroacupuncture. Of these proteins, 21 have been characterized as playing a role in inflammation, enzyme metabolism, and signal transduction, and this study undoubtedly will elucidate other pathways triggered by acupuncture (Sung et al, 2004).

A growing body of evidence suggests that *meditation* alleviates anxiety, fosters a positive attitude, and improves the immune response. A meditation training program known as "mindfulness-based stress reduction" (MBSR), developed by Jon Kabat-Zinn, PhD, in the late 1970s, yielded increased left frontal lobe activation in response to both negative and positive emotion induction. When vaccinated after intervention, the meditation group experienced a significantly increased rise in antibody titers. The correlation between the shift toward left-sided brain activation and the elevated immune response demonstrates the relationship between the PNI system and meditation (Davidson et al, 2003). Similarly, cancer outpatients using the same MBSR technique experienced improved mood, which correlated with a more favorable hormone profile with regard to melatonin, cortisol, dehydroepiandrosterone sulfate (DHEA-S), and the cortisol/DHEA-S ratio, as well as an enhanced immune response (Carlson et al, 2004).

The quasi-experimental study carried out by Robinson et al (2003) using an 8-week structured MBSR intervention in patients with human immunodeficiency virus (HIV) infection showed that NK cell activity and number increased significantly in the MBSR group compared with the controls. In a more recent single-blind randomized controlled trial, Creswell et al assessed the efficacy of an 8-week MBSR meditation program compared with a 1-day control seminar on CD4+ T-lymphocyte counts in stressed HIV-infected adults. Participants in the 1-day control seminar had reduced CD4+ T-lymphocyte counts, whereas counts among participants in the 8-week MBSR program were unchanged from baseline to postintervention. Another study also found an indication that mindfulness meditation training can buffer CD4+ T lymphocyte declines in adults infected with HIV-1 (Creswell et al, 2009).

Beneficial effects of MBSR have also been reported among cancer patients. Quality-of-life, mood, endocrine, immune, and autonomic parameters have been assessed in patients with early-stage breast and prostate cancer enrolled in an MBSR program. In this study the authors carried out preintervention and postintervention as well as 6- and 12-month follow-up measurements of the psychobehavioral and physiological parameters. They found significant general improvements in stress symptoms, which were preserved through the follow-up periods. In addition to a steady decrease in salivary cortisol level throughout the follow-up period, improvements in immune patterns were also maintained as shown by a decrease in the proinflammatory T helper cell type 1 cytokines. Reductions in heart rate and systolic blood pressure were positively correlated with improvements in self-reported stress symptoms. This pilot study data clearly showed the longer-term effects of MBSR on a range of potentially important psychoimmunophysiological biomarkers (Carlson et al, 2007). Another study enrolled women who had been recently diagnosed with early-stage breast cancer and were not currently receiving chemotherapy into an MBSR program. Compared with the levels before MBSR intervention, postintervention and 4-week follow-up assessments in the MBSR group showed an increase in peripheral blood mononuclear NK cell activity and cytokine production accompanied by a decrease in IL-4, IL-6, and IL-10 production, whereas the non-MBSR control group showed reduced NK cell activity and interferon-γ levels and increased IL-4, IL-6, and IL-10 production. Furthermore, the MBSR-intervention group demonstrated reduced cortisol levels, improved quality of life, and improved coping effectiveness (Witek-Janusek et al, 2008).

Among the other mind-body programs is the one developed by Herbert Benson, MD, in the 1970s, in which he emphasized the *relaxation response*. A large body of evidence has been developed showing its beneficial effects on a wide array of diseases and disorders, and it is only recently that a special interest in its *mechanism(s) of action* has been developed. Building upon newly developed hypotheses that nitric oxide plays a role in the immune response and in stress-related diseases (Tripathi, 2007), an association between oxygen consumption, through breathing exercises, and nitric oxide production has been elucidated (Dusek et al, 2006). Furthermore, the new technological approaches of high-throughput genomic analyses have been applied to mechanistic investigations of the relaxation response. Thus, genomic counterstress alterations induced by the relaxation response have been detected using whole blood transcriptional profiles. Genomic profiles were compared in 19 long-term practitioners of relaxation, 20 novice individuals who completed an 8-week relaxation program, and 19 healthy controls. Over 2200 genes in the long-term practitioners and 1561 genes in the novice group were differentially expressed compared with the control group. Among these genes, the long-term practitioners and novices shared 433 genes. The gene analysis revealed changes in gene expression related to cellular metabolism, oxidative phosphorylation, and production of reactive oxygen species and regulation of oxidative stress, especially among the relaxation response practitioners (Dusek et al, 2008).

T'ai chi is a Chinese martial art that emphasizes meditative aerobic activity and relaxation. Its practice in the West is witnessing a great development. Several studies using t'ai chi as intervention in subjects who either had their immune response clinically challenged or had immune-related diseases have recently been published. In a prospective randomized controlled trial 112 healthy adults were vaccinated with Varivax (attenuated varicella-zoster virus) and divided to either t'ai chi or health education groups. The t'ai chi group showed a significant improvement in scores on the Short-Form Health Survey (SF-36); in addition, the cell-mediated immune response to the vaccine not only was higher but also increased at a higher rate than in the control group (Irwin, Olmstead et al, 2007).

Another randomized clinical trial tested whether t'ai chi could improve immune function and psychosocial functioning in 252 HIV-affected individuals compared with a wait-listed control group. Although only modest effects were observed on the psychosocial test results, a significant increase in the lymphocyte proliferation function was found. The investigators concluded that t'ai chi could be considered as an effective alternative intervention in patients with immune-mediated diseases (McCain et al, 2008).

Yoga has become a popular practice in Western culture. Based on the development and balance of psychophysical energies, yoga has proven to be beneficial in pulmonary and cardiovascular conditions, including asthma, chronic bronchitis, and hypertension (Raub, 2002). A study investigating the effects of yoga and meditation on psychological profile, cardiopulmonary performance, and melatonin secretion demonstrated increased well-being, improved performance, and elevated plasma melatonin levels (Harinath et al, 2004).

Yoga has been administered as adjuvant therapy in treatment of other health conditions, in addition to the afore-mentioned disorders. Premenstrual syndrome, or PMS, is considered to be a stress-related psychoneuroendocrine disorder for which the numerous available treatments have not brought satisfactory relief. Fifty healthy women of reproductive age were assigned either to a Hatha Yoga group performing a 61-points relaxation exercise or to a no-intervention control group. Several physiological parameters were measured: heart rate, systolic and diastolic blood pressure, electromyographic activity, electrodermal galvanic activity, respiratory rate, and peripheral temperature. After 10 minutes of Hatha Yoga practice, values of all parameters declined significantly except that temperature increased, which suggests a reduction in sympathetic activity and basal sympathetic tone. Thus, Hatha Yoga could be used as an adjuvant to other medical treatment in alleviating PMS symptoms (Dvivedi et al, 2008).

Psychological outcomes, perceived stress, anxiety, and depression levels as well as radiation-induced DNA damage were assessed in 68 breast cancer patients undergoing radiotherapy and enrolled in an integrated yoga program. The psychological outcomes were significantly improved in the yoga group, but only a slight decrease in DNA damage was seen compared with the no-intervention group (Banerjee et al, 2007).

In another study, 98 outpatients with stage II or III breast cancer were assigned to either yoga or supportive therapy. Data were analyzed only for those who underwent surgery followed by radiotherapy and chemotherapy ($n = 38$). Subjects were assessed using the State Trait Anxiety Inventory (STAI) before and after 60 minutes of daily yoga sessions. Results showed a general decrease in self-reported STAI scores in the yoga group and a positive correlation of these scores with distress during conventional treatment intervals (Rao et al, 2009).

Looking into the neuroendocrine mechanisms underlying the effect of yoga, Madanmohan et al (2002) approached the question of whether shavasan yoga modulates the stress physiological response from a different angle (yes, the pose is indeed from a different angle). They used the cold pressor test (CPT) to trigger a stress response in 10 healthy subjects who were taught shavasan practice and measured the respiratory rate interval variation, deep breathing difference, and heart rate, blood pressure, and rate-pressure-product response to CPT before and immediately after shavasan. A significant increase in deep breathing difference and a close to significant increase in respiratory rate interval variation were observed, which indicate improved parasympathetic activity. Values of the other parameters mirroring sympathetic activity were blunted, which suggests that yoga practice helps reduce the sympathetic load on the heart (Madanmohan et al, 2002).

Biochemical and genomic approaches have also been undertaken to understand the action mechanisms underlying the stress reduction effects of Sudarshan Kriya Yoga. Whole blood drawn from 42 healthy subjects was used to measure glutathione peroxidase levels, and red blood cell lysate was used for superoxide dismutase activity assay as well as to estimate glutathione levels. White blood cells were separated and processed for gene expression. The results showed a better immune status and antioxidant profile both at the enzyme activity and at the RNA level in the yoga intervention group. A prolonged lymphocyte life span supported by the upregulation of antiapoptotic and survival genes was also observed. All together, these results suggest that Sudarshan Kriya has beneficial effects on immunity, cell death, and stress regulation through transcriptional pathways (Sharma et al, 2008).

PLACEBO EFFECT

A *placebo* is an inert substance or a control method used to evaluate the psychological and physiological effects of a new drug or procedure. The response to the placebo should not exceed that to the experimental drug or method, which would otherwise be considered ineffective. The placebo response is unpredictable, unreliable, and mediated by nonspecific mechanisms that are dismissed as immeasurable and irrelevant.

How does the psychoneuroimmunological complex relate to the placebo effect? It has been argued that every therapeutic intervention—whether complementary, integrative, and alternative medicine or allopathic medicine—involves a placebo effect. Most allopathic physicians consider it unethical or even deceitful to actively encourage a placebo response. However, in a recent survey of 1200 practicing internists and rheumatologists in the United States that inquired about behaviors and attitudes regarding the use of placebo treatments, among those who responded ($n = 679$), half reported prescribing placebo treatments on a regular basis in the form of saline, sugar pills, over-the-counter analgesics, and vitamins within the previous year. Most physicians describe these substances to their patients as potentially beneficial or as a treatment not typically used for the patient's condition, and most physicians believe this practice to be common and ethically allowable (de la Rochefordiere et al, 1996).

PNI research demonstrates that an expectation of recovery can alter subjective feelings of well-being and result in ANS activation and pituitary hormone production. Thus, specific verifiable pathways have been identified by which expectation can alter immunity. However, expectation likely has different effects in different individuals, producing large shifts in autonomic balance and hormonal output in some and negligible changes in others, which explains the unpredictability of the placebo response. Together with the idea that complementary therapies affect merely "subjective" measures of disease activity, these observations have formed the platform on which allopathic physicians argue that complementary practices are fundamentally flawed and of limited benefit.

Although fallacious, defeatist, and ultimately counterproductive, these arguments persist. The expectation of recovery that promotes a placebo response is separate from any subjective improvement and, incidentally, is also different from hope. It is possible to feel subjectively better without expecting a full recovery. Similarly, it is possible to expect recovery without feeling better at all. Complementary therapies cannot be dismissed as mere placebos, and it is becoming increasingly obvious that they produce substantial subjective and objective clinical benefits unrelated to the placebo effect.

Individuals differ in their responsiveness to the various activation stimuli, whether expectancy, subjective sensations, or complementary therapies. This would explain why complementary therapies that are supposedly mediated by placebo mechanisms, as in allopathic arguments, could outperform placebos in a double-blind trial (Reilly et al, 1994). It would also explain the need to combine a number of complementary approaches to ensure that these pathways are fully activated.

There is fortunately a growing body of scientific literature published since 2006 from psychoneurologists and neuroscientists addressing the specific issues of placebo and *nocebo,* which is the worsening of symptoms due to a nonspecific response, and their potential biological mechanisms. According to Eccles (2007), the placebo response in clinical medicine could be compared to a component of an allergy treatment that possesses "nonspecific effects" (e.g., natural recovery) and a "true placebo effect" represented as the psychological therapeutic effect of the treatment. Intrinsic positive belief in the efficacy of the treatment characterizes the true placebo effect, which can be enhanced by extrinsic factors such as the interaction with physician. Negative belief, however, can engender a nocebo effect that may elucidate some psychogenic diseases (Eccles, 2007). To examine placebo and nocebo symptoms, college students were recruited into what appeared to be a clinical trial evaluating the effectiveness of an herbal supplement on cognitive performance. Subjects received either an herbal supplement or a placebo (both are placebo inactive pills) and a list of positive and adverse effects. Most participants reported symptoms, and those who believed they were ingesting the herbal supplement reported significantly more symptoms than those who thought they were taking a placebo. In this case the belief may exacerbate the placebo response (Link et al, 2006).

SUMMARY

The medical and scientific communities are showing growing interest in the neurohumoral mechanisms underlying PNI responses to complementary therapies.

The latest research in the biomedical sciences and the social sciences is beginning to demonstrate mechanisms of action by which CAM therapies exert their benefits. The studies published to date have been carried out with relatively small groups of subjects and reflect conventional study criteria and design. Although complementary medicine research currently follows the conventional scientific approach to silence critics, evaluation of the efficacy of various complementary, integrative, and alternative modalities may require the development of additional methodologies based on a new paradigm to overcome foreseeable limitations.

It is noteworthy that the criticism of alternative and integrative therapies as being placebos has moved basic and clinical scientists to question the placebo and nocebo response. There is a call to expand the thinking beyond the "expectation and brain reward circuitry" or Pavlovian conditioning to include other pathways and mechanisms that reflect the psychoneuroimmunoendocrine paradigm. The theoretical framework needs to be redefined, and methodological as well as ethical paradigms should be developed to elucidate the placebo-nocebo response.

⊖ Chapter References can be found on the Evolve website at http://evolve.elsevier.com/Micozzi/complementary/

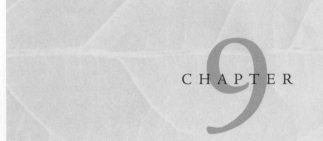
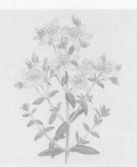

CHAPTER

9

MIND-BODY MODALITIES

DENISE RODGERS
MARC S. MICOZZI

HISTORICAL OVERVIEW

Life and healing are inherently mysterious. The essential "stuff" of the universe, including the universe of the mind and body, remains essentially unexplained. The void inside every atom is pulsating with information or unseen intelligence. Molecular biologists and geneticists locate this intelligence within DNA, primarily for the sake of convenience. Life unfolds as DNA imparts its coded intelligence into a sequence in which energy and information are interchanged for the purpose of building life from matter.

The reality ushered in by quantum physics made it possible to manipulate the invisible intelligence that underlies the visible world. Albert Einstein taught that the physical body, as with all material objects, is like an illusion, and trying to manipulate it can be like grasping the shadow and missing the substance. The unseen world is a real world, and when we are willing to explore the immense creative power that lies within the mind, we can then access the unseen dimensions of the body.

Although mainstream consciousness seems highly aware of the inherent power of the mind, some of the earliest records of certain mind-and-body techniques were found in Babylonia and ancient Sumer well before the rise of experimental science. In the third century BC, Hippocrates was well versed in the art of mental healing. A serpent coiled around a staff is the Hippocratic symbol used today to portray the medical and healing profession. History reveals that the coiled serpent symbolizes the healing energy possessed by each of us, lying dormant at the base of the spine (as literally in Kundalini Yoga), with the staff representing life itself. Eastern philosophy posits that when the serpent is unleashed, healing energy spirals up the spine and out the forehead. This energy, said to be mental in nature, can then be used to heal the physical body.

Most ancient and indigenous medical systems make use of the extraordinary interconnectedness of the mind and body. Native American and Asian Indian cultures believe their members to be in contact with natural healing forces through their dreams, visions, and mystical experiences.

106

The ancient Greeks were also known for their healing temples. These centers existed for more than 800 years and endured until the rise of the Christian era. Patients would travel long distances to experience one of the Aesculapian healing temples. The first step in seeking a cure was to create inner cleanliness by taking a purifying bath. Patients then were put on a special diet or fast. They would attend one of the great dramas of Euripides or Sophocles, observing the tensions and movements of life. Later they were taken to visit one of the shrines, where healers used imagery to visualize the affected part of the body. During sleep the priests entered the patients' rooms and touched the diseased parts. Thereafter, patients would dream and were said to awaken healed.

Philippus Aureolus Theophrastus Bombast von Hohenheim, known as Paracelsus, was a sixteenth-century Renaissance Swiss physician. Although considered the father of modern drug therapy and scientific medicine, he nevertheless opposed the idea of separating the mind from the healing processes of the body. Along with his esteemed medical theories, he held that imagination and faith were the cause of healing power:

> Man has a visible and an invisible workshop. The visible one is his body, the invisible one is the imagination of the mind.... The spirit is the master, imagination the tool, and the body the plastic material. The power of the imagination is the great factor in medicine. It may produce diseases in man and it may cure them. Ills of the body may be cured by physical remedies or by the power of spirit acting through the soul.

Paracelsus believed that physicians could heal by tapping the power of God. He also believed that dreams gave humans clairvoyance and the ability to diagnose illness from long distances.

The philosophies of all these cultures had a common belief in a spiritual center that resides within. They believed in spirit over matter, mind over body. In contrast, modern allopathic medicine has regarded these connections as nonscientific and of secondary importance. Scientific healing, in the form of drug therapy and surgery, has grown to become a dominant Western form of treatment. Since the early 1900s, however, many medical scientists have begun to reinvestigate the role the mind plays in healing. In critical situations, physicians have been known to say, "We've done all we can do—it's in God's hands now," or "It depends on the patient's will to live."

Every physician has witnessed miraculous recoveries unexplainable by scientific understanding. Labeling a recovery as a "spontaneous remission" has become common to describe a healing that cannot be explained by medical standards. Physicians have also long recognized the effectiveness of placebos, substances with no known pharmacological action or benefit. In some cases, placebos can be as much as 70% effective in the treatment of illness, thereby proving the theory that a patient's therapeutic expectation is a contributing factor to healing.

During the past 35 years, the scientific community has made great strides in exploring the mind's capacity to affect the body. This movement has received its impetus from several sources. The rise in the incidence of chronic illness over the past few decades and the rapidly increasing cost of treatment have set the stage for deeper exploration of mind-body therapies. These therapies show great promise for mobilizing the body's inherent power to heal itself.

Recent studies have begun to further deepen our understanding of the effects of stress on the body. Convincing evidence supports the concept that the immune system, along with other organs and systems in the body, can be and is often influenced by the mind. These research efforts and clinical experiments suggest that the separation between mind and body, long taken for granted in Western philosophy, is difficult to quantify. These challenges are all part of a new approach to medical science: the challenge of proving that the mind—along with our thoughts and emotions—has a significant impact on the body's health.

For patients, this new synthesis has very practical significance. It suggests that by paying attention to and exerting some control over mental and emotional states, they may actually contribute to prevention of or recovery from disease. The conscious participation of the patient in the process of healing not only offers new insights but also raises new questions about the nature and reality of consciousness.

The predominant fundamental tenet of mind-body medicine is the concept of *treating the whole person*. Another significant tenet is that people can be active participants in their own health care and may be able to prevent disease or shorten its course by taking steps to manage their own mental processes.

Medical researchers are beginning to rediscover what other cultures have historically used in their healing systems, such as meditation, hypnosis, and imagery. Grounded in ancient philosophy, these interventions are capable of stimulating and often facilitating the mind's capacity to affect the body. Experimentation has given practitioners the opportunity to offer nontoxic therapies while examining the specific links between mental processes and autonomic, immune, and nervous system functioning.

Evidence grows that states of mind can affect physiology. No one is promising that people can cure themselves of disease by adjusting their mental attitudes; this idea is not the message of mind-body interventions. However, mind-body approaches can be used to reduce the severity and frequency of biological symptoms and can potentially help strengthen the body's resistance to disease.

The techniques of mind-body medicine are reasonably well accepted for treating certain chronic and difficult-to-treat medical conditions, from pain syndromes to hypertension. In well-designed studies, relaxation, guided imagery, biofeedback, hypnosis, and related strategies have been proven workable. New evidence is showing that mind-body interventions are consistently effective in improving psychological and medical outcomes after surgery. In a meta-analysis encompassing 191 studies and more than 8600 patients, psychosocial-behavioral interventions showed reliably moderate-sized effects in improving recovery, reducing pain, and decreasing psychological distress (Dreher, 1998). As discussed in this chapter, there is movement on all fronts. Mainstream medical institutions are beginning to take awkward "baby steps" toward implementing these approaches within departments of psychology, psychiatry, oncology, neurology, and rehabilitation. "Mind and body" departments are being established in medical schools and hospitals nationwide. More impressively, both conventional and holistic professionals are beginning to incorporate these approaches into their own personal regimens for greater health and wellness.

This chapter discusses evidence that supports mind-body approaches, describes some of the more widely used techniques, and summarizes the results of some of the most effective interventions. The approaches discussed in this section not only demonstrate dramatic results in specific areas but also help form the basis for a new perspective for medicine and healing. From this perspective, it becomes evident that every interaction between physician and patient has the potential to affect the mind and, in turn, the body of the patient.

ROLE OF CONSCIOUSNESS

DISMISSAL OF THE MIND

Although ancient mystics believed in the power of the human mind, Western science began to question such matters by the mid-1800s. Until that time, physicians believed the prevailing philosophy that the patient's inner life and social being were vital components of all diagnosis and treatment. They generally believed that medicine should take into account not only biological but also behavioral, moral, psychological, and spiritual factors.

These models and methods began to fade by the end of the nineteenth century, however, and a patient-specific model of treatment gave way to a disease-specific model. During the rise of this era of experimental science, four leading German physiologists (Hermann von Helmholtz, Carl Ludwig, Emil du Bois-Reymond, and Ernst Wilhelm von Brücke) pledged themselves to account for all bodily processes in purely physiological terms. They considered that any reported connection between mental states and bodily functions were biased, subjective, nonmeasurable, and scientifically unreliable (Figure 9-1). More than 15,000 American physicians traveled to Germany to study the fascinating laboratory experimentations being introduced at that time. These innovative breakthroughs were in direct contrast with the style of medicine that had been practiced for centuries. It was believed that proper research could be conducted only in laboratories on isolated constituents—microorganisms, components of blood and urine, tissue, and organs—with the focus on devising universal remedies independent of individual patients. This approach has put contemporary medicine in the position of having to learn the scientific basis of something it has known for centuries: that beliefs, thoughts, and feelings affect physiology.

POWER OF PLACEBO

The word *placebo* is Latin for "I please." This concept is well illustrated by an anecdote concerning Sir William Osler. One of North America and England's busiest and most famous physicians, Osler brought new light to the

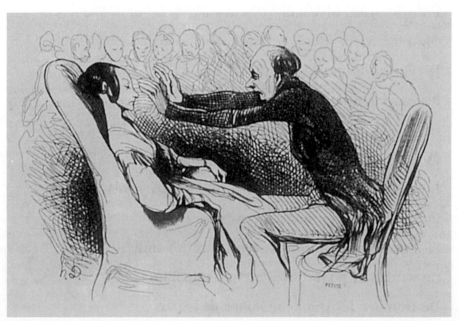

Figure 9-1 Mesmerism and hypnotism were the object of satire and a number of caricatures during the nineteenth century. (Courtesy Bibliothèque Interuniversitaire de Médecine, Paris.)

power of placebo near the turn of the nineteenth century. Dr. Osler made a house call to a dying boy, who had been unresponsive to any previous treatments. Osler appeared at the boy's bedside dressed in magnificent scarlet academic robes. After a brief examination, Osler sat down at the boy's bedside, peeled a peach, sugared it, and cut it into pieces. He then fed it, bit by bit, with a fork to the entranced patient, telling him that it was a most special fruit and that if he ate it, he would not be sick. (Perhaps Osler had read the account of "*Hanuman* Eating the Magic Peach" in the Sanskrit creation epic, *The Ramayana*.)

Osler confided to the boy's father that his son's chances for survival were slim. He continued to visit the boy daily for more than a month, always dressed in his majestic scarlet robes and offering the boy nourishment with his own two hands. This dramatic presentation inspired magic and belief well beyond laboratory science and helped catalyze the boy's unexpected and complete recovery.

Eloquently summing up the placebo's power, Osler wrote the following:

> Faith in the gods or saints cures one, faith in little pills another, hypnotic suggestion a third, faith in a plain common doctor a fourth.... The faith with which we work.... has its limitations [but] such as we find it, faith is the most precious commodity, without which we should be very badly off. (1953)

During World War II the anesthesiologist Beecher noted with surprise, as he examined men with serious shrapnel wounds at Anzio beach, that many of them refused morphine, something that he almost never saw in Boston when he tended to patients with the far less serious wounds produced by controlled surgery. How could such a phenomenon be explained? Under conditions that produce extreme stress or fear, higher emotional centers in the brain can activate a descending system that suppresses incoming pain signals. This descending analgesic system utilizes the body's own endogenous opiate-like neurotransmitters, the endorphins. The threshold for activation of descending analgesia by stress is high; otherwise pain would lose its survival value. But the nervous system appears to be organized so that in circumstances that produce the greatest stress or fear—for example, pursuit by a predator or mortal combat, circumstances in which the survival value of running or fighting far outweighs the risk of using already damaged limbs—pain can be completely suppressed (Hyman, 1998).

Among the early placebo studies documented are those conducted by Dr. Ronald Katz, chairman of the Department of Anesthesiology at the University of California at Los Angeles School of Medicine. Katz reported a series of observations involving patients who were informed that headaches were a complication of spinal anesthesia. At the last minute the patients were told that the choice of anesthesia had been changed from spinal to general. Despite the change, all the patients experienced the symptoms associated with spinal anesthesia (Katz, 1977).

Dr. J.W.L. Fielding conducted a study at the Department of Surgery at Queen Elizabeth Hospital in Birmingham, England, similar to Katz's study investigating expectations. In compliance with informed consent procedures, 411 patients were told they could expect to lose hair as a result of the chemotherapy being administered. Thirty percent of the patients unknowingly received placebos instead of chemotherapy and experienced hair loss even though the pills they had taken contained no medication (Fielding et al, 1983).

Although it has sometimes confounded as much as clarified, the mechanism of pain has provided fascinating clues to investigators of the mind-body healing response. In one landmark study in 1978, dental patients experiencing the aftereffects of an extracted tooth were given a sugar pill and told it was a powerful painkiller. They reported significant pain relief. Then experimenters added another agent: along with the placebo, a separate group of dental patients were given a chemical known to block the action of the brain's own endorphins. The second group experienced significantly less pain reduction than the first group (Levine et al, 1978).

Here was a study that indicated a specific mechanism for placebo—endorphins—without which the magic effect would not have occurred. These studies and many other similar ones led scientists to believe that endorphins mediate much of the mind-body effect, whether that effect is triggered by trauma, placebo, hypnosis, or any other mental agent.

There are likely many mind-body routes, with many mechanisms to create similar effects. Therefore, different states of mind may affect the body along different pathways, or the same substances may have multiple effects. In other words, relief of pain may also stimulate immune function, because pain-relieving endorphins are key messenger molecules that also "talk" to the immune system.

The natural conclusion emerging from placebo research is that expectation or belief affects biology. The emotional responses of individuals to the world around them, stimulating hopes and joys, fears and anguish, has a potential affect on the physical body. This understanding is fundamental to the treatment of illness. It does not mean that conventional medical treatment should be supplanted by psychological or emotional approaches. The most effective and comprehensive strategy of treatment should be expanded to include the awareness of emotional and psychological factors in concert.

MIND AND EMOTION EVERYWHERE

Former chief of the Brain Biochemistry Section of the National Institute of Mental Health, Candace Pert, PhD, co-discoverer of endorphins, made some startling revelations regarding the existence of neuropeptide receptors throughout the entire body. Pert found that the endocrine system and even the immune system all have these messenger molecules. This means that neuropeptide molecules are involved in a psychosomatic communication network and that the biochemistry of emotion could be mediating the transference of information flowing throughout the body. Pert maintains that the emotions are the bridge between the mental and the physical, which makes them prime candidates for a variety of links between thought and healing.

MIND AND IMMUNITY

Psychoneuroimmunology, a term coined by Robert Ader, an experimental psychologist, was first introduced to the scientific community in 1981. Ader had previously conducted experiments with rats which showed that the immune system could be conditioned and therefore did not operate autonomously, but was actually under the influence of the brain (see Chapter 8).

In subsequent research at the University of Rochester, Ader and Nicholas Cohen continued to show that the immune system can be trained, or conditioned, to respond to a neutral stimulus (placebo). They found that the administration of an immune-suppressing drug and placebo together "conditioned" the immune system to respond to the placebo alone after the drug was discontinued. They also found that by alternating the administration of real medication and placebos, thus conditioning the body's physiological response to the placebo, the conditioning effects of a drug can be increased. They believed that side effects of dependence could be reduced in addition to costs (Ader et al, 1991).

Considering the brief time that psychoneuroimmunology has existed as an accepted field of research, a great amount of data has been collected in support of the idea that homeostatic mechanisms are the product of an integrated system of defenses of which the immune system is a critical component. Now that we understand that peptides and receptors are expressed by the nervous system, the digestive system, and the immune system, it is not surprising to learn that immunological reactivity can be influenced by stressful life experiences (Ader, 2003).

It has become increasingly clear that there must be an intricate network behind spontaneous remissions, which are known to occur in cancer more often than any other disease. Research will likely continue to raise more questions about the mechanics of how the power of the mind actually works. How can the anticipation of a physical effect actually bring about physical change? And if anticipation or attitudes do play a role in creating physical change, how can that knowledge be used to enhance medical treatment or promote good health? If we can answer these questions, can we determine how the human mind converts ideas and expectations into chemical realities? Mind-body practitioners and medical researchers alike must answer these questions.

PSYCHOTHERAPY

The word *psychotherapy* is derived from Greek words meaning "healing of the soul" and refers to treatment involving emotional and mental health, which is interwoven with physical health. Psychotherapy encompasses a wide range of specific treatments, including combining medication with discussion, listening to the patient's concerns, and using more active behavioral and emotional approaches. It should also be understood more generally as the matrix of interaction in which all health professionals operate (Box 9-1).

An average of "one in every five people in the United States experiences a major psychological disorder every six months—most commonly anxiety, depression, substance abuse, or acute confusion" (Strain, 1993). The rate is believed to be even higher among patients with a chronic illness and among elderly patients. Approximately three fifths of patients with psychological problems are seen only by primary care physicians, many of whom are not adequately trained in psychotherapy or do not have adequate time to spend with each patient discussing these psychological issues. Despite the enormous need for different forms of psychological care, most people who display the greatest need for such care receive less than adequate screening and treatment for their psychiatric conditions.

Research also indicates that primary care physicians recognize cases of depression in only one fourth to one half of the patients who experience it, and they recognize other types of mental illness in less than one fourth of

---

BOX 9-1

Major Figures in Psychotherapy as Related to Complementary and Alternative Medicine Approaches

Carl Jung
Unconscious
Collective unconscious
Archetypes

Abraham Maslow
Humanistic psychology
Self-actualization
Hierarchy of needs

Carl Rogers
Person-centered psychotherapy
Humanistic psychology

Milton Erikson
Unconscious
Hypnosis
Family system therapy

cases. However, these same physicians write most of the prescriptions for antidepressant and antianxiety drugs and may often prescribe them inappropriately. Clearly, there is a significant need for better recognition and management of the psychiatric conditions that often accompany serious illness.

METHODS OF PSYCHOTHERAPY

Mental health professionals are paying more attention to features shared by all effective forms of psychotherapy, especially collaboration between the therapist and patient in developing an account of the patient's emotional life that promotes confidence, heightens well-being, and suggests ways to overcome cognitive or emotional difficulties. The primary aim of psychotherapy is to transform the meaning of the patient's experience by improving emotional state through an intimate relationship with a helpful person. Conventional psychotherapy is conducted primarily through psychological methods such as suggestion, persuasion, psychoanalysis, and reeducation. Although research suggests that the methods do not differ greatly in effectiveness, several hundred types of psychotherapy are available, used individually or in groups. Generally, most forms of psychotherapy fall in the following general categories:

- **Psychodynamic therapy.** Psychodynamic therapy is derived from psychoanalysis and seeks to understand and resolve emotional conflicts that originate in childhood relationships and repeat themselves in adult life. Sessions usually are devoted to exploring current emotional reactions from past situations. This approach works best if the patient's goal is to make fundamental changes in personality patterns rather than to change one specific behavior. Psychodynamic therapy is often called *interpretive therapy* or *expressive therapy*.
- **Behavior therapy.** Behavior therapy emphasizes changing specific behavior, such as a phobia, by stopping what has been reinforcing it or by replacing it with a more desirable response. Sessions are usually devoted to analyzing the behavior and devising ways to change it, with specific instructions carried out between sessions. Behavior therapy is more effective with focused problems, such as a fear of public speaking.
- **Cognitive therapy.** Cognitive therapy is similar to behavior therapy in changing specific habits; however, it emphasizes the habitual thoughts that underlie those habits. The general strategy is similar to that of behavior therapy, and the two approaches are often used together. Cognitive therapy is effective therapy for treating depression and low self-esteem.
- **Systems therapy.** Systems therapy focuses on relationship patterns, either in couples, between parents and children, or within the whole family.

This approach requires that everyone involved attend therapy sessions and often entails experiential practice aimed at changing problem-causing patterns. Systems therapies work well for a troubled marriage or intense conflicts between parent and child, where the problem is in the relationship between them.
- **Supportive therapy.** Supportive therapy concentrates on helping people who are in an intense emotional crisis, such as a deep depression, and may be used in combination with pharmacological support. It focuses on building tools to handle overwhelming day-to-day situations.
- **Body-oriented therapy.** Body-oriented therapy hypothesizes that emotions are encoded in and may be expressed as tension and restriction in various parts of the physical body. Various methods of therapy, including breathwork, movement, and manual pressure, are used to help release emotions that are believed to have been held in the muscles and tissues.

Recent research indicates that psychotherapeutic treatment can hasten recovery from a medical crisis and in some cases is the best treatment for it. Brief psychotherapy reduced time spent in hospitals for elderly patients with broken hips by an average of 2 days; these patients returned to the hospital fewer times and spent fewer days in rehabilitation (Strain, 1993). Other studies show that psychotherapy is most effective when begun soon after a patient is admitted to a hospital. At present, however, most psychological problems associated with physical illnesses remain undiagnosed or are not identified until near the end of a hospital stay.

One of the most common psychological problems of medical patients is "reactive" anxiety and depression—the emotional distress stemming from a patient's reaction to diagnosis. Those with serious or terminal illnesses are particularly vulnerable. In other cases, psychiatric symptoms are directly caused by the patient's physical disease. Still other patients experience a shift in their mental or emotional status as a direct result of a specific medication. For example, some patients taking high levels of steroids may react psychotically, whereas others may experience severe depression.

ROLE OF GROUP SUPPORT AND PSYCHOLOGICAL COUNSELING

Psychologists have known since World War II that social support and group consciousness greatly aid people in their attitudes and emotional resiliency. Over the past 10 years, clinical studies have shown that social support indeed has a significant influence on symptoms of stress for patients with chronic illnesses.

In an earlier yet still impressive study of patients with established coronary artery disease, group support and psychological counseling were combined with diet and exercise. Symptoms such as angina pectoris rapidly diminished or disappeared, and after 1 year the coronary artery obstructions were smaller. This evidence strongly suggested that the most deadly and expensive U.S. health care problem could potentially be reversible through a complementary, noninvasive, diet and behavioral modification approach that emphasizes group psychotherapy (Ornish, 1990).

A landmark case study was conducted in 1989 by David Spiegel, MD, a professor of psychiatry and behavioral sciences at Stanford School of Medicine, in which he investigated the benefits of group support on women with metastatic breast cancer. The women who participated in the group psychotherapy lived an average of 18 months longer than those who did not participate, doubling their survival time. The added survival time was longer than that any medication or other known medical treatment could be expected to provide for women with advanced breast cancer. The intense social support the women experienced in these sessions appeared to influence the way their bodies coped with the illness, which suggested that quality of life affected longevity (Spiegel et al, 1989).

In 1999, Spiegel conducted a multicenter feasibility study to examine the benefits of a supportive-expressive group psychotherapy intervention for patients with recently diagnosed breast cancer. One hundred and eleven breast cancer patients within 1 year of diagnosis were recruited from 10 geographically diverse sites of the Community Clinical Oncology Program of the National Cancer Institute and two academic medical centers. Each patient who participated in the expressive psychotherapy group met for 12 weekly sessions of 90 minutes each. Results indicated a significant decrease in mood disturbance scores, anxiety, and depression in group participants (Spiegel et al, 1999).

A similar study was conducted involving 102 women with metastatic breast cancer who were randomly selected to receive 1 year of weekly supportive-expressive group therapy and educational materials. Control women received education materials only. Participants who received group therapy showed a significantly greater decline in traumatic stress symptoms and total mood disturbance than did control subjects (Classen et al, 2001).

Recent research suggests that the maintenance of emotional well-being is critical to cardiovascular health. People who feel lonely, depressed, and isolated have been found to be significantly more likely to suffer illnesses and die prematurely of cardiovascular diseases than those who have adequate social support (Williams et al, 1999). Consequently, the development of appropriate interventions to improve the emotional health of people with certain psychosocial risk factors has become an important research goal. It is anticipated that such interventions will increase life expectancy of people at risk and may also save millions of dollars in medical care costs.

A cross-sectional study conducted at Stanford examined whether coping styles of emotional suppression and "fighting spirit" were associated with mood disturbance in 121 cancer patients participating in professionally led, community-based support groups. The investigators concluded that expression of negative affect and an attitude of realistic optimism may enhance adjustment and reduce stress for cancer patients in support groups (Cordova et al, 2003).

Recent studies are beginning to show a convergence of significant psychological, health behavior, and biological effects after a psychological intervention for cancer patients. An Ohio State University study tested the hypothesis that a psychological intervention could reduce emotional distress, improve health behavior, and enhance immune responses; 227 women who had undergone breast cancer surgery were randomly assigned to receive an intervention that included strategies to reduce stress, improve mood, alter health behaviors, and maintain adherence to cancer treatment. The control group received no intervention. The treatment group met in weekly sessions for 4 months. Patients who attended the weekly support group sessions showed significant lowering of anxiety, improvements in perceived social support, improved dietary habits, and reduction in smoking. Immune responses for the intervention group paralleled their psychological and behavioral improvements. T-cell proliferation remained stable or increased in the treatment group, whereas the responses declined in the control group (Andersen et al, 2004).

COST-EFFECTIVENESS OF PSYCHOTHERAPY

Psychotherapy has been shown to speed patients' recovery from illness. Faster recovery leads to reduced costs and fewer return visits to medical practitioners. In one study, patients who frequently visited medical clinics were offered short-term psychotherapy, and significant declines were seen in visits to their doctors, days spent in the hospital, emergency department visits, diagnostic procedures, and drug prescriptions. Their overall health care costs were decreased by 10% to 20% in the years after brief psychotherapy (Cummings et al, 1988).

A more specific example of cost effectiveness was provided by a 1991 study in which participation in 10 group sessions of 90 minutes of psychotherapy and relaxation techniques significantly reduced the severity of pain. In patients with chronic pain, those who participated in the outpatient behavioral medicine program had 36% fewer clinic visits than those who did not (Caudill et al, 1991).

In a 1987 study conducted jointly by Mount Sinai Hospital and Northwestern Memorial Hospital, psychiatrist George Fulop of Mount Sinai and his colleagues observed that patients hospitalized for medical or surgical reasons had significantly longer hospital stays if they also had concurrent psychiatric problems, especially if they were elderly. In other words, a patient who had a heart attack and who was also depressed tended to remain in the hospital for more days than a similar heart attack patient whose mood was normal. Fulop's study suggested that treating a medical patient's psychological conditions with psychotherapy in conjunction with medication could not only improve psychological well-being but also affect the patient's physical condition (Fulop et al, 1987).

Another well-known study, published in 1983 by psychologists Herbert J. Schlesinger and Emily Mumford and their colleagues at the University of Colorado School of Medicine, investigated patients with four common chronic diseases: asthma, diabetes, coronary heart disease, and high blood pressure. The researchers examined a group of Blue Cross/Blue Shield enrollees who underwent some form of psychotherapy after having been identified as having one of these physical conditions, then compared them with a control group who did not receive psychological treatment after similar diagnoses were made (Schlesinger et al, 1983). Three years after they received their medical diagnoses, patients who had undergone 7 to 20 mental health treatment visits had incurred lower medical charges than those who did not have psychological treatment. The total charges for the psychotherapy group, including those incurred for psychotherapy and counseling, were more than $300 less than for the control group. In other words, the savings on medical bills offered by psychotherapy more than compensated for its costs. After 21 sessions the savings began to diminish as the cumulative cost of mental health care increased.

Although this study is often cited as "proof" of psychotherapy's financial advantages for medically ill patients, it was a retrospective study rather than a prospective study. More scientifically controlled studies are needed in which subjects are selected at random from the beginning of treatment and closely followed after treatment. Another limitation of this particular research approach was that the investigators could not clearly define the type of mental health problems the patients experienced or the specific treatment they received. The information gathered encompassed a large variety of psychiatric interventions.

More rigorous research on specific forms of psychotherapy, including precise diagnoses, will be needed to reach firm conclusions about the economic benefits of psychological treatment for medically ill patients. However, there is already sufficient evidence to suggest that this cost-benefit research is important to pursue. For example, during the period from 1965 to 1980 patients who underwent psychotherapy used other medical services significantly less than patients who did not receive psychotherapy.

The concept of what constitutes appropriate areas for psychiatric intervention should be expanded. Many people, including health care professionals and academicians, consider psychotherapeutic intervention in physical illness a peripheral concern. Important research questions regarding unexplained mind-body events have long existed but are generally ignored. However, the studies previously cited suggest that psychological intervention can be most beneficial when used early in the disease process and can affect mortality in certain illnesses.

Although research continues to mount on the effects of psychotherapeutic interventions, further studies are needed to continue researching how the mind and body are interconnected and how these methods can offer genuine opportunity to improve health and limit costs simultaneously.

RESEARCH ON SOCIAL SUPPORT AND MORTALITY

Thanks to a growing number of large-scale studies, evidence of a link between social support and physical well-being has been abundant. This research shows that having many close social relationships is associated with a lower risk of dying at any age. Research that has looked specifically at sick people shows that once serious illness strikes, social support continues to affect their chances of staying alive.

Over 30 years ago, medical researchers were drawn to the tight-knit Italian community of Roseto in eastern Pennsylvania. Its late-middle-aged citizens seemed nearly immune to heart disease, seemingly in defiance of medical logic. The men of the town smoked, and drank wine freely. (This same effect observed in Europe would later become known as the *French Paradox.*) They worked in slate quarries 200 feet down in the earth. At home their tables were laden with Italian food modified in a way that would horrify a dietitian. To save money, they had replaced olive oil with . . . lard! Yet their hefty bodies contained healthy hearts. Why?

Every aspect of their health was examined in a comprehensive series of tests, observations, and interviews; however, traditional medical science did not offer any answer.

The answer lay in social science, not medicine. Stated simply, it was found that people nourish other people. Households contained three generations; everyone had a place. The community had stability and predictability. Everyone had a part in his or her society. Similar "Roseto effects" have been documented from Israel to Borneo, as well as in France (as noted earlier).

The researchers who came to study it also predicted that the Roseto effect would disappear. Indeed, as suburbs appeared, with fences and satellite dishes, the rate of heart attacks in time came to reflect the national averages ("A new 'Roseto Effect,'" 1996). Even the success of the Ornish diet in preventing and reversing heart disease has been thought by some observers to be, at least in part, due to the social support of the dieters' cooking, eating, and interacting together (especially because the diet itself is thought by many to be too high in carbohydrates for optimal health; see Chapter 25) (Egolf et al, 1992).

Internist James Goodwin at the Medical College of Wisconsin studied cancer survival in several thousand patients. The married cancer patients did better medically and had lower mortality rates than the unmarried patients

(Goodwin et al, 1987). Similarly, in a study of 1368 patients with coronary artery disease, Redford Williams at Duke University found that having a spouse or other close confidant tripled the chances that a patient would be alive 5 years later (Williams et al, 1999).

In an overview of research concerning mortality and social relationships, James House observed that the relationship between social isolation and early death is as strong statistically as the relationship between dying and smoking or having a high serum cholesterol level. Therefore the data suggest that it may be as important to one's health to be socially integrated as it is to stop smoking or to reduce one's cholesterol level (House et al, 1988).

In 1990, epidemiologists Peggy Reynolds and George Kaplan at the California Department of Health Services studied the number of social contacts that cancer patients had each day. Women with the least amount of social contact were 2.2 times more likely to die of cancer over a 17-year period than were the most socially connected women (Reynolds et al, 1990).

People who feel lonely, depressed, and isolated have been found to be significantly more likely to experience illnesses and to die prematurely of cardiovascular diseases than those who have adequate social support (Williams et al, 1999). Naturally, many other potential social factors can account for why one patient survives longer than another. Therefore, most such studies have been careful to eliminate the obvious confounding variables, such as smoking and alcohol use, differences in socioeconomic status, and access to health care. In general, however, the studies still consistently show that more and better social support from family and friends is associated with lower odds of dying at any given age.

Although the relationship between social support and health outcome has been largely underestimated by medical science, two studies recently examined social support and its relationship to mortality. The Department of Community and Preventative Medicine at the University of Rochester School of Medicine found that certain aspects of informal caregiving are important factors in enhancing the survival of frail nursing home residents. Several social support variables were statistically significant predictors of mortality. Participants whose caregiver was a spouse had a significantly lower risk of mortality than those whose caregiver was not a spouse (Temkin-Greener et al, 2004). Researchers at the Mayo Clinic recently reaffirmed many of these finding in a systematic overview of recent evidence related to the social support network, specifically the role of social support in cardiovascular disease–related outcomes (Mookadam et al, 2004).

A number of studies have demonstrated a relationship between depression and low perceived social support and increased cardiac morbidity and mortality in patients with heart disease. Evidence also suggests that depression increases the risk of acute myocardial infarction as well as the level of resulting morbidity and mortality (Malach et al, 2004).

RELAXATION
STRESS MANAGEMENT

The popular term *stress* was brought into use by Professor Hans Selye, director of the Institute of Experimental Medicine and Surgery at the University of Montreal. He defined stress as "the rate of wear and tear on the body." Confusion and debate continue as to whether stress is the factor that causes the wear and tear or is the resulting damage. Selye described a "general adaption syndrome," which has three phases: an alarm reaction, a stage of resistance, and a stage of exhaustion. A stress cause, or stressor, activates the sympathetic branch of the autonomic nervous system. Hormones bring about physiological changes in the body, often referred to as the "fight-or-flight response" (Selye, 1978).

The problem of stress has received wide publicity in the media in recent years. The cliché has also been heard that "stress" was the epidemic of the 1980s and 1990s. Consequently, the term *stress* has become a buzzword that has acquired a highly negative connotation. Much advice has also been received over the last few years, from all sorts of sources, about the many different approaches to controlling stress. All the alarmist and negative publicity has stimulated further anxiety and concern in many people's minds—a fear of stress, which in itself can lead to further stress. Having become aware of it, everyone now wants to manage his or her stress, and many cater to this growing demand. This rapidly expanding market is served by various experts, consultants, and therapists. Vitamin regimens, herbal supplements, fitness programs, relaxation techniques, and personal development courses are being offered, all in the name of *stress management*. Numerous experts, both qualified and self-appointed, are convinced that their particular product or service will banish stress for good.

The fact remains that there are no magic cures and no magic bullets. Stress is essentially a result of an interaction between a negative environment, unhealthful lifestyles, and self-defeating attitudes and beliefs. Therefore, in contrast to what is believed by stress management consultants, no one particular technique, method, program, or regimen of vitamins or herbs can reduce long-term stress.

Stress is most often viewed as the outside pressures and problems that encroach on our busy lives: deadlines, excessive workload, noise, traffic, problems with spouse or children, and excessive demands made by others. Stress is the unconscious response to a demand. Stress is not "those things out there," but rather what happens inside the mind and body as we react unconsciously to those things or people. Normally, we experience some degree of stress in everything we do and everything that happens to us.

In *The Magical Child*, Joseph Chilton Pearce states, "Stress is the way intelligence grows." He explains that, under stress, the brain immediately grows massive numbers of new connecting links between the neurons that enable learning. Although the stressed mind/brain grows in ability and the unstressed mind lags behind, the overstressed brain can collapse into physiological shock. Something is essential to maintain the optimal level of stress, and this is relaxation (Pearce, 1992).

When the stress response is minor, we do not notice any symptoms. The greater the stimulation, the more symptoms we notice. Holmes and Rahe's scale of life changes provides a guide to the amount of stress attached to major events, such as marriage, relocation, emigration, loss of a job, death of a spouse, or birth of a child. These significant life events can quickly overload our ability to cope (Holmes et al, 1967).

In *The Human Zoo,* Desmond Morris posits that modern humans are engaged in the "stimulus struggle": "If we abandon it, or tackle it badly, we are in serious trouble." We are trying to maintain the optimal level of stimulation—not the maximum, but the level that is most beneficial, somewhere between understimulation and overstimulation (Morris, 1995).

Stress becomes a problem when it reaches excessive levels, when the demands exceed our ability to respond or to cope effectively. When we are under excessive, prolonged stress and no longer able to cope or adjust, the "stress" becomes "distress." Symptoms then develop that lead to stress-induced illnesses. The physical body "engine" begins to rev at high speed, totally absorbing restricted, unproductive energy. Over extended periods, this wear and tear begins to take its toll, and disease can creep into the body.

We can learn to control our responses to stress by changing the ways that we think. "Stress management" is developing the ability to assert control over our behaviors. When we become aware of our ability to control attitudes and behaviors, we naturally begin to assert control over the life situations that seem to be stressful. It is not the stress itself that is harmful but our reactions to it that create havoc in the body and mind.

The greatest stressor that most people experience daily is *change.* Challenges, frustrations, conflicting demands, and occasional loss, grief, and suffering are among the many unconscious responses to change. These life events are inevitable and require us to adapt to new situations. If we do not adapt to change by altering our attitudes, our minds and bodies suffer. When changes take place in our environment, career, and personal relationships, it becomes essential to learn how to behave, think, and feel differently to cope with the new situation effectively.

We are all continuously adjusting to changing conditions, rather like an air conditioner controlled by a thermostat. As the temperature outside increases, the thermostat turns on the air conditioner, which begins to bring the interior temperature back to a specified normal level of comfort. The greater the changes outside, the harder the machine has to work to keep up with them. If the external temperature moves into extreme ranges, the machine will be pushed to the limit. If it exceeds its specified limit, it will eventually break down, and the motor will burn out.

So it is with the human machine. Our bodies continuously react to whatever is happening around us or inside of us. We respond physically, mentally, and emotionally to even the most minute changes. This process occurs all the time, whether we are consciously aware of it or not.

Different individuals respond differently to stress. We know people who can remain cool, calm, and collected under the most trying circumstances, and we know others who are unable to cope when faced with even minor situations. The differences are mostly a result of the differences in upbringing, past understandings, present experiences, attitudes, belief structures, family values, perceptions, and coping skills developed over years and generations. Furthermore, when different individuals experience distress, the symptoms they develop are also different; different people seem to channel their excessive stress into different parts of the body. The long-term effects of such different responses include physical illnesses such as ulcers, headaches, chronic backaches, and high blood pressure, which ultimately results in heart disease, cancer, or other chronic disorders.

Decades of research have linked stress, either directly or indirectly, to coronary heart disease, cancer, strokes, lung ailments, accidental injuries, cirrhosis of the liver, immune system deficiencies, and suicide. Stress is often a component of chronic illness, either as a precursor of disease or as an outcome. People who manage stress are more resilient, experience fewer symptoms, and experience an improved quality of life (Kabat-Zinn, 1990).

In looking at 26 randomized controlled trials testing the effect of cognitive-behavioral techniques (including meditation) on hypertension, Eisenberg et al (1993) found that no single technique appears to be more effective than any other in treating essential hypertension. When prescribed in the absence of other behavioral interventions, cognitive-behavioral techniques were not nearly as effective as standard antihypertensive pharmacotherapy.

Harvard-trained cardiologist Herbert Benson began investigating the benefits of relaxation in the late 1960s and continues to delve into the effects of stress on various disease-specific populations. Benson's group has examined the stress phenomenon and its effect on cardiovascular diseases and neurodegenerative diseases (Esch et al, 2002a, 2000b). They found that stress has a major impact on the circulatory and nervous systems, playing a significant role in susceptibility, progress, and outcome of both cardiovascular and neurodegenerative diseases. However, they also found that some amounts of stress can actually improve performance and thus can be beneficial in certain cases.

According to the American Institute of Stress in New York, workplace stress leads to $300 billion in health care costs each year as a result of missed work (Schwartz, 2004). The Organizational Science and Human Factors Branch of the National Institute for Occupational Safety and Health claims that stressed workers incur health care costs that are 46% higher, an average of $600 more per person, than other employees (Sauter, 2004).

THE RELAXATION RESPONSE

Convinced that the benefits of meditation could potentially lower high blood pressure, Benson continued his research into a variety of psychological and physiological effects that appear common to many mind-body practices. He later identified the relaxation response, which is similar to the response common to meditation, prayer, autogenic training, and some forms of hypnosis (Benson, 1975). He later described his method in a book of the same name.

Benson's research indicated that excessive stress can cause or aggravate hypertension and the related diseases of atherosclerosis, heart attack, and stroke. He then examined the nature of the relaxation response, showing that physiological changes as remarkable as those seen in the fight-or-flight response also occur during true relaxation, including a decrease in oxygen consumption, metabolic rate, heart rate, and blood pressure, as well as increased production of alpha brain waves. A marked decrease in blood lactate level was also found. Blood lactate has often been linked with anxiety. According to Benson, following these guidelines can help in achieving the relaxation response:

1. Try to find 10 to 20 minutes in your daily routine; before breakfast is generally a good time.
2. Sit comfortably.
3. For the period you will practice, try to arrange your life so that you will have no distractions. For example, let the answering machine handle the phone, or ask someone to watch the children.
4. Time yourself by glancing periodically at a clock or watch (but do not set an alarm). Commit yourself to a specific length of practice.

Expanding on these guidelines, Benson suggests the following as one of several approaches that can be used to elicit the relaxation response:

Step 1: Pick a focus word or short phrase that is firmly rooted in your personal belief system. For example, a nonreligious individual might choose a neutral word such as *one, peace,* or *love*. A Christian person wanting to use a prayer could pick the opening words of Psalm 23, "The Lord Is My Shepherd"; a Jewish person could choose *shalom*.

Step 2: Sit quietly in a comfortable position.

Step 3: Close your eyes.

Step 4: Relax your muscles.

Step 5: Breathe slowly and naturally, repeating your focus word or phrase silently as you exhale.

Step 6: Throughout, assume a passive attitude. Do not worry about how well you are doing. When other thoughts come to mind, simply say to yourself, "Oh, well," and gently return to the repetition.

Step 7: Continue for 10 to 20 minutes. You may open your eyes to check the time, but do not use an alarm. When you finish, sit quietly for a minute or so, at first with your eyes closed and later with your eyes open. Then do not stand for 1 or 2 minutes.

Step 8: Practice the technique once or twice a day.

Benson's subsequent research into the relaxation response investigated several efficient techniques of relaxation training, including Transcendental Meditation, Zen and yoga, autogenic training, progression relaxation, hypnosis, and sentic cycles (Table 9-1). He found that these methods had four common elements: a quiet environment, an object on which to focus the mind, a passive attitude, and a comfortable position. Some practices are more effective than others, and some are easier to learn and practice than others (Benson, 1993).

TABLE 9-1

Relaxation Response

Technique	Oxygen consumption	Respiratory rate	Heart rate	Alpha waves	Blood pressure	Muscle tension
Transcendental meditation	Decreases	Decreases	Decreases	Increase	Decreases*	(Not measured)
Zen and yoga	Decreases	Decreases	Decreases	Increase	Decreases*	
Autogenic training	(Not measured)	Decreases	Decreases	Increase	Inconclusive	Decreases
Progressive relaxation	(Not measured)	(Not measured)	(Not measured)	(Not measured)	Inconclusive	Decreases
Hypnosis with suggested deep relaxation	Decreases	Decreases	Decreases	(Not measured)	Inconclusive	(Not measured)

*In patients with elevated blood pressure.

Benson's group also found that patients with chronic pain who meditated regularly had a net reduction in general health care costs, which suggests that the use of relaxation techniques is cost effective (Caudill et al, 1991).

Deepak et al (1994) found that 11 patients with drug-resistant epilepsy who practiced Benson's relaxation response for 20 minutes each day experienced a decrease in absolute frequency of seizures, and that the decrease became significant at between 6 and 12 months of continued practice. Duration of seizures declined over the 12 months to a more significant degree than did frequency of seizures.

The value of Benson's technique for patients with congestive heart failure was evidenced in a study of 57 veterans with this disorder who received relaxation response training. Approximately half the group reported physical improvements that went beyond disease management and into lifestyle changes and improved relationships (Chang et al, 2004).

EXERCISE FOR STRESS REDUCTION

Michael Sacks, MD, professor of psychiatry at Cornell University Medical College, found that various forms of exercise can be powerful methods of relaxation effective for dealing with the stress of daily life. Researchers have found in various studies that exercise can decrease anxiety and depression, improve an individual's self-image, and buffer people from the effects of stress. Not every study has shown the precise benefits for which researchers were looking, but taken as a whole, the research strongly supports the common experience that exercise can elevate mood and reduce anxiety and stress (Sacks, 1993).

Although most research has focused on the physical benefits of exercise, any exercise can help people feel more focused and relaxed as long as the activity is enjoyable. Regular exercise does seem to affect one aspect in particular: the ability to withstand stress. Exercise and physical fitness can act as a buffer against stress, so that stressful events have a less negative impact on psychological and physical health.

MEDITATION

In 2003 the Centers for Disease Control and Prevention announced that chronic diseases affect more than 90 million Americans and account for one third of the years of potential life lost before age 65. The financial burden of treating chronic diseases now amounts to more than 60% of the total medical care costs in the United States. Evidence is accumulating that chronically ill patients gain much benefit from using meditation, including a decrease in the number of visits to physicians (Sobel, 1992).

Complementary and alternative medicine (CAM) encompasses a broad group of interventions, such as meditation, that are not taught widely at U.S. medical schools or generally available at U.S. hospitals (see Chapter 1). In 1997, however, more than 42% of the adult U.S. population used CAM to manage cancer and other chronic diseases, and meditation is one of the most common practices (Eisenberg et al, 2001).

Although meditation is ancient in its roots, the science of meditation and its physiological effects is in its infancy. Only recently has the concept of meditation been introduced into the realm of modern Western medicine. As a results of the Cartesian split between the mind and body in the early seventeenth century, science emphasized the body and medicine went in the direction of science. The term *mind-body connection* relates to an understanding that the two are not separate (they have always been together) and have an interactive influence on each other. Meditation is said to realign the two, the consciousness with the physical body, creating a more harmonious interaction.

Like the word *medicine,* the word *meditation* suggests something to do with healing. The root in Latin means "to cure" but that its deepest root means "to measure" (Bohm, 1983). But what does medicine or meditation have to do with measure? The ancient Greeks said, "Man is the measure of all things." According to Jon Kabat-Zinn, PhD, founder and director of the Stress Reduction Clinic at the University of Massachusetts Medical Center, meditation has to do with the platonic notion that every shape, every being, every thing has its right inward measure. In other words, a tree has its own quality of wholeness that gives it particular properties. A human being has an individual right inward measure, when everything is balanced and physiologically homeostatic. That is the totality of the individual at that point in time" (1993a, 1993b, 1993c). He believes that medicine is the science and art of restoring right inward measure when it is thrown off balance. From the meditative perspective and from the perspective of the new mind-body medicine, health does not have a finite or static destination. Health is a dynamic energy flow that changes over a lifetime, with health and illness coexisting.

Most meditative practices have come to the West from Asian religious practices, particularly those of India, China, and Japan. Others can be traced to the ancient cultures of the world. Although Western meditators practice a contemplative form of meditation, there are also many active forms of meditation, such as the Chinese martial art t'ai chi, the Japanese martial art aikido, and the walking meditations of Zen Buddhism.

Until recently, the primary purpose of meditation has been religious or spiritual in nature. During the past 20 years, however, meditation has been explored as a means of reducing stress on both mind and body. Many studies have found that various practices of meditation appear to produce physical and psychological changes. Meditation is a self-directed practice for the purpose of relaxing and calming the mind and body. Many methods of meditation include focusing on a single thought or word for a specific time. Some forms of meditation focus on a physical experience, such as the breath or a specific sound or mantra. All forms of meditation have the common objective of stilling the restlessness of the mind so that the focus can be directed inwardly.

Meditation is thus a technique used to calm mental activity, endless thoughts, and ways of reacting to one's circumstances. As long as these accumulated impressions linger in the inner recesses of the mind, pushing for attention, it remains difficult to experience an inner state of peace, calm, and health. Fast-paced Western society, filled with external stimuli, has conditioned us to push our minds and bodies to the point of exhaustion, often to the detriment of our own well-being. To be still, to experience the peace and contentment that lies within, we must free ourselves from this external materiality. Meditation is the process of calming and releasing the distractions from the mind for the purpose of opening up and awakening to our true inner natures.

EASTERN TECHNIQUES AND TRANSCENDENTAL MEDITATION

In the mid-1960s, a popular trend in meditation called *Transcendental Meditation (TM)* began to emerge. The Vedic philosophy and practice was brought from India to the United States by its founder, Maharishi Mahesh Yogi. The Maharishi had eliminated ancient yogic elements that he considered would be unpopular in a contemporary twentieth century western society. Omitting difficult physical postures and mental exercises, his modified version became easily understood, accepted, and practiced by Westerners (see Chapter 32).

TM is relatively simple in application. A student is given a mantra (a word or sound) to repeat silently over and over again while sitting in a comfortable position. The purpose of repeating the sound or word is to prevent distracting thoughts from entering the mind. Students are instructed to be passive and, if thoughts other than the mantra come to mind, to note them and return the attention to the mantra. TM is generally practiced in the morning and in the evening for approximately 20 minutes.

On the Maharishi's first visit to America in 1959, a San Francisco newspaper heralded TM as a "nonmedicinal tranquilizer" and praised it as a promising cure for insomnia. TM soon began to ride a crest of popularity, with almost half a million Americans learning the technique by 1975, and it was embraced by many celebrities of that day, such as the Beatles. It is believed that more than 2 million people currently practice TM.

In 1968, Harvard's Herbert Benson was asked by the Maharishi International University in Fairfield, Iowa, to test TM practitioners on their ability to lower their own blood pressure. Benson initially refused to participate but was later persuaded to do so. Benson's studies and other research showed that TM was associated with reduced health care costs, increased longevity, and better quality of life (Benson et al, 1977); reduced anxiety, lowered blood

pressure, and reduced serum cholesterol levels (Cooper et al, 1978); viable treatment of posttraumatic stress syndrome in Vietnam veterans (Brooks et al, 1985); and reduction in chronic pain (Kabat-Zinn et al, 1986).

In a study aimed at linking TM practice to longevity, 73 elders were randomly assigned to either a TM program, mindfulness training, a relaxation program, or no treatment. Both the TM and mindfulness training groups showed significant reductions in systolic blood pressure compared with those receiving mental relaxation training or no training. As reported by the nursing staff, TM and mindfulness training improved patients' mental health. Longevity was defined as the subjects' survival rate over a 36-month period, which was found to be greater for those using TM than for those receiving mental relaxation training and control subjects (Alexander et al, 1989).

Additional research showed TM's effectiveness in the reduction of substance abuse (Sharma et al, 1991), blood pressure reduction in African Americans (Schneider et al, 1992), and lowering of blood cortisol levels initially raised by stress (MacLean et al, 1992).

In a follow-up study of 127 African American elders, Schneider again found that blood pressure decreased significantly in those practicing both TM and progressive muscle relaxation compared with the control group, and that TM was significantly more effective than progressive muscle relaxation techniques (Schneider et al, 1995).

In a study to examine the effects of TM on nine women with symptoms of cardiac syndrome X, those who practiced TM for 3 months showed an improvement in quality of life, exercise tolerance, and angina episodes (Cunningham et al, 2000). An experiment to determine the effects of TM-based stress reduction on carotid atherosclerosis in 60 hypertensive African Americans used B-mode ultrasound to measure carotid intima-media thickness, a surrogate measure of coronary atherosclerosis. The group practicing the TM technique group showed a significant decrease in thickness, whereas thickness increased in the control group (Castillo-Richmond et al, 2000).

Herron and Hillis broke new economic ground by conducting a quasi-experimental, longitudinal study of the impact of a TM program on government payments to physicians in Quebec. They found that payments to physicians treating practitioners of TM were lower than payments to physicians treating a randomly selected and matched control group over a 6-year period, with a 13.78% mean annual difference in payments. A true experimental design with randomization would be needed to control for social factors that may have confounded study results (Herron et al, 2000).

WESTERN TECHNIQUES AND MINDFULNESS MEDITATIONS

The term *mindfulness* was coined by Jon Kabat-Zinn, known for his work using mindfulness meditation to help medical patients with chronic pain and stress-related disorders

(1993a, 1993b). Like other mind-body therapies, mindfulness meditation can induce deep states of relaxation, at times can directly improve physical symptoms, and can help patients lead fuller and more satisfying lives. Although Asian forms of meditation involve focusing on a sound, phrase, or prayer to minimize distraction, the practice of mindfulness does the opposite. In mindfulness meditation, distractions are not ignored but are focused on. This form of meditation practice can be traced originally to the Buddhist tradition and is about 2500 years old. The method was developed as a means of cultivating greater awareness and wisdom, with the aim of helping people live each moment of their lives as fully as possible.

Kabat-Zinn points out that mindfulness is about more than feeling relaxed or stress free. Its true aim is to nurture an inner balance of mind that allows an individual to face life situations with greater clarity, stability, and understanding and to respond more effectively from that sense of clarity.

An integral part of mindfulness practice is to accept and welcome stress, pain, anger, frustration, disappointment, and insecurity when those feelings are present. Kabat-Zinn believes that acknowledgment is paramount. Whether pleasant or unpleasant, admission is the first step toward transforming that reality.

As noted earlier, Kabat-Zinn founded the Stress Reduction Clinic at the University of Massachusetts Medical Center in Worcester, where he is an associate professor of medicine. The Center for Mindfulness in Medicine, Health Care, and Society established in 1995, is an outgrowth of the clinic. Since the clinic was founded, more than 10,000 medical patients have gone through Kabat-Zinn's mindfulness meditation programs, almost all referred by their physicians.

To date, the Center for Mindfulness has produced 15 peer-reviewed papers on mindfulness-based stress reduction. Current research pursuits of the center include a prostate cancer study funded by the U.S. Department of Defense; a cost-effectiveness study; development of an innovative substance abuse recovery program for young, low income, inner city mothers; and a wide variety of other collaborative research endeavors in various states of development.

Unlike in standard medical and psychological approaches, the clinic does not categorize and treat patients differently depending on their illnesses. Their 8-week courses offer the same training program in mindfulness and stress reduction to everyone. They emphasize what is "right" with their patients, rather than what is "wrong" with them, focusing on mobilizing their inner strengths and changing their behaviors in new and innovative ways. Facilitators maintain that the programs are not held out as some kind of magical cure when other approaches have failed; rather, they provide a sensible and straightforward way for people to experience and understand the mind-body connection firsthand and use that knowledge to better cope with their illnesses.

In the practice of mindfulness, the patient begins by using one-pointed attention to cultivate calmness and stability. When thoughts and feelings arise, it is important not to ignore or suppress them or analyze or judge them by their content; rather, the thoughts are observed intentionally and nonjudgmentally, moment by moment, as events in the field of awareness.

This inclusive noting of thoughts that come and go in the mind can lead to a detachment from them, which allows a deeper perspective about the stresses of life to emerge. By observing the thoughts from this vantage point, one gains a new frame of reference. In this way, valuable insight can be allowed to surface. The key to mindfulness is not the topic focused on but the quality of awareness brought into each moment. Observing the thought processes, without intellectualizing them and without judgment, creates greater clarity. The goal of mindfulness is to become more aware, more in touch with life and what is happening at the time it is happening, in the present.

Acceptance does not mean passivity or resignation. Accepting what each moment offers provides the opportunity to experience life more completely. In this manner, the individual can respond to any situation with greater confidence and clarity.

One way to envision how mindfulness works is to think of the mind as the surface of a lake or ocean. Many people think the goal of meditation is to stop the waves so that the water will be flat, peaceful, and tranquil. The spirit of mindfulness practice is to experience the waves.

The consistent practice of mindfulness meditation has been shown to decrease the subjective experience of pain and stress in a variety of research settings. One study found a 65% improvement in pain symptoms and an approximately 60% improvement in sleep and fatigue levels from before to after the intervention in a sample of 77 patients with fibromyalgia, an illness known to have psychosomatic components (Kaplan et al, 1993).

Dunn et al (1999) used electroencephalographic recordings to differentiate between two types of meditation, concentration and mindfulness, and a normal relaxation control condition. They found significant differences between readings at numerous cortical sites, which suggests that concentration and mindfulness meditations may be unique forms of consciousness and not merely degrees of a state of relaxation.

In a pilot study using mindfulness of movement as a coping strategy for multiple sclerosis, patients attended six individual one-on-one sessions of mindfulness training. Results showed that balance improved significantly in those who underwent the training compared with those who did not (Mills et al, 2000).

Eighty cancer patients were followed for 6 months after attending a mindfulness meditation group for 1.5 hours each week for 7 weeks. They were also asked to practice meditation at home on a daily basis. Results showed significantly lower mood disturbances and fewer symptoms of stress at the 6-month follow-up for both male and female participants. The greatest improvement, however, occurred on subscales measuring depression, anxiety, and anger. Results for various mindfulness meditation techniques are consistent with those for other meditation-based interventions (Carlson et al, 2001).

Nurses are often known to make mindfulness practice part of their continuing education. They find that this technique often prevents compassion fatigue and burnout, enhances health, and increases awareness of holism within the self.

HYPNOSIS

Modern hypnosis is said to have begun in the eighteenth century with Franz Anton Mesmer, who used what he called "magnetic healing" to treat a variety of psychological and psychophysiological disorders, such as hysterical blindness, paralysis, headaches, and joint pains. The famous Austrian neuropathologist Sigmund Freud initially found hypnosis to be extremely effective in treating hysteria and then, troubled by the sudden catharsis of powerful emotions by his patients, abandoned its use.

The word *hypnosis* is derived from the Greek word *hypnos,* meaning "sleep." It is believed that hypnotic suggestion has been a part of ancient healing traditions for centuries. The induction of trance states and the use of therapeutic suggestion were a central feature of the early Greek healing temples, and variations of these techniques were practiced throughout the ancient world.

In more recent years, hypnosis has experienced a resurgence. Initially, this form of therapy became popular with physicians and dentists. At present, hypnosis is widely used by mental health professionals for the treatment of addictions, anxiety disorders, and phobias and for pain control. During hypnosis a patient enters a state of attentive and focused concentration and becomes relatively unaware of the immediate surroundings. While in this state of deep concentration, the individual is highly responsive to suggestion. Contrary to popular folklore, however, people cannot be hypnotized against their will or involuntarily. They must be willing to concentrate their thoughts and to follow the suggestions offered. Essentially, all forms of hypnotherapy are actually forms of self-hypnosis.

Hypnosis has three major components: *absorption* (in the words or images presented by the hypnotherapist), *dissociation* (from one's ordinary critical faculties), and *responsiveness.* A hypnotherapist either leads patients through relaxation, mental imagery, and suggestions or teaches patients to perform the techniques themselves. Many hypnotherapists provide guided audiotapes for their patients so that they can practice the therapy at home. The images presented are specifically tailored to the particular patient's needs and may use one or all of the senses.

Physiologically, hypnosis resembles other forms of deep relaxation. It is known to decrease sympathetic nervous system activity, decrease oxygen consumption and carbon dioxide elimination, and lower blood pressure and heart rate, and it is linked to increase or decrease in certain types of brain wave activity.

Hypnotherapy's effectiveness lies in the complex connection between the mind and the body. It is now well understood that illness can affect one's emotional state and, conversely, that one's emotional state can affect one's physical state. For example, stress, an emotional reaction, can make heart disease worse, and heart disease, a physical condition, can cause depression.

Hypnosis carries this connection to the next logical step by using the power of the mind to bring about change in the body. No one is quite sure how hypnosis works, but with more sophisticated imaging techniques, that is changing.

CLINICAL APPLICATIONS

One of the most dramatic early uses of hypnosis was for treatment of skin disorders. In the mid-1950s an anesthesiologist, Arthur Mason, used hypnosis to effectively treat a 16-year-old patient who had warts. Within 10 days after the youth underwent hypnosis, the warts fell off and normal skin replaced it (Mason et al, 1958). Since that time, hypnosis has been used to dramatically improve other skin disorders, such as ichthyosis, and the importance of the role of the skin in the development of the immune system has been recognized (see Chapter 8).

Depending on the individual's situation, hypnotherapy can be used as a complement to medical care or as a primary treatment. Many people find that hypnotherapy's benefits are enhanced by the use of biofeedback to induce physiological changes. Biofeedback helps patients see that they can control certain bodily functions simply by altering their thoughts, and the added confidence helps them improve more rapidly.

There is little doubt that the regular practice of self-hypnosis is helpful to people with chronic disease. The benefits include reduction of anxiety and fear, decreased requirements for analgesics, increased comfort during medical procedures, and greater stability of functions controlled by the autonomic nervous system, such as blood pressure. Training in self-hypnosis also enhances the patient's sense of control, which is often affected by chronic illness. Hypnotherapy may also have direct clinical effects on certain chronic diseases, such as reducing bleeding in hemophiliac patients, stabilizing blood glucose level in diabetic patients, and reducing the severity of asthmatic attacks.

Irritable Bowel Syndrome

For many years, W.M. Gonsalkorale has been researching the benefits of hypnotherapy for management of irritable bowel syndrome at the University Hospital of South Manchester, United Kingdom. In only 3 months, symptoms such as pain and bloating, as well as the level of "disease interference" with life, improved profoundly for most of

232 patients who underwent hypnotherapy (Gonsalkorale et al, 2002). Good evidence now supports the long-term benefits for up to 6 years following hypnotherapy. In 204 patients, of the 71% who responded to therapy, 81% maintained their improvements, and the remaining 19% claimed that deterioration of symptoms had been slight (Gonsalkorale et al, 2003). Besides improving physical symptoms, hypnotherapy has also been shown to decrease cognitive symptoms such as anxiety and depression, and to improve quality of life (Gonsalkorale et al, 2004).

Preoperative Therapy

In 1997, Mehmet Oz, a cardiothoracic surgeon at Columbia Presbyterian Medical Center, received a great deal of attention for advocating and using complementary medical approaches in his surgical practice. Oz took 32 patients scheduled for coronary bypass surgery and randomly assigned them to two groups. One group received instruction on self-hypnosis relaxation techniques before surgery, and the other group received no instruction. Results showed that patients who practiced the self-hypnosis techniques were significantly more relaxed than the control subjects in the days after surgery (Ashton et al, 1997). There was no significant difference between the two groups in length of hospital stay and postoperative morbidity and mortality.

Postoperative Therapy

Carol Ginandes, a Harvard instructor, investigated how hypnotherapy can help people heal more quickly after surgery. Each of 18 women undergoing breast reduction surgery was placed in one of three groups. One group received standard surgical care. The second group received the same care and also received psychological support. The third group underwent hypnosis before and after surgery in addition to receiving standard care. Those who underwent hypnosis healed more rapidly, felt less discomfort, and had fewer complications (Ginandes et al, 2003).

Pain Control

Hypnosis can also be effective in reducing the fear and anxiety that accompanies pain. It is said that anxiety increases pain, and hypnotherapy helps a patient gain control over the fear and anxiety, thereby reducing the pain. Many controlled studies have demonstrated that hypnosis is an effective way to reduce migraine attacks in children and teenagers. In one experiment, 30 schoolchildren were randomly assigned to receive a placebo or propranolol (a blood pressure–lowering agent) or were taught self-hypnosis. Only the children who used the self-hypnosis techniques experienced a significant decrease in severity and frequency of headaches (Olness et al, 1988). A study of chronically ill patients reported a 113% increase in pain tolerance among highly hypnotizable individuals compared with members of a control group who did not receive hypnosis (Debeneditis et al, 1989).

Researchers at Virginia Polytechnic Institute found that during induction of a hypnotic state aimed at bringing about pain control, the prefrontal cortex of the brain directed other areas of the brain to reduce or eliminate their awareness of pain (Gordon, 2004). A technique used for pain control during surgery in people with little or no tolerance for chemical anesthesia, called "spinal anesthesia illusion," was developed by Philip Ament, a dentist and psychologist from Buffalo, New York. In this method a deep state of relaxation is induced by having the patient count mentally or focus on a specific image. The patient is given the suggestion that he or she will feel a growing numbness begin to spread from the navel to the toes as he or she counts to a higher and higher number. Once the patient feels numb, the surgery can proceed. After the surgery the therapist gives the patient suggestions that lead to the gradual return of normal sensations (Perlman, 1999).

Dentistry

Some people have learned to tolerate dental work (e.g., drilling, extraction, periodontal surgery) using hypnosis as the sole anesthesia. Even when an anesthetic is used, hypnotherapy can also be used to reduce fear and anxiety, control bleeding and salivation, and lessen postoperative discomfort. Used with children, hypnosis can decrease the chances of developing a dental phobia (Perlman, 1999).

Pregnancy and Delivery

It is believed that Lamaze and other popular breathing techniques used during labor and delivery may actually work by inducing a hypnotic state. Women who have used hypnosis before delivery tend to have a shorter labor and more comfortable delivery than other pregnant women. There are even reports of cesarean sections performed with hypnosis as the sole anesthesia. Women are taught to take advantage of their body's natural anesthetic abilities to make childbirth a less painful, more positive experience (Goldman, 1999).

Anxiety

Hypnosis can be used to establish a new reaction to specific anxiety-causing stimuli, such as in the treatment of stage fright, fear of airplane flight, and other phobias. Typically the hypnotherapist helps the patient undo a conditioned physiological response, such as hyperventilation or nausea. This method can also be used to help calm athletes who are preparing to compete. Hypnotherapy can be used to quell almost any fear, whether associated with examinations, public speaking, or social interactions.

Allergies and Asthma

Ran Anbar, a pediatric pulmonologist at the State University of New York's Upstate Medical University in Syracuse, teaches children self-hypnosis to help them control their allergies and asthma (Gordon, 2004).

BIOFEEDBACK

Biofeedback therapies emerged in the 1960s and 1970s, when advances in psychological and medical research converged with developments in biomedical technology. Improved electronic instruments could convey information to patients about their autonomic nervous systems and their muscles in the form of audio and visual signals that patients could understand. The word *biofeedback* became the general term to define the procedures and treatments that make use of these instruments (Green et al, 1977).

Biofeedback therapy uses special instruments and methods to expand the body's natural internal feedback systems. By watching a monitoring device, patients can learn by trial and error to adjust their thinking and other mental processes to control bodily processes previously thought to be involuntary, such as blood pressure, temperature, gastrointestinal functioning, and brain wave activity. In fact, biofeedback can be used to influence almost any bodily process that can be measured accurately.

Biofeedback does not belong to any particular field of health care and is used in many disciplines, including internal medicine, dentistry, physical therapy and rehabilitation, psychology and psychiatry, and pain management. As with other forms of therapy, biofeedback is more useful in addressing some clinical problems than others. For example, biofeedback is a useful treatment in Raynaud disease, a painful and potentially dangerous spasm of the small arteries, and certain types of fecal and urinary incontinence. It has also become an integral part of the treatment of many other disorders, including headaches, anxiety, high blood pressure, teeth clenching, asthma, and muscle disorders.

More recently, researchers have been experimenting with biofeedback treatments for conditions believed to stem from irregular brain wave patterns, such as epilepsy, attention-deficit disorder (ADD), and attention-deficit/hyperactivity disorder (ADHD) in children, with promising results.

Biofeedback is successful in helping people learn to regulate many physical conditions, partly because it puts them in better contact with specific parts of their bodies. For example, biofeedback can help teach people to tighten the muscles at the neck of the bladder to better control impaired bladder function. It can help postoperative patients learn to reuse the muscles of the legs and arms. It can help teach stroke patients to use alternative muscles to move a limb if the primary ones can no longer do the job. Biofeedback is also helpful in training patients to use artificial limbs after amputation.

In a normal biofeedback session, electrodes are attached to the area being monitored. These electrodes feed the information to a small monitoring box that registers the results aurally by a tone that varies in pitch or visually by a light that varies in brightness as the function being monitored decreases or increases. A biofeedback therapist leads the patient in mental exercises to help the patient reach the desired result. Through trial and error, patients gradually train themselves to control the inner mechanism involved. For some disorders, training requires 8 to 10 sessions; however, a single session often can provide symptomatic relief. Patients with long-term or severe disorders may require longer therapy. The aim of the treatment is to teach patients to regulate their own inner mental and bodily processes without the help of a machine.

FIVE COMMON FORMS OF BIOFEEDBACK THERAPY

1. **Electromyographic biofeedback.** Electromyographic feedback measures muscular tension. Sensors are attached to the skin to detect electrical activity related to muscle tension in a given area. The biofeedback instrument amplifies and converts this activity into useful information, displaying the various degrees of muscle tension. This form of biofeedback therapy is most often used for reduction of tension headaches, physical rehabilitation, treatment of chronic muscle pain, management of incontinence, and promotion of general relaxation.

2. **Thermal biofeedback therapy.** In thermal biofeedback therapy skin temperature is measured as an index of changes in blood flow from the constriction and dilation of blood vessels. Low skin temperature usually means decreased blood flow in that area. A temperature-sensitive probe is taped to the skin, often on a finger. The instrument converts information into feedback that can be seen and heard and can be used to reduce or increase blood flow to the hands and feet. Thermal biofeedback is often used for management of Raynaud disease, migraine headaches, hypertension, and anxiety disorders, and to promote general relaxation.

3. **Electrodermal activity therapy.** In electrodermal activity therapy, changes in sweat activity too minimal to feel are measured. Two sensors are attached to the palm side of the fingers or hand to measure sweat activity. They produce a tiny electrical current that measures skin conductance on the basis of the amount of moisture present. Increased sweat can mean arousal of part of the autonomic nervous system. Electrodermal activity devices can be used to measure the sweat output stemming from stressful thoughts or rapid deep breathing. Electrodermal activity therapy is most often used in the treatment of anxiety and hyperhidrosis.

4. **Finger pulse therapy.** In finger pulse therapy, pulse rate and force are measured. A sensor is attached to a finger and helps measure heart activity as a sign of arousal of part of the autonomic nervous system. Finger pulse therapy is most often used for management of hypertension, anxiety, and some cardiac arrhythmias.

5. **Breathing biofeedback therapy.** In breathing biofeedback therapy, the rate, volume, rhythm, and location of breathing are measured. Sensors are placed around the chest and abdomen to measure air flow

from the mouth and nose. The feedback is usually visual, and patients learn to take deeper, slower, lower, and more regular breaths using abdominal muscles. This simple form of biofeedback is most often used for management of asthma and other respiratory conditions, hyperventilation, and anxiety.

GOALS AND APPEAL

The general goal of biofeedback therapy is to lower body tension and change faulty biological patterns to reduce symptoms. Many people can and do reach goals of relaxation without the use of biofeedback. Although biofeedback may not be necessary, it can potentially add something useful to any treatment.

A major reason that many patients find biofeedback training appealing is that, as with behavioral approaches in general, it puts the patient in charge, giving the patient a sense of mastery and self-reliance with regard to the illness. It is believed that such an attitude can play a critical role in shortening recovery time, reducing incidence, and lowering health care costs.

RESEARCH CONSIDERATIONS

Biofeedback-assisted relaxation training has been shown to be associated with a decrease in medical care costs, a decrease in the number of claims and costs to insurers in claims payments, reduction in medication and physician use, reduction in hospital stays and rehospitalization, reduction of mortality and morbidity, and enhanced quality of life (Basmajian, 1989).

An unpublished study involving 241 employees of a Siberian metal company showed promising results for the integration of biofeedback training into occupational medicine as a method to increase workers' ability to work with few errors while increasing labor productivity levels. The employees had psychosomatic disorders presenting with symptoms of headache, sleepiness, and periodic blood pressure fluctuations. Workers attended 10- to 40-minute biofeedback sessions over 2 weeks. The results clearly indicated that the workers were able to control the brain's blood flow. Furthermore, a follow-up biofeedback session was repeated 1 month later and showed that all workers in the initial group could recall their strategies for producing positive change.

In another study, 30 patients with fibromyalgia syndrome received biofeedback and experienced statistically significant improvements in mental clarity, mood, and sleep (Mueller et al, 2001). However, future research using controlled trials is needed to understand disease mechanisms better.

Biofeedback, both sensory and augmented, has been used with some degree of success to treat patients with fecal incontinence. Forty women with fecal incontinence were randomly assigned to receive either augmented biofeedback or sensory biofeedback. After 12 weeks of

treatment the augmented form of biofeedback was found to be superior, although fecal incontinence improved in both treatment groups (Fynes et al, 1999). Another study compared biofeedback to standard care for treatment of fecal incontinence. Results showed that biofeedback was not superior to standard care in improving incontinence, but those who received biofeedback had significantly better scores on tests of hospital anxiety and depression (Norton et al, 2003).

More recently, 92 patients with systemic lupus erythematosus were assigned randomly to receive biofeedback-assisted cognitive-behavioral treatment, a symptom-monitoring support intervention, or usual medical care. Those who received biofeedback experienced significantly greater reductions in pain and psychological dysfunction than those who did not receive the biofeedback-assisted therapy. At 9-month follow-up, the biofeedback group continued to exhibit relative benefit compared with the control group (Greco et al, 2004).

In a randomized United Kingdom study, 38 patients with fecal incontinence were assigned to undergo sphincter repair or sphincter repair plus biofeedback. Although the results were not statistically significant, continence and satisfaction scores improved in the biofeedback group, and these improvements were sustained over time. Quality-of-life measures also improved in the biofeedback group (Davis et al, 2004).

The Department of Psychiatry at Robert Wood Johnson Medical School in New Jersey evaluated the effectiveness of heart rate variability (HRV) biofeedback as a complementary treatment in 94 patients with asthma. Patients in the two groups receiving biofeedback were prescribed less medication than those in the two control groups (placebo and wait list), which indicates that HRV biofeedback may be a useful adjunct to asthma treatment and may help to reduce dependence on steroid medications (Lehrer et al, 2004). Biofeedback techniques have also been used with some success to treat epilepsy and attention problems, such as sleeplessness, fatigue, and body pain.

Research on exactly how biofeedback works is somewhat inconclusive. Some studies link its benefits directly to physiological changes that the patient learns to make voluntarily. Other experiments find benefits even for patients who do not make the desired changes in the physiological measures. Biofeedback appears to help some patients increase their sense of control, heighten their optimism, and lessen feelings of hopelessness triggered by chronic health problems (Hatch et al, 1987). It appears that biofeedback used as adjunct therapy could add something beneficial to an existing therapy.

GUIDED IMAGERY

Since human societies began analyzing human experiences, philosophers have tried to define and explain the interior processes of the mind—all those experiences that are invisible to another person because they do not have physical referents. Philosophers have speculated at length on the nature of mental imagery, and scientists have found the phenomenon difficult to verify or measure. Behavioral psychologists of the 1920s went so far as to say that mental images simply do not exist.

Since 1960, psychologists have done a great amount of work exploring and categorizing mental imagery and inner processes. Contemporary psychologists distinguish several types of imagery. Probably the most common form of imagery that people experience is memory. If a person tries to remember a friend, the bed in his or her room, or the feel of the seats of his or her car, that person immediately perceives an image in his or her mind, the "mind's eye." People refer to this experience as "forming a mental picture." Some people believe that they do not "see" the scene but simply have a strong sense of the scene and "know" what it looks like.

Imagery is both a mental process and a wide variety of procedures used in therapy to encourage changes in attitudes, behaviors, or physiological reactions. As a mental process, it is often defined as "any thought representing a sensory quality" (Horowitz, 1983). In addition to the visual, it includes all the senses: aural, tactile, olfactory, proprioceptive, and kinesthetic. *Imagery* is often used synonymously with *visualization*. However, visualization refers only to "seeing" something in the mind's eye, whereas imagery can use one sense or combination of senses to produce an image.

Creating images with the mind is also a way of communicating with the deeper-than-conscious aspects of the mind. This is apparent when one considers the dream state, which communicates mainly in images that are then interpreted to make a story. This communicative quality of imagery is important, because feelings and behaviors are primarily motivated by subconscious and unconscious factors.

Imagery can be taught either individually or in groups, and the therapist often uses it to accomplish a particular result, such as cessation of addictive behavior or bolstering of the immune system to attack cancer cells. Because it often involves directed concentration, imagery can also be regarded as a form of guided meditation.

Many practices discussed in this chapter use a component of imagery. Psychotherapy, hypnosis, and biofeedback all use various elements of this process. Any therapy that relies on the imagination to stimulate, communicate, solve problems, or evoke a heightened awareness or sensitivity could be described as a form of imagery.

Numerous early studies indicated that mental imagery could bring about significant physiological and biochemical changes. These findings have encouraged the development of imagery as a health care tool. Imagery was found to have the capacity to affect dramatically the oxygen supply in tissues (Olness et al, 1988), cardiovascular parameters (Barber, 1969), vascular or thermal parameters (Green et al, 1977), the pupil and cochlear reflexes, heart rate and galvanic skin response (Jordan et al, 1979), and salivation (Barber et al, 1984; White, 1978).

CLINICAL APPLICATIONS

Communication with the unconscious had previously been the domain of hypnosis, which basically consists of two components: (1) the use of a technique to induce a state of consciousness in which there is freer access to the deeper part of the mind, and (2) a method of communicating with that deeper part of the mind. Often this communication involves making suggestions to the inner depths of the mind, suggesting items or behaviors that the individual desires for his or her betterment. In guided imagery, different techniques are used to induce the necessary state of consciousness, some quite similar to more common relaxation techniques and to meditation techniques (Jordan et al, 1979).

Self-Directed Imagery

Increased attention is being focused on the ability of individuals to use the principles of guided imagery. Through the practice of effective deep relaxation techniques, individuals can bring themselves into a state of consciousness in which they have increased access to deeper parts of the mind. Then, using imagery, they can "reprogram" new healthy images (Achterberg, 1985).

Self-directed imagery is powerful way in which individuals can have more control over their healing processes. Imagery can be used to contribute to the healing of physical problems and has been used extensively in the area of pain control. In one method the individual allows an image for his or her pain to emerge. For example, an individual may create an image that characterizes the area of pain, then create a second image to counteract the pain image. Once the images are formed, the individual uses a relaxation or meditation technique to open access to the levels where his or her self-healing power resides and to imagine the healing image. This process can be repeated as often as necessary, allowing changes in the healing image that either might appear spontaneously or might be appropriate if the image associated with the pain were to change.

Self-directed imagery can also be used to stimulate personal growth and change by repeatedly entering a relaxed or meditative state and strongly imaging a new desired behavior. Similarly, when one repeatedly images oneself as having already achieved a desired goal, the deeper mind gradually accepts this new image and works to bring it into reality.

Carl O. Simonton, MD, often regarded as the grandfather of guided imagery, and his wife Stephanie brought the use of meditation and imagery for cancer self-help to popular attention. They emphasized several aspects characteristic of a powerful healing image: (1) the image is created by the healee himself or herself, (2) it involves as many sense modalities as possible, and (3) it has as much dynamism and energy behind it as possible. The image must be vital, because that vitality is what stimulates the image to take root (Simonton et al, 1978).

RESEARCH CONSIDERATIONS

Early studies suggest a direct relationship between imagery and its corresponding effects on the body. Their findings include the following:

1. Correlations were found between levels of various types of leukocytes and components of cancer patients' images of their disease, treatment, and immune system (Achterberg et al, 1984).
2. Natural killer cell function was enhanced in geriatric patients (Kiecolt-Glaser et al, 1985) and in adult cancer patients with metastatic disease (Gruber et al, 1988) after engaging in a relaxation and imagery procedure.
3. Specificity of imagery training was suggested by a study in which patients were trained in cell-specific imagery of either T lymphocytes or neutrophils. The effects of training, assessed after 6 weeks, were statistically associated with the type of imagery procedure used (Achterberg et al, 1989).

Of all the many mind-body modalities, guided imagery appears to be the most widely used and accepted in many nursing departments. The University of Akron College of Nursing conducted a study demonstrating that guided imagery was an effective intervention for enhancing comfort in women undergoing radiation therapy for early-stage breast cancer. In this study, 53 women were randomly assigned to either a control group or a treatment group. The experimental group listened to a guided imagery tape once a day for the duration of the study. The guided imagery group demonstrated significantly improved comfort compared with the control group, with the treatment group experiencing greater comfort over time (Kolcaba et al, 1999).

A community-based nursing study was recently conducted in Sydney, Australia, where 56 people with advanced cancer experiencing anxiety and depression were randomly assigned to one of four treatment conditions: (1) progressive muscle relaxation training, (2) guided imagery training, (3) both types of training, and (4) no training (control). Patients were tested for anxiety, depression, and quality of life. The guided imagery training led to no significant improvement in anxiety but was associated with significant positive changes in depression and quality of life (Sloman, 2002).

Nurses at Ephrata Community Hospital in Pennsylvania found that offering their patients guided imagery compact discs (CDs) was effective in a variety of ways. They reported that guided imagery (1) helped patients relieve pain and anxiety before and after surgery, (2) helped patients relax and sleep better during evening hours, (3) helped to lower blood pressure, and (4) reduced the need for breathing and respiratory devices. Nurses also reported that the CDs were often more effective than sedation for easing confusion in older patients. Each bedside had a packet of CDs and a CD player with earphones. Each CD focused on a major component of a successful hospital stay (e.g., health and healing, comfort, peaceful rest, courage, serenity). In addition, all the staff nurses, therapists, social workers, and managers were trained in the use of the CDs and employed them for their personal benefit (Miller, 2003).

Differences in pain perception with guided imagery were examined at Kent State's College of Nursing, where 42 patients were randomly assigned to treatment (guided imagery) and control (no imagery) groups. Those who participated in guided imagery experienced decreased pain during the last 2 days of the 4-day trial (Lewandowski, 2004).

In 1993 a study was conducted by Bennett to compare the effectiveness of various types of guided imagery in preoperative patients. Three outcomes were examined: intraoperative blood loss, length of hospital stay, and use of postoperative pain medication. A population of 335 surgical patients were randomly assigned to five groups. Each of the four experimental groups was provided with a guided imagery audiotape created by four different therapists. The control group received an audiotape with a "whooshing" noise that produced no meaningful physiological effect. Results showed that use of three of the four guided imagery audiotapes yielded no significant beneficial effects on any of the medical outcomes examined. By contrast, use of the guided imagery audiotape produced by Belleruth Naparstek, a highly regarded therapist and imagery practitioner, led to highly significant results for two outcomes, reduced postoperative blood loss and length of stay. Bennett found that Naparstek's tape was much more sophisticated than the others. Her imagery had been scored with specially composed music designed to highlight and accompany each image, with an emphasis on spiritual connectedness. Naparstek included visualizations of positive outcomes, faster wound healing, less pain, and no nausea (Bennett, 1996).

In two unpublished studies, guided imagery was used to reduce menopausal symptoms. The University Hospital in Linkoping, Sweden, found that menopausal women using guided imagery averaged 73% fewer hot flashes over 6 months and had a significant reduction in other symptoms. A study at New England Deaconess Hospital involving 33 menopausal women who were not using hormone replacement therapy found that guided imagery strategies produced a significant reduction in hot-flash intensity, tension and anxiety, and depression.

Cleveland Clinic researchers assessed 130 colorectal surgery patients for anxiety levels, pain perceptions, and narcotic medication requirements (Tusek et al, 1997). The treatment group listened to guided imagery tapes for 3 days before their surgery, during anesthesia induction, intraoperatively, after anesthesia, and for 6 days after surgery; the control group received routine perioperative care. Patients in the guided imagery group experienced considerably less preoperative and postoperative anxiety and pain, and they required 50% less narcotic medication after surgery than patients in the control group.

Not only has the use of guided imagery been shown to be effective for reducing pain and anxiety preoperatively and postoperatively, but it is now proving to be cost effective. In 1999 a cardiac surgery team implemented a guided imagery program and compared cardiac surgical outcomes in those who participated in guided imagery and those who did not. Patients who completed the guided imagery program had a shorter average length of hospital stay, a decrease in average direct pharmacy costs, and a decrease in average direct pain medication costs, while overall patient satisfaction with the care and treatment provided remained high (Halpin et al, 2002).

MENTAL HEALING

The idea that consciousness can affect the physical body is a time-honored concept with a respected historical base. The observation that "there is a measure of consciousness throughout the body" is scattered about in the 2000-year-old Hippocratic writings. The ancient Persians expounded on this concept, insisting that a person's mind can intervene not just in his or her own body but also in that of another individual located far away. The great Muslim physician Abu Ali ibn Sina (Avicenna in Latinized form, AD 980-1037) later postulated that it was the faculty of imagination that humans use to make themselves ill or to restore health.

The attitudes of the ancient Greeks and Persians toward the interaction between minds and bodies gave rise to two very different types of healing: local and nonlocal. The Greeks believed that the action of the mind on the body was a "local" event in the here and now. The Persians, however, viewed the mind-body relationship as "nonlocal." They held that the mind was not localized or confined to the body but extended beyond the body. This implied that the mind was capable of affecting any physical body, local or nonlocal.

IMPLICATIONS OF NONLOCALITY

Modern physicists have long recognized the concept of nonlocality. These developments rest largely on an idea in physics called "Bell's theorem," introduced in 1964 by the Irish physicist John Stewart Bell and supported by subsequent experiments. Bell showed that if distant objects have once been in contact, a change thereafter in one causes an immediate change in the other, even were they to be separated to the opposite ends of the universe. Thus it is important to realize that nonlocality is not just a theoretical idea in physics, but that its proof rests on the results of actual experiments.

The idea prevalent in contemporary science is that the mind and consciousness are entirely local phenomenon, localized to the brain/body and confined to the present moment. From this perspective nonlocal healing cannot occur in principle because the mind is bound by the "here and now." Research studies examining distant mental influence challenge these modern-day assumptions. Dozens of experiments conducted over the past 25 years suggest that the mind can bring about changes in nonlocal physical bodies, even when shielded from all sensory and electromagnetic influences. This suggests that mind and consciousness may not be located at fixed points in space (Braud, 1992; Braud et al, 1991; Jahn et al, 1987).

Some physicists believe that nonlocality applies not just to the domain of electrons and other subatomic particles but also to our familiar world consisting of dense matter. A growing number of physicists think that nonlocality may apply to the mind. Physicist Nick Herbert, in his book *Quantum Reality,* states, "Bell's theorem requires our quantum knowledge to be nonlocal, instantly linked to everything it has previously touched" (Herbert, 1987).

For the Western model of medicine, the implications of a nonlocal concept are profound and include the following:

1. Nonlocal models of the mind could be helpful in understanding the actual dynamics of the healing process. They may help to explain why in some patients a cure suddenly appears unexpectedly or a healing appears to be influenced by events occurring nonlocally.

2. Nonlocal manifestations of consciousness may complicate traditional experimental designs and require innovative research methods, because they suggest that the mental state of the healer may influence the experiment's outcome, even under "blind" conditions (Solfvin, 1984).

Nonlocality assumptions give rise to the idea that consciousness could prevail after the death of the body/brain, which suggests that some aspect of the psyche is not bound to points in space or time. This idea in turn leads toward a nonlocal model of consciousness, which allows for the possibility of distant healing exchange.

This nonlocal model of consciousness implies that at some level of the psyche, no fundamental separations exist between individual minds. Nobel physicist Erwin Schroedinger suggested that at some level and in some sense there may be unity and oneness of all minds (Schroedinger, 1969). In the nonlocal model, distance is not fundamental but is completely overcome. In other words, because of the unification of consciousness, the healer and the patient are not separated by physical distance.

For 30 years, psychologist Lawrence LeShan investigated the local and nonlocal effects of prayer and mental healing. He taught these techniques to more than 400 people and ultimately became a healer himself. He maintained that healing changes were observed to have occurred 15% to 20% of the time but never could be predicted in advance of any specific healing (LeShan, 1966).

LeShan found that mental-spiritual healing methods can be categorized into the following two main types:

- *Type I (nonlocal).* The healer enters a prayerful, altered state of consciousness in which he or she views himself or herself and the patient as a single entity. There is no physical contact or any attempt to offer anything of a physical nature to the person in need, only the desire to connect and unite. These healers emphasize the importance of empathy, love, and caring in this process. When the healing takes place, it does so in the context of unity, compassion, and love. This type of healing is considered a natural process and merely speeds up the normal healing processes.
- *Type II (local).* The healer does touch the patient and may imagine some "flow of energy" through his or her hands to the area of the patient receiving the healing. Feelings of heat are common in both the healer and patient. In this mode, unlike type I, the healer holds the intention for healing.

Research into the origins of consciousness and how it relates to the physical brain is practically nonexistent. Although hypotheses purporting to explain consciousness do exist, there is no agreement among researchers as to its nature, local or nonlocal.

SPIRITUALITY AND HEALING

Throughout the ages, ancient mystical traditions have valued the spiritual qualities of humans over the physical, emphasizing the transcendence of one over the other. In the background of most mystical traditions is the idea that the body is somehow at odds with the spirit. A war wages, and one must battle the war to achieve an enlightened status. Still other theologians postulate that the greatest spiritual achievement of all may lie in the realization that the spiritual and the physical are but one, and that perhaps the ultimate spiritual goal is to transcend nothing but to realize the integration and oneness of our being.

A new quality of spiritual awakening has been emerging worldwide over the past 30 years. This innovative approach encourages people to develop faith in their own capacity to create their own reality in partnership with the "God-force within." In many cultures, both Eastern and Western, prayer-based spiritual healing is an integral part of modern religious practices.

The premise of creating our own reality is, in essence, a spiritual one. This concept is sometimes contrary to many fundamental religious positions that embrace God as an external being, because spirituality emphasizes a "God-within" reality. Transcending the boundaries and limitations of specific religions, a spiritual practice honors the relationship between the individual and the God-force as a partnership.

When people consider the possibility that they create their own realities, the question that invariably arises is,

"Through what source? What is the source of this power of creation that runs through my being?" The answer to this question is found not externally but internally. This internal source seeking to understand our own nature is divinity in action, incarnated in each person.

The blending of spirituality with the tenets of alternative and complementary therapies provides individuals with a means of understanding how they contribute to the creation of their illness and to their healing. This understanding does not come from a place of self-blame and does not view illness as a result of the will of God but rather is an attempt to understand a spiritual purpose for suffering in a physical body. The relationship that is cultivated ultimately transcends the human value system of punishment versus reward and grows into a relationship based on principles of co-creation and co-responsibility. Therefore the journey of healing for patients, as well as the journey of life, is freed of the burden of feeling victimized by fate, circumstances, or God, and patients are free to have faith and hope not only in God but in themselves as well.

Research in the last 10 years has made an indelible mark on the way health care professionals think about the role of spirituality and religion in physical, mental, and social health. Hundreds of studies have explored the relationship between body and spirit. Most studies have been cross-sectional, but some have also been longitudinal. Many studies now document an association between religious involvement and lower anxiety, fewer psychotic symptoms, less substance abuse, and better coping mechanisms. A comprehensive review found that 478 of 742 quantitative studies (66%) reported a statistically significant relationship between religious involvement and better mental health and greater social support. The review also found that almost 80% of those who are religious have significantly greater well-being, hope, and optimism compared with those who are less religious (Koenig et al, 2001).

At Duke University, studies were conducted examining the effects of religiousness on the course of depression in 850 hospitalized patients over age 60. Results showed that religious coping predicted lower levels of depressive symptoms at baseline and at 6 months after discharge (Koenig et al, 1992).

Koenig's studies and others have shown that spirituality and religiosity are clearly associated with longer survival, healthier behaviors, and less distress and are believed to have an effect on coping (Pargament et al, 1998; Tix et al, 1997), anxiety (Koenig et al, 1993), success in aging (Crowther et al, 2002), end of life issues (Daaleman et al, 2000), and cortisol levels in patients with human immunodeficiency virus infection and acquired immunodeficiency syndrome (Ironson et al, 2002).

POWER OF PRAYER

The use of prayer in healing may have begun in human prehistory and continues to this day as an underlying tenet in almost all religions. The records of many of the great religious traditions, including the mystical traditions of Christianity, Daoism, Hinduism, Buddhism, and Islam, give the strong impression that enlightenment comes when one begins to explore the dynamic qualities of interrelation and interconnection between the self and the source of all beings.

The word *prayer* comes from the Latin *precarious,* "obtained by begging," and *precari,* "to entreat"—to ask earnestly, beseech, implore. This suggests two of the most common forms of prayer: *petition,* asking something for one's self, and *intercession,* asking something for others.

Prayer is a genuinely nonlocal event, not confined to a specific place in space or to a specific moment in time. Prayer reaches outside the here and now; it operates at a distance and outside the present moment. Because prayer is initiated by a mental action, this implies that some aspect of our psyche also is genuinely nonlocal. Nonlocality implies infinitude in space and time, because a limited nonlocality is a contradiction in terms. In the West, this infinite aspect of the psyche has been referred to as the *soul.* Empirical evidence for the power of prayer therefore may be seen as indirect evidence for the soul.

Scientific attempts to assess the effects of prayer and spiritual practices on health began in the nineteenth century with Sir Francis Galton's treatise "Statistical Inquiries into the Efficacy of Prayer" (Galton, 1872). Galton assessed the longevity of people who were frequently prayed for, such as clergy, monarchs, and heads of state. He concluded that there was no demonstrable effect of prayer on longevity. By current scientific standards, Galton's study was flawed. He was successful, however, in promoting the idea that prayer is subject to empirical scrutiny. Galton did acknowledge that praying could make a person feel better. In the end he maintained that although his attempts to prove the efficacy of prayer had failed, he could see no good reason to abandon prayer.

Those who practice healing with prayer claim uniformly that the effects are not diminished with distance; therefore it falls within the nonlocal perspective discussed earlier. Claims about the effectiveness of prayer do not rely on anecdote or single case studies; numerous controlled studies have validated the nonlocal nature of prayer. Moreover, much of this evidence suggests that praying individuals, or people involved in compassionate imagery or mental intent, whether or not it is called "prayer," can purposefully affect the physiology of distant people without the awareness of the receiver.

The medical community has recently begun to acknowledge the importance of exploring the association between spirituality and medicine. Many medical schools now offer courses in religion, spirituality, and health. According to a 1994 survey, 98% of hospitalized patients ascribe to a belief in God or some higher power, and 96% acknowledge a personal use of prayer to aid in the healing process. In addition, 77% of 203 hospitalized family practice patients believed that their physicians should consider their spiritual needs. In contrast, only 32% of the patients' family physicians

actually discussed spirituality with their patients (King et al, 1994).

Anecdotal accounts of the power of prayer are legendary, and countless books on the subject are available; however, literature of scientific value is still limited.

The now-famous prayer study involving humans was published in 1988 by Randolph Byrd, a staff cardiologist at San Francisco School of Medicine, University of California. Byrd randomly assigned 393 patients in the coronary care unit either to a group receiving intercessory prayer or to a control group receiving no prayer. Intercessory prayer was offered by interventionists outside the hospital. They were not instructed how often to pray but were told to pray as they saw fit. In this double-blind study, the prayed-for patients did better on several counts. Although the results were not statistically significant, there were fewer deaths in the prayer group; these patients were less likely to require intubation and ventilator support; they required fewer potent drugs; they experienced a lower incidence of pulmonary edema; and they required cardiopulmonary resuscitation less often (Byrd, 1988).

In 1999, W.E. Harris attempted to replicate Byrd's findings at the Mid America Heart Institute in Kansas City. Although the study did not produce statistically significant results, the researchers reported that patients received significant benefit from intercessory prayer, as reflected by a coronary care unit outcome measure (Harris et al, 1999). Critics have charged that performing controlled studies on prayer is impossible, because extraneous prayer for the control group cannot be eliminated.

Other studies have been conducted to assess the effect of intercessory prayer on the treatment of alcohol abuse and dependence (Walker et al, 1997), the well-being of kidney dialysis patients (Matthews et al, 2001), and feelings of self-esteem (O'Laoire, 1997). A prospective study of 40 patients with class II or III rheumatoid arthritis compared the effects of direct-contact intercessory prayer with distance intercessory prayer. Persons receiving direct-contact prayer showed significant overall improvement at the 1-year follow-up. The group receiving distant prayer showed no additional benefits (Matthews et al, 2000).

The benefits of spiritual healing were examined in 120 patients with chronic pain at the Department of Complementary Medicine at the University of Exeter, United Kingdom. Patients were randomly assigned to face-to-face healing or simulated face-to-face healing for 30 minutes per week for 8 weeks or to distant healing or no healing for the same time. Although subjects in both healing groups reported significantly more "unusual experiences" during the sessions, the clinical relevance of this is unclear. It was concluded that a specific effect of face-to-face or distant healing on chronic pain could not be demonstrated over eight treatment sessions in these patients (Abbot et al, 2002).

Although research problems will be difficult to overcome in evaluating the power of prayer, Byrd's initial prayer study broke significant ground in medical research. Many questions still remain unanswered, and further study is warranted to define the effects of intercessory prayer on quantitative and qualitative outcomes and to identify end points that best measure efficacy.

Although validated evidence continues to build concerning the efficacy of prayer, Dossey (1993) maintains that some serious questions arise in the wake of these experiments. Evidence shows that mental activity can be used to influence people nonlocally, at a distance, without their knowledge. Scores of experiments on prayer also show that it can be used to great effect without the subject's awareness. The question arises of whether it is ethical to use these techniques if recipients are unaware that they are being used. This question becomes even more compelling as one considers the possibility prayer, or any other form of mind-to-mind communication, may be used at a distance to harm people without their knowledge. Institutional review committees that oversee the design of experiments involving humans to ensure their safety have rarely had to consider these types of ethical questions.

COMBINED APPROACHES

Although evidence continues to mount regarding the efficacy of mind-body approaches used individually, more researchers and clinicians are beginning to combine various approaches to create a synergistic healing process.

Combining hypnosis with guided imagery yielded impressive results in improving the postoperative course of pediatric surgical patients. Fifty-two children were randomly assigned to an experimental group or control group. Children in the experimental group were taught imagery, which included hypnotic suggestions for a favorable postoperative course; children in the control group received no such training. The children in the imagery group had significantly lower postoperative pain ratings and shorter hospital stays than those in the control group. State anxiety was decreased in the guided imagery group but increased in the control group (Lambert, 1996).

A study at the University of Texas (Houston) School of Public Health was conducted to differentiate the effects of imagery and support on coping, life attitudes, immune function, quality of life, and emotional well-being after breast cancer. Forty-seven breast cancer survivors were randomly assigned to (1) standard care only, (2) standard care with six weekly social support sessions, or (3) standard care with guided imagery sessions. For women in both active treatment groups, interferon-γ levels increased, neopterin levels decreased, quality of life improved, and natural killer cell activity remained unchanged. Compared with standard care only, both social support and guided imagery interventions improved coping skills, increased perceived social support, and generally enhanced feelings of meaning in life. Imagery participants had less stress, increased vigor, and improved functional and social quality of life compared with the support group (Richardson et al, 1997).

In another study, Harvard's Mind/Body Institute randomly assigned 128 otherwise healthy college students to an experimental group or a wait-list control group. The experimental group received six 90-minute group training sessions in the relaxation response and cognitive-behavioral skills; the control group received no training. Significantly greater reductions in psychological distress, state anxiety, and perceived stress were found in the treatment group compared with the control group (Deckro et al, 2002).

California Pacific Medical Center conducted a study funded by the U.S. Department of Defense that examined the outcomes for 181 women with breast cancer. Women were randomly assigned to participate in a 12-week "mind, body, and spirit" support group or a standard support group. The women in the mind, body, and spirit group were taught meditation, affirmations, imagery, and ritual. In the standard group, cognitive-behavioral approaches were combined with group sharing and support. Both interventions were found to be associated with improved quality of life, decreased depression and anxiety, and spiritual well-being. Only women in the mind, body, and spirit group, however, showed significant increases in measures of spiritual integration. At the end of the intervention, those in the mind, body, and spirit group showed higher satisfaction and the group had fewer dropouts than the standard group (Targ et al, 2002).

Kinney and Rodgers (2003) conducted a similar intervention for breast cancer survivors using a mind, body, and spirit self-empowerment program. Fifty-one women participated in a 12-week psychospiritual supportive program that included multiple strategies for creating a balance among spiritual, mental, emotional, and physical health. Components included meditation, visualization, guided imagery, affirmations, and dream work. Statistically significant improvements were seen in depression, perceived wellness, quality of life, and spiritual well-being.

Guided imagery and progressive relaxation techniques were the focus of a recent study at New Jersey Goryeb Children's Hospital. Eighteen children between the ages of 5 and 12 with chronic abdominal pain were taught guided imagery and progressive relaxation techniques over 9 months. Abdominal pain improved in 89% of the patients, weekly pain episodes decreased, pain intensity decreased, days missed from school decreased, and physician office contacts decreased. In addition, social activities increased and quality of life improved (Youssef et al, 2004).

A recent Korean study examined the effectiveness of a combination of guided imagery and progressive relaxation techniques in reducing the chemotherapy side effects of anticipatory nausea and vomiting and postchemotherapy nausea and vomiting in 30 patients with breast cancer; the effects on patients' quality of life was also measured. Both therapies combined produced improvements on all measures (Yoo et al, 2005). Mind-body pathways and therapeutic modalities have been difficult to understand and interpret in Western biomedicine.

⊜ Chapter References can be found on the Evolve website at http://evolve.elsevier.com/Micozzi/complementary/

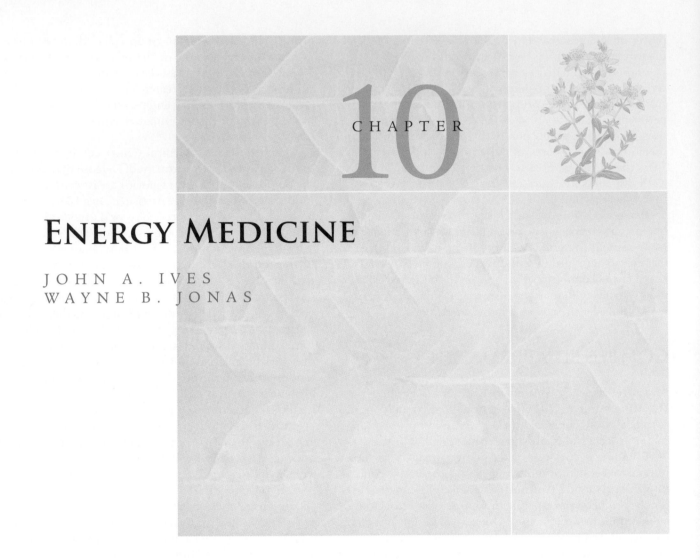

CHAPTER 10

ENERGY MEDICINE

JOHN A. IVES
WAYNE B. JONAS

We live forwards, but we understand backwards.
—WILLIAM JAMES

Nothing is so firmly believed as that which is least known.
—MICHEL DE MONTAIGNE

ENERGY AND ENERGY MEDICINE

Modern definitions for energy are introduced to grade school students. In the United States, high school students are taught formal (mathematical) definitions for energy as part of introductory physics courses. Energy is defined as the ability to do work and has two basic forms, potential and kinetic. Potential energy is stored energy and has the ability to do work. Kinetic energy is, simply put, the movement of things—from air molecules to sound to the splitting of neutrons into atomic nuclei. Underlying these deceptively simple descriptions are several subtleties that have been investigated and understood to such an extent that we can harness the awesome power of atomic energy.

Thus, we can see how putting a venipuncture needle in someone's arm is an example of kinetic energy: the movement of the needle through the skin, the movement of the fluid into the lumen of the vein, and the movement of the pharmaceutical agent to the receptor of the target cell. Then, in a microburst of activity the receptor binds the agent, often releasing potential energy that was stored in the characteristic configuration of the receptor itself. The change in receptor topology releases stored energy and helps to propel or allow the movement of molecules and atoms across the cellular membrane, in the process consuming potential energy stored in the molecule adenosine triphosphate (ATP), the universal coin of energy in the biology of cellular reactions and actions.

It is at this energetic interface that the pharmaceutical industry and much of allopathic medicine have focused their efforts. This is the space where endogenous molecules as well as pharmaceutical agents ultimately interact with our physical selves. These agents cause and modulate cellular responses through interactions with a class of biomolecules called "receptors." Sometimes the agent is

130

harvested and acquired from natural sources (materia medica), sometimes it is synthesized in a laboratory, and nearly always it interacts with a naturally occurring receptor type associated with some tissue or organ, or groups of tissues or organs. The point is that all of these steps and the downstream and sidestream consequences involve the use of energy and its transformation from potential to kinetic and back again with some loss to heat and randomness at every step. All health and healing involve these biochemical, energy-driven reactions, and thus all healing is a form of energy medicine.

Because of our understanding of the nature of these biochemical reactions, we believe that all of life is dependent on these reactions and that when these fail, life ceases. Certainly, life is dependent on these chemical energies, and in allopathic medicine we use the kinetic energy of objects (i.e., pharmaceuticals) to affect biological processes and, hopefully, maintain or improve health and healing.

SUBTLE AND VITAL ENERGY

It is also well known that different types and sources, or packets, of energy may interact, which results in a modulation or change in the energies involved. It is at this interface that energy medicine takes place, and we will describe possible models for understanding this interface.

So far we have described a conventional view of energy in healing. However, the "energy" in so-called energy medicine is not of this nature. First and foremost, it is not directly measurable. Second, it does not appear to fall off in power with distance by the inverse square law. Finally, it is not blocked by barriers that block conventional energy. This distinction in "energies" is important, because often these two very different concepts are used interchangeably and confusion results. Yet both types of "energy medicine" are placed in this single category by the National Center for Complementary and Alternative Medicine (NCCAM). This blindsight may not be a surprise, because when members of Congress were first legislating the funding to create what is now the NCCAM at the National Institutes of Health (NIH), leaders at the NIH told Congress that the NIH "does not believe in bioenergy" (Sen. Arlen Specter R/D-PA, personal communication). It has been suggested to Congress (by the editor of this book) that the U.S. Department of Energy may be a better place to study bioenergy. We will summarize research involving both types of energy, but will make a clear distinction between the two uses of the term. We will also discuss the limits of current standards for evaluating this area and possible models to help improve our understanding of these concepts.

The intriguing and disputed (at least by Western allopathic healers) energy medicines such as qigong, reiki, and therapeutic touch are thought to involve putative forms of energy. That is, not only have there been questions about the efficacy of these energy medicine modalities, but there have not been any unequivocal demonstrations of the involvement of either known or heretofore unknown forms of energy from the healer or between the healer and the patient. These modalities are based on philosophy, historical use, and/ or tradition but without much modern scientific empirical evidence. These energy medicine modalities are thought to involve the interactions between the "energy field" of the patient and the *energy field* or the *intention* of the healer. We will return to this idea of intention and interaction with forms of energy when we discuss the *quantum enigma*. For now, we will consider what is meant by the use of the terms *intention* and *human energy fields* to be related and interdependent.

As hinted at earlier, often what is missing is a rational *mechanism of action* in the practice of energy medicine. The confounding of *mechanism* with *empiricism* in the study of healing has been an ongoing challenge in medicine (see Chapter 6). This mechanism provides a distinction between veritable forms of energy medicine such as magnetic therapy and the putative forms such as reiki (NCCAM, 2007). In spite of this gap in our understanding and knowledge, and the stress placed on understanding mechanism by the biomedical complex, it remains difficult to find funding for basic mechanistic studies. For several years, the NCCAM dedicated over 60% of its budget to clinical research and 20% to applied research at centers, with only the remaining funds allocated to basic research (http://nccam.nih.gov). Further, the NCCAM continues to move more toward clinical trials (although the methodology for such trials is frequently inappropriate; see Chapters 5 and 26), to the further exclusion of basic research and applied research. Thus, basic research on energy (both veritable and putative) medicine is scarce.

Although recent literature on forms of bioenergy—qi, ki, prana—and their biomedical application has significantly increased, the form of energy involved in energy medicine remains largely mysterious. There are some recent examples in the English-language literature of attempts to characterize this energy (Ohnishi et al, 2008), but these studies have not been replicated by other groups. To date, the most complete, criteria-based, systematic review of this area is the book by Jonas and Crawford (2003b). An additional comprehensive survey has been compiled by Benor (2004).

In addition, over the past 30 years considerable work has been done on the measurement of external qi as physical energy. The majority of publications in this field are in Chinese and therefore are not easily accessible to the Western scientific community. The few English-language references dealing with bioenergy include a book by Lu (1997). A more complete review by Zha is found in the proceedings of the Samueli Hawaii meeting of 2001 (Zha, 2001). A thorough review of previous work on physical measurements of external qi is outside the scope of this chapter, and the previous references are included as the most accessible material. It appears from these documents that the previous experiments neither had been done in a rigorously controlled way nor had utilized instruments that are currently state of the art. The documented experiments reveal, at best, very low levels of physical energy associated with external qi emission by qigong practitioners and healers (Hintz et al, 2003).

The lack of solid evidence or an accepted mechanistic explanation for the "energy" in energy medicine presents a fairly large hurdle to acceptance by Western medicine. Although there is no universal agreement as to what is meant by the "energy" in energy medicine—or even what kind it might be—terms such as "subtle energy," "qi energy," and prana are often used. There does seem to be some consensus on both sides of this discussion that, whatever it is, it is not the energy currently identified and described by traditional Western physics (see Chapter 1).

Finally, for a concept of such "energy" to be of value and to be adopted within the scientific community there must be consilience among and with accepted physics, chemistry, and biology. Therefore, any putative bioenergy involved in energy medicine must be internally consistent and allow for consilience with the other known energies. A cybernetic or systems analytic approach consistent with conventional descriptions of electromagnetic energies describing this system is shown in Figure 10-1 and is a level of abstraction based on the concepts of (1) information sources, (2) a medium for carrying the signal, and (3) receivers. In this view, the underlying physical layer of transfer of information is intentionally hidden to allow discussion of the transfer of bioinformation without an a priori decision about what is the physical mechanism for that transfer (Hintz et al, 2003).

In this model, we can define a bioenergy system as one which is comprised of the following:

- A source that generates energy and modulates it in some manner so that it conveys information
- A coupling mechanism connecting the bioenergy source to a transfer medium
- A transfer medium through which the bioenergy flows
- A coupling mechanism connecting the transfer medium to the bioenergy sink
- A terminal sink that includes a mechanism for the perception of information

The input and output coupling depends on properties of the source and the transfer medium, and likewise for the sink. The term *perception* rather than *reception* is used to imply some active process that uses some form of perceptual reasoning in processing the information based on its content.

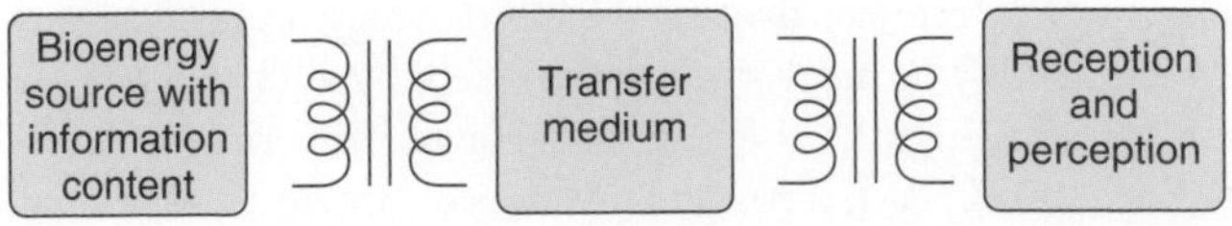

The means by which information is transmitted and interacts with the system, in the sense that physicists understand it, is not clear. Feedback loops in biosystems are examples of information transfer. In most, if not all, cases the physical means by which the feedback is provided to the system is either understood or is assumed to involve interactions among actual physical objects. In the case of the placebo pill and the branding study reported later, it is not self evident how the information is transmitted but, de facto, it appears to be.

Thus, in these studies, information is able to significantly influence a biological system and its response to pain. Although we have some understanding of the biological consequences of energy medicine (Yan et al, 2008), the means by which this is done, the "energy," remains unknown. For example, qigong has been demonstrated to have antidepressive effects in patients, but although the psychological mechanisms underlying this effect have been described, the neurobiological mechanism remains unclear (Tsang et al, 2008). The same may be said of hypnosis, for which the clinical effects are now widely accepted (thanks in part to statistical profiling) but the neurobiological mechanism has remained unclear since the time of Mesmer (see Chapter 6). The authors conclude that further research is needed to elucidate the biology and consolidate its scientific base.

There are examples within the field of veritable energy medicine, however, in which there is a good understanding of the energies and energy fields involved. For example, the magnetic fields employed in transcranial magnetic stimulation (TMS) are well characterized (see Chapter 11). Even so, the biology and biological mechanisms at work and affected by the magnetic fields are only beginning to be understood (Lopez-Ibor et al, 2008). Thus, although TMS has been shown to be an effective alternative for the treatment of refractory neuropathic pain by epidural motor cortex stimulation, the mechanisms at work remain poorly understood (Lazorthes et al, 2007).

STANDARDS AND QUALITY

Although it is facile to recommend that complementary and alternative medicine (CAM) be held to the same standards as conventional medical science, the complexity and intricacies of CAM are reported by the White House Commission on Complementary and Alternative Medicine Policy (2002). This is particularly true for energy medicine.

Studies are conducted in nearly all the CAM disciplines that lend themselves to the hypothesis-driven paradigm, and a search of the literature attests to that. Essentially, CAM scientific research is following the same standards used for conventional research, that is, the use of statistically significant number of subjects, specimens,

Figure 10-1 Block diagram of bioenergy transport mechanism components.

or replicates; the introduction of internal and experimental controls; the definition of response specificity; and the requirement for reproducibility. The last is perhaps the most challenging criterion. In several cases, experiments have shown positive results but when repeated, sometimes in the same laboratory, do not work despite following the precautions of maintaining identical experimental conditions.

This challenge is illustrated in the work published by Yount et al (2004). They investigated the effect of 30 minutes of qigong on the healthy growth of cultured human cells. A rigorous experimental design of randomization, blinding, and controls was followed. Although both a pilot study that included 8 independent experiments and a formal study that included 28 independent experiments showed positive effects, the replication study of over 60 independent experiments showed no difference between the sham (nontreated) and treated cells. This study represents an excellent example of holding basic science research on energy medicine to the highest standard of experimental methodology.

This level of rigor is rarely achieved in energy laboratory research, however. The basic and clinical research in the area of distant mental influence on living systems (DMILS) and energy medicine was reviewed. The quality of research was quite mixed. Although a few simple research models met all quality criteria, such as in mental influence on random number generators or electrodermal activity, much basic research into DMILS, qigong, prayer, and other techniques was poor (Jonas et al, 2003b). In setting up these evaluations, the reviewers established basic criteria that should be met for all such laboratory research (Jonas et al, 2003a; Sparber et al, 2003).

In basic scientific research, formulating the testable hypothesis is sometimes not the major issue; it is setting up and testing the practice itself. In the example of Yount et al (2004), in which they followed the most rigorous methodological and experimental designs, the practice under investigation was not a simple treatment with defined doses of a pharmaceutical compound or an antagonist of a specific receptor. Instead it was an unknown amount of energy of unknown characteristics emanating from the hands of a number of qigong practitioners, with variable skills.

Acupuncture is a CAM application that lends itself to use in animal models for in vivo and ex vivo evaluation of its effects. By applying electroacupuncture, researchers are able to control the amount of energy delivered. However, the challenge here is the placement of the needles. Whereas in humans, needles would be placed based on meridian maps, in rats they must be placed so that they will not be disturbed during normal grooming while still being located along a meridian of relevance. In addition, 20-minute electroacupuncture is what is often used because this is what would be done in humans (Li et al, 2008), but should not the time and dose parameters be adjusted to the animal's body size?

Mind-body–based therapies are often not considered energy medicine, especially when applied to oneself, although they are considered so for the purposes of this book. However, when the goal is to produce a change in an outside entity through meditation, for example, then we claim this is a form of energy medicine and, as such, very challenging to explore in a laboratory setting. Although there are several studies showing the effects of meditation on cell growth (Yu et al, 2003), differentiation (Ventura, 2005), water pH, and temperature change, as well as on the development time of fruit fly larvae (Tiller, 1997), we believe that for these studies the necessary level of methodological rigor has not been met. Independent replication has been especially problematic. On the other hand, some CAM applications, such as homeopathy, phytotherapy, and dietary supplements (Ayurveda or traditional Chinese medicine) are relatively easy to translate to the laboratory setting. This is due to the fact that these practices and their products of use can be thought of as conventional interventions using pharmaceutical compounds, for which dose and time-course experiments can be designed. We will return to homeopathy later in this chapter as a form of energy medicine.

HOW GOOD IS GOOD ENOUGH?

At this point it is appropriate to talk about levels of evidence and how we should catalogue the evidence, and at what point we should consider policy and educational changes to health care training to incorporate new information, knowledge, and understanding.

When evaluating scientific evidence one must carefully consider the nature of the evidence itself. Figure 10-2 shows a way to categorize the types of data associated with

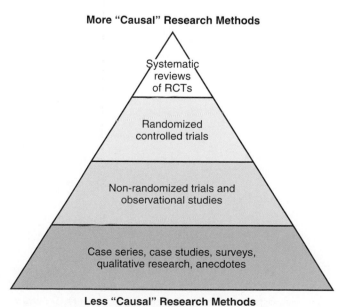

Figure 10-2 "Best" evidence hierarchy.

biomedical research. This evidence pyramid illustrates how to evaluate the "causal" characteristics of the data. Thus, randomized controlled trials are second from the peak or best evidence, which is systematic reviews of randomized controlled trials. At the base are anecdotes, qualitative research, and case studies. Evidence of this type should not be ignored, but it should not be overinterpreted. In cases in which the information is sufficiently compelling, the therapeutic interventions are novel, or the condition has no other remedies available for patients, then further studies are often warranted. The "evidence" may be good enough to indicate the need for further research and the generation of more valid data but may not be good enough to form a basis for medical decisions.

ORTHODOXIES AND PLACEBO

Virtually all the doctor's healing power flows from the doctor's self-mastery.

Healing power consists only in and no more than . . . bringing to bear those forces . . . that already exist in the patient.

—ERIC J. CASSELL, MD,
THE NATURE OF SUFFERING AND THE GOALS
OF MEDICINE, ED 2, 2004

By the same token, we should always examine our orthodoxies and assumptions. For example, it would be reasonable to assume that subjects given a placebo for pain would get little to no relief. In a study reported at the 1979 Society for Neuroscience conference, R.H. Gracely showed evidence that the expectations (*intentions?*) of the physician significantly affected the outcomes (Gracely and al, 1979)

(Figure 10-3). All subjects were given the same placebo, but half were given it by physicians who thought they were giving active medication. The patients of physicians who thought they were giving an active agent experienced a significant reduction in pain, whereas subjects in the other study arm received no relief and in fact their pain got worse.

In 1999 the impact of expectation was further explored in a four-arm study carried out by C.E. Margo (1999). One group was given an "unbranded" placebo, another group was given a "branded" placebo, a third group was given unbranded aspirin, and the fourth group was given branded aspirin. As can be seen from Figure 10-4, there appears to be an analgesic effect just from the act of taking a pill, and this effect is significantly improved if the pill is branded. In this study actual aspirin produced greater analgesia than branded placebo, and branded aspirin was better than unbranded aspirin for analgesia. The author interpreted these data to indicate that taking a pill has significant analgesic effect for patients with pain, whether the pill has any conventionally defined "bioactive" agent or not. Further, branding of the pill enhances the effect whether it is a placebo or active. One can interpret this as a demonstration of the power and efficacy of therapeutic expectation (a form of *intention*) (Kirsch, 1999).

MAGNETIC THERAPY

Before we get into the more exotic forms of energy medicine, and to drive home our point about the need to evaluate the quality and type of information we have on a subject, we discuss the relatively well studied use of magnetic therapy for the treatment of pain (see Chapter 11).

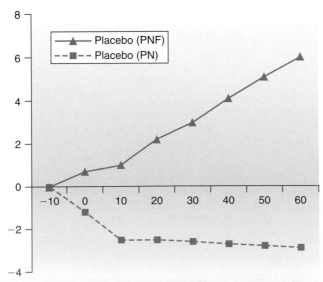

Figure 10-3 Physician knowledge affects outcome. (From Gracely RH et al: The effect of naloxone on multidimensional scales of postsurgical pain in nonsedated patients, *Soc Neurosci Abstr* 5:609, 1979.)

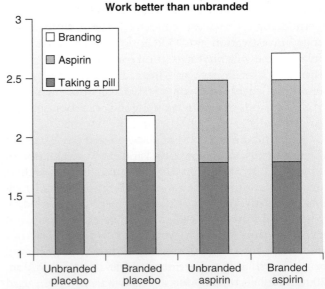

Figure 10-4 Branded aspirin and branded placebo work better than unbranded. (From Margo CE: The placebo effect, *Surv Ophthalmol* 44:31, 1999.)

Magnetic therapy is reportedly a safe, noninvasive method of applying magnetic fields to the body for therapeutic purposes. The use of magnets for relief of pain has become extremely popular, with consumer spending on such therapy exceeding $500 million in the United States and Canada and $5 billion worldwide (Weintraub, Mamtani, Micozzi, 2008; Weintraub et al, 2003). There have been many clinical studies of magnetic therapy. For example, Therion's Advanced Biomagnetics Database claims to contain over 300 clinical studies. However, few of these are randomized controlled trials, and the quality of the research is unknown.

It has been known for a while that magnets can reduce pain in subjects (Vallbona et al, 1997). Table 10-1 shows the data from a 1997 study by Vallbona et al. A highly significant analgesic effect is demonstrated by these data. Overall, the evidence shows that patients with severe pain appear to respond better to magnetic therapy than patients with mild symptoms. There appear to be no adverse effects from application of static or dynamic pulsed magnetic therapy (Harlow et al, 2004; Segal et al, 2001; Weintraub and Cole, 2008; Weintraub et al, 2003). In a randomized, double-blinded, placebo-controlled trial involving 36 symptomatic patients with refractory carpal tunnel syndrome, application of dynamic magnetic fields produced significantly greater pain relief than use of a placebo device as measured by short- and long-term pain scores, and better objective nerve conduction without changing motor strength or sensitivity to electrical current (Weintraub and Cole, 2008; Weintraub, Mamtani, Micozzi, 2008).

The Weintraub study on magnetic therapy (Weintraub et al, 2003) was the first multicenter, double-blind, placebo-controlled study to examine the role of static magnetic fields in treatment of diabetic peripheral neuropathy and neuropathic pain. The results confirmed those of two previous pilot studies showing that the antinociceptive (pain relief) effect was significantly enhanced with long-term exposure to magnetic therapy. Since then the evidence has continued to support magnetic therapy

as an effective tool for dealing with neuropathic pain (Segal et al, 2001).

Overall, 14 of 22 studies reported a significant analgesic effect of static magnets. Of the 19 better-quality studies, 12 found positive results and 6 found negative results, and in 1 there was a nonsignificant trend toward a positive analgesic effect. The weight of evidence from published well-conducted controlled trials suggests that static magnetic fields are able to induce analgesia (Eccles, 2005).

Taken as a whole, the studies of magnetic therapy are of the type required by the evidence pyramid (see Figure 10-2) to qualify as good to best and demonstrate a causal link between magnetic therapy and analgesia.

Clearly there is an interaction of energy with the body. This interaction probably involves electric potentials and action potentials across neuronal membranes with known and measurable forms of energy that we have called "veritable" forms of energy medicine. Veritable energy medicine includes electromagnetic, sound, and light therapies (NCCAM, 2007).

DISTANT HEALING

Let us now look at a set of studies performed to examine the effects of a healer's employing distance healing on cells in culture. This healer explained that he uses intention to focus his mind and channel "Divine love through his heart" to perform healing. This claim and similar energy medicine practices are often called "distant healing" because the practitioners do not place their hands on the patient or subject. Practitioners of this form of healing believe that the distance does not matter, although most, in fact, do their work within a foot or so of their patients. This healer usually placed his hands within inches of the person on whom he was working. As an aside, he also performs diagnosis by placing his hands near the person but without touching the person. We will return to the issue of distance later in the description of the studies' findings. The approach of this healer is typical of the so-called laying on of hands practiced in many cultures and accepted and associated traditionally with healing in Western medicine as well as Judeo-Christine tradition.

The explanation often given for any benefit seen from energy medicine of this kind is that it is a strong placebo effect that results from belief and expectation generated during the encounter (Moerman et al, 2002). The investigators intended to minimize this effect by using cells grown in laboratory culture. The healer came to the laboratories one morning per week throughout much of two sequential winters. The researchers wanted to understand how he "communicated" with cells in the laboratory and influenced them with his "intention" in a positive and healthful way. The study would not involve diagnosis or even a human subject. By working with cultured cells in a

TABLE 10-1

Proportion of Subjects Reporting Improvement of Pain After 45 Minutes of Magnetic Therapy

	Active magnetic device (n = 29)	Inactive device (n = 21)
Pain improved	n = 22 (76%)	n = 4 (19%)
Pain not improved	n = 7 (24%)	n = 17 (81%)

From Vallbona C, Hazlewood CF, Jurida G: Response of pain to static magnetic fields in postpolio patients: a double-blind pilot study, *Arch Phys Med Rehabil* 78:1200, 1997.
χ^2 (1 df) = 20.6, $P <.0001$.

laboratory setting, the investigators increased their power over the experimental and control parameters by comparing the effects of the healer to no treatment or sham treatment, comparing treatments at different doses and time periods, and examining the effects of various other environmentally controlled conditions, including the effects of expectation with blinding.

The healer was asked to alter the calcium flux in such a way as to increase the concentration of calcium ions inside the cells. Any change in cellular calcium was measured by putting the cells in a scintillation counter before and after the healer's "treatments." A demonstration of significant effect would be powerful evidence that something, some form of energy presumably, flowed from the healer to the cells and changed their biochemistry in a targeted, intentional, and specific way.

The studies used Jurkat cells, an immortalized line of T lymphocytes derived from human immune system T cells. They were established as an immortalized line in the late 1970s and are available for purchase and easy to grow and maintain in the laboratory. They have been used extensively to study mechanisms of action for human immunodeficiency virus and anticancer agents. There is, in fact, a vast literature on Jurkat cells, because they are a favorite choice for cellular immunobiologists interested in understanding cellular mechanisms of the immune system.

The setup was quite simple. Jurkat cells were grown in tissue culture dishes to near confluence, then on the day of the experiment the cells were suspended in a balanced salt solution, "loaded" with calcium-sensitive dye (fura-2) and placed inside a square cuvette. Because of the activity of the dye the amount of light emitted by the cells is proportional to the amount of free calcium ions inside the cell. When the light is measured spectrofluorometrically, this technique provides an accurate and objective measure of the amount of free calcium inside the cells.

As noted earlier, the healer was asked to increase the internal concentration of calcium ions inside the cell. He told the investigators that he would need 15 minutes of relative quiet while he placed his hands near the cuvette of cells and concentrated on his intention (Figure 10-5). The experiments were repeated in six independent trials occurring on different days. Internal cellular calcium concentrations were significantly increased by 30% to 35% ($P < .05$, Student t test) compared with controls run in parallel. Varying the distance between 3 and 30 inches did not seem to have an effect on the outcome (Kiang et al, 2005).

Three independent attempts were made by the healer to affect calcium concentration in this system from approximately 10 miles away. He tried first with internal visualization, then with a photograph of the cells to focus his attention, and finally with a video camera display of a "live" version of the cells. None of these tests produced any noticeable change in the calcium concentration. Anecdotally, a few uncontrolled tests were run in

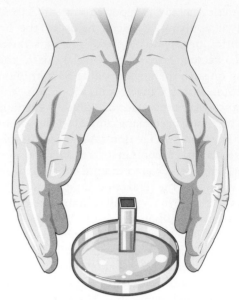

Figure 10-5 Performance of external bioenergy.

which the healer's hands were kept behind his back rather than toward the cuvette of cells. This position seemed to interfere with his ability to affect calcium concentration. This occurred in spite of the fact that the researchers documented a "linger effect" in which cells put on the table where the healer had focused his intention but after he had left showed an increase in calcium concentration similar to that of the cells that had been directly subject to his intention. This linger effect disappeared over time, and within 24 hours cells placed in this way had a calcium concentration no different from that of controls.

Finally, the investigators attempted to block the healer's "energy" or intention by placing a grounded copper Faraday cage around the cuvette containing cells. Thus the healer, although still within 30 inches of the cells, had to keep his hands outside of the wire enclosure surrounding the cells. There was no significant difference in effect on the internal calcium concentration. It was still raised by the healer's 15 minute "treatment." This suggests that, whatever the energy is, it is not blocked by a Faraday cage the way an electric field would be (Box 10-1).

BOX 10-1

Summary of Results of Distant Healing Experiment

30% increase in cellular calcium absorption in 15 minutes

Effect *not* blocked by a Faraday cage

Lingering effect for 24 hours

No effect at a distance of 10 miles

THERAPEUTIC TOUCH, HEALING TOUCH, AND ENERGY THERAPIES

Reiki, healing touch (HT), qigong, and therapeutic touch (TT) are all "energy therapies" that use gentle hand techniques thought to help repattern the patient's energy field and accelerate healing of the body, mind, and spirit. They are all based on the belief that human beings are fields of energy that are in constant interaction with other fields of energy from others and the environment. The goal of energy therapies is to purposefully use the energetic interaction between the practitioner and the patient to restore harmony to the patient's energy system. Western allopathic approaches focus on diseases and their underlying mechanisms. Cure is the end-all and be-all. Most energy therapies are based on a holistic philosophy that places the patient within the context of that patient's life and an understanding of the dynamic interconnectedness with themselves and their environment (Cassidy, 1995; Chapter 5). They are about healing rather than cure (Engebretson et al, 2007).

The most common contemporary touch therapies used in nursing practice are TT, HT, and reiki. The first two were developed by nurses, whereas reiki comes out of pre–World War II Japan and although not targeted for nursing is being used today by many in hospital settings (Engebretson et al, 2007; Krieger, 1993; Mentgen, 2001). Controversy has accompanied the use of these therapies, even after the inclusion of these therapies by the North American Nursing Diagnosis Association (NANDA). The controversy has not prevented their increasing popularity within the profession to promote health by reducing symptoms and ameliorating treatment side effects. Practitioners use TT and HT to improve health and healing by addressing, in the word's of the official NANDA diagnosis, a patient's "Disturbed Energy Field: disruption in the flow of energy surrounding a person's being that results in a disharmony of the body, mind, and/or spirit" (NANDA, 2008).

Like many other energy therapies, TT is not designed to treat specific diseases but instead to balance the energy field of the patient or, through a boosting of energy, improve the patient's energy. TT was developed by Dolores Krieger, PhD, RN, in the 1970s. She borrowed from and mixed together ancient shamanic traditions and techniques she learned from well-known healers of her time. Like acupuncture, qigong, and yoga, HT is based on the idea that illness and poor health represent an imbalance of personal bioenergetic forces and fields that exist around and through a person's body. Rebalancing and boosting of these energies is done through a clear intention to support and harmonize the person with his or her innate energy balance. These practices therefore typically begin with the practitioner performing some form of ritual that clears and focuses the intention to bring harmony and balance to the person who is in need.

In a typical TT session, the practitioner begins with a centering process to calm the mind, access a sense of compassion, and become fully present with the patient. The practitioner then focuses intention on the patient's highest good and places his or her hands lightly on the patient's body or slightly away from it, often making sweeping hand motions above the body. Enough research on TT has been published in peer-reviewed journals to perform a meta-analysis of the combined results from separate studies. Two meta-analyses have determined that TT produces a moderately positive effect on psychological and physiological variables hypothesized to be influenced by TT, primarily anxiety and pain (Peters, 1999; Winstead-Fry et al, 1999). A systematic review of the HT research published in 2000 included 19 randomized controlled trials involving 1122 patients (Astin et al, 2000). The reviewers found 11 studies (58%) that reported statistically significant treatment effects. Another systematic review of the literature on wound healing and TT found only four studies that met the author's criteria for quality. Of these, two showed statistically significant effects, whereas the other two found no effect from TT. The evidence is therefore insufficient to conclude that TT works for wound healing (O'Mathuna et al, 2003).

Applications for which TT and HT seem to work well include reducing anxiety, improving muscle relaxation, aiding in stress reduction, promoting relaxation, enhancing a sense of well-being, promoting wound healing, and reducing pain. In addition, no serious side effects have been associated with these healing modalities (Engebretson et al, 2007). One review of touch therapies looked at studies with outcomes such as pain reduction, improvement of mood, reduction of anxiety, promotion of relaxation, improvement of functional status, improvement of health status, increase in well-being, wound healing, reduction of blood pressure, and increase in immune function. The authors found that the studies were mixed in their quality and the degree of evidence supporting the effectiveness of touch therapies in influencing these outcomes (Warber et al, 2003).

Reiki was originally intended as a self-practice. Today it is often performed by practitioners to help their clients strengthen their wellness, assist them in coping with symptoms such as pain or fatigue, or support their medical care, sometimes in the case of chronic illness or at the end of life. Reiki was developed by Mikao Usui in Japan in the 1920s as a spiritual practice. One of his master students, Chujiro Hayashi, with Usui's help, extracted the healing practices from the larger body of practices. Hayashi began to teach these practices and opened a clinic to treat patients. Reiki practice itself is extremely passive. Practitioners lay their hands gently on the patient or hold them just above the body without moving their hands except to place them over another area. The reiki practitioner does not attempt to adjust the patient's energy field or actively project energy into the patient's body. Also, unlike other forms of energy medicine and more like meditation, reiki does not involve an assessment of the patient's energy field or an active attempt to reorganize or adjust the patient's energy field. Instead reiki practitioners believe that healing energy arises from the practitioner's hand as a response to the patient's needs. It is in this way customized to the patient's needs and condition.

In one study, 23 reiki-naive healthy volunteers participated in standardized 30-minute reiki sessions. They often reported experiencing a "liminal state of awareness." This state is characterized by novel and paradoxical sensations, often symbolic in nature. The experiences run the gamut from disorientation in space and time to altered experience of self and the environment as well as relationships with people, especially the reiki master. In another study, quantitative measures of anxiety and objective measures of systolic blood pressure and salivary immunoglobulin A were altered significantly by the reiki experience; anxiety and systolic blood pressure were lowered, whereas immunoglobulin A level was increased. Skin temperature, electromyographic readings, and salivary cortisol level were all lowered but not significantly. When these results are taken together, it is apparent that in this study reiki induced states of lowered stress and anxiety and should be considered salutogenic in nature. The authors concluded that the liminal state and paradoxical experiences are related to the ritual and holistic nature of this healing practice (Engebretson et al, 2002).

A 2008 systematic Cochrane review of the literature on touch therapy for pain relief included studies of HT, TT, and reiki (So et al, 2008). The authors evaluated the literature to determine the effectiveness of these therapies for relieving both acute and chronic pain. They also looked for any adverse affects from these therapies. Randomized controlled trials and controlled clinical trials investigating the use of these therapies for treatment of pain that included a sham placebo or "no treatment" control arm met the criteria for inclusion. Twenty-four studies, including 16 involving TT, 5 involving HT, and involving 3 reiki, were found that met these criteria. A small but significant average effect on pain relief (0.83 units on a scale of 0 to 10) was found. The greatest effect was seen in the reiki studies and appeared to involve the more experienced practitioners, but the authors concluded that the data were inconclusive with regard to which was more important, the level of experience or the modality of therapy. In spite of the paucity of studies, the authors concluded that the evidence supports the use of touch therapies for pain relief. Application of these therapies also decreased the use of analgesics in two studies. No statistically significant placebo effect was seen, and no adverse effects from these therapies were reported. The authors pointed out the need for higher-quality studies, especially of HT and reiki (So et al, 2008).

LIGHT, HEALING, AND BIOPHOTONS

Light therapy is, of course, a veritable form of energy generally not thought of as a "subtle energy" of the types we have just discussed (NCCAM, 2007) (see Chapter 11). There is good evidence that applied near-infrared (NIR) light (670 and 810 nm) can significantly improving wound healing and even promote neural regeneration in animal models (Byrnes et al, 2005; Whelan et al, 2008). The mechanisms underlying this "photobiomodulation" are not understood. Nonetheless, the therapeutic use of low-level NIR laser light is a promising area. Physiological effects that have been documented include increased rate of tissue regeneration as well as reduction in inflammation and pain. Production of reactive oxygen species by cells put under stress is lowered with NIR treatment. The application of 810-nm NIR light has been tested in an animal spinal cord injury model and has been shown to significantly increase axonal number and distance of regrowth. This light treatment also returned aspects of function to baseline levels and significantly suppressed immune cell activation and cytokine-chemokine expression. The authors concluded that externally delivered NIR light improves recovery after injury and suggested that light will be a useful treatment for human spinal chord injury (Whelan et al, 2008).

To understand more about the role of light in biology and human health, investigators examined the spontaneous emission of ultraweak photons, often called "biophotons," in humans (Van Wijk et al, 2008). Although these photons are in the visible range (470 to 570 nm) they are at too low a level to be seen in normal background light. Thus, a very efficient photomultiplier was developed, and the experiments were run in a completely light-tight environment. Reactive oxygen species are theorized to be the principle source of the photons, because these are very reactive molecules and are involved in interactions with high enough energy to result in spontaneous photon emissions. Measurement of human photon emission (biophotons) may therefore be a noninvasive method for assessing oxidative state, general health, chronic disease, and healing.

The study found that biophotons were emitted in a generally symmetrical pattern from the human body. This was not true for individuals with chronic diseases such as diabetes and arthritis, however. Further, reproducible emission patterns were demonstrated in meditating subjects, and another pattern was identified in sleeping individuals. The investigators believe this approach holds promise as a real-time, continuous, and noninvasive method for monitoring health, wellness, healing, and chronic disease, and perhaps even states of consciousness.

An important focus for future research is whether energy medicine modalities exploit these biophotonic emissions. It is not hard to imagine that some, or perhaps all, of us are able to detect these emissions. If this is possible, it is a small step to imagine that healers "learn" to detect these biophotons and their correlations with health or the lack of it. Finally, is it possible that healers interact with their clients' biophotons and use this system not only to gain information and knowledge but, in fact, to transmit biological information and instructions to their clients through these interactions? Is it possible that healers emit biophotons in patterns to which a patient's biosystems and biophotons respond and with which they interact? At this point, these are all untested hypotheses. Only by further researching these questions will we learn the answers.

THE QUANTUM ENIGMA

I cannot seriously believe in [quantum physics] because . . . physics should represent a reality in time and space, free from spooky actions at a distance.

—ALBERT EINSTEIN

The universe begins to look more like a great thought than a great machine.

—SIR JAMES JEANS

Since its inception quantum mechanics has had a problem with consciousness—this in spite of the fact that it is the most rigorously tested theory in all of science. Furthermore, no test ever performed has ever failed to agree completely with the theory (Rosenblum et al, 2008). So, where is the problem?

Although quantum mechanics is applied in much of our daily lives, from computers to magnetic resonance imaging, there is an aspect of it that is counterintuitive and paradoxical. This enigma is best illustrated with light in what is called the "double-slit experiment." As the reader will recall, light has a dual (and paradoxical) nature. It can be either a wave or a "particle" (photon) (see Chapter 1), and Nobel Prizes have been awarded both for demonstrating that light is a wave and for demonstrating that light is a particle. Which of these it is at any moment is dependent on our conscious observation. How can this be? At this moment in time no one knows, but the evidence has never been refuted, and in fact, the more sophisticated we become in our experiments and tests the more entrenched and mysterious this phenomenon becomes (Walborn et al, 2003).

The double-slit interference experiment is performed in the following way. (Because this is not a text or chapter on quantum mechanics, we will gloss over some of the details.) Light is shined into the back of two open boxes with slits on the front sides. On the wall opposite the slits, on the other side from the light source, is a projection screen. No light can reach this screen except the light that comes through the slits. If the slits are narrow enough and spaced properly, the waves of light come out the slits

and, because they are made of waves with high points (peaks) and low points (valleys), the waves can interact and interfere with each other in a fashion analogous to waves on water. The light spreads out from the two slits and the waves interact where they strike the screen. Where two peaks reach the screen at the same point there is a light band. Where two valleys reach the screen at the same point there is a shadow, because no light has reached this point. What one sees, as demonstrated all the time in physics courses around the world, is a series of light and dark stripes, or "interference pattern." This is considered definitive evidence for the wave nature of light.

Now here is the next part. The experiment can be run so that only a single "packet" of light exists in *both* boxes. (This is the part we are glossing over, but this experiment can be and has been done many times.) When this procedure is followed, the interference pattern is still generated, which demonstrates that light is a wave and that the wave of energy was distributed in both boxes. However, if there are photon detectors in both boxes, and we **observe** them while the experiment is running, only *one* of the detectors will react, and a photon (a quantum of light energy) will be found in only one box. Furthermore, the interference pattern will not appear because there is no longer a wave of light. The wave function is said to collapse and form the photon. If you find this confusing, you are in good company. No one has been able to adequately explain this undisputed phenomenon, called *complementarity*. It is important to note that no physicist disputes this phenomenon, but there is considerable controversy as to how to interpret it. The majority simply ignore it and its implications. (To the extent that the *mechanisms* of much of complementary medicine become understood to be based on this *quantum enigma*, it may some day be labeled *complementarity medicine*.)

If this experiment is repeated many times it always comes out one of two ways. If there is no photon detector, then we see the wave nature of light. If there are photon counters in both boxes that we **observe,** then we only see photons and no wave. Furthermore, the probability of finding the photon in one box or the other is exactly 50:50. It was this phenomenon that drove Einstein to try and wish it away by saying that "God does not play dice." The reader will have noted that we used *italics* when describing the act of **observation.** This is where consciousness comes in. As strange as this sounds, the collapsing of the wave function is dependent not only on the presence of the instruments but on our conscious awareness of their output. This phenomenon is demonstrated elegantly in the recent work of Walborn et al on a phenomenon called *quantum erasure* (Walborn et al, 2002, 2003).

These same papers address another aspect of quantum physics called *entanglement*. It appears that the universe makes most, if not all, things in pairs. Thus, it is possible to entangle two photons such that they have paired aspects of their quantum natures. (This is another case in which we are glossing over the technical details, but entanglement at the photon level has been demonstrated repeatedly.) Two photons thus entangled have a very strange property: without any detectable form of energy transfer or communication and in a distance-independent manner, whatever is done to one photon *immediately,* without time delay and no matter the distance separating them, affects the other entangled photon. This is not a causal effect. Observation and the observer do not cause the effect. Rather, the effect is said to be a *nonlocal connectivity* or nonlocal correlation (Hyland, 2003).

Where does that leave us? Light has a dual nature, and which of its two natures it demonstrates depends on **how we look at it.** When photons, and apparently other very small quanta, are entangled they remain entangled regardless of the distance between them. Furthermore, whatever happens to one is immediately reflected in the other without any time delay and with no detectable or explainable form of energy or information transfer. We conclude, as do some physicists (Rosenblum et al, 2008), that these phenomena demonstrate **interaction among consciousness and energy and matter** that appears to go beyond currently understood principles of physics, and that there are ways to transfer information that are independent of distance and through means that physics has not yet determined.

We feel that the incorporation of quantum physics into the discussion on energy medicine provides a possible explanation for some of the empirical observations, anomalies, and hallmarks of this therapy. In addition to helping to explain the role of consciousness in healing, and in energy medicine in particular, quantum mechanics and physics may explain some of the anomalous observations that have been made in aspects of energy medicine such as *distant healing.*

Most forms of energy obey an *inverse square law.* That is, the effect or force drops as an inverse square of the distance. Quantum effects do not show this drop-off with distance. Furthermore, all other energies exert their influence either at or below the speed of light. Quantum effects, however, like many phenomena in energy medicine, seem to happen immediately without an appreciable time delay. Thus, two of the anomalous aspects of energy medicine, *independence of time* and *independence of distance,* are also observed in quantum effects (Julsgaard et al, 2001). In this way we may explain the exchange of healing information, or "subtle energy," between healer and patient from a distance (Bennett et al, 2000).

We are not alone in making this connection. C.W. Smith (1998) has postulated that the body functions as a macroscopic quantum system. This idea may also be applicable to related fields of energy medicine. The data reported by Smith in his 2003 paper suggest that the acupuncture meridian system is made up of quantum domains and networks. Even the proposition that consciousness and intention are connected through quantum mechanical means to our body's healing potentials has been proposed by others (Jahn et al, 1986).

There are serious problems with this hypothesis, however. Specifically, quantum effects have only been demonstrated at an extremely small scale and are thought by most physicists not to be applicable in domains larger than Planck's constant (i.e., photons and electrons) and that only traditional Newtonian mechanics applies to domains we experience in everyday life. Smith's proposal is that there is a hierarchical series of networks and domains in which quantum effects are transmitted to molecules through their quantum particles, and that molecules transfer this information to cells, and so on, until the intact organism is involved and influenced by quantum effects.

HOMEOPATHY AS ENERGY MEDICINE

Homeopathy is defined as yet another form of energy medicine by the NIH (NCCAM, 2007). This may make sense, because standard pharmacology is surely *not* at work in what are called "high-potency" remedies. These are remedies in which the original active substance is diluted to such an extent that there is no possibility than any of the original constituents are present. Dilutions of 30,000-fold, 100,000-fold, or even a millionfold are quite common in this type of homeopathy. Quantum theory is currently in vogue, and perhaps partly because of its mysterious nature, it is sometimes invoked to explain all aspects of energy medicine, including homeopathy. This is usually not done in a formal mathematical way and is often done by novices to the world of quantum mechanics.

Harald Walach and his colleagues have addressed this gap using a formal mathematical approach, however, and published a paper in *Foundations of Physics* in 2002 in which they describe how quantum mechanics and quantum theory could be applied to macro environments and to nonphysical properties such as intention and thoughts. Their theory, called "weak quantum theory and generalized entanglement," demonstrates that, mathematically at least, transfer of information between consciousnesses in a nonphysical way is possible (Atmanspacher et al, 2002). Walach has also produced experimental data to support this hypothesis that need independent replication.

Walach has also gone on to present a case for the application of weak quantum theory and generalized entanglement to homeopathy (Walach, 2003). He contends that the remedies are entangled with both the system and the condition (symptoms) and that even when the original substance has been diluted out of the solution the entanglement remains. Further, he proposes that this explains both the efficacy of homeopathy when it works and the difficulty conventional researchers have in demonstrating this efficacy in clinical trials. Milgrom has also developed formal models for mapping how quantum mechanics could be used to explain the effects of homeopathy and has made suggestions for testing these models in clinical settings (Milgrom, 2006, 2008a, 2008b).

Because entanglement is not fully understood, may not operate inside the normal boundaries of time and space, and is certainly complex and counterintuitive, conventional, linear, cause-and-effect experiments may not properly test the system as it actually exists: *entangled*. Certainly physicists have demonstrated how counterintuitive and mysterious this property can be, and how difficult it is to show, even when one knows what one is looking for and specifically sets up sophisticated experiments to demonstrate the existence of entanglement. Standard biomedical research methods and study designs, including randomized controlled trials, would not demonstrate entanglement. Walach believes that weak *quantum effects and entanglement underlie much of CAM practices and especially energy medicine* (Walach, 2005). If this supposition is true, it would explain the difficulty in demonstrating the efficacy of energy medicine using conventional experimental approaches and would simultaneously provide an explanation for the effects that are clinically observed empirically but without apparent causal connections. For example, two salient characteristics of energy medicine are the apparent lack of dissipation of the effect of "subtle energy" with distance and our inability to block the effects with conventional energy barriers (Astin et al, 2000). This same pair of phenomena is observed in entangled quantum effects. Thinking in this way and designing tests to support or refute the weak quantum theory and entanglement hypothesis represent important directions for future research.

PLACEBO AND BIOFIELD

We are not so bold as to suggest that we know *the* mechanism for energy medicine. On the contrary, we contend that there is legitimate debate as to whether there even is such a thing as "subtle energy." Our goal in this chapter has been to present some of the discussion that is occurring in the field and the literature around energy medicine. There are at least three theories as to the underlying mechanisms giving rise to the effects of energy medicine: (1) a *conventional energy* explanation, (2) an explanation based on *placebo effects*, and (3) a *quantum entanglement* explanation. Just what the mechanism of the well-established placebo effect may be is not addressed in this distinction. We have spent time in this chapter on the quantum mechanics approach, not because we feel that it is the most correct one, but because it is the most novel and perhaps least understood of the theories, and it also best fits all the best data collected so far regarding all forms of energy medicine.

A mechanism that also might explain the effects of energy medicine is the *placebo* effect. That is, whatever is going on is the result of patients' convincing themselves

that they are healing or being healed—they feel less pain, they have fewer complaints, and so on—but "nothing really happened" between healer and patient. However, this explanation is not really more satisfactory and also does not fit some of the best data. The placebo effect itself is not understood nor well defined and thus still begs the question of mechanism. Second, if patients actually experience healing and/or feeling better, then something "really" is happening *consciously,* and we are back to our first point of still not knowing the underlying mechanism while in fact having authentic healing. Thus, we find invoking the placebo effect to be equivalent to confessing that something really is happening with the patient but that we don't know how, or whether it is coming from within or from without. In addition, the known mechanisms of placebo such as belief, expectancy, and conditioning do not account for some of the best-replicated data on the direct effects of intention in living and nonliving systems and blinded distant effects (Jonas et al, 2003b).

The idea of a "vital force" has been a core aspect of traditional healing practices for millennia and has often been used to explain therapeutic practices in the West such as mesmerism, magnetic healing, and faith healing (see Chapter 6). It has also been part of discussions in Western science at least since 1907 when Henri Bergson proposed it as an explanation for why organic molecules could not be synthesized at the time (Bergson, 1911). This thinking held that electricity—the physics and engineering wonder of the time—was somehow connected with this vital force. Chinese and Indian healers had an equivalent idea many thousands of years older, called "qi" or "prana." Clearly this idea has been around a long time.

The modern expression of this idea is often called the "biofield hypothesis" (Rubik, 2002). For our discussion here the important aspect of the biofield hypothesis is its dependence on classical electromagnetic fields and forces. (See Rubik's paper for a more thorough description of this concept and discussion.) As Rubik points out, "The biofield is a useful construct consistent with bioelectromagnetics and the physics of nonlinear, dynamical, nonequilibrium living systems." Although some aspects of energy medicine may be explained by the biofield and it is completely consistent with and even sufficient to explain magnetic therapy, there are at least two aspects of some forms of energy medicine that it does not adequately explain. One is the apparent distance independence. The other is the apparent instantaneous state change (like quantum entanglement) that is part of some forms of energy medicine. This is the second anomaly of subtle energy medicine: it often happens faster than classical mechanisms could explain.

It is possible that these anomalies, as well as the very fundamental aspects of energy medicine, have their explanation and source in quantum physics. We acknowledge that others disagree with this idea (May, 2003). Still others feel that, although this is not the whole explanation, some aspects of quantum physics may be relevant and may play a role in energy medicine (Dossey, 2003). If it is true that energy medicine is often working through nonclassical and quantum forms of energy, it is now possible to visualize a future in which energy medicine uses a combination of classical and quantum energy fields and forces to target and regulate endogenous processes and fields within the body to affect healing and salutogenesis. If energy medicine and distant healing are fundamentally forms of information transfer, then quantum mechanics may provide the explanation and means for this process. In addition to explaining the transfer of healing energy between people, it may underlie the natural self-healing process itself. Rein (2004) has proposed that this information flow within the body is necessary for health and that when it is impeded ill health and disease result. In this thinking, energy medicine is also the flow of information through quantum effects between healer and patient. In an analogous fashion, salutogenesis and health is the free flow and transfer of information within the body and the interchange of information with the environment to augment this flow. Thus, we believe that the fields of information and quantum models will be important areas of focus for future research and practice. Indeed, if testable theoretical models can be developed that explain data from both veritable and putative forms of energy medicine, a new paradigm of understanding in science and health care may emerge that is as important and revolutionary as our biochemical models were in the twentieth century.

Ⓔ Chapter References can be found on the Evolve website at http://evolve.elsevier.com/Micozzi/complementary/

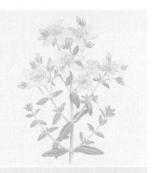

CHAPTER 11

BIOPHYSICAL DEVICES: ELECTRICITY, LIGHT, AND MAGNETISM

MICHAEL I. WEINTRAUB
MARC S. MICOZZI

There is a biophysical aspect to many healing modalities that has long been observed clinically. Contemporary fundamental physics is now in the process of providing explanatory models, mechanisms, and paradigm for the biophysical basis for many healing phenomena. These biophysical characteristics extend beyond the currently established basis of biomedical science in reductionist biochemical, molecular biological, and anatomical terms. Further, biophysics is consistent with many biomedical observations in whole-organism biology, physiology, and homeostasis.

Contemporary biophysics is important for understanding the basis of many contemporary diagnostic and therapeutic approaches. Biophysics, rather than biochemistry or molecular biology, may better provide explanatory mechanisms for the observed effectiveness of such clinical practices as acupuncture, homeopathy, touch, and meditation.

For example, nonthermal, non-ionizing electromagnetic fields in low frequencies have been observed to have the following effects on the physical body: stimulation of bone repair, nerve stimulation, promotion of soft tissue wound healing, treatment of osteoarthritis, tissue regeneration, immune system stimulation, and neuroendocrine modulation.

Contemporary biophysically based modalities include electrodermal screening, applied kinesiology, bioresonance, and radionics. Utilization of these approaches requires the availability of devices and practitioners.

Many well-established historical healing traditions have drawn on diagnostic and therapeutic approaches that may now be interpreted in light of contemporary biophysics. The ancient and complex healing traditions of China and India make reference to and use practices based primarily on biophysical modalities. Acupuncture, acupressure, jin shin do, t'ai chi, reiki, qigong, tui na, and yoga may be seen today to operate on a biophysical basis, but these methods have developed over three millennia in widespread clinical practice and observation. Contemporary outcomes-based clinical trials are demonstrating the efficacy of these modalities in management of many medical conditions (Wootton et al, 2003). In addition, Asian medical systems have used sound, light, and color for their healing properties, which may be viewed in biophysical perspective (see Chapter 2).

U.S. SCHOOLS OF THOUGHT AND PRACTICE

Biophysical medical modalities have also been prominent in the history of American medicine. Several schools of thought were created in the United States, or brought from Europe, that center around healing approaches which we may now associate in whole or in part with emerging biophysical explanations. Such schools and their founders have often influenced each other through time (Box 11-1).

In addition, interpretations of herbal, nutritional, and even pharmacological therapies have been extended to include "vibrational energy" as a mechanism of action.

There have been many adherents, practitioners, and clinical observations of these schools of thought and practice over time. They have been outside the realm of regular medical practice partially because the mechanisms of action of these approaches have not been explained within the biomedical paradigm. Hypnosis is an example of an effective therapeutic modality with widespread effectiveness and acceptance within medicine. However, there remains no explanation for its mechanism of action. An alternative approach to explaining hypnosis has been developed on a statistical basis, describing the profile of clients and conditions likely to benefit and developing

"hypnotic susceptibility scales." This same approach is available for the clinical study of any therapeutic modality with observable outcomes in the absence of an identified "mechanism of action." Mechanism is always bounded by the prevailing scientific paradigm and may not be the most clinically useful question (see Chapter 5). With the development of new scientific observations, a new paradigm emerges that is more inclusive in its explanation of observed phenomena.

INDIVIDUAL PRACTITIONERS

In addition to the fairly widespread, organized schools of thought and practice, there are many intuitive healers whose practices are highly individuated and highly eclectic. These practitioners represent important approaches used by many clients. The knowledge and practices of such gifted healers must be passed on or they will be lost. This represents a situation in the contemporary United States that is analogous to that of herbal remedies in the rain forest. Environmentalists are rightly concerned about the loss of biodiversity when unique plants disappear; ethnobotanists are concerned about the loss of the peoples whose cultural knowledge alone can convert the rain forest plants to cures.

EMPIRICAL ASSUMPTIONS OF BIOPHYSICALLY BASED MODALITIES

1. The human body has a biophysical component.
2. What has been scientifically defined as the "mind" is biophysically linked to the human body.
3. Every part of the human body is biophysically linked to every other part of the body.
4. Mental states (thoughts, emotions) generate physiological responses in the human body through neurological, hormonal, and immunological mechanisms (psychoneuroimmunology).
5. Biophysically based modalities are noninvasive by currently measurable and clinically observable criteria.

MAGNETISM

Human awareness of magnetism extends back in time, with extravagant claims of "magnetic" healing traced back more than 4000 years. In more recent times, attempts to explain the efficacy of this invisible force by invoking unique and unfounded scientific principles and claims, as well as the commercial efforts to sell these products, produced an interesting history of pseudoscience, sensationalism, and controversy. Today in the twenty-first century, despite the fact that permanent magnets and electromagnetic therapies are currently riding the crest of public enthusiasm, it is not surprising

---

BOX 11-1

Schools and Their Founders with Influence on the Development of Biophysical Devices (in Chronological Order)

- Homeopathy (Samuel Hahnemann, Germany, 1830-1860)
- Faith healing (Phineas Quimby, 1830-1860)
- Christian Science (Mary Baker Eddy, 1861-1880)
- Theosophy (Helena Blavatksy/Henry Steel Olcott, 1861-1880)
- Movement therapy (Matthias Alexander, 1861-1880)
- Iridology (Nils Liljequist, Ignaz von Peczely, 1861-1900)
- Zone therapy/reflexology (William Fitzgerald, 1901-1920)
- Anthroposophical medicine (Rudolf Steiner, 1901-1920)
- Polarity therapy (Randolph Stone, 1921-1940)
- Bach flower remedies (Edward Bach, 1921-1940)
- Electromagnetism (Semyon and Valentine Kirlian, 1921-1940)
- Movement therapy (Moshé Feldenkrais, 1941-1960)
- Shiatsu (Tokujiro Namikoshi, 1941-1960)
- Jin shin jyutsu (Jiro Murai, 1941-1960)
- Orgone therapy (Wilhelm Reich, 1941-1960)
- Structural integration (Ida Rolf, 1960-1980)

that the scientific community remains somewhat skeptical of the current widespread claims. A major obstacle has been an inability to determine a mechanism of action. In addition, fundamental questions regarding efficacy can only be resolved by rigorous, randomized, double-blind, placebo-controlled trials, which have only recently come about in the scientific community. The scientific community can now look at this subject objectively and perhaps reverse the entrenched skepticism.

Historical perspectives on magnetism and healing are provided by a number of sources (Armstrong et al, 1991; Geddes, 1991; Macklis, 1993; Markov, 2007; Mourino, 1991; Rosch, 2004; Weintraub, 2001, 2004a, 2004b), which include several excellent reviews of this rich history. According to the Yellow Emperor's Canon of Internal Medicine (or the Yellow Emperor's Inner Classic) magnetic stones (lodestones) were applied to acupressure points as a means of pain reduction. Similarly, the ancient Hindu Vedas ascribed therapeutic powers of ashmana and siktavati (instruments of stone). The term *magnet* was probably derived from Magnes, a shepherd who, according to legend, was walking on Mt. Ida when suddenly the metallic tacks in his sandals were drawn to specific rocks. These rocks were mineral lodestones that contained magnetite, a magnetic oxide of iron (Fe_3O_4). These natural magnetic stones were noted to influence other similar adjacent stones that were brought into close proximity, producing movement. Thus, the ancients called them *alive stones* or *Herculean stones* because they were meant to lead the way. Various powers were attributed to these stones as noted in the writings and artifacts of the ancient Greek and Roman civilizations. For example, Plato, Euripides, and others indicated that these invisible powers of movement could be put to practical use, such as by building ships with iron nails and destroying opposing military ships and navies by maneuvering them close to magnetic mountains or magnetic rock.

Medicinal and healing properties were also attributed to these lodestones. Various magnetic rings and necklaces were sold in the marketplace in Samothrace around AD 200 to treat arthritis and pain. Similarly, lodestones were ground up to make powders and salves to treat various conditions. Numerous claims and anecdotal stories led to the public embrace of these magical devices. In 1289, the first major treatise on magnetism was written by Peter Peregrinus. He ascribed to lodestone curative properties for treating gout, baldness, and arthritis and spoke about its strong aphrodisiac powers. He also described drawing poison from wounds with close application. His work contains the first drawing and description of a compass in the Western world.

The Middle Ages witnessed the emergence of numerous myths that persist in certain segments of society. For example, it was believed that magnets could extract gold from wells and that application or ingestion of garlic could neutralize magnetic properties. The idea that magnets could be used therapeutically resurfaced in the early sixteenth century when Paracelsus (Philippus Aureolus Theophrastus Bombast von Hohenheim), considered to be one of the most influential physicians and alchemists of his time, used lodestones (magnets) to treat conditions such as epilepsy, diarrhea, and hemorrhage. He believed that every person is a living magnet, that they can attract good and evil, and that magnets are an important elixir of life.

Scientific enlightenment in the seventeenth century on this topic began with the work of Dr. William Gilbert, physician to Queen Elizabeth I of England. He wrote his classic text *De Magnete* in 1600 describing hundreds of detailed experiments concerning electricity and also terrestrial magnetism. He debunked many medicinal applications and was responsible for laying the groundwork for future research and study. Despite the fact that Luigi Galvani and Alessandro Volta made significant contributions, for the next 100 years there were no major advancements in the study of magnetism.

In the early eighteenth century, there was significant interest in both magnetism and electricity. Francis Hauksbee, in 1705, invented an electrostatic engine that, by rotating and spinning an attached globe, could transfer an electronic charge to various metallic objects brought close to it, such as chain, wire, and metal. This procedure induced electrical shocks. Refinements in this machine led to more general usage, and in 1743, traveling circuses throughout Europe and the American colonies provided individuals with shocks for a small fee. Legend suggests that Benjamin Franklin witnessed an "electrified boy" exhibition and thus became interested in both electricity and magnetic phenomena. Franklin is famed for his experiments on electricity, using lightning, in which he attached a key to an airborne kite in a thunderstorm (as depicted in the heroic portrait by Benjamin West entitled "Franklin Taming Lightning") (See Chapter 1). In fact, it was actually Franklin's young son who was sent out into the lightning storm with the kite, risking the exhibition of Franklin's own version of an "electrified boy."

Much of the current magnetic terminology regarding electricity originated with Franklin, such as charge, discharge, condenser, electric shock, electrician, positive, negative, plus and minus, and so on. Franklin distinguished himself in studies primarily of electric fluid and charges, and concluded that all matter contained magnetic fields that are uniformly distributed throughout the body. He believed that when an object is magnetized, the fluid condenses in one of its extremities. That extremity becomes positively magnetized, whereas the donor region of the object becomes negatively magnetized. He felt that the degree to which an object can be magnetized depends on the force necessary to start the fluid moving within it.

The scientific revolution came to Europe with the development of carbon-steel magnets (1743 to 1751). Father Maximilian Hell and later his student, Franz Anton Mesmer, applied these magnetic devices to patients, many of whom were experiencing hysterical or psychosomatic symptoms. Specifically in his major treatise "On the

Medicinal Uses of the Magnet" Mesmer described how he fed a patient iron filings and then applied specially designed magnets over the vital organs to generally stop uncontrolled seizures. His cures were not only astounding but also good theater, because they were performed in front of large groups (see Chapter 9). The power of suggestion was clearly being displayed and ultimately transferred to nonferric objects such as paper, wood, silk, and stone. Mesmer reasoned that he was not dealing with ordinary mineral magnetism but rather with a special *animal magnetism*. The term *mesmerization* is often applied to his displays of people overcoming illness and disease by *mesmerizing* their bodies' innate magnetic poles to induce a crisis, often in the form of convulsions. After this crisis, health would be restored. He hailed this animal magnetism as a specific natural force of healing. His claims of success infuriated his conservative colleagues and motivated the French Academy of Sciences under King Louis VI to convene a special study in 1784. The panel for this study included Antoine-Laurent Lavoisier, Joseph-I. Guillotin, and Benjamin Franklin, ambassador to France from the newly independent United States of America. In a controlled set of experiments, blindfolded patients were to be exposed to a series of magnets or sham magnetic objects and asked to describe the induced sensation. Although there remains controversy as to whether and what experimental observations were made, the committee "lost their heads" (a process that was soon to be facilitated by the invention of one of their members, Dr. Guillotin, in the coming French Revolution) in bickering about mechanism of action. They concluded that the efficacy of the magnetic healing resided entirely within the mind of the individual and that any healing was due to suggestion. Based on these conclusions, the medical establishment declared Mesmer's theories fraudulent, and mesmerism was equated with medical quackery. Mesmer left France in disgrace. Some members of the panel who remained in France, such as Lavoisier, literally lost their heads.

Nonetheless, in the United States magnetic therapy flourished, with significant sales of magnets, magnetic salves, and liniments by traveling magnetic healers. Later in the nineteenth century Daniel David Palmer, the founder of chiropractic and self-described "magnetic healer," stated that putting down his hands for physical manipulation of the patient produced better results than the simple "laying on of hands."

In Europe, Hans Christian Ørsted (1777-1851), a physicist, continued studies and noted that a compass needle was deflected when a current flowed through a nearby wire. He also discovered that not only did a current-carrying wire coil exert a force on a magnet, but a magnet exerted a force on the coil of wire, inducing an electrical current. The coil behaved like a magnet, as if it possessed magnetic north and south poles. Magnetism and electricity were somehow connected. Ørsted was instrumental in creating a proper scientific environment that led to further study, with André-Marie Ampère deducing the quantitative relationship between magnetic force and electric current. In the 1820s, Michael Faraday and Joseph Henry (later founding secretary of the Smithsonian Institution in the 1850s) demonstrated more connections between magnetism and electricity, showing that a changing magnetic field could induce an electrical field perpendicularly.

In 1886, the Sears catalogue advertised numerous magnetic products such as magnetic rings, belts, caps, soles for boots, and girdles. In the 1920s, Thacher created a mail-order catalogue advertising over 700 specific magnetic garments and devices and products that he described as a "plain road to health without the use of medicine and was dependent on the magnetic energy of the sun." He believed that the iron content of the blood made it the primary magnetic conductor of the body, and thus the most efficient way to *recharge* the body's magnetic field was by wearing his magnetic garments. The complete set was said to "furnish full and complete protection of all the vital organs of the body." *Collier's Weekly* dubbed Thacher the "king of the magnetic quacks." There was no government regulation of these devices or claims, and thus these types of promotion fueled skepticism. The U.S. Food and Drug Administration (FDA) had no jurisdiction over medical devices at that time and there were no good scientific trials, although problems with the purity of drugs had led to the passage of the Pure Food and Drug Act of 1906 and the subsequent formation of the FDA.

In 1896, Arsène D'Arsonval reported to the Société de Biologie in Paris that when a subject's head was placed in a strong time-varying magnetic field, phosphenes (sensations of light caused by retinal stimulation) were perceived. Some 15 years later, Silvanus P. Thompson (1910) confirmed that not only could phosphenes be induced, but that exposure to a strong alternating magnetic field also produced taste sensation. Various coils were constructed by Dunlap and later Magnusson and Stevens. They noted that magnetophosphenes were brightest at a low frequency of about 25 Hz and became fainter at higher frequencies.

After World War II, there was heightened interest and research in magnetotherapy in Japan and the former Soviet Union. Specifically, in Japan magnetotherapeutic devices were accepted under the Drug Regulation Act of 1961, and by 1976, various devices were commonly and commercially employed to treat various illnesses and promote health. Similar interest in Bulgaria, Romania, and Russia led to development of various therapeutic approaches, so that the physician had available the use of magnetic fields to assist in treating disease. Today, Germany, Japan, Russia, Israel, and at least 45 other countries consider magnetic therapy to be an official medical procedure for the treatment of various neurological and inflammatory conditions (Whitaker et al, 1998). By contrast, magnetotherapy had limited acceptance in Western medicine. Unwarranted claims and its promotion by charlatans only led to further public and scientific skepticism.

The modern era of magnetic stimulation began with the work of R.G. Bickford and colleagues (Bickford et al 1965) who considered the possibility of stimulation of the nervous system (frog nerve and human peripheral nerves). He also discussed the generation of eddy currents in the brain that could reach a certain magnitude to stimulate cortical structures through an intact cranium (Bickford et al, 1965). Barker and colleagues at the University of Sheffield developed the first commercial cranial magnetic stimulator in 1985 (Barker, 1991; Barker et al, 1987). They gave a practical demonstration at Queen's Square by stimulating "Dr. Merton's brain," which caused muscle twitches. As might be expected, the physiological and clinical possibilities became obvious (Merton, 1980). Although there were technical challenges, they were met with the development of devices capable of stimulating the brain focally at frequencies of up to 100 Hz using specific coil configurations (i.e., circular). Adaptations for focal therapy were created. Thus, a new discipline developed using high and low repetitive stimulation frequencies directed to previously inaccessible areas of the brain and body (George et al, 2003; Kobayashi et al, 2003; Pascual-Leone et al, 1994). As of July 1998, over 6000 publications existed that dealt with basic neurophysiology, clinical syndromes, and therapeutic implications. Although most of the initial papers were the results of open-label (nonplacebo) observations, many current publications report on randomized, double-blind, placebo-controlled trials. Thus, when all of this information is pooled, both experimental and clinical, the data strongly suggest that the application of exogenous magnetic fields at low levels does indeed induce a biological effect on a variety of systems, especially pain sensation and the musculoskeletal system.

Essential terms must be defined to understand the role of magnetism. *Biomagnetics* refers to the field of science dealing with the application of magnetic fields to living organisms. Basic research on cells in culture as well as clinical trials have provided a better understanding of mechanisms of action (Adey, 1992, 2004; Adey et al, 1999; Lednev, 1991; Markov, 2004; Markov et al, 2001; Pilla, 2003; Pilla et al, 1997; Timmell et al, 1998). Human tissues are dielectric and conductive and therefore can respond to electrical and magnetic fields that are oscillating or static. Cell membranes consist of paramagnetic and diamagnetic lipoprotein materials that respond to magnetic fields and serve as signaling (transduction) pathways by which external stimuli are sent and conveyed to the cell interior. Calcium ions are very important in transduction coupling at the cell membrane level. Electromagnetic fields can also alter the configuration of atoms and molecules in dielectric and paramagnetic-diamagnetic substances. Thus atoms in these substances polarize, to some degree, when placed in an electromagnetic field and act as a dipole and align accordingly (Adey, 1988, 1992; Blumenthal et al, 1997; DeLoecker et al, 1990; Engstrom et al, 1999; Farndale et al, 1987; Lednev, 1991; Maccabee et al, 1991; Pilla et al, 1997; Repacholi et al, 1999; Rosen, 1992; Rossini

et al, 1994; Timmel et al, 1998). Adey feels that free radicals are important for signal transduction. Chemical bonds are essentially electromagnetic bonds formed between adjacent atoms. The breaking of the chemical bonds of a singlet pair allows electrons to influence adjacent electrons with similar or opposite spins, which thereby become triplet pairs, and so on. Thus, by imposing magnetic fields in this medium, one may influence the rate and amount of communication between cells. At the cell membrane level, free radicals of nitric oxide may play an essential role in this regulation of receptors specifically (Adey, 1988, 1992, 2004). It is known that free radicals are involved in the normal regulatory mechanisms in many tissues and that certain disorders are associated with disordered free radical regulation producing oxidative stress. These include Alzheimer disease, Parkinson disease, cancer, and coronary artery disease. This entire area is still incompletely understood yet under intense research scrutiny.

Magnetic field strength is indicated by magnetic flux density, which is the number of field lines (flux) that cross a unit of surface area. It is usually described in terms of the unit gauss (G) or tesla (T). There are 10,000 G in 1 T. Because there is an exponential decay of field strength with distance from a magnetic source according the inverse square law, the objective is to apply a static magnetic device as close to the skin as possible and to ensure that a magnet of sufficient size and surface field is used when the target is in deep tissue areas. *Magnetotherapy* is defined as the use of time-varying magnetic fields of low-frequency values (3 Hz to 3 KHz) to induce a sufficiently strong current to stimulate living tissue.

Faraday's law (1831) defines the fundamental relationship between a changing magnetic field and a conductor (any medium that carries electrically charged particles). When a wire is used as an example of a conductor, Faraday's law basically states that any change in the magnetic environment of the coil of wire with time will cause a voltage to be induced in the wire. No matter how the change is produced, a voltage will be generated. Thus, magnetic field amplitude may be varied by powering the electromagnet with sinusoidal or pulsing current or by moving a permanent magnet toward or away from the wire, moving the wire toward or away from the magnetic field, rotating the wire relative to the magnet, and so on (DeLoecker et al, 1990; Goodman et al, 2002; Serway, 1998; Smith, 1996; Wittig et al, 2002).

Lenz's law states that the polarity of the voltage induced according to Faraday's law is such that it produces a current whose magnetic field opposes the applied magnetic field (back EMF, or electromagnetic field). Therefore, if a current is passed through a coil that creates an expanding magnetic field around the coil, the induced voltage and associated current flow produce a magnetic field in opposition to the directly induced magnetic field.

Eddy currents are induced by the voltage generated according to Faraday's law in any conducting medium. When the conducting medium does not contain defined current pathways, there is no induced current, only induced voltage. There is movement in a spiral, swirling fashion, and this in turn potentially penetrates the membranes of the neurons. If the induced current is of sufficient amplitude, an action potential or an excitatory or inhibitory postsynaptic potential may be produced.

The Hall effect and the Lorentz force are related to the same physical phenomenon of electromagnetism. In the Hall effect, when charged particles in a conductor move along a path that is transverse to a magnetic field, the particles experience a force that pushes them toward the outer walls of the conductor. The positively charged particles move to one side and the negatively charged particles move to the other side. This produces a voltage across the conductor known as the "Hall voltage." Because the human body is replete with charged ions, the Hall effect would certainly occur to varying degrees when a magnetic field is passed through the body. The strength of the Hall voltage produced depends on three factors: (1) the strength of the magnetic field, (2) the number of charged particles moving transverse to the magnetic field, and (3) the velocity of movement of the charged particles (ions). The pulsing and static magnetic fields in current therapeutic applications are much too weak and the endogenous currents much too small for the Hall effect to be of any significance in magnetic field bioeffects (Pilla et al, 1992, 1993). However, this is somewhat controversial and not universally accepted. Clearly, cellular and neural components in the body provide conductive pathways for ions, so it is reasonable to assume that these components would be prime objects of attention in attempting to observe the Hall effect. It is presumed that this voltage might add to the nerve's resting potential of -70 mV and make it harder to depolarize. Once the resting potential rises from its normal undisturbed voltage of about -70 mV to a voltage of approximately -55 mV (threshold potential), an action potential spike is initiated. When ions move under the influence of a voltage, they become an electric current the magnitude of which is determined by Ohm's law, which states that electric current equals voltage divided by resistance.

This phenomenon predicts the effects of ions exposed to a combination of exogenous AC/DC magnetic fields at approximately 0.1 G and the dynamics of ions in a binding site. A bound ion in a static magnetic field will precess at the Larmour frequency and will accelerate faster to preferred orientations in the binding site with increased magnetic field strength. Thus, an increased binding rate can occur with a resultant acceleration in the downstream biochemical cascade.

Magnetic fields can penetrate all tissues, including epidermis, dermis, and subcutaneous tissue as well as tendons, muscles, and even bone. The specific amount of magnetic energy and its effect at the target organ depends on the size, strength, and duration of contact of the device. Magnetic fields fall into two broad categories: (1) *static (DC)* and (2) *time varying (AC)*.

The strength of *static magnetic* devices varies from 1 to 4000 G. Static fields have zero frequency, because the polarity and field strength do not change with time but rather remain constant. Permanent magnets produce only static fields unless they are rotated or otherwise moved, which causes the magnetic field amplitude to change with time at the tissue target. Static magnetic fields that are either permanent or electromagnetic are in the range of 1 to 4000 G and have been reported to have significant biological effects (Colbert, 2004; Markov et al, 2001; Pilla, 2003; Pilla et al, 2003). The most common static magnets sold to the public are known as refrigerator or flat-button magnets. They are made of various materials and also have different designs. Configuration can be unidirectional so that only one magnetic pole is represented on one side of the surface (whereas the opposite pole is on the opposite side away from the applied surface) or the surface can have a bipolar north-south design that appears repetitively as concentric ring, multitriangular, or quadripolar configurations.

The term *bipolar magnets* refers to a repetitive north-south polarity created on the same side of a ceramic or plastic alloy or neodymium material, whereas the term *unipolar* refers to only one magnetic pole at a given surface, that is, north or south. Multipolar alterations of north and south have also been employed. Each specific manufacturer makes claims as to the superiority of its product. However, the most important characteristic of the magnetic field is the field strength at the target site and also the duration of exposure that leads to biological effects. It is believed that tissues, cells, and other structures have a "biological window" within which they can interact with these invisible fields. Static magnetic fields of 5 to 20 G have been felt to be pertinent. Thus, the gauss rating and field strength at the surface are irrelevant in predicting biological response. Bipolar magnets, using a small arc, are capable of inducing biologically significant fields at a relatively short distance from the surface (1 to 1.5 cm), whereas the penetration of unipolar magnets is much deeper (4 to 8 cm) (Markov, 2007).

As indicated earlier, review of the literature reveals that static magnetic fields in the 1 to 4000 G range have been reported to have significant biological effect. Basic science has demonstrated that static magnetic fields ranging from 23 to 3000 G can alter the electrical properties of solutions. In addition, weak static magnetic fields can modulate myosin phosphorylation at the molecular level in a cell-free preparation (Markov et al, 1997). At a cellular level, exposure to 300 G doubled alkaline phosphatase activity in osteoblast-like cells (McDonald, 1993). Neurite outgrowth from embryonic chick ganglia was significantly increased by exposure to 225 to 900 G (Macias et al, 2000; Sisken et al, 1993). McLean and coworkers, in several experiments using unidirectional and multipolar magnets, demonstrated a blockade of sensory nociceptive neuron action potentials by exposure to a static magnetic field in the 10 mT range. A minimum magnetic field gradient of 15 G/mm was required to cause approximately 80% action potential blockade in isolated nerve preparations (McLean et al, 1995). This blockade reversed when the magnetic exposure was removed. Protection against kainic acid–induced neuronal swelling was also demonstrated with magnetic exposure (McLean et al, 2003). Others have demonstrated a biphasic response of the acute microcirculation in rabbits exposed to static magnetic fields (10 G) (Ohkubo et al, 1997; Okano et al, 1999). Despite all this provocative and promising data in both in vitro and in vivo studies, skepticism prevails because of design flaws (Holcomb et al, 2002; Ramey, 1998). Specifically, a rigorous randomized, placebo-controlled, double-blind design has been lacking; basic mechanisms of action have not been identified; and optimum target dosage and optimum polarity have yet to be determined. The absence of nonmagnetic placebos as controls has also been described as a problem.

Colbert (2004) reviewed 22 therapeutic trials reported in the U.S. literature from 1982 to 2002. Clinical improvement in subjects who wore permanent magnets on various parts of their bodies was demonstrated in 15 studies, whereas 7 reported limited or no benefit. Magnetic field strength varied from 68 to 2000 G and time exposure varied from 45 minutes to constant wearing for 4 months. Thus the optimum treatment duration, as well as the optimal polarity (unidirectional, multipolar, etc.), has yet to be established. Complicating the issue even further is the observation by Blechman et al (2001) that a significant number of the static magnets sold to the public had lower field flux density measurements than the manufacturers claimed. It is known that a large amount of cancellation occurs in multipolar arrays. Similarly, Eccles (2005) conducted a critical review of the randomized controlled trials that used static magnets for pain relief. He found a 73% statistical reduction in pain. He also commented on the difficulty in performing double-blind studies using static magnets because of the obvious interaction with metallic objects.

Specific clinical trials using a double-blind, placebo-controlled design include that of Vallbona et al (1997), who applied 300- to 500-G concentric-circle bipolar magnets over painful joints in patients with postpolio syndrome for 45 minutes and reduced pain by 76%. Carter et al (2002) applied unipolar 1000-G static magnets and placebos over the carpal tunnel for 45 minutes and both groups experienced significant pain reduction. This was felt to represent a placebo effect. Unidirectional magnetic pads (150 to 400 G) were placed over liposuction sites immediately after the procedure and kept in place for 14 days; this treatment produced a 40% to 70% reduction of pain, edema, and discoloration (Man et al, 1999). Brown et al (2002) demonstrated statistical reduction of pelvic pain with magnetic therapy. Patients with fibromyalgia who slept on a unidirectional magnetic mattress pad (800-G ceramic magnets) for 4 months experienced a 40% improvement (Colbert et al, 1999). Weintraub (1999)

noted a 90% reduction in neuropathic pain in patients with diabetic peripheral neuropathy with constant wearing of multipolar 475-G insole devices. There was also a 30% reduction in neuropathic pain associated with nondiabetic peripheral neuropathy (Man et al, 1999; Weintraub, 1999). A nationwide study using placebo controls also confirmed these results in 275 patients with diabetic peripheral neuropathy (Weintraub et al, 2003).

Hinman et al (2002) found a 30% response to short-term application of unipolar static magnets positioned over painful knees. Greater movement was also noted. Holcomb et al (2002), using a quadripolar array of static magnets with alternating polarity, demonstrated analgesic benefit in patients with low back pain and knee pain.

Saygili et al (1992), in an investigation of the effect of magnetic retention systems in dental prostheses on buccal mucosal blood flow, failed to detect changes in capillary blood flow after continuous exposure to a magnetic field for 45 days. Hong et al (1982) had 101 patients with chronic neck and shoulder pain wear magnetic necklaces or placebos for 3 consecutive weeks after baseline electrodiagnostic studies, but no significant improvement was seen in the magnetic therapy group. In a study using a randomized placebo crossover design Martel et al (2002) could not identify any change in forearm blood flow after 30 minutes of exposure to bipolar magnets. Other randomized placebo-controlled trials producing negative results should be mentioned, including Collacott et al's study (2000) of the use of bipolar devices in patients with chronic low back pain and Winemiller et al's study (2003) of the use of magnetic insoles by patients with plantar fasciitis. Weintraub and others commented on design flaws in both of these studies (Weintraub, 2000, 2004a, 2004b). Simultaneous application of static magnets to the back and feet in patient with failed back syndrome was also ineffective (Weintraub et al, 2005). Pilla independently assessed the strength of the magnetic devices and found them to be less than the manufacturer's claims, thereby confirming the observations of Blechman et al (2001) regarding the discrepancy between claimed and measured field flux densities.

It is assumed that the biological benefits from static magnetic fields are similar to those from pulsed electromagnetic fields, but the correlation has been imperfect. The specific mechanism of biological benefit remains to be determined. At present, the most generally accepted theory is that static magnetic fields on the order of 1 to 10 G can affect ion-ligand binding, producing modulation (Pilla, 2003; Pilla et al, 1997, 2003). There may also be physical realignment and translational movement of diamagnetically anisotropic molecules. Despite these theoretical and scientific rationales for benefit, criticism and skepticism prevail. Critics allege that it is all placebo effects, yet a more enlightened and open-minded appraisal would accept the positive in vitro and in vivo observations. Ramey (1998), a veterinarian, has been a noted critic of static magnetic therapy, yet these devices are used extensively in veterinary medicine (e.g., magnetic blankets for race horses).

The World Health Organization has stated that there are no adverse effects on human health from exposure to static magnetic fields, even up to 2 T, which equals 20,000 G (United Nations Environment Programme MF, 1987). Similarly, in 2003 the FDA extended nonsignificant risk status to magnetic resonance imaging (MRI) using flux densities of up to 8 T (U.S. Food and Drug Administration, 2003).

PULSED ELECTROMAGNETIC FIELDS

The generation of pulsed electromagnetic fields (PEMFs) require an electric current to produce a pulsating (time-varying) magnetic field. This is because the coil that produces the magnetic field is stationary. Regardless of how the waveforms are transmitted through the coil, the ensuing magnetic flux lines appear in space in exactly the same manner as the flux lines from a permanent magnet. The magnetic field penetrates biological tissues without modification, and the induced electrical fields are produced at right angles to the flux lines. The ensuing current flow is determined by the tissue's electrical properties (impedance) and determines the final spacial dosimetry. Peak magnetic fields from PEMF devices are typically 5 to 30 G at the target tissue with varying specific shapes and amplitudes of fields.

Cellular studies (in vitro, in vivo) have been most provocative. In reviewing this work, Markov has summarized various cellular and structural changes in response to this PEMF exposure (Markov, 2004; Markov et al, 2001). Specifically, changes in fibrinogen, fibroblasts, leukocytes, platelets, fibrin, cytokines, collagen, elastin, keratinocytes, osteoblasts, and free radicals are noted. In addition, magnetic fields influence vasoconstriction, vasodilatation, phagocytosis, cell proliferation, epithelialization, and scar formation.

Similarly, in a series of reviews, Pilla has summarized the effects of these weak PEMFs on both signal transduction and growth factor synthesis as it relates to fractures (Pilla, 2003; Pilla et al, 1992, 1993, 2003). He noted that there is upregulation of growth factor production, calcium ion transport, self-proliferation, insulinlike growth factor II release, and insulinlike growth factor II receptor expression in osteoblasts as a mechanism for bone repair. He also cited an increase in both transforming growth factor-β1 messenger RNA and protein in osteoblast cultures, producing an effect on a calcium/calmodulin-dependent pathway. Other studies with chondrocytes confirm similar increases in transforming growth factor-β1 messenger RNA and protein synthesis with PEMF exposure, which suggests a therapeutic application for joint repair (Ciombor et al, 2002; Pilla et al, 1996). PEMFs have also been successfully applied to stimulate nerve regeneration. Neurite outgrowth has been demonstrated in cell cultures exposed to electromagnetic fields. Eddy currents are generated that can depolarize, hyperpolarize, and repolarize nerve cells, which suggests that neuromodulation potentially can arise.

In 1979, the FDA approved the use of PEMF as a means of stimulating and recruiting osteoblast cells at a fracture site. Application of coils around the cast induces current flows through the fracture site, producing 80% success. It became apparent after early testing that intermittent exposure, rather continuous exposure, was the optimal technique. Currently, there are four FDA-approved devices for treatment of non-union fractures, and each has specific signal parameters, treatment time, and so on. It is not yet clear how long PEMF exposure must last to trigger a bioelectrical effect. Effective waveforms tend to be asymmetric, biphasic, and quasi-rectangular or quasi-triangular in shape. This indicates that tissues have various windows of vulnerability and susceptibility to PEMF. Based on the high success rate of PEMF therapy, it is currently considered part of the standard armamentarium of orthopedic spine surgeons and is recommended as an adjunct to standard fracture management. In addition, the results are equivalent to those of surgical repair with minimal risk, and the treatment is more cost effective.

PEMF therapy has also been used to treat other orthopedic conditions as well as painful musculoskeletal disorders. These include aseptic necrosis of the hips, osteoporosis, osteoarthritis, osteogenesis imperfecta, rotator cuff dysfunction, and low back pain (Aaron et al, 1989; Binder et al, 1984; Fukada et al, 1957; Jacobson et al, 2001; Linovitz et al, 2000; Mooney, 1990; Pipitone et al, 2001; Pujol et al, 1998; Wilson et al, 1974; Zdeblic, 1993). Markov, in his reviews (Markov, 2004, 2007; Markov et al, 2001), stated that with the exception of periarthritis, for which no difference was reported between treatment and control groups, reduced pain scores were noted in carpal tunnel pain (93%) (Battisti et al, 1998) and rotator cuff tendinitis (83%) (Binder et al, 1984), and 70% of multiple sclerosis patients had reduced spasticity (Lappin et al, 2003). Pilla reports double-blind studies claiming benefit for chronic wound repair (Battisti et al, 1998; Kloth et al, 1999; Mayrovitz et al, 1995; Todd et al, 1991), acute ankle sprain (Ciombor et al, 2002; Pilla et al, 1996), and acute whiplash injuries (Foley-Nolan et al, 1990, 1992).

Pujol et al (1998) targeted musculoskeletal pain using magnetic coils, which produced a benefit compared with placebo. Weintraub and Cole (2004) applied nine consecutive 1-hour treatments to patients with peripheral neuropathy, which induced a greater than 50% reduction in neuropathic pain. This was an open-label, nonplacebo trial.

Pickering et al (2003) demonstrated that gentamicin's effect against *Staphylococcus epidermidis* could be augmented by exposure to a PEMF. In other research with a double-blind, placebo-controlled design, use of pulsed high-frequency (27-MHz) electromagnetic therapy to treat persistent neck pain produced significant improvement by the second week of therapy (Foley-Nolan et al, 1990, 1992).

In 1983 Raji and Boden applied 27-MHz pulsed electromagnetic therapy to the transected common peroneal nerve of rats; 15 minutes of treatment daily produced accelerated healing with reduced scar tissue, increased growth of blood vessels, and maturation of myelin (Fukada et al, 1957). Despite all the convincing data, the use of PEMF therapy does not enjoy universal acceptance. In addition, the large number of different commercially available PEMF devices, which generate low-frequency fields of different shapes and amplitudes, are a major variable in attempting to understand and analyze the putative biological clinical effects. It has been speculated that the target area receives 5 to 30 G and that each tissue has its own biophysical window and specific encoding susceptibility (Pilla et al, 2003).

Despite all these provocative data, there is considerable uncertainty about the specific mechanisms involved as well as the optimal approach in terms of frequency, amplitude, and duration of exposure. Of course, this issue may be moot based on available data, because several different devices generating different frequencies and amplitudes and used for different durations have been successful in producing similar non-union fracture healing. In addition, there is an abundance of experimental and clinical data demonstrating that extremely low frequency and static magnetic fields can have a profound effect on a large variety of biological systems, organisms, and tissues as well as cellular and subcellular structures. It is assumed that the target is the cell membrane with ion and ligand binding and that even small changes in transmembrane voltage can induce a significant modulation of cellular function. In a recent review, Pilla has attempted to provide a unifying approach for static and pulsating magnetic fields, as well as weak ultrasound, which also induces electrical fields comparable to those associated with PEMFs (Pilla, 2003). Pilla has also employed pulsed (nonthermal) radiofrequency fields at 27.12 Hz and has achieved soft tissue healing, reduction of edema, and postoperative pain relief. Pulsed radiofrequency therapy has recently been approved by the FDA (Mayrovitz et al, 1995).

A novel device has now been developed with time-varying, biaxial rotation that generates simultaneous static (DC) and oscillating (AC) fields. The fields are constantly changing and thus produce variable exposure to tissues and varying amplitudes at the target tissue. Weintraub and coworkers have recently found this type of therapy to be effective in reducing neuropathic pain from diabetic peripheral neuropathy and carpal tunnel syndrome (Weintraub and Cole, 2007a, 2007b).

TRANSCRANIAL MAGNETIC STIMULATION

Transcranial magnetic stimulation (TMS) is a specific adaptation of PEMF that creates a time-varying magnetic field over the surface of the head and depolarizes underlying superficial neurons, which induce electrical currents in the brain. High-intensity current is rapidly turned on and off in the electromagnetic coil through the discharge of capacitors. Thus, brief (microseconds) and powerful magnetic fields are produced, which in turn induce current in the brain. Two magnetic stimuli delivered in close sequence to the same cortical region through a single stimulating coil are used. The first is a conditioning stimulus at sub–motor threshold intensity that influences the intracortical neurons and exerts a significant modulating effect on the amplitude of the motor evoked potential induced by the second, supra–motor threshold stimulus. This modulating effect depends on the interval between the stimuli. Cortical inhibition consistently occurs at intervals between 1 and 5 msec, and facilitation is seen at intervals between 10 and 20 msec. TMS is simple to perform, inexpensive, generally safe, and provides useful measures of neuronal excitability. It has also been used along the neuraxis and continues to provide important insights into basic neurological functions, neurophysiology, and neurobiology. Although TMS is generally used as a research tool, it has been proposed that the therapeutic use of TMS be considered. The abnormalities that are revealed by TMS are not disease specific and need clinical correlation. Initially, stimulation directed to the primary motor cortex in individuals with a number of movement disorders helped investigators appreciate the role of the basal ganglia. Specific TMS studies looked at Parkinson disease, dystonia, Huntington chorea, essential tremor, Tourette syndrome, myoclonus, restless legs syndrome, progressive supranuclear palsy, Wilson disease, stiff-person syndrome, and Rett syndrome, among others. The results were promising, which suggests that future large multicenter trials are warranted.

TMS has also proved useful in investigating the mechanisms of epilepsy, and repetitive TMS may prove to have a therapeutic role in the future (Osenbach, 2006).

TMS also is used in preoperative assessment of specific brain areas to optimize the surgical procedure. Both inhibitory and facilitatory interactions in the cortex can be studied by combining a subthreshold conditioning stimulus with a suprathreshold test stimulus at different short (1- to 20-msec) intervals through the same coil. In addition, this paired-pulse TMS approach is used to investigate potential central nervous system–activating drugs, various neurological and psychological diseases, and so on. Left and right hemispheres often react differently (Cahn et al, 2003). The clinical utility of this aspect has not yet been demonstrated. If TMS pulses are delivered repetitively and rhythmically, the process is called "repetitive TMS" (rTMS) and can be modified further to induce excitatory or inhibitory effects. In rare cases seizures may be provoked in epileptic patients as well as in normal volunteers (Abbruzzese et al, 2002; Amassian et al, 1989; Cantello, 2002; Chae et al, in press; George et al, 1999; Kobayashi et al, 2003; Lisamby et al, 2001; Pascual-Leone et al, 2002; Rollnik et al, 2002; Terao et al, 2002; Theodore, 2003; Wasserman, 1998; Walsh et al, 1999).

Repetitive TMS leads to modulation of cortical excitability. For example, high-frequency rTMS of the dominant hemisphere, but not the nondominant hemisphere, can induce speech arrest (Orpin, 1982). This effect also correlates with results of the Wada test. The higher the stimulation frequency, the greater the disruption of cortical function. Lower frequencies of rTMS in a 1-Hz range can suppress excitability of the motor cortex, whereas 20-Hz stimulation trains lead to a temporary increase in cortical excitability. Pascual-Leone and coworkers have been studying these effects in patients with neurological disorders such as Parkinson disease, dystonia, epilepsy, and stroke. Osenbach (2006) provides a comprehensive review of the use of motor cortex stimulation (MCS) to manage intractable pain, concluding "there is little doubt that MCS provides excellent relief in carefully selected patients with a variety of neuropathic pain but leaves many unanswered questions." Tinnitus has been recalcitrant to many therapies, but there has been increasing use of magnetic and electrical stimulation of the auditory cortex with benefit (DeRidder et al, 2004; Whitaker et al, 1998). Psychiatric conditions, including anxiety, mania, depression, and schizophrenia, are also being treated with TMS (George et al, 1999, 2003, 2004). These early observations and data suggest a rich potential therapeutic utility heretofore not known. Elucidation of the underlying neurobiology is still a work in progress in various neuropsychiatric syndromes. Creating sham TMS is difficult, and there is some evidence to suggest that tilting of the coils produces some biological effect on the brain with (George et al, 2004).

A controversial and legitimate concern relates to the possibility that exposure of living tissue to an electromagnetic field may play a causative role in malignancy and birth defects. Specifically, this concern has been raised because of the foci of childhood leukemia cases reported adjacent to high-power lines. During a 5-year period (1991 to 1996), Congress appropriated $60 million for dedicated research to look for such a causal association. The result was that no significant risk from power line frequencies could be confirmed and the fears did not appear justified. *No funding* was made available to explore and expand the beneficial effects of magnetics and electromagnetic fields!! The facts are that there is now a 30-year experience with and history of the approved use of PEMF in promoting repair of recalcitrant fractures with not one adverse effect reported. Similarly, static magnetic fields have been employed for therapeutic uses for centuries, and no adverse effects have been reported.

The FDA has received a number of reports and complaints through its Medical Device Reporting system concerning electromagnetic field interference with a variety of medical devices, such as pacemakers and defibrillators. In addition, the development of advanced magnetic resonance technology using ultra-high magnetic field systems of more than 3 T, although they were considered safe, led to a reassessment of biomedical implant devices, which were previously judged to be safe to use at 1.5 T; of the 109 implants and devices tested, 4% were considered to have a magnetic field interaction at 3 T and were potentially unsafe to use with fields of this magnitude (Shellock, 2002). Because of potential concerns regarding radiofrequency-induced magnetic fields with thermal effects at the cellular and molecular levels, the FDA has limited switching rates for generation of these gradient fields to a factor of three below the mean threshold of peripheral nerve stimulation (Shellock, 2004). Recently, Weintraub, Khoury, et al (2007) looked at the biological effects of 3-T MRI machines compared with 1.5-T and 0.6-T machines and found that 14% of subjects experienced sensory symptoms (new or altered) with both 3-T and 1.5-T systems.

The study of magnetic fields (static and pulsed) has evolved from a medical curiosity into investigation of significant and specific medical applications.

There are at least five major professional and scientific societies involved in the study of the biological and clinical effects of electromagnetic fields (Markov et al, 2001): (1) the Bioelectromagnetics Society (BEMS), (2) the European Bioelectromagnetics Association (EBEA), (3) the Bioelectrochemical Society (BES), (4) the Society for Physical Regulation in Biology and Medicine (SPRBM), and (5) Engineering in Medicine and Biology (IEMB).

That PEMF and TMS can influence biological functions and serve as a therapeutic intervention is not in dispute. However, judging the efficacy of static magnets for treatment of various clinical conditions remains challenging, particularly because the important dosimetry component has not been documented. The ultimate question is what it will take to convince the scientific community of the merits of static magnetotherapy. Although the debate continues, more attention must be focused on creating strong randomized, placebo-controlled designs and looking for biological markers. This step should help reduce the skepticism of the medical community. A major obstacle to future progress has been the lack of research funding, especially National Institutes of Health (NIH) funding. When Senator Arlen Specter (R-Pennsylvania), a senior member of the Senate Appropriations Subcommittee on Health and Education, which had doubled the NIH budget, asked the leadership of the NIH about funding research on bioenergy, he was told that the NIH "does not believe in bioenergy." Perhaps the U.S. Department of Energy should sponsor research in this field. Its leaders cannot respond that they don't believe in energy. The medical device industry has been willing to support many innovative studies, but if major advancement of knowledge is to occur in the field of magnetotherapy, recent history shows that it will require a combination of support by both government and industry.

LIGHT

The application of light for medicinal purposes (healing) has been understood for thousands of years. The ancient Greeks observed that exposure to sunlight induced strength and health. During the Middle Ages, the disinfectant properties of sunlight were used to combat plague and other illnesses, and in the nineteenth century, cutaneous tuberculosis (scrofula) was treated with ultraviolet light exposure. Currently light therapy is used to treat psoriasis, hyperbilirubinemia, seasonal affective disorder, and vitamin D deficiency.

The Light Cure and Vitamin D

Although vitamin D has been understood only relatively recently, it has been a part of biology for a very long time. A microorganism that is estimated to have lived in the oceans for 750 million years is able to synthesize vitamin D, which possibly makes vitamin D the oldest hormone on the planet.

It was recognized over 150 years ago that people, especially children, who lived and worked in dark urban areas where there was little light were susceptible to bone diseases such as rickets. In Boston in 1889 it was estimated that 80% of infants had rickets. This pattern marked a shift away from a U.S. population that was primarily engaged in agriculture (Thomas Jefferson's idea of an agrarian democracy) during the 1800s and exposed to plenty of light on the farms and in the fields. The lack of light in dank, dark urban environments was compounded by the unavailability of fresh foods and lack of food distribution.

At that time it was noted that an extended visit to the country with clean air, clean water, abundant sunlight, and the benefits of nature would often cure medical disorders. Thus the idea of the nature cure was born (see Chapter 2). One of the many famous beneficiaries of the nature cure in the late 1800s was future president Theodore Roosevelt, who was well known for saying that he was literally "Dee-lighted" with any number of things, including the results of his cure for his lung disease. One of the most common lung diseases in the late 1800s was tuberculosis (TB). Sanitoriums and solariums were created in wilderness areas away from the cities so that TB patients could benefit from the nature cure. Although no antibiotic treatments were available at that time, many patients with TB benefitted from exposure to nature, including sunlight.

As early as 1849, cod liver oil was also used in the treatment of TB, according to the *Brompton Hospital Records,* Volume 38 (Table 11-1). We now know cod liver oil to be one of the few dietary sources of vitamin D. We also now know that vitamin D activates the immune system cells that can fight TB. So the nature cure of sun and fish oil (also known to sailors as the "sun-fish" cure), which delivered increased vitamin D, was the right treatment for the times.

The direct connection between sunlight and bone metabolism was also established in 1919 when Huldschinsky treated rickets with exposure to a mercury arc lamp. In 1921, Hess and Unger observed that sun exposure cured rickets.

In the 1930s medicine began to directly appreciate the connection between sunlight and the metabolic activities we now associate with vitamin D. This was also the decade that saw the actual identification and labeling of the many metabolically active constituents we now call vitamins. Vitamin D was discovered in the early 1920s by Windaus, who was later awarded the Nobel Prize for synthesizing vitamin D in the laboratory by replicating the photoactivation process that occurs in the skin.

In the 1930s the federal government set up an agency to recommend to parents, especially those living in the Northeast, that they send their children outside to play and get some sun exposure.

Fortification of milk with vitamin D also began at that time. Unfortunately, the last 40 years have actually seen a reversal of some of the sensible public health recommendations regarding adequate vitamin D and sun exposure. ∾

Vitamin D and Dermatology: There Goes the Sun

Many physicians and public health organizations, including the biomedically oriented World Health Organization, have been trying to go one better on Moby Dick's Captain Ahab, who "would strike the sun if it insulted" him. For 40 years there has been a concerted campaign to make people avoid sun exposure. Because ultraviolet B (UVB) light from the sun is responsible for the photoactivation of vitamin D in the skin, sun blockers that "protect" the skin also virtually eliminate photoactivation of vitamin D. A sunscreen with a sun protection factor (SPF) of 8 is supposed to absorb 92.5% of UVB light, whereas doubling the SPF to 16 absorbs 99%. This essentially shuts down vitamin D production. (It also demonstrates that SPF formulations above 16 have little marginal utility and calls into question the appropriateness of the ever-increasing SPF numbers found on the pharmacy shelves.) People have become photophobic, and dermatologists have been on a campaign to "strike the sun."

A study in Australia, which has high levels of sunlight and high rates of skin cancer, found 100% of dermatologists to be deficient in vitamin D. In fact, most people should go outside in the sun for reasonable periods of time to get the many benefits of sunlight (Box 11-2). It is always wise to protect the face and head with a hat and sunglasses, because less than 10% of UVB light absorption happens above the neck and the face is the most cosmetically sensitive. It is best to expose the entire body in a bathing suit for 10 to 15 minutes at least three times per week. African Americans require more sun exposure

(Continued)

The Light Cure and Vitamin D—cont'd

because their natural skin pigmentation provides an SPF equivalent of 8 to 15. ∾

Global Dimensions of Deficiency

Essentially little or no active vitamin D is available from regular dietary sources. It is principally found in fish oils, sun-dried mushrooms, and fortified foods like milk and orange juice. However, many countries worldwide forbid the fortification of foods. There is potentially plenty of vitamin D in the food chain, because both phytoplankton and zooplankton exposed to sunlight make vitamin D. Wild-caught salmon, which feeds on natural food sources, for example, has available vitamin D. However, farmed salmon fed food pellets with little nutritional value have only 10% of the vitamin D of wild fish. The "perfect storm" of photophobia, lack of exposure to sunlight, and insufficiency of available dietary vitamin D has led to a national and worldwide epidemic of vitamin D deficiency.

Estimates are that at least 30% and as much as 80% of the U.S. population is vitamin D deficient. In the United States, at latitudes north of Atlanta, the skin does not make (photoconvert) any vitamin D from November through March (i.e., essentially outside of daylight savings time; so although we shift the clock around, it does not salvage vitamin D synthesis). During this season the angle of the sun in the sky is too low to allow UVB light to penetrate the atmosphere, and it is absorbed by the ozone layer. Even in the late spring, summer, and early fall, most vitamin D is made between 10 AM and 3 PM when UVB from the sun penetrates the atmosphere and reaches the earth's surface.

It might be expected that vitamin D deficiency would be a problem limited to northern latitudes.

In Bangor, Maine, among young girls 9 to 11 years old, nearly 50% were deficient at the end of winter and nearly 20% remained deficient at the end of summer. At Boston Children's Hospital, over 50% of adolescent girls and African American and Hispanic boys were found to be vitamin D deficient year round. In another study in Boston 34% of whites, 40% of Hispanics, and 84% of African American adults over age 50 were found to be deficient.

Vitamin D deficiency is also a national problem, however. The U.S. Centers for Disease Control and Prevention completed a national survey at the end of winter and found that nearly 50% of African American women aged 15 to 49 years were deficient. These are women in the critical childbearing years. A growing fetus must receive adequate vitamin D from the mother, especially because breast milk does not provide adequate vitamin D. A study of pregnant women in Boston found that in 40 mother-infant pairs at the time of labor and delivery, over 75% of mothers and 80% of newborns were deficient. This observation was made despite the fact that pregnant women were instructed to take a prenatal vitamin that included 400 IU of vitamin D and to drink two glasses of milk per day.

Further, vitamin D deficiency is a global problem. Even in India, home to 1 billion of the earth's people, where there is plenty of sun, 30% to 50% of children, 50% to 80% of adults, and 90% of physicians are deficient. In South Africa, vitamin D deficiency is also a problem even though Cape Town is situated at 34 degrees latitude.

Although there are many new bilateral and multilateral governmental and private efforts to export Western medical technology and pharmaceuticals to the Third World to combat infectious diseases such as acquired immunodeficiency syndrome (AIDS), there is no comparable effort to acknowledge and address the global dimensions of the vitamin D deficiency epidemic. The U.S. Congress and president just deemed it as a great achievement to give $40 billion in tax dollars to U.S. pharmaceutical companies to send expensive drug treatments for AIDS (a preventable disease) overseas. By contrast, addressing the vitamin D deficiency epidemic could be accomplished with much safer and less expensive nutritional supplements together with sunlight, the only source of energy that is still free. ∾

Light has one identity as electromagnetic waves characterized by wavelength but also exists as tiny energy bundles, or photons. Visible light, called the "visual spectrum," is electromagnetic radiation at wavelengths of 400 to 700 nanometers (nm) appreciated by the human eye. The human eye is sensitive to approximately 90% of the spectrum of electromagnetic radiation that propagates through the atmosphere and reaches the earth's surface. As a sensory organ, the eye evolved to detect that portion of the electromagnetic spectrum that is there to be seen in the terrestrial environment.

One nanometer equals one billionth of a meter. The shorter the wavelength, the higher the energy (from Planck's law, the energy level is the inverse of the wavelength multiplied by the Planck constant) and the greater the ability of light to penetrate tissues. For example, a blue-violet light has a shorter wavelength, and a red light has a longer wavelength. Infrared light is even longer in wavelength (lower energy) and ultraviolet light is even shorter in wavelength (higher energy) than the visible spectrum. This is the reason for the concern of dermatologists that DNA-damaging ultraviolet light with a shorter wavelength and higher, "ionizing" energy is dangerous, and for the notion that using infrared light with a longer wavelength and lower energy for tanning is a

TABLE 11-1

Historic Milestones in Recognition of the Relations Among Sunlight, Vitamin D Activity, and Health

Year	Observation/ Milestone	Vitamin D pioneers
1849	Cod liver oil (vitamin D) treats tuberculosis	Brompton Hospital
1889	Nature cure treats rickets	S. Weir Mitchell et al
1919	Mercury arc lamp (ultraviolet B light) treats rickets	Huldschinsky
1921	Sun exposure cures rickets	Hess and Unger
1920s	Vitamin D discovered	Adolf Windaus
1920s	Vitamin D photosynthesized in laboratory	Adolf Windaus (Nobel Prize, 1928)
1940s	Sunlight protects *against* cancer	Apperly
1970	25-Hydroxyvitamin D_3 isolated	Holick
1971	1,25-Dihydroxyvitamin D_3 isolated	Holick
1979	Vitamin D receptors found	De Luca et al
1980	Vitamin D treats psoriasis	Holick et al
2002	Vitamin D regulates blood pressure	Li et al

BOX 11-2

Get Some Sun: Benefits of Sunlight

- Improves bone health
- Improves mental health
- Improves heart health
- Prevents many common cancers
- Alleviates skin disorders
- Decreases risk of autoimmune disorders
- Decreases risk of multiple sclerosis
- Decreases risk of diabetes

"safer" form of exposure. (See the sidebar "The Light Cure and Vitamin D.")

X-rays, gamma rays, ultraviolet rays, cosmic rays, and others all fall below visible light on the electromagnetic spectrum. Longer wavelengths such as infrared rays, microwaves, television signals, and FM/AM radio waves have different characteristics. Laser beams are a particular kind of amplified light. The atomic models that led to the discovery of lasers were conceptualized and developed in 1917 by Albert Einstein. His discovery became known as "LASER" for *l*ight *a*mplification by *s*timulated *e*mission of *r*adiation. When an atom is in an excited state and an incoming light particle reaches it, it may eject an additional photon instead of absorbing the particle. This theory was a revolutionary concept that proved to be true, and Einstein received the Nobel Prize for explaining the photoelectric effect. By 1960, the first practical ruby red laser was developed by T.H. Maiman, who used crystals and mirrors to produce a monochromatic, nondivergent light beam in which all waves were parallel and in phase. These characteristics were subsequently referred to as "monochromaticity," "collimation," and "coherence," respectively. The original ruby red beam was a visible red light with a wavelength of 694 nm. Since then, various crystals and gases have been used to develop lasers in other regions of the electromagnetic spectrum, including infrared and visible-light lasers (Box 11-3).

Every object has optical properties that determine the effectiveness of light and the interaction of light with that object. For example, the light from mid-infrared and far-infrared lasers, such as carbon dioxide, holmium, and yttrium-aluminum-garnet lasers, is primarily absorbed by water in the tissues. This absorption of the infrared light energy produces heat, which leads to local vaporization that does not spread. The light from near-infrared and visible-light lasers such as neodymium and argon lasers is poorly absorbed by water but is rapidly absorbed by pigments such as hemoglobin and melanin. This optical property makes these lasers effective in the destruction of tissues that are rich in pigment, such as retina, gastric mucosa, and pigmented cutaneous lesions. It is easy to see how these so-called high-powered surgical lasers, using heat and energy, lead to specific tissue changes. Over the past 30 years, numerous animal and laboratory experiments were carried out using these high-energy lasers. These experiments produced results that ultimately led to human testing and approval by the FDA of the use of lasers in humans.

Despite more than 30 years of similar experiments using weak or low-level nonthermal lasers, there is still controversy concerning the effectiveness of low-level laser therapy (LLLT) as a treatment modality because of a lack

BOX 11-3

LASER (Light Amplification by Stimulated Emission of Radiation)

When light is directed onto an object, one (or more) of the following occurs:
1. The light is reflected.
2. The light is transmitted.
3. The light is scattered.
4. The light is absorbed.

of randomized, double-blind, placebo-controlled trials and publication of findings in peer-reviewed journals. Various articles have made claims, but the studies reported by many have flawed methodology, use different time and dosage schedules, and do not have a strict placebo-controlled design. Despite all these shortcomings, several investigations were brought to the attention of the FDA, and in 2002 the FDA approved an application for the use of laser light as a therapeutic device for pain relief.

Cold laser therapy, or LLLT, is based on the idea that monochromatic light energy, which depends on wavelength for its penetration, can alter cellular functions. Because the original European studies on wound healing in animals yielded positive results, the technique was described as "biostimulation." Mester et al (1982), and Lyons (1987) found that light could be stimulatory at low power and could elicit an opposite inhibitory effect at higher power. In addition, the cumulative dosages of the radiation could sometimes be inhibitory. Today a variety of lasers are available, but the two most popular are helium-neon (HeNe) (632 nm) and gallium-aluminum-arsenide (GaAlAs) (830 nm). In practice, these visible and infrared lasers have powers of 30 to 90 mW and deliver from 1 to 9 J/cm² to treatment sites. To date, they have been shown to be safe within this range, but they have also been used at higher doses.

Musculoskeletal tissues appear to have optical properties that respond to light between 500 and 1000 nm. Sufficient specific laser dose and the number of treatments needed are still the subject of controversy. It is hypothesized that light-sensitive organelles, or chromatophores, absorb light (Walsh, 1997) and that ultimately the energy produces a biological reaction. It has been suggested that chromatophores are present on the myelin sheath and in mitochondria, and that it is the monochromatic wavelength properties, rather than the coherency and collimation of laser light, that induce biological changes. It is presumed that the collimation and coherency lead to rapid degradation by scatter. Others have theorized that the primary photoreceptors are the flavins and porphyrins and that the therapeutic benefit of pain reduction produced by a combination of red and near-infrared light is caused by an increase in β-endorphins, blocking depolarization of C-fiber afferents, a reduction in bradykinin levels, and ionic channel stabilization.

Tissue penetration depends on the wavelength. The shorter HeNe laser beam (632 nm) penetrates several millimeters into tissue, whereas the GaAlAs (830 nm) at 30 mW allows photons to penetrate more than an inch (3 cm). Several authors have stated that an infrared laser beam travels about 2 mm into tissue and that this represents one penetration depth with a loss of $1/e$ (37%) of beam intensity (Basford, 1998). However, the shorter visible HeNe red beam is attenuated the same amount in 0.5 to 1 mm (Anderson et al, 1981; Basford, 1995; Kolari, 1985). How does one measure the decay in the amount of energy with distance? At the surface of the skin, the laser delivers

from 1 to 9 J/cm². Karu (1987) has demonstrated that light of 0.01 J/cm² can alter cellular processes. As a result, approximately six penetration depths (3 to 6 mm for HeNe red light and about 24 mm for GaAlAs infrared light) are possible before the strength of the beam stream drops from 9 J/cm² to 0.01 J/cm². Thus, the threshold and specific therapeutic amount needed for stimulation differs for the superficial nerves and tissues and for the deeper structures. There is also a scattering of energy that influences nonneural adjacent tissues (i.e., flexor tendons in the forearm and wrist with stimulation at the level of the carpal tunnel).

It has been stated that tissue penetration and saturation with pulsed frequency settings of 1 to 100 Hz influenced pain and neuralgia, whereas setting of 1000 Hz influenced edema and swelling and 5000 Hz influenced inflammation. Light from a superpulsed laser using a gallium arsenide (GaAs) infrared diode provides the deepest penetration in body tissues. It operates at a wavelength of 904 nm. Superpulsing is defined as the generation of continuous bursts of very-high-power pulses of light energy (10 to 100 Watts) that are of extremely short duration (100 to 200 nanoseconds). This allows GaAs penetration to tissue depths of 3 to 5 cm and deeper. Some versions of GaAs therapeutic lasers actually penetrate to tissue depths of 10 to 14 cm (Kneebone, 2007). There have been many claims and studies regarding LLLT, but the varied quality of trials has led to controversy. Basford (1986, 1995, 1998), a major critic of the deficiencies of many studies, notes that LLLT research has developed along the following three separate lines:

1. Cellular function
2. Animal studies
3. Human trials

Perhaps the strongest and most well-established research has been on changes in cellular functions. There is a strong body of direct evidence indicating that LLLT can significantly alter cellular processes. The following are specific areas of treatment in which benefits have been claimed:

- Stimulation of collagen formation leading to stronger scars (Mester et al, 1985), increased recruitment of fibroblasts and formation of granulation tissue (Mester et al, 1973), increased neovascularization (Mester et al, 1982), and faster wound healing (Lam et al, 1986; Lyons et al, 1987; Rochkind et al, 1987)
- Pain relief and reduced firing frequency of nociceptors (Mezawa et al, 1988)
- Enhanced remodeling and repair of bone (Rochkind et al, 1987; Walsh, 1997)
- Stimulation of endorphin release (Yamada, 1991)
- Modulation of the immune system via prostaglandin synthesis (Kubasova et al, 1984; Mester et al, 1982)

Basic animal and cellular research with red-beam low-level lasers has produced both positive and negative results. Passarella (1989) believes that the optical properties of mitochondria are influenced by HeNe laser irradiation, with new mitochondrial conformations produced that ultimately lead to increased oxygen consumption. Walker (1983) has suggested that HeNe laser light affects serotonin metabolism, and Yu et al (1997) has demonstrated an increased phosphate potential and energy charge with light exposure. Further research continues at the cellular level. Fibroblast, lymphocyte, monocyte, and macrophage cells have been studied, and bacterial cell lines of *Escherichia coli* have served as models for investigation (Karu, 1988). The most popular laser in such cellular research has been the HeNe laser with a wavelength of 632.8 nm. However, some major discrepancies are found in the results reported in the existing literature because of the wide variation in the laser parameters employed, particularly dose and treatment time. Because imprecise dosimetry has clouded the issues, the optimal dose for achieving a biological benefit has yet to be determined.

Despite the problems posed by a lack of standardization, lack of controls, and imprecise dose and treatment schedules for in vivo experimental work, results from cellular research were extrapolated to research on animals. Subsequently, a wide variety of animal models were employed to assess the putative biostimulatory effects of laser irradiation on wound healing. Small, loose-skinned rodents such as mice, rats, and guinea pigs have been used most often, but studies using pig models have led to different results. It has been argued that pigskin represents a more suitable model for extrapolation to humans, because it is similar in character to human skin, which has led to its use in human skin grafts, for example (Basford, 1986; Hunter et al, 1984).

Baxter (1997) provides an excellent review of the animal models used in the wound-healing literature. The details of experimental and irradiation procedures are so numerous and variable, however, that reproduction of results and intertrial comparisons are usually not practical. Research groups reported either acceleration in healing or no effect on the healing process. Two criteria frequently used to assess wound healing were collagen content and tensile strength. Rochkind et al (1989) conducted one of the largest series of controlled animal trials, comparing the recovery of LLLT-treated crushed sciatic nerves with that of nonirradiated nerves in rats. Constant low-intensity laser irradiation (7.6 to 10 J/cm² daily for up to 20 days) demonstrated highly beneficial effects as judged from recordings of compound action potentials. Wound-healing rates in both irradiated and nonirradiated wounds were accelerated, but the amplitude of action potentials in crushed sciatic nerves was raised substantially only in the irradiated groups. The laser treatment also greatly reduced the degeneration of motor neurons, which suggested that these results might be extrapolated for application in human research trials.

The information gained from trials of in vivo animal exposure to laser photobiostimulation indicated that, in certain animal models, wound healing could be achieved.

The reader is cautioned to remain both critical and skeptical, however, because variations existed in methodology, techniques, dosimetry, exposure time, and frequency of treatments.

Despite the aforementioned controversy and limitations, many clinicians were persuaded by the cellular and animal data to attempt human trials. A number of disorders, including neurological, rheumatological, and musculoskeletal conditions, have been treated with LLLT with various claims regarding results. The FDA had previously been a major obstacle because of the absence of randomized, placebo-controlled trials and the varying methodology, varying dosages and techniques, and absence of objective parameters. However, as described earlier, in February 2002 it approved the application for the use of LLLT for pain relief.

Carpal tunnel syndrome is a common clinical disorder, seen in 5% to 10% of the population, and is caused by compression of the median nerve at the wrist. Acroparesthesia (numbness, tingling, and burning) in the first three fingers often arises and may interfere with sleep. When resistant to conservative treatment, the disorder often progresses, with weakness and atrophy. There are nine flexor tendons adjacent to the median nerve, and they often intersect the nerve fascicles in the carpal tunnel. Thus, nerve compression or tendinitis may serve as a cause.

Basford et al (1993), using laser light of only 1 J of energy, found that both sensory and motor distal latencies could be significantly decreased in normal volunteers. Basford et al's study was a double-blind controlled trial using a GaAlAs percutaneous laser. Weintraub (1997), who used a similar laser but at higher energy levels of 9 J and measured compound motor nerve action potential/sensory nerve action potential electrophysiological parameters, reported a nearly 80% success rate in resolving the symptoms of carpal tunnel syndrome with laser therapy. There were no control subjects in the study, but almost 1000 sensory and motor nerve latencies were analyzed before and after each treatment. Particularly interesting was the fact that the distal latency was prolonged in 40% of subjects, yet they remained asymptomatic. This prolonged latency suggests that nonneural tissues were stimulated and could be responsible for symptoms of tendonitis. At the dose used, a significant number of individuals showed immediate prolongation of distal latency (nerve conduction). They remained asymptomatic, however, and by the next visit, the distal latency was back to baseline or improved. A similar observation has also been made by others (Snyder-Mackler et al, 1988). Padua et al (1998) have validated Weintraub's study, and currently three placebo-controlled trials are being conducted with preliminary reports of 70% success (Lasermedics, 1999). In addition, several reports of studies using higher doses of 10 to 12 J of infrared laser light (40 to 50 mW) revealed alterations in conduction in both the median and superficial radial nerves (Baxter et al, 1994; Bork et al, 1988; Walsh et al, 1991).

Naeser et al (1996) and Branco et al (1999) used a combination of two noninvasive, painless treatment modalities—red-beam laser and microampere-level transcutaneous electrical nerve stimulation (TENS)—to stimulate acupuncture points on the hand of patients with carpal tunnel syndrome or wrist pain. Sham treatments were used as a control. A significant reduction in median nerve sensory latencies in the treated hand and a 92% reduction in pain were observed. Postoperative failures also decreased with this protocol. Weintraub (n.d.) used his original laser treatment protocol (9 J/cm^2) and also stimulated various acupressure points as did Naeser et al (1996) and Branco et al (1999) as well as the flexor tendons in the upper wrist. Up to 85% improvement in wrist pain was achieved in patients with carpal tunnel syndrome.

Other superficial nerves also respond to laser biostimulation. Disorders such as meralgia paresthetica, cubital tunnel syndrome, tarsal tunnel syndrome, radial nerve palsy, and traumatic digital neuralgias have responded to this treatment (Weintraub, 1998). Because of the small number of individuals treated, these observations are to be considered anecdotal. However, Weintraub believes that his observations that nonneural structures play an important yet unappreciated role in symptomatic carpal tunnel syndrome, and probably other nerve entrapments, are indeed significant. For example, the distal latency of the median nerve could be longer than 5 milliseconds in patients who have become asymptomatic with laser treatment. Either a threshold exists for the median nerve, or the tendons and blood vessels surrounding the median nerve exert some influence. Franzblau and Werner (1999) raised similar issues in a provocative editorial titled, "What Is Carpal Tunnel Syndrome?"

The efficacy of laser therapy in treating various pain syndromes has been investigated by several groups. Preliminary double-blind studies by Walker (1983) demonstrated improvement in seven out of nine patients with trigeminal neuralgia. Two out of five patients with postherpetic neuralgia showed improvement, and five out of six patients with radiculopathy improved. Baxter et al (1991) also believed that laser therapy was effective for postherpetic neuralgia. Moore et al (1988) investigated the efficacy of GaAlAs laser therapy in the treatment of postherpetic neuralgia in a double-blind, crossover trial involving 20 patients. The result was an apparently significant reduction in pain. Hong et al (1990) validated these results in their study, in which 60% of patients with postherpetic neuralgia felt improvement within 10 minutes. Friedman et al (1994) used an intraoral HeNe laser directed at a specific maxillary alveolar tender point to significantly abort atypical facial pain.

Trigeminal neuralgia was successfully treated with HeNe laser by Walker et al (1986). In the 35 patients studied in this double-blind, placebo-controlled trial, a significant difference was found in visual analogue scale pain ratings between patients receiving active laser treatment and placebo-treated patients.

Using an intraoral HeNe laser directed at a specific maxillary alveolar tender point, Weintraub (1996) was able to abort acute migraine headaches in 85% of cases in a study that included a sham-treatment control condition. These findings support the trigeminovascular theory of migraine with a maxillary (V2) provocative site. The results achieved rival those of pharmacotherapy. Interestingly, Friedman (1998) used cryotherapy (cold water) applied to the same maxillary alveolar tender point to treat atypical facial pain and migraine headache. The treatment produced a striking reduction in discomfort.

Several groups have investigated the efficacy of laser therapy in the treatment of radicular and pseudoradicular pain syndromes. Bieglio and Bisschop (1986) and Mizokami et al (1990) reported positive effects in treating these conditions. Low-power laser therapy has also been used successfully to induce preoperative anesthesia in both veterinary practice and dental surgery (Christensen, 1989). In contrast to the numerous clinical human studies of laser-mediated analgesia, there have been relatively few laboratory studies. Most of the experiments have been completed in China in a variety of animals, including rats, goats, rabbits, sheep, and horses. There are no English abstracts or translations of most of these works. Other studies in animals that were published in English and used tail-flick methodology to assess pain have reported variable findings.

Laser acupuncture using an HeNe diode was reported to be successful in the treatment of experimentally induced arthritis in rats. Vocalization and limb withdrawal in response to noxious stimulation were the parameters measured (Zhu et al, 1990). Although it is clear that problems exist in extrapolating the findings of laboratory work to humans, as noted earlier Naeser et al (1996) and Branco et al (1999) were successful in applying this procedure to treatment of carpal tunnel syndrome. Similarly, Weintraub (1997) saw additional improvement when he combined Naeser's acupressure points with his protocol in treating this syndrome.

One of the major economic burdens in the United States has been caused by the high incidence of soft tissue injuries and low back pain and subsequent work disability l. Numerous studies using HeNe and infra-red (IR) laser diodes (830 nm range) have reported varying results (Basford, 1986, 1995; Gam et al, 1993; Klein et al, 1990), but randomized controlled and blinded studies have been difficult to carry out.

Rheumatologists in the United States have found encouraging results in laser treatment of rheumatoid arthritis (Goldman et al, 1980), and similar results have been reported in the Soviet Union/Russia, Eastern Europe, and Japan. Walker et al (1986) reported success after a 10-week course of treatment with HeNe lasers. Using a GaAlAs 830-nm laser, Asada et al 1989 found 90% improvement in an uncontrolled trial in 170 patients with rheumatoid arthritis. Despite these generally positive results, Bliddal et al (1987) did not see any significant change in symptoms of morning stiffness or joint function in such patients. However, slight improvement was noted in pain scale ratings. Similar positive results for laser therapy have been reported for osteoarthritis and other conditions. Critics have argued, however, that because rheumatoid arthritis is a disease of exacerbation and remission, it is difficult to assess the efficacy of the therapy.

A number of reports document the apparent efficacy of laser therapy in reducing pain associated with sports injuries. These reports initially came from Russia and Eastern Europe, but the results were subsequently confirmed by Morselli et al (1985) and Emmanoulidis et al (1986). It is notable that in the latter study improvement was accompanied by a decrease in thermographic readings.

The use of laser therapy to treat tendinopathies, especially lateral humeral epicondylitis (tennis elbow), has been studied by numerous groups. There has usually been a relatively rapid response to therapy; however, Haker and Lundberg (1990) failed to show any effect of laser acupuncture treatment on tennis elbow.

Chronic neck pain is common and is often associated specifically with a herniated disk, degenerative disk disease, degenerative spine disease, spinal stenosis, or facet joint dysfunction. The small C-nociceptive afferents and the larger myelinated A delta fibers usually innervate these areas. Local chemical dysfunction with release of substance P, phospholipase A, cytokines, nitric oxide, and so on is probably also involved. It is theorized that direct photoreception by cytochromes produces elevated production of adenosine triphosphate and changes in cell membrane permeability. Antiedema affects and antiinflammatory responses have been alleged to occur in response to laser therapy through reduction in bradykinin levels and increase in β-endorphin levels. The depth of penetration as well as the total dose influence the success of the laser treatment at the target tissue level. Thus, combinations of high-output (centiwatt) GaAlAs and GaAs (superpulsing) lasers can achieve penetration of 3 to 5 cm and even deeper (10 to 14 cm). In addition, acupressure point stimulation (2 to 4 J of energy) to the ear, hand, or body should be used.

Low back pain syndrome is the most common cause of disability in the United States, affecting 75% to 85% of Americans at some point in their lifetimes. Common causes include herniated disks, spinal stenosis, spondylosis, facet joint dysfunction, and failed back syndrome secondary to surgery. As with chronic neck pain, the small C-nociceptive afferents and A delta fibers are involved, with localized chemical dysfunction producing altered signal transduction. Use of a high-output GaAlAs infrared laser at 9 J/cm and/or a GaAs superpulsed infrared laser may be effective in treating the deeper tissues. Usually the nerve irritation occurs deep, around 60 mm, secondary to a herniated disk. Acupressure point stimulation should also be used.

Naeser et al (1995) improved blood flow in stroke patients using laser acupuncture treatment and noted improvement in symptoms.

Weintraub has achieved benefit by stimulating naguien acupressure points with an 830-nm laser Naeser (1999), in a review of the highlights of the Second Congress of the World Association for Laser Therapy, reported that Wilden treated inner ear disorders, including vertigo, tinnitus, and hearing loss, with a combination of 630- to 700-nm and 830-nm lasers. The total dose was at least 4000 J. Daily 1-hour laser treatments to both ears were performed for at least 3 weeks. The lasers were applied to the auditory canal and the mastoid and petrosal bones. Wilden said that he used this approach for more than 9 years in 800 patients, and except in very severe cases, most patients reported improvement in hearing.

Application of laser light to the hegu point on the side contralateral to the pain may be effective for treating migraine headaches. Treatment with an intraoral HeNe laser directed along the zone of maxillary alveolar tenderness also achieves success in the range of 78%. Stimulation is repeated three times at intervals of 1 to 1½ minutes.

Meralgia paresthetica is an often disabling symptom that is caused by compression of the lateral anterior femoral cutaneous nerve at the level of the inguinal ligament. The author (Weintraub) has treated 10 patients with this condition by applying laser stimulation from the level of the inguinal ligament to the level of the knee anterolaterally. Significant pain reduction was noted in 8 of the 10 patients by the fourth treatment, but there have been recurrences.

The soles of the feet and various acupressure points were stimulated by laser without providing relief in 10 cases of nondiabetic peripheral neuropathy. However, the use of monochromatic infrared and visible light phototherapy to treat diabetic peripheral neuropathy has been reported to be successful in inducing temporary or permanent relief from pain and inflammation (Leonard et al, 2004).

No detrimental effects are produced by low-output nonthermal lasers, although it is obvious that direct retinal exposure is to be avoided. Pregnancy does not appear to be a contraindication with LLLT, but investigators have been advised to avoid treating pregnant women and individuals with local tumors in the area of treatment. Individuals who are taking photosensitizing drugs such as tetracycline or who have photosensitive skin should probably avoid this treatment. It has also been suggested that the use of phototherapy after steroid injections is contraindicated, because antiinflammatory medicine is well documented to reduce the effectiveness of photobiostimulation (Lopes-Martins et al, 2006).

Medicine is faced with many conditions that respond poorly or marginally to pharmacological therapy. Thus, the appeal of noninvasive therapeutic laser and other phototherapy devices that are both effective and safe is evident, and they are a most welcome addition to the physician's armamentarium. Therapeutic laser treatment has been used successfully in a number of fields and is a popular modality worldwide. Critical analysis of the literature indicates that the majority of studies suffer from methodological flaws such as the absence of controls, variable duration and intensity of laser treatment, and poor quality. Consequently, the majority of observations are to be considered anecdotal until appropriate randomized control trials have been undertaken. In the interim, laser therapy appears to be safe and worthy of further investigation for the management of pain and other medical conditions.

NONINVASIVE BIOPHYSICAL DEVICES FOR DIAGNOSIS AND TREATMENT

Practitioners using biophysical modalities employ a number of noninvasive devices (i.e., devices that do not penetrate the skin) to measure electrical charges and magnetic fields of particular low frequencies. Such devices are also believed to promote healing by interacting with the body.

Biophysical properties of the body have long been observed and utilized in healing. For example, these properties have been known as *qi* (*chi*) in traditional Chinese medicine, *prana* in Ayurvedic medicine, and *vital force* in homeopathy. Acupuncturists, homeopathic doctors, chiropractors, and practitioners of biophysical medicine and magnetic field therapy (including medical doctors) are among the practitioners who use noninvasive devices to detect and influence biophysical properties of the body.

Although conventional medicine recognizes the presence of electrical charges and magnetic forces in the body, certain biophysical properties, also referenced as "subtle energy," have not generally been studied or utilized by Western science and medicine.

Unlike other medical devices regulated by the FDA, many of the noninvasive devices used to detect and influence these biophysical properties fall into a gray area from a regulatory standpoint. In 1976 the FDA set standards for the regulation of acupuncture needles as an experimental device, and the needle was reclassified as a therapeutic device in 1996, based partly on clinical evidence published in a series of articles in the new *Journal of Alternative and Complementary Medicine: Research on Paradigm, Practice and Policy* during 1995. The FDA team working on reclassification specifically requested the founding editor of the journal at that time (the editor of this textbook) to provide lists of references to accelerate the review process. That FDA action occurred before the NIH Consensus Conference on Acupuncture in 1997. However, the FDA did not adopt standards for electroacupuncture devices, a major category of biophysical devices. One of the challenges continues to be the inability of Western science to measure these biophysical properties. As a result, such devices, when cleared by the FDA, are generally approved for use for "investigational" purposes, as in research studies, but not in the diagnosis or treatment of illness.

The following sections discuss four categories of devices: (1) electrical and magnetic devices used in conventional medicine for conventional purposes, (2) conventional devices used in innovative applications, (3) conventional devices used for both innovative and conventional applications, and (4) unconventional devices.

ELECTRICAL AND MAGNETIC DEVICES USED IN CONVENTIONAL MEDICINE

Devices that measure the electrical and magnetic properties of the physical body have been used in conventional medicine for many years. These electrical devices include the electrocardiograph (ECG, EKG), electroencephalograph (EEG), and electromyograph (EMG), used to measure heart, brain, and muscle activity, respectively, for diagnostic purposes. The ECG reads the electrical rhythms of the heart, the EEG records electrical brain waves, and the EMG measures electrical properties of the muscles, which may be correlated to muscle performance. The EMG is often used in physical (rehabilitative) medicine to diagnose conditions that cause pain, weakness, and numbness.

In addition to devices that measure electrical charges, conventional medicine has made increasing use of magnetic resonance imaging (MRI) for diagnostic purposes. MRI measures the magnetic fields of the body to create images for the diagnosis of physical abnormalities. Another magnetic device, the superconducting quantum interference device (SQUID), combines magnetic flux quantization and Josephson tunneling to measure magnetic heart signals complementary to ECG signals.

CONVENTIONAL MEDICAL DEVICES USED IN INNOVATIVE APPLICATIONS

Some of the devices just described have also been used in innovative ways (not as originally intended) for treatment purposes, such as the use of the ECG and EEG in biofeedback to monitor subconscious processes and "feed back" this information to support behavioral change. The ECG is also the basis of the Flexyx Neurotherapy System, an innovative approach to the modulation of central perception and the processing of afferent signals from the physical receptors in the body (pressure, pain, heat, cold).

MRI, used to diagnose a variety of medical abnormalities, is also being used in a number of innovative ways, as in neuroscience to show brain activity during performance of different tasks, such as reading or other language tasks, and during acupuncture. At the NIH, basic science researchers are currently investigating innovative uses of MRI to measure physiological changes, such as those involved in eye movement or brain activity.

CONVENTIONAL DEVICES USED FOR TREATMENT IN BOTH CONVENTIONAL AND BIOPHYSICAL MEDICINE

Some devices that utilize electrical charges and magnetic fields are being used by both conventional and biophysical medical practitioners.

Superconducting quantum interference device In addition to its use in conventional medicine, the SQUID has also been used to measure weak magnetic fields of the brain. In other studies, it has been used to measure large, frequency-pulsing biomagnetic fields that emanate from certain practitioners, such as polarity therapists. This biomagnetic field is thought to trigger biological processes at the cellular and molecular levels, helping the body repair itself.

Transcutaneous electrical nerve stimulation unit. Developed by Dr. C. Norman Shealy, the TENS unit is used by both conventional medical and biophysical practitioners for pain relief. The FDA approved the TENS unit as a device for pain management in the 1970s. The electronic unit sends pulsed currents to electrodes attached to the skin, displacing pain signals from the affected nerves and preventing the pain message from reaching the brain.

TENS has been suggested to stimulate the production of endorphins as one proposed mechanism of action. In 1990, TENS was the subject of a study published in the *New England Journal of Medicine.* Although it was found ineffective in this study, other studies have found TENS helpful for mild to moderate pain. TENS may have better results in relieving skin and connective tissue pain than muscle or bone pain.

Electro-Acuscope. Using a lower amplitude electrical current than the TENS unit, the Electro-Acuscope device reduces pain by stimulating tissue rather than by stimulating the nerves or causing muscle contractions. It is thought to relieve pain by running currents through damaged tissues. Medical doctors, chiropractors, and physical therapists use the Electro-Acuscope for treatment of muscle spasms, migraines, jaw pain, bursitis, arthritis, surgical incisions, sprains and strains, neuralgia, shingles, and bruises. As with the TENS unit, the Electro-Acuscope has been approved by the FDA as a device for pain management.

Diapulse. The Diapulse device emits radio waves that produce short, intense electromagnetic pulses which penetrate the tissue. It is said to improve blood flow, reduce pain, and promote healing. The Diapulse is used in a variety of health care settings, especially in the treatment of postoperative swelling and pain.

UNCONVENTIONAL DEVICES USED IN BIOPHYSICAL MEDICINE

The following devices are some of the more popular devices used in biophysical medicine. The FDA has not set standards for these devices, but some may be registered with the FDA as "biofeedback" devices.

Electroacupuncture Devices

Dermatron. Voll, a German physician, introduced the Dermatron in the 1940s. Voll believed that acupuncture points have electrical conductivity, and he used this device to measure electrical changes in the body. This technique became known as "electroacupuncture according to Voll" (EAV) and is currently termed *electroacupuncture biofeedback.* Used for diagnosis, the Dermatron became the basis for a number of devices manufactured in Germany, France, Russia, Japan, Korea, the United Kingdom, and the United States.

Vega. Another modified electroacupuncture device similar to the Voll device, the Vega works much faster and is also used for diagnosis. Based on the belief that the first sign of abnormality in the body is a change in electrical charge, this device records the change in skin conductivity after the application of a small voltage. Computers have been added to recent models using different names, such as the Computron.

Mora. Franz Morel, MD, a colleague of Voll, developed the Mora, another variation of the Voll device. Morel believed that electromagnetic signals could be described by a complex waveform. The Mora reads "wave" information from the body. Proponents believe that the Mora can relieve headaches, migraines, muscular aches and pains, circulation disorders, and skin disease.

Other devices. Modern variations of Voll's electroacupuncture devices include the Accupath 1000, Biotron, Computron, DiagnoMetre, Eclosion, Elast, Interro, LISTEN System, Omega AcuBase, Omega Vision, Prophyle, and Punctos III.

Devices Using Light and Sound Energy

Cymatic instruments. In addition to the electroacupuncture, biofeedback, and other devices that measure electrical charges described earlier, there are also therapeutic *cymatic* devices, in which a sound transducer replaces the electrodes of the EAV devices. Each organ and tissue in the body emits sound at a particular harmonic frequency. The cymatic device recognizes and records the emitted sound patterns associated with each body part and bathes the affected area with sound to balance the disturbance. These devices are used for diagnosis and treatment.

Sound probe. The sound probe emits a pulsed tone of three alternating frequencies. This device is thought to destroy bacteria, viruses, and fungi that are not in resonance with the body.

Light beam generator. The light beam generator is thought to work by emitting photons of light that help to restore a normal energy state at the cellular level, allowing the body to heal. The light beam generator is believed to promote healing throughout the body and to help correct such problems as depression, insomnia, headaches, and menstrual disorders.

Infratronic QGM. The Infratronic QGM uses electroacoustical technology to direct massagelike waves into the body. This device is employed as an effective pain management tool in China, Japan, Taiwan, Singapore, France, Spain, Mexico, and Argentina. The FDA has approved this device for therapeutic massage in the United States.

Teslar watch. Named after the researcher Nikola Tesla, the Teslar watch was developed to modulate the harmful effects of "electronic" pollution from modern sources, such as computers, cell phones, televisions, hair dryers, and electric blankets. It is believed that these products create magnetic energy that may destabilize the body's electromagnetic field. Although this energy is at extremely low frequencies, which range from 1 to 100 Hz, it is believed to affect humans adversely over time.

Kirlian camera. The Kirlian camera records and measures high-frequency, high-voltage electrons using the *gas visualization discharge* technique, also called the "corona discharge technique." The most experienced researchers in this technique are Russian; Seymon and Valentina Kirlian pioneered this research in the 1970s. Other contributors include Nikola Tesla in the United States, J.J. Narkiewich-Jodko in Russia, and Pratt and Schlemmer in Prague. In 1995, Konstantin Korotkov and his team in St. Petersburg developed a new Kirlian camera using a Crown TV.

Chapter References can be found on the Evolve website at http://evolve.elsevier.com/Micozzi/complementary/

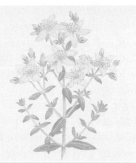

12

THE ARTS IN MEDICINE

RICHARD A. LIPPIN
MARC S. MICOZZI

The capacity for the arts to enhance health has been known since antiquity. We are currently experiencing a resurgence of general interest in this topic based on several megatrends in medicine. For example, on March 31, 2006, the Public Broadcasting System aired a both live and prerecorded broadcast on arts therapy entitled "Circle of Care," produced by SearchLight Productions for WHYY in Philadelphia, which demonstrated these trends. These megatrends include a shift from reductionism to holism and a shift from paternalism to consumerism. Other fundamental factors contributing to the serious study of the relation of the creative and the healing arts are major scientific advances in neuroscience and the concurrent growth of so-called mind-body medicine and the resurgence of interest in the application of physics, including energy concepts, to human health. Passive exposure to the arts, including music, dance, painting, sculpture, poetry, and drama, has proven health-giving properties, and interestingly, passive exposure to live or original arts can be differentiated from exposure to electronic or printed reproductions.

The central theme of this chapter, however, is the relationship of "expressive" or "active" creative arts therapies, in which patients actively engage in one or more of the creative arts, to human health and well-being. This creative process enhances or augments the life force through classic biophysiological responses such as movement, relaxation, and emotional catharsis, as well as through self-discovery and awareness; increased self-esteem, pleasure, hope, and optimism; and the achievement of transcendence, which enhances our spiritual selves. Perhaps most important, the creation of beauty itself is a profound and powerful source of health and well-being.

HISTORY

Contemporary physician Michael Samuels has stated that art, prayer, and healing all come from the same source. Other scholars have said that every child, every adult, and every culture gives form to its feelings and ideas through art. Even before objective language was used in science with conceptual thought, it is believed that early, preliterate humans naturally embodied feelings, attitudes, and thoughts in symbols. Thus, some believe that the metaphorical use of language preceded the literal and scientific use. Many anthropologists who study prehistory have hypothesized that singing and dancing preceded the development of verbal interchange among humans. Eighteenth-century Italian philosopher Giambattista Vico has suggested that humans danced before they walked and that poetry came before prose. This belief was echoed by social theorist Jean-Jacques Rousseau, who believed that musical sounds accompanied or preceded speech as we know it.

The most basic roots of the impact of the arts on health may be traced to the dawn of *Homo sapiens* and humans' unique awareness of themselves. This existential jolt of separateness or aloneness and awareness of mortality has been a driver of artistic expression ever since. The early cave drawings in southern France may have served many purposes for early humans. Through them, for example, humans communicated and thus connected with fellow humans, mastered and taught others about a vast and potentially hostile environment by rendering it in artistic form, recorded their accomplishments and existence, and simply enjoyed the pleasures of beautiful images, rhythmic sound, and elegant movement. All these behaviors represented individual and collective cultural survival mechanisms and were "health giving" in the broadest sense.

The ancient Greeks recognized the connection between healing and the arts by their building of aesculapia, or temples of medicine, constructed in places of natural beauty, where, among other interventions, arts played a prominent role in the healing process. According to Aristotle, Pythagoras began the daily practice of singing and playing as the means by which the soul achieved catharsis. Homer told of his hero Ulysses being treated for hemorrhage with both bandages and incantation. Athaneum reported a cure for sciatica in which flutists were hired to play music in the Pythagorean mode for the affected area. In other non-Western traditions, as early as the Han dynasty, Chinese scholars began to realize that music could affect the human body, not only psychologically but physiologically, and during the Jin (Tsin) dynasty (265 to 420 BC), music was known and used as a means of cultivating a pleasant personality and positive mood.

During the Renaissance, music as one art form pervaded medieval medical practice and theory. Music was prescribed not only for good digestion and for bodily preparation before surgery but also as a stimulus to wound healing, a mood changer, and a critical accompaniment to bloodletting. Specifically composed medical music (the shivaree) graced the wedding chamber to ensure erotic coupling at the astrologically auspicious moment.

In the modern era, although highly creative individuals in the arts and health continue to make individual contributions, the roots of the application of the arts to medical science belong to the professional *creative arts therapy* movement. Stimulated by the growth of modern mental health science after World War II, art therapists, music therapists, dance or movement therapists, poetry therapists, and drama therapists have provided meaningful therapeutic opportunities for people of all ages in a wide variety of settings, but with a particular emphasis on mental health settings.

The creative arts therapists have established a solid professional base through education, training, professional publications (including journals), credentialing mechanisms, and scientific research. There are currently more than 5000 music therapists, 10,000 dance therapists, 3000 art therapists, and several hundred drama and poetry therapists in the United States. The arts therapy movement now includes more than 140 undergraduate and postgraduate degree programs. At least 10 professional associations are in existence for various creative arts therapies, and several professional journals are being published.

The growth of the application of the arts in medicine owes a debt to this creative professional community. It is noteworthy that two hearings were held in 1991 and 1992 under the jurisdiction of the U.S. Senate's Select Committee on Aging dealing with the healing power of music, the visual arts, and dance in the aging population. These hearings led to changes in the Older Americans Act that enhanced insurance coverage for the creative arts therapies and provided increased professional credibility and acceptance of these interventions.

Also, a hospital arts movement continues to grow. This successful movement emphasizes improving the environmental quality of health care institutions through architectural design, interior design, and placement of fine art in strategic health care setting locations and performances in a variety of hospital arts settings, such as lobbies, waiting rooms, patient rooms, and high-tech intervention venues. These individuals and organizations generally do not state that they are engaging in "therapy," but they have a general belief in the salutary effect of aesthetic environments on patients, visitors, family members, staff, and the overall health care institution community. Among the leading organizations in this important new field are the Society for the Arts in Healthcare, the Foundation for Hospital Arts, Art That Heals, Arts as a Healing Force, the British Healthcare Arts Centre, and the Center for Health Design and Aesthetics. Collaboration with the professional architectural and interior design community provides exciting opportunities. Some professionals have begun incorporating not only performance but also specific sounds into the holistic health care environment. For example, Annette Ridenour, president of Aesthetics, Inc., worked with a composer whose music integrates with the architecture, the color, and the intention of the selected space. Patients and staff often participate in the production of such art and performances (Ridenour, 1999). Again, these activities are not categorized as therapeutic per se, but leaders in the field are encouraging at least some outcome measurement studies, which economics may demand.

In recent years there has been a growing interest in the application of the arts to all specialties of medicine, in addition to the previous emphasis on the application of the arts in psychiatry. In part, this trend relates to the recognition of the problems associated with excessive pharmacological and surgical intervention. Calls for the formation of a new medical specialty known as "arts medicine" seek to explore the many synergistic relations among the healing and the creative arts (Lippin, 1985). The arts could be explored for their etiological, diagnostic, educational, therapeutic, and environmental impact on health. Also in recent years, creative arts and expressive arts therapists are expanding their emphasis on applying their work in mental health settings to other medical specialties, most notably pediatrics, gerontology, oncology, cardiology, physical medicine and rehabilitation (physiatry), and thanatology (death and dying). For several reasons, there appears to be differential capacity to apply these interventions to pediatric populations, geriatric populations, and to other "special" populations, as explored later in this chapter.

 Definitions

Arts: For this chapter the definition is limited to music, dance, visual arts, poetry, and drama. (A case can be made that all human activities, such as avocational cooking and gardening or work for pay, can be engaged in artistically when aesthetics becomes an "ontology," or way of being.)

Creativity: Mihaly Csikszentmihalyi (1996) defines creativity as "the ability to produce something that changes the existing patterns and thoughts in a domain."

Creative arts therapy: The National Coalition of Arts Therapies Associations (NCATA) states that creative arts therapies include art therapy, dance and movement therapy, drama therapy, music therapy, psychodrama, and poetry therapy. These therapies use arts modalities and creative processes during intentional intervention in therapeutic, rehabilitative, community, or educational settings to foster health, communication, and expression and promote the integration of physical, emotional, cognitive, and social functioning, enhancing self-awareness and facilitating change.

Arts medicine: The International Arts-Medicine Association states that arts medicine studies the relationship of human health to the arts. Arts and artistic activities are explored for their etiological, diagnostic, educational, therapeutic, and environmental potential.

Expressive therapies: Natalie Rogers, a leader in this field, states that expressive therapies are the use of the expressive arts in a supportive setting to facilitate awareness, growth, and healing. Various art modes interrelate simultaneously in what Rogers (1993) calls the *creative connection.*

Imagery and visualization: Imagery is both a mental process and a wide variety of procedures used in therapy to encourage changes in attitudes, behavior, or physiological reactions. As a mental process, it can be defined as "any thought representing a sensory quality, which might include the visual, oral, tactile, olfactory, proprioceptive and kinesthetic." Whereas *visualization* refers to "seeing something in the mind's eye" only, procedures for *imagery* fall into at least three major categories: evaluation or diagnostic imagery, mental rehearsal, and therapeutic intervention.

Leaders in the creative arts therapies field and others have introduced more recent terms, such as *musicmedicine, medical art therapy,* and *medical dance therapy,* which reflect the increasing use of the creative arts therapies in medical settings other than mental health settings. Of particular note is the pioneering work of Drs. Ralph Spintge and Roland Droh, who founded the International Society for Music in Medicine after studying music's anxiolytic and analgesic properties in thousands of surgical patients in a hospital wired throughout for music in Ludenscheid, Germany (Spingte et al, 1989).

THEORETICAL CONSIDERATIONS AND MECHANISMS OF ACTION

Before the various types, current practices, and research in expressive or creative arts therapies is discussed, consideration of general theory and possible mechanisms of action seems appropriate. Expressive arts therapies are often categorized as "mind-body therapies" or as embracing the "holistic model" of medicine. Fueled by advances in neuroscience, mind-body or holistic medicine recognizes that the entire universe and everything in it, including one's perceptions of it through the human brain, affect human physiology and medical outcomes, ranging from accidents to dysfunction and disease to wellness and peak performance.

One fundamental shift that is gaining credibility is support for a transformation from our current pathology-based health care system to a health care system that embraces a fundamental view of humans as good and empowered to seek and achieve increasingly higher levels of health or wellness. The arts play an essential role in realizing the preceding health care model, because the arts promote the salutary effects of freedom, self-esteem, growth, pleasure, communication, love, a sense of community, and the connectedness to a universal life force.

Another fundamental concept associated with the expressive arts therapies is that humans can deterministically choose to perceive the innate and abundant beauty of themselves and the universe and can incorporate this beauty into their lives through a conscious decision. Therefore, one role of the health professional or healer is to recognize, validate, nurture, support, and facilitate the expression of the innate goodness and beauty of the patient and the universe. In this model, physicians and other health professionals do not direct behavior or provide interventions; instead, they allow or provide permission to enjoy the beauty and bounty of human existence. Thus they do not extinguish negative behaviors so much as they encourage innate positive ones.

Also, humans have an innate ability to counter both individual and collective destructiveness and decay (entropy)—in short, to choose life over death. Engaging in the arts is thus life affirming and life enhancing. Neurosurgeon Michael Salcman (1992) has stated, "at the heart of both the arts and the sciences is a desire to leave the world marginally better than one finds it. Thus the will to create and heal is the moral force and guiding principle of the medical profession."

Another fundamental theoretical consideration is the growing call for the "democratization of the arts." Thus, everyone may engage in the arts without fearing shame, ridicule, derision, or embarrassment and in a safe environment that allows patients to cast off their "inner critic." Such concepts have been described as the emergence of a new paradigm of "medical optimism" (Lippin, 1985, 1991). This paradigm is essentially based on a love of life, self-determination, and responsibility, in contradistinction to our current predominant medical paradigm of pathology and paternalism, which is based on a fear of death, dependency, and victimhood. Once proven and potential biological mechanism of action for arts interventions is muscular movement, which is a central feature of expression in all the arts. Furthermore, engaging in the arts can induce relaxation and pleasure. The arts can also lead to self-knowledge, self-discovery, mood change, and emotional catharsis (e.g., weeping, laughing, sexual activity). Finally, the arts can elicit and augment spiritual and transcendental states and their associated psychological and physiological benefits.

MUSCULOSKELETAL MOVEMENT

Artistic creation involves musculoskeletal movement, which is a reaffirmation and augmentation of life force itself, because movement is central to the living state. To some degree, all expressive arts involve muscular movement. Although the most obvious expression is dance, movement is also involved in music making, singing, painting, sculpting, drama, and even the act of writing. Musculoskeletal movement involved in the creation of art may have special relevance for pediatric and geriatric populations and those categorized as having disorders of movement, regardless of the specific cause.

In addition to the basic musculoskeletal and cardiopulmonary benefits of movement, from a psychiatric perspective, movement "frees up" and allows the discharge of suppressed emotions and trapped energy from psychic and somatic blocks. Such an energy release facilitates new levels of perception that may lead to integration of body, mind, and spirit. Dance therapists have stated that movement is our primary realm of expression on which all other means depend. For example, the movement impulse can be transformed into words, tones, lines, and color. Our inner experience is externalized through movement to some material separate from ourselves.

From a musculoskeletal or exercise perspective, the demands of ballet are said to exceed those of professional football. For example, in dance, the deceleration of the "rigid" body is of the order of 40 g. At the professional level, virtually all forms of art require an extraordinary level of sensorimotor control, precision, speed, endurance, and strength. For example, forearm blood flow changes in pianists increase over basal blood flow rates, and cardiac index increases at the highest stages of piano playing. Increases in heart rate and blood pressure can be achieved, which demonstrate not only that forearm activity is significant in piano playing, but that it is truly a "total body" experience. One of the theories also proposed to explain the noted longevity of orchestral conductors is the amount of musculoskeletal movement or aerobic exercise in which conductors routinely engage as they practice their art.

In singing, so-called classical (opera quality) and "belting" (e.g., Ethel Merman) singing techniques have been analyzed by electromyography to measure both intrinsic and extrinsic muscles associated with the act of singing.

Many studies have demonstrated the antidepressant effect of musculoskeletal movement in exercise. Exercise has been proven to be time efficient and cost effective compared with psychotherapy and drug treatment for depression and is potentially useful as a means of preventing future depressive episodes. Hence exercise, including movement in the arts, may become a primary treatment of choice. Also, exercise is probably safer than a lifelong commitment to pharmacotherapy.

RELAXATION RESPONSE

Herbert Benson's classic description of the relaxation response did not specifically reference the arts. His emphasis was on mental focusing devices and a passive attitude toward distracting thoughts (Benson et al, 1974). However, other authors believe that the arts, either passively experienced or actively pursued, can elicit the relaxation response. Steven Halpern has documented music's impact on the relaxation response through what he calls his "antifrenetic alternative" music, which he contrasts with other forms of New Age music. In Western culture a passive relaxation response can be supplemented with what some have called *active meditation,* in which engaging in the arts produces a timeless experience associated with deep relaxation and neurophysiological changes. Psychiatrist and music therapist John Diamond, for example, refers to the arts as the "royal yoga" or the supreme meditation.

There are three explanations for how music promotes a relaxation response. *Biochemical theory* states that music is the sensory stimulus processed through the sense of hearing. Sound vibrations are transformed into neurological impulses that activate biochemical changes, either through the sympathetic or parasympathetic nervous system. *Entrainment theory* suggests that oscillations produced by music are received by the human energy field, and various physiological systems entrain with or match the hertz or oscillation frequency of the music. *Metaphysical theory* suggests that music is divine in nature and puts us in touch with or augments our spiritual selves, thus inducing a highly relaxed state.

EMOTIONAL CATHARSIS

Among the healing capacities of the arts is its ability to stimulate or augment emotion and the biological and behavioral concomitants of emotions. These range from simple mood alteration to full-blown emotional catharsis. A body of serious psychiatric literature exists on the complex topic of emotional catharsis. In addition, various stress-releasing techniques have been identified, such as the "weep response" (crying), the "mirth response" (laughing), and the "sexual response" (orgasm) (Lippin, 1985).

It is becoming increasingly clear that the arts can both stimulate and augment weeping, laughing, and sexual behaviors. The physiology of all three of these important human behaviors and their benefits are being increasingly studied and validated by the scientific community.

Music, poetry, and photographs can be used to stimulate conscious memories or may subconsciously precipitate sad and wistful mood changes leading to weeping. Laughing can be stimulated through all of the arts, but especially through the joy of dancing, music, theater, clowning, and popular singing (e.g., barbershop quartets).

The capacity for stimulating healthy sexuality through various forms of artistic expression is well known, especially as it relates to the stimulatory effect of visual depictions of sexuality and physical beauty of the human form, as well as the enhanced libido associated with dancing.

SELF-DISCOVERY

Knowledge of oneself has been defined as a cornerstone of health in most cultures. Some authors believe it is the most important goal of any psychotherapeutic intervention. This can be characterized as a lifelong intrapsychic discovery or "self-diagnostic process" for everyone. It is theorized that only through self-knowledge can rational, hence healthy, choices be made.

Carl Rogers, developer of person-centered psychotherapy, incorporated the belief that each individual has worth, dignity, and the capacity for expression and self-direction (Rogers, 1951). Rogers's philosophy is based on a trust in the inherent impulse all human beings have toward growth and his faith in the innate capacity of each person to reach toward his or her full potential. This tenet is a major theoretical foundation for the value of expressive arts therapy as developed by Rogers's daughter, Natalie Rogers. She enhances her father's theory of creativity by using the fundamental person-centered principles as the foundation for expressive arts as a healing process. A critical component to this theory is that individuals or groups must have a safe, accepting, empathetic, and supportive environment to develop this full potential (Rogers, 1993).

Carl Rogers's research revealed that when a person feels accommodated and understood, emotional healing occurs. This basic truth is so simple yet so profound that it is often overlooked or misunderstood. The creative process is easily squashed in a judgmental atmosphere. Creating a nonjudgmental, permissive, stimulating environment for expression of self is essential to emotional healing. Furthermore, Sigmund Freud believed that love and work are central to health ("the purpose of life is to love and to work").

Noted sociologist Jean Houston describes "entelechy," or the discovery and dynamic unfolding of the core of who we are and who we are meant to be, our "essence" (Houston, 1982). It has long been known that the arts can play a key role in the self-discovery process. Engaging in the creative arts can provide a safe, direct path to both the "personal unconscious" and the "universal collective unconscious" as described by Carl Jung. It also provides a path to spiritual discovery. For example, the more one regularly creates, the more one will notice an image often repeated in various ways. This is described as "the true self made visible." Not only specific organs but also physiological processes may have the capacity to stimulate the production of psychic images meaningfully related to the type of physical disturbance and its location. This phenomenon may arise from electrical and chemical messages from the diseased part of the body to the brain, which are interpreted as mental images. We may comprehend that, through wordless communications and in his or her own idiom (the arts), a person can and does convey both somatic and psychological conditions. Somatically, pictures may point to events in the past relevant to anamnesis (recall), early diagnosis, and prognosis. During a former period of creative activity from 1986 to 1995, the National Museum of Health and Medicine in Washington, DC, mounted an exhibition on "headache art" in which headache sufferers depicted their afflictions through visual representations. Psychologically, we may observe what happens deep in the mind (e.g., how drawings can help express hopes, fears, and forebodings through past or ongoing traumas).

Furthermore, drawings can serve as bridges between the health provider and the patient, the family, and the surrounding world. Indeed, their meaning and what it implies could guide the healing professions to assist especially critically ill patients in living as near to his or her essential being as possible, whether in recovery, in the midst of illness, or close to death.

Finally, we may ask how it can be that spontaneous drawings may reflect the total situation of a person (e.g., as dreams may). D'Arcy Hayman (1969) has stated that the expressive arts "give voice to the self," the highest form of individuality. Natalie Rogers, one of the founders of expressive arts therapies, says we express our inner feelings by creating outer forms; "expressive art" refers to using the emotional, intuitive aspects of ourselves in various media. To use the arts expressively means going into our inner realms to discover feelings and to express them through visual art, movement, sound, writing, or drama. In the therapeutic model based on humanistic principles, the term *expressive therapy* has been reserved for nonverbal and metaphorical expressions. *Humanistic* expressive arts therapy differs from the analytical or the medical model of arts therapies, in which the arts are used to diagnose, analyze, and "treat" people. Many have already discovered some aspect of expressive art as being helpful in their daily lives. One may doodle as one speaks on the telephone and find it soothing. One may write or keep a personal journal and find that as one writes, feelings and ideas change, perhaps as one writes down one's dreams and looks for patterns and symbols. One might paint or sculpt as a hobby and realize that the intensity of the experience transports oneself out of everyday problems, or perhaps one sings while in the shower, driving, or going for long walks. These activities exemplify self-expression through movement, sound, writing, and art to alter one's state of being. These are ways to release one's feelings, clear one's mind, raise one's spirits, and bring oneself into higher states of consciousness. This process is indeed therapeutic (Rogers, 1993).

When using the arts for self-healing or therapeutic purposes, the expressive arts therapist is not concerned about the beauty of the visual art, the grammar or the style of writing, or the harmonic flow of the song. The expressive arts therapist uses the arts to encourage the patient to "let go," to express, and to release. We can also gain insight by studying the symbolic and metaphorical messages. Art speaks back to us if we take the time to let in those messages. In regard to music, it may bypass the intellectual defenses and go to the nexus that connects the body, mind, emotion, and spirit. People are often afraid to experience themselves fully because of the possible pain they may discover. Music is a nonverbal form through which we can explore aspects of ourselves on a multisensory level.

The expressive arts thus may lead into the unconscious as they allow us expression of previously unknown facets of ourselves. This brings to light new information and awareness.

CREATIVITY

Because creativity is believed to be increasingly strategic in the business world and is supported by scientific discovery, much has been written recently on the topic. Little is known, however, about the fundamental biology and health impact of creativity. Noted psychologist Abraham Maslow believed that creativity is a fundamental characteristic inherent in humans at birth. Carl Rogers, aforementioned founder of person-centered psychotherapy, stated that from the nature of the inner condition of creativity, it is clear that it cannot be forced but must be permitted to emerge. A limited amount of early childhood research has shown that exposure to and involvement in the arts has a potential trophic or growth influence on the brain and on the body.

In expressive arts therapies, although the expressive product itself may have value and can provide important feedback cybernetically to the individual, it is the process of creation that can be profoundly transformative. Norman Cousins observed cellist Pablo Casals literally transformed from a frail and slow 90-year-old to a vibrant, thoroughly engaged musician while playing the cello, demonstrating extraordinary intellectual and physiological performance. Cousins attributed this to Casals's being thoroughly engaged in his own creativity and his desire to accomplish a specific purpose, not merely in a physical exercise of playing the cello (Cousins, 1979).

Creativity expert Mihaly Csikszentmihalyi references the term *flow* and describes creative individuals as having the personality traits of independence, self-confidence, unconventionality, alertness, ambition, commitment to work, willingness to confront hostility, inquisitiveness, a high degree of self-organization, and the ability to work effectively for long periods without sleep. Their cognitive style, the way they think, rather than their native intelligence, seems to set creative individuals apart from their peers. Intrinsic factors (a passion for pursuing a particular activity for the sake of the activity itself) rather than extrinsic factors (e.g., fame, fortune, status, prizes) seem to motivate creative individuals (Csikszentmihalyi, 1990, 1996).

Some believe that a correlation exists between creativity and mental illness or emotional pain. However, most experts would argue that it is unlikely that mental illness could be routinely advantageous to the creative process, because the concentration required for creative endeavors is likely to be hampered by symptoms of the illness, which would make creative "flow" difficult to achieve. A high rate of psychosis and neurosis among artists and performing artists does not mean that emotional turmoil is the source of creativity. Instead, most people who have serious mental illness, including major mood disorders, show little evidence of creativity.

Neurobiology of the Creative Process

The therapeutic benefits of activities that involve the experience of creativity provide powerful evidence for a biologically adaptive function that may be independent of any specific kinesthetic, visual, or musical art form. University of Tennessee ethologist Neil Greenberg believes that important insights into the nature of creativity can be obtained by looking into its biological causes and consequences. He has drawn on his work into the neuroendocrine aspects of behavior to develop a model of creativity as a highly evolved mechanism for coping with stress. In his view, creativity is part of the ensemble of neurobehavioral mechanisms that enable organisms to respond to real or perceived needs of varying urgency (Greenberg, 1997). In other words, creativity is a key mechanism for coping with possible challenges to the dynamic balance within the organism and between the organism and its environment. The fullest expression of creativity involves contributions from systems that mediate affect, motivation, and cognition and that are orchestrated largely by the neural and endocrine mechanisms of the stress response. The needs that these mechanisms address range from coping with life-threatening emergencies to resolving cognitive dissonance.

The well-studied selective effects of the stress response on different forms of learning and on pathologies associated with creativity (e.g., depression, temporal lobe epilepsy) provide a framework for examining the roles of ancient and recently evolved brain mechanisms in creativity.

Creativity is energized and focused by neural mechanisms linked to hormonal responses that evolved to cope with stress and that are woven throughout the nervous system. Specific patterns of neuroendocrine responses evoked are determined by the duration and intensity of a stressor and apparent prospects for its control. Furthermore, the way the stress response is activated can determine whether creative work will be impaired or enhanced. Specific neural mechanisms involved in creativity thought to be affected by elements of the stress response include heightened reactivity, long-term potentiation, perceptual restructuring, and selective memory.

The study of creativity has been handicapped by its traditional focus on one or another element of the dynamic ensemble of underlying processes. Furthermore, the concept is torn between two points of view: (1) that creativity is expressed only rarely, and then only in gifted individuals, and (2) that it is so ubiquitous as barely to deserve special comment. Drawing on the work of Margaret Boden, and working with Bruce MacLennan, a University of Tennessee computer scientist specializing in neural connectionism, Greenberg is working to bridge the gap and build a framework for understanding when and why creativity is manifest.

Tinnin has written about neurophysiology and the aesthetic response. He puts forth a theory of the aesthetic response to explain why it is so resistant to verbal analysis.

There is a mimetic response to art that is not available for verbal reflection not only because it is automatic and unintended, but also because its nonverbal, cerebral initiative is actively denied by consciousness, which reflexively owns all mental initiative (Tinnin, 1990, 1991, 1992). Human perception of nonverbal communication, including art, is an active, unconscious process in which the receiver creates the perception by active mimicry. The viewer's response to a picture, for example, begins with an active, nonverbal experience that is largely outside of consciousness and involves kinesthetic and visceral mimicry that precedes verbal interpretation. The viewer circumscribes the lines and volumes with movement of the scanning eyes while mimetic movement of other body parts follows the contours of the figure. The listener's response to music is played out with movement by the head, shoulders, and other body parts. Observers of sculpture unknowingly imitate the implied movement of the sculpture. This kinesthetic imitation is automatic and unintended, and it predicts the person's pleasure in the art. Thus, is it the sensation produced by mimetic motor activity combined with an emotional pattern of visceral arousal that constitutes the aesthetic experience? Any inhibition of either kinesthetic or autonomic mimicry determines the pleasure of the response to the artistic stimuli. This resistance is universal and is a necessary consequence of the ego's requisite maintenance of mental unity.

Arieti (1976) defined creativity as the "magic synthesis" of primary process thinking and secondary process thinking into what he called "tertiary process"; thus he built on Freud's topographical model of the mind as consisting of conscious and unconscious portions, each with different systems of logic. In addition to Arieti's magic synthesis, other theorists have put forth proposals to account for creativity in terms of the conscious/unconscious dichotomy, including sexual sublimation, regression in the service of the ego, freedom from neurosis, schizophrenic thinking, and a race against the human awareness of mortality.

PLEASURE AND PLAY

There has been increasing societal awareness in modern Western culture that pleasure is not a sin, although societal values increasingly reward work and not play for most Americans. The role of physicians as "finger waggers," admonishing patients not to succumb to their "basic instincts," is changing. Rather, physicians can trust their patients or even encourage them to engage in responsible pleasures that do not harm others or society. A new role of the physician is to give permission, even encouragement, to enjoy the beauties and bounties of life (including the arts) without guilt. The inclusion of pleasure and creativity into life is part of a prescription for total health.

On an intuitive and anecdotal basis, the capacity for the arts to induce pleasure is well known. Although explanation of the neurophysiology of human pleasure is still in its infancy, this topic is being studied more carefully.

Using research findings in the fields of medicine, biology, and psychology, Robert Ornstein and David Sobel, MDs, in their book *Healthy Pleasures,* have been pioneers in articulating the crucial role of pleasure in health. Dr. Sobel has defined pleasure as having a central role in human evolution in that pleasure can serve as a guide to survival behaviors (Ornstein et al, 1989).

Creativity expert Mihaly Csikszentmihalyi (1990, 1996) notes that eight main elements have been reported repeatedly to describe how it feels when an experience is pleasurable: (1) clear goals exist every step of the way (e.g., a musician knows what note to play next); (2) there is immediate feedback to one's actions (e.g., an artist sees what color he has placed on the canvas); (3) a fine balance and congruence exist between challenge and skills; (4) action and awareness are merged; (5) abstractions are excluded from consciousness, that is, there is total engagement (e.g., a musician becomes the music, a dancer becomes the dance); (6) there is no worry of failure, and self-consciousness disappears; (7) the sense of time becomes distorted (in a positive sense) (e.g., dancers and figure skaters may report that a quick turn seems 10 times as long); and (8) the activity becomes "autotelic," that is, something that becomes an end in itself. Although the arts can provide gains in money and status, most people engaging in the arts do so because of the sheer pleasure.

Related to pleasure is the concept of *play.* Because stress is proven to be linked with ill health, engaging playfully in music, art, dance, poetry, and drama can move a person from puritanical emphasis on "doing something productive" into becoming a receptive being. In this state there is increased activation of the parasympathetic nervous system, which is one of the reasons why play could be so essential to health.

We may seek creative experience because it is pleasurable, but pleasure, like creativity itself, exists not for its own sake but because it serves the needs of organisms to thrive and reproduce. Pleasure is nevertheless an ardently sought emotion. Michel Cabanac (1971) derived the equation *pleasant = useful* from his extensive review of the responses of people to external thermal stimuli when they possess differing internal thermal states. Pleasure, Robert Wright reminds us, is *not* the end purpose of life; contrary to some traditional views, such as that of J.S. Mill, *pleasure is a device for steering the organism in the right direction.* Our seeking of pleasure, Wright believes, is "sponsored by [our] genes, whose primary goal . . . is to make us prolific, not lastingly happy." Pleasure is addictive; "we are designed to feel that the next great goal will bring bliss, and the bliss is designed to evaporate shortly after we get there."

Others emphasize the adaptive function of pleasure in their interpretation of our vulnerability to addiction. Pleasure is an emotional experience, and emotions "are coordinated states, shaped by natural selection, that adjust physiological and behavioral responses to take advantage of opportunities and to cope with threats that have recurred over the course of evolution. . . . Thus, the characteristics and regulation of basic emotions match the requirements of specific situations that have often influenced fitness. Emotions influence motivation, learning and decisions and, therefore, influence behavior and, ultimately, fitness."

OPTIMISM AND HOPE

Hope is currently viewed as a significant determinant of health and health outcomes. Again, however, we are in the early stages of understanding the physiology of these feelings.

In *Learned Optimism* (1990), psychologist Martin Seligman explored the limited research on optimism's impact on the immune system. The relationship of hope and optimism to health is linked also to the concept of meaning in life (Frankl, 1963). Palomore (1995) studied social factors such as work satisfaction and predictors of longevity, and Wong (1989) described the need for personal meaning in successful aging. Engaging in the arts can provide a person with a sense of hope and meaning through actively expression of the self, production of a beautiful product, and the sharing of it with loved ones or the public.

The most important function of the arts from a medical standpoint, however, may be its *revitalization* function, in which the creative process itself reaffirms and augments the desire of humans to choose life over death consciously and deterministically in this critical and tenuous period in the history of human culture and civilization.

SPIRITUALITY AND TRANSCENDENTAL STATES

The arts are playing an increasing role in the spiritual renewal of the Western world. Addressing the National Coalition of Arts Therapies Associations (NCATA) in Washington, DC, in November 1990, renowned psychoanalyst Rollo May described art therapists as "harbingers or sparks of a new world—a new religion based on man's endless search for beauty and the joy of human beings helping other human beings."

The excesses of materialism and alienation, rebellion, and shock seen in modern art (the so-called culture of transgression) may be viewed by some as yielding to a postmodern emphasis and rebirth of arts that connect us to our spiritual selves, with an emphasis on enduring values, including beauty and harmony within ourselves and within the universe. For many, engaging in the arts is fundamentally a spiritual path or transformational process, a way of being, a shift from scientism and materialism to the treatment of the soul. Michael Samuels and colleagues believe that the arts free the body's own internal healing mechanisms, uniting body, mind, and spirit as art is produced; no interpretation or therapy is necessary. The creative process itself is the healer (Samuels, 1991). In music, Reverend Cynthia Snodgrass quotes biblical passages on the need to reclaim our sound traditions. From the Genesis passages of creation to the collapsing walls of Jericho to the healing of King David with the melodies of the harp, we may see revival in those testimonies from the Hebrew scriptures that stand as witness to music's power.

Deep within us, Samuels (1991) believes, we have a memory of the beautiful place where our spirit was given breath by traveling inward, and only through art we can experience this spiritual essence, this loving and healing force. Thus, art is the voice of the spirit and is the energy of healing. The artist and the healer are feeling the rebirth of these ancient traditions. At the source, "they" and "we" are all connected. In the place of birth is a universal land of awesome power and beauty. From it comes painting of stars, of swirls of light, of radiance; from that universal realm comes early movement and the softest sounds: "ohm," "amen," or "mama" (Chapter 32). Closer to the surface we find radiant colors, still abstract, and in the next world we see the birth of archetypal symbols and dream figures; finally, upward we are in "body land" and the so-called material world.

Because art acts at the level of the spirit, energy is involved (Chapter 10). Art therapist Shaun McNiff says that whenever illness is associated with the loss of soul, the arts emerge spontaneously as remedies, or "soul medicine." Creation is interactive, and all the players are instruments of the soul's instinctual process of ministering to the self (McNiff, 1981, 2004). Art historian and psychiatrist Hans Prinzhorn believes that patients' art was a natural antidote to schizophrenic disintegration and alienation. Louise Montello, a music therapist, writes about the loss of self or the loss of one's connection to the "divine child," which she believes is the root of much chronic illness (Montello, 1992, 1994, 2002). "Once the self, however, is awakened through the arts which is some sort of playful and/or prayerful activity, the healing process is awakened from within. Once self is established, then the soul can be consciously cared for," says Montello. The medieval philosopher Thomas Moore, in his famous book *Care of the Soul,* says, "Art is not about the expression of talent or the making of pretty things—it is about the preservation and containment of soul." Art captures the eternal in the everyday, and it is the eternal that seeds the soul. In Montello's description of working with emotionally disturbed ("soul-starved") children, she states that these children hunger for the beauty, love, and goodness that art can provide.

McNiff (1992) notes that art as a medicine is in a postheroic phase in the history of art. Individual heroics are replaced by the individuation of expression within a group that supports each member's natural and spontaneous emanations. Connection exists between our life force, our inner core or soul, and the essence of all things. Therefore, as we journey inward to discover our essence or wholeness, we discover our relatedness to the outer world. The shamanic community of the creator is in our genes, waiting to be released. This collective involvement is yet another shamanic element that survives to manifest itself in every aspect of the current application of art as medicine. Painters influence and stimulate one another with their images, as do musicians improvising with related sounds. Participants become what the romantic poets call "agencies of the flying sparks." Soul moves about through charges and countercharges.

In this world, pathology and health are not limited to patients; they are in all of us. Tribal societies knew how to make use of those who were possessed by emotional upheavals. In contemporary Western society, we do not. By trying to fix them, improve them, eliminate them, drug them, and/or cure them, we are demonstrating that we have not grasped how they can help us. McNiff says that the best medicine one can offer to a troubled person is a sense of purpose, the feeling that what he or she is going through may contribute to the vitality of the community and that the process is reciprocal (McNiff, 1981, 1992, 2004). During the biblical age of prophets, harp players would perform special pieces of music to produce a mental state in which extrasensory powers were thought to be activated, and the Bible says of Elisha, "And it came to pass when the minstrel played that the hand of the Lord came upon him." David played for King Saul to help him recover from depression and paranoia. In this spiritual renaissance, especially among so-called evangelicals, the arts are playing an increasing role in religious services throughout the world. Thus, making a joyful noise unto the Lord becomes increasingly manifest in such phrases as "God respects you when you work. He loves you when you sing." Many believe the basic purpose of the creative or expressive arts therapies is to access the deepest centers of the spirit and bring back the abducted soul from the excesses of a modern, excessively materialistic, and increasingly uncivil society.

CURRENT PRACTICE AND GOALS

The goals of *dance and movement therapy* are numerous and vary according to the population served. For emotionally disturbed persons, the goals are to uncover and express feelings, gain insight, and develop therapeutic bonds and attachments. For physically disabled patients, the goals are to increase movement and self-mastery and esteem, have fun, and heighten creativity. For the elderly population, the goals are to maintain a healthy body, enhance vitality, develop relationships, and express fear and grief. For mentally retarded persons, the goals are to motivate learning, increase bodily awareness, and develop social skills. An underlying goal in dance and movement therapy is for visible movement to affect total biopsychosocial potential and function, promoting healing by altering mood, reawakening stored feelings and memories, organizing thoughts and actions, reducing isolation, and establishing rapport. Total body movement stimulates the functions of body systems such as circulation, respiration, and skeletal and neuromuscular activity, including the use of muscles and joints to reduce body tension and body armoring. Other known clinical effects are the reduction of chronic pain, depression, and suicidal ideation.

Music therapy goals include physical and emotional stimulation for those in chronic pain and those with impaired movement. The neurological mechanisms by which music decreases pain awareness were discussed earlier. Music can evoke a wide range of emotional responses and has both sedative and stimulant qualities. Music is also a unique form of communication. Music can be used with patients who are nonverbal or who have difficulty communicating, such as in autism, in which music can facilitate social interaction. Music has been used effectively in the treatment of eating disorders. Music can be used by the individual to express a wide range of emotions, from anger and frustration to affection and tenderness. Selecting music from an individual's past may evoke memories of times, places, events, and persons. Such memories can contribute additional information to the individual's treatment.

Art therapy can be used effectively as a therapy and especially as a diagnostic tool. Patients may focus on parts of their bodies that unconsciously concern them, a concern that they have been unable to verbalize. Patients may draw images about their disease processes and explore all the medical and psychological manifestations of their disorder.

Poetry therapy uses poetry for the purposes of healing and personal growth. The participant's own creative writings are viewed as avenues toward self-discovery. Poems used as a method of life review and reminiscence have been particularly effective in assisting elderly persons. In a "life review" the person writes his or her own autobiography using photo albums, letters, memoirs, and interviewing techniques to gather and integrate the person's life experiences into a meaningful whole. Telling one's own "story" through poems, songs, and journals produces vital narrative material for the therapeutic process. The special goals of poetry therapy are to increase the patient's spontaneity and capacity for playing with words and ideas; to strengthen communication, particularly listening, speaking, and writing skills; and to help the patient experience the life-giving and nourishing qualities of beautiful writing. Poems serve as catalysts to evoke feelings within and can help in focusing on the other person's reaction to the words. Poetry enables individuals to express experiences they may be unable to relate in any other way, which may be the first step in speaking about shameful and taboo subjects. The most powerful poetic device is symbolic representation through *metaphor*. When patients externalize feelings into poetry, the product is a tangible, literally black-and-white, testament to feelings and thoughts previously without literal form. The externalization gives participants a feeling of mastery and allows them to view their own feelings from a different perspective. Patients often are comforted by a poem, which they can literally carry on their persons as they do with biblical and other quotes. Poetry may have layers of meaning with an ability to conceal and reveal, thus providing both psychological closeness and distance when necessary. Reading poetry aloud with others, as with prayer, can build cohesion, boost ego, and enable individuals and groups to respond to the rhythm and beauty of the poem together.

Practices that use the techniques of imagery include biofeedback, systematic desensitization, counterconditioning, echosynthesis, neurolinguistic programming, Gestalt therapy, rational-emotive therapy, meditation, relaxation techniques, and hypnosis. Procedures for imagery fall into at least three major categories: (1) evaluation or diagnostic imagery, (2) mental rehearsal, and (3) therapeutic interventions. Techniques used in evaluation or *diagnostic imagery* involve asking the patient to describe his or her condition in sensory terms. *Mental rehearsal* is an imagery technique used before medical treatments, usually in an attempt to relieve anxiety, pain, and side effects that are exacerbated by a heightened emotional reaction. Surgery or a difficult treatment is rehearsed before the event so that the patient is prepared and is rid of any unrealistic fantasies.

Imagery as a *therapeutic intervention* is based on the concept that images have either a direct or an indirect effect on human physiology and health outcomes. Patients are taught how to use their own flow of images about the healing process, or they are guided through a series of images that are intended to soothe or distract them to reduce sympathetic nervous system arousal or generally enhance relaxation.

Whether imagery is merely an antidote to feelings of helplessness or whether the image itself has the capacity to induce the desired physiological effect is still unclear. Existing research suggests that both conclusions are justified, depending on the particular situation being studied. Among the research accomplishments in imagery, there is a great emphasis on immunology. Findings include correlations between the action or levels of various types of leukocytes and components of cancer patients' images of their disease, treatment, and immune system, as follows:

- Enhanced natural killer cell function after a relaxation and imagery training procedure in geriatric patients and in adult cancer patients with metastatic disease.
- Altered neutrophil adherence or margination and white blood cell count after an imagery procedure.
- Increased secretion of immunoglobulin A (IgA) after training in location, activity, and morphology of IgA and 6 weeks of daily imaging.

The specificity of imagery training was suggested in patients engaging in cell-specific imagery of either T lymphocytes or neutrophils.

MEDICAL ART THERAPY

A special issue of *Art Therapy* on the topic of art and medicine (1993) noted the term *medical art therapy* and stated that distinct differences exist between art therapy conducted in the psychiatric milieu and art therapy conducted in a medical setting because of the environmental realities and goals of each. Also, the physical conditions of patients determine how often therapy can be presented and used. Healing is defined not only by improved laboratory values, x-ray films, or the eradication of a tumor. Healing is the process of "being made whole," physically, psychologically, and spiritually. Healing can take place even as the body weakens and dies. Thus it is said that, although the body may not be cured, it may be healed.

The greatest impact of engaging in the art of expressive therapies could be their potential to synthesize and integrate patient issues such as pain, loss, and death. The art therapies assist patients through art making and the creative process. *Medical art therapy* is defined as the use of art, expression, and imagery with individuals who are physically ill, experiencing trauma to the body, or undergoing aggressive medical treatment such as surgery or chemotherapy. In some cases, such as when the patient is fragile and susceptible to infection, the therapist must be cognizant of maintaining a sterile environment through the appropriate use of art therapy media and tools. At other times the patient may be unable to participate actively without physical adjustments, such as arranging for the therapist to be at the bedside or developing special devices to assist the patient in the creative act. Other art therapists have discussed necessary adaptations in art experiences for patients with dementia and for pediatric patients who have experienced serious burns. Art therapy with pediatric cancer patients may be offered in the hospital waiting room, where children await chemotherapy and radiation treatments or checkups. Family, including siblings, may be present and may become part of the art therapy. However, confidentiality is not easily maintained in this type of open environment, where patients come and go at will and where art therapy essentially takes place in a quasi-public arena, such as a waiting area or at a bedside.

RESEARCH

Advances in neuroscience, psychoneuroimmunology, and psychoneurocardiology have provided the tools necessary to engage in solid scientific research on creative and expressive arts therapies (see Chapter 8). In particular, the impact of music on human physiology has been well studied and demonstrates great promise. For example, music's capacity as an analgesic or anxiolytic agent is well documented, as is its impact on mood. Use of music in burn patients, terminally ill patients, and those with cerebral palsy, stroke, and Parkinson disease has been studied. The impact of music on the immune system has also been studied, including the impact on patients with acquired immunodeficiency syndrome (AIDS) and other immune disorders.

Bittman et al (2001), for example, demonstrated significant modulation of neuroendocrine-immune parameters in normal subjects through group drumming, a form of music therapy. Furthermore, music has been studied extensively among elderly patients as a means to improve quality-of-life measures. Mickey Hart, one of two drummers with the former San Francisco Bay Area band the Grateful Dead, has advocated this type of work. Other studies have demonstrated the effect of music on physiological measures such as galvanic skin response, vasoconstriction, muscle tension, respiratory rate, heart rate variability, pulse rate, and blood pressure. Music has been used to relieve anxiety and depression in coronary care units and to promote recovery from heart attacks. It has also been shown that listening to different types of music can lower levels of the stress hormones cortisol, adrenaline, and noradrenaline, and natriuretic peptide, a potent antihypertensive hormone produced by the atria of the heart.

Neurophysiology researchers have postulated that music affects brain function in at least two ways: (1) it acts as a nonverbal medium that can move through the auditory cortex directly to the limbic system (an important part of the emotional response system), and (2) it may stimulate the release of endorphins, thereby allowing these polypeptides to act on specific brain receptors. This two-step mechanism is supported by direct recording of neuronal discharge rates while listening to music. Because music can alter mood and emotional states, however, it is also likely that the immune and hormonal changes seen after subjects listen to music are mediated by the autonomic nervous system. The Institute of HeartMath previously investigated the effects of music on autonomic activity with power spectral density analysis of heart rate variability and of immunity, measuring levels of secretory IgA from saliva samples. This work demonstrated a relationship between increased autonomic activity and increased salivary IgA levels.

The term *designer music* was introduced by the music industry to describe a new genre of music designed to affect the listener in specific ways. This term has also been used in the scientific literature to specify this type of music. Research and clinical studies have shown that so-called designer music produces a significant effect on listeners' physiological and psychological status. As mentioned earlier, after U.S. Senate hearings in 1991 on the impact of music on elderly persons, the Older Americans Act Amendments of 1992 listed music therapy as both a supportive and preventive medical service. Furthermore, among the initial grants of the National Institutes of Health (NIH) Office of Alternative Medicine (now the National Center for Complementary and Alternative Medicine) was one to investigate the effects of specific music therapy interactions on empirical measurements in persons with brain injuries.

In the visual or "plastic" art therapy field, research has been done on the use of art therapy with psychiatric and burn patients as well as with patients with eating disorders, chemical addictions, deafness, aphasia, and autism. It has also been studied as a prognosticator in children with cancer, in childhood bereavement cases, and in sexually abused adolescents. The visual arts, because they produce a permanent visual record, lend themselves to high-quality research in art as a diagnostic tool.

Dance therapy research has demonstrated clinical efficacy in ameliorating depression, decreasing bodily tension, facilitating expression of anger, reducing chronic pain, and enhancing circulatory, respiratory, and musculoskeletal function.

Although music and the other arts have been used successfully as treatment modalities for mood and other psychiatric disorders and medical conditions, uncertainty remains as to how such effects are mediated in the brain. There is speculation that benefits are achieved through music's ability to modify directly the neuronal substrates (neurological loci) of affective states, which then have widespread effects on the autonomic, hormonal, and immunological mechanisms of the body. Studies could be undertaken to quantify specific components of dance, including exercise; social contact and bonding; spontaneous versus instructional dance; male-female versus male-male or female-female dancing versus group dancing; touch versus no-touch dancing; and dancing with and without music. Manfred Clynes postulated "essentic (sic) forms," which he describes as "biologically given expressive dynamic forms for a specific emotion" and theorizes that the neurobiological process of recognition of pure emotion essentic forms may release specific substances in the brain, which then act to transmit and activate those specific emotional experiences (Clynes, 1982). The "iso principle," first described in 1948, seeks to match the patient's musical mood in music therapy, which helps the patient gain insight into internal thoughts and memories. These concepts require further research.

Entrainment, as noted earlier, is an aspect of sound that is closely related to rhythm and the way these rhythms affect humans. Powerful rhythmic vibrations of one object will cause the less powerful vibrations of another object to "lock in step" and oscillate at the same frequency. The music potential ("rider") is based on the fact that the hypothalamus has strong connections to the limbic system. Thus the connection between music and health is likely to have a mechanism involving a "neural" hypothalamic–frontal limbic loop and a neuroendocrine hypothalamic-immunological loop.

New research is beginning to explain the physiology of hope and positive expectations. In one series of studies, patients entering the hospital for open heart surgery or surgical repair of a detached retina were evaluated before and after surgery. Those who expressed greater optimism regarding surgical results, confidence in the ability to cope with the surgical outcome, and trust in their surgeon recovered more quickly. Among patients undergoing heart surgery, death rates were lower. Hopeful expectations may also predict who will develop cancer of the cervix. The more optimistic the woman, the less likely she is to have cervical cancer.

A study of patients with advanced breast and skin cancer revealed that a joyful attitude and optimistic style were the strongest psychological predictors of how long patients would remain cancer free before the disease returned. *Webster's Dictionary* defines optimism as "an inclination to anticipate the best possible outcome; a tendency to seek out, remember and expect a pleasurable experience." Optimists have a high level of internal "locus of control" and feel challenged, not threatened, by the current environment and the future. Also related to optimism is the capacity for love. Siegel (1987) noted that if he taught AIDS patients to love themselves and others fully, there was an automatic increase in the levels of immune globulins and killer T cells.

In the aesthetic paradigm, which governs use of the arts, the fundamental goal of the artist is to communicate, share, or even love, unlike in the athletic or militaristic paradigm, in which the fundamental purpose of the athlete or soldier is to compete or kill.

Pennebaker and Francis (1992) of Southern Methodist University in Dallas found that individuals who wrote about upsetting personal events displayed significant changes in psychometric surveys.

 Research issues in creative or expressive arts therapies

1. What is the impact of aesthetic stimuli, including color, form, sound, rhythm, movement, words, and beauty itself, on human physiology?
2. Specifically, how does the human brain perceive, process, integrate, and react to aesthetic stimuli?
3. What is the neurophysiological nature of creativity and its relationship to human health?
4. What are the biopsychosocial characteristics of living and performing and of visual artists as related to a more complete understanding of the limits of human capacities?
5. How can the study of highly successful elderly artists and performers contribute to understanding the role of the arts in the aging process?
6. How can the arts be effectively used to enhance early brain development and early childhood education?
7. How can the arts contribute to the development of individual and cultural self-esteem, in that self-esteem is increasingly viewed as central to the development of mental health and cultural well-being?

Research issues in creative or expressive arts therapies—cont'd

8. How can the arts be used to improve diagnostic and prognostic capabilities in medicine?
9. Which already developed models are most promising for the successful integration of the arts to improve the environmental quality of health care settings?
10. What specific steps must be taken to ensure inclusion of arts medicine topics in formal art or medical curricula?

SPECIAL POPULATIONS

Although the expressive arts therapies can be used with most patients in most medical settings, these therapies are of special value to the following subgroups:

- *Pediatric patients.* Children are more freely expressive and in the early years are less verbal than other medical populations. Children also can engage in creative play more easily.
- *Geriatric patients.* The geriatric population is especially vulnerable to the excesses of pharmacological and surgical interventions. The arts can serve as an alternative or supplement. Also, musculoskeletal movement associated with expressive arts in older persons can be a fundamental therapeutic goal. Disorders of the central nervous system, especially those associated with memory loss (e.g., Alzheimer disease) seem to be differentially benefited by creative or expressive arts therapies. Verghese et al (2003), for example, specifically identified dance as the only primary physical activity to confer some protection against cognitive decline.
- *AIDS patients.* Since the AIDS epidemic became manifest in the early 1980s, the expressive arts have played a key role in assisting patients, their loved ones, and their families in dealing with this devastating disease. Much art has been produced by and for patients with AIDS, partly because of the effect of this syndrome on the artistic workforce sector. The famous AIDS quilt project is an example of this phenomenon.
- *Health professionals.* Health professionals have always been subject to physical and psychological stresses inherent in their profession. Increased incidences of serious forms of psychopathology, sociopathy, and burnout are seen in these populations. Also, disabled or ill health professionals can cause significant harm to patients in their charge. In recent years massive changes in the

enterprise of health care have led to additional transition and career stresses for health professionals. On the positive side, some studies have demonstrated that physicians, in particular, possess differential creative skills. Therefore, health professionals are encouraged to engage in the arts, especially as a stress reduction technique or for stress prevention. Also, when physicians engage in the arts, they share and demonstrate their common humanity with their patients. Contemporary physician-poet John Graham-Pole (1997) stated, "Such self-revealing [writing poetry] opens my vulnerability to others, helps me lick my wounds without leaving a scar, washes me clean, releases my tensions, redresses my balance, captures painful and delicious sense, validates me as a sentient human being."

- *Patients with chronic diseases and chronic pain.* Engaging in the arts provides hope, pleasure, and beauty and enhances the quality of life for individuals coping with chronic disease and chronic pain syndromes.
- *Dying patients.* Faced with the realization of their mortality, dying patients often seek to resolve lifelong psychosocial issues and, importantly, spiritual issues. This can be greatly facilitated and enhanced through artistic expression. Dying patients often express lifelong conflicts and desires through artistic expression. Also, the creation of artistic products allows the dying patient to leave something of value to loved ones, friends, and society. Self-generated art adds beauty, joy, and meaning to the last days of the dying patient's life. Also, dying patients often are depressed and may be in pain, and the arts can assist with these conditions as well.

SUMMARY

As the excesses of the predominant scientific and theoretical paradigm in medicine yield to the new and emerging paradigm, the application of the arts will play an increasing role in *health* in the broadest sense of the term. We are entering into an era in the twenty-first century when art is viewed as a major positive force able to unlock each person's potential for goodness and individual growth, as reflected in a healthier society composed of revitalized, healthier people.

The arts will continue to make a major cost-effective contribution to individual, institutional, and societal health. Researchers, educators, and practitioners, as well as the payers and regulators of these endeavors, will increasingly appreciate the role that the arts can play in producing healthy individuals, healthy families, healthy communities, healthy schools, healthy workplaces, and a healthy planet.

Spiritual Aesthetics—Its Role in the New Twenty-First-Century Medicine

The classical definition of *aesthetics* is "that branch of philosophy dealing with the nature of beauty, art, and taste and with the creation and appreciation of beauty." Spiritual aesthetics can be defined as incorporating the aforementioned definition of aesthetics but would add that spiritual aesthetics is that branch of aesthetics which deals with the transcendent nature of aesthetics and its capacity to provide insight into and a relationship with a universal, loving, divine presence.

Love of the beauty of nature as well as humankind's creations is inclusive. Natural beauty includes the human body in all its manifested shapes and sizes, as well as flowers, birds, and fishes. And love of the great creations of humans, notably words, especially poetry—but also music, the visual arts, song, and dance. We also find beauty in medicine as an art and science and in healing. The true healer neither knows nor seeks boundaries between art and medicine. For this reason, one may view art and medicine as one.

Not only can art and medicine be seen as one, but also as forms of prayer, as a spiritual expression. We are coming to realize how powerful the arts can be as a special path to healing. Engaging in the arts can be such a healing experience because of the arts' capacity to help us realize the divine and the divine within each of us.

Many great thinkers have written eloquently on this topic including Carl Jung, Rollo May, and more recently John Diamond, Shawn McNiff, and Thomas Moore. Michael Samuels says it well and simply: "Art, prayer and healing all come from the same source—the human soul. The energy that fuels these processes is the basic force of life, the force of creativity, of love."

We will perhaps come to see how the new medicine of the twenty-first century must incorporate spiritual aesthetics as possibly its last best hope. As is noted in the Book of Ecclesiastes, "God has made everything beautiful in its time." May the practice of medicine and the art of healing manifest the divine artist within each of you. ❧

—Richard Lippin

Acknowledgments

We wish to acknowledge the following individuals and organizations for their help in the preparation of this chapter: Natalie Rogers, author of *The Creative Connection;* Neil Greenberg, University of Tennessee; Susan Kleinman, chair of NCATA; Alicia Seeger, administrator of the National Association for Poetry Therapy; Eric Miller of Expressive Therapies Concepts; and the creative arts therapy community, on whose shoulders the modern arts-medicine movement stands; our physician colleagues within the arts-medicine movement, including John Graham-Pole, John Diamond, Michael Samuels, Patch Adams, Michael Salcman, Eric Avery, Joel Elkes, Yoshihito Tokuda, and Itzhak Siev-Ner; also, David Hinkamp of the American College of Occupational and Environmental Medicine, Section on Arts-Medicine, and Naj Wikoff of the C. Everett Koop Institute at Dartmouth University; and from the hospital arts movement, Janice Palmer and John Feight.

⊖ Chapter References can be found on the Evolve website at http://evolve.elsevier.com/Micozzi/complementary/

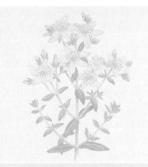

CHAPTER

13

CREATIVE AND EXPRESSIVE THERAPIES

SHERRY W. GOODILL
PAUL NOLAN

INTRODUCTION AND THEORETICAL PREMISES

This chapter describes the creative arts therapies—specifically art, dance/movement, drama/psychodrama, music, and poetry therapies—as separate arts-based integrative medicine health care disciplines. The term *creative arts therapy* refers to an arts-based therapy performed by a creative arts therapist who is credentialed under the auspices of the national organization representing that treatment modality. A creative arts therapist demonstrates aesthetic competencies in his or her respective arts modality and has received education and training in that art form prior to entering into study and clinical training in one of the creative arts therapies.

The chapter covers professional, theoretical, clinical, and research areas, providing brief descriptions and discussing commonalities among the creative arts therapies. Similarities and differences between the creative arts therapies, expressive therapies, and the arts in the health care network are developed; however, the chapter primarily is about the creative arts therapies.

To place the creative arts therapies in the context of complementary and alternative medicine (CAM), one must look back to the early 1990s, when the National Institutes of Health established the Office of Alternative Medicine (OAM; now the National Center for Complementary and Alternative Medicine, or NCCAM). The creative arts therapies were listed under the mind-body intervention category, just as they appear in the mind-body section of this text, and the inaugural round of field investigations funded by the OAM included two creative arts therapy studies (see Goodill, 2005a). Today, the NCCAM references the creative arts therapies in the following statement:

> Some techniques that were considered CAM in the past have now become mainstream (for example, patient support groups and cognitive-behavioral therapy). Other mind-body techniques are still considered CAM, including meditation . . . prayer, mental healing, and therapies that use creative outlets such as art, music, or dance. (NCCAM, n.d.)

These therapies focus on the intrapersonal and interpersonal processes of arts expression and reception within a therapeutic relationship with a creative arts therapist. The actual art product, such as a drawing, song, or dance, although representing a client creation and a statement about the person at a given point in time, is not typically the goal in the creative arts therapies. Searle and Streng (2001) describe the use of the arts product, or artifact, in therapy to "illustrate particular feelings or dynamics, to aid verbal integration, and as tools of assessment" (p. 5). The use of an art product, such as a drawing, a musical theme or song, or a personally symbolized movement, adds a new and unique dimension to psychotherapeutic applications as a "third party" or as a bridge that connects the client's inner and outer worlds. Searle and Streng refer to this as a triangular relationship, in that the art product adds a third point in a client–therapist–art product triangle. This third element in therapy provides for variations in the dynamics of the therapeutic relationship, in which both participants may be active within what Winnicott conceptualized as the "potential space," or that psychic area in which subjectivity and objectivity interact.

HEALING OR TREATMENT

The creative arts therapies continually deal with the relations among "healing" and "treatment" in that they attempt to "retain the healing properties of the Creative Arts while developing a science of Arts Therapies" (Zwerling, 1984, p. 16). Zwerling disagreed that the healing function of the arts defines the creative arts therapies; he also addressed the dangers in obliterating the potential healing impact of the arts modality. In addressing their healing and treatment roles, he believed that the arts therapies needed to address the issue, "How will we use the arts modalities in an organized, systematic, deliberate way to bring about change in somebody who needs change?" (p. 32).

Thus, the healing properties of the creative art therapies, in that their use "attracts that which is well, or healthy, in clients" according to the author (Nolan), may represent their short-term, or therapeutic effect. This effect can be described as a change, usually for a short period of time, of a mental, affective, and/or physical state in the client. These changes seem to be related to the effect of the arts experience itself on the client, in the sense of the *arts as therapy* approach used by many expressive therapists, whereas the use of the arts within a therapeutic relationship to address persistent problems in living in the social, occupational, and self-esteem domains describes the arts psychotherapy model used by most creative arts therapists.

Although the arts have been described as having "healing power," the way that the arts are used within a therapeutic relationship "is a crucial factor that determines whether or not therapeutic transformation can occur" (Karkou & Sanderson, 2006, p. 53). Although one may experience a short-term, healing effect from the arts on a regular basis, within the creative arts therapies the role of the therapeutic relationship is integral to the longer-term healing transformation, as in a psychotherapeutic effect.

CREATIVE ARTS, EXPRESSIVE THERAPIES, ARTS IN HEALTH CARE

Many titles and terms are used in relation to the arts within the health care arena. These include *arts therapies, expressive arts therapies, therapeutic arts, creative arts therapy* (or *in* therapy), *expressive therapies,* and *arts psychotherapy,* to name a few. Until the mid-1990s many of these terms were used interchangeably by expressive and creative arts therapists. Over time the differences began to become reflected in the literature, and the separateness between these two approaches became more apparent. This difference was manifested by a more consistent distinction in the use of the two titles "creative arts therapist" and "expressive therapist/expressive arts therapist." However, the term *expressive therapy* occasionally appears in the psychotherapy literature without a connection to any of the arts. Unfortunately, Internet sites such as Wikipedia undo any attempts at clarity by jumbling up these terms into an interchangeable and incorrect mess.

The creative arts therapies are distinguished from expressive therapies and arts in health care, two other established approaches that invoke the therapeutic uses of the arts. Various professionals and authors use these three terms interchangeably. However, the differences in their purposes and the ways in which they are used are important to understand. The creative arts therapies are perhaps the most clinical in that their history demonstrates that they are most often used in the observation and treatment of medically related diseases and disorders. Although they are not limited to this realm of treatment, it is safe to say that most creative arts therapies are used with individuals who have a clinical or developmental diagnosis or an ongoing somatic or psychological concern. Education and training in the creative arts therapies is centered on the use and integration of the arts within a systematic, clinically focused therapeutic relationship. *Expressive arts therapies* practitioners may draw on many different arts forms (multimodal) and rely primarily on transformation through the arts. *Creative arts therapies* practitioners use only the art form in which the therapists have in-depth artistic skills and understanding. This art proficiency is integrated with education in a specific creative arts therapy modality and supervised training leading to arts psychotherapy practice. Some creative arts therapists extend this mental health–oriented education and training into specific medical, rehabilitative, educational, or community practice.

Creative arts therapists incorporate art products into the therapeutic relationship, but they rely more on the client's inner process of creativity and art making in relation to the client's developmental level and clinical need. The addition of the arts in health care movement, a large umbrella concept that includes all of the aforementioned titles and terms in addition to the use of artists in any field who provide services in health care settings, has added to the number of titles and training differences, as well as raising issues of scope of practice, treatment functions, and boundaries in the multiple uses of the arts in health care settings.

AMBIGUITIES IN HEALTH CARE ARTS PRACTICE

Including the arts in health care has proved attractive to various health care professionals, including physicians, nurses, and occupational therapists, among others, who refer to their own use of music, art, or dance/movement as "therapy." For example, the nursing literature, in particular, contains published reports of many studies in which recorded music was played to achieve a temporary therapeutic effect. This practice is referred to as *music therapy,* although it falls outside of the established definition and ethical practice of music therapy and is used by a noncredentialed person. Although these types of uses of an art form may have positive effects and the research reports are helpful, the good intentions of the practitioner may result in a negative effect as well. Every person not only has a highly personal, subjective response to the arts but also develops mental associations that can trigger powerful emotional responses to the arts. A health care worker untrained in the psychological effects of the arts may rely on his or her own preferences or personal beliefs in presenting arts experiences to health care consumers. It is not unusual for a well-intentioned health care worker to present an arts experience to an unattended seriously ill patient only to have the result be a more anxious or, worse yet, confused and disoriented patient. Patients in medical settings who have anxiety-producing medical problems are sometimes unable to defend against the unexpected emotionally overwhelming experience induced by arts stimuli, especially if the patient is left alone during the arts experience (Nolan, 2006). The use of the arts stimulus by a credentialed creative arts therapist allows for modulation and modification of the arts depending on treatment goals and patient response.

COMMONALITIES AMONG THE CREATIVE ARTS THERAPIES

Nolan, in a 1989 unpublished manuscript, identified the following as some of the commonalities within the different creative arts therapies:

- They all have ancient roots and have been a part of health care since antiquity.
- They all use aesthetically guided arts experiences within a clinically structured therapeutic relationship to invoke a wide range of physical, psychological, and spiritual responses in the client.
- They all rely on nonverbal and verbal processes.
- They all use imagery, associations, metaphor, symbolization, and affective and body processes.
- They all use the arts to stimulate unconscious processes.
- They all use, promote, and nurture creative processes.
- They all follow clinical guidelines, codes of ethics, and educational requirements of a governing body.
- They all work as primary or adjunctive therapies.

Creativity is the basis of all of the *creative arts therapies,* and it is assumed that this human endowment is available as a potential and an actualized tendency, in greater or lesser degree, in all humans. A general assumption of these therapies is that the activation of a client's potential for creativity enhances adaptation, provides motivation, encourages self-actualization, and improves quality of life. Creativity is both a means for conducting therapy and a client goal. Creative art therapists may recognize spontaneous patient/client creative processes and behaviors or employ arts-based techniques to activate creative thinking in patients/clients.

It is important to note that clinical work in the arts therapies is far from strictly nonverbal. Poetry, drama therapy, and psychodrama rely heavily on spoken or written language; music therapy's techniques of song writing engage the poet within for creation of lyrics; dance/movement therapists and art therapists engage their clients in the exchange of words and observations during the movement or art making, and also afterward. Initially, the nondiscursive use of spoken or written language is actually key to the integration of felt, sensory, *unlanguaged* arts experiences. Consequent discussion with the therapy group or with the therapist helps a patient generalize discoveries made in the creative process to everyday life and the treatment concerns that brought him or her to therapy in the first place.

EDUCATION, CREDENTIALING, AND PROFESSIONAL ISSUES

Each creative arts therapy specialty has organized professionally with its own educational standards, credentials, codes of ethics and standards of practice, research, and scholarship. All provide continuing education to members and interested others through national and regional conferences and, increasingly, through online formats. The following sections summarize the state of the various fields from an organizational standpoint. Specific information about training and credentials is provided to assist the reader who seeks clinical services, consultation, or collaboration with a creative arts therapist. Although the information provided here covers the predominant groups in the United States, all six of the identified creative arts therapies are international in scope, with lively collegial and interdisciplinary networking.

AMERICAN DANCE THERAPY ASSOCIATION

The American Dance Therapy Association (ADTA) is the primary national organization for dance/movement therapy. The entry-level degree for dance/movement therapy, also known as dance therapy, is the master's degree. Established in 1966, the ADTA confers professional credentials in a two-tiered system: the R-DMT (Registered Dance/Movement Therapist) for clinicians with new master's degrees, and the BC-DMT (Board Certified Dance/Movement Therapist) for advanced clinicians, supervisors, and instructors of dance/movement therapy. The Dance/Movement therapy Certification Board upholds the standards for these clinical credentials. The ADTA upholds educational standards in masters programs through its regulatory Committee on Approval. The *American Journal of Dance Therapy,* a peer-reviewed journal, has been in regular publication since 1977 (ADTA, n.d.).

AMERICAN ART THERAPY ASSOCIATION

The American Art Therapy Association (AATA) was established in 1969. As with dance/movement therapy, the master's degree is required for entry into the field of art therapy. At career entry, art therapists are credentialed with the designation ATR (Art Therapist Registered), and the Art Therapy Certification Board conducts examination-based certification to confer the designation ATR-BC (Art Therapist Registered—Board Certified) on advanced practitioners. Educational programs are regulated by AATA's Education Program Approval Board, and *Art Therapy: Journal of the American Art Therapy Association* publishes peer-reviewed articles (AATA, n.d.).

AMERICAN MUSIC THERAPY ASSOCIATION

The American Music Therapy Association (AMTA) is now the predominant professional organization for music therapy. The field of music therapy was organized in the United States with the founding of the National Association of Music Therapy in 1950 and the American Association of Music Therapy in 1971. The merger of these in 1998 formed AMTA, which publishes two peer-reviewed journals, the research-oriented *Journal of Music Therapy* and the practice-oriented *Music Therapy Perspectives.*

Music therapists can obtain practice credentials with a bachelor's degree and can sit for the certification examination given by the Certification Board for Music Therapists. Board-certified music therapists are so designated with the MT-BC (Music Therapist—Board Certified) credential (AMTA, n.d.). A graduate degree in music therapy provides for more advanced levels of practice. Doctorate

degrees that are field specific are just beginning to develop.

Currently, creative arts therapists are licensed in many states under various mental health titles including Licensed Professional Counselor, Licensed Mental Health Counselor and Licensed Creative Arts Therapist.

NATIONAL ASSOCIATION FOR POETRY THERAPY

The National Association for Poetry Therapy (NAPT), incorporated in 1981, defines poetry therapy as "the interactive use of literature and/or writing to promote growth and healing" and uses the umbrella term *poetry therapy* to encompass related modalities, including applied poetry facilitation, journal therapy, bibliotherapy, biblio/poetry therapy, and poetry/journal therapy (NAPT, n.d.). Preparation of poetry therapists is regulated by the National Federation for Biblio/Poetry Therapy and is not degree based, but emphasizes specific didactic and supervisory plans of study with practical training. There are separate requirements and credentials for those with a bachelor's degree (the Certified Applied Poetry Facilitator, or CAPF) and those with a mental health master's degree (the Certified Poetry Therapist, or CPT). Requirements include knowledge of psychology, group dynamics, and literature, among other topics. The NAPT also publishes the *Journal of Poetry Therapy: The Interdisciplinary Journal of Practice, Theory, Research and Education.*

NATIONAL ASSOCIATION FOR DRAMA THERAPY

Although drama therapy and psychodrama are often combined in the literature and sometimes in practice, they are distinct disciplines. Each has unique training standards and credentialing bodies, and is organized by a different professional association. Drama therapy has been defined as the "intentional and systematic use of drama/theater processes to achieve psychological growth and change" (Emunah, 1994, p. 3).

The National Association for Drama Therapy (NADT) incorporated in 1979 and has since maintained standards of professional competence in this discipline. Drama therapy training requires a master's or doctoral degree, either in drama therapy or in another related area. A handful of drama therapy graduate degree programs exist, but drama therapists also train through institute and individual plans of study regulated by the NADT (NADT, n.d.). Drama therapy literature is found in various publications, including the journals *Dramatherapy* and *The Arts in Psychotherapy.*

AMERICAN SOCIETY OF GROUP PSYCHOTHERAPY AND PSYCHODRAMA

The American Society of Group Psychotherapy and Psychodrama (ASGPP) is the main professional organization for those who practice psychodrama in the United States.

Psychodrama has its roots in the seminal work of J.L. Moreno and encompasses the use of the therapeutic structures of psychodrama (in which the scene is developed around the needs of an individual) and sociodrama (in which the focus is on the needs and understanding of the group). Training (chiefly institute based) is regulated by the American Board of Examiners in Psychodrama, Sociometry and Group Psychotherapy, with a master's degree required along with specific didactic and practical education in psychodrama. Certification in psychodrama is two tiered with the designations Certified Practitioner (CP) for beginning clinicians and Trainer, Educator, Practitioner (TEP) for advanced practitioners. The peer-reviewed *Journal of Group Psychotherapy, Psychodrama and Sociometry* is one venue for literature in this specialty.

NATIONAL COALITION OF CREATIVE ARTS THERAPIES ASSOCIATIONS

The National Coalition of Creative Arts Therapies Associations (NCCATA) has joined the aforementioned six creative arts therapy specialties together for the primary purpose of educating the public and governmental entities about the creative arts therapies. In terms of scholarship, the journal *Arts in Psychotherapy* publishes research, theory and clinical practice pieces in all of these disciplines. Although many creative arts therapists have doctoral-level preparation, doctoral education is not regulated in these professions. A handful of doctoral programs do exist, and because these programs generate scholarship and research, they are critical to the viability of these professions. NCCATA, founded in 1979, is an alliance of the creative arts therapy professional associations and is dedicated to the advancement of the arts as therapeutic modalities. NCCATA represents over 15,000 individual members of six creative arts therapies associations nationwide. The creative arts therapy members include music therapy, art therapy, dance/movement therapy, drama therapy, poetry therapy, and psychodrama (NCCATA, n.d.).

CLINICAL AND RESEARCH LITERATURE

We now take the reader on a quick tour of the clinical and research literature in the creative arts therapies. This review is by no means exhaustive, but simply illustrative of the range of relatively recent work. The four categories used here are something of a contrivance, because patterns of comorbidity among physical and psychological disorders are many, and distinctions between domains of functioning, treatment settings, and diagnoses are influenced by culture, public policy, institutional structures, and local and regional systems. Nonetheless, we have selected four areas of recent concern in the society: trauma, behavioral and psychosocial problems in children and teens, mental illness, and creative arts therapy

applications in medical illness. Patients' names, when used in vignettes, are pseudonyms.

TRAUMA

Johnson (2009) reports that creative arts therapies have been applied to the treatment of acute trauma, specifically in accessing memories of the trauma or the abuse, treating chronic posttraumatic stress disorder (PTSD), and performing cross-cultural interventions with survivors of war, torture, and disasters. Significant reduction of PTSD symptoms and reduced frequency of nightmares were reported by Morgan and Johnson (1995). Art therapy was found to be the most effective for veterans with PTSD symptoms in a single-session design in which art therapy was 1 of 15 treatment components in an inpatient PTSD program. Art therapy produced significant short-term symptom reduction and lowered distress, possibly related to the focus of attention onto interpersonal or external stimuli, which allowed traumatic material to be processed differently than through verbal means (Johnson et al, 1997). Art therapy has also been used to treat individuals who have experienced mass trauma. One example is the work of Gonzalez-Dolginko. (2002), which had a community focus, after the attack on the World Trade Center in New York City.

Music therapy approaches to trauma include music therapist Austin's vocal holding (Austin, 2001, 2002) and vocal psychotherapy (Austin, 2007b) for adult survivors of sexual and physical assault and abuse, and trauma by neglect. Austin (2007a) also describes an approach used with adolescents who were victims of childhood trauma such as physical, sexual, or emotional abuse, which for many continued in the foster homes. As a result, these adolescents have great difficulty trusting others and forming attachments. They often suffer from intense feelings of anxiety, rage, and depression. Unconsciously they may blame themselves for the situation in which they find themselves. Listening to music, singing, writing songs, and playing improvised music proved effective in facilitating self-expression and nonviolent communication and in creating a safe and playful environment in which relationships could grow and community could flourish.

Amir (2004) used music therapy improvisational methods with adult survivors of childhood sexual abuse. She described a case involving 2 years of therapy with a 32-year-old woman who had difficulty in making and keeping relationships as an adult. Music therapy improvisation was used to develop a supportive therapeutic relationship in which the client was able to re-create memories and gain mastery over the abuse within the musical improvisations.

Loewy and Frisch Hara (2002) edited a book describing a 9-week program that combined music psychotherapy and trauma training used in New York City after the terrorist attacks of September 11, 2001. The book presented several music therapy approaches by various authors that were used to help individuals coping with the events and aftermath of a traumatic experience. Reports of working with a self-selected group of adult caregivers seeking support in dealing with their experiences of the traumatic events of 9/11 stressed the roles of music and music therapy in encouraging self-care.

Lang and McInerney (2002) described a different experience in trauma therapy, working in a postwar environment at the Pavarotti Music Center in Bosnia-Herzegovina. They found that many of their clients "did not have the words to say what was clearly expressed through the non verbal medium of music" (p. 172). The clients were able to reexperience the feelings associated with the traumatic events of war that they had witnessed. The music making served as a support for their feelings, which led to an acknowledgement and acceptance. The therapists observed that, over time, their clients were able gradually to retake control over some aspects of their lives.

Mills and Daniluk (2002) conducted a phenomenological investigation of the experience of five women, all of whom were sexually abused as girls and had been treated using dance/movement therapy for issues related to that early abuse. The researchers were interested in the women's own perceptions of how dance/movement therapy may have played a role in their psychological healing. The six themes that emerged from analysis of in-depth interviews about the therapy were that women felt a sense of *struggle* in the therapy (vulnerability, challenge, discomfort, and efforts to keep from being overwhelmed) yet also reported a sense of *spontaneity, freedom,* and *permission to play;* a sense of *intimate connection* with others; and a *reconnection to their own bodies* as a result of the dance/movement therapy experience. A direct quote captures one participant's appreciation of the mind-body integrative aspect of this modality: "Dance therapy was one of the first experiences of discovering how much was stored in my body.... I discovered that there were whole aspects of my body and my experiences that I hadn't gone into.... it was a powerful way of getting connected to myself" (p. 80).

Gray (2001) presented a case study of dance/movement therapy with an adult survivor of political torture. The story of the therapy, 19 individual sessions given over 6 months, is an impressive narrative of healing and courage. The patient, Rita, began with symptoms of PTSD and in the context of the psychotherapeutic relationship explored her emotional pain, sense of helplessness and disconnection, body-level trauma, depression, and shame. Using images arising from the bodily felt experience, symbolization in posture and gesture, integration of verbal and nonverbal expression, and "titration" of the intensity and pace of the work (p. 35), the therapist guided Rita's recall of the traumatic events, the rebuilding of a capacity to trust, and the rekindling of a will to live. With this, many of the crippling symptoms of PTSD subsided.

Harris (2007) reported two group case studies of dance/movement therapy with children traumatized by war. In the first, he developed culturally sensitive dance groups for teens who had been among the Lost Boys of Sudan and had resettled in the United States. In the second, dance/movement therapy was the primary method used in psychosocial rehabilitation of adolescent boys who had been conscripted as child soldiers in the civil war in Sierra Leone. In both groups, Harris demonstrated through detailed and vivid descriptions of therapeutic methods and patient responses how the integrated focus of dance/movement therapy on embodiment, creativity, and group process brought about healing and recovery for these young people.

Johnson's seminal work in drama therapy for survivors of trauma has focused largely on the needs and treatment of combat veterans. The increasing incidence of PTSD among men and women returning from combat zones has become a growing challenge to the public health care system in the United States. The clinical discoveries made by Johnson and his colleagues constitute an effective way to address the complex ways that trauma interferes with functioning (James et al, 1997). The intensity of the war experience is brought home in the intensity of residual memories—feelings that are difficult to access, much less express verbally. The drama therapy creates a theater in which the stark reality can be visited from a psychologically safer distance in role playing, character, and symbols. It is key, the authors emphasize, that drama therapists working with this population "preserve the playspace, that is, the sense that the group exists within an imaginary, pretend environment in which feelings can be played out" (James et al, 1997, p. 385). In this space, in which reality is suspended briefly, the feelings emerge and are examined as patients move through what the authors term "developmental transformations." There are three necessary and sequential phases to this treatment: the acknowledgment and expression of anger, the working through of shame, and finally the cultivation of an empathic stance toward others. Working through the anger and shame phases may involve actions and interactions that recall unspeakable events, and the therapist must be prepared to work with the passion and the imagery that the veterans carry in to the treatment sessions. As one group entered into the empathic phase, the image of a cauldron formed, and into it the men threw "hate, anger, fear, shame, guilt, sadness and regret" (p. 392). They chanted and stirred the pot until the imaginary substance from the pot splatted out like clay, and the concomitant emotion was labeled "shame." Under the improvisatory guidance of the therapist, the clay was formed into a person, dubbed "Being," who spoke through the voices of the men in the group, confessing to the atrocities of war. As Being was joined in exclaiming, "We have killed! We have all killed! You are not alone!" (p. 393), the men joined each other in weeping and holding. At that point, without the veil of the role or the imaginal, the therapist could support the group members in open interaction focused on sharing one another's pain and burdens. Following this they discussed the process verbally, wrote in their journals, and made the first steps toward translating the gains made through symbols and imagery into their behavioral repertoires and everyday relationships. This example, given here in condensed form, shows vividly how the drama-related methods bring the internal experience out and into a social context where is it accessible to group therapeutic and healing processes.

After the horrific massacre at Columbine High School in Colorado, poetry therapist Catherine O'Neill Thorn and several colleagues worked with surviving students at Columbine. The outpouring of emotion, shaped by the teens' resilient and inherent aesthetic sense in the context of a psychologically safe group writing environment, yielded a collection of heart-wrenching yet beautiful poetry, *Screams Aren't Enough* (O'Neill Thorn, 1999, "Art from Ashes"). More importantly, the teens involved show through their poetry how their process of healing evolved from pure shock to anger and confusion to a search for faith in the face of pain in the world. This collection of poetry by four of the young women in their project attests to the healing power of expressive writing and the poetry form. One excerpt, from a poem by Jocelyn Heckler, age 16, brings this to life (p. 24):

> As I lay my head down
> I feel the brisk coolness of crisp sheets
> Surround my body
> And, as I feel the heat from my body
> Flowing to make my bed of equal warmth
> I remember that I am alive. . . . And in the deepest void
> of darkness
> I take refuge in the melodious song
> Of my pen scratching paper
> As it creates a masterpiece of words
> And I remember
> that I am alive.

MENTAL HEALTH AND EDUCATION IN CHILDREN AND ADOLESCENTS

A study by Harvey (1989) with a repeated measures design investigated the use of art therapy, music therapy, and dance/movement therapy in a classroom-based program intended to provide affective education. Specific goals were to enhance self-concept, creative thinking, intrinsic motivation, and reading comprehension in a sample of second- and fourth-graders (n = 58). Creative arts therapists trained in each of the three disciplines worked together in 30-minute sessions held twice weekly for 12 weeks. Standardized measures were used to assess each target area of child functioning, and statistically significant increases in reading comprehension ($P = .000$), verbal originality ($P = .014$), and figural creative originality ($P = .023$) were seen after intervention. Additional analysis led the researcher to conclude that "interventions designed specifically to address persona/social affective conflict produce positive gains in creative thinking and school achievement" (p. 98) and that "young students can

become aware of their creative abilities and can begin to relate their perceptions of mastery, challenge and cognitive competency to these creative abilities following the use of creative arts therapies" (p. 98).

Hervey and Kornblum (2006) published a mixed-method program evaluation of Kornblum's dance/movement therapy curriculum "Disarming the Playground: Violence Prevention through Movement and Pro-social Skills" (2002). The program served 56 children in three second-grade classrooms, 33% to 50% of whom had special needs or were identified as at risk. Children received weekly group sessions of 45 minutes for either one half, three quarters, or a full school year, depending on the classroom. Mean scores on the Behavior Rating Index for Children, an assessment scale completed by the classroom teachers, showed significant decreases in problematic behaviors over the year that the program was given ($P = .002$). The children themselves described their gains from the program in terms of the prosocial skills that they continued to use independently, at home and in school. These included the skills of ignoring, making "I" statements, slowing and calming oneself, moving away or leaving a tense or provocative situation, and using the "Four Bs," a simple sequence for interrupting escalating energy and reorienting (Hervey et al, p. 125). It is notable that these outcomes are the result of a body-centered intervention using creative movement and dance therapy methods.

In their evaluation of a mixed-method violence prevention program, Koshland and Wittaker (2004) reported on a 12-week dance/movement therapy intervention used with a sample of 54 children. At the end of the dance/movement therapy program, statistically significant decreases were seen in the incidence of several problem behaviors among children participating in the program: instigating fights ($P = .041$), failing to calm down ($P = .029$), being short tempered and quick to anger ($P = .017$), throwing articles ($P = .041$), becoming upset when something desired could not be done immediately ($P = .029$), and acting aggravated or abusive when frustrated ($P = .048$). The number of aggressive incidents that were reported to the principal's office decreased significantly more in the group undergoing the dance/movement therapy program than among children in the same school who did not participate in the program ($P < .001$).

The role theory that informs drama therapy has been articulated by Landy et al (2003) as follows:

> Role is a set of archetypal qualities representing one aspect of a person, an aspect that relates to others and when taken together, provides a meaningful and coherent view of self. . . . A human personality, in turn, is essentially an amalgamation of the roles a person takes on and plays out. According to role theory human beings are motivated to seek balance among their often discrepant roles. Implicit here is the notion that humans have access to an internal system of roles and that they may call upon those roles as they are needed. (p. 152)

As in any mainstream, alternative, or complementary therapy, good practice begins with assessment. Landy's use of his Role Profile Assessment with a 13-year-old girl called Dakota shows how this unique drama therapy assessment can bring out important and previously unacknowledged concerns. In this method the client sorts a stack of 70 cards, each labeled with a role, into four stacks: "I am this," "I am not this," "I am not sure if I am this," and "I want to be this." Dakota's work in completing the assessment caused family issues to surface. A child of divorce, Dakota struggled with the role cards for Orphan and Daughter, exploring how she was indeed a biological daughter, but felt like an orphan in relation to a mother with whom she could neither identify nor share. Working with the Sister card, she revealed a wish for someone who could experience what she did and who could understand her (Landy et al, 2003). It is well known among therapists that it is sometimes difficult to engage adolescents in the therapy process. As illustrated here, this brief drama therapy assessment can indicate clear directions for therapy in a nonthreatening manner and engage teens in exchanges about real issues in their lives.

Music therapy approaches with children with autism and a wide variety of developmental disorders were pioneered in the United States by Nordoff and Robbins (1971). Their approach and results led to the establishment of training centers on four continents. Their music-based approach was founded on the premise that all children, regardless of handicap, are musically sensitive and possess musical capabilities, which in turn can be used to promote communication and a wide range of other developmental improvements. Their work is focused largely on enhancing humanness and improving communication, and relies on clinical case studies.

Another poetry therapy program involving adolescent girls in residential mental health treatment focused on the goals of "uncovering and processing interpersonal conflict, exploring resistance to therapy, and deepening positive support among group members" (Gillespie, 2005, p. 222). Group sessions began with an affirmation of confidentiality by the group and a report by each girl on her current feeling state and any immediate concerns. "Warm-ups" focused on collaboration, with creation of a group story in which each member moved the story line forward by adding a line or two to what had come before. The story built improvisationally, and afterward the therapist helped the group discuss the story and the group or personal issues that might have arisen from the story. From collaborative story creation the group moved to collaborative poem writing, beginning with first lines provided by the therapist and elaborated by the group members as they passed the poems around and contributed line by line. In this way, the group created several poems together, then read them aloud and explored personal meanings. The therapist facilitated the linking of these responses to individual treatment objectives, helping the patients draw analogies to their lives outside the poetry sessions.

MENTAL HEALTH

Mental health populations are the group most served by all creative arts therapy disciplines in the United States. This is linked with their inception as health care disciplines beginning in the post–World War II era.

Art therapy has developed a wide range of clinical approaches in the treatment of mental disorders over the last four decades. In most applications art therapy is informed by psychodynamic orientations. Other orientations being developed more fully are cognitive-behavioral and humanistic perspectives. The art psychotherapy approach has been in use since the publication in 1966 of Naumburg's book on the topic, which further developed the concept that artwork contains both manifest and latent content. Judith Rubin (1987), Cathy Malchiodi (1990), and Helen Landgarten (1981) are some of the developers of current art therapy practice in mental health.

Dally (2008) reported on innovative uses of art therapy in a multidisciplinary team approach to work with eating-disordered adolescents and their families, using clay sculptures to depict the family. This process leads to easier and better awareness and articulation of family struggles. Also, art therapy has been used in prisons to reduce depression among inmates. In Gussak's 2007 study, a significant decrease in depression was seen among inmates participating art therapy as measured by the Beck Depression Inventory.

Erhardt et al (1989) conducted an interesting study involving outpatients who had been in dance/movement therapy as part of multidisciplinary treatment for chronic and persistent mental illness. Through interviews, video review, and the use of a modified Q-sort method, the interviewers were able to determine what aspects of group dance/movement therapy the patients found most beneficial. To test a theoretical model proposed by Schmais (1985) on curative factors in group dance/movement therapy, the researchers followed the well-established wisdom on the effectiveness of psychotherapy, namely, that the patient's perception of change and benefit is a strong predictor of such positive effects. Of the eight factors included—expression, rhythm, synchrony, vitalization, relaxation, exercise, music, and cohesion—patients gave the highest ranking to vitalization, defined here as "an increase of energy that mobilizes the entire body" (Erhardt et al, 1989, p. 49).

Koch et al (2007) investigated the important question of the differential benefits of a circle dance intervention, a music listening session, and exercise. This study, with a three-group repeated measures design, examined mood-related variables (depression, vitality, and affect) in a group of psychiatric patients (n = 31), all of whom carried some diagnosis of depression and who were assigned to one of the three treatment groups. A single session of each intervention was given under well-controlled conditions. As revealed by a comparison of scores on a self-report measure before and after the intervention, the patients in the dance group showed a significant decrease in depression compared with both the music group ($P <.001$) and the exercise group ($P <.05$), and a significant increased in vitality compared with the music group ($P <.05$).

A meta-analysis of studies of dance/movement therapy (Cruz et al, 1998) showed overall effect sizes for dance/movement therapy in the moderate range, a magnitude of change similar to that reported for other approaches such as verbal psychotherapy, meditation methods, cognitive-behavioral therapy, and exercise. The Cruz et al meta-analysis focused on studies with treatment outcomes addressing the variables of anxiety, depression, vitality, and self-concept in psychiatric populations. Since the publication of this meta-analysis, other studies have been completed showing benefits of this modality on various aspects of mood (e.g., Dibbel-Hope, 2000; Erwin-Grabner et al, 1999).

One meta-analysis of the effectiveness of psychodrama techniques has been conducted (Kipper et al, 2003), and it is quite instructive. The researchers gathered data from 25 controlled trials of psychodrama sessions (including some studies of several-session courses of therapy and some of single-session exposure) representing a total combined sample size of 281 study participants. They analyzed for differential effects of four main psychodrama techniques: role reversal, doubling, role playing, and the combination of multiple techniques. The total overall adjusted median effect size for all techniques combined was 0.85, which indicates a large intervention effect, according to Cohen's benchmarks (Kipper et al, 2003, p. 19). Calculating separately the effect sizes for each of the four techniques, the researcher found that the techniques of role reversal and doubling each had large mean effect sizes, whereas the techniques of role playing and combination of multiple techniques had effect sizes in the small to moderate range (again, as defined by Cohen). Importantly, post hoc analyses revealed that these effects were as strong for mental health patients, prisoners, and special needs populations as they were for healthy participants, and that there were no differences in effect for male and female participants. This meta-analysis advanced research in the area by studying the critical question of which creative arts therapy methods are most effective with which populations.

Music therapy uses a wide range of receptive methods, including music-assisted relaxation, song lyric analysis, elicitation of mental imagery for self-management or psychotherapy, and recreational listening. Expressive methods can include singing, song writing, ensemble instrumental playing with or without singing, movement to music, action games using music, instrumental and vocal improvisation, and music composition. Individuals with mental disorders represent the largest clinical population served by music therapists around the world. Much of the literature describes clinical methods or uses case studies to illustrate how outcomes are reached. As more doctoral programs in music therapy are established, additional research designs are being developed, including designs for qualitative and quantitative outcome studies.

Gold et al (2005) compiled a Cochrane review on the effects of music therapy in individuals with schizophrenia. For the four studies that met the inclusion criteria, they found that music therapy improved overall mental functioning and reduced negative symptoms, which are usually medication resistant. In their Cochrane abstract they state, "Music therapy as an addition to standard care helps people with schizophrenia to improve their global state and may also improve mental state and functioning if a sufficient number of music therapy sessions are provided. Further research should address the dose effect relationship and the long-term effects of music therapy."

Music therapy approaches using live and recorded music to help individuals with eating disorders have been developed incorporating a wide range of psychotherapeutic perspectives, including ego psychology (Nolan, 1989a, 1989b), psychodrama (Parente, 1989a, 1989b), object relations (Robarts et al, 1994), behavior therapy (Justice, 1994), Jungian psychology (Sloboda, 1995), and modified cognitive-behavioral approaches (Hilliard, 2001).

Approaches to music psychotherapy that were developed in the 1970s, such as the Bonny Method of Guided Imagery and Music, have since been the subject of increasingly more sophisticated study, from outcomes assessment to the development of specific measuring tools (Bruscia, 2000).

All of the creative arts therapies rely on images, metaphors, and symbols as representations of the inner life and carriers of the therapeutic process, and accept that images can be manifested in words, graphic elements, the kinesthetic sense (Serlin et al, 2000), and sounds. The poetry therapy described by Springer (2006) for those in recovery from substance addictions and for trauma survivors offers examples of metaphor as an agent of insight and change. Springer cautions that in using poetry therapeutically it is important to explicitly relax the rules of poetry writing and recommends the use of "sense poems" when clients are invited to imagine an abstract phenomenon in terms of concrete sensory qualities: "What is the color of addiction? What does it sound like? What does it smell like? What does it look like? What does it feel like?" (p. 74). In setting the stage for behavioral change, the poetry therapist helps the patient enter the imaginal realm where a different life can be envisioned. The imagined then becomes a plan, and the authenticity of plans that spring from the creative process can buoy the recovering person over the sometimes rough seas of therapeutic work.

Poetry therapist Amanda Meunier's case study of George, a 45-year-old man with schizophrenia in short-term treatment, illustrates beautifully the weaving together of patient-created poems, attention to specific treatment goals, dialogue about both the poetry and the individual's life, and study of published works that is poetry therapy. In this case, George articulated his own treatment foci: "gain better identification and acceptance of his negative feelings, particularly anger. . . . [find] constructive outlets for dealing with his anger. . . . [accept] his own morality and discuss parental loss" (Meunier, 2003, p. 231). Meunier described the course of therapy in four phases: the supportive phase, in which goals were set and she used the structured of published poems and directed journaling with George; the apperceptive phase, in which George's poetry and their discussions probed his anger, family relationships and feelings about death; the Action phase, marked by poetry that evidenced an understanding of life's cyclic nature and by intentions to make healthy changes in his life; and the integrative phase, in which George openly worked toward autonomously applying the gains and insights made during this brief therapy.

MEDICAL SETTINGS

When the creative arts therapies are provided as part of wholistic, integrated health care, the goals have to do with increasing quality of life, improving the ability to cope, providing psychosocial support, and sometimes reducing pain.

Art therapy has developed many approaches for working in medical settings. The randomized study by Monti et al (2006) used a mindfulness approach to art therapy in groups of women with breast cancer. Their results showed significant improvement in quality of life and reduction in indicators of distress. Creative arts therapy clinical work for people with neurological disorders is directed at physical problems and symptoms associated with the disorders. An example of the latter is an art therapy study in which people with Parkinson disease (n = 19) and a control group without Parkinson disease (caregivers and volunteers) were asked to mold clay into recognizable shapes. Postreatment scores on the Brief Symptom Inventory indicated a decrease in symptoms in all areas in both groups. The Parkinson group showed improvements that were significant and, overall, higher than those of the control group in somatic and emotional areas, including depression, anxiety, average level of distress, and obsessive-compulsive symptoms. Choice of clay color seemed to be related to creation of human figures and affective response.

Berrol et al (1997) conducted a multisite, mixed-methodology demonstration project showing the impact of group dance/movement therapy in older adults who had experienced stroke, cerebral aneurysm, or traumatic brain injury. The study used a randomized controlled trial design (n = 107) with qualitative analysis of data from videotapes of treatment sessions and content analysis of both patient responses to satisfaction questionnaires and therapists' reports. Compared with patients in the control group, those in the treatment group showed significantly greater positive changes in two dimensions of perceptual-motor functioning, dynamic balance walking backward and walking sideways to the left, and in one range-of-motion item, reaching down from a seated position to cross the midline right to left. The treatment group also showed significant improvement in cognitive performance (decision making, ability to make oneself understood, and short-term memory) (p = .006) and in five components of social interaction (ease with others, involvement in social/group activities as well as planned/structured activities, acceptance of invitations, self-initiated activities, and interaction with others) (p = .0027).

Studies on the benefits of dance/movement therapy for adults with cancer have shown that breast cancer patients in particular seem to profit from this modality. Sandel et al (2005) found significant improvement in breast cancer–specific quality of life (as measured with the Functional Assessment of Cancer Therapy–Breast [FACT-B] questionnaire) in women in the group dance treatment condition compared with a wait-list group. Serlin et al (2000) used patient ratings on the Profile of Mood States inventory as one indicator of treatment effectiveness of a group dance/movement therapy program and reported that "significant improvement was found on the fatigue, vigor and tension subscales, while depression and anxiety decreased" (p. 130). In addition, compelling qualitative findings were noted in the way the women participants described the bodily changes they felt in themselves after existentially oriented supportive dance/movement therapy.

Creative arts therapy programs for medically ill children are sometimes integrated with child life and pediatric psychology services. This is the case at the Hackensack University Medical Center, New Jersey, where dance/movement therapy is part of the holistically oriented treatment for children with hematologic and oncologic diseases. Cohen and Walco (1999) described this work as a developmentally sensitive approach to helping children through the challenges of serious illness by providing creative explorations of feelings, relationships, the body image, and ways of coping. Their goal was to use both structured and improvisational movement expression not only to bring out children's fears and concerns but also to encourage the maintenance or resumption of normal development. This work can be done at the bedside, even when little movement is possible, or in outpatient programs. An example of the latter was the dance/movement therapy–based support group for teens (boys and girls) with cancer. The group called themselves "The Braves," and with the guidance of Cohen, their therapist, they tackled the difficult issues of emerging sexuality, peer dynamics, body image, trust, and mortality in playful yet serious psychophysical expression.

Music therapy studies in medical settings with adults and children have increased greatly in the last decade. This section presents brief examples in the areas of cancer, palliative care, neurological rehabilitation, pain reduction, and neonatal intensive care. Clinical use of music therapy in patients with cancer is well described in empirical and clinical case studies. The literature related to music therapy in hospice and palliative care is fairly large and growing. The primary use of supportive music psychotherapy is to improve the individual's quality of life; decrease pain; reduce anxiety and depression; encourage expression; improve communication, especially between family members; and enhance spiritual well-being. Music therapists often continue to work with families after the patient's death for bereavement support (Dileo et al, 2005; Hilliard, 2003; Magill et al, 2002; O'Callaghan, 1996, 1997).

In Hilliard's 2003 study, 80 individuals living in their homes and receiving hospice care were randomly assigned to receive standard care plus music therapy (live music) or standard care alone. Quality of life was shown to be higher in the music therapy group.

Music therapy has a wide range of applications in pediatric medical environments. Music therapy researchers and educators Jayne Standley and Jennifer Whipple (2003) conducted a meta-analysis of the use of music therapy in pediatric settings. A range of music therapy populations and applications was studied, including all major specializations from the neonatal intensive care unit (NICU) through pediatric hospice care.

Although music has historically been linked with pain reduction, it is only recently that empirical studies by music therapists have been published. Standley, in her 1986 meta-analysis of all empirical studies using music in dental and medical treatments, found that "music conditions enhanced medical objectives whether measured by physiological (ES [effect size] = .97), psychological/self report (ES = .85), or behavioral (ES = 1.10) parameters" (p. 79). Standley added that most of the studies included participant's pain as a variable. Loewy et al (2005) compared the sedating effects of live music to the effects of chloral hydrate in children undergoing electroencephalographic (EEG) testing. Sixty children between the ages of 1 and 5 years were assigned to either the music group or the chloral hydrate group. Of the children in the music group, 97% needed no other intervention to complete the EEG recording, whereas 50% of the children in the chloral hydrate group required additional interventions to finish the EEG testing. Those in the music group achieved sedation more quickly and were able to leave the hospital much sooner than those in the chloral hydrate group.

NICUs employ music therapy to increase nonnutritive sucking (Standley, 2000); to improve physiological measures, including reducing heart and respiration rates and increasing blood oxygen saturation using infant-directed singing and simulated womb sounds; and to alter the overall NICU sound environment (Stewart et al, 2000).

Living with a chronic medical condition impacts all aspects of life—vocational, spiritual, relational, sexual, emotional, and psychological—and when cure is elusive, comprehensive care must equip people to live as full and satisfying a life as possible (Goodill, 2005b, 2006) Baker and Mazza (2004) show how this can be accomplished with poetry therapy and therapeutic writing in their case study of a woman with systemic lupus erythematosus

who was also a breast cancer survivor. Anna struggled with chronic pain and fatigue, but also with a sense of hopelessness and a belief that her own need for therapy was a weakness in herself. The disease had damaged both her marriage and her career. As described in the case study, therapeutic writing, performed in the context of an empathic ongoing therapeutic relationship, enabled her to first accept her limitations and then build into her life the supports she needed to function optimally. Baker and Mazza quote the from the patient's journal: "I have decided to replace my stubbornness with determination. I am determined not to be defined by my disease. It is a part of my life but not all of it" (p. 150).

Consistent with the definition of poetry therapy as including therapeutic writing, some of the work in poetry therapy, as in the case study described earlier, draws on the curative properties of creating a narrative by writing out one's troubling thoughts and feelings. This effect has been extensively researched by psychologist James Pennebaker and his many collaborators. Among the related studies is that by Krantz and Pennebaker (2007) in which dance/movement was shown to confer similar health benefits.

Application of poetry therapy as a crisis intervention tool in a day treatment program for people living with human immunodeficiency virus (HIV) infection was describe by Schweitert (2004). In a descriptive case study, she tells of Wilberto, who despite making good progress in the program nearly relapsed into drug use when frustrated by the challenges of a new employment situation. When Wilberto stormed into the clinic, anxious and angry, the poetry therapist quickly recognized the crisis and the danger this situation presented to Wilberto. Within a few minutes the therapist structured the collaborative writing of a "calm-down" poem using sentence stems. As Schweitert reports, "the finished product was stunning" (p. 191):

Stem (by the Therapist)	Line Completion (by the Patient)
When I get angry	*I need to get away!*
If I can just	*take myself outside*
Then I will	*watch the squirrels having fun*
And maybe	*find a cool, quiet lake*
Where I can	*calm my mind and feel peace*
That would be	*perfect.*

The patient, visibly calmer, kept the poem with him and, as the case study documents, began a new initiative in both therapy and work. Four months later he had avoided relapse and was actively addressing issues related to living with HIV.

Music therapy clinical work and studies have increased in all the rehabilitative sciences in parallel with the rapid growth of neurosciences in the last 25 years. Neuroscientists are very interested in the human response to music, because music is processed in many different areas of the brain. By studying the response to music scientists are learning much more about the way the brain works. Clinicians, educators, and developmental specialists are learning how music affects the individual's physical, cognitive, interpersonal, emotional, and spiritual life in ways that were unimaginable three decades ago. Perhaps the best current examples of the effects of music on the whole person from a neurological perspective come from Oliver Sacks (2007), a strong advocate for the creative arts therapies, who, in working with music therapist and researcher Concetta Tomaino at the Institute for Music and Neurologic Function in New York City, has sparked worldwide interest in the areas of music and memory, neural plasticity, and the reactivation of nerve pathways in people with a wide range of chronic neurological disorders.

Research on the uses of music, specifically rhythmic auditory stimulation (RAS), for gait training in stroke patients is demonstrated in the prolific research of Michael Thaut. In a recent study (Thaut et al, 2007) RAS and neurodevelopmental therapy (NDT)/Bobath-based training were used in two groups of hemiparetic stroke patients. The study included 78 patients who had experienced a stroke 3 weeks earlier (43 in the group receiving RAS, and 35 in the group receiving NDT/Bobath training). Over a 3-week period of daily gait training, the RAS group outperformed the NDT group in velocity, stride length, and steps per minute.

SUMMARY

As can be seen from the array of study topics and methodologies described, practitioners of the creative arts therapies engage in all forms of systematic inquiry, including quantitative, qualitative, mixed-method, and arts-based studies. The research agendas for these disciplines currently identify as priorities the evaluation of clinical outcomes, comparison and refinement of treatment methods, theory testing, derivation of theories, psychosocial assessment using art forms and media, definition of best practices in therapist preparation and education, and investigation of basic research questions linking creative arts therapy practice with findings from other disciplines.

As the creative arts therapies develop and grow as health care professions, the arts remain at the core of practice while creativity remains the underlying drive. Healing, or becoming whole, occurs through a process of activation of the person's creative potential through the arts within a therapeutic relationship. As psychologist Ernest Rossi (1999) posits, creative activity is one way to stimulate endogenous mind-body healing processes.

Ultimately, there are similarities in processes across the creative arts therapies, yet these processes are distinctively crafted by the uniqueness of the art forms. The similarities appear in the innate responses to the arts as well as in the individual's use of creativity and the arts to form human relationships. We can recognize these processes as similar in their effects, yet different in their manifestations, in the following examples: (1) the music therapist's song in the NICU that activates the neonate's inherent creative tendency to "find" the transformational effect in the therapist's voice; (2) the art therapist's facilitation of a client's natural desire to create and show others a visual representation of his or her inner world; (3) the dance/movement therapist's use of an expressive gesture to convey empathy in response to the client's movement depiction of uncovered individuality; (4) the drama therapist's moving a patient out of a role play at precisely the moment when the patient is ready to express authentic feelings; or (5) the poetry therapist's selection of a starter poem that can reflect the as-yet unspoken language of the heart.

The clinical and research discoveries of the creative arts therapies point to future investigations in little explored but increasingly important areas such as the neuroscience and psychological interfaces with the effects of the experience of beauty on health, the spirituality responses to the arts, and the instillation of hope.

⊖ Chapter References can be found on the Evolve website at http://evolve.elsevier.com/Micozzi/complementary/

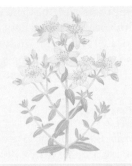

HUMOR

HUNTER "PATCH" ADAMS, with WILLIAM F. FRY,
LEE GLICKSTEIN, ANNETTE GOODHEART,
CHRISTIAN HAGESETH III, RUTH HAMILTON,
ALLEN KLEIN, MARC S. MICOZZI,
VERA M. ROBINSON, PATTY WOOTEN

The arrival of a good clown exercises a more beneficial influence upon the health of a town than of twenty asses laden with drugs.

—THOMAS SYDENHAM, MD
(SEVENTEENTH-CENTURY PHYSICIAN)

Before tackling what humor therapy might be, I [Adams] would like to introduce where I think it fits into complementary and integrative medicine in a discussion on wellness or preventive medicine. Allopathic medicine has generally ignored this field. What could be more complementary to any system of disease care than a sound emphasis on being well? As the economic crisis in medicine worsens, it seems both prudent and inevitable that we focus much greater attention on living healthful lives. **The complementary therapies all have a greater emphasis on health and wellness because they fit into a more holistic approach** (see Chapter 1). Often, when more time is spent with patients, the intimacy that happens leads to a compassionate desire to help the patient feel better. Primary care health providers clearly see the difference between the way healthy people on a wellness program respond to illness and the way people who do not engage in wellness care for their health respond to illness. They also see less frequent illness in people on wellness programs.

WELLNESS—RECOGNIZING WHOLE POTENTIAL

"Exercise and recreation are as necessary as reading. I will say rather more necessary because health is worth more than learning."

—THOMAS JEFFERSON

The practice of medicine can be an exercise in frustration. Current medical education focuses on disease care: a patient comes to the doctor sick, does the prescribed treatment, and returns to the world. Why he or she got sick in the first place is glossed over with a few quick questions, partly because in the short dialogue between physician and patient, there is no time to address the patient's lifestyle. I (Adams) have chosen to spend long hours with patients for these past 35 years to try to understand the processes that lead to illness. In medical school, "health" was defined as the absence of disease, so those not complaining of symptoms were healthy. Yet, so few adults I have spoken with speak of life as a wondrous zestful journey, and most illnesses seen by a family doctor have a huge lifestyle component, frustrating the physician because they could have been prevented with self-care.

HEALTH

Health is obviously so much more than a disease-free interlude. To be healthy is to have a body toned to its maximum performance potential, a clear mind exploding with wonder and curiosity, and a spirit happy and at peace with the world. Most adults, however, exist in a gray area between health and sickness, a zone where people say, "I'm fine," when asked how they feel. This "fine" can be chock full of disease as diverse and inhibiting as (1) the chronic fatigue or "blah" experienced because of those labile fluctuations in blood sugar as a result of a high-sugar diet; (2) the foot problems that come from wearing shoes geared for fashion, not fitness; and (3) the distraction and anger that linger on after poor communication with a spouse or friend. In fact, our lifestyle is assaulting us now and anticipating future expression in disease in hundreds of silent ways.

Because wellness is the summation of all factors leading us to being healthier, this chapter can only touch, ever so briefly, on some of those of paramount importance, ideally stimulating a thirst in each person to discover individual parameters. In the wellness model, patients become responsible for their own health, because health results from an active participation that only the self can give. The health professional's role then shifts from that of a mechanic fixing the breakdowns to that of a gardener nurturing growth.

Much of illness, from minor to profound, has a powerful stress component. The intention of the wellness movement is to offer many insights and paths to eliminate unhealthy stress and make good use of positive stress. It is time to "lighten up" and live life in deepest appreciation of all its gifts.

Wellness is a great investment with many repercussions. A long-term investment in good health opens the door to a lifetime of quality living for the investor. The physical body becomes the vehicle for indulging in every activity one desires, never limited because of being out of shape. However, the benefits of wellness extend far beyond the self. Family life can become a rich, creative, and happy experience on the train of communication and cooperation. The workplace can become a fun place, as a well-dressed attitude and personality help make all employees a team and every task a delight. Separating self, family, and work is arbitrary and possibly even dangerous, because the health of one so obviously has an impact on all the others. People who are at maximum health will be happier and more loving in all their relationships and thus prepared to give their best work performance. An individual striving to be healthy, full of caring and curiosity, brings loving management and creativity to the workplace. A body in tone and at proper weight is ready for the tasks at hand. If any of these areas is ignored in one's pursuit of health, the others will suffer. Studies have shown that emphasizing a human-centered, healthy workplace and providing space and time to exercise and be more personal cuts absenteeism and turnover and increases honesty and productivity.

Unfortunately, one of life's ironies is that wisdom mostly comes with age. By the time we realize that a habit has profoundly hurt us, we feel helpless to change the habit, even justifying it as intrinsic to our nature. Luckily the design of a great organism is such that it can recover remarkably well; in fact, it begins to repair itself as soon as we alter the unhealthy habit. Wellness is not some kind of "end product"; it is a process, a journey, in which each day presents its unique face, and we must choose from many choices which paths to follow. We cannot rest on the health of our past, because it must be renewed each day.

Life is a cascade of choices, and we are an expression of both the short-term and the long-term choices we make. To manage the number of choices we have to make daily, we fall into habits, and a routine substitutes for a choice. These habits can be a double-edged sword: although it is true we do not have to concern ourselves any longer with an immediate choice, once entrenched, a habit is incredibly hard to break. When the habit is an unhealthy one and we want to break it, the task is arduous. Wellness seems like an emerging system to help people restructure or balance habits, so how we live becomes healthy, not as a task of effort but simply as a collection of positive, intentional habits. As medical practitioners focus on the causes and prevention of illness, they are finding that many major diseases could have been prevented or dramatically postponed through lifestyle changes. Most of this information has been reiterated throughout the medical literature from Hippocrates to the present.

NUTRITION

Take nutrition, for example. Simplified, we are a sack of water with chemicals in solution. How these chemicals interact determines what we are to be, but in many of the interactions, chemicals are used up or altered and must be replenished. Nutrition consists of the proper consumption and assimilation of foods containing those necessary chemicals. Because few foods contain all or most of the needed nutrients, we have to obtain them in a variety of foods. As people have moved further from food sources, and as food companies have changed the foods grown to have longer shelf life, our diets have changed dramatically. For about the last 100 years, synthetic chemicals, refined foods, sugar, and salt have replaced many of the natural foods our ancestors ate.

Refined simple sugars so dominate our lives that they are ubiquitous, present even in table salt. In the United States 100 years ago, we consumed 3 lb of sugar per person per year; we now consume 140 to 180 lb. Many believe that this has had a profound effect on our health. Certainly it plays a major role in one of the most devastating diseases—obesity. The federal government has stepped in to encourage some nutritional changes: (1) dramatic cutbacks in sugar and salt consumption, (2) increased consumption of foods containing fiber, and (3) vast decrease in consumption of milk products and other animal fat products. I would expand on this to say: eat mostly whole grains, fresh fruit, and vegetables and, if eating meats, eat mostly fish and poultry.

EXERCISE

If nutrition is the fuel, exercise is the "toner" for the body. Modern civilization has changed few things in our lives as severely as the amount of exercise we get. We have never been as sedentary as we are today, and this, combined with dietary changes, has made much of our adult population overweight and flabby. There is a popular quip that says, "If you do not use it, you lose it." The interplay of muscles, bones, tendons, ligaments, and joints demands consistent stimulation to stay in tone. Being in shape does not mean simply being slender but having all the muscles trained.

There are four types of exercise to consider. The body's internal toner in *heart-lung (aerobic) exercise* strengthens the heart, exercises the bellows to supply oxygen to the body and rid it of carbon dioxide, and tones the muscles used in exercise, all giving the body endurance. Joint *flexibility exercises,* such as stretching or yoga-style exercises, keep the body limber and relaxed. *Strength exercises* are important to tone those muscles not covered in the heart-lung exercises. *Balancing exercises,* such as dance, gymnastics, or circus skills, add another dimension to maximum performance.

Being in shape has obvious rewards in being physically able to do whatever you want to do, and regular exercise has other benefits. It has been shown to lower blood pressure, to have a positive effect on mental health, to diminish stress, and to aid digestion. I believe that regular exercise does such good for the body that it appears to slow the aging process.

EMOTIONAL LIFE

Just as we must exercise our bodies to be fit, so must we exercise our minds to keep awake and alert. The greatest instruments for the mind's stimulation are wonder and curiosity. Boredom is a major disease, eroding the health of many adults who over time narrow their spheres of interest. Wonder and curiosity are the tools that all children carry with them in their interactions with the world. In fact, that wonder and curiosity are what make kids seem so alive. For adults, somewhere along the line, sunsets become routine and life's pace too hectic. But wonder and curiosity can be recaptured. There are no stimulants that begin to awaken a person like a new interest captivating

one's life or consuming ongoing exploration. The next time a person is excited about something, instead of turning it off, jump right into it and share in their interest. Carry your wonder and curiosity into your older years and you take your youth with you. Often, having such a vibrant interest is a major impetus and motivation for staying healthy, so the exploration goes unimpeded.

It goes without saying that love is the most important wellness factor in sustaining a healthy, happy life. Love, that passionate abstract, has captured the arts from the beginning as they attempt to define and elucidate it. As a healing force, *love* can be defined as that unconditional surrender to the overwhelming wonderful feeling experienced in giving to or receiving from an object. We most often express love toward family, friends, God, self, lovers, pets, nature, or hobbies. By "surrender" I mean to lose oneself in awe, trust, respect, fun, and tenderness for the object of surrender. In striving for maximum wellness, one could pursue love in all the parameters just mentioned. It appears that the more one submits to unconditional love toward one object, the easier it is to do so for others. The unconditional aspect is so important, because without it, love is often lost to expectations, doubts, and fears.

If love is the foundation for happiness, then fun, play, and laughter are the vehicles for its expression. The great physician Sir William Osler said that laughter is the "music of life." Humor and laughter are the subjects of this chapter.

FAITH

Faith is the cornerstone of our inner strength. Faith is a personal, passionate, immutable belief in something of inexhaustible power and mystery. Whenever we have to face any kind of devastating change without some kind of solid belief, we become prey to confusion, fear, and panic. Often these crises present questions that have no answers; the discomfort arising from this uncertainty is healed in the domain of our beliefs. Faith has no physical characteristics, no external requirements; it is not a commodity. To acquire a belief, one simply needs to have an interest and a willingness to submit to its mystery. Although there are many great religious traditions that promote a common interpretation of belief, I think the truth is that each person has to find an individual, meaningful faith. Faith is not summarized by a label but expressed by an inner experience of strength that lives in each of us, day by day.

NATURE

Whereas faith is intangible, requiring sweet surrender, nature is a physical, sensual thing. Our relationship with nature has had great historical significance as part of our healthy life. It is of little surprise that most symbols in early religions were from nature. Our moods are often described in terms of nature: a synonym for "happy" is "sunny." The first warm, bright day after winter heightens spirits as few days of the year do. Love has a metaphorical connection to the moon. Most early celebrations grew out of ties with and reliance on the seasons. We have such strong needs to connect with nature that billions of dollars are spent to bring nature into our homes in the form of pets and house plants. Medical literature is currently peppered with the therapeutic significance of putting pets in the lives of elderly and mentally ill patients.

Flowers are a major communication of love at sickbeds, deaths, marriages, and special occasions. The few weeks we take during a year to relax on vacation are mostly spent with a natural setting in mind: the beach or the mountains, for instance. Let's face it—nature is the mother of wonder. If we are to be fully well, we need a daily communion with nature, both in the spectacular sunset and in the tenacious blade of grass as it pushes up through the sidewalk.

CREATIVITY

Our imagination, hands, and senses are the tools for the next major wellness factor—creativity. Life is experienced as a rich journey if we believe we have a creative hand in its passage. Creativity is not just expressed through hobbies and arts but can touch every aspect of life: our work, family, and even how we wait in line. The importance seems to be in the enjoyment of the process rather than in the quality of the final product. Creativity works like our muscles: the more it is exercised, the greater its tone. Explore the next idea, activity, or interest in your life that catches your eye. Whenever exploring, do not settle for one point of view; set it aside and insist on other perspectives. Explore the spontaneous. The key here is to be open and susceptible. Do not catalogue your hobbies and interests as indulgences; respect them as major medicines. Our interests often decline with age, and this can be deadly. Try to see each day as a building block to the next. Be sure to take advantage of all the human creativity in existence, because the arts give such a sense of well-being.

SERVICE

As soon as people recognize how fortunate they are to be well, there arises the urge to give thanks. The healthy expression of that thanks is in service. Unless individuals believe they live a life of service, in whatever form suits them, I believe that they will have a difficult time feeling that life is ultimately fulfilling. John Donne (see the Front Matter) wrote, "No man is an island," acknowledging that we are all connected in some way. It is through helping others that we find this deepest interdependence. It is important that this service be done out of thanks in the joy of giving, because service can easily slide into a debit-and-credit mentality. Service can take many forms, from simply being a loving friend or parent to stopping to help someone in need. These are very personal forms of service.

I suggest that there is also an important wellness connection to our community and our planet.

SYNERGY

To these components of wellness could be added passion, hope, relaxation, wisdom, and peace. In the wellness lifestyle, each of these components suggests a context in which men and women can live their lives so that they can feel healthy, as well as a context that dramatically softens the experience when they do become sick. I think it safe to say that these components of wellness, regularly practiced, are healthy to individuals and families. When these two are healthier, it helps make the community and society healthier.

All these wellness components act uniquely in each person within a specific culture, and they all act together in a person at the same time without a measurement of relative value.

Most of these wellness components are dramatically affected by the others; for example, humor is different in a jolly, friendly person than in an angry, lonely one. If one were to use these components in a therapeutic way, it would make sense to have the medical environment exude these qualities to create a context of love, wonder, curiosity, and humor. This atmosphere would have a positive health effect on patients, staff, and visitors, whether in an office or in a hospital.

The examination of these wellness qualities, until modern times, has not been by science, but rather by art, philosophy, and religions. However, some of the most exciting research in medicine today is finding the connections in biochemistry and physiology between the mind and its thoughts, and the health of the body. This new field is evolving and is now popularly called *mind-body medicine* or *psychoneuroimmunology* (see Chapter 8).

HUMOR

This chapter looks at one component of wellness—humor. Many of the wellness components (e.g., love, passion, faith) are difficult to measure with some scientific precision or standard. Humor is believed to be different because it has a handle to measure it—laughter. Laughter has wide variation within genders, ages, and cultures, which makes actual studies point to a direction rather than establish a fact. This is one area of study in which anecdotal experience may have to count as science. I do not think one who uses humor in therapy does so because he or she found that laboratory studies showed value. Humor therapy is not a static regimen of memorized jokes and numbers of chuckles per hour. Humor therapy comes out when therapists decide to let their humorous parts join the interaction with a patient. This can be in many forms, such as laughter, theater, verbal, and physical play. With humor, the one who practices (whether laugher, funny person, clown, or comic) the craft in the "laboratory of laughter" is the patient, audience, or friend. All of one's past experience in that laboratory is brought to the spontaneous act with the patient, and if it is effective, smiling and laughter occur. This positive feedback is the determining feature in reproducing the gesture, statement, or behavior that elicited the laughter. When a patient says, "My doctor has a good bedside manner," he or she is speaking not about expertise but about qualities of interaction. A friendly, playful sense of humor is at the core of a good bedside manner. The patient's appreciation perpetuates the behavior. Friendship is the safest context for humor to work in, so when humor has missed its mark, instead of offense, forgiveness is felt.

A merry heart doeth good like a medicine.

—PROVERBS 17:22

HISTORY

There is little history of the use of laughter therapy; much of it is being made now (Box 14-1). However, there is a large body of comments on humor and laughter from philosophy, religion, and the arts.

Arthur Koestler (1964) summarizes a fraction of these comments in his book *The Act of Creation:*

> Among the theories of laughter that have been proposed since the days of Aristotle, the "theory of degradation" appears as the most persistent. For Aristotle himself laughter was closely related to ugliness and debasement; for Cicero "the province of the ridiculous . . . lies in certain baseness and deformity"; for Descartes laughter is a manifestation of joy "mixed with surprise or hate or sometimes with both"; in Francis Bacon's list of laughable objects, the first place is taken by "deformity."

The essence of the "theory of degradation" is defined in Hobbes's *Leviathan:*

> The passion of laughter is nothing else but sudden glory arising from a sudden conception of some eminency in ourselves by comparison with the infirmity of others, or with our own formerly.

Bainey, one of the founders of modern psychology, largely followed the same theory:

> Not in physical effects alone, but in everything where a man can achieve a stroke of superiority, in surpassing or discomforting a rival, is the disposition of laughter apparent.

> For Bergson laughter is the corrective punishment inflicted by society upon the unsocial individual: "In laughter we always find an unavowed intention to humiliate and consequently to correct our neighbor." Max Beerbohm found "two elements in the public's humour: delight in suffering, contempt for the unfamiliar." McDougall believed that "laughter has been evolved in the human race as an antidote to sympathy, a protective reaction shielding us from the depressive influence of the shortcomings of our fellow men."

Herbert's Spencer's Laughter as "Survival of the Fittest"

The first to make the suggestion that laughter is a discharge mechanism for "nervous energy" seems to have been Herbert Spencer, a nineteenth century British social scientist who is paradoxically credited with coining the term "survival of the fittest"; he based this term on his interpretation of Charles Darwin's work on evolutionary biology. (Darwin himself never used the term.) Nonetheless, Spencer's concept certainly provided ample reasons for humans in society to be "nervous" and thus have the need to discharge "nervous energy."

Spencer's essay on the "Physiology of Laughter" (1860) starts with the proposition: "Nervous energy always tends to beget muscular motion; and when it rises to a certain intensity always does beget it. . . . Emotions and sensations tend to generate bodily movements, and . . . the movements are violent in proportion as the emotions or sensations are intense." Hence, he concludes, "when consciousness is unawares transferred from great things to small" the "liberated nerve force" will expand itself along the channels of least resistance, which are the muscular movements of laughter.

One wonders where in these descriptions appears something useful in helping patients or caregivers in the delivery of care. For this we turn to research done in the twentieth century.

RESEARCH

According to Ruxton (1988), humor can help establish rapport and verbalize emotionally charged interpersonal events. Using humor, patients may find it easier to express embarrassing or frightening parts of their history, and when nurses use funny anecdotes and are more vulnerable with a patient, it appears to strengthen the staff-patient bond.

Coser (1959) looked closely at a hospital's social structure and found that humor helped relieve tension, reassure, transfer information, and draw people together. Norman Cousins (1979) put humor back on the therapeutic map when he laughed himself well from a profound painful chronic illness, dramatically reducing the pain of his ankylosing spondylitis. He spent the rest of his life working at the University of California School of Medicine investigating the positive emotions and their relationship to health. Dr. William Fry studied humor for 30 years and believes it is an exercise for the body. Mirthful laughter exercises the diaphragm and cardiovascular systems. Initially it causes an increase in heart rate and blood pressure, but after a short while it produces a much longer lasting decrease in heart rate and blood pressure, a relaxation response. Paskind (1932) showed that skeletal muscle tone was diminished during mirthful laughter in muscles not actually participating in the laughter. Lloyd (1938) showed an expiratory predominance with mirthful laughter manifesting in a decrease in residual air in the lungs and increased oxygenation of the blood. Based on work done by Schachter and Wheeler (1962) and Levi (1965), catecholamine levels appear to be elevated with mirthful laughter. Researchers later found the body's immune response to laughter (see Chapter 8).

Sigmund Freud had originally suggested that the psychotherapeutic use of humor causes a release of stress, tension, and anxiety. Psychotherapists use humor to facilitate insight (through metaphor, joke, or story) and offer a sense of detachment or perspective. Humor can build a closer relationship between therapist and patient. Humor can be offered as a tool for coping with life's troubles (Box 14-2).

Mahrer and Gervaize (1974) looked at their review of the research literature on laughter in psychotherapy and found that strong laughter is a valuable indication of the presence of strong feelings and is seen by most therapeutic approaches as a desirable event. Strong laughter seems to correlate with increased self-esteem and heightened experiencing.

Although no research has conclusively shown a release of endorphins with mirthful laughter, the anecdotal literature about laughter's pain-killing properties is massive. Cousins (1979) opened this door. The Clemson nurses' program did a study with elderly residents in a long-term care facility. The residents were divided into two groups. One group watched a comedy video nightly for 6 weeks; the other watched a serious drama. The nurses checked the need for analgesics. There were fewer requests for painkillers from the comedy group. Texas Tech University School of Medicine did another test.

Research participants were shown comedy or serious material for just 20 minutes. Relaxation therapy was given to another group. The researchers then determined the participants' pain thresholds using inflated blood pressure cuffs. The comedy group had the greatest pain tolerance of the three groups.

I (Adams) would like to relate a powerful story of a time when humor quite clearly was a painkiller.

CONTEXT

I (Adams) have been doing street clowning almost daily for 35 years, increasingly all over the world. In my 35 years of being a physician, I have always practiced in a humorous context. With a group called Gesundheit Institute, we are building the first hospital to fully incorporate humor. Although the idea is disconcerting at first, in the many lectures to lay and medical audiences I (Adams) have given for the last 20 years about our work, when asked which ward they would choose—a serious, solemn one or a fun, silly one—more than 85% have chosen the fun one. Few people need more than their personal experience to be completely convinced that humor is necessary for their personal health and the health of their relationships.

The primary practice of medicine is a delicate balance between science and art. Ideally, this relationship is one of friendship in which, although the parties have radically different approaches, there is a mutual appreciation of the value of all parties involved and a thankfulness and a necessity that they can work together in harmony. Science and art play different roles in the healing interaction. Medical science works at tackling the disease (the organ or systems afflicted) using a well mapped out series of thought processes, tests, and treatments. The "art of medicine" is concerned with how the disease affects the patient, the family, and their society—the larger repercussions of the disease. These concepts are beautifully discussed in *The Illness Narratives* (Kleinman, 1988) and *The Nature of Suffering* (Cassell, 1991). The art of medicine comes from the intuition and inherent magic found in compassion, love, humor, wonder, and curiosity. For these reasons, one is hard put to break down the components or mechanics of what is working in the art of medicine. Simply put, science serves reductionism, and art serves holism. For this reason, when I (Adams) do clowning, I am free to explore all these healing abstractions. I use all of these in a multitude of combinations, not because they are well mapped out but because they can more freely arise within the clown persona.

I (Adams) am both a professional clown and a physician. Each discipline took about the same number of years to master. The difficulties in becoming each were also similar. In one I had to master information and the ability to synthesize information to make responsible decisions, and in the other I had to master the art of spontaneity and freedom of behavior. I could never say which parts of my clown persona did the trick in a healing interaction, and I

BOX 14-2

Medical Humor

- The Doctor gave a man 6 months to live. The man couldn't pay his bill, so the doctor gave him another 6 months.
- The Doctor called Mrs. Cohen saying, "Mrs. Cohen, your check came back." Mrs. Cohen answered, "So did my arthritis!"
- *Doctor:* "You'll live to be 60!"
  Patient: "I am 60!"
  Doctor: "See! What did I tell you?"
- A doctor held a stethoscope up to a man's chest. The man asks, "Doc, how do I stand?"
  The doctor says, "That's what puzzles me!"
- *Patient:* "I have a ringing in my ears."
  Doctor: "Don't answer!"

Compiled by Christine Vlahos, MSPT, New York, New York

bet the patient could not either. I can only say that my character brings a blatant expression of love, innocence, fun, joy, and friendliness to which people readily respond.

I believe humor and love are at the core of good bedside manner, burnout prevention, and malpractice prevention, and for these alone, humor deserves a central place in a medical practice. But let us not deny its value in just raw fun. Despite my long, deep experiences with humor, I still can be brought to tears of joy over its power.

This was all brought home to me in November 1991 in a children's burn unit in a hospital in Tallinn, the capital of Estonia.

 Case Study

For many years I (Adams) have taken a group of clowns to the former Soviet Union to promote good relations between our countries, to spread good cheer, and to provide a 2-week seminar in clowning for both beginners and professionals. We clown in hospitals, orphanages, prisons, and schools, and we perform a tremendous amount in the street. Everywhere we go, patients, staff, and clowns are tremendously uplifted; at times it even seems to help their medical problems.

Estonia was the footnote to a trip that normally just visits Moscow and St. Petersburg. I added it in 1991 so that we could explore a new country. We arrived 25 clowns strong at the burn hospital, where right off I noticed a woman crying outside a closed door. My medical training told me that this was a mother crying agonizingly over a severely ill child. I knew that to touch her pain I should not clown with her—but with her child. Against strong protestations from the smiling staff, I went inside the room.

I walked in on three women (one physician and two assistants) who had just begun to change dressings and perform débridement on a 5-year-old boy, Raido, with at least 60% third-degree burns solid from ears to knees on both sides of his body. He was in his third week of recovery. I was first struck by the medical supply and pharmaceutical shortages so devastating in the Soviet Union in the winter of 1991. There were no masks or gloves and no strong painkillers, but the work had to be done. With the utmost in loving tenderness on the staff's part and commanding bravery on the boy's part, I watched the bandages come off his wound, revealing a bloody exudative, meaty field, slowly healing from the edges with no evidence of grafts. The silence was punctuated by Raido's screams with each tug of the bandages. At first I felt the horror of a parent for his suffering. From this came a gushing empathy moving the clown to act instinctively; to love, comfort, care for, and bring forth laughter. Without fear.

I watched only for the first third of removal because I was not sure how to proceed. Raido's neck involvement prevented him from looking up at me. When they took a short break, I went over, dressed in full clown regalia, bent over him, and smiled. Spontaneously he looked surprised and delighted and

said in Estonian, "You look beautiful." My heart was captured. I immediately went around to the head of his stretcher and spent the next hour stroking his face and hair, smiling and laughing and talking with him. We played. He stopped screaming entirely. I was only 1 foot from his small, unburned face, and I fell in love with him (having a 4-year-old son myself). I had never seen humor's power so raw. I kept telling him he was beautiful and strong and that he was going to live.

It is clear that the child is the one who changed himself from being sad to being cheerful. I was my clown self. His response "you're beautiful" came as a surprise. My character is not "beautiful." It was his willingness to let me inside that made me be of value to him. Another child could have been spooked and cried. Unlike an operation, the impact of humor on the patient wholly has to do with the patient.

I cannot say what I did that was, in this case, the catalyst for a pain-free experience. Was it the sparkle in my eye, the duck hat on my head, the soothing stroking of his head, the words of love and encouragement—or was it simply skilled diversion?

Raido asked me to come back to his room, so I wheeled his mummified body (bandages already bloody) back to his bed. There for 1 hour I entertained him with clown silliness, still peering into his sky-blue eyes and stroking his face. I don't know who benefited more, because my whole body shook, thrilled for being there. I left most of my toys with Raido, even dressing up his dad like a clown while Raido laughed heartily. It was hard to leave him; I felt like he had given me so much.

HUMOR AS THERAPY

So what is humor therapy? In its broadest sense it is whatever one does to put mirth into a patient encounter or hospital setting. This is a brand new field, and many are exploring how to add humor to the medical setting.

Ruth Hamilton has been using humor carts at Duke University Medical Center since 1989. Peggy Bushey is a nurse who has used the same carts in the intensive care unit (ICU) at Medical Hospital of Vermont for several years. These carts have comic videos and cassettes, funny and cartoon books, props, makeup, and costumes, and a host of volunteers are called in on consultation for patients or staff who request it. Patients have given wonderful feedback on the painkilling and relaxing results of cart use. There is a suggestion that they improve communication, help visitors to hospitals to relax, and even increase motivation in rehabilitation programs. Greater staff relaxation may also be a factor.

Other hospitals, such as Dekalb Medical Center near Atlanta, have created lively rooms, similar to an expanded cart, with all the same items and a place to use them. Carts and rooms do not make humor, however, so the volunteer becomes the key.

In 1990, Michael Christensen of the Big Apple Circus started taking clowns into children's hospitals to make regular, three-times-a-week rounds to the children. What started out as a whim for him has become a full-time passion. He now has 45 clowns in six hospitals in New York City. Clowns who have worked for him have since set up similar programs in France, Germany, and Holland. The wonderful, positive feedback by staff, patients, and family keeps this program alive.

Others, like Annette Goodheart, insist that they do "laughing therapy," not humor therapy. There are laughter meditations and workshops on laughter and play. For many the decision has simply been how to bring more laughter, play, and levity to the medical setting. I suggest a broader view for humor therapy. In our society, which harbors alienation, depression, anxiety, and boredom, one could decide to be indiscriminately humorous and joyous to try to add these elements to every human encounter. I believe it would help our general societal health.

Humor therapy could include wearing a loud bow tie, singing on the ward, engaging in word play, posting cartoons around the hospital, and even inviting comedians to come into the hospital. One note of caution: some believe humor can be harmful in some situations, especially in psychotherapy. I would certainly suggest humor that is not racist or sexist. I suggest first becoming quite close to your patients and having them be sure of your tenderness and sincerity, so that if a funny situation or joke hurts, someone can simply apologize. It behooves the medical history taker to make an exploration into the patient's sense of humor and act on it. Because humor in therapy is so new to medicine, I asked a half-dozen of the leading voices in humor today to make a few statements about their place in the use of humor. I also encourage people considering putting more humor in their practice to consult the resources at the end of this chapter for greater depth.

HUMOR THERAPY IN PRACTICE

BIG APPLE CIRCUS CLOWN CARE UNIT

The Big Apple Circus Clown Care Unit (CCU) is a community outreach program of the Big Apple Circus, a not-for-profit performing arts organization presenting the finest classic circus in America. The CCU transforms the performance of classic circus arts to aid in the care and healing of hospitalized children and teens, and their parents and caregivers.

Just as classic circus defines a specific body of knowledge, so too does classic clowning. The classic clown types, White, Auguste, and Eccentric, appeared as horsemen, acrobats, jugglers, dancers, musicians, and of course actors and actresses. Using all these skills, they had a singular focus: to make people laugh. To this end, they used parody. They parodied all circus acts, rules, structures, and authority as symbolized in one circus figure: the black-booted, top-hatted, red-coated, riding-cropped ringmaster.

For the Big Apple Circus CCU the hospital room replaces the circus ring; the physician replaces the ringmaster; and all the rules, charts, formulas, procedures, machines, and straight-laced, white-washed corridors of the hospital become the source of endless parody. The focus is still to bring laughter to patients' hearts.

Using juggling, mime, music, and magic, 35 specially trained "doctors of delight" bring the joy and excitement of classic circus to the bedsides of hospitalized children 2 and 3 days each week, 50 weeks a year. The Big Apple CCU makes "clown rounds," a parody of medical rounds in which the healing power of laughter is the chief medical treatment. Using sophisticated medical-clown techniques (including red-nose transplants, rubber chicken soup, and kitty cat scans), professional CCU performers work one-on-one with hospitalized children, their parents, and caregivers to ease the stress of serious illness by reintroducing laughter and fun as natural parts of life.

In the Beginning

The CCU was created in 1986 by Michael Christensen, director of clowning at the Big Apple Circus, in cooperation with the medical staff at Babies and Children's Hospital of New York at NewYork-Presbyterian/Columbia University Medical Center. The first CCU clowns, "Dr. Stubs" and "Disorderly Gordoon," learned that they could reduce children's fears about their hospital experiences by using medical instruments as props (e.g., blowing bubbles through a stethoscope) or performing silly medical procedures that echo real medical procedures (e.g., chocolate milk transfusions). The "red-nose transplant," for example, was created specifically to ease the fears of heart transplant patients at Babies and Children's Hospital.

At every CCU host hospital the medical staff has recognized the healing effect of the CCU—how joy and delight relieve the stress of pediatric patients and their worried parents; how music, magic, and mayhem in the halls make patients easier to treat and enhance the effectiveness of the medical staff; and how a happy child appears to get better faster. Dr. Driscoll, chairman of pediatrics at Babies and Children's Hospital of New York, states "When a child begins to laugh, it means he's probably beginning to feel better. I see the clowns as healers. When someone gets around to studying it, I wouldn't be at all surprised to see a connection between programs like the CCU and shorter hospital stays."

In addition to being the subject of numerous news articles and television features, Michael Christensen and the CCU have received wide public recognition for their innovative work in the field of health and humor, including the prestigious Raoul Wallenberg Humanitarian Award, the Red Skelton Award, and the Northeast Clown Convention's annual Gold Nose Award.

Resident Hospital Programs

The Big Apple Circus currently operates CCU programs in seven prominent metropolitan hospitals: Babies and Children's Hospital of New York at Columbia-Presbyterian Medical Center, Harlem Hospital Center, the Hospital for

Special Surgery, Memorial Sloan-Kettering Cancer Center, Mount Sinai Medical Center, New York University Medical Center, and Schneider Children's Hospital of Long Island Jewish Medical Center. Each CCU clown team works under the direct supervision of the hospital's chief of pediatrics.

In addition, the CCU is resident each summer at Queens Hospital Center and Paul Newman's Hole in the Wall Gang Camp for children with cancer and chronic blood diseases.

Working in close partnership with the medical staff at each hospital, the CCU tailors its activities to meet the special needs of each facility. The supervising clown consults daily with nurses, child life staff, and chief residents on the status of individual children. The clown team visits children in all areas of the hospital, including at their bedsides in wards, in ICUs, and in clinic and acute care waiting rooms. The CCU clowns also visit specialty clinics such as the bone marrow transplant unit at Memorial Sloan-Kettering Cancer Center and the human immuno-deficiency virus/acquired (HIV/AIDS) immunodeficiency syndrome clinic at Harlem Hospital.

All CCU clowns are professional performers who have auditioned and have been selected for their professionalism, artistry, and sensitivity. They undergo a rigorous CCU training program to prepare them to work safely and appropriately in the hospital environment. The CCU continually improves its level of quality through rehearsals, continuing education, and procedural and artistic reviews.

The CCU has plans to expand to preeminent children's hospitals in major cities throughout the country. Affiliate programs begun by Big Apple Circus CCU–trained performers currently operate in Paris, France; São Paulo, Brazil; and Wiesbaden, Germany.

If you would like further information about the CCU, please contact us:

Big Apple Circus Clown Care Unit
35 West 35th Street, 9th Floor
New York, NY 10001
(212) 268-2500

THE GROWING WORLD OF HUMOR

When I (Fry) first started my humor studies in 1953, there was a dearth of scientific investigation of the subject. Literary analyses of humor and comedy abounded, and there was ample hypothesizing and theorizing, particularly about the identity of the crucial element of humor that precipitates the mirthful reaction. Also, a few psychological and anthropological studies had carried out examinations of humor preferences, humor values, interactive uses of humor, communication, and humor; this was as close as we got to science. Mind you, it was not a complete wasteland, but it looked like an Edward Hopper canvas; it certainly was not Times Square at midnight on New Year's Eve.

I had entered the field through the gate of humor and communications, as a member of ethnologist Gregory Bateson's research team (Bateson was married to anthropologist Margaret Mead). The research team had been originally assembled by Gregory to explore the roles of the "paradoxes of logical type" in communication (Fry, 1971). As a psychiatrist, I was the team member with training most closely related to the so-called hard sciences, with university classes in a large variety of chemistries, physics, embryology, bacteriology, laboratory technology, physiology, and biochemistry. The scientific method had been portrayed to me as the criterion for research purity and rigor. I did and still do hold the scientific method in high respect. During my psychiatric residency, I had exercised my understanding of scientific discipline by designing, conducting, and reporting in the literature a postdoctoral psychophysiological study of schizophrenia.

In the 1950s a certain excitement had been stirred in the humor studies field by psychologist D.E. Berlyne, a very talented and innovative scholar. Up to the time of his contributions, humor theory was strongly dominated by the views Freud had adopted from philosopher Herbert Spencer's "discharge of energy" postulate (see Box 14-1). This dominance directed most views of humor to observing it primarily as a cathartic phenomenon, a sudden diminution of repressed psychic energy involving a release from inhibition. Berlyne's contribution shifted emphasis to the state of arousal, which he proposed to be the dominant element of the humor response: "laughter . . . is restricted to situations in which a spell or moment of aversely high arousal is followed by sudden and pronounced arousal reduction" (Berlyne, 1972). Needless to say, this attempt to supplant Freud's doctrine aroused much controversy and energy. Some of the energy was channeled into research procedures aimed at proving or disproving one or another of the main themes and their various corollaries. As these experiments proceeded and were reported in the scientific literature, I became increasingly distressed by what I perceived as defective protocols, in that much of the test ratings were based on subjective, vaguely defined, and arbitrary criteria; in many instances, test results were measured by degrees of humor identified as "much," "moderate," or "slight," or by some similar system. I believed that conclusions based on these studies were flawed by deficiencies of objectivity. I agonized over this scientific design issue for many months, even several years into the 1960s.

I finally came to the conclusion that the best readily available source of objectivity in humor experimentation would be the physiological phenomena that both the Freudians and the Berlynians agreed accompany the perception of humor and the experiencing of reactive mirth. A National Institute of Mental Health small grant in 1963-1964 made it possible for me to develop an answer to the question of whether it is possible to observe experimentally the somewhat ephemeral physiology of mirth in such artificial and rigid environments as those that often develop in scientific pursuits (when the fun of science is lost sight of or is ignored). The outcome of my feasibility exploration was "certainly yes," and after wasting months during the Vietnam War buildup futilely trying to obtain financial support from government scientific agencies (when armaments had so much greater priority than laughter), I got to work on designing and carrying out a series of basic science studies of the physiology of mirth and laughter. That research program continued during the following approximately 15 years.

I (Fry) and my colleagues in those studies were able to perform contributive research in most of the human body's major physiology system areas (Fry, 1994). We have been able to demonstrate significant impacts of mirth and mirthful laughter in the cardiovascular, respiratory, muscular, immune, endocrine, and central nervous systems. With that basic science information established and disseminated, many other professionals subsequently have found it possible and desirable to extend their speculations and practice outside spheres of scholarly study in a number of directions, many of them relating to health issues, both in prevention of disease and in uses of humor as adjunctive therapy to traditional treatment procedures.

During the years in which I was absorbed in that research adventure (the 1960s, 1970s, and early 1980s), several other themes and ventures were forming, developing, building, expanding, and arousing the interest and participation of more and more persons throughout North America, in the United Kingdom, and to a certain extent in Europe, especially in France, the Netherlands, and Belgium. This process was a vital component of a truly revolutionary movement throughout the world. The worldwide movement has been designated by several different titles, depending on the specific location or years being considered. Broader titles identify this movement as a modern renaissance, a new style of life, and the Deconstruction era; more specific titles designate the Hippy Revolution, the Free Speech Movement, and an overturning of old values. The period for a while was called the Age of Aquarius. Other, less enthusiastic designations characterize the new era as being a time of Satan's dominance over humankind or an ascendancy of evil and libertine practices. Whatever the values ascribed, there is little argument over the presence of new beliefs, values, and social practices, over the revolutions of social customs, garb, artistic expression, communication, lifestyles, music, interpersonal interactions of many varieties, and religious practices. This revolution undoubtedly was built on the shoulders of earlier times, as is the way of the world. However, this was a watershed era, a parametric cultural shift (see Chapter 7).

Tons of paper and miles of words have been exchanged during the past 35 years regarding this parametric revolution. Discussion of the underlying implications, dealing with issues of the past and future of humanity, is beyond the scope of this contribution. Suffice it to say that a vast proportion of the revolutionary changes has been associated with what can be called the "pragmatics" of human life and human behavior. Changes brought during these turbulent years have involved more the everyday ways of humans, less so a consideration of the many and deep implications of the turbulence and its innovative consequences. To be sure, these implications have received some attention, but to a large extent in the more traditional manner of analysis and consideration. The changes in lifestyle and performance have been huge and have been little inhibited by the paucity of reflective attention turned toward them. There has been much change in daily ways of life, but not only in so-called developed cultures; the revolution has been universal over the globe, with varied intensities and varied specifics of behavior.

Returning to the issues of humor in health care, it is apparent that a part of the revolution has been a process of reshaping the pragmatics of health care, making it possible to consider many new features of health care, including interrelationships between health care and humor, in which humor takes adjunctive roles such as cited previously. Underlying the pragmatics that predominate with this mutation is new emphasis on the principle of one's personal responsibility for one's own health care (Cousins, 1979). More so than many other products of the revolutionary era, this issue of health care responsibility received more and more attention during the 1970s and 1980s. With this expanding orientation and under the title of "holistic medicine," implementation of adjunctive roles in healing and health care for humor, as well as many other alternative, complementary, and integrative nontraditional medical practices, became not only possible but realized. Many opportunities for using humor and mirthful laughter have been created and taken advantage of successfully. Physician Patch Adams is one of the luminous pioneers in this humor movement. The movement has spread throughout areas of the world where humans attempt to improve the quality of their lives, both in health and at times of disease.

The nature of many humor–health care innovations is such that adjunctive use of humor, mirth, and laughter is having increasingly interesting application. Facilities have been established in hospitals, convalescent homes, day care centers, long-term care units, and rehabilitation centers in which sources of humor are made available. These humor sources are usually intended primarily for the patient or resident, but this practice has also brought forth recognition that benefits of humor can be experienced by others in the broader health care environment. As studies have demonstrated, staff members, patients' family members, volunteers, and community contacts all have benefited by having humor "tonics" available at times when they are beset by the various "negative emotions" so common in such circumstances. Patient benefits are demonstrated to come doubly, both from direct impact and from the energizing and positive effects on those who are participating with the patient in his or her struggle for return to or maintenance of health. It is indicative of this "double value" that much of the encouragement for humor facility establishment in health care institutions has come from nursing staffs, who experience a greater degree of patient-provider interaction, both in terms of quantity and intensity.

This use of humor in health care facilities as adjunctive therapy to other, more traditional medical procedures and practices does not stand alone in the new orientation concerning humor in health care. A rising enthusiasm for humor in wider use, beyond institutional use and beyond the age-old popularity of humor as an important source of entertainment and amusement, is fueling spread of humor forms among populations throughout the world (Berger, 1993). This enthusiasm has broken down many of the customary prejudices against humor, which have previously characterized humor as frivolous, unimportant, or vulgar and reprehensible. People have shaken the sense of guilt or shame or flippancy that earlier restricted their access to their natural, genetically inculcated sense of humor (Morreall, 1983). Individuals in their inner lives, in their relationships with family members, in the workplace, and in their public activities increasingly avail themselves of this element of their biological inheritance to enrich their existence and to make unexpected discoveries about the complexities of life (Blumenfeld et al, 1994; Klein, 1989). Workshops, seminars, lectures, and discussion groups throughout the world explore new and beneficial values of humor and laughter for enabling people to lead healthful lives, for helping patients recover from illness, and for helping patients maintain higher quality of life during illness. Humor has even been admitted into the quiet privacy of psychotherapy and counseling (Fry et al, 1993).

Humor continues to be a major source of entertainment, a major component of the array of pleasures to be enjoyed in this world. All evidence indicates sturdy continuation of that status. Humor and laughter, with new knowledge and new attitudes about their values and benefits, now increasingly spread their magic into areas of human experience not previously visualized as appropriate places for their presence.

LAUGHING SPIRIT LISTENING CIRCLES

The potential for healing laughter bubbles deep within us like natural hot springs. It just is. For *laughing spirit listening circles* humor therapy is about providing the safe space that allows us to erupt in our uniquely unpredictable, often socially unacceptable way, fluidly carrying warm chuckles, hot guffaws, and tender tears to the places within and without that serve our body, our soul, and our community.

The laughter that is the best medicine is that which lies beneath seriousness and respects gravity, sadness,

fear, frustration, and anger. It is not the surface, over-the-counter, diluted gigglery we call "lightening up."

Robust tears are no less potent than lusty laughter, and when "lightening up" is even slightly more valued over "getting heavy," therapy is dead and community is crippled.

Humor therapy in the form called *laughing spirit listening circles* involves participants in a group of 6 to 10, each of whom gets equal time to receive absolute positive, silent attention, first for 3 minutes, then for 5 minutes. The guidelines are "dare to be boring." You do not even have to speak. When you do, just tell the truth without trying to be funny. Stay in connection with individuals when you speak. Receive your support, rather than trying to give. The first time around is often serious, even grave, as people feel the safety and respect and build the integrity of the community. By the second time around, laughter and tears often flow, sometimes interchangeably.

THREE MYTHS ABOUT LAUGHTER THAT KEEP US FROM LAUGHING

The *first major myth* about laughter that prevents us from laughing as much as we need to is that "we must have a reason to laugh." The people who respond to laughter with great seriousness may feel that there is no reason to be laughing, or if there is, they missed it. Not only must we have a reason to laugh, according to this myth, but the reason must be so good that when someone challenges us with "Why are you laughing? What's so funny?" when we explain it, they too will laugh. If they do not laugh, very often we are presented with a puzzled face and a remark, such as, "That was it? Boy, do you have a weird sense of humor!"

Many of us unconsciously censor our laughter because at some level we think our reason for laughing is not good enough. It is important to note here that the reality is that laughter is unreasonable, illogical, and irrational. I propose that we do not need a reason to laugh. When we see a 6-month-old baby laughing, we do not demand, "What's so funny?" but rather delight in the response and often join in. We can do so with adults as well. Insisting on a reason to laugh is an excellent way of stopping someone, or ourselves, from laughing. This is important to remember when we are in situations in which laughter is inappropriate. We may want to ask ourselves, "Why am I laughing right now?" so that we can stop, for example, if we get the giggles when pulled over by a policeman for speeding or some other infraction of the law.

The *second major myth* about laughter is that "we laugh because we are happy," when the reality is that we are happy because we laugh. I ask my groups how many feel better after they have laughed, and there is always a unanimous show of hands. At this point I remark that if laughter came out of happiness, we would not feel better after laughing—we would have already felt better *before* laughing.

Laughter has been assigned the job of indicating happiness because we have been so desperate for some outward sign of this vague, undefined, but treasured state. Actually, most people do not know what happiness is. We know that the U.S. Declaration of Independence (1776) mandates us to pursue it (and in fact, the right to do so is held to be "self-evident"), but judging by our national behavior, we are somewhat confused about where happiness lies. If we feel better after we laugh, laughter must come from a source other than happiness.

Those of us who have laughed until we have cried know that in the middle of the process, we cannot tell which is which. We do not laugh because we are happy and cry because we are sad; we laugh or cry because we have tension, stress, or pain. Laughter and tears rebalance the chemicals our bodies create when these distressed states are present, so we feel better after we have laughed or cried.

The *third major myth* is that "a sense of humor is the same thing as laughter." Although the two terms are used interchangeably, they are very different processes. The reality is that you do not need a sense of humor to laugh. Again, when we see a 6-month-old baby laughing, we do not remark, "Doesn't that baby have a wonderful sense of humor!" A sense of humor is learned; laughter is innate. A sense of humor is an intellectual process, whereas laughter spontaneously engages every major system in the body.

There is absolutely no agreement on what a sense of humor is or what makes something funny. Senses of humor vary according to culture, age, ethnic or economic background, race, gender, and so on. I remarked to one of my groups that women in the ladies' room laugh at different things than men in the men's room. A man raised his hand and said, "Men don't laugh in the men's room." I didn't realize this, having spent very little time in the men's room. (Later on, a man came up to me and said he knew why men didn't laugh in the men's room: it is hard to laugh and aim at the same time.)

Having a sense of humor does not guarantee laughter in the person in whom we identify that trait. Many people with great senses of humor do not laugh. Groucho Marx was known to have laughed only once, publicly or privately. Often, people who make other people laugh do so because they can control when the laughter will occur. The emphasis on humor diverts us from the broad scope of laughter that is available, making laughter a specialty that is then possible only occasionally.

A DEFINITION OF HUMOR

A clear understanding of what constitutes humor and what does not, as listed next, is a necessary starting point to prevent the inevitable misunderstandings that arise when the subject is considered.

1. Humor is *not* the equivalent of laughter. Humor may or may not stimulate laughter; sometimes it is merely a quiet smile or even an inner glow of delight. Laughter may accompany humor, but it also accompanies aggression, surprise, and even grief.
2. Joking makes up a minor percentage of humor experience. Only about 4% of the adult population admit to remembering and telling jokes well, whereas more than 90% consider that they "have a pretty doggone good sense of humor." Humor is conveyed between persons much more nonverbally, such as in the eye twinkle and the smile.
3. Humor is *not* a form of therapy. It is a perspective and an appropriate behavior integrated in the overall conduct of our lives.
4. Humor does *not* cure cancer, baldness, or major depression. Humor is a marvelous adjunct to the overall conduct of one's psychological life, especially when one is confronting illness, tragedy, or death.
5. Although the observational evidence is intriguing, humor as yet has *not* been demonstrated conclusively to release endorphins. ("Endorphins": small children without parents who live in the house all the time.)

Humor is a mature psychological response to stress in which the stressful issue is maintained in consciousness, without distortion, and is responded to with amusement when double meanings, ironies, or some other inconsistency is noted. Humor does not increase the discomfort of the individual nor those in his company.

Until the 1970s, humor was looked down on in the conduct of medicine as being unprofessional or uncaring or even as beneath the standard of care. Such an attitude was in response to immature psychological defenses masquerading as humor (e.g., passive aggression, schizoid fantasy, projection).

Applying humor with kindness, compassion, and empathy is the key. For the most part, humor in medical practice should take the form of gentle amusement, twinkling eye contact, and, only in the rarest situations, jokes.

The following is a short listing of specific guides to the conduct of humor (Hageseth, 1988) in a five, four, three formulation:

- **Five** mature ego mechanisms of defense :
  1. Altruism
  2. Humor
  3. Anticipation
  4. Suppression
  5. Sublimation
- **Four** elements of successful communication of humor:
  1. Relationship
  2. Rapport
  3. Setting
  4. Timing

- **Three** pathways to a humor experience
  1. Nonverbal interaction (e.g., smiling, eye twinkle)
  2. Raising of forbidden subjects
  3. Jokes and other forms of verbal humor

THE LAUGH MOBILE PROGRAM

The Carolina Health and Humor Association (Carolina Ha Ha) is an educational service organization dedicated to promoting humor in health care and for personal growth. As founder and executive director, I (Hamilton) started the Duke Humor Project with the Duke Oncology Recreation Therapy department in 1986. At Duke University Medical Center in Durham, North Carolina, oncology patients may come for as long as 6 weeks for various cancer treatments. One difficulty with recreational programming is that patients must feel well enough to attend a group craft or entertainment program. Often the patient is too ill to leave the room during the intensive treatments. The Laugh Mobile was created to bring humorous media bedside to these patients. Volunteers from Carolina Health and Humor Association use the Laugh Mobile to deliver bedside laughs and to initiate a *humor intervention*. A humor intervention may be described as a plan to promote joy and laughter in the treatment program for patient care.

The Duke Humor Project continues to bring joy bedside to cancer patients at Duke University Medical Center. The Laugh Mobile delivers humorous media bedside to patients and family twice weekly. Humor volunteers engage in yo-yo demonstrations, guitar playing, and practical jokes. For example, the patient may want to set up a "whoopee cushion" under the covers of his or her bed and then invite the doctor "to have a seat and take a load off." Water guns are also dispensed to allow the patient a way to fight back. It is all in the interest of building fun-loving relationships, and the staff is highly receptive to any humor statements from the patient, especially practical jokes.

One of the evolving aspects of the Duke Humor Project and the Laugh Mobile Program is the referral procedure used for targeting the patients. The professional oncology recreation staff attends grand rounds and gathers information about the patients who may be most receptive to humor. Background information is provided in a notebook that goes with the Laugh Mobile. This reports pertinent information on the patient and suggestions for the best approach. For example, the staff may relate that the patient is hard of hearing or that the patient may enjoy learning to juggle scarves. The humor volunteer comes in and sees each patient on referral. The volunteer reports back to the staff about how the humor intervention worked. This gives the hospital staff an opportunity to follow up between Laugh Mobile visits.

As a designer of humor programs such as the Laugh Mobile Program, I see humor and intentional laughter programs expanding to reach patients in all stages of recovery. I believe that to be effective, I must continue to volunteer with the cancer patients and the Laugh Mobile Program weekly. I am now opening new avenues for spreading the humor programming by the design of programs for bone marrow transplant and cardiac care patients. Each illness seems to have its own set of humorous episodes and strategies. It is my challenge to explore with the patient the areas that need more humor and to suggest funny coping strategies. Perhaps my greatest challenge is continually to seek new ways for the "humor impaired" to laugh and to invite the medical staff to enjoy more playfulness. I am confident that community-based groups such as Carolina Ha Ha, which offers both trained volunteers and professional program implementation, will continue to plant the seeds of comic caring and loving laughter.

IT MAY BE SERIOUS, BUT IT NEEDN'T BE SOLEMN

These healing hot springs of holistic "laughtears" are what I'm after in humor therapy.
I try to be playful but others won't respond.
If I ever needed humor it is now.
I want to smile and laugh, but that upsets my family.
—HOSPICE PATIENTS' COMMENTS
(*AMERICAN JOURNAL OF HOSPICE CARE*, 1990)

Salt water is the cure for everything; sweat, tears and the sea
—ISAK DINESEN

A couple of years ago a father-in-law was very ill. Once, when he came home from the hospital, it was his wedding anniversary. The son-in-law suggested that they invite a few friends over for dinner and he would cook a turkey.

He managed to get out of bed to join us. He enjoyed the meal, but the strain of feeding himself and the presence of guests were obviously tiring him. Noticing this and knowing that he could not hear very well, his wife wrote a note and passed it to the son-in-law to give to him. She realized what she just wrote and laughed out loud:

The note said, "Happy Anniversary dear. Do you want to go to bed?"

He read what his wife had written, looked up across the table, and with a twinkle in his eye and a smile on his face slowly said to her, "I would love to dear, but we have company."

It was only a brief moment of levity in his difficult last days, but it was a moment that was long remembered after he was gone.

Looking for humor in the not-so-funny world of serious illness may seem like a disrespectful thing to those who are suffering. However, situational humor, which inevitably arises during stressful times, is very appropriate.

Because of humor's ability to give a new perspective to any situation, it is an important coping tool for everyone involved in the dying process, including the physician.

Laughter is a powerful tool in powerless situations. It can give hope and an upper hand to patients, who are experiencing both physical and mental loss, as well as to physicians, who cannot change that loss or stop the demise of the patient.

The safest way for a physician to find that laughter is first to establish a rapport with the patient, then look for humor by listening to what the patient jokes about. Above all, do not go into a patient's room with a battery of jokes. First, jokes can be offensive, and second, when you enter a patient's room, you have no knowledge of whether they will be receptive to your kidding around. Keep in mind that humor is a wonderful bonding tool, but it can also backfire and create alienation.

Patty Wooten ("Nancy Nurse") once told a story about the time she was bathing a patient who had a rather large surgical scar down her front. The patient said, "Nurse, look at my scar. It looks just like Market Street in San Francisco." Puzzled by this remark, Patty questioned, "What do you mean, 'Market Street in San Francisco?'" "Well," replied the patient, "it goes from Twin Peaks to the waterfront." (Indeed, Market Street in San Francisco does run from Twin Peaks to the waterfront.)

Patty and the patient laughed uproariously together. Then, months later, Patty was bathing another woman who had a similar scar and told her this joke. The patient got highly insulted.

In the first case, humor came from a woman who was comfortable enough to laugh at what she had experienced; the second patient was not.

The best way to find humor when working with seriously ill patients is to listen to what they are saying. The patient is the one who will often give you the laugh lines.

One example comes from a man who had AIDS for 8 years. One day he had put up a Star of David, a crucifix, and a picture of Buddha on the wall.

A friend walked into the house and said, "You're a Quaker, why do you have these opposing religious items around?" The ill man who never missed a moment for some levity, replied, "Well, you never know who's right. I'm covering all bases!"

He was someone who could joke about his illness, because he would be the first one to poke fun at his difficulties. Your patients are the ones who will let you know if it is okay to kid around with them, supply you with laughs, and help you see death as less of a grave matter.

HUMOR IN HEALTH CARE

We think of humor as just fun and play—not serious. Yet, it is one of the most healthy, healing phenomena humans have. It is a cognitive, emotional, and physical response to stress. Humor gives us balance and a perspective and provides a comic relief and survival from all the seriousness of living.

Within the health care arena, which is probably one of the most stressful and craziest areas in which we live, humor is a major coping mechanism for patients and staff and a powerful tool for healing. It is the perfect mind-body connection! The humor, verbal or nonverbal, stimulates the feeling of mirth and the laughter, which researchers have found produces a healthy biochemical response in the body.

As an indirect form of communication, humor facilitates all the relationships and manages all the delicate situations that occur. It conveys messages and helps us get in touch with our feelings. And, when we laugh, we release those associated feelings.

Humor reduces all the social conflicts inherent in health care, and it facilitates change and survival in the system. As a major relief mechanism, humor reduces anxiety, provides a healthy outlet for anger and frustration, and is a healthy denial of all the heaviness of crises, tragedy, and death.

Humor is also a major source of coping for the caregiver and for the prevention of burnout. The health professional who can accept and value his or her need for laughter and comedy can then be comfortable using and encouraging humor with clients.

As a communication tool, humor should be an integral part of the total healing and caring process. Humor conveys our concern, understanding, warmth, and caring. As one patient said, when staff laughed and joked with him, he knew they cared.

For the health professional, the key to the therapeutic use of humor is being sensitive to whose needs are being met and being sensitive to the right time, the right place, and the right amount, like a judicious dose of good medicine. And always, humor must be used in the context of caring, a laughing with and not a laughing at.

HUMOR—ANTIDOTE FOR STRESS

Humor is a perceptual quality that enables us to experience joy even when faced with adversity. Health professionals work in stress-filled environments that place demands on their physical, emotional, and spiritual well-being (Maslach, 1982). Most caregivers are compassionate and sensitive individuals working with people who are suffering. This too can be a source of stress. Caregivers can experience what is known as *compassion fatigue*—feeling that they have very little left to give (Ritz, 1995). Finding humor in our work and our life can be one way to replenish ourselves from compassion fatigue (Ritz, 1995; Robinson, 1991; Wooten, 1995). This can be an effective self-care tool.

In his book *Stress Without Distress,* Selye (1974) clarified that a person's interpretation of stress does not depend solely on an external event, but also on the individual's perception of the event and the meaning he or she gives it; how one looks at a situation determines whether one will respond to it as threatening or challenging (Kobassa, 1983). In this context, humor can be an empowerment tool because it gives us a different perspective on our problems, and with an attitude of detachment, we feel a sense of self-protection and control in our environment (Klein, 1989; McGhee, 1994). As comedian Bill Cosby is fond of saying, "If you can laugh at it, you can survive it."

There is a type of humor called "gallows humor" (McGhee, 1994; Robinson, 1991) that is unique to people who deal with tragedy and suffering. Those outside the caregiving professions often do not understand our sometimes desperate need to laugh and may not appreciate this type of humor. The term *gallows humor* supposedly came into being when two brothers were being executed by hanging. Both were standing on the gallows, and one brother was already hanged when the other brother said, "Look at my brother there, making a spectacle of himself. Pretty soon we'll be a pair of spectacles."

This laughing bravado in the face of death is what caregivers also use to maintain their sanity amidst the horror. It is well documented that there is more laughter in the ICU, emergency room, and operating room than in other places in the hospital setting. Much of the humor is sexual or obscene, or jokes directly about the tragedy and suffering (Ritz, 1995; Rosenburg, 1991; Wooten, 1995). This appears to be a psychological game one plays with oneself and others, in hope of communicating, "See, I'm doing okay amidst all this horror. Really. See? I'm laughing!"

An ICU nurse shared with me a sign that the staff had placed in the visitor waiting area to explain what might be overheard and misunderstood (Box 14-3).

We attempt to maintain balance by offsetting tragedy in our lives with comedy. Another true story of this cathartic activity was shared by Wayne Johnston, an emergency room nurse:

> You saw me laugh after your father died. . . . To you I must have appeared calloused and uncaring. . . . Please understand, much of the stress health care workers suffer comes about because we do care. Sooner or later we will all laugh at the wrong time. I hope your father would understand, my laugh meant no disrespect, it was a grab at

BOX 14-3

Laughter in the Intensive Care Unit

If you are waiting . . .
You may possibly see us laughing; or even take note of some jest;
Know that we are giving your loved one our care at its very best!
There are times when tension is highest;
There are times when our systems are stressed;
We've discovered humor, a factor in keeping our sanity blessed.
So, if you're a patient in waiting, or a relative or friend of one seeing,
Don't hold our smiling against us, it's a way that we keep from screaming.

Sincerely,
The ICU Staff (anon)

balance. I knew there was another patient who needed my full care and attention . . . my laugh was no less cleansing for me than your tears were for you. (Johnston, 1985)

Laughter can provide a cathartic release, a purifying of emotions, and a release of emotional tension. Laughter, crying, raging, and trembling are all cathartic activities that can unblock energy flow (Goodheart, 1996).

An ability to laugh at our situation or problem gives us a feeling of superiority and power. We are less likely to succumb to feelings of depression had helplessness if we are able to laugh at what is troubling us. Humor gives us a sense of perspective on our problems. Laughter provides an opportunity for the release of uncomfortable emotions, which, if held inside, may create biochemical changes that are harmful to the body.

As the famous American humorist Mark Twain once said:

> Humor is the great thing, the saving thing. Afterall, the moment it arises, all our hardnesses yield, our irritations and resentments slip away, and a sunny spirit takes their place. (Klein, 1989)

Ⓔ Chapter References can be found on the Evolve website at http://evolve.elsevier.com/Micozzi/complementary/

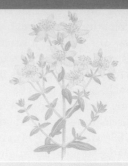

CHAPTER

15

PRINCIPLES OF BODYWORK: MANUAL AND MANIPULATIVE THERAPIES

PATRICK COUGHLIN

Modalities that involve touching, massaging, and manipulating the physical body provide a pathway to healing that are also thought to draw on the connection between body and mind, and have great antiquity. The well known abilities of touch to heal are widely recognized in modern medicine in the tradition of "laying on of hands." These "hands-on" therapies have been well organized and widely available as contemporary systematic therapeutic practice systems. This section presents the basic physiologic principles that underlie the manual therapies, as well as explaining each specific system that makes use of manual and manipulative modalities of healing. ∽

As with other complementary or alternative therapies, bodywork espouses a holistic philosophy that has the following outstanding tenets:

1. The body is a unit.
2. Structure and function are interrelated.
3. The body has an inherent ability to heal itself.
4. When normal adaptability is disrupted, disease may ensue.

Based on these defining principles, bodywork seeks to reverse structural imbalances to optimize the body's ability to self-correct or repair itself, which includes the defense against invasion from foreign substances or organisms.

CONCEPTS APPLICABLE TO MANIPULATION AND BODYWORK PRACTICES

A number of concepts based on physical laws and anatomical principles universally apply to manipulative and bodywork practices. These concepts are briefly described here so that they can be associated with the various forms (styles) of manipulative therapy, providing the reader with a greater understanding of the reasons for applying or seeking this type of treatment.

CONCEPT 1: BILATERAL SYMMETRY

The musculoskeletal system is usually described as being bilaterally symmetrical. That is, if the body is divided in half by a slice made from top to bottom and front to back along the midline (midsagittal plane), the right side should be a mirror image of the left side. This is an idealized assumption, of course, because few if any human bodies are truly symmetrical. Certain behaviors in which we engage, both consciously and unconsciously, are specifically designed to compensate for a lack of bilateral symmetry.

CONCEPT 2: GRAVITY

The human organism is similar to all other organisms in that we are subject to the laws of physics. Thus, the way we interact with planet earth is governed by the pull of the earth on our bodies: the force of gravity. Because of this constant force, and because our bodies have mass, we are given the weight that we must carry as we go about our activities.

CONCEPT 3: TENSEGRITY

Tensegrity was developed as a concept in the late 1940s by the renowned architect Buckminster Fuller and the sculptor Kenneth Snelson. The basic premise of *tensegrity* (tensional integrity) is that in many systems a balance exists between compression and tension. Tensegrity is "an architectural system in which structures stabilize themselves by balancing the counteracting forces of compression and tension which gives shape and strength to both natural and artificial forms." Architectural systems such as suspension bridges employ this concept, but it also is seen in biological systems, including the musculoskeletal system. The muscles and other soft tissues (e.g., joint capsules, tendons, ligaments) act as tensional elements, whereas the bones resist the compression of weight bearing. By maximizing the ratio of tensional elements to compression elements, such a system enables the organism to maintain balance and move with a minimum amount of energy expenditure.

CONCEPT 4: POSTURAL MAINTENANCE AND COORDINATED MOVEMENT

As we evolved from a quadrupedal (four-legged) to a bipedal (two-legged) stance, we became able to "manipulate" our environment because our hands were freed up, but we also became more unstable (visualize the result of removing two legs of a four-legged table; even the Eiffel Tower has four legs). From an architectural point of view, we became a buttressed arch system (the feet, legs, and pelvic girdle) supporting an elongated tower (the spine and head), with two cantilevered upper appendages (the arms) that can assist with balance. However, we are designed for movement (which is necessary for survival) and are rarely stationary, even when seated. Consider the act of walking: for about 40% of the time allotted to the normal gait cycle (the period of two strides), we are moving with only one foot on the ground. Because we engage

in considerable movement, we are constantly adapting to our position relative to the earth, which exerts its gravitational pull. Accordingly, we have programmed into our neuromusculoskeletal system a device that lets us know what that position is at all times and also directs the constant physical adjustments that we make. This is commonly referred to as the "equilibrial triad," which consists of the proprioceptive system, vestibular system, and visual system.

The *proprioceptive* system gives us positional information based on the state of contraction of each muscle in the body, as well as the position of each joint. The *vestibular* system is our "gyroscope," which gives us information on the position of the head and how it and the rest of the body are rotating or accelerating in space. The *visual* system allows us to be well aware of our surroundings and position because we can "see" where we are. In fact, because the visual system is so important in our normal range of activity, the other two parts of the triad act to support it. The proprioceptive and vestibular systems sense the position of the head relative to the body and adjust the posture so that the head is situated with the eyes aligned parallel to the horizon. Together, these three systems act with the motor system to produce coordinated movement, balanced posture, and a properly aligned head.

CONCEPT 5: CONNECTIVE TISSUE (FASCIA)

Connective tissue can be highly organized, as in the case of joint capsules, ligaments, tendons, the meninges of the central nervous system (CNS), intervertebral discs, and articular cartilage, or it can be more diffuse and seemingly less organized. *Fascia* is another name for the connective tissue that surrounds and gives architectural form to the tissues and organs of the body.

Fascia can be divided into two major components: superficial fascia and deep fascia. The *superficial* fascia resides just under the skin (the hypodermis) and serves as a staging center for the immune system (large quantities of antigens from the skin are presented to immune cells in this layer) and as a fat storage depot (the cause of significant attention). The *deep* fascia is much more extensive than the superficial fascia and exists throughout the body, serving to "connect" virtually all the tissues and organs. Skeletal muscles are surrounded by capsules of deep fascia, as are nerves and blood vessels (e.g., neurovascular bundles are wrapped in deep fascia). In this sense the deep fascia forms compartments that separate these tissues, but it also forms a structural continuum, and if physical stress is applied to one area of fascia, this continuity will result in effects' being "felt" in other areas or fascial layers as well (Figure 15-1). The compartmentalization of tissues by the deep fascia also results in the formation of specific pathways for, and limits to, the spread of infection (i.e., along fascial planes), as well as for the accumulation of fluid. Both superficial fascia and deep fascia are richly

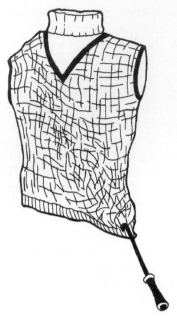

Figure 15-1 A force applied to one part of the fascial continuum affects the entire system.

supplied by blood and lymphatic vessels and by nerves (especially pain fibers).

On the molecular level, fascia is composed of a fibrous component (primarily the macromolecular proteins collagen and elastin) and a soluble, gel-like component, mostly water. The combination of fibrous and soluble components of the fascia creates, in effect, a molecular sieve through which chemical compounds diffuse to and from the cells of the body. Therefore the fascia has a great impact on the function of the organs it surrounds and infiltrates. Cells also reside in the fascia, including fat and immune cells in the superficial fascia. *Fibroblasts,* a major population of connective tissue cells, are responsible for the secretion of fibrous proteins that make up the scaffold of the fascia. Immune cells constantly patrol the fascia, seeking out foreign antigens as well as ingesting and destroying extracellular debris, including used constituents of the fibrous matrix. This creates a significant turnover in the components of the fascia and contributes to its innate adaptability to changing body conditions. The cellular component of the fascia can be significantly altered by a state of inflammation, in which large numbers of immune cells migrate into the area in response to tissue damage or antigenic challenge. Inflammation also stimulates fibroblasts to secrete larger amounts of collagen to reseal any breaches in the continuum, which results in scar formation or fibrosis.

Not only is the fascia very adaptable to the ever-changing internal environment, but it is also significantly affected by the aging process. As the human body ages, the chemical bonds that bind collagen molecules together, known as *cross-links,* become more prevalent. As this occurs, less space is available in the fascia for water and the other soluble components. The end result is a loss of

tissue water and an increase in the fibrous component, which in turn decreases the relative elasticity and physical adaptability of the tissue. In other words, the tissues dry up and become more brittle. This leaves the musculoskeletal system, in particular, significantly more susceptible to microtrauma and macrotrauma.

The physical properties of fascia have stimulated manual therapy practitioners to devise specific techniques to address these properties and the relations among the fascia and the tissue it surrounds. Just as the fascial matrix can become distorted from the forces brought to bear on it, it also can be restored to its original structural relationships by manual means. In addition, because of the continuity of the fascia throughout the body, local fascial distortions can produce distant effects. This is especially true in the case of muscle-associated deep fascia, which, if distorted, can alter the vector and function of that muscle.

The gel-like consistency of the soluble component of the fascia enables it to behave as a colloid, which resists force in direct proportion to its velocity. On the other hand, because of this property, fascia, like a colloid, will respond much more readily if force is applied slowly and gently. In addition, gentle application of force results in gradual yet sustained realignment of the fibrous component of the fascia, which can be palpated in the form of a "release." This is the rationale behind the development of myofascial, craniosacral, and other low-velocity techniques.

CONCEPT 6: SEGMENTATION (FUNCTIONAL SPINAL UNIT)

Anatomically, the human body is arranged lengthwise as a series of building blocks or segments. This can be observed most directly by the looking at the individual vertebrae that make up the spinal column, which extends from the base of the skull to the coccyx ("tailbone"). Just above the coccyx is the sacrum, a single bone resulting from the fusion of five vertebrae. This fusion is significant, because the sacrum articulates with the pelvic bones, which in turn articulate with the femurs. This relationship produces an arch that has the sacrum as its keystone.

Passing between the vertebrae and going from the spinal cord to the periphery are 31 pairs of spinal nerves (one for each side, with the exception of the coccygeal nerve, which is fused at the midline of the body). Each of these spinal nerves contains sensory and motor nerve fibers that are distributed around the body (Figure 15-2).

Most nerves are accompanied by arteries that supply blood to the same region supplied by the spinal nerve. In addition, the *neurovascular bundle* contains veins and lymphatic vessels, which serve to drain away waste products from the same territory. Thus, each segment of the body receives information (and is sending information back to the CNS) as well as nourishment, and each is being drained of waste products. It might appear that each segment functions as a separate entity, but this is not the case. Because of significant overlap both inside and outside the

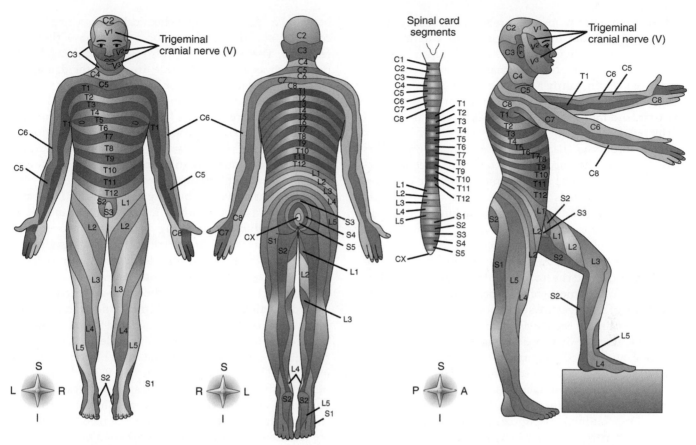

Figure 15-2 Spinal nerves and dermatomes. (Modified from Thibodeau GA, Patton KT: *Anatomy and physiology,* ed 7, St. Louis, 2010, Mosby.)

CNS, each segment is "aware" of what is transpiring in the segments adjacent to it.

The individual spinal nerve and all the tissues that it innervates, called the *segment* or the *spinal segment,* is also referred to as the *functional spinal unit (FSU)*. The FSU thus includes two adjacent vertebrae and the spinal nerves, skeletal muscles, and fascia between them; other bones, muscles, and fascia associated with the segment (e.g., ribs, intercostal muscles); the blood and lymphatic vessels that supply these tissues; and visceral structures within the body cavities that receive innervation from the autonomic portion of the spinal nerves.

CONCEPT 7: REFLEXES AND AUTONOMIC NERVOUS SYSTEM

The CNS, consisting of the brain and spinal cord, can be compared to a computer in that it is designed to integrate and process information. This information basically takes two forms: sensory (input) and motor (output). The most fundamental unit of information processing is the *reflex*. Information enters the CNS through a sensory neuron and is processed in the spinal cord or brain stem through an interaction between the sensory neuron and the motor neuron at a location known as a *synapse*. Motor information then leaves the CNS directly through a motor neuron to effect a response in a skeletal muscle. The most common example of this type of reflex (called *somatic* for the type of tissue involved) is the withdrawal response when a painful stimulus is encountered (e.g., when the hand touches a hot burner). The pain information is relayed through the spinal cord and out to the muscles, which causes the hand's removal before the sensation reaches the cerebral cortex and is perceived.

Although much of the sensory information coming into the CNS reaches consciousness (is perceived), much does not, and we go about our business neither knowing nor feeling what is happening. The same is true of motor activity, which can be voluntary or involuntary (see the discussion of the autonomic nervous system later and Chapter 8). An example of this involuntary phenomenon is the digestive system, which, under normal circumstances, functions without our knowledge (with the important daily exception of elimination). With respect to postural maintenance, if we are asked to attend to our position, we are usually able to do so (a test of this system [conscious proprioception] is to ask an individual to close the eyes and state the location and position of different parts, such as the hands and feet). However, we usually are not particularly attentive to our position (unless we lose our balance), and there is an entire division of the proprioceptive system (unconscious proprioception) that is never perceived. In short, we are constantly adjusting ourselves to adapt to the gravitational pull of the earth and our position relative to it, and most of this activity takes place at the level of the reflex.

The autonomic nervous system has as one of its responsibilities the unconscious control of visceral structures. These structures include smooth muscle (e.g., surrounding blood vessels and the bronchial tubes), cardiac (heart) muscle, glands, and lymphoid (immune) tissue. There are two divisions of the autonomic nervous system that have opposite actions: the *sympathetic* (thoracolumbar) division, responsible for arousal, or the "fight or flight" reaction; and the *parasympathetic* (craniosacral) division, responsible (among other functions) for stimulating the activity of the digestive system, or the "rest and digest" function. Although each division predominates in certain situations, the two divisions normally coexist in balance with one another to maintain a state of homeostasis, which is a form of internal equilibrium. The names "thoracolumbar" and "craniosacral" indicate the origin of the motor nerves of each division. Therefore the spinal nerves of the thoracolumbar region contain both somatic and sympathetic nerve fibers, whereas some of the cranial nerves and sacral nerves contain both somatic and parasympathetic nerve fibers.

Within the CNS, interactions between sensory and motor nerves are constantly taking place through reflexes. Although it has been long known that somatic and visceral reflexes occur, it has only recently been discovered that the two types of reflex loops overlap with one another. That is, stimulation of a visceral structure can produce a somatic response, and stimulation of a somatic structure can elicit a visceral response. This discovery is of extreme importance to the practitioners of manipulation, because it essentially validates the claim that manipulation has global effects on the body, especially with the maintenance or reestablishment of proper blood and lymphatic flow. In fact, it is quite arguable that manipulation of somatic structures (the musculoskeletal system) is entirely capable of restoring proper blood flow to visceral structures through reflexes mediated through the CNS.

CONCEPT 8: PAIN AND GUARDING, MUSCLE SPASM, AND FACILITATION

Patient: "Doc, it hurts when I do this."
Doctor: "Then don't do that!"

Pain is the result of a noxious stimulus that produces tissue damage. This stimulus can come from outside the body, such as a thermal or chemical burn, which is perceived at the skin and produces a classic withdrawal response. The stimulus can also come from inside the body, such as a sprained ankle, in which the damage is perceived at a muscle, joint or ligament.

If pain results from damage to a bone, joint, or ligament, a natural response is for the surrounding muscles to contract reflexively, producing a natural splinting of the area. This is also known as *guarding*. Another result of this type of damage is an altered gait pattern (a limp), which is merely an attempt by the body to "get off" the affected joint, if weight bearing causes additional pain. This can also happen when a paravertebral muscle is overstretched from a bending or lifting maneuver. Proprioceptors in that muscle report the stretch, causing a reflex contraction of that muscle. If the amount of damage is sufficient, the reflex contraction becomes stronger, and other muscles in the area are recruited to "guard" against further stretching and damage. The involved muscles are now considered to be in *spasm*. This reaction can spread (through reflex spread within the CNS) until much of the back musculature is involved. This is what happens when the back "goes out" and the person suffers back spasms. Because of the altered position of the body away from the norm and the prolonged spastic contraction, the involved muscles are required to do much more work than normal, which results in fatigue. When this occurs, muscle contraction results in the compression of local blood vessels, which in turn affects the nutrition of local tissue; this then exacerbates the problem by causing more pain. A downward spiral of pain → spasm → more pain → spasm can result.

Over time, as more and more sensory input is being fed to the CNS, the nerves that are reporting this information, as well as the nerves that are reacting (the motor neurons), become more sensitive. That is, their threshold for activity becomes significantly reduced. This situation is known as *facilitation* and is responsible to a large extent for the downward spiral just mentioned.

Presumably, muscle spasm lasts until the injury is healed and the surrounding muscles are allowed to release their grip on the area. This is why most allopathic physicians prescribe bed rest for back pain (and tell patients, "Don't do that"). Sooner or later the spasm will resolve on its own. However, this is not always the case, and the spasm can persist on a reduced level. This can cause the vertebrae normally moved by that muscle to become fixed in a certain position. The vertebrae may remain in that fixed position even when the muscle spasm is completely resolved. This also creates a need for a compensatory reaction or altered behavior to avoid the generation of more pain, as with a limp (see following discussion). In many patients it is possible to break the cycle of pain → spasm → more pain by the application of manipulative therapy.

CONCEPT 9: COMPENSATION AND DECOMPENSATION

As mentioned, the proprioceptive system is constantly reporting sensory information to the CNS regarding body position so that postural adjustments can be made, primarily to maintain the eyes parallel to the horizon (horizontal gaze). However, such compensatory behavior becomes more prolonged in certain situations. For example, in a person with one leg longer than the other (asymmetry), the pelvis on the "longer" side would be elevated relative to the other side. Because the sacrum is strongly connected to the pelvic bones, the base on which the fifth lumbar vertebra (L5) rests would be tilted toward the short side. This information would be reported by the proprioceptive system, and the FSU above the L4-L5 level would begin a compensatory reaction (through muscular contraction) to move the spine back into vertical alignment, creating a scoliotic curve. These compensatory reactions can occur all the way up the spine, as long as the result is a level head. This creates an overall increased load on the system as a whole and significantly increases the amount of work needed to maintain proper alignment.

In most cases, these responses work well, and no pain or damage is produced. This is especially true in younger people. As persons age, however, changes in body tissues, most notably loss of water and reduced elasticity, alter the mechanical properties of the body as a whole. Eventually the system fails and begins to decompensate. This results in an increase in the amount and number of compensatory reactions as the system becomes further decompensated; this eventually leads to tissue damage (usually on the microscopic level), which ultimately leads to pain, which may be chronic. This scenario explains in part the preponderance of complaints of low back and neck pain in the general population. In fact, musculoskeletal complaints cause about one third of all the office visits to physicians in the United States. On a holistic or preventive level, intervention to correct a musculoskeletal problem or dysfunction before it becomes chronic or debilitating would be sensible and cost effective in the long run. This is where manipulative therapy is indicated and most effective.

CONCEPT 10: RANGE OF MOTION AND BARRIER CONCEPT

Each joint of the body has a normal direction and amount of motion associated with it. This is referred to as *range of motion (ROM)*. When motion is outside of this normal range (a statistical norm that can very considerably), that joint is said to be "hypermobile" or "hypomobile." In addition, joints with a greater ROM are generally less stable than those with less ROM (e.g., hip and shoulder joints). In the spine the lumbar and cervical areas have the greatest ROM, which establishes an increased probability of instability and injury, especially in the lumbar spine,

where significantly greater weight is being borne. This is the principal reason for the relative frequency of lumbar and cervical problems in the general population.

Typically, if there is pain around a joint for any reason, ROM will be decreased or limited. In this case, motion is said to be "restricted." The restriction of motion in a particular direction or plane of space produces a "barrier" to normal motion. However, motion barriers may not necessarily be accompanied by or be the result of pain. In fact, barriers to motion exist under normal circumstances as "anatomical" barriers or "physiological" barriers. A good example of an anatomical barrier is seen in the elbow joint, where the olecranon process of the ulna locks into the olecranon fossa of the humerus, thus preventing overextension of the joint. Therefore the bones themselves present a motion barrier. Joint capsules and ligaments also create anatomical barriers. Physiological barriers are produced by the normal tone of the muscles around a joint, which also act in balance with one another, so that no individual muscle becomes too taut or stretched, producing damage. The proprioceptive system plays an important role in maintaining physiological barriers. If a guarding reaction is present, or if a muscle is in spasm, a temporary physiological motion barrier can be established, in this case referred to as a *restrictive barrier*. In this situation, as previously noted, manipulation can be effective in reducing or eliminating musculoskeletal dysfunction and restoring normal motion.

CONCEPT 11: ACTIVE VERSUS PASSIVE AND DIRECT VERSUS INDIRECT

In treating musculoskeletal disorders with manipulation, two approaches can be used in a variety of techniques. *Active* versus *passive* refers to the activity level of the patient: is the patient actively participating in the treatment, or is the practitioner doing the mechanical work?

Direct versus *indirect* refers to the motion barrier and the practitioner's approach to it. As discussed, a motion barrier is a decrease in normal ROM caused by an increase in the normal physiological motion barrier. The practitioner seeks to remove or release this barrier and restore normal motion. The technique employed can move the affected joint either toward the motion barrier (direct) or away from the barrier (indirect). As a simple example, consider a case in which the flexors of the elbow joint are in spasm, holding the elbow in flexion (bent) and creating a barrier to extension (straightening). A direct technique would be an attempt to move the joint into extension, that is, into or toward the motion barrier. An indirect technique would be to move the elbow joint further into flexion, producing a change in the position of the joint, which would be reported by the muscle and joint proprioceptors. Over a short time, this causes a reflex release of the spastic contraction of the flexor muscles, thereby eliminating the motion barrier.

The various techniques and healing traditions relating to manual and physical manipulations described in this section have their effects based on these eleven principles that describe the movement of the human body as an object in space and living on earth. In addition, many of these "hands-on" techniques consider the human body to have an energetic component whereby physical manipulations also affect the energy of the body, as well as the "mind-body." It is useful to keep in mind this duality of human beings both as physical bodies and as energetic bodies when reading the chapters of this section.

In summary, the practitioner of manual therapy seeks to restore proper anatomical and physiological balance in the patient. At least three types and subtypes of balance are potential targets of the various styles and techniques employed, as follows:

1. The restoration of proper joint range of motion and body symmetry
2. The restoration of balance of nervous activity
   a. Between sensory and motor systems
   b. Between somatic and autonomic nerves
   c. Between the sympathetic and parasympathetic divisions of the autonomic nervous system
3. The restoration of proper arterial flow and venous and lymphatic drainage for proper nutrition of all tissues of the body

Chapter References can be found on the Evolve website at http://evolve.elsevier.com/Micozzi/complementary/

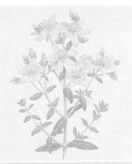

CHAPTER 16

MASSAGE AND TOUCH THERAPIES

JUDITH DELANY
PATRICK COUGHLIN

Manipulation as a therapeutic practice has existed for thousands of years. Although the date of origin of the earliest forms of manipulative therapy is unknown, it has been recorded that Hippocrates was skilled in the use of manipulation and taught it in his school of medicine, more than 2000 years ago. In China the history of manual therapy (tui na) predates the development of the technology necessary to produce the needles used for acupuncture, 3000 to 5000 years ago (Figure 16-1).

All the world's cultures can demonstrate the use of manipulation as a form of therapy. However, much of this information has been passed on as an oral rather than a written tradition, so documentation is difficult or impossible to obtain in many cases. Consequently, the types of manipulative therapy presented here are those for which information is readily available. Although this chapter describes the basic principles and theories of many well-known modalities, it is not totally inclusive of all that exist, nor does it include an extensive discussion of those that are mentioned.

THE BODY'S MATRIX—FASCIA

Whether the modality targets the osseous, muscular, visceral, or even acupuncture structures, it affects, in one way or another, a common integral component—fascia, the colloidal matrix of the body. Fascia comprises one integrated and totally connected network, from the soles of the feet to the attachments on the inner aspects of the skull, and divides the body by diaphragms, septa, and sheaths. However, fascia is so much more than just a background element with an obvious supporting role. It is a ubiquitous, tenacious, living tissue that is deeply involved in almost all of the body's fundamental processes, including its structure, function, and metabolism.

When any part of the fascial network becomes distorted, resultant and compensating adaptive stresses can be imposed elsewhere on the structures that it divides, envelopes, enmeshes, and supports, and with which it connects. The consequences of a structural cascade are not limited to the structural elements of

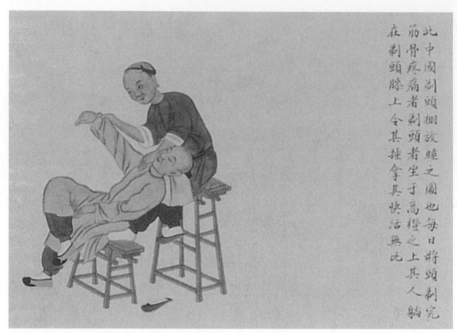

Figure 16-1 A patient receiving manipulation of the shoulder. Joint manipulation has always been an important feature of Chinese medical treatment. (Courtesy The Wellcome Trustees, London.)

muscle, tendon, ligament, bone, and disk. Pressure can also be imposed on the neural, blood, and lymph components, which course alongside and through them, and on the visceral organs and glands. Varying degrees of fascial entrapment of neural structures can, in turn, produce a wide range of symptoms and dysfunctions, such as by triggering the neural receptors within the fascia that report to the central nervous system (CNS) as part of any adaptation process. The sources of such signaling might include the pacinian corpuscles, which inform the CNS about the rate of acceleration of movement taking place in the area; the highly specialized, sensitive mechanoreceptors and proprioceptive reporting stations contained in the tendons and ligaments; or the hormones excreted by the glands, which serve as the chemical messengers of metabolism.

Massage and other manual techniques can be used to manipulate the connective tissues, affecting the fascia by altering its ground substance, elongating shortened tissues, and improving the biochemical environment of the cells. A diverse array of massage techniques and systems of application can offer a variety of affects on isolated tissues, overall structural integrity, and general well-being of the individual.

MASSAGE APPLICATION

As with other manipulative forms of therapy, the use of massage predates written history (Figure 16-2). The Greek physician Aesculapius, credited as the inventor of the art of gymnastics (Nissen 1889), became perhaps the first practitioner of the "one cause, one cure" approach when he abandoned the other forms of contemporary medical treatment in favor of massage to restore the free movement of body fluids and return the patient to a state of health. During the Renaissance the physician Ambroise Paré, author of a widely used surgery text, espoused the application of massage and manipulation and was reportedly the first to use the term *subluxation*. In 1813, Pehr Henrik Ling, a gymnastics instructor, founded the Royal Gymnastic Central Institute, where his theory of massage as passive gymnastics was developed. This work was the genesis of what is now referred to as "Swedish massage," and Ling is now considered by many to be the father of massage.

Johann Georg Metzger, a Dutch physician and student of Ling, developed a basic classification of massage techniques. Although Metzger's work was never published, his students von Mosengeil and Helleday wrote and published descriptions of the techniques. In the late nineteenth century the prominent French physician Marie Marcellin Lucas-Champonnière advocated the use of massage therapy in the treatment of fractures, arguing the case for consideration of soft tissue union in the healing process. His students, the English physicians William Bennett and Robert Jones, effectively brought massage to England. Bennett incorporated the use of massage at St. George's Hospital in London around 1899, and Jones used massage therapy at the Southern Hospital in Liverpool. Jones taught both James Mennell, author of the text *Physical Treatment by Movement, Manipulation, and Massage* (1917) and a tireless advocate of massage, and Mary McMillan, who was very influential in the introduction and promotion of massage in the United States.

There are many others who contributed both to the development of massage techniques and to documentation of massage through research and writing. Early in the twentieth century, several made significant and long-lasting contributions:

- Albert Hoffa's techniques, described in his text *Technik der Massage,* published in 1900, are still in use today. Hoffa advocated the limitation of massage to 15-minute treatments, with no pain experienced by the patient. Like Ling, Hoffa stated that massage should be applied from distal to proximal, with the point of reference being the heart. His adaptations included knuckling and circular effleurage, two-finger pétrissage, and other forms.
- Mary McMillan is credited with the categorization of massage into its five basic techniques. In each of those categories, she introduced innovative variations. She advocated the use of olive oil as a lubricant for its nutritional value when absorbed through the skin. Her influence in the development of massage is universally recognized, and her techniques have been widely adopted by massage therapists in the United States and elsewhere.
- Elisabeth Dicke, proponent of Bindegewebsmassage ("binding webs" massage) was a student of Hoffa who described massage based on the connective tissue system of the body. She described areas of referred pain on the back that indicate internal pathology but do not necessarily correspond to segmental distribution. Areas of tenderness do correspond to certain acupuncture points. Treatment is given with the middle finger in a series of sequenced strokes without lubricant.
- James Cyriax was a strong advocate of friction as the most effective technique in massage. He developed the "transverse friction massage" technique, which is widely used by manual therapists. Deep friction massage is used to stimulate increased circulation to the affected area. It can be applied to muscles, tendons, ligaments, and bones. Cyriax described these methods in detail in his book *Textbook of Orthopaedic Medicine,* volume II.

DEVELOPMENT OF ESSENTIAL THEORIES OF MASSAGE

As awareness of this form of treatment grew, so did the science of physiology, and the two entities became intertwined with the growth of the scientific basis of medicine. Some authors attribute the development of the physical therapy profession as being an outgrowth of massage. Many other forms of so-called bodywork, an assortment of which are discussed in this chapter, are also outgrowths of massage and its various techniques and styles.

One essential theory of massage therapy is based on the principle that the tissues of the body will function at optimal levels when arterial supply and venous and lymphatic drainage are unimpeded ("rule of the artery"). When this flow becomes unbalanced for any reason, muscle tightness and changes in the nearby skin and fascia will ensue, which may result in pain. The basic techniques of massage are designed to reestablish proper fluid dynamics and are directed at the skin, muscles, and fascia, although nerve pathways occasionally are included. In general, articulations are not directly addressed in this form of therapy, although they certainly may be affected by the applied techniques.

Obvious contraindications to massage or areas to avoid during the application of massage include skin infections or melanoma, bleeding (especially within 48 hours of a traumatic event causing bleeding into tissues), acute inflammation (e.g., rheumatoid arthritis, appendicitis), thrombophlebitis, atherosclerosis, varicose veins, and immunocompromised state (to avoid transmission of infection from massage practitioner to patient). In addition, a number of endangerment sites require that extra caution be exercised, such as the region of the carotid artery, supraclavicular fossa, posterior knee, femoral triangle, and abdominal cavity. Specific training may also be required, such as for intraoral applications or for work with lymphedema and cancer patients.

The techniques of massage are generally applied in the direction of the heart to stimulate increased venous and lymphatic drainage from the involved tissues. Muscles are addressed in groups, with one group being treated before advancing to the next. Different combinations of techniques are used depending on the objectives of treatment. Treatment typically begins with more gentle, superficial techniques before progressing to deeper, more aggressive applications. Massage is usually performed with a powder, oil, or other type of lubricant applied to the skin of the patient (or client), who lies prone, supine, or laterally on a table, or who may be seated in a massage chair. Verbal communication between the practitioner and patient is important, because the practitioner will use the cues given by the patient as a guide during the treatment.

The visceral effects of massage include general vasoactivity in somatic tissues as regulated by the autonomic nervous system. Also, effects on blood pressure and/or heart rate (usually decreases in both) can be observed as the person relaxes during the treatment.

MASSAGE TECHNIQUES

There are five basic techniques of massage, and all are of the passive variety (i.e., the practitioner does the work). These techniques are effleurage, pétrissage, friction, tapotement, and vibration. There are numerous variations of these basic techniques, which may create different outcomes within the tissue. For instance, effleurage applied at a moderate pace with lubrication increases blood flow and lymphatic drainage. However, effleurage applied with

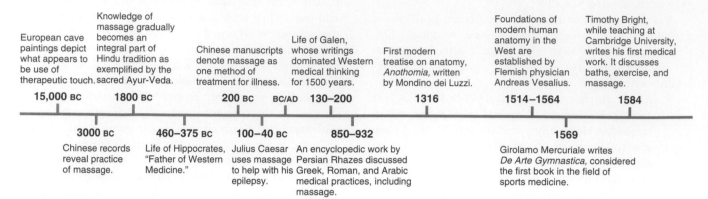

Figure 16-2 Massage timeline. (Modified from Salvo S: *Massage therapy: principles and practice*, ed 3, St. Louis, 2007, Saunders.)

almost no lubrication at a very slow pace produces a shearing force on the tissue that focuses more on changing the ground substance of the fascia. These variations in application provide a vast array of styles, methods, and versions of massage, each with its own foundational platform, despite their common roots in the basic techniques.

- Effleurage is the most frequently used massage technique and is typically used to begin a treatment session and introduce the patient to the process of touching (Figure 16-3). Effleurage is a gliding stroke applied with light to moderate pressure (superficial or deep), serving to modulate the arterial supply and venous and lymphatic drainage of the tissues contacted. The amount of pressure applied determines the layer of the body contacted; very light pressure affects only the skin, deeper pressure the superficial fascia, even deeper pressure the deep fascia, and so on. The thumbs, fingers, or entire palmar surface of the hand is used. A "knuckling" technique may be employed, or the proximal half of the ulna can provide a very broad surface of application. When used during the initial stages of treatment, effleurage is also used as a palpation diagnostic tool, as the practitioner searches for areas of altered texture, asymmetry, or tenderness. Specific long strokes are often used at the conclusion of treatment, especially if sleep induction is desired.
- Pétrissage is somewhat more aggressive than effleurage, with the thumb and fingers working together to lift and "milk" the underlying fascia and muscles in a kneading motion. Care is taken not to pinch or produce bruising. The effect of pétrissage is to increase venous and lymphatic drainage of the muscles and to break up adhesions (small areas of local fibrosis) that may be present in the fascia. Depending on the direction of application and vector of motion restriction (if any), this technique can be considered direct or indirect.

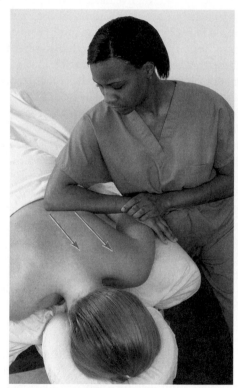

Figure 16-3 Effleurage can be applied with thumbs, fingers, palms, or forearm (as shown here). (Modified from Salvo S: *Massage therapy: principles and practice*, ed 3, St. Louis, 2007, Saunders.)

- Friction can be the most deeply applied massage technique (Figure 16-4). The tips of the fingers or thumb are used in a circular or back-and-forth movement. If deeper pressure is desired, or if the practitioner is easily fatigued, the heel of the hand, or sometimes even the elbow, can be used. Friction can be employed when production of heat is desired, when adhesions are present, or when the target tissue is too deep for pétrissage. Cyriax developed the

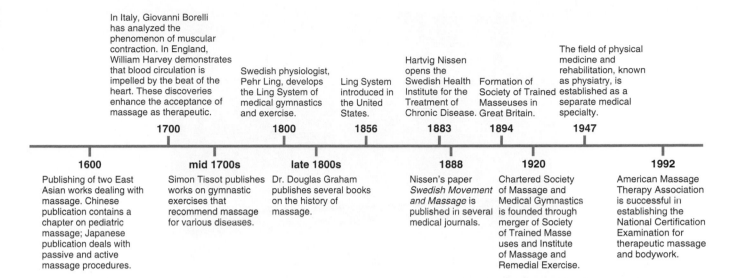

In Italy, Giovanni Borelli has analyzed the phenomenon of muscular contraction. In England, William Harvey demonstrates that blood circulation is impelled by the beat of the heart. These discoveries enhance the acceptance of massage as therapeutic.
1700

Swedish physiologist, Pehr Ling, develops the Ling System of medical gymnastics and exercise.
1800

Ling System introduced in the United States.
1856

Hartvig Nissen opens the Swedish Health Institute for the Treatment of Chronic Disease.
1883

Formation of Society of Trained Masseuses in Great Britain.
1894

The field of physical medicine and rehabilitation, known as physiatry, is established as a separate medical specialty.
1947

1600
Publishing of two East Asian works dealing with massage. Chinese publication contains a chapter on pediatric massage; Japanese publication deals with passive and active massage procedures.

mid 1700s
Simon Tissot publishes works on gymnastic exercises that recommend massage for various diseases.

late 1800s
Dr. Douglas Graham publishes several books on the history of massage.

1888
Nissen's paper *Swedish Movement and Massage* is published in several medical journals.

1920
Chartered Society of Massage and Medical Gymnastics is founded through merger of Society of Trained Masseuses and Institute of Massage and Remedial Exercise.

1992
American Massage Therapy Association is successful in establishing the National Certification Examination for therapeutic massage and bodywork.

technique of transverse friction massage, which is widely used by physical therapists. As with pétrissage, the direction of the applied technique, relative to any motion restriction, will determine whether the application is direct or indirect.

- Tapotement, often seen in classic fight films, involves rapid, repeated blows of varying strength delivered with the sides or palms of the hands, with the hands cupped, or with the fists. Occasionally, rapid pinching of the skin is done. The purpose of tapotement is to stimulate arterial circulation to the area; however, its ability to inhibit reflexive spasms should not be underestimated. Again, the technique should not produce bruising and is not applied over the area of the kidneys or on the chest, or over any recent incisions or areas of inflammation or contusion.

- Vibration that is manually applied is usually considered to be one of the more difficult of the massage techniques to master or to perform without becoming fatigued. The modern application of vibration typically employs a mechanical vibrator or oscillator of some type. When the hands are used, a light, rhythmic, quivering effect is achieved. Brisk snapping or strumming across certain tissues, such as erector spinae muscles, can also be considered a form of vibration, an effect that is similar to the vibration of a guitar string when strummed.

In addition, forces may be applied to the tissue that alter its length, mobility, and density. For instance, a shear force can be applied to a superficial muscle layer to slide it laterally across the underlying muscle and disengage it from a deeper layer, which results in more mobility between the two (Figure 16-5). Stretching a muscle's fibers can elongate the muscle and result in decompression of the associated joint(s). Elongation of a fascial plane might alter postural alignment and result in

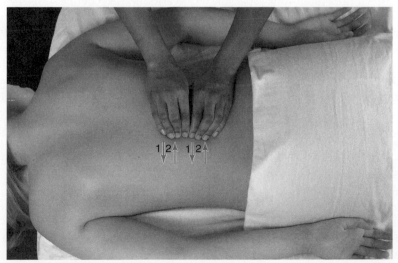

Figure 16-4 Friction applied to paraspinal muscles. (Modified from Salvo S: *Massage therapy: principles and practice*, ed 3, St. Louis, 2007, Saunders.)

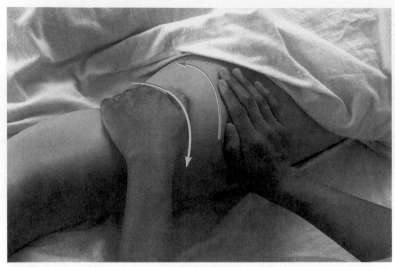

Figure 16-5 Shearing forces applied to the fascia of the anterior thigh. (Modified from Salvo S: *Massage therapy: principles and practice*, ed 3, St. Louis, 2007, Saunders.)

improved biomechanics of the region or of the structure body as a whole.

VARIATIONS IN APPLICATION OF TECHNIQUES

As mentioned previously, variations of these basic techniques produce different outcomes within the tissue. As a result, a multitude of methods, versions, and styles of massage have emerged, with many having broad perspectives regarding application. Although some of the concepts discussed later in the synopsis of various types of massage may seem foreign to the reader, it is worth remembering that many of these applications are centuries, if not millennia, old, far exceeding the experience in the practice of modern medicine. In particular, the Eastern theoretical platforms may contain concepts that do not appear to relate to Western understanding, especially those involving energy, meridians, and mysterious acupuncture points. However, with open and curious minds, even those most academically rooted in Western philosophy can find evidence to support the Eastern principles. The following discussion (after Chaitow and DeLany 2008) provides one example of how Eastern ideas can fit easily into a Western model when research provides physiological support.

Many experts believe that trigger points (see neuromuscular therapy discussion) and acupuncture points are the same phenomenon (Kawakita et al, 2002; Melzack et al, 1977; Plummer, 1980). When traditional and ah shi acupuncture points are both included, approximately 80% of common trigger point sites have been claimed to lie precisely where traditional acupuncture points are situated on meridian maps. (Wall and Melzack, 1990). Some (Birch, 2003; Hong, 2000) find the percentage to be flawed, particularly when the

trigger points are correlated with acupuncture points that are seen to be "fixed" anatomically, as on myofascial meridian maps. However, they agree that so-called acupuncture points may well represent the same phenomenon as trigger points. Ah shi points do not appear on the classical acupuncture meridian maps, but refer to "spontaneously tender" points that, when pressed, create a response in the patient of, "Oh yes!" (*ah shi*). In Chinese medicine ah shi points are treated as "honorary acupuncture points" and, when tender or painful, are addressed in the same way as regular acupuncture points (see Chapter 27). This would seem to make them, in all but name, identical to trigger points.

It is clearly important therefore, in attempting to understand trigger points more fully, to pay attention to current research into acupuncture points and connective tissue in general. Ongoing research at the University of Vermont, led by Dr. Helene Langevin, has produced remarkable new information regarding the function of fascia/connective tissue as well as its relationship to the location of acupuncture points and energy meridians (Langevin et al, 2001, 2002, 2004, 2005).

Langevin and colleagues present evidence that links the network of acupuncture points and meridians to a network formed by interstitial connective tissue. Using a unique dissection and charting method for location of connective tissue (fascial) planes, acupuncture points and acupuncture meridians of the arm, they note that overall, more than 80% of acupuncture points and 50% of meridian intersections of the arm appeared to coincide with intermuscular or intramuscular connective tissue planes (Langevin et al, 2002).

Langevin's research further shows microscopic evidence that when an acupuncture needle is inserted and rotated (as is classically performed in acupuncture treatment), a "whorl" of connective tissue forms around the needle, thereby creating a tight mechanical coupling between the tissue and the needle. The tension placed on the connective tissue as a result of further movements of the needle delivers a mechanical stimulus at the cellular level. They note that changes in the extracellular matrix may, in turn, influence the various cell populations sharing this connective tissue matrix (e.g., fibroblasts, sensory afferents, immune and vascular cells).

Chaitow and DeLany (2008) summarize the key elements of Langevin's research as follows:

- Acupuncture points, and many of the effects of acupuncture, seem to relate to the fact that most of these localized "points" lie directly over areas where there is fascial cleavage, where sheets of fascia diverge to separate, surround, and support different muscle bundles (Langevin et al, 2001).
- Connective tissue is a communication system of as yet unknown potential. Ingber and Folkman (1989) and Ingber (1993) demonstrated integrins (tiny projections emerging from each cell) to comprise a cellular signaling system that modify their function depending on the relative normality of the shape of cells. The structural integrity (shape) of cells depends on the overall state of normality (e.g., deformed, stretched) of the fascia as a whole.
- Langevin et al (2004) report: "'Loose' connective tissue forms a network extending throughout the body including subcutaneous and interstitial connective tissues. The existence of a cellular network of fibroblasts within loose connective tissue may have considerable significance as it may support yet unknown body-wide cellular signaling systems. . . . Our findings indicate that soft tissue fibroblasts form an extensively interconnected cellular network, suggesting they may have important, and so far unsuspected integrative functions at the level of the whole body."
- Perhaps the most fascinating research in this remarkable series of discoveries is that cells change their shape and behavior following stretching (and crowding or deformation). The observation of these researchers is that "the dynamic, cytoskeleton-dependent responses of fibroblasts to changes in tissue length demonstrated in this study have important implications for our understanding of normal movement and posture, as well as therapies using mechanical stimulation of connective tissue, including physical therapy, massage and acupuncture" (Langevin et al, 2005).

As more researchers seek to understand the overlap of Eastern and Western platforms, the parallels between the two will likely become more evident. In addition, as one can readily see, there are many "less than ideal" outcomes in modern patient care. It is important to consider that the following methods often offer significant relief to the suffering patient, with virtually no risk for potential injury or death. In an environment in which the costs of health care are out of control and the potential for medical error is seriously increasing, consideration for their use would seem to be practical, prudent, and economical.

The various massage styles and methods included in the following discussion are arranged alphabetically, with no indication as to which is most useful or more popular. The method's inclusion in the list and the length of any particular discussion only indicates the authors' familiarity and/or fascination with the method and implies nothing regarding its success, value, or appropriate use. Similarly, exclusion from this list simply indicates the restrictions applied in writing a brief chapter for this book, one that only begins to touch on the value, range, and scope of manual techniques. All appropriate touch therapies have intrinsic value, the degree of which is likely to be dependant on the practitioner's degree of mastery.

ACUPRESSURE AND JIN SHIN DO

Acupressure is the application of the fingers to acupuncture points on the body, or "acupuncture without needles." It is based on the meridian or channel system, which permeates Asian medical arts and philosophy. According to this system, there are 12 major channels through which the body's energy, or qi (or *chi*), flows. Although most of the channels are named for specific organs, they do not necessarily correspond to the anatomical body part, but rather are more functional in nature. Interruptions in the flow of qi (prana, ki, vital energy, as described in other cultures) cause functional aberrations associated with that particular channel. These interruptions can be released by specific application of needles or fingers.

Jin shin do, or the "way of the compassionate spirit," was developed by psychotherapist Iona Teeguarden (1978). It is a form of acupressure in which the fingers are used to apply deep pressure to hypersensitive acupuncture points. Jin shin do represents a synthesis of Taoist philosophy, psychology, breathing, and acupressure techniques. In accordance with this philosophy, the body is linked to the mind and spirit, and tender points found in the body can represent expressions of emotional trauma or locked memories (i.e., the somatoemotional component) (Figure 16-6).

The theory of jin shin do states that various stimuli cause energy to accumulate in acupuncture points. Repeated stress in turn causes a layering of tension at the point, known as *armoring*. The most painful point is termed the *local point* as a frame of reference. Other related tender points are referred to as *distal points*. Deep pressure applied to the point ultimately causes a release, and the tension dissipates. The overall effect is to reestablish flow in the channel and balance body energy. The context of the jin shin do treatment is as much psychological as

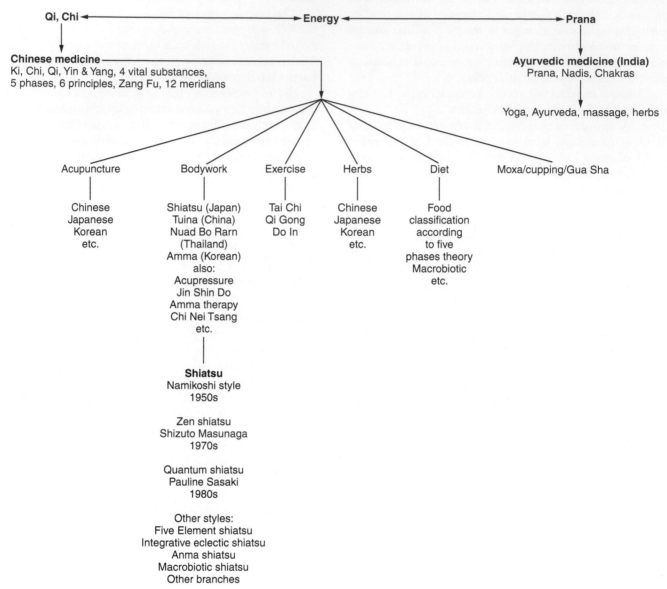

**Traditional Asian Medicine
2500 to 4000 years old**

Figure 16-6 Traditional Asian medicine focuses on the assessment and balancing of energetic systems. (Modified from Salvo S: *Massage therapy: principles and practice*, ed 3, St. Louis, 2007, Saunders.)

physical and reiterates the importance of the body-mind-spirit philosophy of this treatment form.

During the treatment session the practitioner identifies a local point and asks permission nonverbally to treat it. A finger is placed on the local point while another finger is applied to a distal point. Gradually increasing pressure is applied to the local point. After 1 or 2 minutes the practitioner feels the muscle relaxing, followed by a pulsation (practitioners of craniosacral therapy refer to this phenomenon as the "therapeutic pulse"). When the pulsing stops, the patient usually reports a decreased sensitivity at the point, indicating a successful treatment. Myofascial releases are sometimes accompanied by emotional releases as painful memories are brought to consciousness.

AYURVEDIC MANIPULATION

In Sanskrit, *Ayurveda* means "the study or science of life." As a healing art, Ayurveda is one of the world's oldest and, like the Indian culture, probably predates traditional Chinese medicine (TCM). As with TCM, Ayurveda has many concepts and components, as discussed elsewhere in this book. However, several principles pervade Ayurveda (as they do in TCM) and apply to the manual component of Ayurvedic treatment.

Both Ayurvedic and Chinese theory present five basic elements. In contrast to those of Chinese theory (fire, water, earth, wood, metal), however, Ayurveda defines space (ether), air, fire, water, and earth as the five basic elements. These elements flow through the body with one or more predominating in certain areas, corresponding to specific organs, emotions, and other categories. *Prana,* or the life force (qi, ki), also flows through the body, permeating the organs and tissues, and is especially concentrated at various points along the midline of the body, known as *chakras.*

The unity and balance of body, mind, and spirit have deep cultural roots in Ayurveda. Body structure and a person's actions, feelings, and beliefs all reflect his or her constitution. The human constitution is based on the relative proportions and strengths of these three constituents (mind, body, spirit) and the five elements. Three basic types of constitutions *(doshas)* are recognized, which are based on different combinations of the five elements. The first, *vata,* is a combination of air and space and is reflected in kinetic energy. The second, *pitta,* combines fire and water and reflects a balance between kinetic and potential (stored) energy, which is expressed in the third constitution, *kapha,* a combination of earth and water.

The manipulative treatment developed within the Ayurvedic tradition offers three types of touch. *Tamasic* is strong and solid, firmly rooted in the earth (and might be well suited for a kapha constitution). The application is fast, and time is needed for the mind and spirit to "catch up." Tamasic might correspond to high-velocity low-amplitude technique (osteopathy, chiropractic), tapotement (massage), or rubbing and thumb rocking (TCM). The second type of touch, *rajasic,* is slower and is used to expand and integrate initial manual explorations and findings. It is more in resonance with the mind and spirit. As mentioned earlier, greater depth can be achieved with less tissue resistance due to the makeup of the body fascia. Effleurage (massage) and myofascial release (osteopathy) might correspond to this type of touch, which in turn might be more suited to a pitta constitution. The vata constitution might benefit from the third type of touch, *satvic,* in which the application is very slow and gentle and can follow the intention of the mind and spirit. This might correspond to cranial osteopathy, sacro-occipital technique (chiropractic), counterstrain (osteopathy), Trager work, the Feldenkrais method, or healing or therapeutic touch.

In a massage-oriented treatment, different oils are used as lubricants according to the constitution of the individual and the problem to be treated. The patient is prone or supine, lying on either side, or sitting up, with the positions arranged in a specific sequence. Strokes are applied either toward or away from the heart, also in a specific sequence. Another technique, which is rarely encountered, uses the feet to perform the manipulation.

The practitioner stands above the patient, who is lying prone on a reed mat, and applies the technique with the feet. Oils again are used as lubricants, and to maintain balance, the practitioner holds onto a cord strung lengthwise above the patient. The strokes go from the sacrum up the spine and out to the fingers, then back down to the feet. One side is done, then the other. The patient then lies supine, and the process is repeated.

Techniques can be direct or indirect relative to motion barriers. They can also be active or passive. Both the patient and the practitioner act as partners during treatment, exploring tissue and motion in an attempt to unlock the body and restore the unimpeded flow of prana and constitutional balance. Visualization, nonverbal communication, and mind intent are elements of treatment, regardless of the technique employed.

ENERGY WORK

Energy work refers to the techniques that have developed either as part of ancient traditions (e.g., qigong, Qi Gong) or as recently "discovered" methods in which the practitioner manipulates the bioenergy of the patient. The theory of bioenergy basically states that a life force, or vital energy, permeates the entire universe. This energy flows through all living things in distinct patterns. These patterns of flow are reflected in the meridian system (where *qi,* or *chi,* is the name of the life force) originally conceived by the Chinese and in the chakra system of Hindu tradition (where the word *prana* is used to indicate this force). Various forms of exercise have been developed for the cultivation of bioenergy, including yoga, internal qigong, and t'ai chi.

Three basic concepts are important in understanding energy work: intent, cooperation, and the tripartite nature of the human. *Intent* is important in that the practitioner projects his or her mind intent to heal into the patient. For this reason, that intent must go one step further than the "do no harm" doctrine of Western therapeutics to an attitude of love and concern. Intent also assumes a high level of visualization. *Cooperation* implies the partnership between the practitioner and patient as participants in the healing process, with neither being exclusively active or passive. The *tripartite concept* refers to the acceptance of three parts of the human: body, mind, and spirit. This concept is envisioned in the much older Asian cultures as going beyond religion, whereas Western cultures rely on belief systems driven by faith. In addition, the "scientific," reductionist approach of conventional Western medicine is rather dismissive of spiritual aspects and has only recently acknowledged the mind-body connection. Although there are many systems of energy work, four are included here, two rooted in Eastern teachings and two developed in Western application.

The Chinese term *qigong* (or qi gong, Qigong, Qi Gong) refers to the manipulation of bioenergy and loosely translated means "qi work." Qigong can be internal, in which an individual can strengthen and balance the flow of qi within the self, or external, in which a trained practitioner can project his or her qi into a patient to induce a therapeutic effect.

Although the vast majority of the vital energy of an organism is contained within the body, some of it radiates off the skin, the "aura," which has been visualized using Kirlian photography. The qigong practitioner is able to palpate the meridian system through this aura, locate points of blockage, and free these blockages by projecting his or her qi into the patient, using intent and visualization. As in Trager work, the Feldenkrais method, and yoga, specific "external qigong" exercises have been developed that, when performed by an individual, serve to cultivate qi within the self. Qigong is also a natural result of long-term "internal" martial arts training, in which practitioners are capable of seemingly superhuman feats of strength and balance.

Reiki (literally "universal energy") is a method that most likely originated from qigong as practiced by the Chinese Taoists and Buddhists. It probably disappeared from practice in Japan at some point, only to be "rediscovered" by Dr. Mikao Usui in the mid-nineteenth century. Usui was interested in determining the nature of spiritually oriented healing power, as expressed through such individuals as Jesus Christ and the Gautama Buddha. After much study, including a doctorate from the University of Chicago, he began an extended period of fasting and meditation. At the end of this period, he reportedly received a vision and the ability to channel "reiki" through his body to effect healing in others. From that point, he continued healing, eventually training others in his method. Usui handed the title of Grand Master to Dr. Hiyashi Chugiro, who in turn passed it to Hawayo Takata, a Hawaiian woman of Japanese descent. In this way, reiki was exported from Japan to the West.

For practitioners, reiki must be "received" from a master or teacher. Only then is an individual able to effect healing. There are three degrees of reiki training. The first-degree practitioner is capable of giving a basic treatment with the hands on the patient, or about 1 inch away from the skin if touching is not possible. The second-degree practitioner can effect healing with the hands removed from the body, and treatments can be given at a faster rate. The third-degree practitioner is referred to as a "master" and is qualified to teach reiki.

The objective of reiki treatment is to restore internal harmony to the body and to release any blockages, which may be physical or emotional. The five principles of reiki are as follows:

1. Today I give thanks for my many blessings.
2. Just for today, I will not worry.
3. Today I will not be angry.
4. Today I will do my work honestly.
5. Today I will be kind to my neighbor and to every living thing.

During a reiki treatment the hands of the practitioner are placed with the fingers together on the patient. As energy is transferred from giver to receiver, the hands and the area treated become warm, which indicates a release of tension in the area and an increase in the blood flow. The head of the patient is treated first (four locations or positions), followed by the front (five positions) and back (five positions) of the body. Each position is held for 8 to 10 minutes (or less, if the practitioner is above first degree). Problem areas may be held longer until a result is sensed. The hand positions correspond to the energy points or chakras, identified in Hindu tradition, as well as other points. The treatment is completed with a series of general myofascial techniques, including kneading, counterforce, and stroking (effleurage), to close the energy channels.

As with other energy-oriented manipulative techniques, reiki requires significant verbal and nonverbal communication between the giver and receiver, who act in partnership. Permission must be granted both consciously and subconsciously for healing to be successful. Somatoemotional release is quite possible in this treatment.

Therapeutic touch, another form of energy work, was developed by Dr. Dolores Krieger (1992) and Dora Kunz in the late 1960s and early 1970s. In this style of bodywork, energy is directed through the hands of the "giver" (either on or off the body, usually off) to activate the healing process of the "receiver." The therapist essentially acts as a support system to facilitate the process. Therapeutic touch treatments typically last 20 to 25 minutes and are accompanied by a relaxation response and a decrease in perceived pain. Although skeptics have claimed that this technique merely elicits a placebo effect (an interesting concept in itself), successes have been reported with comatose patients, patients under anesthesia, and premature infants.

Therapeutic touch posits that humans are open energy systems, bilaterally symmetrical, and that illness is the result of an imbalance in the patient's energy field. The healer places himself or herself between the patient's illness and the patient's energy field to effect the healing process. The receiver must accept the energy of the healer and the necessity of change for the healing to occur. This should happen both consciously and subconsciously.

There are two phases of the treatment: assessment and balancing. Before balancing the practitioner "centers" himself or herself, entering a state of relaxation and awareness. The hands are moved around the patient's body at a distance of 2 to 3 inches. The patient's energy field is encountered and assessed by feeling for changes in temperature, pressure, rhythm, or a tingling sensation. Simultaneously, the practitioner nonverbally requests the permission of the patient to enter the patient's field and effect a change. During the balancing phase the healer (sometimes referred to as the "sender") then attempts to bring the two energy fields into a harmonic resonance through intent and visualization.

The attitude of the sender is one of empathy and compassion. The intent of the treatment is to facilitate the flow of vital energy, to stimulate it, to dissipate areas of congestion, and to dampen any areas of increased activity. In addition, the concept of rhythm and vibration is used, with color observed as a product of different frequencies within the field. At the beginning of the treatment, at the end of the treatment, or at both times, the practitioner "smoothes" out the patient's energy field by running the hands from head to toe. This sometimes has a cooling effect and is referred to as *unruffling*.

Healing touch, as developed by Barbara Brennan (1988), is similar to therapeutic touch in that the healer seeks to balance the energy field of the patient. A specific sequence of techniques is used in which the healer encounters, assesses, and treats different layers of the patient's visible "aura," correcting any imbalances and smoothing out the field. Healing touch is somewhat more spiritually oriented that therapeutic touch, using techniques such as channeling and employing colors and crystals to assist in the process.

These "energy-based" techniques (in addition to many of the other techniques mentioned) emphasize the importance of psychoemotional cooperation and participation by the patient (i.e., the mind-body connection) for successful application. In addition, the mind intent of the manipulator comes into play as the director of his or her internal energy outward and into the patient. This concept is quite controversial by Western standards of scientific analysis.

Although critics refer to these and other manipulative techniques as "pseudoscience" because of a lack of supportive evidence, the power of the technique and of the mind are not to be undervalued. Clinical outcomes studies have indicated that the intent of both the patient and the clinician have a demonstrable effect in determining treatment outcome. This evidence sheds new and interesting light on the placebo effect as a real phenomenon (especially in light of the fact that placebos are "effective" in randomized drug trials about 30% of the time). It also indicates that treatment of the somatic component of disease can be approached effectively through acknowledgment of the "three-legged stool" model of the human: body, mind, and spirit.

FELDENKRAIS METHOD (AWARENESS THROUGH MOVEMENT, FUNCTIONAL INTEGRATION)

Moshé Feldenkrais (1904-1985) was an Israeli physicist who developed a system of movement and manipulation over several decades (Feldenkrais, 1991). The Feldenkrais method is divided into two "educational" processes. The first, *awareness through movement,* is a sensorimotor balancing technique that is taught to "students" who are active participants in the process. The students are verbally guided through a series of very slow movements designed to create a heightened awareness of motion patterns and to reeducate the CNS to new patterns, approaches, and possibilities (as in learning t'ai chi).

The second process is referred to as *functional integration.* This is a passive technique using a didactic approach, not at all unlike Trager table work (see discussion later in this chapter). The practitioner acts as "teacher" and the patient as "student." The teacher brings the student through a series of manipulons to reestablish proper neuromotor patterning and balance. *Manipulons* are a manipulative sequence of information, action (as initiated by the practitioner), and response. They are gentle and are treated as exploratory, with the therapist introducing new motion patterns to the patient. Manipulons are referred to as "positioning," "confining," "single," or "repetitive." They can also be "oscillating." In all cases the teacher plays a supportive and guiding role while creating a nonthreatening environment for change. Functional integration can be considered a combination of passive, articulatory, or functional techniques.

LYMPH DRAINAGE TECHNIQUES

Manual lymph drainage techniques incorporate application of light pressure to the skin and superficial fascia in a particular pattern that encourages an increase in the movement of lymph. In addition, lymphatic pumps are rhythmic techniques applied over organs, such as the liver and spleen, to increase drainage. The thoracic diaphragm is also sometimes used as a lymphatic pump, because movement of this structure creates increased abdominal pressure, which "pumps" the nearby cisterna chyli, a dilated portion of the thoracic lymph duct that serves as a temporary reservoir for lymph from the lower half of the body (Figure 16-7).

The hand stroke used in lymph drainage is distinctly different from effleurage. Effleurage that is applied in the direction of the heart can also increase the venous and lymphatic drainage of the involved structure(s). However, deeply applied effleurage can inhibit lymph movement and even result in damage to the lymphatic vessels, particularly if the region is already engorged with excessive lymph. Using very light pressure, lymph drainage applies a rhythmic short stroke that creates a short pulling action on the skin and superficial fascia, which is then abruptly released. A turgoring effect encourages the movement of lymph into the lymph capillary. The lymph then moves along the vessels, which empty into progressively larger lymph vessels, until the lymph eventually rejoins the vascular system at the subclavian veins.

Lymph drainage therapy is useful in a variety of clinical settings to encourage overall health and is profoundly useful in postsurgical and posttrauma care. The edema

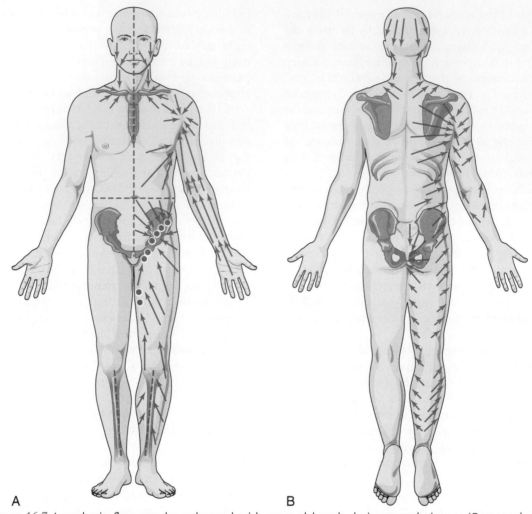

A   B

Figure 16-7 Lymphatic flow can be enhanced with manual lymph drainage techniques. (Borrowed with permission from Chaitow L, DeLany J: *Clinical application of neuromuscular techniques: practical case study exercises,* Edinburgh, 2006, Churchill Livingstone.)

associated with sprains, strains, and a variety of sport injuries can often be quickly reduced with these techniques. The Vodder method of lymph drainage therapy and the Chikly method of manual lymph drainage are the two most popular methods in this highly effective and broadly applicable modality. Although the aims of the two methods are similar, the styles of application and of teaching are moderately different. Developers of both methods have published textbooks and journal articles to support their concepts.

MUSCLE ENERGY TECHNIQUE

Muscle energy technique (MET) can be applied directly or indirectly to individual muscles as well as to muscle groups (Chaitow, 2006). When MET is applied *directly* (i.e., toward the motion barrier, or in an attempt to lengthen a shortened or spastic muscle), the technique is based on the principle of *reciprocal inhibition,* which states that a muscle

(e.g., flexor) reflexively relaxes as its antagonist (the associated extensor) contracts. Conversely, if a muscle in spasm is contracted against resistance and then relaxed, the effect often results in increased range of motion (ROM), or reduction of the motion barrier. This *indirect* application is based on the principle of *postisometric relaxation* (also known as *postcontraction relaxation*) (Lewit and Simons 1984).

This technique is one of the few "active" techniques in manual therapy, that is, the patient does the work. A distinction of MET is the amount of effort exerted by the patient. Usually, less than 20% of the total strength of the muscle is brought to bear during the interval of contraction. Another way of showing this is through the "one-finger rule," in which the amount of force necessary is the force needed to move a single finger of the practitioner when the practitioner lightly resists the contraction. This is in contradistinction to the proprioceptive neuromuscular facilitation technique often used in physical therapy, which employs a maximal muscle contraction and may expose the patient to risk of injury. A thorough knowledge of muscle attachments and their motion vectors is necessary to apply MET effectively and efficiently.

MYOFASCIAL RELEASE

Myofascial release is a gentle technique that uses knowledge of the physical properties of the fascia as it relates to muscles (Figure 16-8). Although some skill is necessary to apply this technique effectively, it is simple to learn and easily applied. The practitioner uses light and deep pressure, depending on the target structures, to palpate motion restriction within the fascia and moves toward or away from the restriction. The position is held until a "release," or softening, is felt, the perception of which is the most difficult aspect of application. The tissues are then slowly returned to their original position. The release can be the relaxation of muscles, changes in the viscosity of the ground substance of the fascia, the slow breaking of fascial adhesions, or the realignment of the fascia to a more appropriate orientation.

MYOFASCIAL–SOFT TISSUE TECHNIQUE

The myofascial–soft tissue technique is a combination direct-indirect massage technique for reducing muscle spasm and fascial tension. It is similar to pétrissage, except that more parts of the hand are typically employed. This technique can be used as a prelude to the high-velocity low-amplitude technique.

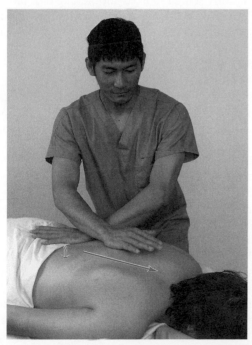

Figure 16-8 A crossed-arm myofascial release (MFR) can be applied broadly to the tissues to alter the ground substance of the fascia. (Modified from Salvo S: *Massage therapy: principles and practice,* ed 3, St. Louis, 2007, Saunders.)

NEUROMUSCULAR THERAPY (NEUROMUSCULAR TECHNIQUES)

Neuromuscular therapy (NMT) is a precise and thorough examination and treatment of the soft tissues of a joint or region that is experiencing pain or dysfunction. As a medically oriented technique, it is primarily used for the treatment of chronic pain or as a treatment for recent (but not acute) trauma; however, it can also be applied to prevent injury or to enhance performance in sports.

NMT emerged on two continents almost simultaneously, but the methods had little connection to each other until recent years. In the early twentieth century, European "neuromuscular technique" emerged, primarily through the work of Stanley Lief and Boris Chaitow. For the last several decades, it has been carried forward through the writing and teaching skills of Leon Chaitow, DO. The protocols of North American "neuromuscular therapy" also derived from a variety of sources, including chiropractic (Raymond Nimmo), myofascial trigger point therapy (Janet Travell, David Simons), and massage therapy (Judith DeLany, Paul St. John). Over the last decade, Chaitow and DeLany (2002, 2008) combined the two methods in a two-volume text that comprehensively integrates the European and American™ versions. NMT continues to evolve, with many individuals teaching the techniques worldwide.

One of the main features of NMT is step-by-step protocols that address all muscles of a region while also considering factors that may play a role in the presenting condition. Like osteopaths, neuromuscular therapists use the term *somatic dysfunction* when describing what is found during the examination. Somatic dysfunction is usually characterized by tender tissues and limited and/or painful range of motion. Causes of these lesions include, but are not limited to, connective tissue changes, ischemia, nerve compression, and postural disturbances, all of which can result from trauma, stress, and repetitive microtrauma (stress due to work and recreationally related activities). Consideration is also given to nutrition, hydration, hormonal balance, breathing patterns, and numerous other factors that impact neuromusculoskeletal health. A distinct focus of treatment is the identification and treatment of *trigger points,* noxious hyperirritable nodules within the myofascia that, when provoked by applied pressure, needling, and so on, radiate sensations (usually pain) to a defined target zone (Figure 16-9).

Although the European and American versions have unifying philosophical threads, there are subtle, yet distinct, differences in the palpation methods. Both methods examine for taut bands that are often associated with trigger points and both use applied pressure to treat the pain-producing nodules. However, European NMT uses a slow-paced, thumb-drag method, whereas and NMT American™ version uses a medium-paced thumb or finger gliding

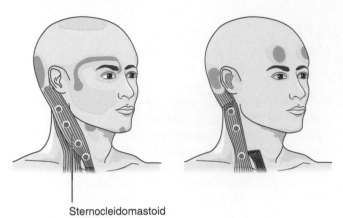

Sternocleidomastoid
muscle

Figure 16-9 Neuromuscular therapy (NMT) focuses attention on locating and treating trigger points (TrPs). TrP referrals from sternocleidomastoid can produce a variety of symptoms, including facial neuralgia, headache, sore throat, voice problems, hearing loss, vertigo, ear pain, and blurred vision. (Borrowed with permission from Chaitow L, DeLany J: *Clinical application of neuromuscular techniques*, vol 1, ed 1, Edinburgh, 2008, Churchill Livingstone.)

stroke. There is also a slightly different emphasis on the manner of application of trigger point pressure release (specific compression applied to the tissues) for deactivation of trigger points. In addition, American NMT offers a more systematic method of examination and treatment, whereas European methods use less detail in palpation of deeper structures, preferring to incorporate positional release and other methods for the deeper treatment. European methods also focus significantly more on superficial tissue texture changes than their American counterparts.

Both European and American NMT support the use of hydrotherapies (hot and cold applications), movement, and self-applied (home care) therapies. Both suggest homework to encourage the patient's participation in the recovery process, which might include stretching, changes in habits of use, and alterations in lifestyle that help to eliminate perpetuating factors. Patient education may also be offered to increase awareness of static and dynamic posture in work and recreational settings, and to teach the value of healthy nutritional choices. Referral to another health care practitioner may also be considered, especially when visceral pathology is suspected.

A successful foundation includes taking a thorough case history, including the patient's account of the precipitating factors, and performing a complete examination of the soft tissues. Although many decisions will be individual to each case, the NMT protocols are performed while keeping a few basic rules in mind. Superficial tissues are treated before deeper layers, and proximal areas are treated before distal regions. Every palpable muscle in the region is assessed, not just those whose referral patterns are consistent with the person's pain or which are thought by the practitioner to be the cause of the problem.

The first aim is to increase blood flow and soften fascia. Although gliding strokes are often the best choice, sometimes tissue manipulation (sliding the tissues between the thumb and finger to create shear) works better. Depending on the stiffness of the tissues, hot packs might be used to further encourage softening. Then the gliding strokes and manipulation can be repeated, alternating with the application of heat, or a few moments can be allowed in between for fluid exchange.

Once the tissues have become softer and more pliable, the practitioner palpates for taut bands. These bands, in which select fibers are locked in a shortened position, vary in diameter from as small as a toothpick to larger than a finger. At the center of the band there is often a thicker, denser area that is associated with trigger point formation.

Once the fiber center is located, it is evaluated for a trigger point, to which pressure is applied until a degree of resistance (like an "elastic barrier") is felt. Sufficient pressure is applied to match the tension, which provokes or intensifies the referral pattern to the target zone. The applied pressure should be monitored, so that what is felt by the patient is no more than a moderate level of discomfort (7 on a scale of 1 to 10). Although the patient may feel some tenderness in the area that is being pressed, usually the focus is on the pain, tingling, numbness, burning, or other sensation in the associated target zone of the trigger point. The common target zones are usually distant from the area and are predictable. They have been well illustrated in numerous books and charts.

As the pressure is sustained, within 8 to 12 seconds the sensations being reported should begin to fade as the practitioner feels a softening of the compressed nodule or (rarely) a profound release. The pressure can be sustained for up to approximately 20 seconds, but longer than this is not recommended because this "ischemic compression" reduces blood flow.

Trigger point treatment (by pressure, needling, spray and stretch, or other method) can be repeated several times within the therapy session, with a few moments between each application to allow fluid exchange to occur. Each time treatment is reapplied, the practitioner should notice the need to increase the level of applied pressure to stimulate the same level of sensation. In some cases, the tenderness and referred sensations will be completely eliminated within one session.

As the final step, the fibers associated with the taut band should be lengthened. This might include passive or active stretching if the associated attachment sites are not too sensitive. If the attachments are moderately tender, inflammation should be suspected and elongation performed manually to avoid putting stress on the attachments. This can be achieved by using a precisely applied myofascial release or a double-thumb gliding stroke in which each thumb simultaneously slides from the central nodule to a respective attachment, applying tension to the band as the thumbs slide away from each other.

Specific training in the use of NMT protocols is necessary, because many contraindications and precautions are associated with NMT use. The protocols can be incorporated into any practice setting and are particularly useful when interfaced with medical procedures. Many complex conditions can benefit from the thorough protocols and treatment strategies used in NMT.

REFLEXOLOGY

In the Asian meridian system of the body, all the major meridians or channels are represented in the hands and feet. Because acupuncture is usually not done on the soles of the feet because of their sensitivity, a system of foot massage was developed in China. William H. Fitzgerald, who called it "zone therapy," introduced this system to the United States in 1913. Now referred to by Dwight Byers and others as *reflexology,* the technique involves the application of deep pressure to various points on the hands and feet by the thumbs and fingers of the practitioner. The feet receive the preponderance of attention in this method, with various identified points not only corresponding to the energy channels of the body but also to specific organs and systems. When treatment is given, areas of tenderness or texture change are identified and pressure is applied. This has the effect of opening that channel and allowing body energy to flow unimpeded through its entirety. When all points are successfully treated, the energy system is flowing and balanced (see Chapter 19).

ROLFING AND OTHER STRUCTURAL INTEGRATION METHODS

Rolfing, a form of structural integration, was developed in the middle of the twentieth century by Ida Rolf. Rolf, who had a PhD in biochemistry, sought help from an osteopath after being dissatisfied with conventional medical treatment of her pneumonia. After this experience, Dr. Rolf embarked on a lengthy period of study, including yoga study, which resulted in the manipulative system that now bears her name (Rolf, 1975, 1997, Rolf and Thompson, 1989). In 1971, she founded the Rolf Institute of Structural Integration in Boulder, Colorado, which now trains and certifies practitioners of this style.

The theory of *Rolfing* is based primarily on physical consideration of the interaction of the human body with the gravitational field of the earth. As a dynamic entity, the human body moves around and through this field in a state of equilibrium, storing potential energy and releasing kinetic energy. In this system, form (potential energy) is in direct proportion to function (kinetic energy), and the balance between the two is equivalent to the amount of energy available to the body. In simple terms, the worse

the posture, the more energy we consume on a baseline level, and thus the less we have available for normal activity. Furthermore, the physical energy of the body is in direct proportion to the "vital energy" of the person. Ideally, the body is always in a position of "equipoise," but this is seldom, if ever, the case.

Rolfing traditionally involves a 10-session treatment protocol designed to integrate the entire myofascial system of the body. Photographs are taken of the patient before and after each session or at the beginning and end of a series of treatments to evaluate progress. The body is treated as a system of integrated segments consolidated by the myofascial system. Attempts are made through "processing," as the treatment is called, to lengthen and center through the connective tissue system by a series of direct myofascial release techniques. As distortions in the system are released, the patient may experience pain. The pain experienced is not merely structural, however. It is thought that emotions are expressed through the musculoskeletal system as behavior, which is reflected in various postures and movement patterns (i.e., the widely accepted psychological concepts of pavlovian conditioning and body language). In other words, the musculoskeletal system is viewed as a link between the body and mind. Emotional or physical traumas are stored in the body as postures, which mirror a withdrawal response from the offending or painful agent. Over time, compensatory reactions occur, but the body ultimately decompensates (fails in adaptation to the imposed stresses), which results in somatic or visceral dysfunction. The direct technique seeks to put the energy of the practitioner into the system of the patient in an attempt to overcome the resistance to change embodied in the withdrawal response. As releases are effected through the treatment, the emotional component may also be expressed (i.e., a somatoemotional release).

The result of the treatment is a feeling of balance and "lightness" experienced by the patient. In addition, the patient should experience a heightened sense of well-being, because the treatment releases the effects of emotional trauma. Thus the feeling of lightness is more than simply an increase in the basal physical energy in the body; it is an increase in the body's vital energy as well.

From Rolf's work sprang a number of other systems of structural integration. Among those who developed their own styles, several stand out with innovative thinking. One of these, Tom Myers, a distinguished teacher of structural integration, suggests that we consider the body to be a tensegrity structure. *Tensegrity,* a term coined by architect-engineer Buckminster Fuller, describes a system characterized by a discontinuous set of compressional elements (struts) that are held together, and/or moved, by a continuous tensional network. The muscular system supplies the tensile forces that erect the human frame by using contractile mechanisms embedded within the fascia to place tension on the compressional elements of the skeletal system, thereby providing a tensegrity structure capable of maintaining varying vertical postures, as well as carrying out significant and complex movements.

Myers (1997) has described a number of clinically useful sets of myofascial chains. He sees the fascia as continuous through the muscle and its tendinous attachments, blending with adjacent and contiguous soft tissues and with the bones, providing supportive tensional elements between the different structures, and thereby creating a tensegrity structure. These fascial chains are of particular importance in helping to draw attention to (for example) dysfunctional patterns in the lower limb that may impact structures in the upper body via these "long functional continuities."

Chaitow and DeLany (2008) note, "The truth, of course, is that no tissue exists in isolation but acts on, is bound to and interwoven with other structures. The body is inter- and intra-related, from top to bottom, side-to-side and front to back, by the inter-connectedness of this pervasive fascial system. When we work on a local area, we need to maintain a constant awareness of the fact that we are potentially influencing the whole body."

SHIATSU (ZEN SHIATSU)

Shiatsu means "finger pressure" in Japanese. It originally developed as a synthesis of acupuncture and anma, traditional Japanese massage. During the eighteenth and nineteenth centuries, anma became more associated with carnal pleasure and subsequently lost its place as a therapeutic practice. Shiatsu further diverged and became systematized in the twentieth century, with the Nippon Shiatsu School opening in the 1940s. Today, shiatsu is practiced worldwide in a multitude of practice settings. Although it has a strong root in energy-based medicine, the physical nature of its practice offers a quality more similar to massage than energy work.

As with other Asian-derived systems, shiatsu employs the meridian or channel concept of the human body. The points along the channels are referred to as *tsubos* (Japanese for "vase"). Shiatsu theory states that when a channel becomes blocked, the tsubos along it can express a "kyo" state (weak energy, low vibration, cold, open) or a "jitsu" state (strong energy, high vibration, heat, closed). The hands are used for three purposes: for diagnosis, for treatment, and for maintenance (to strengthen the newly attained balance).

During a shiatsu treatment the practitioner (or "giver") uses acupressure to open or close jitsu or kyo tsubos, respectively. The technique is applied using the thumb, elbow, or knee, positioned perpendicular to the skin of the "receiver." The body part used by the practitioner and the duration of application depend on the state of the tsubo. Acupressure is combined systematically with passive stretching and rotation of the joints to stimulate the flow of *ki* through the channels. Treatments are described for the whole body (basic) and for each of the 12 major meridians.

Several issues have been raised in this chapter in discussing the Asian styles of manual therapy that are also relevant here to shiatsu. The intertwining of body-mind-spirit is evident as a holistic method of treatment born of an ancient philosophy. The practitioner-patient (giver-receiver) relationship is one of partnership, because each is a participant in the healing process. This is born of the yin-yang principle (giver = yang, receiver = yin). The intention of the practitioner plays a major role in the effectiveness of the treatment; the giver is a nonjudgmental observer or plays an empathetic role. As opposed to the more neutral "do no harm" principle of Western caregivers, there appears to be more of a natural expression of love as a defined part of these systems (as with reiki). Intuition is also an important part of the treatment, because each session is an exploration of the process of healing and of the individuals involved (see Chapter 20).

SPORTS MASSAGE

Sports massage has emerged throughout the world as a valuable tool in prevention of and recovery from injury and for enhancing performance and increasing skills in the sport. Professional sports teams have long recognized the values of sports massage applications, employing athletic trainers, physical therapists, and massage therapists who often travel with the teams to administer care during the season and also work on team members during off-season. The practitioners are responsible for assessing the tissues using manual techniques, but also must consider the habits of use during the associated sport, determine which dysfunctional mechanics are actually useful adaptations by the body in response to stresses imposed by the sport, and incorporate particular strategies and methods of treatment and prevention of injury, depending on what is discovered.

It is important that the practitioner understand the biomechanics of the sport and the way in which the body might adapt to the imposed stresses. What might seem like a dysfunctional mechanic to be released in a nonsporting body might be a necessary or normal occurrence for that athlete. For instance, the external and internal ROM is often displaced posteriorly in a pitcher's shoulder. This possibly occurs in the humeral shaft as a result of the torsional forces imposed on it through years of windup movements, particularly when these forces are placed on the youthful bone. If normal ROM tests are used, the external rotation would appear to be excessive and the internal would appear to be reduced, although overall the degree of ROM is the same as in a nonpitching shoulder. The uninformed practitioner might attempt to increase internal ROM, believing this to be reduced, and thereby destabilize the joint and overstretch the joint capsule, making the shoulder more vulnerable to injury.

Sports massage therapists often appear at neighborhood sport events to provide pre- and post-event massage. The techniques used warm up the tissues close to the time of event participation are significantly different from those used after the event to enhance recovery. Likewise, those used in the off-season to alter mechanics or those used in injured players differ from those used to prepare participants for play. It is important that the practitioner understand when to use which techniques, when ice and heat are appropriate, and just how much therapy is enough without overtreating the tissues. Professional sports massage training is suggested for all practitioners who work with athletes, whether in the field or in the clinic.

STRAIN-COUNTERSTRAIN

Strain-counterstrain (SCS) technique, originally called "positional release technique (PRT)," is a very gentle, passive technique developed by Lawrence Jones, DO. The practitioner usually palpates a muscle in spasm (often associated with strain) while the patient reports on his or her sense of discomfort. The patient is next brought into a position that shortens the muscle or eases the dysfunctional joint (*counterstrain*), which exaggerates the motion restriction. The patient then reports on the level of ease. This position is held usually for 90 to 120 seconds, and the patient is then slowly returned to the original position. The technique is designed to interrupt the reflex spasm loop by altering proprioceptive input into the CNS and can be followed by gentle stretching of the involved muscle. Tender points are also treated in this manner: the patient is brought to a position of ease, held in the position until a "softening" or change in tissue texture is felt or the tenderness subsides, then slowly returned to the original position.

Similar to SCS/PRT just discussed is functional technique (functional positional release), but the latter relies a little more on the practitioner's palpation skills than on the patient's reporting. The practitioner places a hand or finger on a tender area and searches for the most distressed tissue. The patient is then positioned until a "position of ease" is produced or until the discomfort is significantly reduced, and the patient holds this position for a certain period, usually at least 90 to 120 seconds and sometimes considerably longer. The patient is then brought slowly back to the original position. It is possible that as the position of ease reduces nociceptive and aberrant proprioceptive input to the CNS, an interruption of facilitation associated with pain and spasm is achieved. Realignment of fascia is also a result of the functional technique, and it is possible that the actin and myosin filaments are able to "unlatch" due to approximation of the two ends of the fibers.

TRAGER WORK (PSYCHOPHYSICAL INTEGRATION AND MENTASTICS)

Milton Trager, MD, was originally a boxer and gymnast and developed (almost by accident) his technique of psychophysical integration more than 50 years ago (Trager, 1994). To obtain the credentials he believed were necessary to bring his technique to the medical community, he obtained a medical degree from the University of Guadalajara in 1955. While there, he was able to demonstrate his technique and treat polio patients with a relatively high degree of success. After developing the technique over many years in his medical practice, he began to teach the method in 1975. The Trager Institute (Mill Valley, California) was founded shortly thereafter and is responsible for dissemination of information and certification programs.

Trager work is a two-tiered approach, along the lines of the Feldenkrais method (see previous discussion). The psychophysical integration phase, also known as "table work," consists of a single treatment or a series of treatments. Mentastics, as described later, is an exercise taught to patients so that they may continue the work on their own.

Psychophysical integration is essentially an indirect, functional technique. The patient lies on a table, and the practitioner applies a very gentle rocking motion to explore the body for areas of tissue tension and motion restriction. No force, stroking, or thrust is used in this technique, merely a light, rhythmic contact. The purpose is to produce a specific sensory experience for the patient, one that is positive and pleasurable. Any discomfort serves to break the continuum of "teaching" and "learning."

The focus of the treatment, however, is not on any specific anatomical structure or physiological process, but rather on the *psyche* of the patient. An attempt is made to bring the patient into a position (or motion) of ease, in which a sensation of lightness or freedom is experienced. This sensation is "learned" by the patient during the process of sensorimotor repatterning. In the words of Dr. Trager, the patient learns "how the tissue should feel when everything is right." This mind-body interaction is the core of the treatment, in which the patient's psyche is brought to bear on the CNS to break the feedback loop of pain → guarding → muscle spasm and induce a change. The result is deep relaxation and increased ROM (i.e., the sense of lightness).

Patterns of behavior and posture are learned during a person's lifetime in part as reactions to trauma or withdrawal from pain, either physical or emotional (see discussion on structural integration). Initially, the body may be able to compensate for such reactions, but it will eventually decompensate, which results in various somatic or visceral symptoms. The Trager treatment "allows" the patient to reexperience what is normal through this exploratory process.

The practitioner seeks to integrate with the patient by entering a quasi-meditative state of awareness referred to as the "hookup." This allows the practitioner to attend acutely to the work at hand and feel very subtle changes in tissue texture and movement, not unlike the level of attention necessary to practice cranial osteopathy (see later discussion). Without any specific anatomical protocol, the work is very intuitive, and "letting go" is necessary by both parties. The practitioner maintains a position of "neutrality" and makes no attempt to "make anything happen," because it is actually the patient who is sensing and learning. The practitioner's role is one of a facilitator, in which he or she seeks to provide a safe and nurturing environment for the patient to explore new and pain-free patterns of motion.

Mentastics, the continuing phase of Trager work, is short for "mental gymnastics" and follows table work. A basic exercise set is taught, and patients are instructed to practice on their own. These exercises consist of repetitive and sequential movements of all the joints, designed to relieve tension in the body. They are to be performed in an effortless, relaxed state of awareness, in which the individual "hooks up" with the self. The basic principles of Hatha Yoga and t'ai chi are used in these exercises. Once the set is learned, individuals can then continue to explore independently, creating their own custom-designed series.

Practitioners of Trager work have reported success (not necessarily cures) in patients with multiple sclerosis, muscular dystrophy, and other debilitating diseases. Athletes have also reported significant improvements in performance as a result of applying Trager techniques.

TUI NA

Tui na is a manipulative practice within TCM. The literal translation is "pushing and grasping." Tui na, the forerunner of shiatsu in Japan, is more than 4000 years old and predates the manufacture of acupuncture needles. Tui na may be practiced by TCM physicians as part of their general practice, or they may specialize in it, as do members of the osteopathic profession.

As with the other Chinese medical arts, tui na is based on the meridian or channel view of the human body, the yin-yang principle, and the five elements theory. The organs of the body exist not only as anatomical structures, but also in a functional context (e.g., the "triple burner"), as well as in relation to one another. Yin and yang, as opposite forces, coexist in equilibrium with one another. Of the 12 major meridians of the body that correspond to the organs, six are yin, the others yang.

Qi, or vital energy, is a universal force that permeates everything. It is manifest as five separate elements: fire, wood, metal, water, and earth. The organs of the body are categorized accordingly. Qi flows through all the meridians once each day in 2-hour cycles. Therefore each meridian, and thus its associated organ, has its daily strong and weak periods. When the flow of qi is impeded in any channel, that organ or function may become dysfunctional, resulting in disease.

The techniques of tui na combine soft tissue, visceral, and joint manipulation. Typically, the patient is lying on a table or is seated. Soft tissue techniques, which are applied to the limbs, trunk, and head, precede joint mobilization to prepare the joint for movement and to relax the surrounding musculature. The techniques are designed to stimulate local blood flow, venous and lymphatic drainage, and the flow of qi (see previous discussion on shiatsu). These soft tissue techniques include the following:

- *Pressing,* using the thumbs, elbows, or palms
- *Squeezing,* using the whole hand or finger-thumb combination
- *Kneading,* a circular pressing technique, using the thumbs, heel of the hand, elbow, or forearm
- *Rubbing,* a high-frequency technique, using the palms, heels of the hands (chafing), or forearms
- *Stroking* (see effleurage), moving the hand over the skin in a long stroke, in one direction only
- *Vibration,* similar to that used in massage
- *Thumb rocking,* for deep penetration of acupuncture points
- *Plucking,* a transverse friction type of technique
- *Rolling,* using the back of the hand to roll over the skin and underlying tissue
- *Percussion* (see tapotement), which includes pummeling with the fists, hacking with the heels of the hands, and pounding with cupped hands

Included in the joint manipulative techniques are the following:

- *Shaking,* in which traction is applied to the limb and it is shaken with high-velocity low-amplitude movements from 10 to 20 times.
- *Flexion and extension,* primarily applied to the elbow and knee joints (i.e., the hinge joints). These are both high- and low-velocity techniques designed to engage a motion barrier but not to challenge it. In addition, in some of these techniques a thumb is simultaneously applied to an acupuncture point to open a meridian.
- *Rotation,* an articulatory technique used for the ankles, wrists, hips, and shoulders. Practitioners of tui na do not apply this technique to the neck.
- *Pushing and pulling,* a low-velocity technique designed to directly engage a motion barrier, with a counterforce applied by the opposing hand in the opposite direction.
- *Stretching,* a general, low-velocity flexion-extension technique used to loosen the joints of the spine.
- *Thrust,* used on the spinal joints in a manner similar to that in osteopathic and chiropractic methods.

Tui na can be applied to virtually anyone and has few contraindications. The existing contraindications are similar to those for massage, including skin lesions or infection, skin or lymphatic cancer, and osteoporosis. In addition, it is recommended that the low back and abdomen be avoided during pregnancy.

Anatomically, tui na is applied to the musculoskeletal system and viscera, with attention being paid to the meridians and flow of qi (as specific meridians flow through specific joints, muscle groups, and visceral structures). As with other forms of manipulative treatment, tui na seeks to produce a feeling of well-being and health in the patient. In addition, as the emotional and spiritual components of the patient are addressed, emotional release can also be produced.

VISCERAL MANIPULATION

Visceral manipulation generally involves specific placement of gentle manual forces to encourage tone, mobility, and motion of the abdominopelvic viscera and their supporting connective tissue. Although not indicated in patients with tumors or inflammatory disease, visceral manipulation can be useful in stabilizing and balancing blood flow and autonomic innervation and can even dislodge certain obstructions of the gastrointestinal system.

Methods that address manual manipulation of the viscera have been a component of some therapeutic systems in Oriental medicine for centuries and are now practiced extensively by European osteopaths, physical therapists, and other manual practitioners throughout the world. Osteopath and physical therapist Jean-Pierre Barral developed a system of training and practice of this technique that is available to all manual practitioners. Contact the Barral Institute in West Palm Beach, Florida.

OSSEOUS TECHNIQUES

In addition to methods applied to the soft tissues, a variety of techniques can be used to normalize the position of the osseous structure. Although some are discussed elsewhere in this book, the following are often used in conjunction with the afore-listed myofascial methods. Their inclusion as a supporting modality here is meant to encourage the synergistic integration of manual modalities.

ARTICULATORY TECHNIQUE

In the articulatory technique, the practitioner moves the affected joint through its ROM in all planes, gently encountering motion barriers and gradually moving through them to establish normal motion. This low-velocity moderate- to high-amplitude method would be considered a passive, direct/indirect, oscillatory technique

used to restore as much motion as possible to a dysfunctional joint.

CRANIAL OSTEOPATHY AND CRANIOSACRAL THERAPY

Cranial osteopathy (osteopathic techniques applied to the cranium) was developed by W.G. Sutherland in the mid-1900s. His work was based on the observation that the joints between the skull bones are meant to permit motion just as do joints in other areas of the body. While palpating these bones and joints, he discovered the existence of a very subtle rhythm in the body unrelated to respiration or cardiovascular rhythms. Sutherland named this rhythm the cranial rhythmic impulse (CRI). This impulse, he learned, was capable of moving the cranial bones through an ROM that, although very small, was palpable to well-trained hands (Figure 16-10). Cranial theory posits that

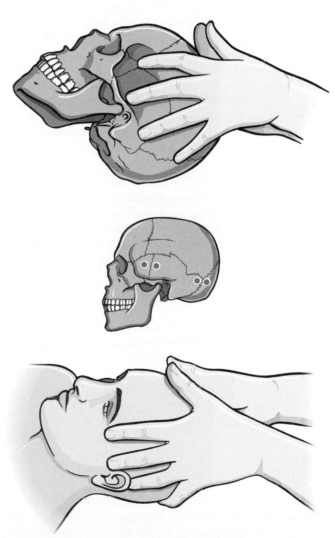

Figure 16-10 Vault hold for cranial palpation. (Borrowed with permission from Chaitow L, DeLany J: *Clinical application of neuromuscular techniques,* vol 1, ed 1, Edinburgh, 2008, Churchill Livingstone.)

there is inherent motility of the CNS, resulting in fluctuations of the cerebrospinal fluid, which bathes the brain and spinal cord. This fluctuation, in turn, moves the cranial bones through their small yet palpable ROM.

These concepts were expanded further in the 1970s by the findings of a research team at Michigan State University supervised by Dr. John Upledger. They discovered that the motion associated with this rhythm is not restricted to the cranial bones and proposed that, because the cranium is linked to the sacrum by the dural membranes, which cover the CNS, the motion is palpable in the sacrum as well. In addition, through the fascial-fluid system, this has effects all over the body. Motion restrictions in this system can be palpated and corrected (either directly or indirectly) through very gentle manipulation, also with global effects. Based on these concepts, craniosacral therapy emerged as a separate and distinct modality.

As releases are produced in this fascial system and throughout the body, memories (sometimes emotionally painful) can be reawakened and produce "somatoemotional release," a form of mind-body connection. Clinical experience suggests that these experiences occur frequently, although it is not understood at this time whether this is due to the proximity of the membranes to the brain, stimulation of associated neural circuitry in peripheral tissues, or some other mechanism.

Cranial osteopathy has been controversial from its inception because of the lack of definitive, objective experimental evidence. Because research studies that could conclusively evaluate the effectiveness of cranial therapies have not been performed to date, evidence of effectiveness comes almost exclusively in the form of clinical case reports and testimonials. Successes have been reported in improving a variety of conditions, including chronic headache, cerebral palsy, autism, and behavioral disturbances. Data are now being gathered through outcome-based studies that lend credence to its effectiveness (Mehl-Madrona et al, 2007; Raviv et al, 2009).

Because of the time and effort necessary to develop this skill, relatively few osteopaths in the U.S. practice cranial osteopathy. The practice of craniosacral therapy, however, has expanded to other manual therapy fields, including chiropractic, physical therapy, massage therapy, and dentistry, with training being offered by the Upledger Institute (Palm Beach Gardens, Florida) and others.

HIGH-VELOCITY LOW-AMPLITUDE TECHNIQUE

The high-velocity low-amplitude (HVLA) technique is probably the most publicly recognized technique of the osteopath or chiropractor. This is a thrust-oriented technique designed to aggressively break through a motion barrier. More often than not, an audible pop is heard, the result of a brief cavitation of the involved joint. The HVLA technique can be applied directly (toward the barrier) or

indirectly (away from the barrier), using short or long levers. Although often associated with manipulation of the spine, the HVLA technique can also be performed on the extremities.

Use of the HVLA technique is contraindicated in patients with osteoporosis, bone tumors, or severe atherosclerosis, and in those who are taking certain medications that make bones more brittle, such as many forms of chemotherapy. Recently, much discussion has focused on the safety of the HVLA technique when performed in the high cervical (neck) region due to potential risk to the vertebral artery. Controversy has expanded to include questions regarding the safety and accuracy of manual screening tests for vertebral artery insufficiencies (such as George's Test and the DeKlynes Test). In March 2004, all U.S. chiropractic schools agreed to abandon the teaching and use of provocation tests such as these due to the inherent risks and high level of false data. An extensive PowerPoint presentation regarding these concerns is available (Clum, 2006).

MASSAGE THERAPY PRACTICE SETTINGS

Massage therapy is used in a variety of clinical settings, spas, private practices, and sport arenas. The expertise of the massage therapist or practitioner is essential in determining which techniques may or may not be appropriate and how the massage may be delivered. Application choices will also be based on the case presentation and may be influenced by the environment, such as a hospital or spa, as well as the allocation of time, prescribed therapy, or other associated modalities (e.g., stretching, exercise, biofeedback) that may be needed or desired. Massage is routinely applied to pediatric, adolescent, and geriatric patients. Frequently, massage therapists expand their therapeutic horizons by taking postgraduate study in other forms of bodywork or specific methods for application to certain pathologies. It is not uncommon to find a therapist who not only does Swedish massage but also employs Trager work, the Feldenkrais method, and craniosacral therapy, moving seamlessly from one to the other, as indicated by the response of the tissues and recipient.

The application of massage therapy in medical settings has recently expanded at a dramatic rate, perhaps because of the growing use of "multidisciplinary approaches" to patient care. Massage therapists and other manual practitioners now render their skills in hospitals, physical therapy clinics, rehabilitation centers, and the offices of physicians, osteopaths, chiropractors, dentists, and multidisciplinary clinics. In professional sport arenas, Olympic competitions, and college, high school, and Little League teams, massage and manual techniques have emerged as valued tools for rehabilitation, enhancement of performance, and prevention of injury. These professions are no longer considered to be on the outskirts of medicine, but are now incorporated as an integral part of treatment options. All manual medicine modalities are areas that are ripe for research, with much being done worldwide to validate them and explore their breadth of application in patient care.

SUMMARY

In closing, it is important to note the value of the preventive aspect of manipulation as a holistic practice. Manipulative treatment can be used for proactive general maintenance as well as for reactive treatment of dysfunction. To use an automobile analogy, most consumers think nothing of periodically getting a car tuned up and paying considerable sums for the privilege. Why not do the same for their own bodies? In addition, the value of manual treatment for young persons cannot be overstated. Structural corrections can be made before fascial distortions become relatively locked in or before continuous aberrant sensory input results in facilitated sensorimotor patterning. Corrections can be made before compensatory reactions in muscles, fascia, and behavior can create unbalanced anatomy and physiology that function poorly and eventually lead to a decreased resistance to disease (pathology). As Alexander Pope once proclaimed, "Just as the twig is bent, the tree's inclined."

The importance given to this information should be tied to the awareness that, as the body ages, adaptive forces cause changes in the structures of the body, with the occurrence of shortening, crowding, and distortion. With this, we can see—in real terms within our own bodies and those of our patients—the environment in which cells change shape. As they do so they change their potential for normal genetic expression, as well as their abilities to communicate and to handle nutrients efficiently.

Reversing or slowing these undesirable processes is the potential of appropriate bodywork and movement approaches. It is yet to be precisely established to what degree functional health can be modified by soft tissue techniques, such as those discussed in this chapter. However, the normalizing of structural and functional features of connective tissue by addressing myofascial trigger points, chronic muscle shortening and fibrosis, as well as perpetuating factors such as habits of use, has clear implications. Well-designed research to assess cellular, structural, and functional changes that follow the application of manual techniques is clinically relevant and sorely needed.

⊖ Chapter References can be found on the Evolve website at http://evolve.elsevier.com/Micozzi/complementary/

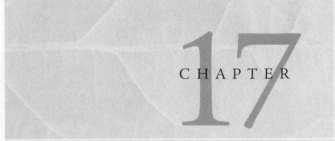

CHAPTER

17

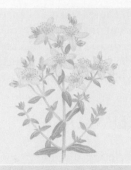

OSTEOPATHIC MEDICINE

JOHN M. JONES III

To find health should be the object of the doctor. Anyone can find disease.

—ANDREW TAYLOR STILL, MD, DO,
FOUNDER OF OSTEOPATHY

HISTORY

Osteopathic medicine began as an offshoot of the standard, "regular" medical practices of the 1800s when one innovative physician became disenchanted with the inadequate and harmful effects of the medicines being used by the doctors of that era.

Andrew Taylor Still, MD, DO, was born in 1828 in Jonesboro, Virginia, when this part of the country was still on the American frontier. His life experiences and observation led him to question the entire system of medicine that existed in nineteenth-century America.

Most medications used in that era were unresearched remedies passed on through tradition from the Middle Ages of Europe. Bleeding and leeching were major components of treatment when Still was trained, as were "purging and puking." One of the most common medications was calomel, a mercuric compound used as a purgative. It was extremely toxic, often causing patients' gums to be resorbed, teeth to fall out, and sores to break out in the mouth. Calomel undoubtedly contributed to many deaths and disfigured many more. Surgery was primitive and performed without antisepsis; anesthetics were just beginning to be used in the mid-1800s. No antibiotics had been identified, and no microbial cause of infectious illness was proven until 1872. There was no knowledge of the immune system, and heart disease and cancer were not understood. Physicians were capable of diagnosing empirically recognized patterns of illness and, in many cases, predicting outcomes. Medical treatment was often more dangerous than doing nothing. In fact, the famous French mathematician and philosopher Descartes (see Chapter 6) was reputed to have said, "Before, when I knew I was sick, I thought I might die; now that they are taking me to the chirurgeon, I know I shall" (Schiowitz, 1997).

Still was seeking a philosophy of medicine and system of treatment based on scientific principles as they could be observed in nature. In one of his books, he stated that in

232

April 1855, he began to discuss reasons "for my faith in the laws of life as given to men, worlds, and beings by the God of Nature" (Still, 1902). He was not alone in his disillusionment with the contemporary state of affairs and quest for a scientifically based philosophy of medicine. The great physician and author Oliver Wendell Holmes, for example, was often quoted from his presentation to the Massachusetts Medical Society (publisher of today's *New England Journal of Medicine*) that "if the whole of *materia medica* as now used could be sunk to the bottom of the sea, it would be all the better for mankind—and all the worse for the fishes" (Holmes, 1892). (The jurist Oliver Wendell Holmes, Jr., Supreme Court chief justice, was his son.)

By the time of the Civil War, a large number of American physicians were homeopathic or eclectic (nonstandard) practitioners. In addition, many people on the frontier took care of their own medical needs (see Chapter 1). Medical education was offered in two ways, one by university degree and one by "reading medicine." At university-affiliated medical schools during the early and mid nineteenth century, students attended a course of 4 months of morning lectures to obtain their degrees. If students voluntarily attended a second year, it was for a repeat of the same lectures. The alternate pathway was used by many American physicians on the frontier, who learned by becoming an apprentice to an established physician. Under the physician's supervision, they read medical and scientific textbooks and accompanied him and possibly other of his colleagues on home and office visits. More specialized studies could be undertaken by arranging to work with an established expert, but most doctors did not pursue such studies. These two systems were later combined and evolved into the current system of medical education (2 years of basic science and medical didactics, followed by 2 years during which students continue to read medical books and journals while shadowing and assisting physicians in hospital and ambulatory care settings, after which the graduate physicians do an additional 3 to 7 years of supervised postgraduate hospital residencies).

Andrew Taylor Still (Figure 17-1) was the son of Abram Still, a circuit-riding Methodist minister who was also a physician, tending to his flock both spiritually and medically. Shortly after Andrew Taylor was born, the family moved from Virginia to Missouri, further out on the nineteenth-century frontier, so that his father could serve the needs of the church in the west. Abram Still was an ardent abolitionist who sided with the small minority of Methodist ministers in Missouri who were opposed to slavery. There were terrible insurrections in the Kansas and Missouri territories over whether they would be admitted to the Union as slave or free states. When the church split over the issue, the elder Still moved the family to Kansas, where they supported the cause of freedom.

Like many pioneer boys, the younger Still grew up contributing to the family food supply by hunting and did much of the butchering of the animals himself. He later

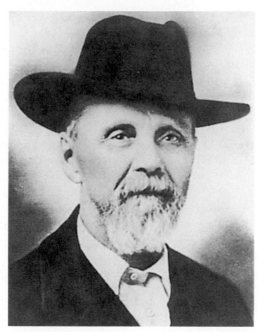

Figure 17-1 Portrait of Andrew Taylor Still, the founder of osteopathy, ca. 1900. (Courtesy Kirksville College of Osteopathy, A.T. Still Memorial Library, Archives Department, Kirksville, Mo.)

stated that his studies of anatomy began this way. In his autobiography, he described an intense headache that occurred when he was 10 years old. To alleviate his discomfort by taking a nap, he placed his jacket over a rope swing to construct a pillow and then lay down with the base of his skull over the other side of the rope. He fell asleep and a short time later awoke to find his headache gone. This phenomenon impressed him, and when he became a physician, the memory of it led him to think about the relationship between the body's anatomy and the disease process. He was perhaps engaging in an early form of craniosacral therapy or myofascial release.

Still obtained his medical education through the process of apprenticeship under an established physician (in Still's case, assisting his father), combined with reading the medical texts of that time. He later attended a medical school in Kansas City, but he did not complete a degree, stating that the school had little to teach him that he did not already know.

The younger Still began his medical career by serving the local community and working with his father with the Shawnee Indian tribe. Ironically, many years earlier his maternal grandmother had been kidnapped by the Shawnee, who had also killed numerous members of that generation of her family. Still had a standard general medical practice, employing the usual medications and involving the full range of available treatment, including obstetrics and minor surgery.

Dr. Still became a battalion surgeon in the Kansas militia during the Civil War; he also served as an officer and led men into battle. He returned to his family in 1864 at the end of the western campaigns, when the Kansas militia was disbanded after the Union victory.

Believing that his family was safe now that the war was over in that part of the country, he was stunned when three of his children died in an epidemic of spinal meningitis. There were no effective medications to treat such an illness. He called other physicians to attend to his family, rather than manage their cases himself, and called ministers to pray for the children as well. Nothing availed, and the children died. This event caused him to question the entire foundation of medical care in his era. He wrote, "It was when I gazed at three members of my own family—two of my own children and one adopted child—all dead from the disease, spinal meningitis, that I propounded to myself the serious questions 'In sickness has God left man in a world of guessing? Guess what is the matter? What to give, and guess the result? And when dead, guess where he goes?'" (Singer et al, 1962).

Seeking a more enlightened practice of medicine, Still based his reasoning on the Methodist philosophy of working to attain perfection, which seemed to have something in common with the new idea of natural evolution. The early evolutionists suggested that there existed a natural process of working toward perfection of the organism and that the human being was the highest naturally evolved life form. Still felt that the human being was perfectly constructed by the one he later referred to in his writings as the God of Nature, the Great Architect, the Great Engineer, and the Great Mechanic. If the human body was perfectly constructed as the highest form of machine, he felt it should simply need fuel and, if something went wrong, adjustment.

Like the general population of the nineteenth century, he had a tremendous admiration for engineering and all things mechanical. Still was also an inventor; during his life he invented a thresher and obtained patents for a new type of churn and stove. He would eventually tell the students at the American School of Osteopathy that they were to become human engineers who knew every part and function of the body. They were to find engineering solutions to human illness and dysfunction.

Even before the Civil War, in the 1850s, Still experimented with manual treatment of patients. But this was in addition to the use of standard medical practices. It was after the war, and the death of his children, that his ideas came together into a complete philosophy regarding the etiology of illness and how to treat it. By 1897, Still wrote in his autobiography that it was on June 22, 1874, that he "flung to the breeze the banner of osteopathy" (Singer et al, 1962). Apparently it was by that date that he was able to define the principles on which his philosophy and practice of medical care would be based. His new methods involved hands-on treatment adjusting the positions of joints and levels of muscle tone; enhancing the circulation of blood, lymphatic, and cerebrospinal fluids; improving the efficiency of respiration; and therefore improving host response to disease.

Still was ostracized in Kansas for leaving the medical fold and denied the opportunity to teach his new ideas at Baker University in Baldwin, Kansas, a Methodist university where he had hoped at least to be able to discuss his ideas. He and his family had donated land to start the university, and he and his brothers had built a mill and sawed timbers for the original building. The local minister, however, indicated to the congregation that his practice was of the devil, because only Jesus was supposed to be able to lay hands on the sick and heal them.

After a period of time and a severe illness, he moved to back to Missouri, finally settling in Kirksville, where he said he found a few people who were willing to listen to reason. He set up a circuit practice of medicine in outlying communities. After Still had been in practice for a while so many people began coming to Kirksville looking for him that he was able to stay in one place. He was not sure what to call his clinical practice. At first he thought his new methods, being hands on, might have something in common with magnetic healing, which was a popular nineteenth-century practice following on Mesmer's concepts of "animal magnetism" and energetic healing (see Chapter 6). Thus for a short time Still called himself a "magnetic healer." Later, he used a business card on which he called himself a "lightning bonesetter." The use of this term implies that he had heard of the folk healers who called themselves by that name. There is no evidence, however, that he ever studied with anyone who had learned this art in the usual way (i.e., it was passed from one person to the next, such as from father to son).

Still coined the term *osteopathy* (from the Greek roots *osteon* and *pathos*) sometime prior to founding the American School of Osteopathy (ASO) in 1892. This nomenclature followed the tradition of naming medical approaches after what was considered the central issue in pathology or cure (e.g., homeopathy, hydropathy, naturopathy). In the case of osteopathy, Still reasoned that malpositioning of bones and joints, especially in the spine, affected both circulation and nerve function, providing the opportunity for the development of disease in the tissues. William Smith, educated in Scotland, was another reform-minded MD who offered to teach anatomy in the new school if Still would teach him his methods. About 10 students began the first year. The school expanded rapidly, and it became impossible for Still to personally instruct all the students in his methods; thus over the next few years his first students became the new professors. Other physicians and college graduates joined the faculty as the curriculum and number of students expanded.

To further disseminate his ideas, Still wrote four books. The *Autobiography of Andrew T. Still* (1897) describes his life and how he developed osteopathy. *The Philosophy of Osteopathy* (1899) and *The Philosophy and Mechanical Principles of Osteopathy* (copyrighted in 1892 but published in 1902) describe his philosophical ideas and contain a great deal of then-current simple knowledge as well as speculation about physiology, a subject poorly understood at the time. In *Osteopathy, Research and Practice* (1910), Still continued to expand on his ideas and described some of his treatment techniques.

These books reveal that he still, on occasion, used some medications—although extremely rarely. He was opposed to the use of opiates and alcohol, having seen much abuse (especially in Civil War injured and disabled), and specifically stated that it was foolish for physicians to dissolve most medications in alcohol, because this practice could lead to dependency. Throughout his books he recommended the use of manipulation to relieve anatomical and therefore physiological stress on the system, and return the body to a state in which it could cure itself through normal physiological processes. Still's original philosophical principles are summed up in "Our Platform," which was published in *Osteopathy, Research and Practice,* and adopted by the ASO as the foundation of its educational program.

The allopathic profession, which was becoming successful in establishing a monopoly on medical training and licensure, vigorously fought the new osteopathic profession. Still's followers, however, achieved great success in their treatment of illness in comparison with their MD counterparts, effecting cures in some "hopeless" cases and treating all types of illnesses. The new doctors also had special expertise in neuromusculoskeletal conditions at a time when no physical medicine, rehabilitation, or physical therapy was available to the public. The ASO rapidly expanded, and new schools founded by graduates helped build the osteopathic profession, which attracted supporters such as Teddy Roosevelt, President William Howard Taft, and Mark Twain (who testified to the New York State Assembly in favor of osteopathic licensure). Osteopaths graduated with the title *Doctor of Osteopathy (DO),* which was changed at the end of the twentieth century to *Doctor of Osteopathic Medicine (DO).*

The 1910 Flexner Report, sponsored by the Carnegie Foundation, compared all American medical schools against a standard represented by the new Johns Hopkins University School of Medicine. Criticism was so devastating that about three quarters of American medical schools closed, including many osteopathic medical schools. The surviving osteopathic medical colleges were located in Kirksville, Missouri; Kansas City, Missouri; Des Moines, Iowa; Philadelphia, Pennsylvania; Chicago, Illinois; and Los Angeles, California. None of these schools received public funding at the time. The osteopathic profession was on its own for further development.

Still's central idea was that structural abnormality causes functional abnormality, leading to illness. To restore health, treatments were designed to use the body's own resources. He theorized that manipulation would increase the body's efficiency, promoting appropriate delivery of blood, return of blood and lymph, delivery of neurotrophic substances, and transmission of neural impulses. Physicians had relatively few medications of value for the patient in the preantibiotic era (during the early 1900s). Osteopathic manipulation, on the other hand, was a technique that a physician could use to effect physiological changes and help stimulate a host response against illness. In addition, osteopathy directly addressed a number of needs with which the medical profession had not successfully dealt: joint pain, physical rehabilitation, and soft tissue injuries.

Soon after Still's death in 1917, his new osteopathic physicians were put to the test during the Spanish influenza pandemic of 1919. The results were excellent. The medical profession had little to offer patients other than antitussives, opiates, and strychnine to stimulate the heart. Osteopathic treatment targeted autonomic changes, blood delivery, lymphatic drainage, and biomechanical improvement in respiration. Osteopathic physicians reported dramatically lower morbidity and mortality rates among their influenza patients.

Between the death of Still in 1917 and World War II, osteopathic colleges, like allopathic colleges, gradually improved standards. In the early 1900s, increasing practice of antiseptic procedure helped improve the safety of surgery, as did the development and use of the sulfa antibiotics by the 1930s. Penicillin, although developed in 1927, was not available for practical use until it was mass produced by Florey and Chain for soldiers and sailors during World War II. Even after the problems of mass production were solved, it was not readily available for the American public until after the war.

Still's students had included MDs who were less opposed to standard medications but integrated his ideas on enhancing the body's own self-healing abilities by treating the structure (anatomy) to enhance the function (physiology) and restore health. By 1928, *materia medica* (the part of medicine concerned with formulation and use of remedies or natural pharmacological preparations, taught in allopathic medical schools before the development of modern medications) was taught at all of the osteopathic medical colleges. In addition, the newly researched and efficacious antibiotics were discussed as they were developed. Osteopathic physicians, along with their MD peers, increasingly had available medications that actually worked, which they used in their general practice of medicine. From Still on, early osteopathic physicians had included surgery in their complete practice of medicine (although, like their counterparts, not all personally performed the surgeries). DOs believed that osteopathic manipulation before and after surgery helped patients tolerate procedures better and reduced the incidence of complications, such as pneumonia, thereby resulting in a shorter recovery time.

As medical specialties and subspecialties were being developed, most osteopaths were general practitioners. American postgraduate training programs were not generally open to DOs. A number of osteopathic specialists obtained their training in Europe from physicians who did not concern themselves with distinctions between types of American physicians; some of these osteopathic physicians returned and set up specialty training programs in their own professions.

During World War II, osteopaths were not allowed to serve in the armed forces as physicians. Although some volunteered and served in other capacities, many stayed home and took care of patients whose MDs were overseas. Although DOs were not allowed to serve during World War II, a benefit was that, while MDs were overseas serving, many families in the United States began to receive treatment from DOs. Patients were unable to see their regular physicians, and this situation helped the growth of osteopathy.

In the postwar period, as returning soldiers attended universities in record numbers on the GI Bill, osteopathic colleges enrolled record numbers of students.

By 1953 the president of the American Medical Association (AMA) had called for and received a report on the status of osteopathic medicine, which indicated that DO training was equivalent to MD training. MDs in general became less concerned with whether their osteopathic colleagues used osteopathic manipulative treatment (OMT) in the care of back pain, in sports medicine, and in rehabilitation, as long as they also prescribed new medications that were proven to be effective.

Two other events in the middle to late twentieth century helped the osteopathic profession gain acceptance. One was the merger, by government regulation, of the osteopathic profession with the allopathic medical profession in California. A second was the establishment of 10 additional osteopathic medical colleges between 1969 and 1981, soon followed by others in the 1990s.

In 1961, California had more DOs than any other state. The state government, however, felt that the American Osteopathic Association (AOA) was unresponsive to its influence and decided to support a merger with the allopathic medical profession. The state osteopathic medical association worked with the California Medical Association to lobby with the public in support of this merger of professions. It was difficult at the time for DOs to obtain admission privileges in most allopathic hospitals, although osteopathic physicians had built their own hospitals. Voters were convinced to support a plan under which new osteopathic licenses would no longer be issued, with the provision that any DO who wished to do so could trade the DO degree and $65 for an MD degree and license. More than 2000 DOs accepted MD degrees and licenses. Benefits to the new MDs included new access to hospital privileges. The largest and arguably most modern osteopathic medical school, the College of Osteopathic Physicians and Surgeons at Los Angeles, was transformed into an MD-granting institution, which shortly thereafter affiliated with the University of California at Irvine.

The rest of the osteopathic profession was immediately concerned that the medical establishment, unable to eliminate the osteopathic profession, was attempting to absorb it. Although there was talk of offers similar to California's

in other states, there was no continuation of the process. Instead, the developments in California paved the way for further acceptance of the osteopathic medical profession. California MDs had seemingly indicated that the main differences between the two types of physicians were the letters of the degree and $65, and the osteopathic medical profession used this ammunition to approach state legislatures and other authorities in defense of osteopathic medical practice rights. Some state legislatures became convinced that it was in their interest to fund colleges of osteopathic medicine when statistics revealed that most DOs practiced general medicine and that a large proportion did so in underserved areas (small towns, rural areas, and inner cities).

The osteopathic medical profession rapidly approved the founding of numerous new osteopathic medical colleges, both public and private. Included among the state-funded colleges were schools in Michigan, Texas, Ohio, West Virginia, and Oklahoma. This rapid expansion continued the trend toward assimilation into the medical mainstream. In the latter part of the twentieth century there were insufficient numbers of osteopathic physicians to serve as role models, as well as a shortage of postgraduate training positions in osteopathic hospitals, and different interest levels in osteopathic student matriculants. The number of osteopathic graduates entering allopathic residencies increased, and young osteopathic physicians began dispersing throughout other hospitals rather than remaining concentrated in osteopathic hospitals.

In the meantime, the development of the osteopathic profession continued around the world and differed markedly from the American evolution of the profession.

OFFSHOOTS OF THE OSTEOPATHIC PROFESSION

As osteopathic techniques were adapted and used by others who had become convinced of their efficacy, offshoots of the osteopathic profession developed. The first person to investigate osteopathy and found another profession was D.D. Palmer, who originated chiropractic. Palmer also initially called himself a "magnetic healer" after Mesmer with his principles of animal magnetism. In his book *The Lengthening Shadow of Dr. Andrew Taylor Still*, Arthur Hildreth, one of the first students at the ASO, mentions that Palmer was a guest of Still's, who often hosted students for dinner (Hildreth, 1942). According to Hildreth, Palmer accompanied a friend in the pioneer class who returned for his second year of instruction and appeared to be interested in becoming a student at the ASO. After learning some manipulation from Still's students, he returned to Davenport, Iowa, and later "discovered" what he called chiropractic.

Stories passed down in families in the profession suggest that Palmer may even have registered as a student for a period of time, but written evidence of this has not been discovered. What is clear and indisputable is that Still, a physician, practiced in northern Missouri as a magnetic healer for almost 20 years before founding his school in 1892. Davenport, Iowa, is not far from Kirksville, Missouri, and Still's reputation was attracting attention from near and far. Whether or not Palmer was a student of Still, it would not be surprising if his "serendipitous discovery" of manipulation in 1895 was based on what he had heard of Still's methods. Palmer founded his own school in 1897.

Still's original students attempted to practice as Still himself had practiced. However, he told his students that they did not have to do exactly as he did provided they could achieve the same results. Granted this freedom to explore, they quickly developed high-velocity manipulative techniques that were passed on at the school. The original chiropractic techniques resembled the high-velocity joint-resetting techniques used and described by some of Still's original students more than the techniques Still himself used, which would support the notion that Palmer learned from the osteopathic students. By 1915, Edyth Ashmore, DO, who was in charge of teaching manipulative technique at the ASO, recommended in her published manual that the students not be taught the original methods of Still, because they were too hard for the students to learn.

Ida Rolf, the founder of *rolfing* (see Chapter 16), a method of bodywork, was clear in her writings that she learned techniques from a blind osteopath and combined them with a knowledge of yoga to create a systematic protocol for whole-body structural integration.

Other adapters of osteopathic technique (and partially of osteopathic philosophy) include John Barnes, a physical therapist who studied myofascial release offered in postgraduate programs at Michigan State University (MSU) and then taught it to physical therapists; and John Upledger, a DO who mixed cranial and other manipulative techniques taught by Still's student William Garner Sutherland, DO, with light trance work and other techniques to develop what he called *craniosacral therapy*, which is generally practiced by nonphysicians.

In addition, because of the availability of postgraduate programs such as those offered by MSU and courses offered by other osteopathic physicians, physical therapists in the United States began using osteopathic techniques such as muscle energy, myofascial release, counterstrain, and even high-velocity low-amplitude thrust. The effect of osteopathic manipulation on physical medicine, rehabilitation, sports medicine, and family practice throughout the United States has been considerable, with many health care professionals and lay personnel learning osteopathic methods of alleviating pain and enhancing physical function.

OSTEOPATHIC PHILOSOPHY

Andrew Taylor Still developed a unified philosophy of medicine in the last half of the nineteenth century, which he called *osteopathic philosophy*. The word *philosophy*

often engenders an immediate visceral response in the scientific or technological mind. The scientific mind is theoretically open to processing all new ideas. The technological mind tends to reject that which has not been statistically demonstrated. Thus the connotation of "philosophy" as an organization of vague or general thoughts about the meaning of life has often been antithetical to the technological mind of the twentieth century. However, some of our greatest scientists, including Einstein, spoke of the importance of ideas that are not yet statistically demonstrated.

Osteopathic philosophy is best described as a background reference system that identifies the nature of the patient, defines the physician's mission, and establishes the basic premises of the logic of diagnosis and treatment. There remains in the general medical community, which has not been exposed to this organizing system, a poor understanding of exactly what is meant by osteopathic philosophy and why doctors of osteopathic medicine consider it important.

Osteopathic medical philosophy is centered on a profound respect for the inherent ability of the human being, and particularly the body, to heal itself. This philosophy has deep roots through recorded medical history. Over time, all ideas evolve as new information is discovered. Osteopathic philosophy is no exception: time has produced a distinction between classical osteopathy, which was taught by Still, and contemporary osteopathic medical philosophy, which integrates the basic elements of Still's ideas with subsequent scientific discoveries (Box 17-1).

CLASSICAL OSTEOPATHIC PHILOSOPHY

Classical osteopathic philosophy identifies the human being as a trinity, including body, mind, and spirit. However, Still speaks in his writings very little about how to deal with the spirit or mind, leaving that up to the individual, and confines himself in general to dealing with the body. The osteopathic perspective is that the body is a marvelous machine that will function perfectly if the structure is perfect. If a patient is sick but his body has sufficient recuperative power, the anatomy can be adjusted to the structural ideal, which assists a return to normal physiology. Surgery and obstetrics are included in this philosophy. Interestingly, Still believed that the diet of his time (completely organic in that era) was sufficient and that the body (the machine) could handle any fuel as long as the machine was working correctly.

The triune nature of the human being that Still so often mentioned dates back to at least the Greeks and probably to the Egyptians. The body is obvious and needs no further definition. The mind, however, has been described both as an epiphenomenon of the brain and its biochemistry and as something that is more than the product of chemical interactions. Emotions are generally identified with the mind, but does a third factor actually exist? Although science openly questions the existence of

BOX 17-1

Traditional Versus Contemporary Osteopathy

Our Platform*

It should be known where osteopathy stands and what it stands for. A political party has a platform that all may know its position in regard to matters of public importance, what it stands for and what principles it advocates. The osteopath should make his position just as clear to the public. He should let the public know, in his platform, what he advocates in his campaign against disease. Our position can be tersely stated in the following planks:

First: We believe in sanitation and hygiene.

Second: We are opposed to the use of drugs as remedial agencies.

Third: We are opposed to vaccination.

Fourth: We are opposed to the use of serums in the treatment of disease. Nature furnishes its own serums if we know how to deliver them.

Fifth: We realize that many cases require surgical treatment and therefore advocate it as a last resort. We believe many surgical operations are unnecessarily performed and that many operations can be avoided by osteopathic treatment.

Sixth: The osteopath does not depend on electricity, X-radiance, hydrotherapy or other adjuncts, but relies on osteopathic measures in the treatment of disease.

Seventh: We have a friendly feeling for other non-drug, natural methods of healing, but we do not incorporate any other methods into our system. We are all opposed to drugs; in that respect at least, all natural, unharmful methods occupy the same ground. The fundamental principles of osteopathy are different from those of any other system and the cause of disease is considered from one standpoint, viz: disease is the result of anatomical abnormalities followed by physiological discord. To cure disease the abnormal parts must be adjusted to the normal; therefore other methods that are entirely different in principle have no place in the osteopathic system.

Eighth: Osteopathy is an independent system and can be applied to all conditions of disease, including purely surgical cases, and in these cases surgery is but a branch of osteopathy.

Ninth: We believe that our therapeutic house is just large enough for osteopathy and that when other methods are brought in just that much osteopathy must move out.

Contemporary Differences with "Our Platform"

Addressing each of the planks of the platform, today's osteopathic physicians would have the following comments.

1. Hygienic and sanitary measures have, in fact, decreased mortality and morbidity in modern society far more than other medical measures.

2. Much of Still's criticism of the medicine of his day was provoked precisely because it was not researched and therefore, to him, without logic and not scientifically valid. However, there have been only a very few osteopathic physicians, most of them at the end of the nineteenth or beginning of the twentieth century, who were completely opposed to all medicines. Contemporary medications are often overused; there may be a higher annual number of deaths caused by medication errors and side effects than are caused by highway accidents.

3. Immunization is now achieved with standard purified doses and is better understood. Statistics have demonstrated that the morbidity and mortality rates associated with not using immunizations are considerably worse than those found when immunizations are used. Although it is impossible to predict the outcome of immunization in an individual case, assuming that the patient who succumbs to an idiosyncratic reaction to a vaccine did not have that reaction because of the sensitivity to the medium (e.g., egg protein), that patient may be the one who would have had a similar or worse reaction to the disease in an epidemic if the population were not immunized.

4. Serums or other blood parts in Still's day were much more dangerous than those found today. However, AIDS and other blood-borne diseases have demonstrated that body fluids, cells, and cell parts must be used with appropriate caution.

5. Surgery is necessary but may remain overused in the United States. Twentieth century medicine has improved diagnostic testing, and more conservative approaches have decreased the number of unnecessary surgeries. The use of aseptic technique, improved anesthesia, and microscopic and endoscopic surgery has diminished many negative consequences.

6. All therapies that are statistically demonstrated to aid patients are completely acceptable. Still was apparently never opposed to the use of x-rays studies for diagnostic purposes, because the ASO had the second diagnostic x-ray machine west of the Mississippi River. The use of radiation therapy as we know it was unknown in his time, as was the use of lasers for therapeutic purposes.

7. We recognize that disease has multiple causes that were unknown in Still's day (e.g., genetic abnormality, nutritional deficiencies, radiation damage [including sunlight], psychosomatic effects) and that his unifactorial description of the cause of illness is no longer tenable.

8. The therapeutic house of the osteopathic profession, except for a few of its founding members, has always included the latest of research on medications and the expansion in medical knowledge through this past century. However, the incorporation of this expanded knowledge into medical school curricula has resulted in less available instructional time for osteopathic manipulation, leaving some physicians less skilled and neglecting its use in appropriate cases.

*"Our Platform" from Korr IM, Ogilvie CD: Health orientation in medical education, U.S. The Texas College of Osteopathic Medicine, *Prev Med* 10:710, 1981.

spirit, it is perhaps easiest to say that throughout history, a possible third factor of human existence has been universally recognized by human societies. This factor is sometimes regarded as the most potent but the most unpredictable. Although osteopathic philosophy recognizes this factor and respects it, Still did not spend a lot of time on this interesting question in his writings or medical practice.

Still focused on what could be seen and demonstrated, particularly on the relations between structure (anatomy) and function (physiology). His methods included taking a history, observing and palpating the body, and adjusting the body's constituent parts so that they were in normal positions, with normal motion, thereby promoting normal physiology. At that point, the innate self-regulating powers of the body would accomplish what was necessary for healing to take place. Surgery and obstetrics were considered to be a normal part of osteopathic practice. Thus, Still in his writings presents osteopathic philosophy as depending on science, and not on the idea of vitalism.

EVOLUTION OF THE OSTEOPATHIC PHILOSOPHY

All philosophies that survive must be capable of incorporating newly discovered information. Striking differences from Still's original platform are found in contemporary osteopathic medical philosophy and practice.

Still died in 1917. But by 1911, while he was still alive, the ASO had incorporated instruction in vaccines, serum therapy, and antitoxins into the bacteriology course (Trowbridge, 1991). Also by 1911 the first modern antibiotic, the arsenic compound Salvarsan, which had been developed by Paul Erlich, had been successfully used against syphilis (infection with *Treponema pallidum*) (Singer et al, 1962). Following the success of Salvarsan, the sulfa drugs were developed by the 1930s. As new medicines were created and researched, the faculty and students at the ASO and other osteopathic medical colleges adopted and used them. By the 1930s, the osteopathic philosophy had been expanded to include medicines that had proven their value through research, as illustrated in the following introductory quote from the 1935 edition of the "Sage Sayings of Still":

Osteopathy is not a drugless therapy in the strict sense of the word. It uses drugs which have specific scientific value, such as antiseptics, parasiticides, antidotes, anesthetics or narcotics for the temporary relief of suffering. It is the empirical internal administration of drugs for therapeutic purposes that osteopathy opposes, substituting instead manipulation, mechanical measures and the balancing of the life essentials as more rational and more in keeping with the physiological functions of the body. The osteopathic physician is the skilled engineer of the vital human mechanism, influencing by manipulation and other osteopathic measures the activities of the nerves, cells, glands and organs, the distribution of fluids

and the discharge of nerve impulses, thus normalizing tissue, fluid and function. (Webster, 1935)

Antiseptic surgical technique was developed at about the same time as osteopathy and was included in surgical procedures practiced by the new profession. One difference between the allopathic and osteopathic approaches was that patients received OMT before and after surgery. Postsurgical treatment focused on soft tissue manipulation and *rib raising*, an articulatory treatment designed to increase the efficiency of breathing while calming the sympathetic nervous system.

The development of the sulfa antibiotics (and their increased use in hospitalized patients in the 1930s) and the advent of penicillin (as noted earlier, developed in 1927 but not commercially available until after World War II in 1945) significantly changed the practice of all medicine. Except for a very few older DOs who believed manipulation was the only answer, osteopathic physicians adopted these "miracle" medicines immediately. By accepting the use of thoroughly researched, effective medicines, classical osteopathic philosophy expanded to a more comprehensive contemporary osteopathic medical philosophy.

As an indication of the evolution of osteopathic thought, George W. Northup, DO, was quoted in 1996 as saying the following:

It is now better understood that a given "disease" is not so easily defined as was once believed. The search for a single cause for a single disease has produced disillusionment. Even the "germ theory" is not sufficient to provide a "simple" explanation for infectious diseases. All of us live in a world of potential bacterial invasion, but relatively few become infected. There are multiple causes, even in bacterially induced diseases. Disease is a total body response. It is not merely a stomach ulcer, a broken bone, or a troublesome mother-in-law. It is a disturbance of the structure-function of the body and not an isolated or local insult. Equally important is the recognition that disease is multi-causal. The understanding that multiple causes of disease can arise from remote but interconnected parts of the body will ultimately emerge into a unifying philosophy for all of medicine. When this occurs, it will embrace many of the basic principles of osteopathic medicine.

The shift in osteopathic thought embraced the progress of the scientific development of medications in the twentieth century but maintained the belief that it is not the physician who heals, but the body itself, which heals through its homeostatic mechanisms. Contemporary osteopathic medical philosophy also maintains a belief in the efficacy of manipulation to diminish or eliminate pain, improve motion, and decrease physiologic and sometimes psychological stress, thereby helping the body regain optimal homeostatic levels.

Still's original opposition to the medication of his time was due to their obvious negative effects and the lack of research to support them. One of his better-known quotes is, "Man should study and use the drugs compounded in his own body" (Still, 1897). This is increasingly the method of study today: finding out how the body works and then using medicines that interact with the body's cellular receptors and that mimic or, in some cases, are identical to the compounds found in the body.

CONTEMPORARY OSTEOPATHIC MEDICAL PHILOSOPHY

The official definition of the term *osteopathic philosophy* at the start of the twenty-first century, published in the "Glossary of Osteopathic Terminology" section of the AOA *Yearbook*, 2000, is the following:

> Osteopathic philosophy: Osteopathic medicine is a philosophy of health care and a distinctive art, supported by expanding scientific knowledge; its philosophy embraces the concept of the unity of the living organism's structure (anatomy) and function (physiology). Its art is the application of the philosophy in the practice of medicine and surgery in all its branches and specialties. Its science includes the behavioral, chemical, physical, spiritual and biological knowledge related to the establishment and maintenance of health as well as the prevention and alleviation of disease. (American Osteopathic Association, 1998)

Osteopathic concepts emphasize the following principles (American Osteopathic Association, 1998):
1. The human being is a dynamic unit of function.
2. The body possesses self-regulatory mechanisms that are self-healing in nature.
3. Structure and function are interrelated at all levels.
4. Rational treatment is based on these principles.

Contemporary osteopathic medical philosophy begins with classical osteopathy and integrates additional knowledge. Rather than application of the choice *either/or* to manipulation or medicine, *both/and* is often more appropriate. Other evolved changes include recently developed knowledge of nutrition, exercise, environmental factors, genetics and molecular biology, neuroimmunology, and psychology.

For instance, nutrition is now considered important. Still did not consider it significant and often recommended that patients just "eat what they want of good, plain nutritious food" (Still, 1897). The importance of nutrition was later added to Still's original philosophy because, although Still commented on avoiding fad diets, the food Americans ate in his age was very different from the average American diet of our times (see Chapter 25). During Still's lifetime all crops were grown organically, by definition, and most of the population of the United States was still in a rural environment. Although he mentioned good food several times, he assumed that the average diet of that era was sufficient for nourishment.

For exercise, Still occasionally mentioned walking or horseback riding. In the preautomotive society of his time, there was little need to recommend these—all people in the United States walked or rode horseback to get where they were going. A great many labor-saving devices had not yet been invented, so normal daily living took care of most of the exercise needs of the population.

Likewise, the dangers of excessive solar radiation to health had not yet become apparent in a society in which tanning was not considered attractive, sun exposure being more commonly experienced as a "red neck" than as a Hollywood tan (see Chapter 11). Farmers often wore long-sleeved shirts and hats, and even swimsuits provided practically full covering of the body and, for women, were paired with a parasol (meaning literally, from the Spanish, "against the sun") for protection from the sun. Air pollution, water pollution, and noise pollution were not specifically identified as causes of illness, nor were workplace toxins. Radiation damage was undiscovered. However, there was a general sense that densely populated, dark, dirty urban environments were unhealthy, which led to the "nature cure" and the "west cure" meant to provide benefit from exposure to recreation in the wilderness away from civilization (see Chapter 1).

Genetic mutations and deficiencies also were unknown. Physicians were virtually ignorant of the science of genetics at the end of the nineteenth century. The current hopeful promotion of "biotech" research promises multiple benefits from our expanding knowledge of molecular biology. Although this knowledge has great potential for both good and harm, its application may also be seen to fit with osteopathic philosophy.

Mind-body approaches have shown considerable potential for patient applications. Biofeedback and the relaxation response have been validated by research as ways of manipulating homeostatic mechanisms to improve psychological, neurological, and immune system functions (see Section II of this book). Psychological counseling techniques have advanced the possibilities for patients to address the stresses in their psychosocial milieu.

All of these etiological factors of illness have accordingly been integrated into an expanding contemporary osteopathic philosophy while it has retained the profound respect for the body's ability to function in the face of many challenges and its inherent capacity for self-healing when injury or illness is present.

Still thought the body was basically perfect as it was and could process environmental and nutritional input without damage unless there was an injury resulting in structural damage. We now know that the human organism is continuous with the environment, and on more than one level (body: physical; mind: thought and emotion; spirit: belief). Illness is seen by the twenty-first-century osteopathic physician as having multiple causes, any one of which can be the initiator or promoter. Nonetheless, all of these factors potentially affect the structure of the body, whether at a gross (neuromusculoskeletal) level or at a microscopic (stereochemical-bioelectrochemical) level.

Wellness therefore lies along a continuum with illness, across the time frame between the points of conception and death. Illness begins as wellness declines. Wellness indicates that the individual is capable of accepting multiple challenges without the decompensation of homeostasis to the point of interference with normal activities. As the system loses optimal homeostatic balance, less of an environmental-emotional insult is needed to precipitate a state of illness.

Early in the continuum lie problems such as nutritional deficiency, insufficient exercise or rest, and inappropriate levels of stress. If these problems are addressed while they are simple, the organism recovers and retains adaptability. On an overlapping or interactive continuum lies gross structural integrity through *tensegrity*, which involves bilateral muscle tone, balance, and function. This tensegrity system is also interactive with neural activity levels (especially in the autonomic nervous system), particularly as these factors affect the rest of the body through the respiratory, circulatory, lymphatic, endocrine, and immune systems.

When nothing is done, our homeostatic mechanisms may effect a recovery from illness without aid. Sometimes, however, the body does not have the ability to recover on its own. In such cases, structural dysfunction at either the gross or the microscopic level can be compounded by the sequelae of inflammation, pain, and tissue congestion. These negative changes in the biochemical environment of the body can cause many variables in the endocrine and immune systems to swing to wider extremes and destabilize one or more of the body's systems, leading to illness. Simple problems can sometimes be solved with manipulation, lifestyle changes (e.g., exercises), or nutrition to reestablish optimal homeostatic set points.

Ideas such as these are not easily understood by a reductionistic approach to the body, in which each variable is analyzed by itself or perhaps in conjunction with one or two other variables (e.g., the balance between insulin and glucagon). Current understanding recognizes much more complexity in the interactions between many more subtle variables, such as homeostatic hormonal systems that control many body functions.

The use of a complex adaptive systems model, with *chaos theory* mathematics, has enabled greater understanding of the complexity of dynamic medical systems. Chaos theory mathematics allows us to understand how altering a single or even a few variables in one system (e.g., cardiovascular) can affect the function of other systems, and thereby the entire human being. One factor that has been noted is that a complex system has *sensitive dependence on initial conditions*. This concept has been popularized as the *butterfly effect,* which suggests that the simple motion of a butterfly's wings in the Amazon may affect the weather patterns in Moscow 3 months later (Gleick, 1987). Although this extreme example may makes us chuckle, or marvel, the mathematical models following chaos theory principles appear to be closer to predicting what actually happens in the natural world than are any previous analyses. Mathematicians now use similar models to explain, for example, a decompensating cycle of cardiac arrhythmia leading to fatal fibrillation (Gleick, 1987). Understanding new concepts such as point attractors, strange attractors, triviality, nontriviality, and degeneracy leads to a better understanding of the processes of homeostasis and the way in which manipulation of anatomical relations and tissue tensions may promote physiological adaptability.

Each of the body's systems is understood to be integrated with the entire body, functioning in a bidirectional manner as part of the whole person. The neuromusculoskeletal system is the largest single system in the body; it reflects the state of health of the other systems, yielding diagnostic clues for systemic or organic function or dysfunction. It can also be used as an access for treatment, using manipulation to change the motion possible at the joints and the set points of muscle length and tone, and thereby affecting vascular and lymphatic flow and neural (particularly autonomic) tone.

OSTEOPATHIC PRINCIPLES

To an osteopathic physician, osteopathic principles are common-sense ideas that provide a milieu in which to diagnose and treat a patient. At some level, the physician should always be aware of the following considerations:

- Who is the patient? The patient is a human being like the physician, a functional unity of body (a genetically constructed grouping of cells and systems), mind (thoughts and emotions), and a third factor (identified by some as spirit), which is interactive with the environment at physical, psychosocial, and energetic levels. The human being functions by transforming thought into action through the neuromusculoskeletal system.
- Where does health arise? Health comes from within the patient.
- What is the goal of the osteopathic physician? The physician seeks health in the patient. Wellness and illness exist on a continuum, or on an interactive multidimensional group of continua. It is the physician's job to help the patient seek the highest possible level of homeostatic balance and performance within the patient's individual limitations and the current circumstances.
- How does the osteopathic physician seek health in the patient? Prevention is the best medicine; the

physician encourages and teaches the patient to follow healthful practices (e.g., appropriate rest, nutrition, exercise, breathing exercises, positive thoughts and emotions, relaxation, social interaction) and to avoid that which is self-destructive (e.g., tobacco, radiation, toxins, excessive alcohol, drugs, overeating).

If the patient has entered the illness end of the continuum, the osteopathic physician must take a careful history, perform a physical examination, and formulate a differential diagnosis. The neuromusculoskeletal system is included as an access point for diagnostic signs that may indicate systemic problems (and later, an access for imparting information to the other systems). Tests may be needed. After arriving at a diagnosis, the physician decides on necessary treatment, bearing in mind all factors that affect the physiology and performance of the patient. The medical standard of care is included in this process, but osteopathic physicians retain a holistic rather than reductionistic focus, and include OMT when it is indicated, whether as primary or adjunct treatment.

What factors affect the physiology of the patient? Physiology can be affected by air, water, and food; nutritional supplements; prescription and over-the-counter medications; physical forces and impacts on the system (ranging from the effects of any movement, including exercise, to trauma); thoughts, emotions, stress, or relaxation; and energy (from gravity to sunlight to magnetic fields to energies of which we may not yet be aware). All of the body's systems are integrative, but five are more easily seen as unifying systems of global body communication (cardiovascular and lymphatic, respiratory, neurologic, endocrine, and immune systems).

The host has control of vulnerability to illness through the immune system and homeostatic mechanisms (the true *vis medicatrix naturae*). When host control decreases and the system downgrades into illness, intervention is necessary. Intervention is designed to support a system that is no longer functioning at an appropriately high level of homeostasis.

How does the osteopathic physician intervene? Just as wellness, injury, and illness exist along a continuum, so do treatment approaches. When physical or emotional force has distorted anatomical or physiological performance, the physician addresses the problems with physical approaches ranging from manipulation to surgery. When genetic limitations or illness make it impossible for the body to perform appropriate functions on its own or with the speed required, the physician uses exogenous substances such as medication, nutritional supplementation, or other proven therapies. (From the point of view of chaos mathematics and dynamical systems, the physician seeks to reverse abnormal trivial point attractors to strange attractor status.) The physician does this in a conservative manner, bearing in mind the body's innate intelligence and the wisdom of using the least possible intervention (least invasive) for the greatest possible results.

OSTEOPATHIC TECHNIQUES

Osteopathy is not just a system of techniques, but a philosophy that is often applied through techniques of osteopathic manipulative medicine, which were developed by osteopathic physicians. Several of the more commonly recognized osteopathic diagnosis and treatment systems are described here. There are, of course, many others. Multiple techniques may be used to achieve a single objective as part of a complete osteopathic treatment. Although some procedures relate more to joint surface apposition, others address muscle and connective tissue tension imbalances, promote vascular and lymphatic flow, or modulate autonomic nervous system tone. Most techniques affect more than one of those functions when applied. One technique may lead to the use of another, depending on the patient's problem, the perception and skill of the osteopathic physician, and the difficulty level in achieving the desired outcome.

Some osteopathic physicians have said that there are only two types of techniques, direct and indirect. *Direct treatment* is treatment that confronts restriction of motion, in which the body part is taken directly toward restricted motion. *Indirect treatment* is treatment in which the body part is taken in the direction of ease of motion. Once the body part is appropriately positioned, activating forces are applied to induce changes in muscle and connective tissue length and tone; central, peripheral, or autonomic nervous system tone (level of activation); joint surface apposition and motion; or vascular-lymphatic function. Treatment goals include tissue relaxation, increased physiological motion, decrease in pain, and optimization of homeostasis.

The following are examples of the more common systems of OMT. Like any form of medical treatment, manipulation in any form has both indications and contraindications, which are not discussed here because they are well outlined in other texts.

SOFT TISSUE AND LYMPHATIC TREATMENTS

Soft tissue treatment, generally a direct treatment, was developed by Still and his early students and is sometimes confused with massage. The techniques focus on altering the tone (and length) of muscle and connective tissue. Soft tissue treatment relaxes muscles and connective tissue, decreases or removes tissue tension impediment to arterial delivery, and alters the tone of the autonomic nervous system. Whereas soft tissue treatment definitely affects the lymphatics, there are also other specific lymphatic techniques that focus on increasing lymphatic return.

HIGH-VELOCITY LOW-AMPLITUDE THRUST

In the direct method of treatment referred to as *high-velocity low-amplitude (HVLA) thrust*, the restrictive barrier is engaged by precise positioning of the body. The thrust when the body part is at the restrictive barrier is very rapid (high velocity) but operates over a very short distance (low amplitude), gapping the articulation by approximately ⅛ inch or less. This allows a reset of both joint position and muscle tension levels, which causes related neural and vascular readjustment.

ARTICULATORY TECHNIQUE

The original general articulatory technique, developed by Still and his students, takes the body part being treated to the end portion of its restricted range of motion in a gentle, repetitive fashion. The repeated motion directly diminishes the restrictive barrier. Movements within one or more planes of motion are treated at one time. This technique can be used to treat individual joints or regions (e.g., shoulder, cervical spine).

Still also used specific articulation techniques that began with diagnosis, placing the body parts in the direction of ease of motion and rotating them into the direction of restriction. These specific articulation techniques have been called the *Still technique* (Van Buskirk, 1996). *Facilitated positional release* (Schiowitz, 1997) is also a variation of the type of work Still himself did.

MUSCLE ENERGY TECHNIQUE

Muscle energy treatment was developed by Fred Mitchell, Sr., DO. It is most commonly used as a direct treatment, and the term *muscle energy* means that the patient uses his or her own energy through directed muscular cooperation with the physician. Reflexive changes in muscle tension are used in a variety of ways to allow dysfunctional, shortened muscles to lengthen; abnormally lengthened muscles to shorten; weakened muscles to strengthen; and hypertonic muscles to relax. Commonly, voluntary isometric contraction of a patient's muscles is followed by a gentle stretch of the dysfunctional, contracted tissue, which decreases abnormal restriction of motion. Other muscle energy techniques use traction on the muscle to pull an articulation back into the appropriate position, reciprocal inhibition to relax antagonists, cross-extensor reflexes to affect an opposite limb, or oculocervical reflexes (using eye motion to relax neck muscles).

COUNTERSTRAIN TECHNIQUE

Counterstrain is a passive positional technique that places the patient's dysfunctional joint (spinal or other) or tissue in a position of ease. This position arrests the inappropriate mechanoreceptor activity or nocifensive reflexes that maintain the somatic dysfunction. Marked shortening of the involved muscle or connective tissue is maintained for 90 seconds. An inappropriate strain reflex (a result of injury) is therefore inhibited by application of counterstrain. Diagnosis is primarily by palpation of areas of tenderness mapped by the originator of this system, Lawrence Jones, DO. This form of diagnosis can also be integrated with positional, movement, or tissue texture abnormalities. The tender point is indicative of inappropriate neurological balance. This system is ideal for the patient who may not respond well to articulatory techniques, such as the postsurgical patient.

MYOFASCIAL RELEASE

Myofascial release is actually a renaming of original osteopathic techniques developed by Still, which early osteopathic physicians called "fascial techniques." Anthony Chila, Robert Ward, and John Peckham developed a course in these techniques at MSU, in which they also acknowledged the importance of the muscle tissue to the treatment. This technique may be performed by either lengthening the contracted tissue (direct myofascial release) or shortening it (indirect myofascial release) and allowing the nervous and respiratory systems to facilitate changes, which remain after the treatment is completed. Two physiological biomechanical tissue processes, creep and hysteresis, also play a role. Compression, traction, torsion, respiratory cooperation, or a combination may be included to facilitate treatment.

OSTEOPATHY IN THE CRANIAL FIELD

Osteopathy in the cranial field, also referred to as *OCF*, *cranial osteopathy*, and *craniosacral osteopathy*, was developed by William G. Sutherland, DO. It is usually done as a mixture of indirect and direct procedures that work with the body's inherent rhythmic motions. It is commonly used in adults as a treatment for headaches or temporomandibular joint dysfunction syndrome and in infants (whose skulls are more flexible) for treatment of symptoms related to cranial nerve compression (e.g., vomiting, poor sleep, poor feeding) or in cases in which mechanical factors can affect fluid drainage (otitis media). Although OCF techniques often focus on the skull and the sacrum, where the dura mater attaches, they can be and are commonly used throughout the body.

John Upledger, DO, taught many nonphysicians a simpler variant of the technique, which included elements not generally practiced by osteopathic physicians, and called his version *craniosacral therapy*. Because application of this technique is not medically licensed and regulated, lay people using this therapy are often doing something considerably different from and less specific than what a licensed osteopathic physician would do in practice.

VISCERAL TECHNIQUES

A variety of techniques have been developed from the beginning of the profession to address imbalance in the viscera. These include stretching and balancing techniques related to ligamentous attachments, as originated by Still, and may involve use of inherent visceral motion. More recently, Jean-Pierre Barral, a nonphysician osteopath from France, has developed and taught an entire system of visceral techniques.

DIAGNOSIS AND TREATMENT IN OSTEOPATHIC MEDICINE

Osteopathic diagnosis and treatment are determined by the osteopathic philosophy, which makes the practice of osteopathic medicine distinctive and different. This philosophy and OMT should not be viewed as merely the addition of something extra to the contemporary Western medical approach (the cherry on top of the ice cream sundae). Osteopathic philosophy serves as an organizer of thought that helps the physician understand what is going on in the entire organism, allows concurrent reductionistic analysis, and then reassembles the parts into the totality of the human being, who is more than the sum of the parts.

Osteopathic diagnosis differs in that the osteopathic physician performs the standard orthopedic and neurological portions of the physical examination, but also includes additional tissue palpation, as well as testing of muscle and joint motion. The musculoskeletal system is examined as an access point for additional diagnostic information, not only on muscle tension but on fluid distribution and autonomic levels of activity. Well-known neurological reflex interactions permit a physician to conclude from musculoskeletal evidence that an underlying visceral problem may exist and should be investigated. When abnormalities are noted, *somatic dysfunction* is diagnosed. It is important to note that somatic dysfunction is not tissue damage, which the body must heal. Rather, somatic dysfunction is a disorder of the body's programming for length, tension, joint surface apposition affecting mobility, tissue fluid flow efficiency, and neurological balance.

Osteopathic diagnosis expands the standard medical differential diagnosis in a number of ways. For example, consider the standard medical diagnosis of lumbalgia or lumbar pain. After examination, the osteopathic physician who finds the appropriate objective criteria will diagnose *lumbar somatic dysfunction,* and the physician's note will include more specific information about which of the lumbar spinal segments is(are) unable to function normally.

Four criteria are used to diagnose somatic dysfunction: tissue texture abnormalities (T), static or positional asymmetry (A), restriction of motion (R), and tenderness (T). These have been referred to by the diagnostic mnemonic *TART.* When these signs are noted at particular spinal segmental levels, knowledge of reflex relationships also guides reflection on their cause. They may be evidence of viscerosomatic, somatovisceral, viscerovisceral, or somatosomatic reflexes. Is the problem simply mechanical, or is it evidence of underlying visceral problems as well? The osteopathic physician then pays more attention to both the history and physical examination of the internal organs related to spinal cord segmental levels. These reflexes show palpatory evidence of autonomic nervous system influence at segmental levels and may produce abnormalities of tissue texture and muscle tone.

The fourth tenet of osteopathic philosophy states that treatment will be based on this knowledge of structure and function. With a primary musculoskeletal problem involving restricted motion and abnormally high muscle tone, it is common sense to decrease the tone and increase the motion to regain normal function. However, when the neuromusculoskeletal system is used as a clue in uncovering visceral dysfunction, it is recognized by the profession that lowering muscle tone related to visceral dysfunction will at the very least decrease one portion of what is now a vicious cycle from which the body is then likely to recover more rapidly. The concept includes lowering inappropriate sympathetic nervous system tone and thereby enhancing homeostatic balance and adaptability. In addition, making it easier for the patient with pneumonia, for example, to breathe more easily by treating the mechanical aspects of breathing makes good sense.

Medication or surgery may be unnecessary, depending on the severity of the problem. OMT may be used as a primary means of treatment for a problem that appears to be of nonsevere, musculoskeletal origin; as primary treatment for simple illness that requires no medication (e.g., viral upper respiratory illness); or as adjunctive therapy along with medication or surgery—again, to enhance homeostatic recovery and adaptability. Medications for symptomatic relief may or may not be used, depending on the case and the preference or needs of the patient.

Two simple case examples are presented here. These are not complete cases, but are designed to illustrate some of the osteopathic differences in approach to diagnosis and treatment. In each example, the techniques chosen did not challenge the patients with muscular effort and were selected with homeostatic effects in mind (decrease of edema, mobilization of fluids, enhancement of respiration). In many other ambulatory cases, any of the listed treatments (e.g., HVLA thrust) could be selected based on four factors: the condition of the patient, the nature of the complaint, the goals of treatment, and the skills of the physician.

Case Example 1

A 67-year-old African American woman with a 30 pack-year history of smoking comes to the office with a productive cough that she has had for 2 weeks. She now has a fever, and the sputum is greenish. She has pain in the ribs on the left side of the thorax and audible rhonchi when examined with the stethoscope. After a careful history taking and physical examination, the physician concludes that although the differential diagnosis includes a possible tumor, this is less likely than a community-acquired pneumonia. Radiographic studies indicate a left lingular pneumonitis, and there is an increased white blood cell count with a left shift. The physician has noted on examination that pulmonary viscerosomatic reflexes are activated in the corresponding thoracic spinal region, which is causing limitation in range of motion and tenderness, along with tissue texture changes, at several thoracic vertebral segments. Several ribs on the left have diminished mobility, and the diaphragm has decreased excursion on the left.

The physician decides to start antibiotics immediately and treats the thoracic segments and ribs with OMT, in this case choosing counterstrain because it requires no muscular effort on the part of the patient and poses minimal risk of injury to bones that may be osteoporotic. In patients who are coughing frequently, breathing mechanics are often disturbed. Treating the thoracic segments and ribs helps normalize the sympathetic nervous system activity and increases the efficiency and ease of breathing. The thoracic outlet, where the thoracic lymphatic duct has passage, is treated, which allows for less tissue compression that impedes the flow of lymphatic fluid. The diaphragm (which often has impaired motion from the spasmodic motion of coughing) is treated with myofascial release, and the cervical region is treated with counterstrain to decrease any problems with the phrenic nerve (which innervates the diaphragm for respiration). A lymphatic pump procedure concludes the treatment. Antitussives are prescribed along with the antibiotics and an expectorant. Acetaminophen may be used for fever and pain. The patient is seen again in 3 days, at which time she is greatly improved.

The rationale behind the medical treatment is obvious: kill the bacteria, decrease the viscosity of the mucus that holds them so that they can be coughed out, and give the patient a painkiller to decrease pain. This type of treatment relies on the body to recover its optimal performance once certain negatives are canceled out. The osteopathic treatment is designed to aid normal physiological processes that augment the body's natural systems in killing the bacteria and reducing pain. OMT may enable a faster recovery for the patient—or increase the odds of survival. The osteopathic physician takes advantage of both possibilities, aiding the host's natural defenses while fighting the bacteria directly through use of antibiotics. The patient's comfort level is also increased by the use of the osteopathic manipulation.

Case Example 2

A 19-year-old white male college student comes for treatment of an apparent sprained ankle. The injury occurred during a soccer game when he reached for the ground with his foot and made a sudden turn. There is no other relevant history. The ankle is swollen, and the patient applied ice immediately after the injury. He can walk, but he keeps most of his weight off the ankle. There is pinpoint tenderness at the posteroinferior right lateral malleolus.

The physician chooses to treat with superficial indirect myofascial release and, afterward, lymphatic techniques to decrease the edema. Treatment is specifically limited to a minimal approach, which causes the patient no pain. The patient is given a set of crutches to use for a couple of days and goes to the hospital to get a radiographic study, the results of which are negative. He is to use ice at least three times a day and to keep his weight off the ankle, which is wrapped after the treatment with an elastic bandage. He is to keep the ankle elevated when possible and to use acetaminophen for pain if needed. Because the radiographic study shows no fracture, the physician continues the treatment 2 days later with counterstrain and lymphatic treatment, and the patient is allowed to discontinue use of the crutches.

Draining excess fluid and decreasing the overabundance of proinflammatory neuropeptides and other biopeptides through the use of OMT allows the hypertonic and injured tissues to return to normal more quickly. The decrease or elimination of muscle spasm allows the ankle and foot to have more normal mechanics, therefore promoting more normal lymphatic and venous drainage. Again, the osteopathic treatment is designed to enhance the body's own methods of healing, promoting a rapid return to more normal homeostatic balance by removing dysfunction.

MANIPULATION AS A CRITICAL ASPECT OF OSTEOPATHIC PHILOSOPHY

If osteopathy is a philosophy, why is the use of manipulation in the practice of medicine considered a hallmark and a necessary, integral part of osteopathic medicine? The answer lies in the original osteopathic philosophy, which relates to the interaction between structure (anatomy) and function (physiology) in the human species, and how we can effect changes in the human body. It can be found at two levels, the macroscopic and the microscopic.

At the macroscopic level, it is easy to see that if there is abnormal pressure on a joint, nerve, or blood vessel, there may be resulting changes in tissue over time. For instance, if there is more pressure on the medial aspect of the right knee, over time there will be changes in the cartilage and bone to compensate. There will also be gait changes as the body attempts to rebalance itself to use the least amount of energy for posture and locomotion. Thus local dysfunction can induce global dysfunction. Manipulation, which has the local effects of adjusting the balance in the musculoskeletal system, also has global effects at a gross level.

At a microscopic level, cellular physiology depends on fluid flow. The original one-celled organisms were bathed in a solution of ancient seawater, which delivered oxygen and nutrients and also took away toxic waste products and carbon dioxide as they were produced and ejected from the cell (see Chapter 25). Multicellular organisms such as the human being contain an internal ocean, which preserves the contents of this ancient seawater, with the same functions. This internal fluid system is the cardiovascular system, delivering oxygen and nutrients to each individual cell and clearing carbon dioxide and waste products (as well as excessive proteins through lymphatic drainage).

If this system is impeded in any way, cells, followed by tissues, organs, and entire systems, decrease their level of function. This form of physiological stress then makes the organism vulnerable to disease. To offer an analogy, a good fluid delivery and clearance system is like an open, clean, flowing stream or river. If the flow is blocked, we have the potential for developing a swamp. Stagnant water allows the buildup of noxious products, and the local environment is completely changed. If the blockage is cleared through manual effort, the stream reestablishes good flow and removes the toxic elements that had begun to build up. When osteopathic treatment is used to adjust tissue tensions toward the norm, the body's own elimination systems can clear toxic waste products produced by cellular damage and allowed to build up by suboptimal fluid flow.

Osteopathic manipulation is therefore a means not only of decreasing or eliminating pain, but also of adjusting the involved structures toward an optimal adaptability level of the body's *tensegrity* system. This adjustment helps prevent noxious stimulus (through compression or excessive stretching of nociceptors) at a macroscopic level, and toxic conditions (through lack of appropriate oxygen and nutrient delivery and inadequate waste clearance) in cells at a microscopic level. Manipulation is therefore a central issue for osteopathic medicine: although it cannot cure all illness, manipulation is used to help the body function at an optimal level, enhancing its ability to heal itself. The body is capable of amazing feats of self-recovery and may perform these feats more quickly and thoroughly if assisted.

Manipulation, like all forms of medical treatment, has limitations. It is possible that the body's functional levels have been so negatively altered that the use of manipulation alone will not enhance the body's self-adjusting systems enough (or perhaps not within an acceptable time) for it to regain good health without the additional assistance of medication or surgery. It may

also be necessary to integrate direct psychosocial intervention to achieve recovery.

Medicines and surgery are used to effect changes in two circumstances, which occur commonly: (1) when the physician believes that preventive measures or manipulation alone will not be able to accomplish the total goal of health (e.g., when use of insulin in a patient with type 1 diabetes or narcotics in a terminally ill cancer patient is necessary), or (2) when speed is of the essence and it would be dangerous to the patient to rely solely on manipulation and/or other conservative measures and wait for the body's self-healing responses (e.g., use of antibiotics to treat infection).

Osteopathic physicians who do not use manipulation or refer patients to have it done but who treat patients in a holistic manner are ignoring a main premise of osteopathic philosophy: elimination of structural impediments that diminish normal physiological function to promote the body's self-healing capabilities.

LEVELS OF IMPLEMENTATION

There have been conspicuous differences between the evolution of Still's ideas in the United States and in other parts of the world. In the United States, there is a vast spectrum of application of osteopathic principles in the practice of medicine by DOs. Internationally, the application of osteopathic philosophy through manipulative techniques has been different from that in the United States and involves multiple pathways and levels of training.

In the United States, DOs have always been physicians. Current practitioners implement the osteopathic medical philosophy at various levels along a continuum of medical care. Initially, all osteopathic physicians believed in the efficacy of manipulation to affect the physiology of the body in a positive way. In fact, this has been the hallmark of the osteopathic profession, and Still's development of osteopathic structural diagnosis and treatment was the original reason for the osteopathic profession's existence.

At one end of the continuum, the earliest osteopathic practitioners implemented a pure, classical form of osteopathy, using either manipulation or surgery but recommending against virtually all medications (which at the time did much harm and little good). This type of practitioner is a historical footnote in the development of osteopathic practice in America; this author knows of no such practitioners at this time. Some physicians accept the importance of manipulation for treatment of musculoskeletal pain but do not see it as having any value in systemic illness.

A small number of osteopathic physicians have chosen to specialize in neuromusculoskeletal medicine (osteopathic specialty: NMM). Some of their patients have primary musculoskeletal complaints, and for others, they are giving adjunctive treatment for medical cases in conjunction with treatment by other physicians. Some of these specialists use a minimum of medications, preferring to refer patients who need medication or surgical care to primary care or specialty physicians.

Within the ranks of primary care osteopathic physicians, some use osteopathic techniques in a reductionistic manner (e.g., treating only the neck if there is neck pain). This limited application ignores the fact that pain may be more noticeable in a body region that is compensating for a problem, rather than in the region that is the primary source of the problem. The physician would be neglecting the many muscle and connective tissue connections between the thoracic region and the neck, as well as the sympathetic chain ganglia in the upper thoracic region that help set the tone for the cervical musculature. In addition, any other restricted region of the body may alter the body's tensegrity relationships, which can result in the complaint of pain in the neck. Such an approach will be successful only if the primary problem is being addressed. It is important to address the primary problem, not just compensation or annoying symptoms.

A majority of osteopathic physicians continue to work in primary care specialties, although that proportion is decreasing. There is a great range in the amount of OMT that these physicians use with their patients. Some who believe in the efficacy of OMT, but feel that they do not have time to use it in a busy day of patient care, may use it to treat a friend or relative and will refer patients who need manipulation to physicians who specialize in its use.

Remarkably, there are a number of DOs who have no belief in the clinical efficacy of OMT. Some never accepted the osteopathic philosophy nor intended to use OMT, but attended an osteopathic medical college because it was a pathway to an unrestricted medical license. A subset of this group believes that the laying on of hands is, however, valuable for evoking either a mind-body or a placebo effect. There are also osteopathic physicians who do not want to be confused with chiropractors and believe that manual therapeutics are best left to doctors of chiropractic, physical therapists, and other manual therapists.

Whether or not they use OMT, virtually all osteopathic physicians in the United States share a profound respect for the body's self-healing ability. They have been taught to approach their patients in a holistic manner, viewing each as a unique human being whose current circumstances are also unique to the person and interact with his or her own psychosocial and environmental milieu.

CURRENT STATUS

PRACTICE RIGHTS

Osteopathic physicians in all 50 of the United States of America have the same practice rights as MDs. At the end of the nineteenth and beginning of the twentieth century,

this was not the case. Some states immediately gave full practice rights to DOs; others gave partial practice rights, which varied from the right to diagnose and treat with manual medicine without prescription of medication, to the inclusion of obstetric privileges, to full medical and surgical privileges. Most states in which osteopathic licensure was possible gave full practice rights.

Although the right to practice was guaranteed by law, it was not always easy for DOs in the early to mid twentieth century to obtain hospital privileges. Even at the time of the Kline Report to the AMA (1953), many MDs were unaware that osteopathic medical education was equivalent to their own and therefore blocked access to hospital privileges. Younger MDs were influenced in this regard by older physicians, whose opinions were formed at a time when DOs did not use the available but highly toxic medications. There was poor understanding among MDs of the rationale behind osteopathy's early rejection of medicines: that medicines in the preantibiotic era were poor in quality and generally toxic, and that use of medications at that time was based on tradition or conjecture rather than research. Some skepticism about new medications is also warranted by all.

This conflict spurred DOs to build their own hospitals, thus forming a network of their own for accreditation standards. At times they used a wing of another hospital, such as the osteopathic wing of the Los Angeles County Hospital (which became the women's wing of the hospital after the osteopathic-allopathic amalgamation in 1962). Osteopathic hospitals expanded in number and size in the 1960s and 1970s. At the end of the twentieth century, many hospitals closed or merged under the purely economic pressures of managed care and health maintenance organizations. The number of osteopathic hospitals, many of which were small community hospitals, declined in the face of these changing economic conditions. Another factor contributing to this decrease was that DOs were freely granted privileges in MD hospitals, which made independent osteopathic hospitals less necessary for patient care. However, this meant a decrease in osteopathic influence in graduate medical education, as an increasing number of graduates of osteopathic medical schools began choosing residencies accredited by the Accreditation Council for Graduate Medical Education (ACGME) rather than the AOA.

REQUIREMENTS FOR MATRICULATION

Prospective students who wish to apply to osteopathic medical schools should have completed a bachelor's degree with a high grade point average and successful scores on the Medical College Aptitude Test (MCAT). Interviewers at the osteopathic colleges look for students who are successful at academic tasks. Preference is given to those who also have sought relevant medical experience, such as working as a volunteer in a hospital or other medical facility, shadowing physicians, holding a job in a related field (e.g., at a hospital laboratory), or participating in medical research. Such experience suggests that an applicant has observed the work of physicians and is able to deal with the sight of blood, sick patients, and patients in pain.

The interview at an osteopathic medical school generally includes informal assessment on the part of the interviewers of the student's ability to empathize with patients. Because most osteopathic physicians are in general or family practice, it is a cultural value of the osteopathic profession to look for applicants who are "people persons," meaning individuals who can interact easily with others. It is believed by DOs that this characteristic enables a physician to communicate with patients in ways that elicit information relevant to diagnosis more easily and elicit better compliance. This does not mean that only extraverts are accepted as students. Interviewers recognize that it is not a favor to accept a student who has good people skills but insufficient academic strength.

Interviewers often also pay attention to whether a student has been interested enough to study the history and philosophy of osteopathic medicine.

CURRENT STATUS OF U.S. OSTEOPATHIC MEDICAL SCHOOLS

All AOA-accredited osteopathic medical schools are listed by the World Health Organization (WHO) in its official list of United States medical schools. Table 17-1 provides additional information about these institutions.

As of 2008, 25 U.S. osteopathic medical colleges or schools (plus three branch campuses) were open and in operation. Five original private osteopathic schools form a core that dates back to the late nineteenth and beginning twentieth century (having opened from 1892 to 1916). Ten new colleges of osteopathic medicine opened their doors between 1970 and 1981. This second wave included six state-funded (public) colleges, as the states involved moved to fill a shortage of physicians, particularly primary care physicians in underserved and rural areas. A third wave of private school development began in 1992 and continues to expand. For the first time, outside entrepreneurs began to found osteopathic medical colleges for their own reasons. Touro University, a Jewish institution, founded Touro University College of Osteopathic Medicine–California in 1992, opened a branch campus in Nevada (Touro University Nevada College of Osteopathic Medicine) in 2004, and started a separate college of osteopathic medicine in Harlem in 2007. This was the first time a private religious university had opened an osteopathic college in the United States. In 2008, the first and only for-profit college of osteopathic medicine since publication of the Flexner Report in 1910 was opened, Rocky Vista University College of Osteopathic Medicine in Parker, Colorado. This was extremely controversial in the osteopathic profession, but there were no rules against it for the AOA to enforce.

POSTGRADUATE EDUCATION

Medical and surgical postgraduate education consists of internships and residencies, which are training programs for general medicine, such as internal medicine or family practice, or for specialty medicine, such as cardiothoracic surgery. Throughout the twentieth century, generalists have increased the time they spend in postgraduate programs and demanded recognition for the practice of general medicine as a specialty itself, distinguishing their practices from those who did only an internship.

The rotating internship was a hallmark of the osteopathic medical profession in the twentieth century. The common understanding among osteopathic physicians was that the best specialist has a good foundation as a generalist. Competence in general medicine was believed to allow more integrated assessment of a patient's needs and to decrease the amount of "falling through the cracks" that is possible when the patient is seeing only a series of specialists. This concept remained in effect for osteopathic postgraduate programs through the last half of the twentieth century, a time when most MD specialists entered their specialty training directly after medical school. A number of states required candidates for licensure as an osteopathic physician to complete a rotating internship.

Increasingly in the last two decades, however, osteopathic medical graduates have favored omitting a year of general internship in favor of immediate pursuit of postgraduate education in a field of specialty. The AOA has responded to perceived needs of graduates by creating *tracking internships,* or internships that retain a level of general training while decreasing some of the previous requirements to allow more time within the internship for specialization. The internship is then credited as the first year of postgraduate training in the appropriate specialty. The end result is that there is still an extra requirement of general medicine and surgery in the AOA tracking internships compared with the ACGME postgraduate year 1 programs in most specialties.

Throughout the twentieth century, the osteopathic profession maintained that most physicians should be family doctors practicing general medicine and attracted students who implemented this philosophy in their choice of specialties. The profession's promotion of family medicine encouraged a number of state legislatures to fund an osteopathic medical college in the interest of their citizens, to supply more generalists and family physicians to underserved and rural areas.

One result of the mix of students favored during recruitment (e.g., students who had osteopathic physicians as role models, applicants screened in informal assessment for their people skills) and the encouragement given to medical school students to choose primary care specialties has been that fewer students were recruited who showed interest in pursuing a career of medical research.

Although the osteopathic medical profession has participated marginally in medical research from its inception, the bulk of its contribution to American health care has been through patient care. With the recent rapid increase in the number of osteopathic medical colleges, development of some state-funded institutions, and the rapid increase in the raw number of osteopathic physicians, attention to the profession's responsibility for contributing to medical research is growing.

Research at osteopathic medical schools falls into three categories. Most of the research is in either basic science or standard medical care. A small amount of research has been conducted on the scientific basis of and effects of osteopathic structural diagnosis and treatment. This third category has historically been poorly funded, because pharmaceutical companies were not inclined to sponsor research that might prove that the use of less medication is better or that use of natural practices is more likely to prevent side effects of medication. Until recently, the government was not interested in funding aspects of medicine with which the medical establishment did not concern itself.

In the early to mid twentieth century, individuals such as Louisa Burns, Irvin Korr, Steadman Denslow, Beryl Arbuckle, and Viola Frymann represented a significant portion of the effort of the profession to validate the scientific and clinical basis of osteopathic manipulation. A group of researchers also came together at MSU's College of Osteopathic Medicine, which was productive from the 1970s forward.

Aside from the commercial and political nature of award grants, other factors have interfered with sufficient accumulation of research in the osteopathic profession. Only five osteopathic medical colleges continued in existence from 1916 to 1968, and all of these were private and had very limited if any endowment funds. Prior to 1969, no state institutions funded an osteopathic college. The colleges focused on producing physicians for the people, not researchers. Although small amounts of research were ongoing at the colleges, few researchers interested themselves in uniquely osteopathic issues. In this research, another factor was the initial difficulty of performing double-blind studies on the use of manual medicine. Eventually this problem was solved by the use of naive subjects, blinded physicians, and sham treatments. The increasing use of outcome and cost-effectiveness studies in the field of medicine has promoted additional interest in doing research on the unique contribution of the osteopathic profession, OMT.

In the 1980s, the AOA passed a special annual assessment that was included in membership dues to build up funds for research. Small pilot grants were distributed to the existing osteopathic colleges that applied. More recently, an Osteopathic Research Center has been funded at the University of North Texas Health Science Center at the Texas College of Osteopathic Medicine in Fort Worth for the purpose of

conducting osteopathically oriented basic science bench research, clinical research, and transitional research that bridges the gap between the two. The AOA Commission on Osteopathic College Accreditation requires institutions, as a part of the undergraduate accreditation process, to "make contributions to the advancement of knowledge and the development of osteopathic medicine through scientific research."

INTERNATIONAL IMPACT AND EVOLUTION OF OSTEOPATHIC CONCEPTS

Osteopathy began as a unique American contribution to the science and art of health care. The international evolution of osteopathy became complex and diversified, as Americans and internationals trained in the United States around 1900, at the inception of the osteopathic medical profession, emigrated or returned to their own native countries. The early osteopath who had the most to do with spreading Still's original discovery internationally was John Martin Littlejohn, a Scotland-educated MD who served for 2 years as dean of faculty at the American School of Osteopathy while obtaining his American DO degree. Leaving Kirksville in 1900, he moved to Chicago and founded the American College of Osteopathic Medicine and Surgery, which is now Midwestern University. Littlejohn was a native of the United Kingdom, and he returned to the United Kingdom in 1913.

In 1918, Littlejohn opened the British School of Osteopathy (BSO), founding an osteopathic profession in which the practitioners did not use surgery, medicine, or obstetrics, and it has not evolved into a profession with an unlimited medical license (Van Buskirk, 1996). The BSO's first diplomates graduated in 1925, but the practice of osteopathy in the United Kingdom remained unregulated until the last decade of the twentieth century. Based on this model, the nonphysician practice of osteopathic philosophy and manipulation spread through the British Commonwealth, was copied in other western European nations, and was disseminated from them to much of the rest of the world. Australia regulated the practice of osteopathy in 1978, and the United Kingdom in 1993.

The British government regulated the practice of osteopathy in 1993 with the Act of Osteopaths and later included nonphysician osteopathic practitioners in the national health care system. These practitioners are generally perceived as specialists in treatment of musculoskeletal pain and adjunctive treatment. They are also sometimes consulted if the patient has vague complaints and continuing physician efforts do not produce an organic diagnosis. Management of medical conditions is left to the physician. Incorporation of a limited amount of medical knowledge has increased in the education of osteopathic practitioners in the past two decades. Their diploma does not give them the education or the right to prescribe medicine or to perform or assist at surgery or childbirth.

TABLE 17-1

Current Status of U.S. Osteopathic Medical Colleges*

College	Location	Affiliated university	First class matriculated	Public, private nonprofit, or for profit	Web address
Kirksville College of Osteopathic Medicine	Kirksville, Mo.	Andrew Taylor Still University (ATSU)	1892	Private	http://www.atsu.edu
DMU-COM	Des Moines, Iowa	Des Moines University	1898	Private	http://www.dmu.edu/com
Philadelphia College of Osteopathic Medicine (PCOM)	Philadelphia, Pa.	Freestanding	1899	Private	http://www.pcom.edu
Chicago College of Osteopathic Medicine	Downer's Grove, Ill.	Midwestern University	1900	Private	http://www.midwestern.edu/ccom
KCUMB-COM	Kansas City, Mo.	Kansas City University of Medicine and Biosciences	1916	Private	http://www.kcumb.edu
Texas College of Osteopathic Medicine	Fort Worth, Tex.	University of North Texas Health Science Center, Fort Worth	1970	Public	http://www.hsc.unt.edu/education/tcom
MSUCOM	East Lansing, Mich.	Michigan State University	1970	Public	http://www.com.msu.edu
OSUCOM	Tulsa, Okla.	Oklahoma State University	1972	Public	http://www.healthsciences.okstate.edu/college
West Virginia School of Osteopathic Medicine	Lewisburg, W.Va.	Freestanding	1974	Public	http://www.wvsom.edu
OUCOM	Athens, Ohio	Ohio University	1976	Public	http://www.oucom.ohiou.edu
New York College of Osteopathic Medicine	Old Westbury (Long Island), N.Y.	New York Institute of Technology	1977	Private	http://www.nyit.edu/nycom
UMDNJSOM	Cherry Hill, N.J.	University of Medicine and Dentistry New Jersey	1977	Public	http://www.som.umdnj.edu
College of Osteopathic Medicine of the Pacific	Pomona, Calif.	Western University of Health Sciences	1978	Private	http://www.westernu.edu
UNECOM	Biddeford, Me.	University of New England	1978	Private	http://www.une.edu/com
NSU-COM	Ft. Lauderdale-Davie, Fla.	NOVA/Southeast University	1981	Private	http://www.medicine.nova.edu

College	Location	Affiliation	Year	Type	URL
Lake Erie College of Osteopathic Medicine (LECOM)	Lake Erie, Pa.	Freestanding	1993	Private	http://www.lecom.edu
Arizona College of Osteopathic Medicine	Phoenix, Ariz.	Midwestern University	1996	Private	http://www.midwestern.edu/azcom
TUCOM-CA	Vallejo, Calif.	Touro University	1996	Private	http://www.tu.edu
PCSOM	Pikeville, Ky.	Pikeville College	1997	Private	http://www.pc.edu/pcsom
Edward Via Virginia College of Osteopathic Medicine	Blacksburg, Va.	Virginia Polytechnic Institute and State University	2003	Private	http://www.vcom.vt.edu
LECOM-B	Bradenton, Fla.	Branch of LECOM	2004	Private	http://www.lecom.edu
TUNCOM	Henderson, Nev.	Branch of TUCOM, Touro University–Nevada	2004	Private	http://www.tu.edu
PCOM Georgia	Suwanee, Ga.	Branch of PCOM	2005	Private	http://www.pcom.edu
ATSU-SOMA	Mesa, Ariz.	ATSU	2007	Private	http://www.atsu.edu/soma
LMU-DCOM	Harrogate, Tenn.	Lincoln Memorial University	2007	Private	http://www.lmunet.edu/dcom
TOUROCOM	New York, N.Y.	Touro University	2007	Private	http://www.touro.edu/med
PNWU-COM	Yakima, Wash.	Pacific North West University of Health Sciences	2008	Private	http://www.pnwu.org
RVU-COM	Parker, Colo.	Rocky Vista University	2008	For Profit	http://www.rockyvistauniversity.org

NOTE: The table lists the colleges in the order in which they began to matriculate students.

COM, College of Osteopathic Medicine; SOM, School of Osteopathic Medicine.

*As of 2008, 25 U.S. osteopathic medical colleges or schools (plus three branch campuses) are currently operating. Five original private osteopathic schools form a core that dates back to the late nineteenth and beginning twentieth century (having opened from 1892 to 1916). Ten new colleges of osteopathic medicine opened their doors between 1970 and 1981. This second wave included six state-funded (public) colleges, as the states involved moved to fill a shortage of physicians, particularly primary care physicians in underserved and rural areas. A third wave of private school development began in 1992 and continues to expand. For the first time, outside entrepreneurs began to found osteopathic medical colleges for their own reasons. Touro University, a Jewish institution, founded TUCOM-CA in 1992, and followed that by opening a branch campus in Nevada (TUNCOM) in 2004 and opening a separate college of osteopathic medicine in Harlem in 2007. This was the first time a private religious university had opened an osteopathic college in the United States. In 2008, the first for-profit college of osteopathic medicine since publication of the Flexner Report in 1910 was opened, Rocky Vista University College of Osteopathic Medicine in Parker, Colorado. This was extremely controversial in the osteopathic profession, but there were no rules against it for the American Osteopathic Association to enforce.

Generally, the public easily identifies this profession and respects the practitioners.

Although practitioners outside the United States are often called DOs, their degree means *Diploma in (or of) Osteopathy,* as opposed to the American degree of DO (which means *Doctor of Osteopathic Medicine*). The level of training and requirements for the diploma in osteopathy are not standardized in most countries, and there is certainly no international standard. Schools in some countries offer a series of weekend courses over several years for physical therapists and others who wish to become osteopaths, whereas there are only a few international 4- to 5-year full-time programs.

A number of part-time osteopathic schools in France began to train physical therapists in osteopathic technique and philosophy sometime after World War II, granting them a diploma of osteopathy. These diplomates continued to practice outside the law by tolerance. Although they organized and formed a national registry, they were not sanctioned by the government. As their numbers grew, they lobbied for and obtained the legal right to practice in 2002. The law specified that they could practice osteopathic diagnosis and techniques; however, the official decrees issued later specified limitations in their practice of osteopathic techniques. The Décret 2007-437 established new educational standards that are required for the practice of osteopathy in France, allowing a time period for those already practicing to fill their deficiencies.

Returning after many years to the North American continent by way of France, osteopathy came full circle when one French citizen opened a part-time osteopathic school in Quebec. American nonphysician health care practitioners were allowed to enroll as students, and a number have made the journey to Canada. The graduates of this school are known as *Diplomates of Osteopathy Manual Practice (DOMPs).*

The laws that govern the practice of physical therapy allow a great deal of leeway in choice of manual techniques. A few physical therapists have claimed that they are the "true osteopaths" because of their part-time training in osteopathic techniques and philosophy. When challenged by law, however, it is clear that they do not have the right to the title *osteopath* in the United States, because this title is reserved by law for American DOs.

A unique international forum was held in Atlanta, Georgia, in 1995 by the American Academy of Osteopathy (AAO), the AOA's specialty college focused on the osteopathic philosophy and osteopathic manipulative medicine. For some years, the AAO had been receiving an increasing number of letters and contacts from international diplomates of osteopathy. A few international practitioners of osteopathy wanted to visit the birthplace of osteopathy, as well as to take courses or arrange for American DOs to offer instruction abroad. As the world increased its movement toward globalization, this trend grew stronger. Many internationals also requested advice

about obtaining practice rights in their own countries that did not have laws permitting osteopathic practice of any type.

The forum allowed presentations by individuals from numerous countries, and at the end certain things had become clear:

- The majority of osteopathic education outside of the United States and the United Kingdom was on a part-time basis and not at the doctoral level.
- The vast majority of international osteopathic education was for profit and entrepreneurial.
- Australia and the United Kingdom were the only countries present that had created national laws allowing the practice of osteopathy (Australia, 1978; United Kingdom, 1993), but not osteopathic medicine as a full licensure including medicine and surgery.
- There were very few registries of osteopaths; in some countries there were competing registries with no government-approved status.
- Great rivalries existed in several countries as to who were the *real* osteopaths, and some competitors sought AAO validation.
- The United States was the only country with strict and extensive national standards set by a government-approved accrediting agency regarding osteopathic education for the award of a doctoral degree, national board examinations, and medical licensure (the latter granted by states).
- The United States was the only country with osteopathic physicians who were trained at the predoctoral level with the goal of full medical and surgical practice rights after graduation.
- The general population of U.S. doctors of osteopathic medicine was very different from the general population of the international diplomates of osteopathy; they have a much broader interest and training in medicine, surgery, and obstetrics.

Subsequently, the International Affairs Committee of the AAO undertook the process of creating an annual international forum. Any international DO was able to come; there were no elected delegates. The AAO realized that it would be difficult if not impossible to set up a representative group from each country, because many had more than one organization claiming its own legitimacy. In initial meetings, the focus was on reports regarding legal status and schools in the various countries. A group of cooperating individuals from various nations remained over the years to work on topics of common interest.

The AAO realized that it was not up to the United States to tell the other countries what to do in their own jurisdictions, but recognized that many were clamoring for guidance on establishing practice rights, educational standards, the vocabulary to use when discussing unique osteopathic concepts, and osteopathic research. As a result, later international forums came to include workshops and discussions on these topics. Competing groups from individual nations were encouraged to cooperate with each other in obtaining practice rights and education.

The following years provided much international progress in the field of osteopathy. The AAO International Affairs Committee also encouraged the participants to think about starting a truly international organization with its own agenda. The result was the founding of the World Osteopathic Health Organization (WOHO). WOHO held its first meeting in conjunction with the AAO annual convocation in 2004, elected officers, founded an international charity, and scheduled its next meeting outside the United States. Later meetings have alternated U.S. and international locations. WOHO's members are individual members, rather than delegates or elected representatives. (A list of members, goals, meetings and additional information may be accessed at the WOHO website at http://www.woho.org.)

The parent organization of the AAO, the AOA, began at the dawn of the twenty-first century to explore communication with practitioners of osteopathy on common interests, but focused on the example of a complete osteopathic medical, surgical, and obstetrical practice and on obtaining the right for U.S. DOs to practice with full medical and surgical rights in other countries.

A move toward higher standards and full-time schools for the nonphysician osteopaths is currently in process internationally, but there still are no international standards requiring full-time schooling to obtain a diploma of osteopathy. The European Union has been developing legislature to give practice rights to and set standards for alternative medical practices, including osteopathy, throughout the member nations in Europe. Currently, WHO has a committee developing suggestions for international osteopathic educational standards.

The Osteopathic International Alliance (OIA) was also founded in 2004. Its goals are somewhat similar to those of WOHO but relate more to international health care policy, fostering improved international health care by promoting osteopathic medicine and osteopathy. The members of the OIA are groups, who send delegates to discuss and vote on issues as specified in the adopted bylaws. (A list of member organizations as well as the goals, bylaws, and other information can be seen on the OIA website at http://www.oialliance.org.)

There is another tier of international osteopathic education, in which MD equivalents from various countries (e.g., United Kingdom, France, Russia, Japan) have taken postgraduate training in osteopathic diagnosis and manipulation. These practitioners have an unlimited medical license, but may have less exposure to osteopathic medical philosophy and/or a focus on a limited range of techniques. However, they have many similarities with American DOs. Many of these physicians integrate osteopathic care into general practice, rehabilitation medicine, sports medicine, rheumatology, or neurology, or focus on the conservative treatment of musculoskeletal conditions as well as preoperative and postoperative care.

France is one country where postgraduate training in osteopathic technique exists for MDs, in large part due to teaching groups inspired by the work of Robert Maigne, MD. French physicians have long enjoyed the right to use osteopathy as part of their practice. In Russia, several osteopathic schools exist in St. Petersburg and Moscow as postgraduate training sites for physicians, including a school at the state university in St. Petersburg. The London School of Osteopathy has also had a postgraduate training program for physicians for many years. Several organizations have existed in Japan for decades that have trained both physicians and nonphysicians in osteopathic techniques and philosophy.

Opinions on the evolution of osteopathy as a nonmedical practice vary. American DOs are aware of the dangers in having an expert in manipulation who is not well trained in differential medical diagnosis. Pain might not be recognized as symptomatic of a serious underlying treatable medical or surgical condition, and appropriate treatment may be delayed until it is too late to obtain a favorable outcome. When all that one has is a hammer, too often every problem begins to look like a nail.

International nonmedical osteopathic practitioners, however, would be quick to point out that a significant number of American DOs who have an excellent knowledge of medical diagnosis and treatment lack sufficient manipulative skills to effectively treat a patient with a problem for which manipulation is clearly indicated.

SUMMARY

Osteopathic medicine is based on a philosophy, a system of logic for medical diagnosis and care with rich roots extending back to Hippocrates and beyond. Andrew Taylor Still, MD, DO, a pioneer physician in Kansas and Missouri, developed the basic tenets of osteopathy and elaborated on them in his writings, which were adopted by the ASO (now Andrew Taylor Still University/Kirksville College of Osteopathic Medicine).

The development of scientifically validated, efficacious medicines aided in the evolution of classical osteopathic philosophy to its current form, contemporary osteopathic medical philosophy. The work of Irvin Korr, PhD, a medical physiologist, further elaborated and explained osteopathic theory in the mid-twentieth century. Korr personally benefited from—and in addition to his basic science research, elaborated on—the preventive care and healthful practices promoted by the original philosophy.

Osteopathic philosophy uses a holistic approach to begin the evaluation of the patient, continuing with a reductionistic approach to focus on aspects of anatomical and physiological dysfunction. One goal of this system of logic is for the osteopathic physician to remember throughout diagnosis and treatment that it is a fellow human being with whom he or she works, even as the physician uses tests that zoom in on the smallest microscopic details of that person. No cell or system in the body is seen as acting in isolation, and the importance of structure and function at each level is always kept in mind. Central to this philosophy is a tremendous respect for the innate capacity of the human being to heal. The physician works with the patient's physiological and psychological processes to obtain an optimal level of homeostasis and function.

OMT, the hallmark of osteopathic treatment as developed by Still, is used in patient care either alone or in conjunction with medicines and surgery, as appropriate. OMT is recognized as having beneficial effects not only in treating pain and restricted motion, but also in decreasing physiological stress and assisting the body's self-healing mechanisms.

The application of contemporary osteopathic medical philosophy varies from physician to physician and, outside of the United States, from country to country.

As the osteopathic profession has evolved both in and outside of the United States, it has changed significantly. The original osteopaths practiced in a distinctive manner very different from that of the allopathic physicians at the end of the eighteenth century. Still developed the osteopathic approach because the medications of his time were not only ineffective but also toxic and were based on tradition or conjecture rather than research. His important contribution to medicine was the idea that by adjusting (normalizing) anatomical functional abnormality, a physician could enhance natural physiological function; that by enhancing the delivery and clearance of blood, lymphatic fluid, and neurotrophic elements, a physician could promote delivery of endogenous substances; and that these endogenous substances were able to do more than the medicines of his time to normalize physiology, eliminate illness, and reestablish health. His development and teaching of OMT were designed not only to do this, but also to eliminate pain and improve biomechanical (physiologic) function in body systems other than the neuromusculoskeletal system, such as the respiratory system.

American osteopathic physicians continued to address the full medical, obstetric, and surgical care of patients. Each succeeding generation of DOs adopted the use of researched medications and decreased the use of OMT for anything but neuromusculoskeletal complaints, so that at the present time, a significant number of American DOs do not use the manipulative skills they learned in osteopathic medical school. Internationally, osteopathy developed in a manner that did not incorporate surgery, obstetrics, or the use of medication. This form of osteopathy continues to rely on endogenous substances for treatment, and the presenting complaints of its patients are generally neuromusculoskeletal pain or movement problems.

The twentieth century saw the development of scientifically researched, efficacious medications with fewer but significant accompanying side effects. As these medications became the standard of allopathic care, they were also adopted by osteopathic physicians. Increasing numbers of osteopathic medical students were attracted to the profession, not by the difference that OMT could make in patient outcomes but by the availability of the full scope of medical and surgical possibilities and a full license to practice as they saw fit. The osteopathic medical profession in the United States ceased to have a distinct identification in the mind of much of the American public, and many patients were unaware that their doctors came from a different tradition. This evolution has followed a standard sociological pattern in which an offshoot of a main group initially diverges, makes a contribution by developing an idea or skill that fills a vacuum not addressed by the main group, then reconverges with the mainstream as changes in both groups make them more similar. As the osteopathic physicians evolved, so did the allopathic physicians. Both sets of licensed physicians practice very differently than their predecessors, relying on research and progress unforeseen in Still's time, and in today's medical milieu, practice cooperatively.

Other factors affecting the evolution of osteopathic medicine have included student recruitment demographics, postgraduate training trends, advances in technology, government, and medical economic factors. The development of a specialty in osteopathic neuromusculoskeletal medicine, as well as widespread dispersion of osteopathic treatment methods through a number of health care professions, has helped to meet patients' perceived medical needs that remain poorly addressed by today's standard medical education.

Chapter References can be found on the Evolve website at http://evolve.elsevier.com/Micozzi/complementary/

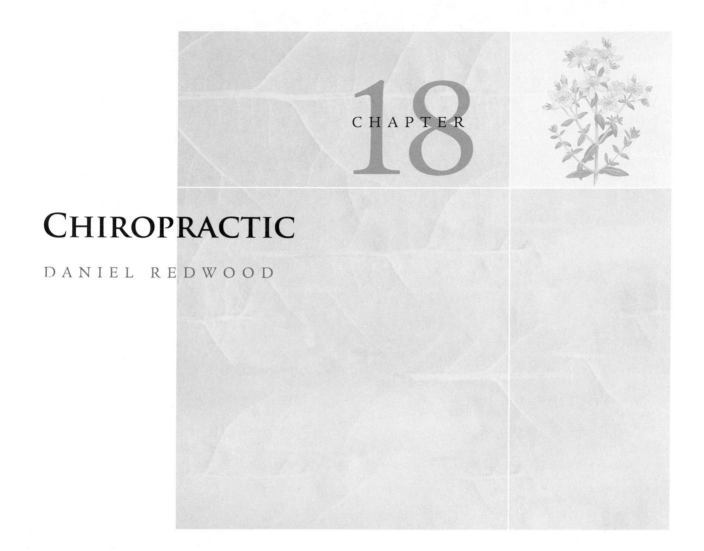

CHAPTER

18

CHIROPRACTIC

DANIEL REDWOOD

orn in the American Midwest in the late nineteenth century, chiropractic has evolved and matured toward mainstream status while largely preserving its essential principles. The contemporary chiropractic profession is in the unique position of having scaled many walls of the health care establishment (with licensure, an increasingly strong scientific research base, widespread insurance coverage, and approximately 30 million patients per year in the United States), while at the same time maintaining strong roots in the complementary and alternative medicine (CAM) community, with a philosophy that emphasizes healing without drugs.

Chiropractic is the third largest independent health profession in the Western world, following conventional (allopathic) medicine and dentistry. Its practitioners are "portal of entry" providers, licensed for both diagnosis and treatment. Unlike dentistry, podiatry, and optometry, chiropractic practice is limited not by anatomical region but by procedure. The chiropractor's scope of practice excludes surgery and the prescription of pharmaceuticals; its centerpiece is the manual adjustment or manipulation of the spine.

The United States is home to approximately 65,000 of the world's 90,000 chiropractors (Chapman-Smith, 2000). Chiropractors are licensed throughout the English-speaking world and in an increasing number of other nations (Box 18-1). Rigorous educational standards are supervised by government-recognized accrediting agencies, including the Council on Chiropractic Education in the United States. After fulfilling college science prerequisites analogous to those required to enter medical or osteopathic schools, chiropractic students must complete a 4-year chiropractic school program, which includes a wide range of courses in anatomy, physiology, pathology, and diagnosis, as well as spinal adjusting, physical therapy, rehabilitation, public health, and nutrition.

Almost 90% of chiropractic patients come to the chiropractor with neuromusculoskeletal complaints (Plamondon, 1995), principally back pain, neck pain, and headaches, the conditions for which spinal adjustment (also known as spinal manipulation) is most effective. As described later, current chiropractic research seeks to define further the role of adjustment/manipulation in the management of various musculoskeletal conditions,

255

BOX 18-1

Countries where Chiropractors are Recognized by National Health Authorities*

African Region	Guam†	Colombia‡	Portugal§
Botswana†	New Caledonia‡	Costa Rica‡	Russian Federation‡
Ethiopia‡	New Zealand†	Ecuador‡	Slovakia‡
Kenya‡	Papua New Guinea‡	Guatemala‡	Sweden†
Lesotho†		Honduras‡	Switzerland†
Mauritius‡	**Eastern Mediterranean**	Mexico†	
Namibia†	**Region**	Panama†	**North American Region**
Nigeria†	Cyprus†	Peru‡	Bahamas‡
South Africa†	Egypt‡	Venezuela‡	Barbados†
Swaziland†	Greece‡		Belize‡
Zimbabwe†	Israel‡		Bermuda‡
	Jordan‡	**European Region**	British Virgin Islands‡
Asian Region	Lebanon‡	Belgium†	Canada†
China/Hong Kong†	Libya‡	Croatia‡	Cayman Islands‡
Japan‡	Morocco‡	Denmark†	Jamaica‡
Malaysia‡	Qatar‡	England†	Leeward Islands†
Philippines†	Saudi Arabia†	Finland†	Puerto Rico†
Singapore‡	Turkey‡	Germany‡	Trinidad and Tobago‡
Taiwan‡	United Arab Emirates‡	Hungary‡	United States†
Thailand§		Iceland†	U.S. Virgin Islands‡
	Latin American Region	Ireland‡	
Pacific Region	Argentina‡	Italy§	
Australia†	Brazil‡	Liechtenstein†	
Fiji‡	Chile‡	Netherlands‡	
		Norway†	

From Chapman-Smith DA: *The chiropractic profession*, West Des Moines, Iowa, 2000, NCMIC Group. p 25.
*Listed according to the seven world regions adopted by the World Federation of Chiropractic. In most other countries, there are no chiropractors in practice, and national health authorities have not considered recognition or lack of recognition.
†Recognized pursuant to legislation.
‡Recognized pursuant to general law.
§De facto recognition.

as well as to evaluate its effectiveness in treating visceral organ disorders, including hypertension, infantile colic, otitis media, dysmenorrhea, and asthma.

HISTORICAL ROOTS, EVOLUTIONARY PROCESS

PRECURSORS IN WESTERN TRADITIONS

Spinal manipulation has been practiced for millennia in cultures throughout the world. Chiropractors' forebears have included prominent figures in the history of medicine.

Hippocrates was an early practitioner of spinal manipulation (Withington, 1959), and according to some scholars, he used manipulation "not only to reposition vertebrae, but also thereby to cure a wide variety of dysfunctions" (Leach, 1994). Galen, a Greek-born Roman physician who lived in the second century AD and whose approach to healing set the officially recognized standard in Western medicine for 1500 years after his death, also used spinal manipulation and reported the successful resolution of a patient's hand weakness and numbness through manipulation of the seventh cervical vertebra (Lomax, 1975).

As Europe endured the Dark Ages, these healing traditions were preserved in the learning centers of the Middle East by the ascendant Arabic civilization. Later, this body of knowledge returned to Europe, and the works of Hippocrates and Galen helped form the foundations of Renaissance medicine. Ambroise Paré, sometimes called the "father of surgery," used manipulation to treat French vineyard workers in the sixteenth century (Lomax, 1975; Paré, 1968).

In the centuries that followed, up to the dawn of the modern era, manipulative techniques were passed down from generation to generation within families. These "bonesetting" methods, transmitted not only from father to son but often from mother to daughter, played an important role in the history of nonmedical healing in Great Britain, and similar methods are common in the folk medicine of many nations (Bennett, 1981).

In the second half of the nineteenth century, the United States was a vibrant center of natural healing theory and practice. Two manipulation-based healing arts, osteopathy and chiropractic, trace their origins to that era. Both began in the American Midwest.

BEGINNINGS OF A NEW PROFESSION

Daniel David Palmer, a self-educated healer in the Mississippi River town of Davenport, Iowa, founded the chiropractic profession in 1895 with two fundamental premises: (1) that vertebral subluxation* (spinal misalignment causing abnormal nerve transmission) is the primary cause of virtually all disease, and (2) that chiropractic adjustment (manual manipulation of the subluxated vertebra) is its cure (Palmer, 1910). This "one cause–one cure" philosophy played a central role in chiropractic history, first as a guiding principle, then later as a historical remnant, providing a target for the slings and arrows of organized medicine (Figure 18-1).

Although few if any contemporary chiropractors would endorse such a simplistic and all-encompassing formulation, it nonetheless remains true that the raison d'être of the chiropractic profession is the detection and correction of spinal subluxations. Chiropractors may do much more, but it is their ability to do this one thing well that has allowed the chiropractic art to survive for a century under a barrage of medical opposition, some of it justified, most of it not.

---

*This differs from the medical definition of subluxation, which is an incomplete or partial dislocation, according to *Dorland's Illustrated Medical Dictionary*. Palmer's use of the term refers to more subtle malposition with neural involvement.

The one cause–one cure adherents among the early chiropractors had two major political effects on the development of the profession. First, their deep faith in the truth of their message, combined with the positive results of chiropractic adjustments, created a strong and steadily growing activist constituency of chiropractic patients and supporters. In their zeal, they generated a grassroots movement that ensured the survival of the profession through stormy years in the first half of the twentieth century. Civil disobedience was an integral part of the early development of the chiropractic profession, as it would later become in the American civil rights movement. Hundreds, including the founder himself, went to jail, charged with practicing medicine without a license.

That chiropractic would prove controversial was evident from its inception. In the first chiropractic adjustment the patient sought treatment for deafness and attained results that greatly exceeded his expectations. Harvey Lillard, a deaf janitor in the building where Palmer had an office, came to him for help. Noting an apparent spinal misalignment in the patient's upper back, Palmer administered the first chiropractic adjustment, after which Lillard is reported to have been able to hear for the first time in nearly two decades.

At first there was hope that Palmer had discovered a cure for deafness, but similar results were not forthcoming when other deaf people sought his assistance. There have been other reports through the years of restoration of hearing through spinal manipulation, including one by a Canadian orthopedist (Bourdillion, 1982), but these have been rare. The story of Lillard's dramatic recovery

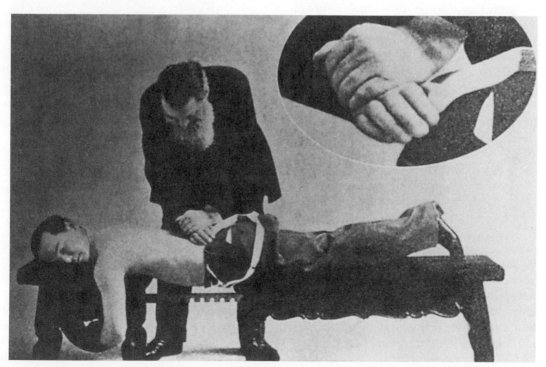

Figure 18-1 Daniel David Palmer, the founder of chiropractic, performing an adjustment on a patient (ca. 1906). (Courtesy Palmer College of Chiropractic.)

has been used to disparage chiropractic, with charges that such an event is impossible, because no spinal nerves supply the ear (which is supplied by cranial nerves).

Current knowledge of neurophysiology provides a credible theoretical basis for this and other apparent visceral organ responses to chiropractic adjustments. The underlying physiological mechanism is the *somatoautonomic* (or *somatovisceral*) reflex. Chiropractors and osteopaths assert that signals initiated by spinal adjustment/manipulation are transmitted through autonomic pathways to internal organs. In the case of Palmer's first adjustment, the relevant nerve pathway begins in the thoracic region, coursing up through the neck and into the cranium along sympathetic nerves that eventually lead to the blood vessels of the inner ear. Normal function of the hearing apparatus depends on an adequate blood supply, which in turn depends on a properly functioning sympathetic nerve supply.

A key question is unresolved: why are there sometimes dramatic positive somatovisceral responses to chiropractic adjustments in such patients, whereas in most cases there appears to be no response?

LEGACY OF CONTENTION: CHIROPRACTIC AND ALLOPATHIC MEDICINE IN THE UNITED STATES

All nascent healing arts face serious challenges, particularly the need to maintain the enthusiasm generated by positive therapeutic results while clearly and consistently distinguishing among the proven, the probable, and the speculative findings. Some of the harshest criticism of chiropractic has been in reaction to the tendency of some chiropractors to "globalize" (Gellert, 1994), making broad, overarching claims on the basis of limited though powerful anecdotal evidence.

Whatever the validity of these medical critiques (some of which mirror intensive self-criticism within the chiropractic profession), the American medical establishment's policy on chiropractic has never been that of a disinterested group solely seeking to serve the public good. Its century-long campaign against chiropractic impeded chiropractic's advancement and at times posed a severe threat to its survival. Until very recently, allopathic medical students were taught that chiropractic is harmful, or at best worthless, and they in turn inculcated these prejudices in their patients.

That such a fiercely antichiropractic policy was pursued by the American Medical Association (AMA) is no longer in dispute. In 1990, the U.S. Supreme Court affirmed a lower court ruling in which the AMA was found liable for antitrust violations for having engaged in a conspiracy to "contain and eliminate" (the AMA's own words) the chiropractic profession (*Wilk v AMA*, 1990). The process that culminated in this landmark decision began in 1974 when a large packet of confidential AMA documents was left anonymously on the doorstep of the International Chiropractors Association's headquarters. As a result of the ensuing *Wilk v AMA* case, the AMA

reversed its longstanding ban on interprofessional cooperation between medical doctors and chiropractors, agreed to publish the full findings of the court in the *Journal of the American Medical Association*, and paid an undisclosed sum, most of which was earmarked for chiropractic research.

This has not completely undone the effects of organized medicine's antichiropractic boycott, but it is nonetheless a laudable milestone on the long road toward reconciliation. Although the swords of contention have not yet been beaten into plowshares of amity, the pace of progress has accelerated substantially in the years since the *Wilk* decision, as men and women of goodwill in both professions strive to inaugurate a new era in which their patients are the beneficiaries of their mutual cooperation (Figures 18-2 and 18-3).

INTERPROFESSIONAL COOPERATION

Relations between the medical and chiropractic professions outside the United States have historically also been less than cordial. In certain instances, however, these

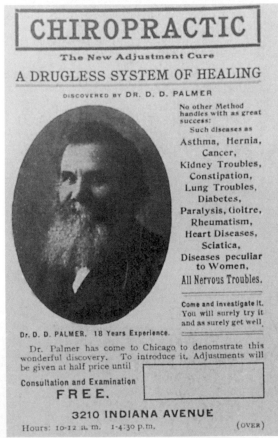

Figure 18-2 In this 1904 advertisement, Dr. Palmer touted chiropractic as a cure for virtually all human ailments. Such claims engendered great controversy. The emphasis on "drugless healing" was appealing to patients in an era in which arsenic, calomel, lead, mercury, and other poisons were used as mainstream therapies by physicians. (Courtesy Palmer College of Chiropractic.)

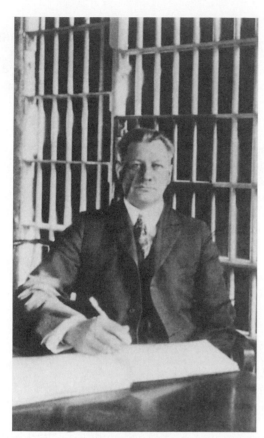

Figure 18-3 Dr. D.S. Tracy behind bars in Los Angeles. Hundreds of chiropractors served time in jail to secure the right to practice their healing art freely. (Courtesy Palmer College of Chiropractic.)

relations have been sufficiently productive to permit closer collaboration between chiropractors and allopathic physicians. This cooperation has had particularly salutary effects in the research arena. Many of the key clinical trials that first established chiropractic's scientific credibility were conducted in Europe and Canada. Gradually, the tide turned in the United States as well. Research projects funded by the federal government have encouraged an atmosphere of growing medical-chiropractic cooperation, and multidisciplinary organizations such as the American Back Society also reflect a newfound common ground. The recent incorporation of chiropractic into the health care system serving the U.S. military has provided an exceptional opportunity for interprofessional cooperation.

AGENCY FOR HEALTH CARE POLICY AND RESEARCH GUIDELINES: HISTORIC BREAKTHROUGH

The 1994 guidelines for treatment of acute lower back pain, developed for the Agency for Health Care Policy and Research (AHCPR; now the Agency for Healthcare Research and Quality) of the U.S. Department of Health and Human Services by a blue-ribbon panel composed primarily of medical physicians and chaired by an orthopedic surgeon (2 of the 23 members were chiropractors), included a powerful endorsement of spinal manipulation (Bigos et al, 1994).

Based on an extensive literature review and consensus process, the AHCPR guidelines concluded that spinal manipulation "hastens recovery" from acute low back pain (LBP) and recommended it either in combination with or as a replacement for nonsteroidal antiinflammatory drugs (NSAIDs). At the same time, the panel rejected as unsubstantiated numerous methods (including bed rest, traction, and various other physical therapy and pharmaceutical modalities) that for many years constituted the foundation of conventional medicine's approach to acute LBP, while endorsing the use of such self-care measures as exercise, use of ergonomic seating, and wearing of low-heeled shoes. In addition, the panel cautioned against lumbar surgery except in the most severe cases.

Perhaps most significantly, the AHCPR guidelines stated that spinal manipulation offers both "symptomatic relief" and "functional improvement." Because none of the other recommended nonsurgical interventions offers both, one might reasonably infer that for patients with acute LBP who show none of the guidelines' diagnostic "red flags" (e.g., fractures, tumors, infections, cauda equina syndrome), manipulation is now the treatment of choice.

The release of the AHCPR guidelines was a landmark event in chiropractic history. Federal standards for the treatment of LBP, the most prevalent musculoskeletal ailment in the United States and the most frequent cause of disability for persons under age 45, now assign a pivotal role to spinal manipulation, of which 94% is provided by chiropractors (Shekelle et al, 1991). This may be the quintessential contemporary example of an "alternative" health care method's achieving entry into the health care mainstream.

Assessment by government agencies in Canada (Manga et al, 1993), Great Britain (Rosen, 1994), Sweden (Commission on Alternative Medicine, 1987), Denmark (Danish Institute for Health Technology Assessment, 1999), Australia (Thompson, 1986), and New Zealand (Hasselberg, 1979) has brought similar approval of spinal manipulation for treatment of LBP. Guidelines jointly issued in 2007 by the American College of Physicians and the American Pain Society similarly recommended spinal manipulation. (Chou et al, 2007).

INTELLECTUAL FOUNDATIONS

The history of chiropractic, as that of all healing arts, is largely one in which empirical process has preceded theoretical formulation. From the earliest days, practitioners have applied new treatment methods on an intuitive, empirical basis, noted that some appeared to be more effective than others, and then theorized on the basis of these findings as to the underlying physiological mechanisms. The resultant body of chiropractic theory, philosophy, and practice draws from principles in the common domain shared by all natural healing arts. In addition, it contains unique chiropractic contributions to the cumulative sum and substance of health knowledge.

Common Domain Principles

Fundamental principles of natural healing, which have been part of chiropractic from the beginning and are incorporated into the curricula at chiropractic training institutions, include the following:

1. Humans possess an innate healing potential, an "inner wisdom of the body."
2. Maximally accessing this healing system is the goal of the healing arts.
3. Addressing the cause of an illness should take precedence over suppressing its surface manifestations in most cases.
4. Pharmaceutical suppression of symptoms can sometimes compromise and diminish the body's ability to heal itself.
5. Natural, nonpharmaceutical measures (including chiropractic spinal adjustments) should generally be an approach of first resort, not last.
6. A balanced, natural diet is crucial to good health.
7. Regular exercise is essential to proper bodily function.

These principles, endorsed and elucidated by chiropractors for more than a century, are currently recognizable as foundations of the emerging holistic health or wellness paradigm. ❧

Core Chiropractic Principles

In addition to precepts shared with other natural healing arts such as acupuncture and naturopathy, core theoretical constructs that form the underpinning of chiropractic are as follows:

1. Structure and function exist in intimate relation with one another.
2. Structural distortions can cause functional abnormalities.
3. Vertebral subluxation is a significant form of structural distortion and dysfunction and leads to a variety of functional abnormalities.
4. The nervous system occupies a preeminent role in the restoration and maintenance of proper bodily function.

5. Subluxation influences bodily function primarily through neurological means.
6. The chiropractic adjustment is a specific and definitive method for the reduction or correction of the vertebral subluxation.

These chiropractic principles reveal something unexpected: although chiropractic is best known for its success in the relief of musculoskeletal pain, its basic axioms do not directly address the question of pain relief. Instead, they focus on the correction of structural and functional imbalances, which in some cases cause pain. This fundamental paradox—that a profession renowned for the relief of musculoskeletal pain does not define its basic purpose in those terms—has been a persistent and sometimes discordant theme in chiropractic history.

DIVERGENT INTERPRETATIONS: TRADITIONALISTS AND MODERNISTS

Historically, a dichotomy has existed within the chiropractic profession between what have sometimes been called "straights" and "mixers," although most chiropractors are part of a broad middle ground between the extremes. Central to this controversy is the degree to which chiropractic practice should focus on symptom relief. Traditionalist, "straight" chiropractors see their approach as being subluxation based rather than symptom driven; they largely confine their role to analyzing the spine for subluxations, then manually adjusting the subluxated vertebrae. A minority within the profession, they generally reject the use of symptom-oriented ancillary therapies such as heat, electrical stimulation, and dietary supplementation. A few jurisdictions limit chiropractors to this circumscribed scope of practice.

Both groups agree that spinal adjusting is the paramount feature of chiropractic practice and that advising patients on exercise, natural diet, and other aspects of evidence-based prevention (Redwood et al, 2008) is appropriately within the chiropractor's scope. The chief philosophical difference between them is that whereas traditionalists seek to treat the cause and not the symptom (some even reject the term *treat* as excessively allopathic), broad-scope modernists seek to treat both the cause *and* the symptom. Although broad-scope chiropractors share their traditionalist colleagues' appreciation of spinal adjusting, they contend that patient care is sometimes enhanced by such adjuncts as electrical physical therapy modalities, hands-on muscle therapies, acupuncture, and nutritional regimens, including supplementation with vitamins, minerals, and herbs.

THEORETICAL CONSTRUCTS AND PRACTICAL APPLICATIONS

BONE-OUT-OF-PLACE THEORY

Pioneer-era chiropractors, following Palmer's lead, assumed that their adjustments worked by moving misaligned vertebrae back into line, which thereby relieved pressure caused by direct bony impingement on spinal nerves. The standard explanation given to patients was the analogy of stepping on a garden hose: if you step on the hose, the water cannot get through, and then if you lift your foot off the hose, the free flow of water is restored. Similarly, the chiropractic adjustment removes the pressure of bone on nerve, thus allowing free flow of nerve impulses.

Based on the information available at the time, such nineteenth-century concepts were plausible. Chiropractors were able to feel interruptions in the symmetry of the spinal column with their well-trained hands, and in many cases they could verify this on radiographic examination. More often than not, when they adjusted the subluxated vertebrae with manual pressure, patients reported significant functional improvements and healing effects.

Problems exist with this theory, however, as best illustrated by noting that, after an adjustment resulting in dramatic relief from headaches or sciatica, a radiographic study rarely shows any immediate, discernible change in spinal alignment. (The American Chiropractic Association Council on Diagnostic Imaging now considers making such comparative radiographic films inappropriate because of the unnecessary radiation exposure.) Positive health changes have not consistently correlated with vertebral alignment. This issue has not been fully resolved, however. A 2007 randomized clinical trial, the first to demonstrate significant benefit from chiropractic in cases of hypertension, used a technique that places great reliance on radiographic analysis of upper cervical vertebral alignment (Bakris et al, 2007).

MOTION THEORY AND SEGMENTAL DYSFUNCTION

Alternative hypotheses have been proposed to replace the bone-out-of-place concept. Chief among these is the theory of *intervertebral motion* and *segmental dysfunction (SDF)*, the dominant chiropractic model of this era. Advocated by a small minority of chiropractors for many decades, this model first achieved profession-wide attention among chiropractors in the 1980s and now has broad acceptance in chiropractic college curricula throughout the world. This theory also allows a coherent explanation of chiropractic and the *vertebral subluxation complex (VSC)* to be communicated in familiar terms to medical practitioners and researchers.

Motion theory contends that loss of proper spinal joint mobility, rather than positional misalignment, is the key factor in the VSC. It posits that the subluxation always involves more than a single vertebra and that subluxation mechanics involve SDF, an interruption in the normal dynamic relationship between two articulating joint surfaces (Schafer et al, 1989).

Anatomically, the vertebral motor unit (or motion segment) consists of an *anterior segment*, with two vertebral bodies separated by an intervertebral disk, and a *posterior segment*, comprised of two adjacent articular facets, along with muscles, ligaments, blood vessels, and nerves, interfacing with one another. Restriction of joint motion, a common feature of the manipulable lesion or subluxation, is termed a *fixation*. Fixations-subluxations are the clinical entity most amenable to spinal manipulation (Box 18-2).

Leach (1994) cites a triad of signs classically accepted as evidence for the existence of SDF:
1. Point tenderness or altered pain threshold to pressure in the adjacent paraspinal musculature or over the spinous process
2. Abnormal contraction or tension within the adjacent paraspinal musculature
3. Loss of normal motion in one or more planes

Chiropractic education includes extensive training in the development of the psychomotor skills necessary to diagnose the VSC or SDF and to perform the manipulative maneuvers best suited to its correction.

Much more problematic than fixations are subluxations involving joint hypermobility, characterized by ligamentous laxity, frequently of traumatic etiology. Hypermobility may be clinically diagnosed by eliciting a repeated click when a joint is moved through its normal range of motion. Hypermobile joints should not be forcibly manipulated, because this can further increase the degree of

BOX 18-2

A Visual Model of Spinal Motion Principles

Former college president and American Chiropractic Association spokesperson, J.F. McAndrews, DC, an early advocate of motion theory and practice, described a visual model of spinal motion principles (Figure 18-4), as follows:

View it as a mobile hanging from the ceiling, with many strings on which ornaments are suspended. As the mobile hangs there, it is in a state of dynamic equilibrium. Then, if you cut one of the strings, the whole mobile starts moving, because its balance has been upset. Eventually, it slows down and reaches a new state of dynamic equilibrium. But things have changed. It doesn't look the same. All those ornaments have shifted, in relation to the central axis and also in relation to each other.

The body's musculoskeletal system works in much the same way. If its normal balance is disrupted, it must compensate. Structural patterns will be altered to a greater or lesser degree, depending on the nature and intensity of the forces that threw off the old pattern of balance.

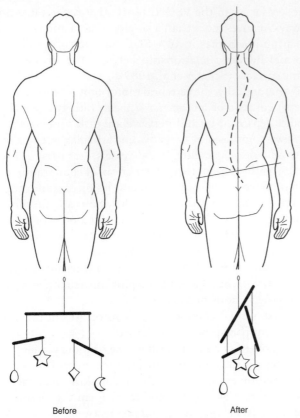

Figure 18-4 Visual model of spinal motion principles comparing a mobile hanging from the ceiling to the body's musculoskeletal system before and after imbalance is introduced.

hypermobility. However, nearby articulations that have become fixated to compensate for the hypermobile joint should be manipulated, and muscles in the area should be strengthened and toned to minimize the workload of the overstressed hypermobile joint.

The motion segment is the initial focus of chiropractic therapeutic intervention and is the site where the most direct and immediate effects of adjustment/manipulation are likely to be noted. More far-reaching effects are possible, however, through neural facilitation.

SEGMENTAL FACILITATION

Segmental facilitation has been defined as a lowered threshold for firing in a spinal cord segment, caused by afferent bombardment of the dorsal horn associated with spinal lesions (Korr, 1976).

Once a segment has become facilitated, the effects can include local somatic pain or visceral organ dysfunction. Segmental facilitation is the dominant hypothesis proposed as the neurophysiological mechanism by which the VSC or SDF influences autonomic function.

Some models of the specific mechanisms of facilitation postulate that inflammation is a key factor (Dvorak, 1985; Gatterman et al, 1990; Mense, 1991); others have proposed neurological models through which such facilitation could occur even in the absence of inflammation

(Korr, 1975; Patterson et al, 1986). When present, inflammation alters the local milieu of the nerve, causing chemical, thermal, and mechanical changes. Inflammation surrounding a nerve is likely to compromise its function. Such aberrant nerve activity, researchers theorize, can disrupt the homeostatic mechanisms essential to normal somatic or visceral organ function.

A facilitated segment may result in either parasympathetic vagal dominance or excessive sympathetic output. As Leach (1994) concluded, "It appears that SDF is capable of initiating segmental facilitation and that certainly this is the most logical explanation for the use of [chiropractic] adjustment . . . for other than pain syndromes; certainly the segmental facilitation hypothesis is gaining greater acceptance and is based upon a large body of acceptable scientific research."

RATIONALE FOR CHIROPRACTIC ADJUSTMENT

INDICATIONS AND CONTRAINDICATIONS

The central focus of chiropractic practice is the analytical process for determining

1. when and where spinal manipulative therapy (SMT) is appropriate, and
2. the type of adjustment most appropriate in a given situation.

Proposed algorithms for this process detail procedures whereby the chiropractor, after arriving at an overall diagnostic impression (not limited to the spine) and methodically ruling out pathologies that contraindicate SMT, proceeds to evaluate SDF to arrive at a specific chiropractic diagnosis (Leach, 1994). This diagnostic process takes into account subluxations that are present, along with other clinical entities (e.g., degeneration, disk involvement, carpal tunnel syndrome), which in certain cases require additional treatment besides SMT or affect the style of SMT that is appropriate.

For example, the presence of advanced degenerative joint disease would not render SMT inappropriate but would rule out all forms of SMT that introduce substantial amounts of force into the arthritic joint. According to the *Guidelines for Chiropractic Quality Assurance and Practice Parameters* (Haldeman et al, 1993), the high-velocity low-amplitude (HVLA) thrust adjustment, the most common form of chiropractic SMT, is "absolutely contraindicated" in anatomical areas where the following occur:

- Malignancies
- Bone and joint infections
- Acute myelopathy or acute cauda equina syndrome
- Acute fractures and dislocations, or healed fractures and dislocations with signs of ligamentous rupture or instability
- Acute rheumatoid, rheumatoid-like, or nonspecific arthropathies, including ankylosing spondylitis

characterized by episodes of acute inflammation, demineralization, and ligamentous laxity with anatomical subluxation or dislocation
- Active juvenile avascular necrosis
- Unstable os odontoideum

These guidelines also classify conditions into the following categories, in descending order of severity: "relative to absolute contraindication," "relative contraindication," and "not a contraindication." Listing all conditions in each category is beyond the scope of this chapter. The key point is that chiropractic diagnosis is geared toward evaluating where each case falls on this spectrum, then proceeding with appropriate medical referral, chiropractic treatment, or concurrent care.

TYPES OF MANUAL INTERVENTIONS USED BY CHIROPRACTORS

The HVLA technique, also known as *osseous adjustment,* is performed by manually moving a joint to the end point of its normal range of motion, isolating it by local pressure on bony prominences, and then imparting a swift, specific, low-amplitude thrust. This thrust is frequently accompanied by a clicking sound indicating joint cavitation, as the joint moves into the "paraphysiological space" between normal range of motion and the limits of its anatomical integrity. Properly applied, the adjustment usually involves little or no discomfort.

Other adjusting methods with wide application in the chiropractic profession include the following:
- High-velocity thrust with recoil
- Low-velocity thrust
- Flexion-distraction (originally an osteopathic technique for lumbar disk syndrome)
- Adjustment with mechanically assisted drop-piece tables
- Adjustment with compression-wave instruments
- Various specific light touch techniques

Some of these procedures are "low-force" methods, developed to assist chiropractors in managing cases in which standard HVLA adjustment is either contraindicated or otherwise undesirable. Also, a minority of chiropractors choose to use these low-force methods as the sole form of manual intervention. Nonadjustive manual measures are also employed by most chiropractors, generally to supplement rather than replace SMT, and include trigger-point therapy, joint mobilization, and massage (Figure 18-5).

CLINICAL SETTINGS AND METHODOLOGIES

INDEPENDENCE BORN OF NECESSITY

Chiropractic's long-time role as a dissenting wing of the Euro-American healing arts has meant that its practitioners have functioned almost entirely within the context of freestanding private practice. Similarly, chiropractic educational facilities have been private institutions, functioning almost entirely without public funding.

This outsider status is changing. Chiropractors now serve on the staffs of a small but growing number of hospitals, and universities in Quebec, Australia, Denmark, Wales, and the United States now include chiropractic departments. Chiropractors have served in official capacities at the Olympic Games since 1980 and play an increasingly prominent role in the treatment of sports and workplace injuries. Virtually all professional athletic teams (along with many collegiate and amateur teams) make chiropractic services available to their members. In 1993, J.R. Cassidy became the first chiropractor to be named research director of a university hospital orthopedics department, at the University of Saskatchewan in Canada. In 1994, John Triano became the first member of the profession to join the staff of the Texas Back Institute, where he worked in the dual role of staff chiropractic physician and clinical research scientist. In 2007, Michael Reed became the first chiropractor to serve as medical director of the Performance Services Division of the United States Olympic Committee and was one of four chiropractors sent to Beijing to treat American athletes at the 2008 Olympic Games (Redwood, 2008a, 2008b).

Among the most promising developments in the mainstreaming of chiropractic is the recent (post-2000) inclusion of chiropractic in the health care systems serving veterans and active-duty military personnel in the United States.

Such developments bode well for the future but are still more the exception than the rule. Evolving outside the mainstream has been a struggle, although it has strengthened many practitioners committed to chiropractic. By far the most serious negative effect of chiropractic's peripheral status has been that the majority of patients who could benefit from chiropractic care have not received it, because referrals from allopathic physicians to chiropractors remain much rarer than referrals to other medical practitioners or physical therapists.

The most salient positive aspect of operating outside the establishment for so many years is that the creative impulses and capacities of individual chiropractors were encouraged rather than quashed. One of the greatest challenges currently facing the profession is developing uniform practice standards—the *Guidelines for Chiropractic Quality Assurance and Practice Parameters* (Haldeman et al, 1993), or "Mercy Guidelines," is an initial effort—while simultaneously maintaining the innovative atmosphere that has characterized the profession since its inception. Ongoing practice standards development continues under the auspices of the Council on Chiropractic Guidelines and Practice Parameters (http://www.ccgpp.org), formed in 1995 at the behest of the Congress of Chiropractic State Associations.

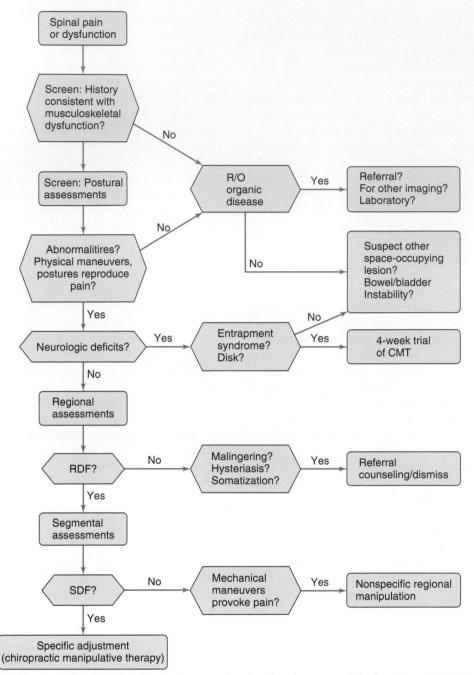

Figure 18-5 Proposed algorithm for the assessment of regional and segmental dysfunction. *CMT,* Chiropractic manipulative therapy; *RDF,* regional dysfunction; *R/O,* rule out; *SDF,* segmental dysfunction. (Modified from Leach RA: *An algorithm for chiropractic management of spinal dysfunction. In The chiropractic theories: principles and clinical applications,* ed 3, Baltimore, 1994, Williams & Wilkins.)

DIAGNOSTIC LOGIC

In the clinical setting the chiropractic model demonstrates both similarities to and differences from the standard medical approach. Foremost, chiropractors seek to evaluate individual symptoms in a broad context of health and body balance, not as isolated aberrations to be suppressed. This holistic viewpoint shares much with both ancient and emerging models elsewhere in the healing arts.

Chiropractors recognize the need for thorough evaluation of symptoms, and they are trained to take histories and perform physical examinations in a manner similar to that used in the typical medical office. However, the chiropractic paradigm does not hold the elimination of symptoms to be the sole or ultimate goal of treatment. Health is more than the absence of disease symptoms. The true goal is sustainable balance, a fact recognized by chiropractors and other holistically oriented health practitioners.

Chiropractors are trained in state-of-the-art diagnostic techniques, and chiropractic examination procedures overlap significantly with those used by orthodox medical physicians. However, chiropractors evaluate the information gleaned from these methods from a perspective that places greater emphasis on the intricate structural and functional interplay between different parts of the body.

CHIROPRACTIC AND MEDICAL APPROACHES TO PAIN

In my experience, conventional medical physicians engage in symptom suppression much more than do chiropractors and also more frequently assume that the site of a pain is the site of its cause. Thus, knee pain is generally assumed to be a knee problem, shoulder pain is assumed to be a shoulder problem, and so forth. This pain-centered diagnostic logic frequently leads to increasingly sophisticated and invasive diagnostic and therapeutic procedures. For example, if physical examination of the knee fails to define the problem clearly, the knee is radiographed. If the x-ray film fails to offer adequate clarification, magnetic resonance imaging (MRI) of the knee is performed, and in some cases a surgical procedure follows.

As do their allopathic colleagues, chiropractors use diagnostic tools such as radiography and MRI (Figure 18-6). The point here is not to criticize these useful technologies but to present an alternative diagnostic model. Chiropractors are familiar with patients in whom this entire high-tech diagnostic scenario, as in the previous knee example, is played out, after which the knee problem is discovered to be a compensation for a mechanical disorder in the lower back, a common condition that too often remains outside the medical diagnostic loop.

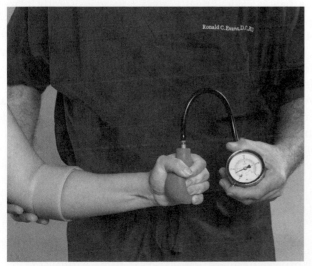

Figure 18-6 Contemporary chiropractors use state-of-the-art diagnostic and therapeutic methods. (Modified from Evans RC: Illustrated orthopedic physical assessment, ed 3, St. Louis, 2009, Mosby.)

If the lower back is mechanically dysfunctional and in need of spinal adjustment/manipulation, this can often place unusual stress on one or both knees. In these patients, medical physicians can and often do spend months or years medicating the knee symptoms or performing surgery, never addressing the source of the problem.

REGIONAL AND WHOLE-BODY CONTEXT: NEUROLOGY AND BIOMECHANICS

The chiropractic approach to musculoskeletal pain involves evaluating the site of pain in a regional and whole-body context. Although shoulder, elbow, and wrist problems can be caused by injuries or pathologies in these areas, pain in and around each of the shoulder, elbow, and wrist joints can also have as its source SDF in the cervical spine. Similarly, symptoms in the hip, knee, and ankle can also originate at the site of the pain, but in many cases the source lies in the lumbar spine or sacroiliac joints. Besides pain, other neurologically mediated symptoms (e.g., paresthesia) can have a similar etiology. The need to consider this chain of causation is built into the core of chiropractic training.

Chiropractors since Palmer have intentionally refrained from assuming that the site of a symptom is the site of its cause. They assume instead that *the source of the pain should be sought along the path of the nerves leading to and from the site of the symptoms.* Thus, pain in the knee might come from the knee itself, but tracing the nerve pathways between the knee and the spine reveals possible areas of causation in and around the hip, in the deep muscles of the buttocks or pelvis, in the sacroiliac joints, and in the lumbar spine.

Furthermore, if joint dysfunction does exist, for example, at the fourth and fifth lumbar levels, it might have its primary source at L4-L5, or it might represent a compensation for another subluxation elsewhere in the spine, perhaps in the lower or middle thoracic vertebrae or in a mechanical dysfunction of the muscles and joints of the feet. Such an integrative, whole-body approach to structure and function is of great value.

For patients whose presentation includes visceral organ symptoms, chiropractic diagnostic logic includes (once contraindications to adjustment/manipulation have been ruled out) evaluation of the spine, with particular attention to spinal levels providing autonomic nerve supply to the involved area, as well as consideration of possible nutritional, environmental, and psychological factors.

CRITERIA FOR REFERRAL TO ALLOPATHIC PHYSICIANS

Chiropractic practice standards mandate timely referral to an allopathic physician for diagnosis and treatment of conditions beyond the chiropractor's domain, or when a reasonable trial of chiropractic care (current standards in most cases limit this to about 1 month) fails to bring satisfactory results (Haldeman et al, 1993).

In addition, chiropractors frequently seek second opinions in less dramatic cases if chiropractic treatment, although helpful, fails to bring full resolution. Referrals from chiropractors to neurologists, neurosurgeons, orthopedic surgeons, internists, and other medical specialists are common. Referrals to complementary practitioners such as acupuncturists, massage therapists, and naturopaths also occur when appropriate, in areas where such practitioners are available.

ETHICS OF REFERRAL

The medical profession has long had a clearly defined set of ethics for *intraprofessional* referral: a report is sent to the referring physician, and the patient remains the patient of the referring physician. In the era when the medical establishment prohibited collegial relations with chiropractors, physicians receiving referrals from chiropractors frequently failed to extend such professional courtesies to them. This now occurs far more rarely.

The most insidious effect of this remnant of the old antichiropractic boycott is that it exerts a subliminal, if not overt, pressure on chiropractors *not* to refer. Ethical chiropractors resist the pressure, but such a vestige of the old order has no place in the modern health care arena and must be eliminated. At a time when many chiropractic patients still elect not to inform their allopathic physicians that they are seeing a chiropractor, the need for breaking down all such barriers should be readily apparent.

RESEARCH

For years, chiropractors were attacked for offering only anecdotal evidence in support of their methods. Since the early 1990s, only those ignorant of the scientific literature can still make such claims. As summarized by Meeker and Haldeman (2002), reports of 43 randomized trials of spinal manipulation for treatment of acute, subacute, and chronic LBP have been published. Thirty trials favored manipulation over the comparison treatments in at least a subgroup of patients, and the other 13 found no significant differences. None of these LBP studies has shown SMT to be less effective than the comparison approaches or a control condition. Eleven randomized, controlled trials of spinal manipulation for neck pain have been conducted; four had positive findings, and seven yielded equivocal results. Seven of nine randomized trials of manipulation for various forms of headache showed positive results.

UNIVERSITY OF COLORADO PROJECT

Contemporary chiropractic research began at the University of Colorado in the 1970s. First with grants from the International Chiropractors Association and later with added financial support from the American Chiropractic Association and the U.S. government, Chung Ha Suh and colleagues at the Biomechanics Department undertook a series of studies that provided an extensive body of chiropractic-related basic science research.

Suh, the first American college professor willing to defy the AMA boycott to pursue chiropractic research, was a native of Korea, where he was not subjected to the same antichiropractic bias as the American health care academics of his era. In launching this research, he had to withstand intense pressure from powerful political forces within the American medical and academic establishments, which condemned chiropractic for lack of scientific underpinning while striving to prevent chiropractors from obtaining the funding and university connections necessary for the development of such a research base (*Wilk v AMA*, 1990).

The University of Colorado team pursued research in two major areas. First, Suh (1974) developed a computer model of the cervical spine that allowed a deeper understanding of spinal joint mechanics and their relationship to the chiropractic adjustment. Second, a range of studies was performed on nerve compression and various aspects of neuron function (Kelly et al, 1975; Luttges et al, 1976; MacGregor et al, 1973, 1975; Sharpless, 1975; Simske et al, 1994; Triano et al, 1982). Sharpless, for example, demonstrated that minuscule amounts of pressure (10 mm Hg) on a nerve root resulted in up to a 50% decrease in electrical transmission down the course of the nerve supplied by that root.

MANUAL ADJUSTMENT FOR LOW BACK PAIN

A substantial body of research has addressed the efficacy of SMT in the treatment of LBP. As referenced earlier, consensus panels evaluating the data have consistently placed spinal manipulation on the short list of recommended procedures for management of acute, uncomplicated LBP.

In an influential trial involving more than 700 patients, British orthopedic surgeon T.W. Meade compared chiropractic manipulation with standard hospital outpatient treatment for LBP, which consisted of receiving physical therapy and wearing a corset (Meade et al, 1990, 1995). He concluded, "For patients with low-back pain in whom manipulation is not contraindicated, chiropractic almost certainly confers worthwhile, long-term benefit in comparison to hospital outpatient management." He described the applicability of these findings for primary care physicians as follows:

> Our trial showed that chiropractic is a very effective treatment, more effective than conventional hospital outpatient treatment for low-back pain, particularly in patients who had back pain in the past and who [developed] severe problems. So, in other words, it is most effective in precisely the group of patients that you would like to be able to treat.... One of the unexpected findings was

that the treatment difference—the benefit of chiropractic over hospital treatment—actually persists for the whole of that three-year period [of the study]. . . . the treatment that the chiropractors give does something that results in a very long-term benefit. (Meade, 1992)

Meade's study was the first large randomized clinical trial to demonstrate substantial short-term and long-term benefits from chiropractic care. Because it dealt with patients with both acute LBP and chronic LBP, Meade's data support the use of SMT for both populations.

Acute Versus Chronic Low Back Pain

Consensus panels and meta-analyses have not fully resolved the question of whether the literature supports recommending spinal manipulation for both chronic and acute LBP. In general, strong agreement exists that the literature supports the appropriateness of SMT for many acute LBP cases, but some debate still surrounds its use in chronic LBP. Nonetheless, the use of spinal manipulation as a treatment for acute, subacute, and chronic LBP received the rating "A—Supported by good evidence from relevant studies" from the Council on Chiropractic Guidelines and Practice Parameters" (Globe et al, 2009; Lawrence et al, 2009). Moreover, recent joint guidelines from the American College of Physicians and the American Pain Society, noted earlier, endorsed manipulation for both chronic and acute LBP (Chou et al, 2007).

Evidence for Benefit of Manual Methods in Chronic Cases

Because a primary care physician's decision about whether and where to refer patients with LBP hinges on which treatments are expected to yield the most satisfactory outcomes, a summary of studies on spinal manipulation for chronic LBP may aid the decision-making process. Besides Meade's work (1990, 1995), an impressive prospective study of LBP was performed at the University of Saskatchewan hospital orthopedics department by Kirkaldy-Willis, a world-renowned orthopedic surgeon, and Cassidy, the chiropractor who later became the department's research director (1985). The approximately 300 subjects in this study were "totally disabled" by LBP, with pain present for an average of 7 years. All had gone through extensive, unsuccessful medical treatment before participating as research subjects. After 2 to 3 weeks of daily chiropractic adjustments, more than 80% of the patients without spinal stenosis had good to excellent results, reporting substantially decreased pain and increased mobility. After chiropractic treatment, more than 70% were improved to the point of having no work restrictions. Follow-up a year later demonstrated that the changes were long-lasting. Even those with a narrowed spinal canal, a particularly difficult subset, showed a notable response. More than half the patients improved, and about one in five were pain free and on the job 7 months after treatment.

In a randomized trial of 209 patients, Triano et al (1995) compared SMT to educational programs for management of chronic LBP, which they defined as pain lasting 7 weeks or longer, or more than six episodes in 12 months. These investigators found greater improvement in pain and activity tolerance in the SMT group, noting that "immediate benefit from pain relief continued to accrue after manipulation, even for the last encounter at the end of the 2-week treatment interval." They concluded, "There appears to be clinical value to treatment according to a defined plan using manipulation even in LBP exceeding 7 weeks' duration."

Koes et al (1992) compared manipulation to physical therapy and treatment by a general practitioner (GP) in a randomized trial involving 256 patients with chronic back or neck pain. Physical therapy included exercises, massage, heat, electrotherapy, ultrasound, and short-wave diathermy. GP care included medication (analgesics, NSAIDs) and advice about posture, rest, and activity. Data indicated that both manipulation and physical therapy were much more effective than GP treatment, with SMT marginally surpassing physical therapy. This advantage was sustained at 12-month follow-up.

Another randomized trial compared the effects of SMT and NSAID treatments, each combined with supervised trunk exercise, in 174 patients with chronic LBP (Bronfort et al, 1996). Both regimens were found to produce similar and clinically important improvement over time that was considered superior to the expected natural history of longstanding chronic LBP. The SMT/trunk-strengthening exercise group showed a sustained reduction in medication use at 12-month follow-up. Also, continuation of exercise during the follow-up year was associated with better outcomes for both groups.

In a study of 115 patients with chronic spinal pain, Giles and Muller (2003) compared the effects of medication (NSAID or analgesic not previously ineffective for the individual patient), spinal manipulation, and acupuncture. Treating practitioners were told to follow their normal office procedures to determine whether manipulation or acupuncture was appropriate, as well as which adjustive/manipulative procedures or acupuncture points should be used. Electrical stimulation was not applied to the acupuncture needles. The highest proportion of patients experiencing early recovery (asymptomatic status) was found for manipulation (27.3%), followed by acupuncture (9.4%), and medication (5%). Manipulation also outperformed the other interventions on a variety of other measures, with one notable exception: acupuncture achieved the best results on the visual analogue scale measurement for neck pain improvement (50% for acupuncture vs. 42% for manipulation).

Recently, a study by Wilkey et al (2008) featured a head-to-head comparison of chiropractic care (pragmatically defined to allow all procedures the participating chiropractors would normally employ) versus medical care in the British National Health Service hospital's pain clinic (defined in similar pragmatic terms). The chiropractic and pain clinic groups started at baseline with similar levels of pain, although patients in the chiropractic group were on average a decade older than those in the pain clinic group and chiropractic subjects had endured their pain for a mean of 3 years longer (7.34 vs. 4.04 years) than the pain clinic group.

Nevertheless, reduction in pain intensity at week 8 was 1.8 points greater (on a 0 to 10 scale) for the chiropractic group than for the pain clinic group, a dramatic difference. Disability scores (which assess the impact of pain on daily activities) measured with the Roland Morris Disability Questionnaire also demonstrated a far larger benefit from chiropractic care, with a greater than fivefold difference in the degree of improvement. This trial measured effects through the end of the 8-week treatment period. A follow-up to this study (with a larger cohort and at least 6-month follow-up) could prove of major value not only for chiropractic but for the broader field of chronic pain management (Redwood, 2008a, 2008b).

Preventing Acute Cases from Becoming Chronic

Because the prognosis for patients with acute LBP is better than that for patients with chronic pain, high priority must be accorded to preventing acute cases from becoming chronic. However, a key factor leads physicians to minimize this concern: the conventional wisdom that 90% of LBP resolves on its own within a short time. Findings published in the *British Medical Journal* call for urgent reassessment of the assumption that most LBP patients seen by primary care physicians experience resolution of their complaints. Contrary to prevailing assumptions, Croft et al (1998) found that *at 3-month and 12-month follow-up, only 21% and 25%, respectively, had completely recovered in terms of pain and disability.* However, only 8% continued to consult their physicians for longer than 3 months. In other words, the oft-quoted 90% figure actually applied to the number of patients who stopped seeing their physicians, not the number who recovered from their back pain. Their dissatisfaction with conventional medical care was also reminiscent of Cherkin's earlier work (Cherkin et al, 1989, 1991). Croft et al (1998) stated the following:

> We should stop characterizing low-back pain in terms of a multiplicity of acute problems, most of which get better, and a small number of chronic long-term problems. Low back pain should be viewed as a chronic problem with an untidy pattern of grumbling symptoms and periods of relative freedom from pain and disability interspersed with acute episodes, exacerbations and recurrences. This takes account of two consistent observations about low-back pain: firstly, a previous episode of low-back pain is the strongest risk factor for a new episode, and, secondly, by the age of 30 years almost half the population will have experienced a substantial episode of low-back pain. These figures simply do not fit with claims that 90 percent of episodes of low-back pain end in complete recovery.

The patients in Croft et al's study were not referred for manual manipulation, and most developed chronic LBP. Based on the AHCPR guidelines, which emphasize the functionally restorative qualities of SMT, it seems reasonable to expect that early chiropractic adjustments could have prevented this progression in many patients. Recall that follow-up in both the Meade (1 year and 3 year) and Kirkaldy-Willis (1 year) studies showed that the beneficial effect of manipulation was sustained for extended periods (Kirkaldy-Willis et al, 1985; Meade et al, 1990, 1995). The decision not to refer patients to chiropractors may mean that many patients with LBP will develop long-standing problems that could have been avoided.

Low Back Pain Patients with Leg Pain

Differential diagnosis is crucial for cases in which LBP radiates into the leg. Specifically, motor, sensory, and reflex testing should be used to screen for signs of radicular syndromes and cauda equina syndrome. However, a British study of primary care practitioners found that a majority of these physicians do not routinely examine for muscle weakness or sensation, and 27% do not regularly check reflexes (Little et al, 1996). Such factors play a central role in determining which patients should be referred directly for surgical consultation and which should be referred for manual manipulation.

The AHCPR guidelines state that manipulation is appropriate for acute LBP cases that include nonradicular pain radiating into the lower extremity (Bigos et al, 1994). In cases in which radicular signs such as muscle weakness or decreased reflex response are present, however, preliminary evidence now suggests that chiropractic can yield beneficial results. In a study involving a series of 424 consecutive cases, Cox and Feller (1994) reported that 83% of 331 patients with lumbar disk syndrome who completed chiropractic treatment (13% of whom had had previous low back surgeries) experienced good to excellent results. ("Excellent" was defined as more than 90% relief of pain and return to work with no further care required, and "good" as 75% relief of pain and return to work with periodic manipulation or analgesia required.) A median of 11 treatments and 27 days were required to attain maximal improvement.

BenEliyahu (1996) followed 27 patients who received chiropractic care for cervical and lumbar disk herniations, the majority being lumbar cases. Pretreatment and posttreatment MRI studies were performed; 80% of the patients had a good clinical outcome, and 63% of the post-MRI studies showed that herniations either were reduced in size or completely resorbed.

In a study of 14 patients with lumbar disk herniation, Cassidy et al (1993) reported that all but one obtained significant clinical improvement and relief of pain after a 2- to 3-week regimen of daily side-posture manipulation of the lumbar spine, directed toward improving spinal mobility. All patients underwent computed tomography (CT) before and 3 months after treatment. In most patients the CT appearance of the disk herniation remained unchanged after successful treatment, although a small decrease was seen in the size of the herniation in five patients, and a large decrease in one patient.

HEADACHES: CHIROPRACTIC COMPARED WITH CONVENTIONAL MEDICINE

Noteworthy chiropractic research to emerge from the United States includes studies on headaches conducted at Northwestern College of Chiropractic in Minnesota (Boline et al, 1995), in which chiropractic was shown to be more effective than the tricyclic antidepressant amitriptyline for long-term relief of headache pain.

During the treatment phase of the trial, pain relief among those treated with medication was comparable to that in the SMT group. Revealingly, however, the patients receiving chiropractic care maintained their levels of improvement after treatment was discontinued, whereas those taking medication returned to pretreatment status in an average of 4 weeks after its discontinuation. This strongly implies that although medication suppressed the symptoms, chiropractic addressed the problem at a more causal level.

A subsequent trial by this group of investigators employing a similar protocol to treat patients with migraine headaches demonstrated that migraines were similarly responsive to chiropractic and that adding amitriptyline to chiropractic treatment conferred no additional benefit (Nelson et al, 1998).

NECK PAIN

Chiropractors have treated acute and chronic neck pain and related upper extremity symptoms since the profession's beginnings, but research on this subject is not extensive, which is also the case for nonmanual methods of treating neck pain (e.g., medications). As noted earlier, Meeker and Haldeman (2002) found that of the 11 randomized controlled trials of spinal manipulation for neck pain conducted, four demonstrated positive findings, seven equivocal findings, and none negative results. Rosner (2003) notes that "the RAND literature review (Coulter et al, 1995) suggested that short-term pain relief and enhancement of range of motion might be accomplished by manipulation or mobilization in the treatment of subacute or chronic neck pain; literature describing acute neck pain was regarded as extremely scanty, and remains so."

SOMATOVISCERAL DISORDERS

Although the bulk of recent and current chiropractic research still focuses on musculoskeletal disorders, research on somatovisceral disorders is also underway. A recent systematic review by Hawk et al (2007) summarizes the literature on chiropractic treatment of nonmusculoskeletal disorders, applying both conventional methods of analysis and a whole systems perspective.

Infantile Colic

In late 1999 a breakthrough study in visceral disorders was published in the *Journal of Manipulative and Physiological Therapeutics*. This randomized controlled trial by chiropractic and medical investigators at Odense University in Denmark showed chiropractic spinal manipulation to be effective in treating infantile colic (Wiberg et al, 1999). An estimated 22.5% of newborns suffer from colic, a condition marked by prolonged, intense, high-pitched crying. Numerous studies have explored a possible gastrointestinal (GI) etiology, but the cause of colic has long remained a mystery.

Health visitor nurses from the National Health Service recruited 50 participants for this study, whose parents consented to a 2-week trial of either dimethicone or spinal manipulation by a chiropractor. Dimethicone, which decreases foam in the GI tract, is prescribed for colic, even though several controlled studies have shown it to be no better than a placebo (Illingworth, 1985; Lucassen et al, 1998).

The infants in the Wiberg study were 2 to 10 weeks of age and had no symptoms of diseases other than colic. Inclusion criteria included at least one violent crying spell lasting 3 hours or longer for at least 5 of the previous 7 days. Mothers of infants in both groups also received counseling and advice on breastfeeding technique, mother's diet, air swallowing, feeding by bottle, burp technique, and other advice normally given to parents by health visitor nurses. The main outcome measure was the percentage of change in the number of hours of infantile colic behavior per day as registered in the parental diary, an instrument with validated reliability.

For the 25 infants randomly assigned to the chiropractic group a routine case history was taken and a physical examination was performed that included motion palpation of the spinal vertebrae and pelvis. The articulations restricted in movement were manipulated (mobilized) with specific light pressure with the fingertips for up to 2 weeks (three to five sessions) "until normal mobility was found in the involved segments" (Wiberg et al, 1999). The areas treated were primarily in the upper and middle thoracic regions, the source of sympathetic nerve input to the digestive tract.

All 25 infants in the chiropractic group completed the 13 days of treatment, whereas the dimethicone group had 9 dropouts. Those who dropped out before submission of the parental diary at the end of week 1 were omitted from the study's statistical analysis. Because some of these infants were reported by their mothers to have dropped out due to a significant worsening of symptoms, the relative benefit of spinal manipulation vis-à-vis dimethicone is understated in the final statistical analysis.

Nonetheless, the mean daily hours of colic in the chiropractic group were reduced by 66% on day 12, which is virtually identical to the 67% reduction in a previous prospective trial. In contrast, the dimethicone group showed a 38% reduction.

The Danish study on infantile colic is the first randomized controlled trial to demonstrate the effectiveness of chiropractic manipulation for a disorder generally considered nonmusculoskeletal. Addressing this issue, the authors conclude that their data lead to two possible interpretations: "Either spinal manipulation is effective in the treatment of the visceral disorder infantile colic or infantile colic is, in fact, a musculoskeletal disorder" (Wiberg et al, 1999).

A contrasting view is provided by a study performed under the auspices of a university pediatrics department in Norway (Olafsdottir et al, 2001). In this study, 86 infants with colic were randomly assigned to chiropractic care or placebo (being held for 10 minutes by a nurse, rather than given a 10-minute visit with a chiropractor). In the chiropractic group, adjustments were administered by light fingertip pressure. The methods used to identify involved segments were not described, and no mention was made of which regions were most frequently involved. Both groups experienced substantial decreases in crying, the primary outcome measure; 70% of the chiropractic group improved versus 60% of those held by nurses. However, no statistically significant differences were found between the two groups in terms of the number of hours of crying or the score as measured on a five-point improvement scale (from "getting worse" to "completely well"). The researchers concluded that "chiropractic spinal manipulation is no more effective than placebo in the treatment of infantile colic." This conclusion raises a significant methodological issue regarding the role of control or placebo interventions in chiropractic research, described in detail later.

Hypertension

In a recent example of medical-chiropractic collaboration, Dickholtz, a Chicago chiropractor, and Bakris, a medical hypertension specialist at the University of Chicago and director of the Rush University Hypertension Center, published a study (Bakris et al, 2007) in which upper cervical chiropractic adjustments led to sustained improvement in chronic hypertension "similar to that seen by giving two different antihypertensive agents simultaneously," with 88% of subjects in the treatment group experiencing more than an 8 mm Hg drop in diastolic blood pressure. Of particular note was the fact that all subjects were taken off their hypertension medications prior to the study, and 85% of the patients in the chiropractic treatment group required only one adjustment to yield these benefits through the full 8 weeks of the study.

Other Visceral Disorders

A pilot study by Fallon, a New York pediatric chiropractor, evaluating chiropractic treatment for children with otitis media demonstrated improved outcomes compared with the natural course of the illness. Both parental reports and tympanography were used to assess improvement in a cohort of more than 400 patients, and data suggest a positive role for spinal and cranial manipulation in the management of this challenging condition (Fallon, 1997; Fallon et al, 1998).

Two small controlled clinical trials evaluating the effects of chiropractic adjustment/manipulation on primary dysmenorrhea showed encouraging results, with both pain relief and changes in certain prostaglandin levels noted (Kokjohn et al, 1992; Thomasen et al, 1979). However, a larger randomized controlled trial addressing this issue did not conclude that there were significant benefits from manipulation (Hondras et al, 1999). The validity of this larger trial's comparison group intervention has been criticized on methodological grounds (Hawk et al, 2007).

A small study at the National College of Chiropractic showed a marked increase in the activity levels of certain immune system cells (polymorphonuclear leukocytes, monocytes) immediately after thoracic spine manipulation (Brennan et al, 1991). These increases were significantly higher than in control groups, who were given either sham manipulation or soft tissue manipulation. To date, no large trials investigating possible effects of manipulation on the immune system have been reported.

METHODOLOGICAL CHALLENGES IN CHIROPRACTIC RESEARCH

The most challenging methodological issues in chiropractic research are the following:

1. What constitutes a genuine control or placebo intervention?
2. How can CAM practitioners properly interpret data collected in trials that compare active and control treatments?

These questions apply not only to chiropractic but to a broad range of procedures, particularly those involving nonpharmaceutical modalities such as massage, acupuncture, physical therapy, and therapeutic touch. Depending on how one defines the placebo, the same set of research data can be interpreted as supporting or refuting the value of the therapeutic method under study (Redwood, 1999).

WHAT CONSTITUTES AN APPROPRIATE PLACEBO?

Two widely publicized studies illustrate the potential difficulties of defining the placebo or control too broadly. In their research on children with mild to moderate asthma, Balon et al (1998) randomly assigned individuals to either active manipulation or simulated manipulation groups. Both groups experienced substantial improvement in symptoms and quality of life, reduction in the use of β-agonist medication, and statistically insignificant increases in peak expiratory flow. Because these two groups did not differ significantly with regard to these improvements, however, the researchers concluded that "chiropractic spinal manipulation provided no benefit."

If the simulated manipulation had no therapeutic effect, this is a reasonable conclusion, but a closer reading of the article's text reveals the following:

> For simulated treatment, the subject lay prone while soft-tissue massage and gentle palpation were applied to the spine, paraspinal muscles and shoulders. A distraction maneuver was performed by turning the patient's head from one side to the other while alternately palpating the ankles and feet. The subject was positioned on one side, a nondirectional push, or impulse, was applied to the gluteal region, and the procedure was repeated with the patient positioned on the other side; then the subject was placed in the prone position, and a similar procedure was applied bilaterally to the scapulae. The subject was then placed supine, with the head rotated slightly to each side, and an impulse applied to the external occipital protuberance. Low-amplitude, low-velocity impulses were applied in all these nontherapeutic contacts, with adequate joint slack so that no joint opening or cavitation occurred. Hence, the comparison of treatments was between active spinal manipulation as routinely applied by chiropractors and hands-on procedures without adjustments or manipulation (Balon et al, 1998).

The validity of this study's conclusion hinges entirely on the assumption that these procedures are therapeutically inert. The following questions may be helpful in evaluating this claim:

1. Would massage therapists view these hands-on procedures as "nontherapeutic"?
2. Would acupuncturists or practitioners of shiatsu concur that direct manual pressure on multiple areas rich in acupuncture points is so inconsequential as to allow its use as a "placebo"?
3. Perhaps most significantly for this study on chiropractic, would the average chiropractor agree that these pressures, impulses, and stretches are an appropriate placebo, particularly in light of the fact that they overlap with certain "low-force" chiropractic adjustments and mobilization procedures?

The authors of the study dismiss these concerns as follows: "We are unaware of published evidence that suggests that positioning, palpation, gentle soft-tissue therapy, or impulses to the musculature adjacent to the spine influence the course of asthma" (Balon et al, 1998). A reasonable alternative interpretation of this study's results, however, is that various forms of hands-on therapy, including joint manipulation and various forms of movement, mobilization, and soft tissue massage, appear to have a mildly beneficial effect for asthmatic patients (Redwood, 1999).

ACTIVE CONTROLS

Another study that raises similar questions is Bove and Nilsson's work (1998) on use of manipulation to treat episodic tension-type headache (ETTH). Patients were randomly divided into two groups; one received soft tissue therapy (deep friction massage) plus spinal manipulation,

and the other (the "active control" group) received soft tissue therapy plus application of a low-power laser to the neck. All treatments were applied by one chiropractor. Both groups had significantly fewer headaches and decreased their use of analgesic medications. As in the asthma study, differences between the two groups did not reach statistical significance. Thus the authors concluded that "as an isolated intervention, spinal manipulation does not seem to have a positive effect on tension-type headache."

Unlike in the asthma study (Balon et al, 1998), Bove and Nilsson's carefully worded conclusion is justified by their data. But would it not have been more informative to affirm an equally accurate conclusion—that hands-on therapy, whether massage or manipulation plus massage, demonstrated significant benefits? Shortly after his paper's publication, Bove noted in a message to an Internet discussion group, "Our study asked one question [whether manipulation as an isolated intervention is effective for ETTH] and delivered one answer, a hallmark of good science.... We stressed that chiropractors do more than manipulation, and that chiropractic treatment has been shown to be somewhat beneficial for ETTH and very beneficial for cervicogenic headache. The message was that people should go to chiropractors with their headaches, for diagnosis and management."

The mass media's reporting on Bove and Nilsson's headache study provides a telling illustration of why defining the placebo or control correctly is more than an academic curiosity. Media reports on this study put forth a message quite different from Bove's nuanced analysis, with headlines concluding that chiropractic does not help headaches. Media reports on the asthma study were similar. Moreover, future MEDLINE searches will include the authors' tersely stated negative conclusions, with no mention of any controversy surrounding their interpretation.

The best way to avoid such confusion in the future is to emphasize increased usage of other valid methodologies, particularly direct comparisons of CAM procedures and standard medical care. Some comparative studies have shown adjustment/manipulation to be equal or superior to conventional medical procedures, with fewer side effects (Boline et al, 1995; Meade et al, 1990, 1995; Nelson et al, 1998; Wiberg et al, 1999; Winters et al, 1997). If fairly constructed, such studies will yield data that allow health practitioners and the general public to place CAM procedures in proper context. Comparing chiropractic and other nonpharmaceutical procedures to highly questionable placebos confuses the issue and delays the advent of a level playing field.

SAFETY OF ADJUSTMENT/ MANIPULATION

All health care interventions entail risk, which is best evaluated in relation to other common treatments for similar conditions (i.e., adjustment/manipulation vs. anti-inflammatory medications for neck pain). Medications with a safety profile comparable to that of spinal manipulation are considered quite safe. Although minor, temporary soreness after a chiropractic treatment is not unusual, major adverse events resulting from chiropractic treatment are few and infrequent. As a result, chiropractic malpractice insurance premiums are substantially lower than those for medical and osteopathic physicians.

The potential reaction to chiropractic treatment that has raised the greatest concern is vertebrobasilar accident (VBA), or stroke, following cervical spine adjustment/manipulation. Stroke following manipulation occurs so rarely that it is virtually impossible to study other than on a retrospective basis, because the cohort necessary for a prospective study would involve hundreds of thousands of patients, at a minimum. The question of whether spinal manipulation is capable of causing a stroke has not yet been resolved. Statistical correlation does not equal causation. Moreover, when such correlation is based on events involving numbers of stroke patients in single digits interspersed among millions of chiropractic visits, conclusions about direct causation not possible.

Lauretti (2003) provided a summary of chiropractic safety issues based on the information available several years ago, putting forth the following key points:

- Every reliable published study estimating the incidence of stroke from cervical adjustment/manipulation agrees that the risk is less than 1 to 3 incidents per 1 million treatments and approximately 1 incident per 100,000 patients.
- Haldeman et al (2001) found the rate of stroke to be 1 in 8.06 million office visits, 1 in 5.85 million cervical adjustment/manipulations, 1 in 1430 chiropractic practice years, and 1 in 48 chiropractic practice careers.
- NSAIDs, which are also widely used for neck pain and headaches, have a much less desirable safety record than adjustment/manipulation.

Since that time, relevant analysis of an unusually large database in Canada has been completed. The two most important and revealing studies exploring the possible relationship between chiropractic and stroke were based on a retrospective review of hospital records in the province of Ontario.

Rothwell et al (2001) reviewed all records from 1993 to 1998 and found a total of 582 VBA cases. Each was age and sex matched to four control cases from the Ontario population with no history of stroke at the event date. Public health insurance billing records were used to document utilization of chiropractic services during the year prior to VBA onset. Because health care in Canada is publicly funded, these data were presumed to be comprehensive.

Slightly more than 90% of the entire VBA cohort (525 of 582 individuals) had no chiropractic visits in the year preceding their VBA. Of the 57 individuals with VBAs who did visit a chiropractor in the 365 days preceding the

VBA (out of 50 million chiropractic visits during the 5-year period studied), 27 are believed to have had cervical manipulation. Of these, 4 individuals visited a chiropractor on the day immediately preceding the VBA, 5 in the previous 2 to 7 days, 3 in the previous 8 to 30 days, and 15 in the previous 31 to 365 days.

Compared with the controls, there was an increased rate of VBA among patients who saw a chiropractor 1 to 8 days before the VBA event, but a decreased incidence of cerebrovascular accident among patients who saw a chiropractor 8 to 30 days before the event. Parsing their data for age-related differences, Rothwell et al found no positive association between recent chiropractic visits and VBAs in patients over age 45. However, patients under age 45 were five times more likely to have visited a chiropractor within the week prior to the VBA and five times more likely to have had three or more visits with a cervical diagnosis in the month preceding the VBA.

"Despite the popularity of chiropractic therapy," the authors wrote in their conclusion, "the association with stroke is exceedingly difficult to study. Even in this population-based study the small number of events was problematic. Of the 582 VBA cases, only 9 had a cervical manipulation within one week of their VBA. Focusing on only those aged <45 reduced our cases by 81%; of these, only 6 had cervical manipulation within 1 week of their VBA." Regarding incidence, they add, "Our analysis indicates that, for every 100,000 persons aged <45 years receiving chiropractic, approximately 1.3 cases of VBA attributable to chiropractic would be observed within 1 week of their manipulation." Recognizing that such a temporal relationship does not imply causation, Rothwell et al "caution that such rate estimates can easily be overemphasized.... this study design does not permit us to estimate the number of cases that are truly the result of trauma sustained during manipulation."

Several years later, Cassidy et al (2008) completed a review of the same records evaluated by Rothwell's group and extended the time period covered in the review by 3 years. They performed additional analyses to determine whether patients who had seen a chiropractor were more likely to have had a stroke than patients who had seen a medical physician. This question, which had not been part of the earlier Rothwell et al (2001) review, was crucial because patients in the early stages of stroke commonly experience symptoms (headache, neck pain) that may lead them to consult either a chiropractor or a medical doctor. Cassidy et al found that it was no more likely for a stroke patient to have seen a chiropractor than a primary care medical physician. The authors concluded, "The increased risks of VBA stroke associated with chiropractic and PCP visits is likely due to patients with headache and neck pain from VBA dissection seeking care before their stroke. We found no evidence of excess risk of VBA stroke–associated chiropractic care compared to primary care."

CHIROPRACTIC IN HEALTH CARE

The greatest issue facing chiropractic in its first century was survival: whether it would remain a separate and distinct healing art, succumb to the substantial forces against it, or be subsumed into allopathic medicine. The question of survival has been resolved.

The key question for the new century, or at least the next generation, is: How can chiropractic best be integrated into the mainstream health care delivery system so that chiropractic services are readily available to all who can benefit from their application? A corollary follows as well: How can such integration be achieved without diluting chiropractic principles and practice to the point where chiropractic becomes a weak shadow of its former self?

It appears that an overwhelming majority of chiropractors do not want to pursue the path toward becoming full-scope allopathic physicians. Moreover, they will not willingly opt for any system in which chiropractic services are available only on medical referral. Chiropractors will function as contributing members of the health care team, but they will voluntarily surrender neither their political independence nor the holistic, wisdom-of-the-body worldview that has always been the core of their concept. How, then, can the desired integration be achieved for the benefit of many millions of current and future patients?

To answer this question in a manner satisfactory to chiropractors, conventional physicians, and the general public, a mutually agreed-on framework based on common goals is essential. Fortunately, a common purpose does exist: all parties seek to create the most effective, efficient health care system possible for the greatest number of people. A framework for implementation also exists, at least in theory: one based on the "level playing field" concept, which embodies a synthesis of two principles, democracy and hierarchy, coexisting in dynamic harmony.

The *democracy* of science is one in which equal opportunity is enjoyed by all, and all hypotheses are "innocent until proven guilty." Blind prejudice on the part of allopathic physicians, chiropractors, or anyone else has no place in this environment. All methods, whether presently considered conventional or alternative (integrative), must prove themselves effective and cost effective, and they must also demonstrate minimal iatrogenic effects. Approaches presently enjoying the imprimatur of the mainstream medical establishment should not be exempt from this scrutiny.

Hierarchy also has a place on the level playing field, as long as it is based on demonstrable skills and proven methods. In areas in which conventional Western medicine has clearly established its superior quality (e.g., trauma care, certain surgeries, treatment of life-threatening infections), this expertise should be honored and deferred to, but this is a two-way street. In areas in which a complementary method such as chiropractic is proved superior (LBP is the first sphere in which this has occurred), chiropractors must be accorded a similar role. Hierarchy in this sense does not imply a "control and domination" model. This is a lateral conception of hierarchy rather than a vertical one, a relationship among equals in which precedence is based on quality, which in turn is determined through adherence to agreed-on standards.

To continue the integration of chiropractic into the mainstream, there is an immediate and pressing need to broaden lines of communication between the chiropractic and medical professions, on a one-to-one basis and in small and large groups, with the goal of offering to all patients the gift of their physicians' cooperation. Each side must learn to recognize its own strengths and weaknesses, as well as the strengths and weaknesses of the other side. No one has all the answers, and humility befits our common role as seekers after truth.

At present, even though chiropractors have clear guidelines for when to refer to medical doctors, neither the medical profession as a whole nor its various specialty groups has developed formal guidelines as to when to refer patients for chiropractic care. Given the legacy of contention surrounding chiropractic, this is not surprising. In the post–AHCPR guidelines era, however, such criteria are essential for informed decision making. The time for creating these criteria is now. At a bare minimum, these guidelines should recommend referral to chiropractors of patients with LBP who do not meet the AHCPR's tightly circumscribed criteria for surgical referral.

The future need not mirror the worst aspects of the past. It is incumbent on all health care providers, as well as wholly consonant with their role as healers, that they heal not only sickness but old rifts among themselves. They now have an unprecedented opportunity to do so.

⊖ Chapter References and Resources can be found on the Evolve website at http://evolve.elsevier.com/Micozzi/complementary/

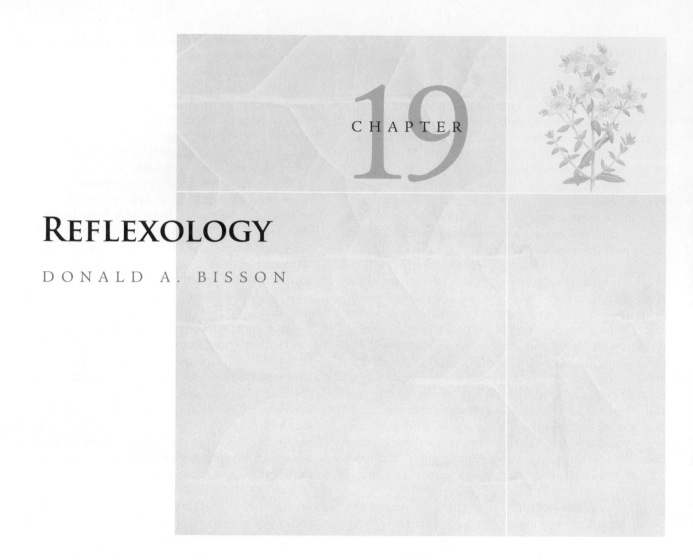

CHAPTER

19

REFLEXOLOGY

DONALD A. BISSON

Reflexology is a focused pressure technique, usually directed at the feet or hands. It is based on the premise that there are zones and reflexes in different parts of the body that correspond to all organs of the body (Bisson, 1999). Stimulation of these reflex areas helps the body to correct, strengthen, and reinforce itself by returning to a state of homeostasis. In Asian countries, some reflexologists also use electrical or mechanical devices. However, these approaches are discouraged in North America.

The oldest documentation of the use of reflexology can be found in Egypt, in an ancient Egyptian papyrus depicting medical practitioners treating the hands and feet of their patients in approximately 2500 BC. (Issel, 1990). William H. Fitzgerald, MD (1872-1942), is credited with being a founder of modern reflexology (Marquardt, 2000). His studies brought about the development and practice of reflexology in the United States.

Dr. Fitzgerald's studies found that application of pressure to various locations on the body deadened sensation in definite areas and relieved pain. These findings led to the development of zone therapy. In the early years, Dr. Fitzgerald worked mainly on the hands. Later, the feet

became very popular as a site for treatment. In his book on zone therapy in 1917, Dr. Fitzgerald spoke about working on the palmar surface of the hand for any pains in the back of the body, and working on the dorsal aspect of the hands and fingers for any problems on the anterior (front) part of the body. Dr. Fitzgerald claimed to relieve pain in a patient by applying pressure to the patient's hands and feet (Fitzgerald et al, 1917).

Joe Shelby Riley, MD, was taught zone therapy by Dr. Fitzgerald. He developed the techniques out to finer points, making the first detailed diagrams and drawings of the reflex points located on the feet and hands (Riley, 1924).

THEORY

As noted earlier, reflexology is based on the premise that there are zones and reflexes in different parts of the body that correspond to all parts, glands, and organs of the entire body. Manipulating specific reflexes removes stress, activating a parasympathetic response to enable the blockages to be released by a physiological change in the body. With stress removed and circulation enhanced, the body is allowed to return to a state of homeostasis (Bisson, 1999).

CONVENTIONAL ZONE THEORY

Conventional zone theory (CZT) is the foundation of hand and foot reflexology. An understanding of CZT and its relationship to the body is essential to understand reflexology and its applications (Bisson, 1999, 2000; Kunz et al, 1987).

Zones are a system for organizing relations among various parts, glands, and organs of the body, and the reflexes. There are 10 equal longitudinal or vertical zones running the length of the body from the tips of the toes and the tips of the fingers to the top of the head. From the dividing center line of the body, there are five zones on the right side of the body and five zones on the left side. These zones are numbered 1 to 5 from the medial side (inside) to the lateral side (outside). Each finger and toe falls into one of the five zones; for example, the left thumb is in the same zone as the left big toe, zone 1.

The reflexes are considered to pass all the way through the body within the same zones. The same reflex, for example, can be found on the front and also on the back of the body, and on the top and on the bottom of the hand or foot. This is the three-dimensional aspect of the zones.

Reflexology zones are not to be confused with acupuncture or acupressure meridians.

Pressure applied to any part of a zone will affect the entire zone. Every part, gland, or organ of the body represented in a particular zone can be stimulated by working any reflex in that same zone. This concept is the foundation of zone theory and reflexology.

In addition to the longitudinal zones of CZT, reflexology also uses the transverse zones (horizontal zones) on the body and feet or hands. The purpose is to help fix the image of the body by mapping it onto the hands or feet in a proper perspective and location. Four transverse zone lines are commonly used: transverse pelvic line, transverse waistline, transverse diaphragm line, and transverse neck line. These transverse zone lines create five areas: pelvic area, lower abdominal area, upper abdominal area, thoracic area, and head area.

INTERNAL ORGANS AND THE THREE-DIMENSIONAL BODY

It is important to remember that internal organs lay on top of, over, behind, between, and against each other in every possible configuration. The reflexes on the hands and feet corresponding to the parts, organs, and glands, overlap as well. For example, the kidney reflexes on the foot chart (Figure 19-1) or hand chart (Figure 19-2) overlap with many other reflexes, just as the kidneys overlap

other organs and parts of the body when viewed from the back or the front.

EXCEPTION TO THE ZONE THEORY

The basic concept of CZT is that the right foot or hand represents the right side of the body, and the left foot or hand, the left side. However, in the central nervous system, the right half of the brain controls the left side of the body and vice versa. In any disorders that affect the brain or the central nervous system, a reflexologist will emphasize the reflexes or areas of the disorder on the opposite hand or foot (Bisson, 1999). For example, the brain reflexes will be worked on the left foot or hand for strokes that caused paralysis on the right side of the body.

ZONE-RELATED REFERRAL AREAS

It is a common assumption that the hands and feet are the only areas to which reflexology can be applied. However, there are reflexes throughout the 10 zones of the body, and they may present unlikely relations within these zones (Kunz et al, 1987). For example, there is a zonal relationship between the eyes and the kidneys, because both lie in the same zone. Working the kidney reflexes can affect the eyes.

If there is an injury on the foot, the area should be avoided and should not be worked. Alternate parts of the body in the same zones may be worked instead. For example, the arm is a reflection of the leg, the hand of the foot, the wrist of the ankle, and so forth. If any part of the arm is injured, the corresponding part of the leg can be worked and vice versa. Common problems such as varicose veins and phlebitis in the legs can be helped by working the same general areas on the arms.

This approach can be used to find other referral areas by identifying the zone(s) in which an injury has occurred and tracing it to the referral area. Tenderness in the referral area will usually help the reflexologist find it.

Referral areas can give insights into problem areas by showing the relationships to the areas in the same zone(s) that may be at the root of the problem. For example, a shoulder problem may be caused by a hip problem, because the shoulder lies in the same zone as the hip.

NEGATIVE FEEDBACK LOOP

A reflexology session usually begins on the right foot or hand and finishes on the left foot or hand. In addition, the reflexes on both feet and hands are worked from the base of the foot or hand up to the top, with the toes or fingers worked last.

To aid the body's self-regulation, a highly complex and integrated communication control system or

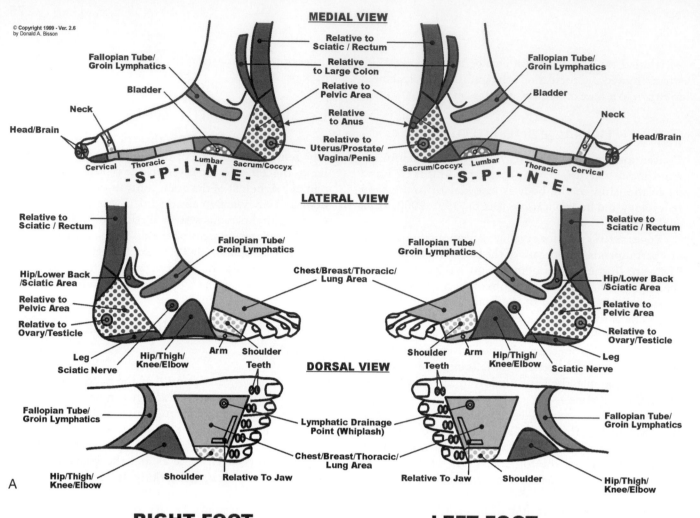

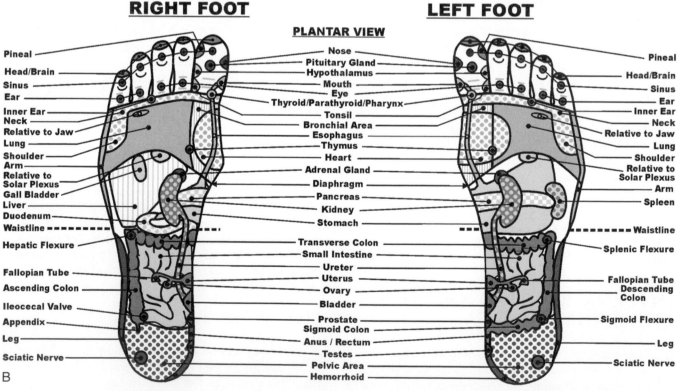

Figure 19-1 Foot reflexology chart. All charts are based on the premise that there are zones and reflexes on different parts of the body that correspond to and are relative to all parts, glands, and organs of the entire body. Reflexologists do not diagnose, prescribe for, or treat specific conditions. Reflexologists do not work in opposition to the medical or other fields, but instead complement and enhance them. (Copyright © Donald A. Bisson, 1999, Version 2.6.)

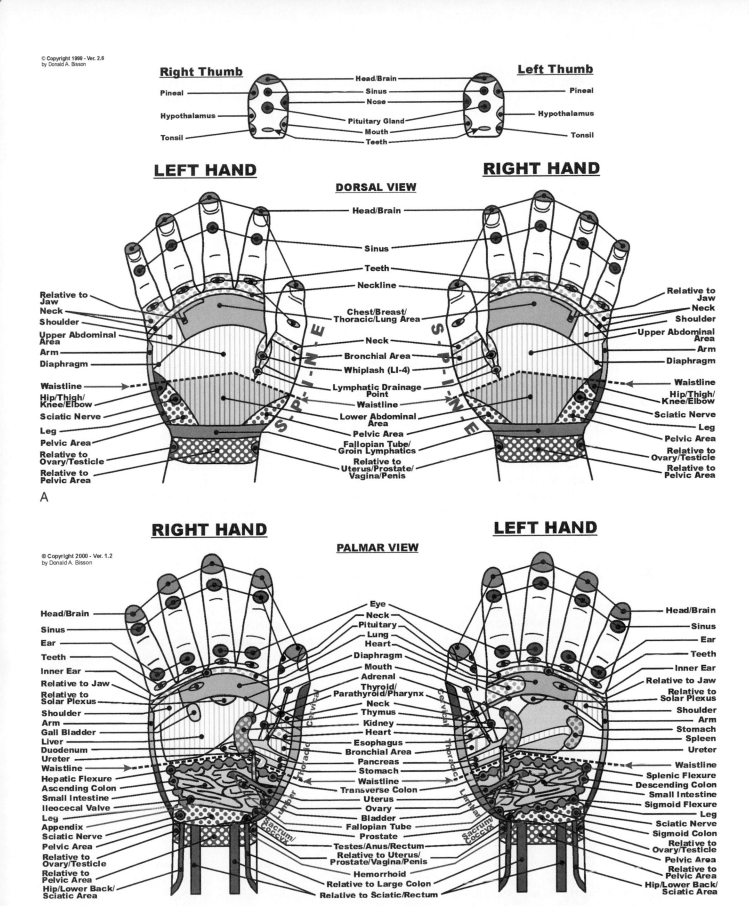

Right Thumb

Pineal

Hypothalamus

Tonsil

Head/Brain
Sinus
Nose
Pituitary Gland
Mouth
Teeth

Left Thumb

Pineal

Hypothalamus

Tonsil

LEFT HAND

RIGHT HAND

DORSAL VIEW

Head/Brain

Sinus

Teeth

Neckline

Chest/Breast/
Thoracic/Lung Area

Neck

Bronchial Area

Whiplash (LI-4)

Lymphatic Drainage
Point

Waistline

Lower Abdominal
Area

Pelvic Area

Fallopian Tube/
Groin Lymphatics

Relative to
Uterus/Prostate/
Vagina/Penis

Relative to
Jaw
Neck
Shoulder
Upper Abdominal
Area
Arm
Diaphragm

Waistline
Hip/Thigh/
Knee/Elbow
Sciatic Nerve
Leg
Pelvic Area
Relative to
Ovary/Testicle
Relative to
Pelvic Area

Relative to
Jaw
Neck
Shoulder
Upper Abdominal
Area
Arm
Diaphragm

Waistline
Hip/Thigh/
Knee/Elbow
Sciatic Nerve
Leg
Pelvic Area
Relative to
Ovary/Testicle
Relative to
Pelvic Area

S-P-I-N-E

S-P-I-N-E

A

RIGHT HAND

LEFT HAND

PALMAR VIEW

Eye
Neck
Pituitary
Lung
Heart
Diaphragm
Mouth
Adrenal
Thyroid/
Parathyroid/Pharynx
Neck
Thymus
Kidney
Heart
Esophagus
Bronchial Area
Pancreas
Stomach
Waistline
Transverse Colon
Uterus
Ovary
Bladder
Fallopian Tube
Prostate
Testes/Anus/Rectum
Relative to Uterus/
Prostate/Vagina/Penis
Hemorrhoid
Relative to Large Colon
Relative to Sciatic/Rectum

Head/Brain
Sinus
Ear
Teeth
Inner Ear
Relative to Jaw
Relative to
Solar Plexus
Shoulder
Arm
Gall Bladder
Liver
Duodenum
Ureter
Waistline
Hepatic Flexure
Ascending Colon
Small Intestine
Ileocecal Valve
Leg
Appendix
Sciatic Nerve
Pelvic Area
Relative to
Ovary/Testicle
Relative to
Pelvic Area
Hip/Lower Back/
Sciatic Area

Head/Brain
Sinus
Ear
Teeth
Inner Ear
Relative to Jaw
Relative to
Solar Plexus
Shoulder
Arm
Stomach
Spleen
Ureter
Waistline
Splenic Flexure
Descending Colon
Small Intestine
Sigmoid Flexure
Leg
Sciatic Nerve
Sigmoid Colon
Relative to
Ovary/Testicle
Pelvic Area
Relative to
Pelvic Area
Hip/Lower Back/
Sciatic Area

Cervical
Thoracic
Lumbar
Sacrum/
Coccyx

Cervical
Thoracic
Lumbar
Sacrum/
Coccyx

B

Figure 19-2 Hand reflexology chart. All charts are based on the premise that there are zones and reflexes on different parts of the body that correspond to and are relative to all parts, glands, and organs of the entire body. Reflexologists do not diagnose, prescribe for, or treat specific conditions. Reflexologists do not work in opposition to the medical or other fields, but instead complement and enhance them. (Copyright © Donald A. Bisson, 1999, Version 2.6.)

network is required. This type of network is called a "feedback control loop." Different networks in the body control diverse functions such as blood carbon dioxide levels, temperature, and heart and respiratory rates. Homeostatic control mechanisms are categorized as negative or positive feedback loops. Many of the important and numerous homeostatic control mechanisms are negative feedback loops.

Negative feedback loops are stabilizing mechanisms; that is, they maintain homeostasis of blood carbon dioxide concentration. As blood carbon dioxide increases, the respiration rate increases to permit carbon dioxide to exit the body in increased amounts through expired air. Without this homeostatic mechanism, body carbon dioxide levels would rapidly rises to toxic levels, and death would result.

The blood circulation loop is from the left side of the body to the right side—fresh oxygenated blood enters the aorta from the left ventricle of the heart and travels to the body, and venous blood with carbon dioxide enters the vena cava on the right side of the heart. By beginning a reflexology session on the right foot or hand, the reflexologist is helping to boost the loop by pushing venous or deoxygenated blood into the heart and lungs so that fresh oxygenated blood will be available to the body cells. The same rationale applies to the direction that the reflexologist works on the foot or hand—from the bottom of the foot upward, to bolster the homeostatic loop (Bisson, 1999, 2000).

BENEFITS AND SCOPE

Reflexology demonstrates four main benefits: (1) it promotes relaxation with the removal of stress; (2) it enhances circulation; (3) it assists the body to normalize the metabolism naturally; and (4) it complements all other healing modalities.

When the reflexes are stimulated, the body's natural electrical energy works along the nervous system to clear any blockages in the corresponding zones.

A reflexology session seems to break up deposits (felt as a sandy or gritty area under the skin), which may interfere with the flow of the body's electrical energy in the nervous system.

Reflexologists do not diagnose medical conditions unless qualified to do so. The only diagnosis made is that of a tender reflex. A reflexologist will refer to other qualified health care practitioners when the services required are outside the reflexologist's scope of practice (Bisson, 1999).

Similarly, reflexologists do not prescribe medications unless qualified to do so. The therapeutic intervention is limited to working the reflexes.

In randomized controlled trials, reflexology has been found to be effective in reducing pain in women with

severe premenstrual symptoms (Oleson et al, 1993) and in patients with migraine and tension headaches (Launso et al, 1999). It has also demonstrated benefit in alleviating motor, sensory, and urinary symptoms in patients with multiple sclerosis (Siev-Ner et al, 2003). Recent systematic reviews on the efficacy of reflexology in cancer patients found positive improvements in anxiety and pain (Andersen et al, 2007; Solà et al, 2004; Stephenson et al, 2003).

Reflexology is a useful complementary or alternative therapy to decrease anxiety and pain in patients with cancer (Lacey, 2002).

ADVERSE EFFECTS

The adverse effects of reflexology are minor and may include fatigue (increase in parasympathetic activity), headache, nausea, increased perspiration, and diarrhea.

CREDENTIALING AND TRAINING

No formal or standardized credentialing exists for reflexology in North America. Certification is provided by certain educational institutions specializing in this training. A patient should look for a therapist who is certified and/or registered as a qualified reflexologist by a reputable organization.

There are many schools of reflexology that can provide adequate training, ranging from 100 to 1000 hours of instruction. The interested individual should look for a school that is established and, if possible, recognized by a local governing body.

In the United States and Canada, there are regulations for practicing reflexology, and individual states and provinces (though not all) have their own sets of educational or licensing requirements.

SUMMARY

Reflexology is a form of manipulative therapy that has been used successfully to treat various disorders and provide pain management. There are many conditions for which reflexology can assist in healing, especially in pain management, as confirmed by recent studies and publications.

Reflexology impacts the autonomic nervous system more directly than many other therapies, balancing the parasympathetic nervous system and the sympathetic nervous system, the two subdivisions of the autonomic nervous system that exert opposite effects on the end organs, to maintain or restore homeostasis (Crane, 1997).

Many of the benefits of reflexology come from the relief of tension and stress (Andersen et al, 2007; Stephenson et al, 2003). As with many alternative medical approaches, good scientific studies to confirm the benefits of reflexology are relatively sparse, and more research is required. Reflexology does appear to relieve stress, which in turn could reduce or minimize physical symptoms (Stephenson et al, 2003). Reflexology can be used as an adjunct to proven therapies in the treatment of disease. The profession of reflexology also needs to be regulated and standardized.

⊜ Chapter References can be found on the Evolve website at http://evolve.elsevier.com/Micozzi/complementary/

SHIATSU

KERRY PALANJIAN

Simple yet profound, the experience with shiatsu, whether a single session or an ongoing therapeutic relationship between therapist and client, brings the wisdom of ancient civilizations to our Western model of life, thought, and medicine. Shiatsu, which is reinforced by Western and Eastern clinical research and receives official Japanese government sanction, is regarded by many as a life-changing experience. Shiatsu's practice as a modality for fully clothed recipients is allowing its growth not only as a therapy in the private sector, but more importantly as an easy-to-implement research tool in numerous clinical settings and hospitals.

HISTORY

The literal meaning of the Japanese word *shiatsu* (she-AAHT-sue) is "finger pressure" or "thumb pressure." Over the centuries, Asian medicine, massage therapy, and twentieth-century advancements have combined to yield "modern" shiatsu.

The word *massage* comes from the Arabic word for *stroke*. The practice of massage dates back 3000 years to China. A tomb found in modern Egypt, determined to be from 2200 BC, depicts a man receiving a foot massage. In the fourth century BC, Hippocrates, known as the father of modern medicine, wrote that "the physician must be experienced in many things, but most assuredly in rubbing" (Ballegaards et al, 1996). Further support for the use of touch and massage as healing tools is noted in ancient Egyptian, Greek, Persian, Roman, and Asian manuscripts (Yamamoto et al, 1993).

During the Middle Ages, there was decreased visibility of massage as a healing tool in the West, principally because of the position of the church, which viewed the manipulation of the body as the work of the devil. Massage was often depicted as a tool of prostitution, a prejudice that still lingers today among uninformed people. In the thirteenth century the German emperor Frederick II seized a number of newborns and did not allow caretakers to cuddle or talk to the infants. All died before they were able to talk. The historian Salimbene described this "experiment" in 1248 when he wrote, "They could not live without petting" (Colt et al, 1997).

People instinctively recognize the need for human touch and contact. From the rubbing of a painful shoulder to the physical act of intimacy, connection and human touch not only feel good but yield many physical and psychological benefits. These benefits are gaining increased recognition among laypeople and are enjoying a substantial increase in support from scientific studies that document numerous broad-based positive effects (see later section on research). The University of Miami Medical School's Touch Research Institute (TRI) is gaining widespread acceptance as a pioneer of research supporting the medical benefits of massage therapy. TRI has published numerous studies and review articles, with more in progress (Colt et al, 1997). Evidence presented in these studies supports the clinical use of massage therapy for a wide range of ailments. Massage therapy has been shown to facilitate weight gain in preterm infants, reduce stress hormone levels, alleviate symptoms of depression, reduce pain, positively increase measurable immune system functions, and alter electroencephalogram readings in the direction of heightened awareness. Research studies also suggest benefits for patients with conditions such as Alzheimer disease, arthritis, cancer, depression, fibromyalgia, job stress, and premenstrual syndrome (PMS), while in addition documenting benefits related to maternity and labor (Colt et al, 1997; Touch Research Institute, n.d.).

Shiatsu's history lies within the antecedents of Asian medicine, as was clearly stated 2000 years ago in *The Yellow Emperor's Classic of Internal Medicine*, a text discussed in *The Art of Shiatsu* (Cowmeadow, 1992). Others suggest that Chinese medical practice was derived from techniques originally developed in India and adapted to China.

Shiatsu has evolved within the genre of touch and massage therapies, as well as within Asian medicine's juxtaposition of ancient and modern Japanese culture. As a healing art or treatment, shiatsu grew from earlier forms of *anma* in Japan (*anmo* or *tui na* in China) (Lundberg, 1992). *An* denotes "pressure" and "nonpressure," and *ma* means "rubbing" (Yamamoto et al, 1993). This method, which was well known 1000 years ago in China, found its way to Japan and was recognized as the safest and easiest way to treat the human body (Masunaga et al, 1977). In Japan, shiatsu was used and taught by blind practitioners who relied on their hands to diagnose a patient's condition (Cowmeadow, 1992). Anma was recognized by the medical authorities in Japan in the Nara period (AD 710-784) but subsequently lost its popularity before gaining more widespread use in the Edo era (1603-1868) (Yamamoto et al, 1993), during which doctors were actually required to study anma. During the Edo period, most practitioners were blind and provided treatments in their patients' homes. An extensive handbook on anma was published in 1793, and anma was considered one component of the Asian healing arts, a reputation it enjoys today. Anma's "understanding and assessment of human

structure and meridian lines" were and are believed to be important distinctions that separate shiatsu therapy from other healing models and massage therapies (Yamamoto et al, 1993). One author states that European physicians and missionaries from the sixteenth century onward introduced Western anatomy and physiology to Japan (Young, 2004), whereas others suggest that Western massage was introduced into Japan in the late 1880s, when the many vocational schools that taught anma were dominated by blind instructors. However, this very limitation stopped the further development of anma and led to the evolution of what we recognize today as shiatsu therapy (Yamamoto et al, 1993). The practitioner Tamai Tempaku is credited with developing shiatsu as a separate therapy in the early 1900s (Young, 2004).

Modern shiatsu, as noted previously, is therefore a product of twentieth-century refinements and evolution that produced the form of therapy used today. Shiatsu began its modern evolution in the 1920s (the Taisho period) when anma practitioners adopted some of the West's hands-on techniques, including those of chiropractic and occupational therapy (Yamamoto et al, 1993), as well as with the merging of *ampuku* (abdominal massage), *do-in* (breathing and self-massage practices), and Buddhism. Tamai Tempaku is credited with establishing shiatsu in Japan and worldwide. The Shiatsu Therapists Association was formed in 1925 (Annussek, 2004).

The practice of shiatsu received much attention from studies conducted after World War II, as described in the following quotation from Saito, and these studies also sparked its growth:

> After World War II, U.S. General Douglas MacArthur directed the Japanese Health Ministry. There were more than 300 unregulated therapies in Japan at that time. MacArthur ordered all 300 to be researched by scientists at the Universities, to document which ones had scientific proof of merit; and which did not. At the end of eight years, the Universities reported back; and "Shiatsu" was the only one therapeutic practice which received scientific approval. (Saito, 2001).

In 1955 the Japanese parliament adopted a bill on "revised anma," which gave shiatsu official government endorsement. This endorsement allowed shiatsu to be legally taught in schools throughout Japan (Yamamoto et al, 1993). Shiatsu received further official Japanese government recognition as a therapy in 1964 (Harmon et al, 1999) through the efforts of Tokujiro Namikoshi and his son Toru, who emphasized the application of pressure on neuromuscular points to release pain and tension (Young, 2004). In the early 1970s, shiatsu began spreading to the West and rapidly gained widespread acceptance (Cowmeadow, 1992). Although shiatsu and its distant cousin acupuncture are considered medically sound and are "accepted methods of treatment for over one-quarter of the world's population," the United States and many other Western nations consider both techniques experimental (Yamamoto et al, 1993). This is interesting, considering that these "experiments" have been conducted successfully for more than 2500 years (Cowmeadow, 1992). However, several U.S. hospitals now allow the use of acupuncture, and medical and nursing students are beginning to be taught the theory and practice of acupuncture, shiatsu, and macrobiotics. These gains suggest that an environment has been established for rapid, ongoing change in the West. There is a growing acceptance and use of these practices among Western-trained physicians and health care providers.

Shiatsu can be described as a synthesis of Eastern and Western medicine, quickly gaining recognition for its success as an adjunctive healing therapy. "The foundations for modern ideas and techniques in the healing realm come from ancient civilizations. In the West it was Greece and Rome. And in the East it was China, India, and Persia. These foundations are the basis of present scientific methods [of healing]" (Yamamoto et al, 1993). Shiatsu's foundations, and therefore shiatsu itself, are a part of the growing trend and movement toward complementary and alternative medicine.

PRINCIPLES AND PHILOSOPHY

Many followers of Eastern traditions believe that the natural state of humanity is to be healthy. Yamamoto and McCarty (1993) describe it this way:

> With observation we can see that there is a definite and distinct order in nature. Nature's power guides all things. When we do not follow nature's order we can become sick. We are often reminded of nature's order by the presence of sickness. Sickness can be our teacher. From a traditional point of view the specific name of an illness is not so important. Physical ailments such as headache, gallbladder pain; emotional states such as anger, depression, irritability; and mental conditions such as paranoia, lack of concentration, and forgetfulness; are all various states of disequilibrium or disease. Theoretically there is no disease that is incurable, if we are able to change the way we think, eat, and live. Of course this is easier said than done.

They also write, "The simple understanding that humans are equipped to heal themselves and that [they] can also help others, [forms] the underlying foundation of Shiatsu. Shiatsu [simply] acts like a spark or catalyst to the human body [and] the combination of treatment and way of life suggestions form the basis of total care" (Yamamoto et al, 1993).

The major underlying principle of shiatsu, derived from the tenets of Asian medicine, is actually a reflection of scientific thought. Simply stated, "Everything is energy." When considered in the context of molecular structure, all matter is a manifestation of energy. Shiatsu interacts directly with this energy, and therefore with life itself.

From the perspective of classic Asian medicine, energy moves along 14 distinct pathways in the body; these pathways are called *meridians* or *channels* (*kieraku* in Japanese, *jing* in Chinese) (Yamamoto et al, 1993). The meridians were discovered by accident when certain acupoints (specific locations along the meridians) were stimulated and beneficial results were observed. For example, asthmalike symptoms caused by certain types of battle wounds were relieved when the corresponding acupoint was touched, and menstrual pain was reduced when a heated rock from a fireplace accidentally brushed against a point on the inner thigh (Schlager et al, 2000). Although many in the West may attempt to deny or discount the existence of the meridian network, modern research conducted by biophysicists in Japan, China, and France has documented its existence. Yamamoto and McCarty (1993) describe some of this research in the following excerpt from *Whole Health Shiatsu:*

> Many studies have been conducted by biophysicists in Japan, China, and France. They postulated that a measurement of acu-point electricity would be a biophysical index that would illustrate the objective existence of the meridian system. They discovered that acu-points have a lower skin resistance. When an electrical current is passed through a classical acu-point, it has a higher electrical conductance, which is a lower resistance, than the surrounding area. They also discovered that when disease or illness is present, pathological changes take place in the body while changes are found in the resistance of relevant meridians and acu-points. Similar internal changes are also reflected by the acu-points. In other words, imbalance in the organs affect the acu-points, imbalance in the acu-points affect the organs. Researchers also found that the external environment, such as temperature, season, and time of day, changed the resistance of acu-points.
>
> In the Lanzhou Medical College in China a test of the acu-points of the Stomach meridian showed significant variations in conductance when the stomach lining was stimulated by cold or hot water, either before or after eating. In Beijing, ear acu-point research learned that low resistance points on the outer rim of the ear were elevated either in the presence of disease or following long-term stimulation of a corresponding internal organ.

In addition to the scientific support developed thus far, support for the benefits of shiatsu comes from the experiences of clients and practitioners alike. Asthmatic clients experience volatility (pain and sensitivity) along the lung meridian. Clients with lower digestive track symptoms such as constipation experience this same sensitivity along the large intestine meridians. Women with PMS symptoms are sensitive on the lower leg along both the bladder and the kidney meridians, which, according to Shiatsu theory and literature, are associated with reproductive energy. When clients experience these connections, which are common in shiatsu, they are quick to convert or more readily accept the principles of Asian medicine and to accept the validity of the meridian network. Not only has research documented scientific evidence to support the theory behind shiatsu, but the body's own level of pain along related organ meridian lines makes clients' enlightenment regarding the existence of meridians, based on their own personal experience with shiatsu therapy, difficult to deny.

It is believed that meridians evolved from energy centers in the body called *chakras* (SHOCK-ras) and that our organ systems subsequently evolved from the meridian network. There are 10 meridians directly related to internal organs, two indirectly related, and two related to systems not recognized by Western medicine.

Along the meridian lines are points called *tsubos* (SUE-bows), or *acupuncture points,* of which there are believed to be about 600 (Annussek, 2004). Yamamoto and McCarty (1993) describe tsubos in the following excerpt from *Whole Health Shiatsu:*

> The word *Tsubo* or *acu-point* derives from the Oriental characters meaning hole or orifice, and position—the position of the hole. Traditionally, the word hole was combined with other terms such as hollow, passageway, transport, and Ki [KEY, or energy, also described in other cultures as chi, qi, and prana]. This suggests that the holes on the surface of the body were regarded as routes of access to the body's internal cavities. The acu-points are spots where Ki comes out.
>
> There are three phases in the historical development of the concept of these holes or acu-points. In the earliest phase people would use any body location that was painful or uncomfortable. Because there were no specific locations for the points, they had no names.
>
> In the second phase, after a long period of practice and experience, certain points became identified with specific diseases. The ability of distinct points to affect and be affected by local or distant pain and disease became predictable. . . .
>
> In the final phase, many previously localized points, each with a singular function, became integrated into a larger system that related and grouped diverse points systematically according to similar functions. This integration is called the *meridian* or *channel system.*

Although the analogy is not completely accurate, shiatsu is often called "acupuncture without needles." To alter a client's internal energy system or pattern, an acupuncturist inserts needles in the same tsubos that are used by a shiatsu practitioner. The most significant difference between the two disciplines is that whereas acupuncture is invasive and is performed by extensively trained doctors, shiatsu is noninvasive and can be practiced by either a professional therapist or a layperson. Shiatsu is also a whole-body technique versus one that is limited to the insertion of needles at specific tsubos. Acupuncture is generally considered more symptom oriented, in that people are much less likely to go to an acupuncturist without a specific complaint, whereas clients often equate shiatsu with health maintenance and go for treatments in the absence of particular "problems." Although some consider shiatsu a

cousin to acupuncture, others suggest a "distant cousin" relationship. The distinctions between the two disciplines are worth noting (Table 20-1). It is also important to note that simple shiatsu can be practiced with little or no understanding of the underlying principles. The practitioner does not have to agree with the principles or understand them to provide shiatsu; however, the techniques are part of a more complicated healing system that, when adhered to and studied, provides more effective results.

Although not all acupuncturists agree with all these distinctions, they form a basis for comparison. All shiatsu practitioners and acupuncturists practice according to their own interpretations and belief systems, so Table 20-1 should not be interpreted as a rigid, fixed framework.

A simple and accurate analogy for understanding the meridian pathways and tsubos in relation to the body's internal organ systems is that tsubos are similar to a system of volcanoes on the earth's surface. We know that a volcano's real energy is not at the surface, but rather is found deep inside the earth. A volcano is a superficial manifestation of the underlying energy. Similarly, a tsubo can be thought of as a manifestation of the underlying energy of the organ system. This does not imply that the therapist should ignore the area of pain a shiatsu client may describe. However, a classically trained shiatsu practitioner looks past sore shoulders, ligaments, and tendons (unless the cause of the pain is trauma to these structures) and focuses on the related organ system through the meridian network. Philosophically, shiatsu practitioners would have a tendency to relate health to the condition of the related "vital" organs (i.e., those associated with the meridian system). Although shiatsu is noninvasive and

TABLE 20-1

Distinctions Between Shiatsu and Acupuncture

Category	Shiatsu	Acupuncture
Movement	Free flowing	Systematic
Focus	Intuitive	Adheres to laws
Theoretical inclination	Daoist	Confucian
Quality	Feminine	Masculine
Tools	Practitioner's body	Needles
Treatment goal	Balance by becoming whole	Balance by alleviating symptoms
Patient interacts with treater	Yes	No
Encourages independence	Yes, immediately	Yes, after treatment series
Physically strengthens		
Receiver	Yes	Sometimes
Treater	Yes	No

appears to deal with external or surface pain, according to shiatsu theory and the experience of those who practice and receive the art, it stimulates, sedates, and balances energy *inside* the body as a way to address the root causes of surface and bodily discomfort.

The principles of Asian medicine evident in shiatsu theory and practice state that two types of energy exist in the universe. These two types of energy, called *yin* and *yang,* exist side by side and are considered both complementary and opposing. Unlike Western medicine, which uses more dualistic terms such as "good and bad," Eastern or Asian medicine looks at health more as a manifestation of balance between yin and yang and considers that an imbalance may *allow* infection or disease to become manifest. An effective way to comprehend this internally is to apply the principles of yin and yang to diet through macrobiotics. When a person's health and metabolism adjust to what Eastern medicine and macrobiotic practitioners consider universal guidelines, natural harmony occurs "from the inside out." Varying states of yin and yang are experienced by the body but are not necessarily comprehended by the mind. This experience can be made manifest by dedication (not necessarily lifelong) to the practice of using food according to the various energetic principles long understood by the Chinese, Japanese, and followers of macrobiotic theory.

In defining yin and yang, one should bear in mind that a continuum exists between the extremes of each. In shiatsu, major organs are paired together under one of the five major elements. Each pair includes both a yang and a yin organ. One organ is more compact and tighter (yang), whereas the other is more open and vessel-like (yin). The five elements—wood (tree), fire, earth (soil), metal, and water—proceed in a clockwise manner within the five-element wheel used in Asian medicine (Table 20-2).

According to shiatsu principles, an organ is fed by its opposite energy. For the shiatsu practitioner, pressing and rubbing movements proceed in the direction that energy travels along each respective meridian. Shiatsu texts often use the term *structure* to describe an organ, whereas acupuncture texts may describe the same organ in terms of the energy that *feeds* it through the meridian. A yang organ is fed by yin energy. A shiatsu practitioner generally describes the compact kidney as yang because of its *structure* (compared with its paired, more hollow and open yin

organ, the bladder). A classically trained acupuncturist generally describes the kidney as yin because it is *fed* by yin energy that flows *up* the body on the kidney meridian. Such differences between the two disciplines in terms of descriptive language can be confusing, although little difference in application of goals, practice, or theory really exists.

Another major principle applied to the practice of shiatsu involves the concepts of *kyo* (KEY-o) and *jitsu* (JIT-sue). Kyo is considered *empty* or *vacant,* whereas jitsu is considered *full, excessive,* or *overflowing.* A jitsu condition along the gallbladder meridian may be a manifestation of a gallbladder imbalance, resulting perhaps from recent consumption of a large pizza and two dishes of ice cream. A kyo or empty condition along the lung meridian (and within the lung itself) may exist in an individual who does not exercise and rarely expands his or her chest cavity or heart. Understanding and finding these energy manifestations is critical to diagnosis in shiatsu practice and is an ongoing, lifelong learning experience for the serious shiatsu practitioner. Although it is generally easy to find jitsu, or excess, it may be much more difficult to find emptiness or vacancy (kyo) within the meridian network. One of the keys to performing highly successful or refined shiatsu is the ability to find specific kyo within the body or the organ's meridian network and then to manipulate it effectively.

Shiatsu practitioners may follow the practice of macrobiotics, a set of universal dietary and spiritual guidelines originally brought to the attention of the modern world by George Ohsawa. As David Sergel (1989) writes:

> The ultimate goal of macrobiotic practice is the attainment of absolute freedom. The compass to reach this goal is an intimate understanding of the forces of Yin and Yang; a comprehension of an order common to all aspects of the infinite universe. The foundation of this freedom lies in our daily diet.... Since the same cultural soil gave form to both shiatsu and macrobiotics, we might expect to see strong possibilities of a harmonious integration between the two. In fact as we delve deeper, we see evidence that shiatsu arose from a macrobiotic mind and is thus according to this view, from its foundation, a macrobiotic practice.

It would be more accurate to state that shiatsu developed out of a society whose dietary pattern reflected the modern perspective and application of macrobiotics. Shiatsu evolved as a result of day-to-day living and thinking in terms of yin and yang, as did almost everything else in these earlier Asian societies, such as feng shui, art, and even politics.

Macrobiotics is a philosophical practice that incorporates the universal guidelines of yin and yang into daily life. With diet as its cornerstone, macrobiotic theory posits that these guidelines can be applied to all people, subject to their condition, constitution, lifestyle, environment, and, most notably, the latitude at which they live. Food

TABLE 20-2

Five Elements of Asian Medicine

Element	Yin	Yang
Wood (tree)	Gallbladder	Liver
Fire	Small intestine	Heart
Earth (soil)	Stomach	Spleen
Metal	Large intestine	Lungs
Water	Bladder	Kidney

choices are governed by season. Macrobiotics is *not* a diet; it is a philosophy that advocates cooked whole grains as the predominant staple food, to be supplemented by other yang foods such as root vegetables and occasional fish, and yin foods such as leafy greens and occasional seasonal fruit. Extreme yin foods include white sugar, honey, caffeine, most drugs, and alcohol. Examples of extreme yang foods are animal proteins such as red meat, chicken, tuna, and shellfish. Dietary choices are adjusted according to an individual's constitution, environment, work, lifestyle, the season, and the place where the person lives (especially global latitude). When used indiscriminately, extreme yin and yang foods are more difficult to balance and affect energy, as manifested along the meridian network. For example, eating tropical fruit in Pennsylvania in January when the temperature is 10° F on a daily basis is seen as "eating out of balance."

Macrobiotic philosophy therefore relies on nature, from which it finds ample support. Although we are able to ship foods thousands of miles from where they are grown, nature may not have intended us to consume such foods regularly in an environment that does not support their growth or cultivation. When applied in this way, the philosophies of shiatsu and macrobiotics touch on and address what is viewed as human arrogance by suggesting that when clear-cut guidelines presented by nature are ignored, health consequences can result. Nature demonstrates that the foods that grow and *can* grow in the latitudes where we live are the foods that support our health most fully. This philosophy also states that consumption of root vegetables (i.e., those that produce more heat in the body) is important in the winter, whereas leafy greens and occasional fruit (foods that cool the body) are needed in summer. Interestingly, we intuitively follow this practice to some extent. People who live in locations where the climate varies from season to season tend to eat more salads and fruit in the summer and more cooked and salty foods in the winter. However, macrobiotic philosophy examines this practice more closely and looks at these specific distinctions of yin and yang as being crucial to creating balance in the body, as well as the cornerstone of addressing such imbalance issues as cancer.

Shiatsu incorporates macrobiotic philosophy into its theory and philosophy regarding the movement of energy along the meridian pathways. A simple explanation of shiatsu philosophy states that the meridians can be seen as circulatory or "plumbing" channels. As long as energy moves freely (i.e., is not too weak or too strong and is not stagnant), health is maintained. If there is a blockage along the channel, the resulting disturbance can lead to minor aches and pains or a major health imbalance. It is possible to observe imbalances of energy flow in specific meridian lines and acupuncture points or tsubos. By applying pressure to a blocked meridian line or tsubo, an overactive or underactive organ system can be directly sedated or stimulated.

Shiatsu massage is not viewed by its practitioners as a panacea. Shiatsu philosophy is very clear in reinforcing the need for dietary and lifestyle guidance and changes to complement and support a shiatsu session (or series of sessions). The choices made by the recipients of treatment are their choices. Many recipients are content to stay at the level at which shiatsu is simply used for decreasing pain and for producing a "calmed sense of revitalization." However, others who are open to the underpinnings of shiatsu philosophy may be willing to take additional steps suggested by a classically trained shiatsu practitioner regarding diet and behavior modification.

With sufficient training, the shiatsu practitioner learns to view the energy manifesting at major tsubos on the surface of the skin as indicative of the underlying condition of the organ to which the tsubo is related and connected. For example, a client may think shoulder pain is caused by how he or she sleeps or sits at a desk. A classically trained shiatsu practitioner does not ignore these factors but looks *past* them to the underlying organ system and the foods that affect that organ system. The practitioner attempts to change the energy pattern not just by working at the proximate points of client complaint and distress, but also by working along the entire meridian (or set of meridians). Dietary suggestions may be offered. If the concept that "everything is energy" can be accepted, it may be possible to accept not only that the specific energies of foods can have an effect on organ systems and ultimately on health, but that this effect can produce effects formerly believed to be unrelated to the internal metabolic state as well as the related surface pain or discomfort.

Shiatsu training touches on the principles of Asian medicine because the nature of the organ systems and their related energy should be understood for effective treatment to occur, although, as mentioned previously, this knowledge is not an absolute requirement to practice shiatsu. How far this education goes, particularly in relation to the underlying effects of specific foods and their yin and yang effects on various organs and the body as a whole, depends on the quality of the school, the knowledge of the instructor, and the interest of the student.

The Japanese Ministry of Health and Welfare demonstrated its support of shiatsu's efficacy when it stated, "Shiatsu therapy is a form of manipulation administered by the thumbs, fingers, and palms, without the use of any instrument, mechanical or otherwise, to apply pressure to the human skin, correct internal malfunctioning, promote and maintain health, and treat specific diseases" (Masunaga et al, 1977).

DIAGNOSIS

The art of Asian diagnosis is a lifelong learning process in the practice of shiatsu. Subtle yet specific, Asian diagnosis is an ongoing and evolving pursuit that a practitioner is continually mastering and learning again from scratch. Modern diagnostic techniques are a relatively recent development in the history of medicine. Powerful, precise, and accurate to a large extent, the contribution of these techniques to the improvement of the human condition cannot be denied. However, diagnostic procedures in Western medicine use a disease-oriented model and tend to focus on parts (e.g., cells, tissues, organs) rather than on the whole organism. For example, Louis Pasteur (1822-1895) believed that microbes were the primary cause of disease. Although this theory has proved correct and is applicable to a large number of cases, germs are not the sole cause of disease. Although Asian diagnosis has been practiced for thousands of years, Western medicine has largely ignored its value. However, this is changing with the increased integration of Eastern and Western diagnostic methods.

In Asian medicine and shiatsu, there are two underlying levels of diagnosing humans: constitutional and conditional. Simply stated, an individual's *constitution* is what he or she was born with. Along with inherited traits, the quality of life, energy, and food intake experienced by the mother while a person is in utero are all considered factors that make up a person's constitution. A person's *condition* is the sum of his or her experience, which includes diet. In classic shiatsu diagnosis, both constitution and condition are assessed according to the methods listed next.

The following four methods of observing "phenomena" are used in Asian medicine (Masunaga et al, 1977):

1. *Bo-shin:* diagnosis through observation
2. *Bun-shin:* diagnosis through sound
3. *Mon-shin:* diagnosis through questioning
4. *Set su-shin:* diagnosis through touch

Each day, whether we realize it or not, we use the first three methods of observation extensively in our interactions with others and the environment. We all have experienced a funny feeling in our stomachs when we enter a room that has recently been the site of some tension related to human interaction. We choose partners based on many factors, including some innate sense of *energy* recognition we find compatible with our own. Although we are unaware that we use aspects of Asian diagnosis in our everyday lives, we nonetheless make assessments and judgments based on these principles. Without these "diagnostic skills," we would not survive. Shiatsu uses the first three methods liberally, while also relying heavily on the fourth.

In a traditional shiatsu session, diagnosis begins with the first contact between client and practitioner, whether in person or on the telephone. The client's tone of voice, speed of delivery, and choice of words give clues to the trained ear regarding the condition and constitution of the shiatsu client.

On meeting a client for the first time, constitutional and conditional assessments are made. How did the client enter the room? Did she walk upright? Did he smile or frown? Was her handshake strong or weak? Was his hand wet, damp, dry, hot, or cold? The client is often unaware that a classically trained shiatsu therapist begins work with the first contact and continues the assessment as a face-to-face meeting begins. Visual diagnosis and verbal questioning continue as the first meeting between client and therapist proceeds.

To arrive at a constitutional diagnosis, the therapist looks at various physical attributes. No single factor observed gives a total picture, but a *macro* assessment takes the various *micro* elements into account. Size of ears, shape and size of head, distance between the eyes, size of mouth, and size of hands are fundamental observations made in constitutional diagnosis before any physical treatment begins.

Factors considered in conditional assessment are slightly different but work in tandem with the overall assessment. The stated reason for the visit is a factor. In addition, tone and volume of the client's voice, pupil size, eye color, color and condition of the tongue, condition of the nails, and response to palpation along specific points on the hands and arms may be used. Pulse diagnosis, the act of reading distinctly differently levels of heartbeats near the wrists on both hands, may be used, depending on the practitioner's level of training. Generally, pulse diagnosis is more the tool of an acupuncturist, but it has been and can be used by a properly trained shiatsu provider.

The four diagnostic methods (observation, sound, questioning, and touch) are used to develop a singular yin-yang analysis (Ballegaards et al, 1996). At its basic level, Asian diagnosis sets out to determine whether a person is *vibrationally,* or *energetically,* more yin or more yang, because these two opposing but complementary states of energy affect each of us.

The diagnostic assessment process continues along specific lines, as follows:

> Yang diagnosis: Excess body heat and desire for coolness; great thirst and desire for fluids; constipation and hard stools; scanty, hot, dark urine
> Yin diagnosis: Cold feeling and desire for warmth; lack of thirst and preference for hot drinks; loose stools; profuse, clear urine; flat taste in mouth; poor appetite. (Yamamoto et al, 1993)

The key is not being able to see the yin and yang extremes described in the excerpt. The key lies in determining not only what tendency within an individual may be contributing to his or her state, but also the particular organ or organs that have a jitsu or kyo condition, and then working those organs' meridians to change that state. This is the point at which the movement from external or initial diagnosis of constitution and condition ends and treatment begins.

At this point, the practitioner's hands become the primary diagnostic tools. Although diagnosis is an ongoing process during treatment, traditional shiatsu first assesses by palpation of the major organs located in the client's hara, or abdomen. Alternatively, some styles of shiatsu begin a treatment session with touch diagnosis on the upper back, an area that also yields a vast amount of information regarding a person's condition. Assessment and diagnosis include observations through palpation that describe the following physical properties: tightness or looseness, fullness or emptiness, hot or cold, dry or wet, resistant or open, and stiff or flexible.

Diagnosis in a shiatsu session does not cease after an initial assessment. Diagnosis is an ongoing process of observation, listening, feeling, and changing focus based on continuously revealed information. The ability to make an accurate diagnosis quickly can be extremely helpful to a practitioner and client in their mutual attempt to create energetic change for the receiving partner. However, shiatsu can be effective in the hands of a relatively unskilled diagnostician. By following the simple concept of paying attention to what is going on underneath one's hands, a layperson with relatively little training can provide an effective, relaxing, and enjoyable shiatsu treatment for family and friends in a nonprofessional setting.

PRACTICES, TECHNIQUES, AND TREATMENT

Unlike some disciplines, shiatsu is easy to learn. It is not possible for a layperson to practice chiropractic, acupuncture, or osteopathy, because medical professionals need not only training but also time and continuing education to master techniques and improve skills. Shiatsu also requires a disciplined approach, constant practice, and continuing study to develop in-depth understanding. However, the *basic* practice remains simple, effective, and safe. Shiatsu techniques can be learned and safely applied by anyone and typically result in positive effects for both the recipient and the provider. It can be performed anywhere, takes place with the recipient fully clothed, and requires no special tools, machines, or oils.

Sergel (1989) states, "While ki may indeed emanate from the giver's fingertips it may not be in this way or only in this way that shiatsu works. Masunaga's approach is to emphasize another side, that the healing ki of *shiatsu lies within the quality or spirit of the touch in itself,* as compared with the idea of some invisible current that emanates from the touch." More than 150 years ago Shinsai Ota, in a book on ampuku (hara, or abdominal) shiatsu, emphasized that "honest, sincere, and simple Shiatsu is much better than merely technique-oriented professional Shiatsu" (Masunaga et al, 1977). Indeed, shiatsu training often emphasizes that the most important element is to be in touch with what is going on *under one's hands.* Experts agree, indicating that when a practitioner applies pressure and stimulation, he or she should then react and follow up based on an intuitive sense of and reaction to internal changes within the recipient (Yamamoto et al, 1993). A traditionally trained shiatsu practitioner, knowledgeable in the food-energy fundamentals of yin and yang and applying those principles in his or her life, is

arguably better suited to respond intuitively to the client. It is believed that *intuition* is enhanced by being in harmony with nature, a condition achieved by following the guidelines of living within nature's principles—earth's rhythms of yin and yang. Harmony in the body is achieved by being in harmony with the universe. Eating large amounts of animal protein and simple carbohydrates, which in their cultivation and processing exploit and pollute the earth, does not yield a calm and focused mind that can easily tap into human intuition. If a person is not in harmony with the natural order, the theory states, he or she is less likely to be able to tap into his or her intuition and tune in to another person's needs and internal energies (Sergel, 1989). Experienced shiatsu practitioners would typically agree.

Although a successful shiatsu session may be based more on intuition than technical understanding, it still is necessary to outline the techniques and preparation needed for a successful shiatsu treatment. Shiatsu recipients are fully clothed. Although shiatsu techniques can be adapted to other massage styles and may be performed on bare skin, traditional shiatsu is applied to a fully clothed person. Clients should be dressed in loose-fitting cotton fiber clothing. Blends containing polyester or other synthetics are thought to block or interrupt the natural transmission of energy between the caregiver and the recipient. Static electricity builds up around synthetic fibers. Because, from an Asian perspective, *everything is energy,* unnatural fibers, which may produce unnatural energies, should not be worn during a shiatsu session.

Because shiatsu requires no special tools or environment, it can be performed anywhere at any time. However, traditional shiatsu is generally performed on a cotton floor futon or shiatsu mat. Shiatsu techniques may be adapted to a table, but this is considered a deviation from the classic perspective. Although shiatsu can take place at any time of day, because the energetic effects of shiatsu differ dramatically in many ways from those of other methods, practitioners may encourage new clients to schedule a session early in the day, preferably before noon. Because shiatsu can yield a "calmed sense of revitalization," the combination of being relaxed and energized is an experience that should be savored throughout the day. Americans often equate "calm and relaxed" with an *inactive* state. Although shiatsu yields different results for different people, one of the most unique effects experienced by most clients is indeed this calmed sense of revitalization. When treated by a competent practitioner, a new shiatsu client may report that "I never felt this way before."

One reason for the difference in the energetic effects of shiatsu as opposed to those of other techniques (often called *regular massage* by the general public) is easy to explain. In many forms of therapeutic massage a technique described as *effleurage* or *stroking* (sweeping the skin with the hands) is used. The many benefits of this type of movement on the skin include stimulation of blood flow and the movement of lymph. Although this technique is beneficial, one of its effects is often a feeling of lethargy as cellular waste is moved through the lymphatic system. Because the effects of shiatsu are realized more on the underlying blockage of energy related to the body's organ systems than on the lymphatic system, a shiatsu session can yield a feeling of increased short-term and long-term energy. This is why chair massage using shiatsu techniques is so appropriate and considered by many superior to other techniques in the corporate setting. Employees do not experience the short-term negative energetic effects (lethargy) of effleurage, but rather the energetic boost, the *calmed sense of revitalization,* often associated with effective shiatsu technique. Masunaga and Ohashi (1977) described this difference in the following way:

> Anma and European massage directly stimulate blood circulation, emphasizing the release of stagnated blood in the skin and muscles and tension and stiffness resulting from circulatory congestion. On the other hand, Shiatsu emphasizes correction and maintenance of bone structure, joints, tendons, muscles, and meridian lines whose malfunctioning distort the body's energy and autonomic nervous system causing disease.

Shiatsu, like other methods, is best received with an empty stomach. This may not always be possible, and recent food consumption is no reason not to receive shiatsu. However, practitioners and recipients should bear in mind that when the body's energies are focused *inward* toward digestion, a shiatsu session, with its attempt to change the body's energies, is somewhat compromised and therefore will be less effective.

In some ways the beginning of a shiatsu session is similar to that for other massage styles. The room used should be simple, clean, and quiet. A thorough history of the client and his or her concerns should be taken. Questions may relate to sleep patterns, lifestyle, eating habits, and work history. A high level of trust should be established quickly. Often a client is seated in a chair or on a floor mat as the shiatsu practitioner observes and asks questions regarding the client's expectations and level of understanding. Diagnostic techniques to determine the client's constitution and condition are undertaken. The hands, eyes, tongue, and coloration along the upper and lower limbs may be examined. Several deep breaths to begin the process may be suggested. A well-trained shiatsu practitioner obtains a complete history to uncover any risk factors affecting the appropriateness of shiatsu treatment. Clinical experience and training, coupled with good references regarding a therapist's skills and practice, should be the determining factors in selecting a shiatsu practitioner.

A shiatsu session usually begins in one of two ways. In classic shiatsu, the practitioner may use hara, or abdominal massage, to determine which organ or organ system meridians may require treatment. Because this type of probing may not be appropriate or well received by many new shiatsu clients, some practitioners start with the client seated in a chair or on a floor mat and make an initial assessment of the client's energies from the upper back and shoulder region. This gives the practitioner immediate feedback on the client's condition and also helps the client relax. Most people are aware of tension in their upper back, shoulder, and neck and respond rather quickly to the process of relaxation so necessary for successful shiatsu.

These early assessments of client condition, coupled with a practitioner's best understanding and synthesis of the client's overall constitution, dictate the direction in which the therapist moves. Classic shiatsu texts state that "kyo and jitsu must first be found in the meridian lines by touching or kneading" to allow the direction of the shiatsu to be most effective (Masunaga et al, 1977). However, even when kyo or jitsu is not accurately determined at the outset, effective treatment may still be provided; these conditions can be addressed during the session without any specific perception or awareness of these qualities.

Whether treatment begins in a chair or on a floor mat, most of the session takes place with the client lying down. Applying various techniques along the meridian network, the practitioner attempts to create a better energy balance for the shiatsu recipient. Techniques used include rocking, tapotement (pounding), rubbing, and stretching. A shiatsu practitioner employs his or her entire body to apply pressure. Feet, elbows, knees, fingers, and palms are used as appropriate. A client may be face down or face up or may lie on the side, as directed or moved by the practitioner.

Although certain techniques such as rubbing and kneading may be used at this point and throughout a shiatsu session, the application of more stationary pressure by the palms, thumbs, forearms, and elbows usually begins early in a session. The muscles at the base of the occiput may be kneaded with the fingers and thumbs. Often the head is rotated with one hand while a stationary base of support at the neck is maintained with the other hand. Although shiatsu providers generally use similar methods, every practitioner is different.

When the techniques applied to the upper back, shoulders, and neck are completed, the client generally reclines to the floor mat in a position the therapist deems most beneficial. This may be the prone, supine, or side position. Certain individuals may use the side position exclusively because of size, pregnancy, or specific issues.

If the client is placed in a prone position, the therapist may use his or her feet to rock the client's hips or to apply graduated pressure to the legs and feet. This "barefoot shiatsu" technique is used extensively by Shizuko Yamamoto and is a very powerful adjunct to the use of the hands, knees, elbows, and forearms. The stretching of the arms and legs and their rotation at the shoulders and hips, respectively, is not uncommon.

Depending on their relative sizes, the practitioner may also walk on the client. Caution is clearly in order when using this rarely practiced technique, but it is sometimes appropriate and beneficial.

Shiatsu sessions typically take place with the provider on his or her knees next to the client. Pressure is applied along distinct meridian lines with the palms and thumbs. Knees, elbows, and forearms may also be used along these specific channels. To access the energy of the various organs through their respective meridians, the client's position changes to side or supine as the session proceeds.

Generally, conversation is minimized or absent during a shiatsu treatment. Music may be played based on the joint needs and desires of giver and receiver. Blood pressure and breathing rates generally decrease during a session. A shiatsu recipient may feel some cold sensations as he or she begins to relax, a natural reaction of the body's autonomic nervous system. Shiatsu can be performed through a cotton blanket, which most practitioners have available. A shiatsu session can be of any length, although a 60-minute duration is common. Sessions often end where they began, at the base of the client's neck or head with gentle kneading or massaging of neck or facial muscles. Shiatsu recipients are generally asked to remain quiet and still for several minutes after a session.

Most people can receive shiatsu. People with sprains and sports injuries who are seeking *direct* treatment of specific areas of trauma are best referred to massage therapists specifically trained to address these issues. However, gentle and focused shiatsu for these types of injuries can be applied to areas not directly related to the affected area to produce positive results by removing pressure and tension that the body may have created by compensating for the injury. Shiatsu can be used during pregnancy if provided by a practitioner trained in the specific meridians and tsubos that should be *avoided* during a session. Shiatsu is effective during pregnancy as long as common sense and the specific training and experience of the therapist are taken into account. Both supine and side positions are typically used, as appropriate and comfortable during pregnancy.

Because stationary and perhaps deeper application of pressure is a major part of shiatsu technique, caution should be exercised when treating people who bruise easily, have low platelet counts, or have leukemia, lymphoma, or extensive skin or other cancers. Clients who have an acute or chronic cystic condition must clearly communicate their complete history to reduce any potential risk. Although burn victims have benefited from massage therapy, the application of shiatsu at or near a burn site is not appropriate. In theory or in practice, however, shiatsu should not be considered a painful massage therapy; quite the opposite is the norm.

The previous description of a shiatsu session should be considered generic. There are many variations to the basic techniques, and numerous schools that teach specific shiatsu practices offer a more distinct focus to the underlying themes presented. For a more thorough description and expansion on the practice of Shiatsu, readers are directed to *Shiatsu: Theory and Practice* (Beresford-Cooke, 2001).

The American Organization of Body Therapies of Asia (AOBTA) notes 12 specific areas of Asian technique. Six major schools of Asian practice often described by shiatsu practitioners are discussed in the following sections, as noted on the AOBTA website.

ACUPRESSURE

Acupressure is a system of balancing the body's energy by applying pressure to specific acupoints to release tension and increase circulation. The many hands-on methods of stimulating the acupressure points can strengthen weaknesses, relieve common ailments, prevent health disorders, and restore the body's vital life force.

FIVE-ELEMENT SHIATSU

The primary emphasis of five-element shiatsu is to identify a pattern of disharmony through use of the four examinations and to harmonize that pattern with an appropriate treatment plan. Hands-on techniques and preferences for assessment vary with the practitioner, depending on individual background and training. The radial pulse usually provides the most critical and detailed information. Palpation of the back and/or abdomen and a detailed verbal history serve to confirm the assessment. The client's lifestyle and emotional and psychological factors are all considered important. Although this approach uses the paradigm of the five elements to tonify, sedate, or control patterns of disharmony, practitioners of this style also consider hot or cold and internal or external symptoms and signs.

JAPANESE SHIATSU

Shiatsu literally means finger *(shi)* pressure *(atsu)*, and although shiatsu is primarily pressure, usually applied with the thumbs along the meridian lines, extensive soft tissue manipulation and both active and passive exercise and stretching may be part of the treatments. Extensive use of cutaneovisceral reflexes in the abdomen and on the back is also characteristic of shiatsu. The emphasis of shiatsu is the treatment of the whole meridian; however, effective points are also used. The therapist assesses the condition of the patient's body as treatment progresses. Therapy and diagnosis are one.

MACROBIOTIC SHIATSU

Founded by Shizuko Yamamoto and based on George Ohsawa's philosophy that each individual is an integral part of nature, macrobiotic shiatsu supports a natural lifestyle and heightened instincts for improving health. Assessments are through visual, verbal, and touch techniques (including pulses) and the five transformations.

Treatment involves noninvasive touch and pressure using hand and barefoot techniques and stretches to facilitate the flow of qi and to strengthen the body-mind. Dietary guidance, medicinal plant foods, breathing techniques, and home remedies are emphasized. Corrective exercises, postural rebalancing, palm healing, self-shiatsu, and qigong are included in macrobiotic shiatsu.

SHIATSU ANMA THERAPY

Shiatsu anma therapy uses a unique blending of two of the most popular Asian bodywork forms practiced in Japan. Dr. Kaneko introduced traditional anma massage therapy based on the energetic system of traditional Chinese medicine in long form and contemporary pressure therapy, which is based on the neuromusculoskeletal system, in short form. *Ampuku,* abdominal massage therapy, is another foundation of anma massage therapy in Kaneko's school.

ZEN SHIATSU

Zen shiatsu is characterized by the theory of kyo-jitsu, its physical and psychological manifestations, and its application to abdominal diagnosis. Zen shiatsu theory is based on an extended meridian system that includes as well as expands the location of the traditional acupuncture meridians. The focus of a Zen shiatsu session is on the use of meridian lines rather than on specific points. In addition, Zen shiatsu does not adhere to a fixed sequence or set of methods that are applied to all. It uses appropriate methods for the unique pattern of each individual. Zen shiatsu was developed by Shizuto Masunaga.

The extended meridian network described and taught by Masunaga is a highly regarded part of shiatsu education. It is taught in quality schools as an integral part of shiatsu theory, diagnosis, and style. A practitioner often learns the extended meridian network toward the end of shiatsu education as an *extension* to the classic meridian network, in the same manner that Master Masunaga explored this expansion in shiatsu thinking, theory, and practice (AOBTA, n.d.).

TRAINING AND CERTIFICATION

There are currently no federal regulatory standards in the United States for shiatsu practitioners or any massage therapists. As of December 2008, *Massage Magazine* indicated that 40 states, plus the District of Columbia and four Canadian provinces, will soon have regulations governing massage therapy, and the American Bodywork and Massage Professionals states that there are over 278,000 credentialed practitioners.

Numerous schools of massage offer certificate programs in shiatsu or more broad-based programs that include

shiatsu massage. These programs may be weekend seminars of 1 or 2 days or may provide 600 or more hours of training particular to shiatsu. Schools may offer 350 to 500 hours of training in classic shiatsu with an additional 150 hours in anatomy and physiology. There appears to be a growing trend toward internships in all schools of massage.

The American Organization for Bodywork Therapies of Asia (AOBTA; formerly the American Asian Body Therapy Association) is the largest and most widespread organization specific to the practice of shiatsu. Applicants who wish to earn the title of Certified Practitioner must complete a 500-hour program, preferably at a school or institution recognized by the AOBTA.

The American Massage Therapy Association (AMTA) is a general association of massage practitioners; it does not actively focus on shiatsu therapy. This association meets regularly with the AOBTA as a federated massage-supporting organization. The AMTA's mission is to develop and advance the art, science, and practice of massage therapy in a caring, professional, and ethical manner to promote the health and welfare of humanity.

The American Bodywork and Massage Professionals (ABMP) is another highly respected association of massage professionals. Unlike the AOBTA and the AMTA, the ABMP is a for-profit organization.

The National Certification Board for Therapeutic Massage and Bodywork (NCBTMB) is a nationally recognized credentialing body formed to set high standards for those who practice therapeutic massage and bodywork. It accomplishes this through a nationally recognized certification program that evaluates the competency of its practitioners. Since 1992, more than 40,000 massage therapists and bodyworkers have received their certification. The NCBTMB examination is now legally recognized in more than 20 states and in many municipalities. The NCBTMB represents a diverse group of massage therapists, not just shiatsu practitioners. A minimum of 500 hours of formal massage education and successful completion of a written examination are the basic requirements for certification. Practitioners must be recertified every 4 years.

A person considering the use of any massage therapy as an adjunct to health maintenance should carefully select the provider of that therapy. In addition to obtaining personal references, it is important to evaluate the practitioner's training, experience, professional affiliations, and certification. Due to the diversity of massage practices available, a seeker of shiatsu therapy should not evaluate a potential therapist based on certification standards applicable to those who practice nonshiatsu techniques.

RESEARCH

The results of a number of randomized controlled trials of shiatsu therapy have recently been published. The following sections provide a brief listing of these shiatsu studies, grouped by category.

CANCER AND SLEEP DISTURBANCES

A study was recently completed at the Joan Karnell Cancer Center at Pennsylvania Hospital to evaluate the effectiveness of shiatsu therapy for treating sleep disturbances in cancer patients. Results are forthcoming. Preliminary data suggest that Shiatsu therapy effectively increased both the quality and the hours of sleep in patients with cancer.

CARDIOVASCULAR SYSTEM

A blind randomized controlled trial at a university-affiliated hospital documented a decrease in systolic, diastolic, and mean arterial pressure, as well as heart rate and skin blood flow, when acupoints were stimulated by pressure. Researchers concluded that acupressure can significantly and positively influence the cardiovascular system (AOBTA, n.d.).

A single-blind pretest-posttest crossover study in which patients were taught how to self-administer acupressure concluded that real acupressure was more effective than sham acupressure in reducing dyspnea (Felhendler et al, 1999).

Sixty-nine patients with severe angina pectoris were treated with acupuncture, shiatsu, and lifestyle adjustments. Invasive treatment was postponed in 61% of patients because of clinical improvement, and the annual number of in-hospital days was reduced 90%, which was calculated to be an annual savings of $12,000 for each patient in the study. The researchers concluded that this combined treatment may be highly effective for patients with advanced angina (Ballegaards et al, 1996).

MATERNITY

In a Boston study, postterm women who used shiatsu were more likely to undergo labor spontaneously than those who did not. The shiatsu group had a significantly lower rate of inductions and slightly fewer cesarean births and instrumental deliveries (Yates, 2004).

NAUSEA WITH BREAST CANCER CHEMOTHERAPY

Finger pressure applied bilaterally to two "major" acupressure points during the first 10 days of a chemotherapy cycle reduced the intensity and experience of nausea among women undergoing therapy (Maa et al, 1997).

NAUSEA AND VOMITING

The use of acupressure at the P6 acupoint was shown to reduce the incidence of nausea and vomiting within 24 hours of anesthesia from 42% to 19% compared with placebo (Dibble et al, 2000).

The use of acupressure at the P6 point was shown to reduce the incidence of nausea and vomiting after cesarean birth compared with placebo (Harmon et al, 1999, 2000).

Placement of acupressure bands at the P6 points on patients receiving general anesthesia for ambulatory surgery led to reduced nausea (23%) compared with the control group (41%), which suggests that this method can be used as an alternative to conventional antiemetic treatment (Harmon et al, 1999, 2000).

Children who received stationary acupressure applied to the Korean K-K9 point for 30 minutes before and 24 hours after strabismus surgery showed a significantly lower incidence of postoperative vomiting (20%) than children in the placebo group (68%) (Fan et al, 1997).

As compared to stimulation of the K-K9 point, stimulation of the P6 (neiguan) acupoint was determined to prevent nausea and vomiting in adults, although no antiemetic effects were noted in children undergoing strabismus surgery. However, it was determined that prophylactic use of bilateral acuplaster in children reduced the incidence of vomiting from 35.5% to 14.7% in the early emesis phase, 58.1% to 23.5% in the late emesis phase, and 64.5% to 29.4% overall. Researchers concluded that the use of acuplaster reduced vomiting in children undergoing strabismus correction (Schlager et al, 2000).

Shiatsu as developed in Korea and Japan is increasingly popular in the United States and stands at the intersection of hands-on therapy, massage and manipulative therapy, and energy healing as representing an ancient Asian healing tradition—thus appropriately placed at a crossroads in this book.

⊖ Chapter References, Suggested Readings, and Resources can be found on the Evolve website at http://evolve.elsevier.com/Micozzi/complementary/

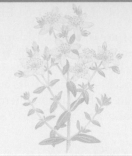

CHAPTER

21

NATUROPATHIC MEDICINE

JOSEPH E. PIZZORNO, JR.
PAMELA SNIDER
JOSEPH KATZINGER

This section describes the background, context, and clinical approaches of select alternative therapeutic systems as developed throughout European and American history. These chapters describe individual approaches as suggested from contemporary Western research, both within and beyond the biomedical paradigm. Where these systems and approaches can be understood in light of the contemporary biomedical paradigm, this view is examined; where they cannot be understood in these terms, this paradox is addressed. When and how these medical systems are embedded in the natural curative environment is clarified, as well as when and how they are embedded in technology. In each case, these medical practices are presented as products of history that make sense in terms of that history.

For example, homeopathy is a highly systematized method of healing that utilizes the principle of "use likes to treat likes" practiced by licensed physicians and other health care professionals throughout the world. In the United States, homeopathic medicines are protected by federal law, and most are available over the counter. The greatest challenge that homeopathy may pose to conventional medicine and science is the common use of extremely diluted medicinal substances. ∽

The doctor of the future will give no medicine, but will interest his patient in the care of the human frame, in diet and in the cause and prevention of disease.

—THOMAS EDISON

Thomas Edison's insightful prediction is proving true today, as natural medicine finds itself in the midst of an unprecedented explosion into mainstream health care. Consumers are spending more annually out of pocket for alternative medicine than for conventional care. In particular, naturopathic medicine as the model for integrative primary care natural medicine is undergoing a powerful resurgence. With its unique integration of vitalistic, scientific, academic, and clinical training in medicine, the naturopathic medical model is a potent contributing factor to this health care revolution.

HISTORY OF "REGULAR" MEDICINE AND NATUROPATHIC MEDICINE*

"REGULAR" MEDICINE

Conventional or "regular" medicine and natural medicine have shaped and helped to define each other throughout history, often in reaction, and perhaps nothing has had as much influence on naturopathic medicine as the rise of regular medicine. Much as naturopathic doctors today may trace some of their roots to Hippocrates, regular physicians also generally consider his view of health and disease to have contributed to the basis of today's medicine, primarily because of his rejection of supernatural or divine forces as the cause of illness, which resulted in the transition to a more physiological and rational approach to wellness. However, in contrast to naturopathic medicine, for which it is a core belief, regular medicine has come to reject Hippocrates' concept of the healing power of nature, a principle that may have done more to define and shape naturopathic medicine than anything else.

Of course regular medicine has made extraordinary leaps since the time of Hippocrates, particularly during the last century, and many aspects of today's education, scientific understanding, and therapeutic modalities would be unrecognizable to an MD only 100 years ago. We have also seen an unprecedented explosion in the size and role of the health care system in the United States, with over 600,000 MDs practicing as of the year 2000 (American Medical Association, n.d.), and $2.1 trillion spent on health care in 2006 (U.S. Department of Health and Human Services, n.d.). By comparison, in the year 1800 there were only 200 graduates of the elite medical

schools in the United States, along with 300 immigrants with European diplomas (Kaptchuk et al, 2001). The consistent thread that ties the regular doctors of the past to those practicing today may be a philosophy of allegiance to scientific principles and adoption of a basic biomedical orientation to illness, but coupled with disregard for the body's innate healing capacity.

In the European countries from which American medical education was derived, medicine first became institutionalized in the twelfth and thirteenth centuries, following a low ebb during the Dark Ages of AD 500 to 1050. Sarleno, Italy, was one of the earliest centers of medical training, followed by universities in Paris and England, where some of the first hospitals were built (Cruse, 1999). Although a graduate from Oxford in the 1500s had received up to 14 years of university education, very poor training was offered in the practice of medicine and patient care (Magee, 2004). When the Enlightenment arrived at the far reaches of Europe in Scotland it was a mature intellectual movement emphasizing observation (empiricism) and reason (rationality). The Scottish Enlightenment of the eighteenth century produced advancements in thinking about economics (Adam Smith, *The Wealth of Nations,* 1776) and law (David Hume) as well as the roots of the Industrial Revolution with the application of the steam engine (James Watt), based on principles used for the steam distillation of scotch whiskey. The "rational medicine" movement was embodied in the school of medicine at the University of Edinburgh from whence Drs. James Hutchison and John Morgan came to establish the first school of medicine in the United States in 1767 at the College of Philadelphia (now the University of Pennsylvania), following the establishment of the first hospital in the nation by Benjamin Franklin and Dr. Thomas Bond during the prior decade in 1752 (Figure 21-1).

In general, however, in the 1700s little had improved—doctors had limited diagnostic ability, and aside from feeling the pulse, inspecting the tongue, and examining the urine and stool, physicians did not touch their patients

---

* The authors express their appreciation to George Cody, whose chapter "History of Naturopathic Medicine," in *A Textbook of Natural Medicine* (JE Pizzorno and MT Murray, editors, St. Louis, 2004, Elsevier), provided the basis for much of this section.

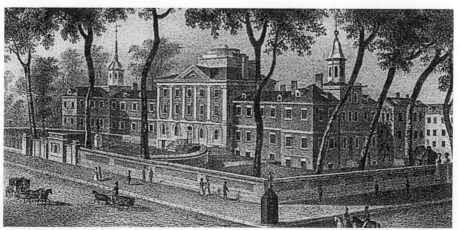

Figure 21-1 Pennsylvania Hospital, the nation's first hospital, founded in 1752. (Courtesy the Pennsylvania Hospital, Philadelphia.)

and often did not even see them (Magee, 2004). There were no consistent theories to explain the cause of illness, nor could the modalities used to treat them be agreed upon. As a result the medical landscape in the 1800s remained incredibly diverse.

This situation was not inconsistent with the political climate at the time, however. Like today, the cultural values of the early nineteenth century greatly influenced the practice of medicine. In the era of "Jacksonian democracy," beginning in the late 1820s, American society had begun to reject any form of "elitism," and the "elites" often included physicians, in large part because regular doctors were mostly available only to the wealthy in society (see Box 1-2). Much of the public harbored a fervent antiintellectualism coupled with belief in the tenet of economic freedom. As a consequence, laws controlling medical practice were viewed by the public as a form of class legislation; a general belief that citizens should have the right to choose their own medical care was combined with a distrust of the motives of "regular physicians" (Ober, 1997). Medical licensing became effectively irrelevant. For most of America's Colonial period, anyone could practice medicine, without a license, regardless of qualification or training. By 1850, all but two states had removed medical licensing statutes from the books (Whorton, 2002). Numerous conflicting claims of efficacy were made by a variety of practitioners, and an intense and heated competition often left patients confused by and dissatisfied with their experience with all types of physicians. The result has been described as both "medical anarchy" (Ober, 1997) and "a war zone" (Kaptchuk, 2001). Because regular medicine was often ineffective and frequently toxic, many patients and physicians defected to other "alternatives."

Partially in response, and after prior attempts, in 1847 a group of physicians founded an organization to serve as the unifying body for orthodox medical practitioners, the American Medical Association (AMA). Physicians who belonged to the AMA considered themselves regular practitioners and adhered to therapeutics termed *heroic medicine* (Rutkow, 2004). It was their treatments that may have most distinguished these regular doctors to their patients, because these often consisted of bleeding and blistering in addition to administering harsh concoctions to induce vomiting and purging, treatments that at the time were considered state of the art. The motivation behind such harsh treatments was a commitment to medical theory and a move away from empirically based medicine. Also, because regular doctors did not share belief in the concept of the healing power of nature (the *vis medicatrix naturae*), they felt that a physician's duty was to provide active, "heroic" intervention. Because the majority of patients recovered notwithstanding their treatments, this had the ironic effect of encouraging both regular doctors' belief in heroic treatments and irregulars' belief in the inborn capacity for self-healing, despite the further injuries caused by many regular treatments. Much like physicians today are pressured to provide an active treatment that

may sometimes be unnecessary (such as an antibiotic for a viral infection), regular doctors of the 1800s also felt pressure to give the heroic treatments for which they were known. As James Whorton (2002) writes, "it was only natural for MDs to close ranks and cling more tightly to that tradition as a badge of professional identity, making depletive therapy the core of their self-image as medical orthodoxy."

Although the AMA initially held no legal authority, it began a major push during the second half of the nineteenth century to create legislation and standards of medical education and competency. This process culminated in 1910 with the publication of *Medical Education in the United States and Canada,* compiled by Abraham Flexner (Figure 21-2), also known as the Flexner Report. It has been described as "a bombshell that rattled medical and political forces throughout the country" (Petrina, 2008). It criticized the medical education of its era as a loose and poorly structured apprenticeship system that generally lacked any defined standards or goals beyond commercialism (Ober, 1997). In some of his specific accounts, Flexner described medical institutions as "utterly wretched . . . without a redeeming feature" and as "a hopeless affair" (Whorton, 2002). Many of the regular medical institutions were rated poorly, and most of the irregular schools fared the worst. After this report, nearly half of the medical schools in the country closed, and by 1930 the remaining schools had 4-year programs of rigorous "scientific medicine."

Following the Flexner Report a tremendous restructuring of medical education and practice occurred. The remaining medical schools experienced enormous growth: in 1910 a leading school might have had a budget of $100,000; by 1965 it was $20 million and by 1990 it could

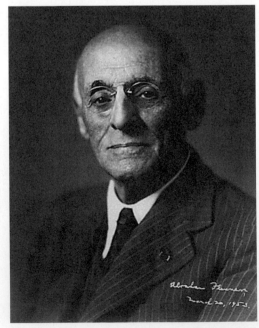

Figure 21-2 Abraham Flexner. (Courtesy National Library of Medicine, Bethesda, Md.)

have been $200 million or more (Ludmerer, 1999). Faculty were now called upon to engage in original research, and students not only studied a curriculum with a heavy emphasis on science, but also engaged in active learning by participating in real clinical work with responsibility for patients. Hospitals became the locus for clinical instruction. As scientific discovery began to accelerate, these higher educational standards helped to bridge the gap between what was known and what was put into practice, and more stringent licensing provided a greater degree of confidence in the competence of the nation's doctors. During this same time period, the suppression and decline of alternative schools of health care occurred, as both public and political pressure increased.

The post-World War II era has been one of undeniable and astonishing achievements by scientific medicine, which has coincided with great strides in public health, sanitation, and living conditions. As understanding of basic clinical science has grown, the biomedical model has continued to evolve, and so has the capacity to make accurate diagnoses and interventions. Today's physician faces new challenges, however, and some of the deficiencies of regular doctors in the past have reared their heads once again. In an era of managed care and health maintenance organizations, it has become increasingly difficult for physicians to spend quality time with patients or to focus on preventative medicine, and the treatment of chronic disease has suffered. Also, physicians must be vigilant against the constant and insidious efforts of the pharmaceutical industry to corrupt medical science, education, and practice for commercial gain. In addition, the increase in specialization and the decline of primary care is a growing problem that shows no sign of slowing. Today's regular doctors are also not easily defined—they have been referred to as "mainstream," "orthodox," "conventional," "allopathic," "scientific," and "authoritarian," all of which have their own positive and negative connotations, and none is universally accepted or accurate as individual MDs are more and more becoming receptive to developing new "integrative" models of health care (Berkenwald, 1998; Kaptchuk, 2001). It is also increasingly being recognized that although regular doctors have presented themselves as the "scientific" branch of medicine throughout recent history, the mantle of science cannot be claimed or exclusively worn by any one field of medicine, and integration of various medical specialties and philosophies benefits all.

A pluralistic health care setting is reemerging. Optimally, it will value the organization, structure, and science-based approach of regular medicine, along with qualities regular medicine has typically been lacking, including a patient-centered and individualized care that reaffirms the importance of the relationship between practitioner and patient, recognition and support of innate healing systems, and a broadening of the scientific approach to allow for the evaluation and incorporation of traditional and natural medicines into current health care delivery in a way that makes use of all appropriate therapeutic approaches, health

care professionals, and disciplines. "We find ourselves," John Weeks, the editor of *The Integrator,* wrote recently, "in an era beyond the polarization of alternative medicine and conventional medicine," with "an opportunity to become a seamless part of an integrated system that might rightfully be called, simply, *health care*" (The Integrator Blog, n.d.).

Although naturopathic medicine traces its philosophical roots to many traditional world medicines, its body of knowledge derives from a rich heritage of writings and practices of Western and non-Western nature doctors since Hippocrates (circa 400 BC). Modern naturopathic medicine grew out of healing systems of the eighteenth and nineteenth centuries. The term *naturopathy* was coined in 1895 by Dr. John Scheel of New York City to describe his method of health care. However, earlier forerunners of these concepts already existed in the history of natural healing, both in America and in the Austro-Germanic European core. Naturopathy became a formal profession after its creation by Benedict Lust in 1896. The profession has now celebrated its 115th birthday.

Over the centuries, natural medicine and conventional medicine have alternately diverged and converged, shaping each other, often in reaction. During the past hundred years the naturopathic profession progressed through several fairly distinct phases, as follows:

1. Latter part of the nineteenth century: *The founding by Benedict Lust.* Origin in the Germanic hydrotherapy and nature cure traditions.
2. 1900 to 1917: *The formative years.* Convergence of the American dietetic, hygienic, physical culture, spinal manipulation, mental and emotional healing, Thomsonian/eclectic, and homeopathic systems.
3. 1918 to 1937: *The halcyon days.* During a period of great public interest and support, the philosophical basis and scope of therapies diversified to encompass botanical, homeopathic, and environmental medicine.
4. 1938 to 1970: *Suppression and decline.* Growing political and social dominance of the AMA, lack of internal political unity, and lack of unifying standards, combined with the American love affair with technology and the emergence of "miracle" drugs and effective modern surgical techniques perfected in two world wars, resulted in legal and economic suppression.
5. 1971 to present: *Reemergence of naturopathic medicine.* Reawakened awareness in the American public of the importance of health promotion and prevention of disease, concern for the environment, and the establishment of modern, accredited, physician-level training reignited public interest in naturopathic medicine, which resulted in rapid resurgence. Current projections predict a continuing increase in the number of licensed naturopathic physicians.

The per capita supply of alternative medicine clinicians (chiropractors, naturopaths and practitioners of Oriental medicine) will grow by 88% between 1994 and

2010, while allopathic physician supply will grow by 16%. . . . The total number of naturopathy graduates will double over the next five years. The total number of naturopathic physicians will triple" (Cooper et al, 1996).

FOUNDING OF NATUROPATHY

Naturopathy, as a generally used term, began with the teachings and concepts of Benedict Lust. In 1892, at age 23, Lust came from Germany as a disciple of Father Sebastian Kneipp (the greatest practitioner of hydrotherapy) to bring Kneipp's hydrotherapy practices to America. Exposure in the United States to a wide range of practitioners and practices of natural healing arts broadened Lust's perspective, and after a decade of study, in 1902 he purchased the term *naturopathy* from Scheel of New York City (who coined the term in 1895) to describe the eclectic compilation of doctrines of natural healing that he envisioned was to be the future of natural medicine. Naturopathy, or "nature cure," was defined by Lust as both a way of life and a concept of healing that used various natural means (selected from various systems and disciplines) of treating human infirmities and disease states. The earliest therapies associated with the term involved a combination of American hygienics and Austro-Germanic nature cure and hydrotherapy.

In January 1902, Lust, who had been publishing the *Kneipp Water Cure Monthly* and its German-language counterpart in New York since 1896, changed the name of the journal to *The Naturopathic and Herald of Health* and began promoting a new way of thinking of health care with the following editorial:

> We believe in strong, pure, beautiful bodies . . . of radiating health. We want every man, woman and child in this great land to know and embody and feel the truths of right living that mean conscious mastery. We plead for the renouncing of poisons from the coffee, white flour, glucose, lard, and like venom of the American table to patent medicines, tobacco, liquor and the other inevitable recourse of perverted appetite. We long for the time when an eight-hour day may enable every worker to stop existing long enough to live; when the spirit of universal brotherhood shall animate business and society and the church; when every American may have a little cottage of his own, and a bit of ground where he may combine Aerotherapy, Heliotherapy, Geotherapy, Aristophagy and nature's other forces with home and peace and happiness and things forbidden to flat-dwellers; when people may stop doing and thinking and being for others and be for themselves; when true love and divine marriage and prenatal culture and controlled parenthood may fill this world with germ-gods instead of humanized animals.
>
> In a word, Naturopathy stands for the reconciling, harmonizing and unifying of nature, humanity and God.
>
> Fundamentally therapeutic because men need healing; elementary educational because men need teaching; ultimately inspirational because men need empowering.

Benedict Lust

According to his published personal history, Lust had a debilitating condition in his late teens while growing up in Michelbach, Baden, Germany, and had been sent by his father to undergo the Kneipp cure at Woerishofen. He stayed there from mid-1890 to early 1892. Not only was he "cured" of his condition, but he became a protégé of Father Kneipp. He emigrated to America to proselytize the principles of the Kneipp water cure (Figure 21-3).

By making contact in New York with other German Americans who were also becoming aware of the Kneipp principles, Lust participated in the founding of the first "Kneipp Society," which was organized in Jersey City, New Jersey, in 1896. Subsequently, through Lust's organization and contacts, Kneipp societies were also founded in Brooklyn, Boston, Chicago, Cleveland, Denver, Cincinnati,

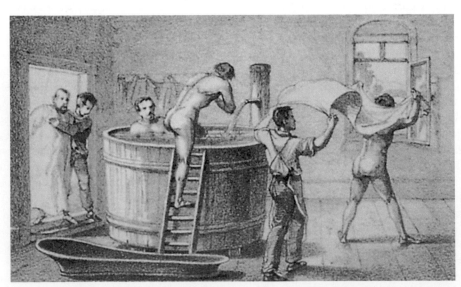

Figure 21-3 Curative baths, one form of hydrotherapy, were a popular form of natural healing in the late nineteenth century. (Courtesy Wellcome Institute Library, London.)

Philadelphia, Columbus, Buffalo, Rochester, New Haven, San Francisco, the state of New Mexico, and Mineola on Long Island. The members of these organizations were provided with copies of the *Kneipp Blatter* and a companion English publication Lust began to put out called *The Kneipp Water-Cure Monthly.* In 1895 Lust opened the Kneipp Water-Cure Institute on 59th Street in New York City.

Father Kneipp died in Germany, at Woerishofen, on June 17, 1897. With his passing, Lust was no longer bound strictly to the principles of the Kneipp water cure. He had begun to associate earlier with other German American physicians, principally Dr. Hugo R. Wendel (a German-trained "Naturarzt") who began, in 1897, to practice in New York and New Jersey as a licensed osteopathic physician. Lust entered the Universal Osteopathic College of New York in 1896 and became licensed as an osteopathic physician in 1898.

Once he was licensed to practice as a health care physician in his own right, Lust began the transition toward the concept of "naturopathy." Between 1898 and 1902, when he adopted the term *naturopath,* Lust acquired a chiropractic education; changed the name of his Kneipp Store (which he had opened in 1895) to "Health Food Store" (the first facility to use that name and concept in the United States), specializing in providing organically grown foods and the materials necessary for drugless cures; and founded the New York School of Massage (in 1896) and the American School of Chiropractic.

In 1902, when he purchased and began using the term *naturopathy* and calling himself a "naturopath," Lust, in addition to operating his New York School of Massage and American School of Chiropractic, issuing his various publications, and running his Health Food Store, began to operate the American School of Naturopathy. All these activities were carried out at the same 59th Street address. By 1907, Lust's enterprises had grown sufficiently large that he moved them to a 55-room building. It housed the Naturopathic Institute, Clinic, and Hospital; the American School of Naturopathy and American School of Chiropractic; the establishment now called the Original Health Food Store; Lust's publishing enterprises; and the New York School of Massage. The operation remained in this four-story building, roughly twice the size of the original facility, from 1907 to 1915.

From 1912 through 1914, Lust took a sabbatical from his operations to further his own education. By this time he had founded his large estatelike sanitarium at Butler, New Jersey, known as Yungborn after the German sanitarium operation of Adoph Just. In 1912 he began attending the Homeopathic Medical College in New York, which granted him a degree in homeopathic medicine in 1913 and a degree in eclectic medicine in 1914. In early 1914, Lust traveled to Florida and obtained an MD's license on the basis of his graduation from the Homeopathic Medical College.

From 1902, when he began to use the term *naturopathy,* until 1918, Lust replaced the Kneipp societies with the Naturopathic Society of America. Then in December 1919, the Naturopathic Society of America was formally dissolved because of insolvency, and Lust founded the American Naturopathic Association. Thereafter, the association was incorporated in some additional 18 states. Lust claimed at one time to have 40,000 practitioners practicing naturopathy. In 1918, as part of his effort to dissolve the Naturopathic Society of America (an operation into which he invested a great deal of his funds and resources in an attempt to organize a naturopathic profession) and replace it with the American Naturopathic Association, Lust published the first *Yearbook of Drugless Therapy.* Annual supplements were published in either *The Naturopath and the Herald of Health* or its companion publication, *Nature's Path* (which began publication in 1925), with which *The Naturopath* at one time merged. *The Naturopath and Herald of Health,* sometimes printed with the two phrases reversed, was published from 1902 through 1927, and from 1934 until after Lust's death in 1945.

Benedict Lust's principles of health are found in the introduction to the first volume of the *Universal Naturopathic Directory and Buyer's Guide,* a portion of which is reproduced in Box 21-1. Although the terminology is almost a century old, the concepts Lust proposed have provided a powerful foundation that has endured despite almost a century of active political suppression by the dominant school of medicine.

SCHOOLS OF THOUGHT THAT FORMED THE PHILOSOPHICAL BASIS OF NATUROPATHY

Because of the eclectic nature of naturopathic medicine, its history is by far the most complex of any healing art, which explains the unusually large portion of this chapter devoted to this subject. Although the following discussion is divided into distinct schools of thought, this is somewhat artificial, because those who founded and practiced these arts (especially the Americans) were often trained in, influenced by, and practiced several therapeutic systems or modalities. It was not until Benedict Lust, however, that the many threads were woven together into a unified professional practice, which makes naturopathic medicine the *first* Western system of full-scope *integrative* natural medicine based on the vis medicatrix naturae. Organized around this principle of the human capacity for healing, naturopathic medicine has been able to discriminately integrate diverse therapeutic systems and modalities into a cohesive framework, acknowledging the biomedical model of health and illness, but also supporting the whole person, including the psychological, social, and spiritual aspects of wellness. It has consistently promoted a patient-centered relationship, as well as collaboration with other health care professionals and disciplines, and today is poised as a model for integrative medicine. Although it draws from the eclectic tradition (see later), it does not do so randomly or indiscriminately. Rather, core principles, such as the vis medicatrix naturae,

BOX 21-1

Principles, Aim, and Program of the Nature Cure System

Since the earliest ages, medical science has been of all sciences the most unscientific. Its professors, with few exceptions, have sought to cure disease by the magic of pills and potions and poisons that attacked the ailment with the idea of suppressing the symptoms instead of attacking the real cause of the ailment.

Medical science has always believed in the superstition that the use of chemical substances that are harmful and destructive to human life will prove an efficient substitute for the violation of laws, and in this way encourages the belief that a man may go the limit in self-indulgences that weaken and destroy his physical system, and then hope to be absolved from his physical ailments by swallowing a few pills, or submitting to an injection of a serum or vaccine, that are supposed to act as vicarious redeemers of the physical organism and counteract life-long practices that are poisonous and wholly destructive to the patient's well-being.

The policy of expediency is at the basis of medical drug healing. It is along the lines of self-indulgence, indifference, ignorance and lack of self-control that drug medicine lives, moves and has its being.

The natural system for curing disease is based on a return to nature in regulating the diet, breathing, exercising, bathing and the employment of various forces to eliminate the poisonous products in the system, and so raise the vitality of the patient to a proper standard of health.

Official medicine has, in all ages, simply attacked the symptoms of disease without paying any attention to the causes thereof, but natural healing is concerned far more with removing the causes of disease, than merely curing its symptoms. This is the glory of this new school of medicine that it cures by removing the causes of the ailment, and is the only rational method of practicing medicine. It begins its cures by avoiding the uses of drugs and hence is styled the system of drugless healing.

The Program of Naturopathic Cure
1. ELIMINATION OF EVIL HABITS, or the weeds of life, such as over-eating, alcoholic drinks, drugs, the use of tea, coffee and cocoa that contain poisons,

meat eating, improper hours of living, waste of vital forces, lowered vitality, sexual and social aberrations, worry, etc.
2. CORRECTIVE HABITS. Correct breathing, correct exercise, right mental attitude. Moderation in the pursuit of health and wealth.
3. NEW PRINCIPLES OF LIVING. Proper fasting, selection of food, hydropathy, light and air baths, mud baths, osteopathy, chiropractic and other forms of mechano-therapy, mineral salts obtained in organic form, electropathy, heliopathy, steam or Turkish baths, sitz baths, etc.

Natural healing is the most desirable factor in the regeneration of the race. It is a return to nature in methods of living and treatment. It makes use of the elementary forces of nature, of chemical selection of foods that will constitute a correct medical dietary. The diet of civilized man is devitalized, is poor in essential organic salts. The fact that foods are cooked in so many ways and are salted, spiced, sweetened and otherwise made attractive to the palate, induces people to overeat, and over eating does more harm than under feeding. High protein food and lazy habits are the cause of cancer, Bright's disease, rheumatism and the poisons of autointoxication.

There is really but one healing force in existence and that is Nature herself, which means the inherent restorative power of the organism to overcome disease. Now the question is, can this power be appropriated and guided more readily by extrinsic or intrinsic methods? That is to say, is it more amenable to combat disease by irritating drugs, vaccines and serums employed by superstitious moderns, or by the bland intrinsic congenial forces of Natural Therapeutics, that are employed by this new school of medicine, that is Naturopathy, which is the only orthodox school of medicine? Are not these natural forces much more orthodox than the artificial resources of the druggist?

From Lust B: *Principles of health,* vol 1, *Universal naturopathic directory and buyer's guide,* Butler, NJ, 1918, Lust Publications.

guide its flexible but solid structure, allowing it to navigate, perhaps uniquely, today's medical world.

The following presents the formative schools of Western thought in natural healing and some of their leading adherents. Although the therapies differ, the philosophical thread of promoting health and supporting the body's own healing processes runs through them all. These threads are derived from centuries of medical scholarship, both Western and non-Western, concerning the self-healing process.

After a brief overview of Hippocrates' seminal contribution to the natural medicine way of thought, the basic

themes are presented in the following order: healthful living; natural diet; detoxification; exercise, mechanotherapy, and physical therapy; mental, emotional, and spiritual healing; and natural therapeutic agents. Hippocrates and centuries of nature doctors' writings remain empirically rich repositories of observations for future research.

Hippocrates

Prehistoric people believed that disease was caused by magic or supernatural forces, such as devils or angry gods. Hippocrates, breaking with this superstitious belief, became the first naturalistic doctor in recorded history.

Hippocrates regarded the body as a "whole" and instructed his students to prescribe only beneficial treatments and refrain from causing harm or hurt.

Hippocratic practitioners assumed that everything in nature had a rational basis; therefore the physician's role was to understand and follow the laws of the intelligible universe. They viewed disease as an effect and looked for its cause in natural phenomena: air, water, food, and so forth. They first used the term *vis medicatrix naturae,* the "healing power of nature," to denote the body's ability and drive to heal itself. One of the central tenets is that "there is an order to the process of healing which requires certain things to be done before other things to maximize the effectiveness of the therapeutics" (Zeff, 1997). The step order used by Tibetan medicine is also an example of the representation of this tenet in traditional world medicines.

Hydrotherapy

The earliest philosophical origins of naturopathy were clearly in the Germanic hydrotherapy movement: the use of hot and cold water for the maintenance of health and the treatment of disease. One of the oldest known therapies (water was used therapeutically by the Romans and Greeks), hydrotherapy began its modern history with the publication of *The History of Cold Bathing* in 1697 by Sir John Floyer. Probably the strongest impetus for its use came from Central Europe, where it was advocated by such well-known hydropaths as Priessnitz, Schroth, and Father Kneipp. They were able to popularize specific water treatments that quickly became the vogue in Europe during the nineteenth century. *Vinzenz Priessnitz* (1799-1851), of Graefenberg, Silesia, was a pioneer natural healer. Unfortunately, he was prosecuted by the medical authorities of his day and was actually convicted of using witchcraft because he cured his patients by the use of water, air, diet, and exercise. He took his patients back to nature—to the woods, the streams, the open fields—treated them with nature's own forces, and fed them on natural foods. His cured patients numbered in the thousands, and his fame spread over Europe. *Father Sebastian Kneipp* (1821-1897) became the most famous of the hydropaths, with Pope Leo XIII and Ferdinand of Austria (whom he had walking barefoot in new-fallen snow for the purposes of hardening his constitution) among his many famous patients. He standardized the practice of hydrotherapy and organized it into a system of practice that was widely emulated through the establishment of health spas or "sanitariums." The first sanitarium in this country, the Kneipp and Nature Cure Sanitarium, was opened in Newark, New Jersey, in 1891.

The best-known American hydropath was J.H. Kellogg, a medical doctor who approached hydrotherapy scientifically and performed many experiments trying to understand the physiological effects of hot and cold water. In 1900 he published *Rational Hydrotherapy,* which is still considered a definitive treatise on the physiological and therapeutic effects of water, along with an extensive discussion of hydrotherapeutic techniques. Drs. O.J. Carroll, Harold Dick, and John Bastyr, among others, brought the use of hydrotherapy techniques forward into modern naturopathic practice.

Nature Cure

Natural living, consumption of a vegetarian diet, and the use of light and air formed the basis of the nature cure movement founded by *Dr. Arnold Rickli* (1823-1926). In 1848 he established at Veldes Krain, Austria, the first institution of light and air cure or, as it was called in Europe, the *atmospheric cure.* He was an ardent disciple of the vegetarian diet and the founder, and for more than 50 years the president, of the National Austrian Vegetarian Association. In 1891, *Louis Kuhne* (ca. 1823-1907) wrote the *New Science of Healing,* which presented the basic principles of "drugless methods." *Dr. Henry Lahman* (ca. 1823-1907), who founded the largest nature cure institution in the world at Weisser Hirsch, near Dresden, Saxony, constructed the first appliances for the administration of electric light treatment and baths. He was the author of several books on diet, nature cure, and heliotherapy. *Professor F.E. Bilz* (1823-1903) authored the first natural medicine encyclopedia, *The Natural Method of Healing,* which was translated into a dozen languages, and in German alone ran into 150 editions.

Nature cure became popular in America through the efforts of *Henry Lindlahr,* MD, ND, of Chicago, Illinois. Originally a rising businessman in Chicago with all the bad habits of those in the Gay Nineties era, he became chronically ill while only in his thirties. After receiving no relief from the orthodox practitioners of his day, he learned of nature cure, which improved his health. Subsequently, he went to Germany to stay in a sanitarium to be cured and to learn nature cure. He went back to Chicago and earned his degrees from the Homeopathic/Eclectic College of Illinois. In 1903 he opened a sanitarium in Elmhurst, Illinois; established Lindlahr's Health Food Store; and shortly thereafter founded the Lindlahr College of Natural Therapeutics. In 1908 he began to publish *Nature Cure Magazine* and began publishing his six-volume series of *Philosophy of Natural Therapeutics.*

One of the chief advantages of training in the early 1900s was the marvelous inpatient facilities that flourished during this time. These facilities provided in-depth training in clinical nature cure and natural hygiene in inpatient settings. Nature cure and natural hygiene are still at the core of naturopathic medicine's fundamental principles and approach to health care and disease prevention.

The Hygienic System

Another forerunner of American naturopathy, the "hygienic" school, amalgamated the hydrotherapy and nature cure movements with vegetarianism. It originated as a lay movement of the nineteenth century and had its genesis in the popular teachings of *Sylvester Graham* and *William Alcott*. Graham began preaching the doctrines of temperance and hygiene in 1830 and in 1839 published *Lectures on the Science of Human Life,* two hefty volumes that prescribed healthy dietary habits. He emphasized a moderate lifestyle, a flesh-free diet, and bran bread as an alternative to bolted or white bread. The earliest physician to have a significant impact on the hygienic movement and the later philosophical growth of naturopathy was *Russell Trall*, MD. According to Whorton (1982) in his *Crusaders for Fitness,*

> The exemplar of the physical educator-hydropath was Russell Thatcher Trall. Still another physician who had lost his faith in regular therapy, Trall opened the second water cure establishment in America, in New York City in 1844. Immediately, he combined the full Priessnitzian armamentarium of baths with regulation of diet, air, exercise and sleep. He would eventually open and or direct any number of other hydropathic institutions around the country, as well as edit the *Water-Cure Journal,* the *Hydropathic Review,* and a temperance journal. He authored several books, including popular sex manuals which perpetuated Graham-like concepts into the 1890's, sold Graham crackers and physiology texts at his New York office, was a charter member (and officer) of the American Vegetarian Society, presided over a short-lived World Health Association, and so on.

Trall established the first school of natural healing arts in this country to have a 4-year curriculum and the authorization to confer the degree of MD. It was founded in 1852 as a "Hydropathic and Physiological School" and was chartered by the New York State Legislature in 1857 under the name New York Hygio-Therapeutic College.

Trall eventually published more than 25 books on the subjects of physiology, hydropathy, hygiene, vegetarianism, and temperance, among many others. The most valuable and enduring of these was his 1851 *Hydropathic Encyclopedia,* a volume of nearly 1000 pages that covered the theory and practice of hydropathy and the philosophy and treatment of diseases advanced by older schools of medicine. The encyclopedia sold more than 40,000 copies.

Martin Luther Holbrook expanded on the work of Graham, Alcott, and Trall and, working with an awareness of the European concepts developed by Priessnitz and Kneipp, laid further groundwork for the concepts later advanced by Lust, Lindlahr, and others. According to Whorton (1982), Holbrook proposed the following:

> For disease to result, the latter had to provide a suitable culture medium, had to be susceptible. As yet, most physicians were still so excited at having discovered the causative agents of infection that they were paying less than adequate notice to the host. Radical hygienists, however, were bent just as far in the other direction. They were inclined to see bacteria as merely impotent organisms that throve only in individuals whose hygienic

carelessness had made their body compost heaps. Tuberculosis is contagious, Holbrook acknowledged, but "the degree of vital resistance is the real element of protection. When there is no preparation of the soil by heredity, predisposition or lowered health standard, the individual is amply guarded against the attack." A theory favored by many others was that germs were the effect of disease rather than its cause; tissues corrupted by poor hygiene offered microbes, all harmless, an environment in which they could thrive.

The orthodox hygienists of the progressive years were equally enthused by the recent progress of nutrition, of course, and exploited it for their own naturopathic doctors, but their utilization of science hardly stopped with dietetics. Medical bacteriology was another area of remarkable discovery, bacteriologists having provided, in the short space of the last quarter of the nineteenth century, an understanding, at long last, of the nature of infection. This new science's implications for hygienic ideology were profound—when Holbrook locked horns with female fashion, for example, he did not attack the bulky, ground-length skirts still in style with the crude Grahamite objection that the skirt was too heavy. Rather he forced a gasp from his readers with an account of watching a smartly dressed lady unwittingly drag her skirt "over some virulent, revolting looking sputum, which some unfortunate consumptive had expectorated."

Trall and Holbrook both advanced the idea that physicians should teach the maintenance of health rather than simply provide a last resort in times of health crisis. Besides providing a strong editorial voice denouncing the evils of tobacco and drugs, they strongly advanced the value of vegetarianism, bathing and exercise, dietetics and nutrition along with personal hygiene.

John Harvey Kellogg, MD, another medically trained doctor who turned to more nutritionally based natural healing concepts, also greatly influenced Lust. Kellogg was renowned through his connection, beginning in 1876, with the Battle Creek Sanitarium, which was founded in the 1860s as a Seventh Day Adventist institution designed to perpetuate the Grahamite philosophies. Kellogg, born in 1852, was a "sickly child" who, at age 14, after reading the works of Graham, converted to vegetarianism. At the age of 20, he studied for a term at Trall's Hygio-Therapeutic College and then earned a medical degree at New York's Bellevue Medical School. He maintained an affiliation with the regular schools of medicine during his lifetime, more because of his practice of surgery than because of his beliefs in that area of health care (Figure 21-4)

Kellogg designated his concepts, which were basically the hygienic system of healthful living, as "biologic living." Kellogg expounded vegetarianism, attacked sexual misconduct and the evils of alcohol, and was a prolific writer through the late nineteenth and early twentieth centuries. He produced a popular periodical, *Good Health,* which continued in existence until 1955. When Kellogg died in 1943 at age 91, he had had more than 300,000 patients through the Battle Creek Sanitarium, including many celebrities, and the "San" became nationally known.

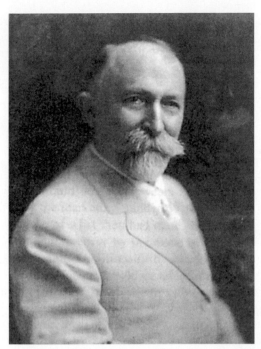

Figure 21-4 Dr. John Harvey Kellogg, brother to the Kellogg of breakfast cereal fame and a physical culture movement proponent. (Courtesy Historical Society of Battle Creek, Battle Creek, Mich.)

Kellogg was also extremely interested in hydrotherapy. In the 1890s he established a laboratory at the San to study the clinical applications of hydrotherapy. This led to his writing of *Rational Hydrotherapy* in 1902. The preface espoused a philosophy of drugless healing that came to be one of the bases of the hydrotherapy school of medical thought in early-twentieth-century America.

INFLUENCE ON PUBLIC HEALTH

It is a little-known fact that most of our current and accepted public hygiene practices were brought into societal use by the early hygienic reformers. Before their efforts, neglect of these basic physiological safety measures was rampant. The hygienists had a great influence on decreasing morbidity and mortality and increasing life span, as well as on the adoption of public sanitation. Orthodox medicine is typically credited with these advances.

Currently, certified professional Natural Hygienists are advocates of the highest standards of training and supervised clinical fasting and participate in the training of naturopathic physicians. Naturopathic medicine uses the precepts of natural hygiene in reestablishing the basis of health, the first step in the therapeutic order.

Autotoxicity

Lust was also greatly influenced by the writings of *John H. Tilden*, MD (who published between 1915 and 1925). Tilden became disenchanted with orthodox medicine and

began to rely heavily on dietetics and nutrition, formulating his theories of "autointoxication" (the effect of fecal matter's remaining too long in the digestive process) and "toxemia." He provided the natural health care literature with a 200-plus-page dissertation entitled *Constipation,* with a whole chapter devoted to the evils of not responding "when nature called."

Elie Metchnikoff (director of the prestigious Pasteur Institute and winner of the 1908 Nobel Prize for his contribution to immunology) and Kellogg wrote prolifically on the theory of autointoxication. Kellogg, in particular, believed that humans, in the process of digesting meat, produced a variety of intestinal self-poisons that contributed to autointoxication. As a result, Kellogg widely advocated that people return to a more healthy natural state by allowing the naturally designed use of the colon. He believed that the average modern colon was devitalized by the combination of a low-fiber diet, sedentary living, the custom of sitting rather than squatting to defecate, and the modern civilized habit of ignoring "nature's call" out of an undue concern for politeness.

Although the concept of toxemia is not a part of the body of knowledge taught in conventional medical schools, all naturopathic students are presented with this concept. Some of that presentation relies on outdated materials, such as the naturopathic texts of 75 and 100 years ago (e.g., Lindlahr, Tilden). However, modern research and textbooks are beginning to investigate this phenomenon. Drasar and Hill's *Human Intestinal Flora* (1974) demonstrates some of the biochemical pathways involved in the generation of metabolic toxins in the gut through dysbiotic bacterial action on poorly digested food (Zeff, 1997). In the last 20 years, our understanding of the concept of toxemia has been significantly updated by practitioners in the newly emerging field of *functional medicine,* a health care approach that focuses attention on biochemical individuality, metabolic balance, ecological context, and unique personal experience in the dynamics of health. Maldigestion, malabsorption, and abnormal gut flora and ecology are often found to be primary contributing factors not only to gastrointestinal disorders but also to a wide variety of chronic, systemic illnesses. Laboratory assessment tools have been developed that are capable of evaluating the status of many organs, including the gastrointestinal tract. These cutting-edge diagnostic tools provide physicians with an analysis of numerous functional parameters of the individual's digestion and absorption and precisely pinpoint what in the colonic environment is imbalanced, thus promoting dysbiosis.

Thomsonianism

In 1822, *Samuel Thomson* published his *New Guide to Health,* a compilation of his personal view of medical theory and American Indian herbal and medical botanical lore. Thomson espoused the belief that disease had one general cause—derangement of the vital fluids by "cold" influences on the human body—and that disease therefore had one general remedy—animal warmth or "heat." The name of the complaint depended on the part of the body that was affected. Unlike the conventional American heroic medical tradition that advocated bloodletting, leeching, and the substantial use of mineral-based purgatives such as antimony and mercury, Thomson believed that minerals were sources of "cold" because they come from the ground and that vegetation, which grew toward the sun, represented "heat" (Figure 21-5).

Thomson's view was that individuals could self-treat if they had an adequate understanding of his philosophy *and* a copy of *New Guide to Health*. The right to sell "family franchises" for use of the Thomsonian method of healing was the basis of a profound lay movement between 1822 and Thomson's death in 1843. Thomson adamantly believed that no professional medical class should exist and that democratic medicine was best practiced by laypersons within a Thomsonian "family" unit. By 1839 Thomson claimed to have sold some 100,000 of these family franchises, called "friendly botanic societies."

Despite his criticism of the early medical movement for its heroic tendencies, Thomson's medical theories were heroic in their own fashion. Although he did not advocate bloodletting or heavy metal poisoning and leeching, botanical purgatives—particularly *Lobelia inflata* (Indian tobacco)—were a substantial part of the therapy.

Eclectic School of Medicine

Some of the doctors practicing the Thomsonian method, called *botanics,* decided to separate themselves from the lay movement and develop a more physiologically

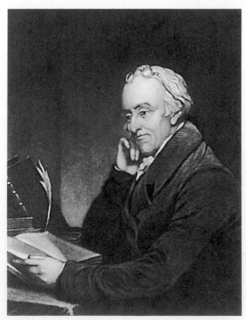

Figure 21-5 Samuel Thomson (1769-1843). (Courtesy National Library of Medicine, Bethesda, Md.)

sound basis of therapy. They established a broader range of therapeutic applications of botanical medicines and founded a medical college in Cincinnati. These Thomsonian doctors were later absorbed into the "eclectic school," which originated with Wooster Beach of New York.

Wooster Beach, from a well-established New England family, started his medical studies at an early age, apprenticing under an old German herbal doctor, Jacob Tidd, until Tidd died. Beach then enrolled in the Barclay Street Medical University in New York. After opening his own practice in New York, Beach set out to win over fellow members of the New York Medical Society (into which he had been warmly introduced by the screening committee) to his point of view that heroic medicine was inherently dangerous and should be reduced to the gentler theories of herbal medicine. He was summarily ostracized from the medical society. He soon founded his own school in New York, calling the clinic and educational facility the United States Infirmary. Because of political pressure from the medical society, however, he was unable to obtain charter authority to issue legitimate diplomas. He then located a financially ailing but legally chartered school, Worthington College, in Worthington, Ohio. There he opened a full-scale medical college, creating the eclectic school of medical theory based on the European, Native American, and American traditions. The most enduring eclectic herbal textbook is *King's American Dispensary* by *Harvey Wickes Felter* and *John Uri Lloyd*. Published in 1898, this two-volume 2500-page treatise provided the definitive work describing the identification, preparation, pharmacognosy, history of use, and clinical application of more than 1000 botanical medicines. The eclectic herbal lore formed an integral core of the therapeutic armamentarium of the naturopathic doctor (ND).

Homeopathic Medicine

Homeopathy, the creation of an early German physician, *Samuel Hahnemann* (1755-1843), had four central doctrines: (1) that like cures like (the "law of similars"); (2) that the effect of a medication could be heightened by its administration in minute doses (the more diluted the dose, the greater the "dynamic" effect); (3) that nearly all diseases were the result of a suppressed itch, or "psora"; and (4) that healing proceeds from within outward, above downward, from more vital to less vital organs, and in the reverse order of the appearance of symptoms (pathobiography), known as Hering's law.

Originally, most U.S. homeopaths were converted orthodox medical doctors, or *allopaths* (a term coined by Hahnemann). The high rate of conversion made this particular medical sect the archenemy of the rising orthodox medical profession. The first American homeopathic medical school was founded in 1848 in Philadelphia; the last purely homeopathic medical school, based in Philadelphia, survived into the early 1930s (see Chapter 24).

Manipulative Therapies: Osteopathy and Chiropractic

In Missouri, *Andrew Taylor Still*, originally trained as an orthodox practitioner, founded the school of medical thought known as *osteopathy*. He conceived a system of healing that emphasized the primary importance of the structural integrity of the body, especially as it affects the vascular system, in the maintenance of health. In 1892 he opened the American School of Osteopathy in Kirksville, Missouri.

In 1895, Daniel David Palmer, originally a magnetic healer from Davenport, Iowa, performed the first spinal manipulation, which gave rise to the school he termed *chiropractic*. His philosophy was similar to Still's except for a greater emphasis on the importance of proper neurological function. He formally published his findings in 1910, after having founded a chiropractic school in Davenport (see Chapter 18).

Less well known is "zone therapy," originated by *Joe Shelby Riley*, DC, a chiropractor based in Washington, D.C. Zone therapy was an early forerunner of acupressure. In zone therapy, pressure to and manipulation of the fingers and tongue and percussion of the spinal column were applied according to the relation of points on these structures to certain zones of the body.

Christian Science and the Role of Belief and Spirituality

Christian Science, formulated by *Mary Baker Eddy* in 1879, comprises a profound belief in the role of systematic religious study (which led to the widespread Christian Science Reading Rooms), spirituality, and prayer in the treatment of disease. In 1875 she published *Science and Health with Key to the Scriptures*, the definitive textbook for the study of Christian Science.

Lust was also influenced by the works of *Sidney Weltmer*, the founder of "suggestive therapeutics." Weltmer's work dealt specifically with the psychological process of desiring to be healthy. The theory behind Professor Weltmer's work was that whether it was the mind or the body that first lost its grip on health, the two were inseparably related. When the problem originated in the body, the mind nonetheless lost its ability and desire to overcome the disease because the patient "felt sick" and consequently slid further into the diseased state. Alternatively, if the mind first lost its ability and desire to "be healthy" and some physical infirmity followed, the patient was susceptible to being overcome by disease (see Chapter 6).

Physical Culture

Bernarr Mcfadden, a close friend of Lust's, founded the "physical culture" school of health and healing, also known as *physcultopathy*. This school of healing gave birth across the United States to gymnasiums where exercise programs were designed and taught to allow individual men and women to establish and maintain optimal physical health.

Although many theories exist to explain the rapid dissolution of these diverse healing arts (the practitioners of which at one time made up more than 25% of all U.S. health care practitioners) in the early part of the twentieth century, low ratings in the infamous Flexner Report (which rated all these schools of medical thought among the lowest), allopathic medicine's anointing of itself with the blessing "scientific," and the growing political sophistication of the AMA clearly played the most significant role.

All these healing systems and modalities were naturally unified in the field of naturopathic medicine because they shared one common tenet: respect for and inquiry into the self-healing process and what was necessary to establish health.

HALCYON DAYS OF NATUROPATHY

In the early 1920s the "health fad" movement was reaching its peak in terms of public awareness and interest. Conventions were held throughout the United States, one of which was attended by several members of Congress, culminating in full legalization of naturopathy as a healing art in the District of Columbia. Not only were the conventions well attended by professionals, but the public also flocked to them, with more than 10,000 attending the 1924 convention in Los Angeles.

During the 1920s and up until 1937, naturopathy was in its most popular phase. Although the institutions of the orthodox school had gained ascendancy, before 1937 the medical profession had no real solutions to the problems of human disease.

During the 1920s, *Gaylord Hauser*, later to become the health food guru of the Hollywood set, came to Lust as a seriously ill young man. Lust, through application of the nature cure, removed Hauser's afflictions and was rewarded by Hauser's lifelong devotion. His regular columns in *Nature's Path* became widely read among the Hollywood crowd.

The naturopathic journals of the 1920s and 1930s provide much valuable insight into the prevention of disease and the promotion of health. Much of the dietary advice focused on correcting poor eating habits, including the lack of fiber in the diet and an overreliance on red meat as a protein source. As in the 1990s, we now hear the pronouncements of the orthodox profession, the National Institutes of Health (NIH), and the National Cancer Institute that the early assertions of the naturopaths that such dietary habits would lead to degenerative diseases, including colon cancer and other cancers of the digestive tract, were true.

The December 1928 issue of *Nature's Path* contained the first American publication of the work of *Herman J. DeWolff*, a Dutch epidemiologist. DeWolff was one of the first researchers to assert, on the basis of studies of the incidence of cancer in the Netherlands, that there was a correlation between exposure to petrochemicals and various types of cancerous conditions. He contended that the use of chemical fertilizers and their application in some soils (principally clay) led to their remaining in vegetables after they had arrived at the market and were purchased for consumption. It was almost 50 years before orthodox medicine began to see the wisdom of such assertions.

SUPPRESSION AND DECLINE

In 1937 the popularity of naturopathy began to decline. The change came, as both Thomas and Campion note in their works, with the era of "miracle medicine." Lust recognized this, and his editorializing became, if anything, even more strident. From the introduction of sulfa drugs in 1937 to the release of the Salk vaccine in 1955, the American public became used to annual developments of miracle vaccines and antibiotics. The naturopathic profession adhered to its vitalistic philosophy and a full range of practice but unfortunately was poorly unified at this time on other issues of standards. This made the profession vulnerable to interguild competition.

Lust died in September 1945 in residence at the Yungborn facility in Butler, New Jersey, preparing to attend the 49th Annual Congress of his American Naturopathic Association. Although a healthy, vigorous man, he had seriously damaged his lungs the previous year saving patients when a wing of his facility caught fire; he never fully recovered. On August 30, 1945, writing for the official program of that congress, held in October 1945 just after his death, he noted his concerns for the future. He was especially frustrated with the success of the medical profession in blocking the efforts of naturopaths to establish state licensing laws that would not only establish appropriate practice rights for NDs but also protect the public from the pretenders (i.e., those who chose to call themselves naturopaths without ever bothering to undergo formal training). As Lust (1945) stated:

> Now let us see the type of men and women who are the Naturopaths of today. Many of them are fine, upstanding individuals, believing fully in the effectiveness of their chosen profession—willing to give their all for the sake of alleviating human suffering and ready to fight for their rights to the last ditch. More power to them! But there are others who claim to be Naturopaths who are woeful misfits. Yes, and there are outright fakers and cheats masking as Naturopaths. That is the fate of any science—any profession—which the unjust laws have placed beyond the pale. Where there is no official recognition and regulation, you will find the plotters, the thieves, the charlatans operating on the same basis as the conscientious practitioners. And these riff-raff opportunists bring the whole art into disrepute. Frankly, such conditions cannot be remedied until suitable safeguards are erected by law, or by the profession itself, around the practice of Naturopathy. That will come in time.

In the mid-1920s, *Morris Fishbein* came on the scene as editor of the *Journal of the American Medical Association (JAMA)*. Fishbein took on a personal vendetta against what he characterized as "quackery." Lust, among others, including Mcfadden, became Fishbein's epitome of quackery. Unfortunately, he proved to be particularly effective politically and in the media.

The public infatuation with technology, the introduction of "miracle medicine," World War II's stimulation of the development of surgery, the Flexner Report, the growing political sophistication of the AMA under the leadership of Fishbein, intraprofession squabbles, and the death of Lust in 1945 all combined to cause the decline of naturopathic medicine and natural healing in the United States. In addition, these years, called the years of *the great fear* in David Caute's book by the latter name, were the years during which to be unorthodox was to be un-American.

U.S. courts began to take the view that naturopaths were not truly doctors because they espoused doctrines from "the dark ages of medicine" (something American medicine had supposedly come out of in 1937) and that drugless healers were intended by law to operate without "drugs" (which came to be defined as anything a physician would prescribe for a patient to ingest or apply externally for any medical purpose). The persistent lack of uniform standards, lack of insurance coverage, lost court battles, a splintered profession, and a hostile legislative perspective progressively restricted practice until the core naturopathic therapies became essentially illegal and practices financially nonviable.

Although it was under considerable public pressure in those years, the American Naturopathic Association undertook some of its most scholarly work, coordinating all the systems of naturopathy under commission. This resulted in the publication of a formal textbook, *Basic Naturopathy* (Spitler, 1948) and a significant work compiling all the known theories of botanical medicine, *Naturae Medicina* (Kuts-Cheraux, 1953). Naturopathic medicine began splintering when Lust's American Naturopathic Association was succeeded by six different organizations in the mid-1950s.

By the early 1970s, the profession's educational institutions had dwindled to one: the National College of Naturopathic Medicine, with branches in Seattle and Portland, Oregon.

NATUROPATHIC MEDICINE REEMERGES

The combination of the counterculture years of the late 1960s, the public's growing awareness of the importance of nutrition and the environment, and America's disenchantment with organized institutional medicine (which began after the miracle era faded and it became apparent that orthodox medicine has its limitations and is prohibitively expensive) resulted in the emergence of new respect for alternative medicine in general and in the rejuvenation of naturopathic medicine. At this time, a new wave of students were attracted to the philosophical precepts of the profession. They brought with them an appreciation for the appropriate use of science, modern college education, and matching expectations for quality education.

Dr. John Bastyr (1912-1995) and his firm, efficient, professional leadership inspired science- and research-based training in natural medicine to begin to reach toward its full potential. Dr. Bastyr, whose vision was of "naturopathy's empirical successes documented and proven by scientific methods," was "himself a prototype for the modern naturopathic doctor, who culls the latest findings from the scientific literature, applies them in ways consistent with naturopathic principles, and verifies the results with appropriate studies." Bastyr also saw "a tremendous expansion in both allopathic and naturopathic medical knowledge, and he played a major role in making sure the best of both were integrated into naturopathic medical education" (Kirchfield et al, 1994).

In response to the growth in public interest during the late 1970s, naturopathic colleges were established in Arizona (Arizona College of Naturopathic Medicine, 1977), Oregon (American College of Naturopathic Medicine, 1980), and California (Pacific College of Naturopathic Medicine, 1979). None of these three survived. In 1978 the John Bastyr College of Naturopathic Medicine (later renamed Bastyr University) was formed in Seattle by founding president Joseph E. Pizzorno, Jr., ND; Lester E. Griffith, ND; William Mitchell, ND; and Sheila Quinn to teach and develop science-based natural medicine. They believed that for the naturopathic profession to move back into the mainstream, it needed to establish accredited institutions, perform credible research, and establish itself as an integral part of the health care system. Bastyr University not only survived but thrived, and it became the first naturopathic college ever to become regionally accredited. In 1993, Michael Cronin, Kyle Cronin, and Konrad Kail, NDs, founded the Southwest College of Naturopathic Medicine and Health Science in Scottsdale, Arizona. In 1997 the University of Bridgeport, with the leadership of Jim Sensenig, ND, founded the University of Bridgeport College of Naturopathic Medicine.

With five credible colleges (including the Canadian College of Naturopathic Medicine in Ontario), active research, an appreciation of the appropriate application of science to natural medicine education, and clinical practice, naturopathic medicine is well on the road to recovery.

A sixth promising naturopathic college, the Boucher Institute of Naturopathic Medicine, was established in January 2000 in Vancouver, British Columbia. Boucher Institute graduated its first class in May 2004.

RECENT INFLUENCES

A tremendous amount of research providing scientific support for the principles of naturopathic medicine has been conducted at mainstream research centers and increasingly at naturopathic medical schools. In fact, allopathy is turning more to the use of naturopathic methods in the search for effective prescriptions for diseases that are currently intractable and expensive to treat (Werbach, 1996). It is now well established that nutritional factors are of major importance in the pathogenesis of both atherosclerosis and cancer, the two leading causes of death in Western countries, and studies validating their importance in the pathogenesis of many other diseases continue to be published. Much of the research now documenting the scientific foundations of naturopathic medicine practices and principles can be found in *A Textbook of Natural Medicine* (Pizzorno et al, 1985-1995). This two-volume, 200-chapter work contains 7500 citations to the peer-reviewed scientific literature documenting the efficacy of many natural medicine therapies.

Although the naturopaths were astute clinical observers and a century ago recognized many of the concepts that are now gaining popularity and are being supported by scientific data, the scientific tools of the time were inadequate to assess the validity of their concepts. In addition, as a group they seemed to have little inclination for the application of laboratory research, especially because "science" was the bludgeon used by the AMA to suppress the profession. This has now changed. In the past few decades a considerable amount of research has now provided the scientific documentation of many of the concepts of naturopathic medicine, and the new breed of scientifically trained naturopaths is using this research to continue development of the profession. The following sections describe a few of the most important trends.

Therapeutic Nutrition

Since 1929, when Christiaan Eijkman and Sir Frederick Hopkins shared the Nobel Prize in medicine and physiology for the discovery of vitamins, the role of these trace substances in clinical nutrition has been a matter of scientific investigation. The discovery that enzyme systems depended on essential nutrients provided the naturopathic profession with great insights into why an organically grown, whole-foods diet is so important for health. Formulation of the concept of "biochemical individuality" by nutritional biochemist Roger Williams in 1955 further developed these ideas and provided great insights into the unique nutritional needs of each individual and the way to correct inborn errors of metabolism and even treat specific diseases through the use of nutrient-rich foods or large doses of specific nutrients. Linus Pauling, the two-time Nobel Prize winner, originated the concept of "orthomolecular medicine" and provided further theoretical substantiation for the use of nutrients as therapeutic agents.

Functional Medicine

In 1990, Jeff Bland, PhD, coined the term *functional medicine* to describe a putatively science-based development of therapeutic nutrition for the prevention of illness and promotion of health. Focusing on biochemical individuality, metabolic balance, and the ecological context, functional medicine practitioners avail themselves of recently developed laboratory tests to pinpoint perceived imbalances in an individual's biochemistry that are thought to cause a cascade of biological triggers, paving the way to suboptimal function, chronic illness, and degenerative disease. A broad range of functional laboratory assessment tools in the areas of digestion (gastrointestinal system), nutrition, detoxification and oxidative stress, immunology and allergy, production and regulation of hormones (endocrinology), and the heart and blood vessels (cardiovascular system) provide physicians with a basis to recommend nutritional interventions specific to the individual's needs and to monitor their efficacy.

Environmental Medicine and Clinical Ecology

Although recognition of the clinical impact of environmental toxicity and endogenous toxicity has existed since the earliest days of naturopathy, it was not until the environmental movement and the seminal work of Rachel Carson and others that the scientific basis was established. Clinical research and the development of laboratory methods for assessing toxic load have provided objective tools that have greatly increased the sophistication of clinical practice. Clinical and laboratory methods were developed for the assessment of idiosyncratic reactions to environmental factors and foods.

Spirituality, Health, and Medicine

Naturopathic medicine's philosophy of treating the whole person and enhancing the individual's inherent healing ability is closely aligned with its mission of integrating spirituality into the healing process. Scientific evidence is growing on the part spirituality can play in healing. René Descartes has been accused of separating mind from body back in the seventeenth century, and medical science has attempted to explain disease independently of mind, in terms of germs, environmental agents, or wayward genes. At present, however, the evidence on the link between mind and body is not just clinical observation but chemical fact. An explosion of research in the new and rapidly expanding field of psychoneuroimmunology is revealing physical evidence of the mind-body connection that is changing our understanding of disease (see Chapter 8). Scientists no longer question whether but rather *how* our minds have an impact on our health, and the implications of the connections uncovered in only the last 20 years are extraordinary.

In his book *Healing Words* (1993), Larry Dossey, MD, pulls together what he describes as "one of the best kept secrets in medical science": the extensive experimental evidence for the beneficial effects of prayer. Dossey reviews studies that provide evidence for a positive effect of prayer on not only humans but mice, chicks, enzymes, fungi, yeast, bacteria, and cells of various sorts. He emphasizes, "We cannot dismiss these outcomes as being due to suggestion or placebo effects, since these so-called lower forms of life do not think in any conventional sense and are presumably not susceptible to suggestion" (Pizzorno, 1995).

"Cutting-Edge" Laboratory Methods

A final significant influence has been the development of laboratory methods for the objective assessment of nutritional status, metabolic dysfunction, digestive function, bowel flora, endogenous and exogenous toxic load, liver detoxification and other system functions, and genomics. Each of these has provided ever more effective tools for accurate assessment of patient health status and effective application of naturopathic principles.

Genomics

One of the most exciting recent advances is genomic testing, the ability to evaluate each individual's template for making the enzymes of life. This technology is now providing a level of objective evaluation of biochemical individuality never before available, greatly strengthening the naturopathic doctor's ability to practice personalized medicine. The ability to assess each individual's unique nutrient needs as well as susceptibilities to environmental toxins promises to change fundamentally the practice of medicine (Pizzorno, 2003).

During the last several years, as America's staggering health care debt accumulates because of the increase in chronic disease, these core, traditional naturopathic principles are surfacing widely as central to creating an effective health care system, as follows:

> Current medical education inculcates many of the dominant values of modern medicine: reductionism, specialization, mechanistic models of disease, and faith in a definitive cure.... What is needed is a model of care that addresses the whole person and integrates care for the person's entire constellation of comorbidities.... Nothing short of a fundamental redesign of primary care systems is required. (Grumbach, 2003)

PRINCIPLES

Although in many ways, modern medicine resembles a science, it continues to be criticized for its lack of unifying theories, and for this reason alone its claim to being a science has remained suspect.

—BLOIS (1988)

What physicians think medicine is profoundly shapes what they do, how they behave in doing it, and the reasons they use to justify that behavior.... Whether conscious of it or not, every physician has an answer to what he thinks medicine is, with real consequences for all whom he attends.... The outcome is hardly trivial.... It dictates, after all, how we approach patients [and] how we make clinical judgments.

—PELLEGRINO (1979)

Medical philosophy comprises the underlying premises on which a healthcare system is based. Once a system is acknowledged, it is subject to debate. In naturopathic medicine, the philosophical debate is a valuable, ongoing process which helps the understanding that disease evolves in an orderly and truth-revealing fashion.

—BRADLEY (1985)

Naturopathic medicine is a distinct system of health-oriented medicine that, in contrast to the currently dominant disease-treatment system, stresses promotion of health, prevention of disease, patient education, and self-responsibility. However, naturopathic medicine symbolizes more than simply a health care system; it is a way of life. Unlike most other health care systems, naturopathy is not identified with any particular therapy but rather is a way of thinking about life, health, and disease. It is defined not by the therapies it uses but by the philosophical principles that guide the practitioner.

Seven powerful concepts provide the foundation that defines naturopathic medicine and create a unique group of professionals practicing a form of medicine that fundamentally changes the way we think of health care. In 1989 the American Association of Naturopathic Physicians unanimously approved the definition of *naturopathic medicine,* updating and reconfirming in modern terms its core principles as a professional consensus. "The definition and principles of practice provide a steady point of reference for this debate, for our evolving understanding of health and disease, and for all of our decision making processes as a profession" (Snider et al, 1988).

The seven core principles of naturopathic medicine are as follows, with "wellness and health promotion" emerging into the forefront of the scholarly discussion of naturopathic clinical theory:

1. The healing power of nature *(vis medicatrix naturae)*
2. First do no harm *(primum non nocere)*
3. Find the cause *(tolle causam)*
4. Treat the whole person *(holism)*
5. Preventive medicine
6. Wellness and health promotion (emerging principle)
7. Doctor as teacher *(docere)*

THE HEALING POWER OF NATURE (VIS MEDICATRIX NATURAE)

Belief in the ability of the body to heal itself—the vis medicatrix naturae (the healing power of nature)—if given the proper opportunity, and the importance of living within the laws of nature is the foundation of naturopathic medicine. Although the term *naturopathy* was coined in the late nineteenth century, its philosophical roots can be traced back to Hippocrates and derive from a common wellspring in traditional world medicines: belief in the healing power of nature.

Medicine has long grappled with the question of the existence of the vis medicatrix naturae. As Neuberger stated, "The problem of the healing power of nature is a great, perhaps the greatest of all problems which has occupied the physician for thousands of years. Indeed, the aims and limits of therapeutics are determined by its solution." The fundamental reality of the vis medicatrix naturae was a basic tenet of the Hippocratic school of medicine, and "every important medical author since has had to take a position for or against it" (Neuberger, 1932).

When standard medicine soundly rejected the principle of the vis medicatrix naturae at the turn of the twentieth century, nature doctors, including naturopathic physicians in the United States from 1896 on, diverged from conventional medicine. Naturopathic physicians recognized the clinical importance of the inherent self-healing process; embraced it as their core academic and clinical principle; and developed an entire system of medical practice, training, and research based on it and on related principles of clinical medicine.

Naturopathic medicine is therefore "vitalistic" in its approach (i.e., life is viewed as more than just the sum of biochemical processes), and the body is believed to have an innate intelligence or process (the vis medicatrix naturae), which is always striving toward health. Vitalism maintains that the symptoms accompanying disease are not typically caused by the morbific agent (e.g., bacteria); rather, they are the result of the organism's intrinsic response or reaction to the agent and the organism's attempt to defend and heal itself (Lindlahr, 1914a; Neuberger, 1932). Symptoms are part of a constructive phenomenon that is the best "choice" the organism can make, given the circumstances. In this construct the physician's role is to understand and aid the body's efforts, not to take over or manipulate the functions of the body, unless the self-healing process has become weak or insufficient.

Although the context and life force of naturopathic medicine is its vitalistic core, both vitalistic and mechanistic approaches are applicable to modern naturopathic medicine. Vitalism has reemerged in current terms in the body-mind-spirit dialogue. Matter, mind, energy, and spirit are each part of nature and therefore are part of medicine that observes, respects, and works with nature. Much of modern biomedicine and related research is based on the application of the theory of mechanism (defined in *Webster's Dictionary* as the "theory that everything in the universe is produced by matter in motion; materialism") in a highly reductionistic, single-agent, pathology-based, disease care model. Applied in a vitalistic context, mechanistic and reductionistic interventions provide useful techniques and tools to naturopathic physicians. The unifying theory of naturopathic medicine, as discussed later, provides clinical guidance for integrating both approaches.

FIRST DO NO HARM (PRIMUM NON NOCERE)

Naturopathic physicians prefer noninvasive treatments that minimize the risks of harmful side effects. They are trained to use the lowest-force and lowest-risk preventive, diagnostic, therapeutic, and co-management strategies. They are trained to know which patients they can safely treat and which ones they need to refer to other health care practitioners. Naturopathic physicians follow three precepts to avoid harming the patient:

1. Naturopathic physicians use methods and medicinal substances that minimize the risk of harmful effects and apply the least possible force or intervention necessary to diagnose illness and restore health.
2. When possible, the suppression of symptoms is avoided because suppression generally interferes with the healing process.
3. Naturopathic physicians respect and work with the vis medicatrix naturae in diagnosis, treatment, and counseling because, if this self-healing process is not respected, the patient may be harmed.

FIND THE CAUSE (TOLLE CAUSAM)

Every illness has an underlying cause or causes, often in aspects of the lifestyle, diet, or habits of the individual. A naturopathic physician is trained to find and remove the underlying cause(s) of disease. The therapeutic order helps the physician remove them in the correct "healing order" for the body (see later discussion). As the new science of psychoneuroimmunology is explicitly demonstrating, the body is a seamless web with a multiplicity of brain–immune system–gut–liver connections (see Chapter 8). Not surprisingly, chronic disease typically involves a number of systems, with the most prominent or acute symptoms being those chronologically last in appearance. As the healing process progresses and these symptoms are alleviated, further symptoms then resurface that must then be addressed to restore health. To paraphrase David Jones, MD, on the "tack rules": "If you're sitting on a tack, it takes a lot of aspirin to feel better. If you're sitting on two tacks, removing one does not necessarily lead to a 50% improvement or reduction in symptoms."

TREAT THE WHOLE PERSON (HOLISM)

As noted previously, health or disease comes from a complex interaction of mental, emotional, spiritual, physical, dietary, genetic, environmental, lifestyle, and other factors. Naturopathic physicians treat the whole person, taking all these factors into account. Naturopathically, the body is viewed as a whole. Naturopathy is often called *holistic medicine* in reference to the term *holism,* coined by philosopher Jan Christian Smuts in 1926, to describe the *gestalt* of a system as greater than the sum of its parts. A change in one part causes a change in every part; therefore the study of one part must be integrated into the whole, including the community and biosphere.

Naturopathic medicine asserts that one cannot be healthy in an unhealthy environment, and it is committed to the creation of a world in which humanity may thrive.

In contrast to the high degree of specialization in the present medical system, which reflects a mechanistic orientation to single organs, the holistic model relegates specialists to an ancillary role. Emphasis is placed on the physical, emotional, social, and spiritual integration of the whole person, including awareness of the impact of the environment on health.

PREVENTIVE MEDICINE

The naturopathic approach to health care helps prevent disease and keeps minor illnesses from developing into more serious or chronic degenerative diseases. Patients are taught the principles for living a healthful life, and by following these principles, they can prevent major illness. Health is viewed as more than just the absence of disease; it is considered a dynamic state that enables a person to thrive in, or adapt to, a wide range of environments and stresses. Health and disease are points on a continuum, with death at one end and optimal function at the other. The naturopathic physician believes that a person who goes through life living an unhealthful lifestyle will drift away from optimal function and move relentlessly toward progressively greater dysfunction. Genotype, constitution, maternal influences, and environmental factors all influence individual susceptibility to deterioration, and the organs and physiological systems affected. Box 21-2 lists these and other determinants of health addressed by the naturopathic physician in both treatment and prevention.

The virulence of morbific agents or insults also plays a central role in disturbance, causing decreasing function and ultimately serious disease.

In our society, although our expected life span at birth has increased, our health span has not, nor has our health expectancy at age 65. We are living longer but as disabled individuals (Pizzorno, 1997). Although such deterioration is accepted by our society as the normal expectation of aging, it is not common in animals in the wild or among those fortunate peoples who live in an optimal environment (i.e., no pollution, low stress, regular exercise, and abundant natural, nutritious food).

In the naturopathic model, death is inevitable; progressive disability is not. This belief underscores a fundamental difference in philosophy and expectation between the conventional and naturopathic models of health and disease. In contrast to the disease treatment focus of allopathic medicine, the health promotion focus of naturopathic medicine emphasizes the means of maximizing health span.

WELLNESS AND HEALTH PROMOTION (EMERGING PRINCIPLE)

Establishing and maintaining optimal health and balance is a central clinical goal. Wellness and health promotion go beyond prevention. This principle refers to a proactive

BOX 21-2

Determinants of Health and Other Factors in Naturopathic Preventive Medicine

---

Determinants of Health

Inborn
- Genetic makeup (genotype)
- Constitution (determines susceptibility)
- Intrauterine/congenital factors
- Maternal exposures
  - Drugs
  - Toxins
  - Viruses
  - Psychoemotional influences
- Maternand paternal genetic influences
- Maternal nutrition
- Maternal lifestyle

Disturbances
- Illnesses: pathobiography
- Medical intervention (or lack of)
- Physical and emotional exposures, stresses, and trauma
- Toxic and harmful substances

Hygienic/Lifestyle Factors
- Nutrition
- Rest
- Exercise
- Psychoemotional health
- Spiritual health
- Community
- Culture
- Socioeconomic factors
- Fresh air
- Light
- Exposure to nature
- Clean water
- Unadulterated food
- Loving and being loved
- Meaningful work

---

state of being healthy, characterized by positive emotion, thought, intention, and action. Wellness is inherent in everyone, no matter what disease is being experienced. The recognition, experience, and support of wellness through health promotion by the physician and patient will more quickly heal a given disease than treatment of the disease alone.

DOCTOR AS TEACHER (DOCERE)

The original meaning of the word *docere* is "teacher." A principle objective of naturopathic medicine is to educate the patient and emphasize self-responsibility for health. Naturopathic doctors also recognize the therapeutic potential of the physician-patient relationship. The patient is engaged and respected as an ally and a member of her or his own health care team. Adequate time is spent with patients to diagnose, treat, and educate them thoroughly (see Chapters 1 and 2).

NATUROPATHIC PRACTICE TODAY

Current naturopathic physicians are licensed primary care providers of integrative natural medicine and are also recognized for their clinical expertise and effectiveness in preventive medicine. NDs are trained as family physicians, regardless of elective postdoctoral training or clinical emphasis. This is intentional and consistent with naturopathic principles of practice. NDs are trained to assess causes and develop treatment plans from a systems perspective and with systems skills on the basis of naturopathic principles and, specifically, the principle of "treating the whole person," as follows:

> Naturopathy, in fact, is typically *meta-systematic*.... The organism [is] always seen in the context of its physical and social environment.... Beyond this, naturopathy ultimately might even be considered *cross-paradigmatic*, touching inevitably on the economics, politics, history, and sociology of the various healing alternatives, ultimately penetrating to the contrasting philosophies underlying naturopathy and allopathy. Naturopathy results from a guiding philosophy at odds with the dominant mechanistic philosophy undergirding Western industrialized society. Allopathy, in contrast, is clearly derived from these same premises. Or in Eisler's terms, naturopathy embraces a *partnership* model of relationship, while allopathy falls within the *dominator* model.... [T]his partnership/dominator model extends not only to the treatment process but to the healer/patient relationship itself. (Funk, 1995)

NDs may also practice as specialists, after postdoctoral training in botanical medicine, homeopathy, nutritional medicine, physical medicine, acupuncture, Ayurvedic medicine, Oriental and Chinese herbal medicine, counseling and health psychology, spirituality and healing, applied behavioral sciences, or midwifery. Some NDs choose to focus their practice on population groups such as children, the elderly, or women, or in clinical areas such as cardiology, gastroenterology, immunology, or environmental medicine. These diverse practices are consistent with the eclectic origins of naturopathic medicine and are part of its strength.

In addition to NDs with these specialties, at one end of the spectrum are practitioners who adhere to the nature cure tradition and focus clinically only on diet, detoxification, lifestyle modification, hydrotherapy, and other self-healing modalities. At the other end are those whose practices appear to be similar to the average conventional medical practice, with the only apparent difference being the use of pharmaceutical-grade botanical medicines instead of synthetic drugs. However, fundamental to all styles of naturopathic practice is a common philosophy and principles of health and disease: the unifying theory in the hierarchy of therapeutics, or the therapeutic order described in the following section. The therapeutic order is derived from all of the principles and guides the ND's choice of therapeutic interventions.

UNIFYING THEORY: THE HEALING POWER OF NATURE AND THE THERAPEUTIC ORDER

In facilitating the process of healing, the naturopathic physician seeks to use those therapies and strategies that are most efficient and that have the least potential to harm the patient. The concept of "harm" includes suppression or exhaustion of natural healing processes, including inflammation and fever. These precepts, coupled to an understanding of the process of healing, result in a therapeutic hierarchy. This hierarchy (or therapeutic order) is a natural consequence of how the organism heals. Therapeutic modalities are applied in a rational order, determined by the nature of the healing process. The natural order of appropriate therapeutic intervention is as follows:

1. Reestablish the basis for health.
2. Stimulate the vis medicatrix naturae.
3. Tonify and nourish weakened systems.
4. Correct deficiencies in structural integrity.
5. Prescribe specific substances and modalities for specific conditions and biochemical pathways (e.g., botanicals, nutrients, acupuncture, homeopathy, hydrotherapy, counseling).
6. Prescribe pharmaceutical substances.
7. Use radiation, chemotherapy, and surgery.

This appropriate therapeutic order proceeds from least to most force. All modalities can be found at various steps, depending on their application. The spiritual aspect of the patient's health is considered to begin with step 1 (Zeff, 1997; steps 5 through 7 added by Snider).

The concepts expressed in the therapeutic order are derived from the writings of Hippocrates and those of medical scholars since Hippocrates concerning the function and activation of the self-healing process. Dr. Jared Zeff (1997) expresses these concepts as the hierarchy of therapeutics in his article "The Process of Healing: A Unifying Theory of Naturopathic Medicine." These concepts are further explored, refined, and developed in *The Textbook of Natural Medicine*, third edition (Pizzorno, 2006) in a chapter written by Zeff, Snider, and Myers entitled "A Hierarchy of Healing: The Therapeutic Order—the Unifying Theory of Naturopathic Medicine."

The philosophy represented in the therapeutic order does not determine what modalities are good or bad. Rather, it provides a clinical framework for all approaches and modalities, used in an order consistent with that of the natural self-healing process. It respects the origins of

disease and the applications of care and intervention necessary for health and healing with the least intervention.

The therapeutic order exemplifies the concept of using the least force, one of the key tenets of the naturopathic principle "Do no harm." The therapeutic order schematically directs the ND's therapeutic choices so that they are implemented in an efficient order rather than in a "shotgun" approach. This common philosophy and theory both distinguishes the field of naturopathic medicine and enables it to consider and incorporate new therapies.

Naturopathic medicine's philosophical approach to health promotion and restoration requires that practitioners possess a broad range of diagnostic and therapeutic skills and accounts for the eclectic interests of the naturopathic profession. Obviously, at times the body needs more than just supportive help. The goal of the ND in such situations is first to use the lowest-force and lowest-risk clinical strategies (i.e., the least invasive intervention that will have the most effective therapeutic outcome) and, when necessary, to co-manage or refer to specialists and other health care professionals.

Because the goal of the ND is to restore normal body function rather than to apply a particular therapy, virtually every natural medicine therapy may be used. In addition, to fulfill their role as primary care family physicians, NDs may also administer vaccines and use therapies such as office surgery and prescription drugs when less invasive options have been exhausted or found inappropriate. In the restoration of health, prescription drugs and surgery are a last resort but are used when necessary. As Kirschner and Brinkman (1988) noted, "The use of petroleum by-products and the removal of body parts is a poor first line of defense against disease."

Naturopathic medical school curricula are continually revised in light of these principles. Curriculum integration is built on the science-based educational structure already in place in these colleges. Basic science, ND, and non-ND physician faculty are trained in naturopathic philosophy and principles and the therapeutic order as core assumptions that invite scholarly inquiry. Discussion and inquiry concerning the philosophy and theory are stimulated and supported in interdisciplinary faculty teams. The fruits of these endeavors are brought into the classroom to enhance students' critical thinking concerning clinical values and assumptions. Naturopathic research on these principles themselves is a widely embraced priority for the naturopathic profession. In 2004 the Naturopathic Medical Research Agenda, a 2-year research project sponsored by the NIH's National Center for Complementary and Alternative Medicine, identified three key hypotheses as central to the future and the foundations of naturopathic medical research. The third hypothesis states: "The scientific exploration of naturopathic medical practices and principles will yield important insights into the nature of health and healing" (Standish et al, 2004).

DIAGNOSIS

In the naturopathic medicine program at Bastyr University, for example, the principles just discussed and the therapeutic order are translated into a series of questions that drive curriculum development and case analysis and provide guidance to students learning the art and science of naturopathic medicine. These Naturopathic Case Analysis and Management questions (see next section) are integrated with conventional SOAP (*subjective, objective, assessment, plan*) algorithms as the process of naturopathic case analysis and management, the clinical application of philosophy to patient care. For example, although a conventional pathological diagnosis is made through the use of physical, laboratory, and radiologic procedures, it is done in the context of understanding the underlying causes of the pathology and the obstacles to recovery.

NATUROPATHIC CASE ANALYSIS AND MANAGEMENT

I. The Healing Power of Nature (vis medicatrix naturae)

1. What is the level of the disease process? What is the direction of the disease process? What is the purpose of the disease process?
2. How is the healing power of nature supported in the case? What therapeutic interventions allow/respect, palliate, facilitate, or augment the self-healing process? How does the therapeutic intervention do this?
3. Is the person in balance with nature?
4. What is being in balance with nature?
5. Is this person in balance with his or her environment?
6. How are you assessing the healing powers of this individual?
7. What is the prognosis for this individual?
8. What is the patient's metaphor for healing? What moves or will move this patient toward healing or recovery?
9. How does the patient see himself or herself healing (the patient process)?
   - Are people helping him or her?
   - Is he or she doing it on his or her own?
   - How long will it take?
   - Is the doctor doing the healing?
   - Is the patient doing the healing?
   - Are the doctor and patient working together?
   - What else is important in this patient's healing process?

II. First Do No Harm (primum non nocere)

1. What is the potential for harm with this particular treatment plan?
2. Are you doing no harm? How?
3. How are you avoiding suppression? Is suppression necessary? Why?
4. What is the appropriate course of action? Is it waiting?
5. What is the appropriate level and force of intervention? Why? How is the least force applied?
6. Identify the appropriate treatment:
   - Level of therapeutic order
   - Modality/substance
   - Dosage
   - Frequency
   - Duration
   Justify the timing of the treatment in terms of short- and long-term management.
7. Are there any obstacles to the patient's recovery? Explain.
8. What referral or co-management strategies are required to ensure patients' optimal outcome?

III. Find the Cause (tolle causam)

1. What level of healing are you aiming toward (i.e., suppression, palliation, cure)?
2. Where and/or what are the limiting factors in this person's life (concept: health is freedom from limitations)?
3. Where is the center of this person's disease (i.e., physical, mental, emotional, spiritual)?
4. What are the causative factors contributing to this patient's condition or state? What is the central cause or etiology? What are other contributing causes? Of these causative factors, which are avoidable or preventable?

IV. Treat the Whole Person (Holism)

1. How are you working holistically?
2. Can you see the person beyond the disease?
3. What aspects of the person are you addressing?
4. What aspects of the person are you not addressing?
5. Would a referral to another health care practitioner assist you in working holistically? When? To whom? If not, why not?
6. What are the patient's goals and expectations in relation to his or her health and treatments?
7. What are your goals and expectations for the patient? What are the differences between yours and the patient's? How are they similar?
8. How will the treatment plan help the patient take more responsibility for his or her health and healing?
9. Are you empowering the patient? How?
10. What is the vitality level of this patient?
11. Identify cultural, community, and environmental issues and concerns that need to be included in the assessment.
12. What family/psychological/spiritual/social systems issues need to be included in the assessment?

V. Preventive Medicine

1. What is being done or planned in regard to prevention?
2. "Doctor" means "teacher"—what are you teaching this person about his or her health?
3. Have you done a risk factor assessment for this patient? Have all preprimary, primary, secondary, and tertiary interventions and education relevant to life span or gender been identified and addressed?
4. Does this patient do regular health screening self-examinations?

VI. Wellness and Health Promotion (emerging principle)

1. What is being done to cultivate wellness?
2. How are you contributing to optimal health in this individual?
3. How can you contribute to optimal health in this individual?
4. What are the patient's goals and expectations in relationship to his or her own wellness (e.g., creativity, energy, enjoyment, health, balance)?

5. How can these goals be achieved? Are the expectations realistic?
6. How can achievement of these goals be measured?
7. Once these goals are achieved, how can the patient maintain an optimal level of wellness?
8. Are you stimulating wellness or treating disease, or both?
9. Is the patient demonstrating positive emotion, thought, and action? If not, why not?
10. Can the patient recall or imagine a state of wellness?
11. Is the patient able to participate in his or her own process toward a state of wellness?

VII. Doctor as Teacher (docere)

1. What type of patient education are you providing? Assess wellness issues and prevention issues for this person. Identify educational needs of this patient regarding (a) therapeutic goals, (b) prevention, and (c) wellness.
2. How can you determine the level of the patient's responsibility?
3. In what ways do you cultivate and enhance your role as teacher?
4. How have you listened to and respected the patient?
5. In what ways are you working to draw out the patient's vital force and vitality through the physician-patient relationship?

THERAPEUTIC MODALITIES

Naturopathic medicine is a vitalistic system of health care that uses natural medicines and interventionist therapies as needed. Natural medicines and therapies, when properly used, generally have low invasiveness and rarely cause suppression or side effects. This is because, when used properly, they generally support the body's healing mechanisms rather than taking over the body's processes. The ND knows when, why, and with what patient more invasive therapies are needed based on the therapeutic order and appropriate diagnostic measures. The ND also recognizes that the use of natural, low-force therapies; lifestyle changes; and early functional diagnosis and treatment of nonspecific conditions is a form of preprimary prevention. This approach offers one viable solution for cost containment in primary health care.

Traditional health care disciplines such as traditional Chinese medicine (TCM), Unani medicine, and homeopathic medicine each have a philosophy, principles of practice, and clinical theory that form a system for diagnosis, treatment, and case management. A philosophy of medicine is, in essence, the rational investigation of the truth and principles of that medicine. The principles of practice form an outline of or guidelines to the main precepts or fundamental tenets of a system of medicine. Clinical theory provides a system of rules or principles explaining that medicine and applying that system to the patient by means of diagnosis, treatment, and management. The specific substances and techniques, as well as when, why, and to whom they are applied and for how long, depend on the system. Modalities (e.g., botanical medicine, physical medicine) are not systems but rather therapeutic approaches used within these systems. One modality may be used by many systems but in different ways.

The importance of systems is that the efficacy, safety, and efficiency of diagnostic and treatment approaches depend as much on the system as on the effects of the substance on physiology or biochemical pathways. This is exemplified by data in the TCM Work Force Survey conducted by the Department of Human Services in Victoria, New South Wales, and Queensland, Australia. In this study, Bensoussan and Myers (1996) assessed adverse events and length of TCM training for practitioners, as follows:

> The number of adverse events reported were compared to the length of TCM training undertaken by the practitioner. It appears from these findings that shorter periods of training in TCM (less than one year) carry an adverse event rate double that of practitioners who have studied for four years or more.... These practitioners were asked to respond to two questions regarding the theoretical frameworks they used to guide their TCM practice. TCM philosophy is adopted more readily as the basis for practice by primary TCM practitioners than by allied health practitioners using TCM as part of their practice. In answer to the question, "Do you rely more predominantly on a TCM philosophy and theoretical framework for making your diagnosis and guiding your acupuncture or Chinese herbal medicine treatments?" 90% of primary TCM practitioners answered yes in contrast to 24% of non-primary practitioners.

Nonprimary practitioners were typically educated for less than 1 year and were medical doctors.

It is the system used by each of these disciplines that makes it a uniquely effective field of medicine rather than a vague compendium of complementary and alternative medicine (CAM) modalities. Techniques from many systems are used in naturopathic medicine because of its primary care integrative approach and strong philosophical orientation.

Clinical nutrition, or the use of diet as a therapy, serves as the therapeutic foundation of naturopathic medicine. A rapidly increasing body of knowledge supports the use of whole foods, fasting, natural hygiene, and nutritional supplements in the maintenance of health and treatment of disease. The recognition of unique nutritional requirements caused by biochemical individuality has provided a theoretical and practical basis for the appropriate use of megavitamin therapy. Controlled fasting is also used clinically.

Botanical medicines are also important. Plants have been used as medicines since antiquity. The technology now exists to understand the physiological activities of herbs, and a tremendous amount of research worldwide, especially in Europe, is demonstrating clinical efficacy. Botanical medicines are used for both vitalistic and pharmacological actions. Pharmacological effects and contraindications, as well as synergetic, energetic, and dilutional uses, are fundamental knowledge in naturopathic medicine (see Chapters 5 and 22).

Homeopathic medicine derives etymologically from the Greek words *homeos,* meaning "similar," and *pathos,* meaning "disease." Homeopathy is a system of medicine that treats a patient and his or her condition with a dilute, potentized agent, or drug, that will produce the same symptoms as the disease when given to a healthy individual, the fundamental principle being that *like cures like.* This principle was actually first recognized by Hippocrates, who noticed that herbs and other substances given in small doses tended to cure the same symptoms they produced when given in toxic doses. Prescriptions are based on the totality of all the patient's symptoms and matched to "provings" of homeopathic medicines. Provings are symptoms produced in healthy people who are unaware of the specific remedy they have received. Large numbers of people are tested and these symptoms documented. The symptoms are then added to toxicology, symptomatology, and data from cured cases to form the homeopathic materia medica. Homeopathic medicines are derived from a variety of plant, mineral, and chemical substances and are prepared according to the specifications of the *Homeopathic Pharmacopoeia of the United States.* Approximately 100 clinical studies have demonstrated the clinical efficacy of homeopathic therapies (see Chapter 24).

Traditional Chinese medicine is analogous to naturopathic medicine to the extent that it is a system with principles corollary to working with the self-healing process. According to Bensoussan and Myers (1996),

> TCM shares some common ideas with other forms of complementary medicine, including belief in a strong inter-relationship between the environment and bodily function and an understanding of illness as starting with an imbalance of energy.... The TCM diagnostic process is ... particularly holistic in nature [again similar to that in naturopathic medicine] and is usually contrasted to a reductionistic approach in western medicine. Western medicine often defines disease at an organ level of dysfunction and is increasingly reliant on laboratory findings. In contrast, TCM defines disease as a whole person disturbance.

Quiang Cao, ND, LAc, Bastyr University, explains as follows:

> TCM never treats just the symptom, but the individual's whole constitution and environmental conditions; all are considered in a holistic context. The symptom signals constitutional excess or deficiency. The goal is not just to alleviate the symptom but to balance yin and yang, hot and cold, excess and deficiency, internally and externally.

Acupuncture is an ancient Chinese system of medicine involving the stimulation of certain specific points on the body to enhance the flow of vital energy (qi) along pathways called *meridians.* Acupuncture points can be stimulated by the insertion and withdrawing of needles, the application of heat (moxibustion), massage, laser,

electrical means, or a combination of these methods. Traditional Chinese acupuncture implies use of a very specific acupuncture technique and knowledge of the Oriental system of medicine, including yin-yang, the five elements, acupuncture points and meridians, and a method of diagnosis and differentiation of syndromes quite different from that of Western medicine. Although most research in this country has focused on its use for the pain relief and the treatment of addictions, it is a complete system of medicine effective for management of many diseases (see Chapter 27).

Hydrotherapy is the use of water in any of its forms (e.g., hot, cold, ice, steam) and with any method of application (e.g., sitz bath, douche, spa and hot tub, whirlpool, sauna, shower, immersion bath, pack, poultice, foot bath, fomentation, wrap, colonic irrigation) in the maintenance of health or treatment of disease. It is one of the most ancient methods of treatment and has been part of naturopathic medicine since its inception. Nature doctors, before and since Sebastian Kneipp, have used hydrotherapy as a central part of clinical practice. Hydrotherapy has been used to treat disease and injury by many different cultures, including the Egyptians, Assyrians, Persians, Greeks, Hebrews, Hindus, and Chinese. Its most sophisticated applications were developed in eighteenth-century Germany. Naturopathic physicians today use hydrotherapy to stimulate and support healing, to detoxify, and to strengthen immune function in many chronic and acute conditions.

Physical medicine refers to the therapeutic use of touch, heat, cold, electricity, and sound. This includes the use of physical therapy equipment such as ultrasound, diathermy, and other electromagnetic energy devices; therapeutic exercise; massage; massage energy, joint mobilization (manipulative), and immobilization techniques; and hydrotherapy. In the therapeutic order, correction of deficiencies in structural integrity is a key factor; the hands-on approach of naturopathic physicians through physical medicine is unique in primary care.

Detoxification, the recognition and correction of endogenous and exogenous toxicity, is an important theme in naturopathic medicine. Liver and bowel detoxification, elimination of environmental toxins, correction of the metabolic dysfunction(s) that causes the buildup of non–end-product metabolites—all are important ways of decreasing toxic load. Spiritual and emotional toxicity are also recognized as important factors influencing health.

Spirituality and health measures are central to naturopathic practice and are based on the individual patient's beliefs and spiritual orientation; put simply, what moves the patient toward life and a higher purpose than himself or herself. Because total health also includes spiritual health, naturopathic physicians encourage individuals to pursue their personal spiritual development. As a plethora of studies in the newly emerging field of psychoneuroimmunology have demonstrated, particularly those examining both the placebo and the nocebo effect, the body is not a mere collection of organs, but rather a body, mind, and spirit in which the mind-spirit part of the equation marshals tremendous forces promoting health or disease.

Counseling, health psychology, and *lifestyle modification techniques* are essential modalities for the naturopathic physician. An ND is a holistic physician formally trained in mental, emotional, and family counseling. Various treatment modalities include hypnosis and guided imagery, counseling techniques, correction of underlying organic factors, and family systems therapy.

THERAPEUTIC APPROACH

RESPECT NATURE

We are natural organisms, with our genomes developed and expressed in the natural world. The patterns and processes inherent in nature are inherent in us. We exist as a part of complex patterns of matter, energy, and spirit. Nature doctors have observed the natural processes of these patterns in health and disease and have determined that there is an inherent drive toward health that lives within the patterns and processes of nature.

The drive is not perfect. At times, when unguided, unassisted, or unstopped, the drive goes astray, causing preventable harm or even death; the healing intention becomes pathology. The ND is trained to know, respect, and work with this drive and to know when to wait and do nothing, act preventively, assist, amplify, palliate, intervene, manipulate, control, or even suppress, using the principle of the least force. The challenge of twenty-first-century medicine is to support the beneficial effects of this drive and come to a sophisticated application of the least-force principle in mainstream health care. This will prevent the last 20 years of life from being those of debility from chronic, degenerative disease for the average American and extend the health span throughout the life span.

Because the total organism is involved in the healing attempt, the most effective approach to care must consider the whole person. In addition to physical and laboratory findings, important consideration is given to the patient's mental, emotional, and spiritual attitude; lifestyle; diet; heredity; environment; and family and community life. Careful attention to each person's unique individuality and susceptibility to disease is critical to the proper evaluation and treatment of any health problem.

Naturopathic physicians believe that most disease is the direct result of the ignorance and violation of "natural living laws." These rules are summarized as consuming natural, unrefined, organically grown foods; ensuring adequate amounts of exercise and rest; living a moderately paced lifestyle; having constructive and creative thoughts and emotions; avoiding environmental toxins; and maintaining proper elimination. During illness, it is also important to control these areas to remove as many unnecessary stresses as possible and to optimize the

chances that the organism's healing attempt will be successful. Therefore, fundamental to naturopathic practice is patient education and responsibility, lifestyle modification, preventive medicine, and wellness promotion.

NATUROPATHIC APPROACHES TO DISEASE

The ND's therapeutic approach is therefore basically twofold: to help patients heal themselves and to use the opportunity to guide and educate the patient in developing a more healthful lifestyle. Many supposedly incurable conditions respond very well to naturopathic approaches.

A typical first office visit to an ND takes 1 hour. The goal is to learn as much as possible about the patient using thorough history taking and review of systems, physical examination, laboratory tests, radiology, and other standard diagnostic procedures. Also, the patient's diet, environment, toxic load, exercise, stress, and other aspects of lifestyle are evaluated, and laboratory tests are used to determine physiological function. Once a good understanding of the patient's health and disease status is established (making a diagnosis of a disease is only one part of this process), the ND and patient work together to establish a treatment and health promotion program.

Although every effort is made to treat the whole person and not just his or her disease, the limits of a short description necessitate discussing typical naturopathic therapies for specific conditions in a simplified, disease-oriented manner. The following sections provide examples of how the person's health can be improved through naturopathic approaches, resulting in alleviation of the disease.

Cervical Dysplasia

The only traditional medical approach to treating cervical dysplasia, a precancerous condition of the uterine cervix, is surgical resection. Nothing is done to treat the underlying causes. The typical naturopathic treatment would include the following:

1. *Education.* The patient should be educated about factors that increase the risk of cervical cancer, such as smoking (risk = 3.0), multiple sex partners (risk = 3.4), and the use of oral contraceptives (risk = 3.6) (Clarke et al, 1985).
2. *Prevention.* Because 67% of patients with cervical cancer are deficient in one or more nutrients (Orr et al, 1985) and the level of serum β-carotene (critical for prevention of cancer of cells such as those in the cervix) is only half that of normal women (Dawson et al, 1984), the woman's nutritional status would be optimized in general (through diet, especially by increasing intake of fruits and vegetables) and with regard to those nutrients known to be deficient (often as a result of oral contraceptive use) in women with cervical dysplasia and the deficiencies of which may promote cellular abnormalities: folic

acid (Van Niekerk, 1966), β-carotene (Dawson et al, 1984), vitamin C (Romney et al, 1985), vitamin B$_6$ (Ramaswamy et al, 1984), and selenium (Dawson et al, 2984).

3. *Treatment.* The vaginal depletion pack (a traditional mixture of botanical medicines placed against the cervix) would be used to promote sloughing of the abnormal cells.

The advantages of this approach are that (1) the causes of the cervical dysplasia have been identified and resolved, so the problem should not recur; (2) no surgery is used, thus no scar tissue is formed; and (3) the cost, particularly considering that many women with cervical dysplasia have recurrences when treated with standard surgery, is reasonable. More important, however, is that the woman's health has been improved, and other conditions that could have been caused by the identified nutritional deficiencies have now been prevented.

Migraine Headache

The standard medical treatment for migraine heachache is primarily to use drugs to relieve symptoms, a costly and recurrent practice. Nothing is done to address the underlying causes. In contrast, the naturopath recognizes that most migraine headaches are due to food allergies, and abnormal prostaglandin metabolism caused by nutritional abnormalities results in excessive platelet aggregation. The approach is straightforward, as follows:

1. Identify and avoid the allergenic foods, because 70% or more of patients have migraines in reaction to foods to which they are intolerant (Natero et al, 1989).
2. Supplement with magnesium, because migraine patients have significantly lowered serum and salivary magnesium levels, which are even lower during an attack (Sarchielli et al, 1992). In one study, 42% of 32 patients with an acute migraine had low serum magnesium levels (Mauskop, 1993). In another report, magnesium levels in the brain, as measured by nuclear magnetic resonance spectroscopy, were significantly lower in patients during an acute migraine than in healthy individuals (Weaver, 1990). Several studies have shown the importance of magnesium in reversing the causes of migraine (Johnson, 2001).
3. Reestablish normal prostaglandin balance by decreasing consumption of animal fats (high in platelet-aggregating arachidonic acid) and supplementing with essential fatty acids such as fish oils (Woodcock et al, 1984). Omega-3 supplementation has proven effective in adolescents with migraine (Harel et al, 2002).
4. Supplement with riboflavin. "Forty-nine individuals with recurrent migraines were given 400 mg/day of the B-vitamin riboflavin for at least 3 months. The average number of migraine attacks fell by 67% and migraine severity improved by 68%" (Gaby, 1998).

Hypertension

Patients with so-called idiopathic, or essential, hypertension can be treated very effectively if they are willing to make the necessary lifestyle changes, as follows:

1. *Diet.* Numerous studies have shown that excessive dietary salt in conjunction with inadequate dietary potassium is a major contributor to hypertension (Fries, 1976; Khaw et al, 1984; Meneely et al, 1976). Further, dietary deficiencies in calcium (Belizan et al, 1983; McCarron et al, 1982), magnesium (Dyckner et al, 1983; Resnick et al, 1989), essential fatty acids (Rao et al, 1981; Vergroesen et al, 1978), and vitamin C (Yoshioka et al, 1981) all contribute to increased blood pressure. Also, increased consumption of sugar (Hodges et al, 1983), caffeine (Lang et al, 1983), and alcohol (Gruchow et al, 1985) are all associated with hypertension. Many studies have shown the antihypertensive effects of increasing consumption of fruits and vegetables, key to the dietary recommendations of NDs for over a hundred years (John et al, 2002).
2. *Lifestyle.* Smoking (Kershbaum et al, 1968), obesity (Havlik et al, 1983), stress (Ford, 1982), and a sedentary lifestyle are all known to contribute to the development of high blood pressure.
3. *Environment.* Exposure to heavy metals such as lead (Pruess, 1992) and cadmium (Glauser et al, 1976) increase blood pressure.
4. *Botanical medicine.* Many herbal medicines are used when necessary for the patient's safety initially to lower his or her blood pressure rapidly until the slower, but more curative, dietary and lifestyle treatments can have their effects. Included are such age-old favorites as garlic *(Allium sativa)* and mistletoe *(Viscum album).*

The causes of high blood pressure are not unknown, but they are generally unheeded.

Lifestyle modification is crucial to the successful implementation of naturopathic techniques—health does not come from a doctor, pills, or surgery but rather from patients' own efforts to take proper care of themselves. Unfortunately, our society expends considerable resources to induce disease-promoting habits. Although it is relatively easy to tell a patient to stop smoking, get more exercise, and reduce his or her stress, such lifestyle changes are difficult in the context of peer, habit, and commercial pressure. The ND is specifically trained to assist the patient in making the needed changes. This involves many aspects: helping the patient acknowledge the need; setting realistic, progressive goals; identifying and working through barriers; establishing a support group of family and friends or of others with similar problems; identifying the stimuli that reinforce the unhealthy behavior; and giving the patient positive reinforcement for his or her gains.

ACCOUNTABILITY IN NATUROPATHIC MEDICINE

Acceptance of a profession typically is seen to derive from sanctions associated with educational institutions, professional associations and licensing boards.

—ORZACK (1998)

It is extremely important to realize that the establishment of standards and especially credentialling standards is critical for the public to know . . . whatever the discipline is.

—LEVENDUSKI (1991)

Although naturopathic medicine in the early part of the twentieth century was unique, clinically effective, and powerfully vitalistic, it suffered because it had not reached maturity in terms of professional unification, scientific research, and other recognizable standards of public accountability. These goals have finally been achieved during the two decades of 1978 to 2000.

Naturopathic medicine has responded to the need not only to integrate the best that conventional and natural medicine have to offer, but also to address the issues of public safety, efficacy, and affordability through the following mechanisms:

- Fully accredited naturopathic medical training (regional and professional)
- Standardized science-based naturopathic medical education
- Broad-scope licensing laws
- Nationally standardized licensing examinations
- Professional standards of practice and peer review
- Credentialing and quality improvement plans
- Documentation of scientific research and efficacy

These are well-accepted mechanisms for public accountability in all forms of licensed health care. Naturopathic medicine's credibility has resulted in part from these important achievements by a unified profession.

SCOPE OF PRACTICE, LICENSING, AND PROFESSIONAL ORGANIZATIONS

NDs practice as primary care providers. They see patients of all ages, from all walks of life, with every known disease. They make a conventional Western diagnosis using standard diagnostic procedures, such as physical examination, laboratory tests, and radiological examination. However, they also make a pathophysiological diagnosis using physical and laboratory procedures to assess nutritional status, metabolic function, and toxic load. In addition, considerable time is spent assessing the patient's mental, emotional, social, and spiritual status.

Therapeutically, NDs use virtually every known natural therapy: dietetics, therapeutic nutrition, botanical medicine (primarily European, Native American, Chinese, and Ayurvedic), physical therapy, spinal manipulation, lifestyle counseling, exercise therapy, homeopathic medicine, acupuncture, psychological and family counseling, hydrotherapy, and clinical fasting and detoxification. In addition, according to state law, NDs may perform office surgery, administer vaccinations, and prescribe a limited range of drugs. Because NDs consider themselves an integral part of the health care system, they meet public health requirements and work within a referral network of specialists in much the same way as a family practice medical (allopathic) doctor. This network includes the range of conventional and nonconventional providers.

NDs (or NMDs) are licensed in 13 states (Alaska, Arizona, California, Connecticut, Hawaii, Kansas, Maine, Montana, New Hampshire, Oregon, Utah, Vermont, and Washington), the District of Columbia, and the two U.S. territories of Puerto Rico and the Virgin Islands. NDs have a legal right to practice in Idaho and Minnesota. Because no licensing standards exist in these two states and NDs also practice in other states without government approval, individuals with little or no formal education are still able to proclaim themselves NDs, to the significant detriment of the public and the profession. The American Association of Naturopathic Physicians (AANP, Washington, DC) assists consumers in identifying qualified NDs (http://www.naturopathic.org).

The scope of naturopathic practice is stipulated by state law. Legislation typically allows standard diagnostic privileges. Therapeutic scope is more varied, ranging from only natural therapies to vaccinations, limited prescriptive rights, and office surgery. In addition, some states allow the practice of natural childbirth. Many states identify NDs as primary caregivers in their statutes.

In addition to the Council on Naturopathic Medical Education (CNME), two key organizations provide leadership and standardization for the naturopathic profession. The AANP, founded in 1985 by James Sensenig, ND, and others, was established to provide consistent educational and practice standards for the profession and a unified voice for public relations and political activity. Most licensed NDs in the United States are AANP members. The Naturopathic Physicians Licensing Examination (NPLEx) was founded under the auspices of the AANP in 1986 by Ed Hoffman-Smith, PhD, ND, to establish a nationally recognized standardized test for licensing. NPLEx is recognized by all states licensing NDs. All states licensing NDs and all states in the process of attaining licensure have state professional naturopathic associations. The Alliance for State Licensing is an ongoing state licensure effort.

INTEGRATION INTO THE MAINSTREAM

The American public has increasingly turned to alternative practitioners in search of healing for a variety of conditions not ameliorated by conventional medical practices. Such conditions include otitis media, cardiovascular disease, depression, chronic fatigue syndrome, gastrointestinal disorders, chemical sensitivities, recurrent infectious diseases, rheumatoid arthritis, general loss of vitality and wellness, and many other chronic and acute conditions.

> Unquestionably, the health care system is undergoing profound change.... Many...current aspects of health care have resulted from a period of rapid change in the early part of this century. We are returning to a period of rapid change.... What is less certain is exactly where that change will lead. The task...is to identify and understand the forces of change and describe these forces so that [we] can make [our] decisions more wisely. (Bezold, 1986)

EXAMPLES OF INTEGRATIVE STEPS

Naturopathic medicine has accomplished important steps in integrating into mainstream delivery systems.

Reimbursement: "Every Category of Provider" Law

In 1993, during health care reform in Washington State, the "every category of provider" law was passed. This law mandated that insurance companies include access to every category of licensed provider in all types of plans in insurance systems for the treatment of all conditions covered in the basic health plan. Washington State Insurance Commissioner Deborah Senn, who vigorously enforced this law, formed the Clinician Working Group on the Integration of Complementary and Alternative Medicine, bringing together medical directors, plan representatives, and conventional and CAM providers to identify issues and solutions to integration barriers in insurance systems. This step has been important in increasing consumers' access to the health care providers of their choice, including licensed CAM professionals, as well as providing a solution focus to valid integration challenges.

Other reimbursement initiatives have also been successful. NDs throughout the United States are being integrated as primary care providers and specialists in traditional and managed care systems. The Pacific Northwest has emerged as a testing ground or model for integration because of the legislative and regulatory environment in the region.

Health Professional Loan Repayment and Scholarship Program

In 1995, Washington State's Department of Health made naturopathic physicians eligible for student loan repayment in the state's Health Professional Loan Repayment and Scholarship Program. Grants are awarded for student scholarships and student loan reimbursement to health care providers qualified and willing to provide health care in underserved areas or to underserved populations. The first and second naturopathic physician grants for loan repayment were awarded in 1998 and 2000.

King County Natural Medicine Clinic

No conventional model or infrastructure now exists in mainstream medicine for the systematic delivery of care that integrates natural and conventional providers. This integrative model is fundamental to naturopathic medicine. The King County Natural Medicine Clinic in Kent, Washington, is the first publicly funded integrative care clinic in the United States and has been a collaboration between Bastyr University and Community Health Centers of King County with funding provided by the Seattle King County Department of Public Health. This project forms an unprecedented union between three health forms: conventional medicine, natural medicine, and public health. The clinic has successfully applied a co-management model by using an interdisciplinary health care team co-led by naturopathic physicians and medical doctors, including nurse practitioners, acupuncturists, and dietitians. The clinic serves the medically underserved.

The Centers for Disease Control and Prevention and independent investigators have conducted research to study the provider-to-provider interactions and their effect on health care, patient satisfaction, and cost effectiveness. Other studies have compared results from natural and conventional therapies on specific conditions treated using this model.

Co-management

In *The Emerging Integrative Care Model,* Milliman and Donovan (1996) describe co-management as follows:

> Naturopathic medical [co-management] is the practice of medicine by a naturopathic physician (N.D.) in concert with other care givers (N.D., M.D., D.O., L.Ac., D.C., etc.) wherein each care giver operates:
>
> - In communication with others, according to established convention
> - Within his licensed scope of practice and acknowledged domain of expertise
> - With respect for the other care giver's autonomy, but with recognition of the ultimate responsibility and, therefore, authority of the patient's primary care giver (PCP)
> - With respect for the other care giver's expertise, but with recognition of the ultimate responsibility and, therefore, final authority of the informed patient's choices and decisions.

Co-management presents an opportunity to educate other providers to naturopathic medicine as well as a chance to learn from them and expand one's information base and diagnostic and therapeutic potential. Most importantly, however, it greatly increases the therapeutic choices and quality of care to patients, often resulting in more supportive and less invasive therapies (minimizing iatrogenic diseases), while promoting healthier lifestyles and overall reduction in health-care dollars spent.

CONTINUOUS QUALITY IMPROVEMENT

In 1996 the Washington Association of Naturopathic Physicians developed a quality assurance program consistent with national accreditation standards. This plan, known as *Continuous Quality Improvement (CoQI)*, was completed and adopted by the Washington State Department of Health and was the first naturopathic CoQI plan approved in the United States. This process is used by all health care professions and enables the profession to define and continuously update its own standards of care. Jennifer Booker and Bruce Milliman, NDs, led this effort.

Residencies

Utah is the first state to require a 1-year residency for naturopathic licensure. Residency opportunities for NDs are growing rapidly through sites established by the naturopathic colleges. Cancer Treatment Centers of America offers a growing number of residencies and staff positions to naturopathic physicians. The National College of Naturopathic Medicine and Bastyr University offer a growing number of residencies throughout the United States. All naturopathic colleges also offer on-site residencies.

Hospitals and Hospital Networks

A number of hospitals across the United States continue to employ NDs as part of their physician staff in both inpatient and outpatient settings. Examples of the types of treatment centers established over the last 10 years are the following:

- HealthEast Healing Center, a clinic that is part of a larger "hospitals plus provider networks delivery system," employs MDs, an ND, an acupuncturist, and bodyworkers, using a "learning organization" model (*Alternative Medicine Integration and Coverage,* 1997).
- The Alternative and Complementary Medical Program at St. Elizabeth's Hospital in Massachusetts has a credentialed ND on staff. "The hospital is a teaching center for Tufts University Medical School" (*Alternative Medicine Integration and Coverage,* 1998).
- Centura Health (CH), the largest health care system in Colorado, is composed of an association of Catholic and Adventist hospitals. CH owns preferred provider organization Sloans Lake Managed Care. NDs are credentialed along with ND homeopaths and many other CAM providers in this hospital-based network (*Alternative Medicine Integration and Coverage,* 1998).
- American Complementary Care Network has recently placed two NDs in key positions: medical

director of naturopathic medicine and chair of quality improvement (*Alternative Medicine Integration and Coverage,* 1998). Other networks, such as Wisconsin-based CAM Solutions and Seattle-based Alternare, have integrated ND-credentialed medical directors on staff.

When health systems, insurers, and health maintenance organizations decide to cover alternative medicine, NDs are sought out in states with licensure. Even in states without naturopathic licensure, health systems and managed care organizations exploring integration have come to understand and value the depth of training of naturopathic physicians (Weeks, 1998).

EDUCATION

The trend of modern medical research and practice in our great colleges and endowed research institutes is almost entirely along combative lines, while the individual, progressive physician learns to work more and more along preventive lines.

—LINDLAHR (1914)

The education of the ND is extensive and incorporates much of the diversity that typifies the natural health care movement. The training program has important similarities to conventional medical education (science based, identical basic sciences, intensive clinical diagnostic sciences), with the primary differences being in the therapeutic sciences, enhanced clinical sciences, clinical theory, and integrative case management. Naturopathic training places the pathology-based training of conventional physicians into the context of the broader naturopathic assessment and management model inclusive of nature, mind, body, and spirit in health care. To be eligible to enroll, prospective students must first successfully complete a conventional premedicine program that typically requires a college degree in a biological science. The naturopathic curriculum then takes an additional 4 years to complete. Residency opportunities are increasing rapidly throughout the United States, at the National College of Naturopathic Medicine, Bastyr University, and Southwest College of Naturopathic Medicine and Health Sciences. As noted previously, residency is now required for licensure in the state of Utah.

The first 2 years concentrate on the standard human biological sciences, basic diagnostic sciences, and introduction to the various treatment modalities. The conventional basic medical sciences include anatomy, human dissection, histology, physiology, biochemistry, pathology, microbiology, immunology and infectious diseases, public health, pharmacology, and biostatistics. The development of diagnostic skills is initiated with courses in physical diagnosis, laboratory diagnosis, and clinical assessment. The program also covers natural medicine subjects such as environmental health, pharmacognosy (pharmacology of herbal medicines), botanical medicine, naturopathic philosophy and case management, Chinese medicine, Ayurvedic medicine, homeopathic medicine, spinal manipulation, nutrition, physiotherapy, hydrotherapy, physician well-being, counseling and health psychology, and spirituality and health.

The second 2 years are oriented toward the clinical sciences of diagnosis and treatment while natural medicine subjects continue. Not only are the standard diagnostic techniques of physical, laboratory, and radiological examination taught, but what makes the diagnostic training unique is its emphasis on *preventive* diagnosis, such as diet analysis, recognition of the early physical signs of nutritional deficiencies, laboratory methods for assessing physiological dysfunction before it progresses to cellular pathology and end-stage disease, assessment and treatment of lifestyle and spiritual factors, and methods of assessing toxic load and liver detoxification efficacy. The natural therapies, such as nutrition, botanical medicines, homeopathy, acupuncture, natural childbirth, hydrotherapy, fasting, physical therapy, exercise therapy, counseling, and lifestyle modification, are studied extensively. Courses in naturopathic case analysis and management integrate naturopathic philosophy into conventional algorithms using the therapeutic order.

During the last 2 years, students also work in outpatient clinics, where they see patients first as observers and later as primary caregivers under the supervision of licensed NDs.

As previously mentioned, four schools currently exist in the United States and two in Canada: Bastyr University, National College of Naturopathic Medicine (NCNM), the Southwest College of Naturopathic Medicine and Health Sciences (SCNM), the University of Bridgeport College of Naturopathic Medicine (UBCNM), and, in Canada, the Canadian College of Naturopathic Medicine (CCNM) and the Boucher Institute of Naturopathic Medicine. The oldest institution is NCNM, which was established in 1965 in Portland, Oregon. The largest institution and first to receive accreditation is Bastyr, established in Seattle, Washington, in 1978. Over the years Bastyr has broadened its mission also to include accredited degree and certificate programs in nutrition, acupuncture and Chinese medicine, midwifery, applied behavioral sciences, health psychology, exercise, and spirituality and health. SCNM, established in 1993, has developed an active research department. The UBCNM, established in 1997, is the most recent addition. Like its counterparts in the United States, CCNM in Toronto, Ontario, has a rapidly increasing enrollment. Naturopathic education is accredited by the CNME, recognized by the U.S. Department of Education. The CNME has granted accreditation to the naturopathic medicine programs at NCNM, Bastyr, SCNM, and UBCNM. Bastyr and NCNM also have institutional accreditation by the Northwest Commission on Colleges and Universities, SCNM has institutional accreditation by the Higher Learning Commission of the North Central Association of Colleges and Schools, and UBCNM has institutional accreditation by the New England Association of Schools and Colleges. All states licensing naturopathic physicians recognize the CNME as the official accrediting agency for naturopathic medicine. The offices of the CNME are located in Portland, Oregon.

RESEARCH

Science clearly is an essential condition of a right decision.
—PELLEGRINO (1979)

However, clinical decisions cannot be solely dependent on science, when, with the best of efforts and with billions of public and private dollars spent, medical research has yielded twenty percent (and in some narrow areas up to fifty percent) of medical procedures and practices as scientifically proven and efficacious.
—OFFICE OF TECHNOLOGY ASSESSMENT (1978)

There is a paucity of theories of medicine.... The theory of medicine has lagged seriously behind theories of other sciences... any unitary theory of medicine which identifies it exclusively with science is doomed to failure.
—PELLEGRINO (1979)

The primary intellectual problem facing medicine today is that the information base of medicine is so poor. For a profession with a 2,000 year history which is responsible in the United States for 250 million lives and spends over $600 billion a year, we are astonishingly ignorant. We simply do not know the consequences of a large proportion of medical activities. The ... task is to change our mind set about what constitutes an acceptable source of knowledge in medicine.
—EDDY (1993)

The relationship between scientific research and the study of the healing power of nature, a traditionally vitalistic principle, is important. The scientific method is a well-accepted approach to communicating what we learn about medicine's mysteries to others; however, it has been limited in its development by conventional medicine's approach to research. Orthodox research appears to turn on the premise that the universe functions without *telos* or purpose. Connections are mechanistic. Clinical investigation is directed toward pharmaceutical disease management based on a single-agent, placebo-controlled, double-blind crossover trial.

What distinguishes naturopathic medicine's clinical research from that of *biomedicine* (a term coined to refer to the currently dominant school of medicine) is not the presence or lack of science. It is a collective confidence in the perception of a vital force or life force. The arguments then follow. What is it? What exactly does it do and how? As Dr. John Bastyr noted in an interview in August 1989, "We all have an innate ability to understand that there is a moving force in us, that doesn't necessarily need to be understood mechanistically." Future scientific work and naturopathic medical research on this principle is bound by the shared perception that (1) there is a pattern in health and disease, (2) there is order in the healing process, and (3) order is based on the life force, which is self-organized, intelligent, and intelligible. Within this paradigm, we can research the life force.

Confirming and challenging clinical perceptions and even disproving core assumptions is fundamental to naturopathic medicine's core values. Scientific methods must be challenged to find new approaches to test large quantities and types of clinical data, outcomes, and systems from naturopathic practices. So far, the reality of the healing power of nature (vis medicatrix naturae) has not been proved or disproved by the single-agent double-blind study. New models (e.g., outcomes research, field- and practice-based research, multifactorial models) provide fruitful methods for researching the validity of nonconventional medicine and offer new opportunities for research on conventional practices.

Until recently, original research at naturopathic institutions has been quite limited. The profession has relied on its clinical traditions and the worldwide published scientific research, as follows:

> Research in whole practices [is] only recently gaining interest with the development of methodologies in practice-based and outcomes research. There is a lack of research in whole practices like naturopathy, Oriental medicine, or Ayurveda compared to conventional practice whether in a particular disease or in overall health outcomes. Biomedical research methods which are considered gold-standard by the scientific community have been typically developed to provide reliable data on a single therapeutic intervention for a specific Western disease entity. The requirements of these research methods distort naturopathic practice and may render it apparently less effective than it may actually be. The measures may not take account of residual benefits in a patient's other health problems nor on future health and health care utilization.
>
> Compounding the methodological difficulties of research in this medical variant, there are structural obstacles as well. Distinct from the situation in conventional medicine, there is only the beginning of a research infrastructure at the profession's academic centers. Practitioners expert in naturopathic medicine and the individualization of treatment are typically not trained in rigorous comparative trials. Even if the infrastructure and training were in place, sources of funding remain few and small, and most funding agencies make their decisions on the basis of biomedical theories which naturopathy may directly challenge. When research is done on aspects of naturopathic treatment, more studies are done on substances rather than procedures or lifestyle changes. Without the economic incentives which favor the in-depth study of patentable drugs, trials in naturopathic therapeutics, often derived from a long history of human use, are smaller and with fewer replications. Many practices present special methodological or ethical problems for control, randomization, blinding, etc., perhaps making it impossible to perform a study as rigorous as some might wish. Nevertheless, there are numerous studies which yield indications of the effectiveness of individual treatments. (Calabrese et al, 1997)

As mentioned earlier, a comprehensive compilation of the scientific documentation of naturopathic philosophy and therapies can be found in *A Textbook of Natural Medicine,* coauthored and edited by Joseph Pizzorno, ND, and Michael Murray, ND. First published in 1985, the textbook was, until 1998, in a loose-leaf, two-volume set, published by Bastyr University Publications and updated regularly. The third edition (2006, Churchill Livingstone) consists of more than 200 chapters and references more than 7500 citations from the peer-reviewed scientific literature.

In the past 20 years, Bastyr University, NCNM, SCNM, and CCNM have developed active research departments, which has resulted in expanding publication of original research in peer-reviewed journals, both alternative and mainstream. In 1994, Bastyr University was awarded a 3-year, $840,000 grant by the NIH Office of Alternative and Complementary Medicine to establish a research center to study alternative therapies for human immunodeficiency virus infection and acquired immunodeficiency syndrome (HIV/AIDS). Of particular importance has been the approval and funding by the federal government's National Center for Complementary and Alternative Medicine of numerous research studies as well as fellowships and postdoctoral study positions at the naturopathic institutions. The result has been a growing number of naturopathic physicians with strong research training and credentials.

THE FUTURE

We could have a significant and immediate impact on costly health care problems if the complementary and alternative medicine disciplines and interventions were widely available.
—DOSSEY AND SWYERS (1992)

Naturopathic medicine is enabling patients to regain their health as NDs effectively co-manage and integrate care with pertinent providers, to their patients' and the public's benefit. Today's ND, an extensively trained and state-licensed family physician, is equipped with a broad range of conventional and unconventional diagnostic and therapeutic skills. This modern ND considers himself or herself an integral part of the health care system and takes a full share of responsibility for common public health issues. NDs are healers and scientists, policy makers, and teachers and are active in industry and environmental issues.

The scientific tools now exist to assess and appreciate many aspects of naturopathy's approach to health and healing. Conventional medical organizations that spoke out strongly against naturopathic medicine in the past now often endorse techniques such as lifestyle modification, stress reduction, exercise, consumption of a high-fiber diet rich in whole foods, other dietary measures, supplemental nutrients, and toxin reduction.

These changes in perspective signal the paradigm shift that is occurring in medicine. Emerging knowledge, high health care costs, and unmet health care needs continue to force this shift in perspective into changes in our current health care system. What was once rejected is now becoming generally accepted as effective. In many situations, it is now recognized that naturopathic alternatives offer benefit over certain orthodox practices. In the future, more concepts and practices of naturopathic medicine will undoubtedly be assessed and integrated into mainstream health care.

Historically, emerging bodies of knowledge in health care have formed into schools of thought and professions (with standards) as the public's need for their services increased. Naturopathic medicine's reemergence is no accident or anomaly. Naturopathic medicine has followed the developmental stages that health care professions typically undergo while becoming accountable to the public. Access has increased with increasing research, conceptual unity, and standards.

These models and standards in emerging CAM fields, including naturopathic medicine, hold answers to issues in health care, its delivery, and the health care system that are as significant as the interventions. With accreditation, licensure, reimbursement, ongoing research, and widespread public acceptance, the naturopathic clinical model is reaching professional maturity today.

⊖ Chapter References can be found on the Evolve website at http://evolve.elsevier.com/Micozzi/complementary/

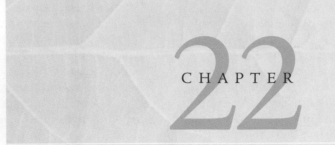

22

WESTERN HERBALISM

VICTOR S. SIERPINA
SUSAN M. GERIK
RADHESHYAM MIRYALA
MARC S. MICOZZI

Plants have been used by humans for food, medicine, clothing, and tools, as well as in religious rites, since before recorded history, more than 60,000 years ago, as evidenced by pollen from plants placed in Neanderthal cave burials found in modern-day Iraq (Solecki et al, 1975). Indeed, the art of herbal medicine probably predates *Homo sapiens.* Catalogues of remedies in pharmacopoeias date back 5000 years (Inamdar et al, 2008). No continent, island, climate, or geography that is home to human culture lacks a formal tradition of incorporating local flora into daily and ceremonial life as a means of enhancing health and well-being. Prehistoric plant life prepared the earth to be a viable and hospitable habitat for *Homo sapiens,* and plant ecology continues to help maintain the oceans, continents, and atmosphere today. Only recently have many Western health care providers recognized the number of remedies that had their origin in herbal medicine (Inamdar et al, 2008).

Herbal products have gained increasing popularity in the last decade. When questioned, approximately one fourth of adults reported using an herb to treat a medical illness within the past year (Bent, 2004, 2008). The most common herbs used included ginkgo, garlic, St. John's wort, soy, kava, echinacea, and saw palmetto (Bent, 2008). The global market for herbal products is over $60 billion annually (Inamdar et al, 2008).

DEFINITIONS

Herbalism is the study and practice of using plant material for food, medicine, and health promotion. This includes not only treatment of disease but also enhancement of quality of life, both physically and spiritually. A fundamental principle of herbalism is to promote preventive care and guided, simple treatment for the general population. An *herbalist,* or *herbal practitioner,* is someone who has undertaken specific study and supervised practical training to achieve competence in treating patients. Herbal medicines are recommended by physicians in the practice of integrative medicine and by other practitioners within the pharmacopeia of their traditions (see Chapter 4).

There is also an eclectic practice of herbal medicine in Europe and North America that draws on herbs from

BOX 22-1

Common Themes of Herbalism

- *Optimization of health and wellness.*
- *Emphasis on the whole person.* This includes body, mind, and soul; past, present, and future; and community.
- *Emphasis on the individual.*
- *Emphasis on the community.* The illness or recovery of a member might influence the community itself, beyond emotional group empathy.
- *Attention to finding and treating the root cause of a problem,* not only the manifestations and symptoms. However, as with most healers and medicine suppliers, even if the cause remains unidentified or untreatable, symptomatic treatment is offered.
- *Application of the principle of duality* between both the healing and the life-threatening forces of nature. The fundamental assumption of this principle is that natural law is greater than the will of the individual or community, and that healing requires the healer, the patient, and the community be in alignment with natural forces.
- *Belief in the reality of the unmeasurable and abstract.* Although dual, the abstract and physical worlds are inseparable. An herbalist as healer devotes himself or herself to maintaining balance and communication between the visible and invisible. This goal might be accomplished through connecting with spirituality or by adjusting activities to natural cycles (e.g., in Tibetan medicine, blending a formula during a specific season, moon phase, or auspicious date).
- *Premise of recycling.* Nature is inherently circular and repetitive; generally sequential, but not predominantly linear; and predictable, but seldom certain. This leads to the common traditional practice of offering an object or prayer in return for healing plants and for addressing requests for healing to both the physical and the spiritual world.
- *Openness to exchange of knowledge.* Most traditions incorporate new medicinal plants and new herbal uses and preparations that have been learned about through trade or travel.
- *Regulation of the herbalist's practice* through local accountability to his or her community. Success and prestige arise primarily from professional reputation that grows by word of mouth, not from image, business acumen, or material wealth (see Chapter 5).
- *Humility* generated from the healer's recognition of his or her own limits and skills. Because reputation generally depends on treatment efficacy and community standing, an herbalist would be reluctant to take on a case without reasonable confidence that he or she could succeed. Complex or incurable cases would be referred to another kind of practitioner, or the patient would be advised that no treatment was available other than palliation of suffering.

many healing traditions and has been called *Western herbalism.*

An herb can be an angiosperm (i.e., a flowering plant), shrub, tree, moss, lichen, fern, algae, seaweed, or fungus. The herbalist may use the entire plant or just the flowers, fruits, leaves, twigs, bark, roots, rhizomes, seeds, or exudates (e.g., tapped and purified maple syrup), or a combination of parts. Botany defines an *herb* as a nonwoody, low-growing plant, but herbalists use the entire plant kingdom. In many herbal traditions, nonplants including animal parts (organs, bone, tissue), insects, animal and insect secretions, worm castings, shells, rocks, metals, minerals, and gemstones are used as healing agents. These examples are recorded in ancient and contemporary materiae medicae and formal manuscripts of healing agents with their indications and uses. Egyptian, Chinese, Tibetan, European, American, and other worldwide materiae medicae are important references for herbal practitioners. This chapter addresses only plant herbal agents.

Herbalism may be a misleading term because it implies that a single hidden "root" gives rise to the diverse ways in which all human cultures across the millennia have used plants for food, medicine, and ritual. The use of herbs by the peoples of the Americas, Europe, Africa, the Middle and Far East, the Pacific Islands, and other regions is specific to each society and paradigm. For example, contemporary Western scientists have been restricted until recently by the Western mechanistic premises of biology and physics (see Chapter 1).

Although there is no single, worldwide system of herbalism, all herbal traditions share certain themes (Box 22-1).

 ### "Herb" and Other Words

erb as a word has an ancient pedigree, originating with the Latin word *herba,* which refers to green crops and grasses and could also mean the same as we mean by *herb* today (*Oxford English Dictionary,* or *OED*). The word entered English through Old French. The English use of "herb" in the sense of a plant whose stem does not become woody and persistent but remains more or less soft and succulent, dying down to the ground (or entirely) after flowering, can be traced to the thirteenth century. In the thirteenth century it was also understood that an "herb" (with variant spellings, e.g., "erbe") is a plant whose leaves and stems (and sometimes roots) could be used as food or medicine or for scent or flavor.

Herbarium, in the sense of a collection of dried plants, has its origins in the eighteenth century. A source for the association of "herbarium" with the medicinal properties of plants is that the idea for drying plants for study originated with a professor in sixteenth-century Italy who also held a chair in "simples," in which he studied medicinal and other plants.

(Continued)

"Herb" and Other Words—cont'd

Herbalist has shifted meaning. Originally (in the sixteenth century) an "herbalist" was one versed in the knowledge of herbs and plants—a collector of and writer about plants, more what we mean by "botanist" today. Usually, however, "herbalist" is now used to refer to early writers about plants, as well as persons who use alternative medical therapy, although the *OED* does not mention this.

Herbal meaning a book containing names and descriptions of herbs (or other plants in general) that provides properties and virtues came into use in the early sixteenth century. "Herbal" meaning belonging to, consisting of, or made from herbs has its origins in the early seventeenth century.

Early botanical gardens started in Renaissance Italy. These should properly be called "physic gardens," because they were used to help educate medical students, that is, to teach people—in this case medical students—about medicinal plants. Physic gardens appeared in England in the sixteenth century, in private hands. The Oxford Physic Garden began in 1621. (The Chelsea Physic Garden was begun in 1673 by the Society of Apothecaries.) The Oxford Physic Garden became the Botanic Garden in 1840, an important and representative change. There was no real difference between a "physic garden" and a "botanic garden," because botany and the study of the medicinal properties of plants were not distinct fields. William Turner (1510-1568) was a physician, was the author of an herbal, and is considered the father of English botany. For Turner, taxonomy was not separate from pharmacology in the study of plants.

Although the process was gradual, by the nineteenth century the study of plants for their own sake—botany—was a clearly separate field. Pharmacopoeias and botanical atlases grew in importance as the need for herbals waned.

There are clear ways to classify types of gardens. In the 1790s, Dr. Benjamin Rush called for the establishment of a "botanic garden" at the College of Physicians of Philadelphia. In Rush's time this would have meant a garden to study the properties of plants, in this case, medicinal properties. Rush suggested, however, that the garden could also be a source of medical preparations, as well as a place to grow plants that might be lost as Europeans settled North America. Although it was not the only purpose of Rush's garden, study was a component, and research lies at the heart of any botanical garden's purpose. (Botanical gardens are not limited strictly to taxonomy.)

Therefore, *medical botany* would be the study of the medicinal properties of plants, for example, chemical analysis to find new medically important compounds.

A *medical botanical garden* would be the source of plants for studying their medical properties.

A *medicinal herb garden* would, in a technical sense, be a place that has examples of plants, from which samples could be taken to make medicinal preparations. Also, the garden would contain only herbaceous plants, not plants with woody stems and branches.

CLASSIFICATIONS OF HERBALISTS

Each cultural or medical system has different types of herbal practitioners, all consistent with its paradigm. However, most paradigms identify professional herbalists, lay herbalists, plant gatherers, and medicine makers. (Professional and lay herbalists often collect their own plants and prepare their own medicines.)

PROFESSIONAL HERBALIST

A professional herbalist undergoes formalized training or a long apprenticeship in plant and medical studies or, alternatively, in plant and spiritual or healing studies. This knowledge includes extensive familiarity—often a relationship—with specific plants, which involves their identification, habitat, harvesting criteria, preparation, storage, therapeutic indications, contraindications, and dosing. A professional herbalist is not necessarily the primary healer (Iwu, 1993). A professional herbalist might follow a family tradition or might be selected at a young age as being endowed with the potential for mastering the use of plants as healing aids. In Europe and the United States, this group includes officially trained medical herbalists, clinical herbalists, licensed naturopathic doctors specializing in botanical medicine, licensed acupuncturists with training in Chinese herbal medicine, licensed Ayurvedic doctors, Native American herbalists and shamans, Latin American curanderos, and other lineage-recognized or culturally recognized professional herbalists. The shaman from Madagascar who—although never acknowledged or compensated for his contribution—revealed the usefulness of *Caranthas roseus,* the periwinkle plant from which vinblastine and vincristine were developed in the West for treatment of certain cancers, exemplifies the spirit and expertise of a professional healer and herbalist. Furthermore, the herbal practitioner's familiarity with each medicinal plant or herbal formula usually is greater than the medical practitioner's familiarity with each individual pharmaceutical. This permits the herbalist to select precisely a particular plant or formula for each individual patient. Three different patients with a chief complaint of headache would likely each receive a different herbal prescription. The approach that an herbalist uses to determine which herbs to prescribe is distinct from that used by a conventional Western physician to prescribe a pharmaceutical.

LAY HERBALIST

A lay herbalist has a broad knowledge of plants useful for health problems but does not have extensive training in medical and spiritual diagnosis and management. He or she may be an herb vendor with a sensitivity to the needs and desires of the marketplace, whose livelihood has been passed down as a family business. Evaluation of medicinal plant quality, strength, uses, and dose is included in the lay herbalist's domain. The Irish herbalist who uses specific herbal treatments for certain skin or stomach symptoms is an example.

PLANT GATHERER, PLANT GROWER, AND MEDICINE MAKER

Plant gatherers, plant growers, and medicine makers might consider themselves herbalists; actually, they are to the practicing herbalist what the contemporary pharmacist is to the clinical physician. In Chinese medicine, there is one specialist who produces and collects plants, one who processes and stores plants, and a clinical herbalist/doctor who prescribes the medicines. In some systems, preparing and handling medicines is considered a spiritual privilege and responsibility. Therefore, certain herbal medicines are prepared only by the herbalist or healer or by a designated assistant.

HERBS AND MEDICINAL PLANTS

Physicians in the United States studied and relied on plant drugs as primary medicines through the 1930s until World War II. Until then, medical schools taught basic plant taxonomy and pharmacognosy and medicinal plant therapeutics. The term *drug* derives from an ancient word for *root*, and the roots and rhizomes of many medicinal plants continue to provide alkaloids, steroidal saponins, and many active constituents that are clinically useful today. The *United States Pharmacopeia* listed 636 herbal entries in 1870; only 58 were listed in the 1990 edition (Boyle, 1991). Although some plants were dropped because they were found to be weak or unsafe, the majority of clinically useful plants were replaced with pharmaceuticals, which generated profits from patented drugs and contributed to the standardization and industrialization of medicine.

CHARACTERISTICS AND COMPOSITION

In many traditional systems the characteristics of a medicinal plant are emphasized without attention to its composition, because techniques and equipment for plant analysis are relatively new.

Preanalytical, chemical knowledge of medicinal and food plants is derived from direct perception through the five senses; from the herbalist's attentive, empirical observation of plants' effects on animals and humans; and, in some traditions, from sacred teachings and "sixth sense" intuition.

More recently, attention is being paid to standardizing the product, that is, to providing a consistent, measured amount of product per unit dose, and one ingredient is selected as the marker, usually the presumed active ingredient. Although research may reveal different or additional active ingredients, for convenience the designated constituent will usually remain the accepted marker. Over the years, more and more sophisticated methods of analysis to detect the marker have been developed, including such techniques as high-performance liquid chromatography and dioxide array detection. Perhaps a disadvantage to identifying, categorizing, and researching molecular constituents from plants is the risk of equating the plant's therapeutic efficacy to its composition. Analysis is reductionist in paradigm, and data cannot exist beyond the limits of the technology (and available funding to apply it) or the paradigm from which it arises (Cheng et al, 2008).

Food, medicinal, and healing plants may contain digestible fiber (carbohydrates and hemicellulose) and indigestible fiber (cellulose and lignins), nutritives (calories, vitamins, minerals, trace elements, amino acids, essential fatty acids, and water), and inert and active constituents.

When a Western paradigm is followed, plant constituents can be classified according to their morphology, source plant taxonomy, therapeutic (pharmacological) applications, or chemical constituents (Tyler et al, 1988) (Box 22-2).

BOX 22-2

Classic Organization of the Active Chemical Constituents in Plants

1. *Carbohydrates:* sugars, starches, aldehydes, gums, and pectins
2. *Glycosides:* cardiac glycosides in *Digitalis purpurea* leaf, anthraquinone glycosides in *Aloe* species latex and rhubarb *(Rheum officinale)* root and rhizome, flavinol glycosides (rutin and hesperidin, used to reduce capillary bleeding), and other glycoside types
3. *Tannins:* present in coffee and tea
4. *Lipids:* fixed oils and waxes
5. *Volatile oils:* essential oils such as peppermint and eucalyptus
6. *Resins*
7. *Steroids:* including the steroidal saponins from Mexican yam *(Diocorea* species), the original source of early oral contraceptives
8. *Alkaloids:* atropine from *Atropa belladonna*, quinine from cinchona, morphine from *Papaver somniferum*
9. *Peptide hormones*
10. *Enzymes:* bromelain from pineapple

PHYSIOLOGICAL ACTIVITIES

Activities and corresponding indications for the use of plants are, again, paradigm specific (see the sidebar "Influences on Plant Activities and Their Therapeutic Properties"). In the United States alone, opinions vary regarding a particular plant's full spectrum of physiological action because of the complex nature of plants and their uses.

Influences on Plant Activities and Their Therapeutic Properties

- Specific plant species, variety, and sometimes the individual plant itself
- Habitat, including latitude, longitude, exposure, humidity, rainfall, sun, shade, wind, temperature and daily and seasonal variation, soil, soil microorganisms, insects, birds, animals, companion plants, pests, plant diseases, and interaction with humans (damage, cultivation, harvesting, and pollution)
- Composition and constituents (presence of active and inert ingredients)
- How and when the plant is collected, stored, processed; how the herb is dispensed and dosed
- Presence of adulterants, pests, or disease
- The prescriber; many traditional systems in Africa and Asia ascribe the ability to potentiate the plant's healing properties only to initiated healers or shamans
- The patient's health status, disease, age, and receptivity to healing
- The symbolic or cultural significance of the plant
- The placebo effect

A sample of some classic herb categories based on plant actions—often associated with identifiable nutritives or active constituents—are adaptogens (balance body systems), anticatarrhals (eliminate mucus), carminatives (antigas), demulcents (reduce inflammation), galactogogues (promote milk production), nervines (reduce stress), and tonics (promote optimal organ function) (Sierpina, 2001).

These examples illustrate a few of the many actions ascribed to herbs viewed from the classic Western paradigm. Often, contemporary research explains the constituents, mechanisms of action, and clinical responses that justify traditional uses. Occasionally, some plants are found to be inactive or ineffective or to contain potential toxins, which results in their discontinuance or necessitates special methods of preparation and dosing. As with most current prescription medications, some strong herbs must be dosed carefully to render them safe and effective.

There are other limitations to the direct association of active constituents with in vivo and clinical medicinal actions. Many times the active compounds remain unidentified, or the physiological response to the medicinal part of the whole plant is distinct from the actions of the individual active constituents (e.g., *Valeriana, Echinacea*). In addition, ingredients that appear inert are sometimes later found to be active when a more accurate mechanism of action or bioassay associated with the plant's effects is discovered.

When a nonreductionist paradigm is used, plant composition alone offers an incomplete explanation of the full scope of the properties and actions of food and healing plants. Traditional herbalists, nineteenth-century vitalists (see Chapter 6), naturopathic doctors, and many contemporary medical doctors and practitioners share a belief in a "life force" that is yet to be fully understood. Many herbalists hold that healing energy is inherent to plants; it is this energy, in addition to nutritive or chemical constituents, that promotes healing. Shamans, traditional healers, and alchemists use their skills, knowledge, and power to instill certain plants with special healing properties, in this view.

HERBAL THERAPEUTICS

Different cultural paradigms use plants for healing in a manner founded on each paradigm's premises (Box 22-3).

Herbal medicines can be delivered in many forms. Some plants are best when used fresh but are seldom marketed fresh because they are highly perishable, and improper storage will affect quality. Dried, whole, or chopped herbs can be prepared either as *infusions* (steeped as tea) or *decoctions* (simmered over low heat). Typically, flowers, leaves, and powdered herbs are infused (e.g., chamomile or peppermint), whereas fruits, seeds, barks, and roots require decocting (e.g., rose hips, cinnamon

BOX 22-3

Herbal Practices

Herbal practitioners in the United States may rely primarily on one of the following, or a combination:
1. *The plant's pharmacological actions:* in some cases enhanced by specific processing and extractive solvents and techniques or formulation of plant medicines into standardized extract products to concentrate and guarantee unit doses of active constituents
2. *Individual plant pharmacokinetics:* best preserved by using single, whole plants or their extracts
3. *Synergistic formulating:* blending of a number of medicinal plants together to achieve specific therapeutic effects unachievable by using a single herb alone
4. *Nutritional value:* as when *Urtica repens,* or nettles, is recommended as a tea rich in absorbable iron
5. *Energetics:* Vibrational energy, as for example with Bach Flower remedies, and various flower essences

bark, licorice root). Many fresh and dried herbs can be tinctured as medicines preserved in alcohol. Some plants are suited to acetracts (vinegar extracts), whereas others are active and well preserved as syrups, glycerites (in vegetable glycerine), or miels (in honey). Powered or freeze-dried herbs are available in bulk and as tablets, troches, pastes, and capsules. Fluid and solid extracts—strong concentrates (four to six times the crude herb strength)—and fresh plant juices preserved in approximately 25% alcohol (as with the fresh plant *Echinacea succus*) are other forms.

Nonoral delivery forms include herbal pessaries, suppositories, creams, ointments, gels, liniments, oils, distilled waters, washes, enemas, baths, poultices, compresses, moxa, snuffs, steams, and inhaled smokes and aromatics (volatile oils). The predominant plant delivery forms vary among different herbal traditions. Tinctures are widely used in Britain and the United States; tablets of standardized extracts of certain herbs (e.g., *Ginkgo biloba*) are popular in Germany and the United States; decoctions are common in Tibetan, Chinese, and African traditions; therapeutic oils are used topically and internally in Ayurvedic treatments; and teas, smokes, and compresses are used in the Native American tradition.

Capsules and tablets are the most common delivery system. Gelatin or vegetable-based capsules are filled with powdered dried herbs. Tablets are powdered herbs compressed into a solid pill, often with a variety of inert ingredients as fillers.

Herbs are supplied in a variety of sizes and strengths, so it is important to read the label carefully. The label also usually gives an average suggested dose as a guideline, based on research and clinical use. It is recommend to start at the low end; watch for a response, including unwanted effects; and adjust the dose accordingly.

SAFETY

Side effects of drugs can be serious or fatal; the worst is death by overdose. According to one report, overdoses are associated with an annual rate of 30.1 deaths per 1 million prescriptions of antidepressants. On the other hand, to quote Norman Farnsworth, PhD, professor of pharmacognosy at the University of Illinois, Chicago, "Based on published reports, side effects or toxic reactions associated with herbal medicines in any form are rare.... In fact, of all classes of substances ... to cause toxicities of sufficient magnitude to be reported in the United States, plants are the least problematic."

Herbal products are often considered safe because they are "natural" products (Kuruvilla, 2002). Nonetheless, the quality of products may be affected by species differences, seasonal variations, environmental factors, collection methods, transport and storage, manufacturing practices, or contamination with foreign plant material, toxins, heavy metals, or environmental pollutants. One must also remember that any substance that has biological activity has the potential to cause adverse

effects. Dangerous and lethal side effects related to direct toxic effects, allergic reactions, effects from contaminants, and interaction with drugs or other herbs have been reported (Chan, 2003; Dobos et al, 2005; Hu et al, 2005; Izzo et al, 2001).

Groups have assembled to look at special circumstances of herb use in the context of dental procedures, in the perioperative period, and with concurrent use of particular prescribed drugs. Some cautions identified through these inquiries include the following: bromelain, cayenne, chamomile, and feverfew interact with aspirin; aloe latex, ephedra, ginseng, and licorice interact with corticosteroids; kava, St. John's wort, and valerian interact with central nervous system depressants; chamomile, horse chestnut, and fenugreek enhance the risk of bleeding; ginseng can produce hypoglycemia; and ephedra may lead to cardiovascular instability (Abebe, 2002, 2003; Ang-Le et al, 2001; Bent, 2004, 2008; Izzo et al, 2001).

Quality control is essential, with assurance that the product contains ingredients and quantities as labeled, and without such contaminants as bacteria, molds, or pesticides. Selection of plant material based on quality, standardization of methods of preparation, and enforcement of regulations regarding labelling improve the quality and safety of herbal preparations as therapeutic agents.

In traditional medicine systems, herbs are prepared to obtain the most active ingredient for use in the specific preparation discovered to be most effective for the particular herb and tailored to the unique characteristics of the patient (Khalsa, 2007).

In 2004, Europe enacted legislation designed to improve the protection of public health by setting up a registration scheme for manufactured traditional herbal medicines. The evidence of 30 years of traditional use was relied upon to establish a European list of herbal substances that includes indication, strength, dosing recommendations, and route of administration. The list is now being compiled by the Committee on Herbal Medicinal Products at the European Medicines Agency (Routledge, 2008). The European Agency for the Evaluation of Medicinal Products has drafted test procedures and acceptance criteria for herbal drug preparations (Rousseaux et al, 2003).

The Therapeutic Goods Administration in Australia created a Complementary Medicines Evaluation Committee to address the issue of regulation of herbal products (Rousseaux et al, 2003).

In the United States, trade and professional organizations such as the American Herbal Products Association are setting standards including good agricultural practice, good laboratory practice, good supply practice, good manufacturing practice, and standard operating procedures which can help control environmental factors that may contribute to contamination (Chan, 2003; Fong, 2002; Routledge, 2008). Most herbal products are regulated as "dietary supplements." In 1994 the U.S. Dietary Supplement Health and Education Act (DSHEA) set new guidelines with regard to quality, labeling, packaging, and marketing of supplements. It also sparked a surge of interest in herbal products. DSHEA allows manufacturers to make "statements of nutritional support for conventional vitamins and minerals." Because herbs are not nutritional in the conventional sense, DSHEA allows manufacturers to make only what are called "structure and function claims," but no therapeutic or prevention claims. Thus a label can claim that St. John's wort "optimizes mood," but it cannot call it a "natural antidepressant," which would be a therapeutic claim.

General Guidelines for the Use of Herbal Medicines

1. The clinician should take a careful history of the patient's use of herbs and other supplements.
2. An accurate medical diagnosis must be made before herbs are used for symptomatic treatment.
3. *Natural* is not necessarily *safe;* attention should be paid to quality of product, dosage, and potential adverse effects, including interactions.
4. Herbal treatments should, for the most part, be avoided in pregnancy (and contemplated pregnancy) and lactation.
5. Herbal use by children should be done with care, using the appropriate dosage based on weight.
6. Adverse effects should be recorded, and the dosage reduced or the product discontinued. It can be carefully restarted to ascertain whether or not it is the source of the problem.

The regulatory authority of the U.S. Food and Drug Administration (FDA) over herbs is frequently misrepresented as "absent," including by the FDA commissioner, according to hearings of the U.S. House of Representatives Committee on Government Reform in 2001. Nonetheless, the health care system must rely on vigilance by the medical profession and voluntary compliance by industry to safeguard patients against adverse reactions. Although legislative efforts are periodically made to alter the regulatory environment, changes are not anticipated in DSHEA, which regulates herbs as dietary supplements, not as drugs. Senator Orrin Hatch (R-Utah), co-chair of the Congressional Caucus on Complementary and Alternative Medicine and Dietary Supplements, has documented the unprecedented involvement of a coalition of citizens and commercial groups in the passage of this bill (Hatch, 2002). It is likely that better information and education of consumers and health professionals will help to achieve what more regulation cannot achieve (see the sidebar "Legislative and Regulatory Environment for Herbal Medicines").

Legislative and Regulatory Environment for Herbal Medicines

Under the U.S. Dietary Supplement Health and Education Act (DSHEA) of 1994, as amended 1998, the U.S. Food and Drug Administration (FDA) presently has power to regulate herbal remedies and dietary supplements in the following ways:
1. Institute "good manufacturing practices" (GMPs), including practices addressing identity, potency, cleanliness, and stability (although the FDA did not promulgate GMPs until 13 years after passage of DSHEA)
2. Refer for criminal action for the sale of toxic or unsanitary products
3. Obtain injunction against the sale of products making false claims
4. Seize products that pose an unreasonable risk of illness and injury
5. Sue any company making a claim that a product "cures" or "treats" disease
6. Stop sale of an entire class of products if they pose an imminent health hazard
7. Stop products from being marketed if the FDA does not receive sufficient safety data in advance (under "generally recognized as safe" [GRAS] provisions)

Further abuses involving herbal products adulterated with therapeutic drugs and contaminants (especially a problem with imports from overseas, particularly China) are a serious safety issue. Many times the adulteration is inadvertent, but sometimes undeclared prescription drugs may be fraudulently added, allegedly for medicinal purposes (Chan, 2003). Consumers, health professionals, and responsible elements of the U.S. natural products industry all suffer when irresponsibly adulterated products are imported from abroad. The National Institutes of Health (NIH) clinical trial investigating the Chinese herbal formulation PC-SPES for prostate cancer was undermined by the unwitting use of adulterated herbs. Some natural products from China have even been contaminated with chloramphenicol (Micozzi, 2007).

Improvements in manufacturing and marketing standards in the natural products industry will be required for effective integrative medical practice (Fong, 2002).

PREGNANCY AND BREASTFEEDING

Most of the deleterious effects of natural products on the unborn baby are likely related to hormonal effects and drug interactions rather than to direct teratogenicity. Many herbs have not been approved for use by pregnant and nursing women in the guidelines of the German Commission E, a regulatory agency in some ways comparable to the

U.S. FDA. Commission E has published a collection of reports based on safety and efficacy data on more than 200 herbs that are now available in English translation (Blumenthal et al, 2000).

CHILDREN

Herbs may often be a treatment of choice for children. Despite lack of modern research, centuries of use have shown many products to be safe when dosed appropriately according to children's weight, although there is a general bias in medicine against using CAM treatments in children that many may consider "experimental" despite centuries of use.

Although concerns exist about safety, efficacy, and appropriate dosing in the pediatric population, families do offer herbs to their children. A group in Canada interviewed 1804 families who came to an emergency department. They found that 20% of the families used natural health products concurrently with drugs. A quarter of those paired agents had the potential to cause interactions (Goldman et al, 2007).

Another study was conducted at an emergency department at Emory University in Atlanta, Georgia. Over a 3-month period, 142 families with children aged 3 weeks to 18 years were interviewed. Forty-five percent of caregivers reported giving their children herbal products. Of those 45%, 53% had given one type and 27% had given three or more types in the previous year. The most common therapies were aloe, echinacea, and sweet oil. The most dangerous combination reported was ephedra given concomitantly with albuterol for asthma. Seventy-seven percent of the caregivers did not suspect potential side effects. Only two thirds of the families anticipated interactions with other herbal products or with medications (Lanski et al, 2003).

AGING

Considering the phenomenon of polypharmacy in elderly persons and problems of impaired metabolism and clearance, herbs may offer an alternative to drugs. On the other hand, the practitioner also must be aware of herb-drug interactions. St. John's wort can be very useful for managing depression in the elderly patient, ginkgo for cognitive decline, and kava for sedation, without the adverse effects of the benzodiazepines. These herbs can be used in combination with each other as well.

GENERAL CONSIDERATIONS FOR THE USE OF HERBS IN INTEGRATIVE MEDICINE

As health care providers, we have a responsibility to act as informed intermediaries for patients and families seeking information about the use of herbal products. We must consider issues of quality, safety, and efficacy.

The role of herbalism in contemporary Western society is not to serve as a substitute for the pharmaceutical advances of the last decades but to provide access to an ancient paradigm that is less mechanistic and more holistic and humane in scope and that, if responsibly reclaimed and integrated, can greatly benefit future health care worldwide. This is illustrated in the following statement by Paiakan, a contemporary Kayapo Indian leader.

> I am trying to save the knowledge that the forest and this planet are alive, to give it back to you who have lost the understanding (Odum, 1971).

Changes in the practice of medicine are causing a shift to increasing self-care with more benign, less invasive treatments. Patients prefer to take personal control over their health, such as through the use of herbal remedies not only for therapeutic benefit, but also for prevention of disease. Herbal remedies are commonly used by patients with chronic medical conditions such as cancer, liver disease, immunodeficiencies, asthma, and rheumatological disorders (Inamdar et al, 2008). Because of this, it is critical that practicing clinicians (and, in turn, patients) be made aware of the indications, actions, and drug interactions of herbal remedies.

The World Health Organization (WHO) estimates that 80% of the world's population relies on herbal medicine. Meanwhile, the use of herbs in the United States is expanding rapidly; herbal products are readily found in most pharmacies and supermarkets. From 1990 to 1997, as the use of complementary and alternative (integrative) medicine rose from 34% to 42% of those surveyed, herbal use quadrupled from 3% to 12% (Eisenberg et al, 1998). The growth of complementary and alternative medicine has continued apace in the years since then.

Importantly, these rapid changes have occurred because of popular demand. The public has discovered that natural medicines often provide a safe, effective, and economical alternative, and research is increasingly validating this finding. Many of those who use herbal and high-dose vitamin products fail to tell their physicians. Either they assume that "natural" products are harmless and not worth mentioning, or they fear telling health professionals who may be skeptical about their use. Health professionals, however, are beginning to familiarize themselves with the subject. Aside from some advantages of natural products, herb-drug interactions are a growing concern: almost one in five prescription drug users is also using supplements (Eisenberg et al, 1998).

Reliance on the appropriate use of nutrients and herbs is a critical and fundamental component of many integrative medical practices. Presently in the United States, these natural products are widely available. Unlike for pharmaceuticals, information about the health effects cannot be provided on the product label or with the product as a product insert.

As observed by WHO, herbs are essentially "people's medicine." In many parts of the world, traditional systems of herbalism generally make little distinction between food and medicinal plants, and local accessibility of food, spices, and therapeutic herbs generally is assumed in traditional agrarian, nonindustrialized societies. Before the twentieth century, most people everywhere generally had closer personal contact with food and medicinal plants.

A restoration of the personal and symbolic relationship to food and medicine plants could be linked with contemporary scientific knowledge of herbal applications. Appropriate self-care could be encouraged with public education, access to consultation with professional herbalists and physicians, and access to fresh herbs and high-quality, processed herbal medicines when needed. This improved patient involvement in the self-care of the body and its signals might then improve the use of professional medical care.

Many herbalists consider the patient's direct involvement in his or her own healing and the summoning of the patient's intellectual, emotional, physical, and spiritual attention to the process as critical. Partly for this reason, and because of traditional herbalism's emphasis on "right relationship," social context, and self-responsibility, many herbal practitioners deliberately prescribe elaborate rather than convenient herbal therapies. For example, on returning home to Ghana, a merchant developed an infected leg ulcer. Instead of being supplied an herbal medicine by the herbalist, he was directed to the nearby live plant source (a local tree bark). He collected and prepared the antimicrobial and vulnery poultice and applied it daily until his wound healed. Although self-collection and medicine preparation are generally impractical in the United States, self-involvement in the healing process is possible in many ways and parallels the complex lifestyle changes now routinely recommended to patients with chronic ailments such as cardiovascular disease.

Because of the increasing availability of credible third-party research on the efficacy of herbal and nutritional ingredients, as well as the increasing recognition by the medical profession of the importance of dietary supplementation for optimal health and for the prevention and management of many medical conditions (see *Journal of the American Medical Association,* July 2002), it is incumbent on practitioners of integrative medicine to maintain a medical standard of information and practice about herbal and nutritional ingredients. One approach to this requirement is to develop and maintain capability for clinic-based or hospital-based formularies of appropriate, effective, and high-quality herbs and nutrients.

The current regulatory environment is coupled with the reality that much of the natural products industry does not operate to medical and scientific standards, that many irresponsible marketing claims are made, and that many medical and scientific professionals are not knowledgeable about the science behind herbal and nutritional medicine. For practitioners new to the medicinal use of herbs, dose selection can be confusing. This volatile mix produces much confusion and misinformation on both sides, documented periodically by such sources as the *New England Journal of Medicine.* Medical professionals presently are largely on their own in trying to understand the proper indications, ingredients, and dosages for the appropriate scientific use of herbal and nutritional remedies, and consumers can only look to practitioners for guidance.

New information technologies are being brought on line to provide distributors, consumers, and practitioners fair and accurate information about the appropriate use of dietary supplements. The authors do not, however, recommend any one particular website alone nor advise using websites without confirmation by a knowledgeable practitioner.

In any case, to adequately guide patients, it is essential to obtain a complete drug and herbal history from the patient using an open and nonjudgmental approach.

RESEARCH IN FOOD AND MEDICINAL PLANTS

Although there is a relatively extensive contemporary literature on medicinal and healing plants, much of it exists outside the United States and often in languages other than English. In addition, there is little consistency in standard research designs and protocols among various countries.

Currently the National Center for Complementary and Alternative Medicine (NCCAM) is funding the following centers for botanical research: Botanicals Research Center for Age Related Diseases (Indiana), Botanical Research Center: Metabolic Syndrome (Louisiana), Center for Botanical Dietary Supplements Research in Women's Health (Illinois), Center for Botanical Immunomodulators (New York), Center for Botanical Lipids (North Carolina), and Center for Research on Botanical Dietary Supplements (Iowa). More information regarding this research can be obtained by visiting the NCCAM website and clicking on the links.

The need for more research on food, spice, and medicinal plants is great, especially with regard to their potential use in syndromes and conditions not well recognized or treated by conventional Western medicine. The challenge is to conduct the research in a holistic context. This requires creative funding of research that is unlikely to provide high-profit returns to a single source.

Many medicinal plants eliminated from the *United States Pharmacopeia* over the years were dropped because contemporary research documentation of their efficacy was lacking, not because they were proved to be ineffective (although some plants proved less useful clinically than newly developed drugs).

Retaining a holistic context in medicinal plant research also involves addressing differences in paradigm. Involving traditional herbalists as research design consultants would protect against inadvertently eliminating a critical element of the paradigm within which the herb is used. In the past, plant collection for research has sometimes proved an environmental threat (habitats, species, or traditional knowledge was lost or threatened). A holistic approach to contemporary plant collection and research must be implemented to conserve the traditional knowledge and ecology of the source plant and to avoid transgression of intellectual property rights, destruction of the plant habitat, or an imbalance of economic or intellectual returns to the source habitat and community.

Simple, well-documented analysis and outcomes-based research of crude and whole plant medicines are needed to determine their greatest potential applications and benefit to human health. Increasing contemporary research on medicinal plants is critical, but the importance of documenting and incorporating the empirical knowledge of healing plants cannot be overemphasized. Information gleaned from research should be linked with empirical knowledge (usually derived from hundreds of years of human use across many generations and ethnic groups), along with contemporary clinical reporting from patients and practitioners on tolerance and efficacy. Then herbal therapeutics and preventive protocols can be better targeted to enhance the health of future generations.

PUBLIC POLICY ISSUES

The modern era has brought many advantages in human health and sanitation, but one potential disadvantage of economic and occupational specialization is the loss of contact with the source of plant medicines. The marketplace has become multileveled, so the consumer usually has no direct or personal relationship with the herb producer. Sometimes, because of costs of production, taxes, and marketing, the packaged herbal product costs 20 times the price of the crude herb. There are undeniable advantages to certain prepackaged or concentrated herbal products, but two disadvantages are accountability and economic access. If the sale of fresh or bulk crude herbs is abandoned in the marketplace for the sale of less perishable and higher-return products, the patient has access to only highly processed products, and the cash-poor patient loses access altogether. This is particularly ironic in the case of medicinal plants; most traditional systems considered healing plants a gift of nature and access to them a basic human right.

State governments have developed a traditional role in regulating medical practice and in supporting medical education. The federal government maintains a unique and critical role in stimulating and supporting medical research, regulating medical products and devices, protecting the public health, and helping build health care infrastructure, and it is now paying approximately one third the costs of health care in America.

Policy makers at the state and federal levels should become more knowledgeable about the needs and opportunities related to integrative medicine. The bipartisan Congressional Caucus on Complementary and Alternative Medicine and Dietary Supplements was organized for this purpose. The Integrative Healthcare Policy Consortium, Policy Institute for Integrative Medicine, and other groups are working with members of the caucus and other elected representatives to broaden and deepen federal support for appropriate analyses and programs in integrative medicine. It is unlikely that the current regulatory legislation governing dietary supplements (DSHEA of 1994, as amended in 1998) will be changed. Although funding for NCCAM has increased commensurate with the multiyear doubling of the overall NIH budget, it is critical that other federal agencies charged with programs related to health resources and services, primary care, health professions training and workforce development, consumer education, health services research, and other areas be brought to bear on the important challenge and opportunity of integrative medicine. Integrative medicine has an important role that requires further articulation in current congressional actions on medical liability insurance reform and the national patient safety and quality assurance initiative. Public support together with private innovation has been the hallmark for medical advancement in the twentieth century and should continue to be the case for integrative medicine in the twenty-first century.

SUMMARY

Herbalism clearly offers potential benefit for the treatment of disease as well as promotion of wellness. Going forward, efforts should focus on more standardization of quality control, development of an official compendia that encompasses the content of the various pharmacopoeias currently available, clear and honest communication and sharing of information, and more inclusive research regarding safety and efficacy in all populations.

⊖ See the Evolve site at http://evolve.elsevier.com/Micozzi/complementary for the Common Herbs for Integrative Care Appendix and Image Collection.

⊖ Chapter References can be found on the Evolve website at http://evolve.elsevier.com/Micozzi/complementary/

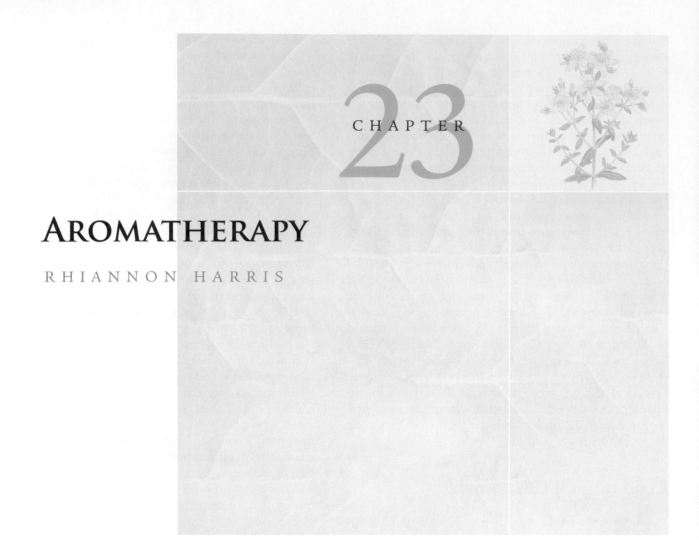

CHAPTER 23

AROMATHERAPY

RHIANNON HARRIS

The versatile nature of essential oils leads to a wide range of potential uses, and their therapeutic value is being harnessed, evaluated, and appreciated in a number of health care settings worldwide. This chapter explores the use of essential oils and aromatherapy with particular reference to clinical practice. By the end of the chapter, the reader will have a global overview of the potential of essential oils as therapeutic agents as well as an appreciation of the particular benefits and challenges of using these powerful substances in clinical environments.

Modern-day aromatherapy has origins spanning sacred and ritual use, perfumery, aesthetics, and medical applications, and these aspects continue to be relevant today when we consider the psychophysiological benefits that essential oils bring to the therapeutic encounter. For a historical overview of the therapy the reader can refer to specialist aromatherapy texts and articles that include accounts of the history and development of modern British aromatherapy by Bensouilah (2005) and Harris (2003) and the development of aromatherapy in the United States by Buckle (2003a, 2003b). This chapter focuses on the current situation and future potential of this versatile therapy.

THEORETICAL FOUNDATIONS

Aromatherapy may be defined as the selected use of essential oils and related products of plant origin with the general goal of improving health and well-being. The word *aromatherapie* was first used in 1937 by the French perfumer and chemist René Maurice Gattefossé (1881-1950), who, along with pioneers Jean Valnet (1920-1995) and Marguerite Maury (1895-1968), is largely credited with the modern revival of interest in the use of essential oils for therapeutic purposes.

In modern-day aromatherapy, the therapist uses these fragrant and active substances to affect the body-mind via a number of administration methods (external, inhalational, internal), usually in dilution and with a focus on a holistic approach to health in cooperation with the patient or client. The concept of the "individual prescription" as stressed by Maury in her seminal work *Secret of Life and Youth: Regeneration Through Essential Oils—A Modern Alchemy* (1964) (originally published in 1961 in French as *La capitale jeunesse*) remains key in contemporary aromatherapy practice.

Essential oils are the main active tools of aromatherapy. These highly concentrated and fragrant substances of plant origin have a complex chemical composition, the totality of which determines the essential oil's aroma and therapeutic potential. The concept of the "whole oil" as opposed to one that has been rectified, concentrated by deterpenation, or otherwise chemically altered is fundamental to most aromatherapists, who believe that there is an inherent synergy between the chemical components that needs to be preserved as much as possible. This concept does have some weight behind it, at least in terms of antimicrobial and antiinflammatory effects, because a number of studies have demonstrated synergy between main active components and minor, less active components in an individual essential oil (Harris, 2002), similar to the observed synergic effects of herbal remedies taken internally.

Essential oils themselves are clearly defined by the industry that uses them. The International Organization for Standardization (ISO) defines them as follows:

> Products obtained from natural raw materials by distillation with water or steam or from the epicarp of citrus fruits by a mechanical process or by dry distillation. The essential oil is subsequently separated from the aqueous phase by physical means.

This criterion sets essential oils apart from other plant extracts, such as those produced with solvents (e.g., hexane or supercritical fluid extraction), which can have quite different chemical compositions and organoleptic properties (Kotnik et al, 2007; Pourmortazavi et al, 2007). These differences mean that the therapeutic effects of these two types of extracts cannot always be compared. Newer advanced technology, however, such as microwave hydrodiffusion with gravity, offers the potential for new extraction methods that yield products of composition similar to that obtained with distillation (Vian et al, 2008), while economizing on time and energy for extraction.

While aromatherapists use predominantly essential oils as defined earlier, they may also use aromatic extracts (e.g., absolutes, resinoids, carbon dioxide extracts), because these products often have a fragrance that is very close to that of the original plant. These extracts are thus frequently used more to confer fragrance benefits than to produce specific physiological or pharmacological benefits.

Other related natural products at the aromatherapist's disposal include the following:

- Hydrolats (also known as hydrosols), fragrant waters that are the second product of distillation and are used predominantly for their therapeutic benefits in topical preparations.
- Fixed/vegetable oils of varying origin and fatty acid composition chosen for their benefits for skin applications or simply as fatty vehicles for essential oil dilution and administration.

- Macerated or infused oils such as arnica, calendula, or St. John's wort incorporated into blends as active bases to complement essential oil efficacy.
- Creams, lotions, gels, and other bases, which are also used as required.

AN EVER-EVOLVING THERAPY

Over the past 20 years as the use of essential oils has grown in popularity and potential, their versatility has led to different styles of aromatherapy, the main ones of which are shown in Figure 23-1. As can be seen, the aromatic medicine style is usually considered to be a branch of herbal medicine rather than purely associated with aromatherapy as it is most commonly perceived.

HOLISTIC AROMATHERAPY

Holistic aromatherapy usually combines essential oils with body massage (see Chapters 16 and 17), and this application remains the main form of aromatherapy as taught and practiced worldwide, with at least 6000 aromatherapists practicing in the United Kingdom alone (Walker et al, 2002). Characteristics of this form of aromatherapy include the following:

- Low doses (0.5% to 2%) of essential oils are blended into lipophilic bases such as vegetable oil or lotion and applied to the body with massage.
- The concept of the "individual prescription" with client participation in essential oil selection is regarded as an important part of the therapy process.
- Essential oils are usually blended together (between two and four essential oils), and the fragrance of the overall combination is a main consideration.
- More than one aromatherapy session is usually necessary, with between four and six sessions being the norm.
- A holistic approach is taken with thorough consultation and focus on balance to the body-mind.
- Self-care and home use of essential oils between therapy sessions is usually actively promoted.

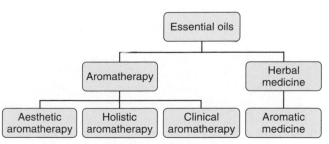

Figure 23-1 Different styles of aromatherapy.

- The main risks to the client relate to the methods of administration used; thus dermatitis (irritant, photocontact, or allergic) along with mucous membrane irritation are the key hazards.

The Holistic Aromatherapist

A profile of the average aromatherapist was compiled from a U.K.-based survey conducted in 2001 (Osborn et al). Obviously these trends are not necessarily representative of all countries where aromatherapy is practiced, but in the author's opinion they do reflect an international profile of holistic-style aromatherapists. Key profile points include the following:

- Most holistic aromatherapists are women.
- Most are middle aged.
- Most are from the middle to upper income bracket.
- Most also practice other complementary therapies, including reflexology, massage, Indian head massage, and energy therapies such as reiki.
- Most are in private practice, although aromatherapy might not be their main source of income.
- Most are working from home or providing domiciliary visits.
- Many also volunteer their aromatherapy services in the community (in rehabilitation centers, hospice settings, residential facilities).
- They liaise with and actively refer to other health care professionals.

AROMATIC MEDICINE OR MEDICAL AROMATHERAPY

As can be seen in Figure 23-1, aromatic medicine, or medical aromatherapy, has its origins in phytotherapy and largely arises, is taught, and is practiced in European countries such as Germany and France where only those who are licensed medical professionals are legally permitted to practice. This more intensive and often internal use of essential oils is now being increasingly taught and practiced in other countries such as the United Kingdom where there may be greater freedom to practice by nonlicensed medical professionals such as herbalists, traditional Chinese medicine practitioners, and practitioners of aromatic medicine (these are usually qualified aromatherapists who have pursued supplementary training in this discipline). This style of aromatherapy is characterized by the following:

- Essential oils are prescribed to treat a range of predominantly physical disorders (e.g., infection, pain, inflammation, specific pathologies).
- Administration methods include topical, oral, sublingual, rectal, vaginal, and inhalational.
- Dosages vary widely according to requirements but are generally higher or more intensive than those employed in holistic aromatherapy.
- Essential oils and other active agents such as herbal tinctures might be used in combination, and they

are usually administered by the patient himself or herself rather than by the practitioner.
- It is usually the pharmacological activity of the essential oils that determines their selection rather than aroma or psychophysiological effects.
- The overall formulation takes into account the chemistry of each active ingredient along with the pathologies concerned as the main considerations.
- Selection of essential oils is usually made by the practitioner with little patient participation.
- Risks to the client are mainly related to the administration methods employed, and thus dermatitis, mucous membrane irritation, and toxicity and drug–essential oil interactions are all possible.

The Medical Aromatherapist

A profile of the medical aromatherapist has not yet been determined, but because of the more allopathic approach, it is hardly surprising that trends resemble those among orthodox practitioners, especially in terms of gender. Having worked closely with medical aromatherapists over a number of years, the author has the following observations.

- There is a larger representation of male practitioners than among holistic aromatherapists.
- Practitioners combine essential oil prescriptions with other orthodox care methods for diagnosis and treatment.
- They are more likely to combine prescriptions with alternative forms of medicine such as homeopathy, acupuncture, and herbal medicine.
- They are more likely to be in private practice than employed in a national health service.
- They are less likely to practice other therapies that involve direct care delivery such as massage.

CLINICAL AROMATHERAPY

When essential oils are integrated into medical environments to address particular patient challenges alongside mainstream care, the practice is often termed *clinical aromatherapy*. It effectively represents a merging of both holistic and medical styles that are adapted to individual needs. While most interventions in medical environments still tend toward use of the lower-dose and external and inhalational methods, as in holistic aromatherapy, there is an increasing trend toward and acceptance of using more intensive interventions where necessary for particular clinical challenges, such as pain management, malodor control, wound care, oral care, and treatment of infection. This style of aromatherapy is characterized by the following:

- A holistic approach, especially with regard to well-being and anxiety reduction, remains a key feature of the clinical aromatherapist's role.

- Interventions are often brief and specifically focussed (e.g., anxiety management, relief of nausea, oral care, wound care, pain relief).
- Most interventions involve topical (including buccal) application or inhalation. Ingestion or rectal administration is less frequent.
- Clinical aromatherapy is usually delivered by a trained practitioner as part of regular health care provision.
- Involvement of the caregiver or the patient's immediate family is often a key element in care provision.
- There is active liaison with other health professionals.

The Clinical Aromatherapist

The development of essential oil use in the clinical environment was and remains largely nurse driven, although in many settings it is not a prerequisite that the practitioner be medically qualified (e.g., nurse, midwife); indeed, many aromatherapists working in hospitals and hospice settings are not nurses. They are often qualified therapists who have a good understanding of pathology and experience in their specialist area. For example, before working in the cancer care or hospice setting, aromatherapists often pursue supplementary training to prepare them specifically for this field. A range of specialist texts and articles exist for clinical aromatherapy integration (Buckle, 2003a, 2000b; Dunning, 2007; Price et al, 2007; Smith et al, 2008; Tiran, 2000).

As yet there has been no survey of clinical aromatherapists, but based on the author's experience in working and training in this style, a typical profile becomes apparent:

- Most clinical aromatherapists are women.
- Many but not all have current or prior medical training in disciplines such as nursing, midwifery, physiotherapy, and occupational therapy.
- Many are able to use essential oils within their full or part-time employment as part of their role (e.g. nurse-aromatherapists or midwife-aromatherapists).
- Others are employed as aromatherapists in a specialized health sector such as midwifery, cancer care or geriatric care.
- Many have education to a higher level (e.g., university).
- More aromatherapy research is conducted by or supported by clinical aromatherapists than by either holistic or medical aromatherapists.
- They are more likely to critically evaluate their work, conduct research and document their findings in professional publications.

AESTHETIC AROMATHERAPY

Aesthetic aromatherapy has its origins in the Anglo-Saxon holistic style of aromatherapy in which pioneers of the art and science of aromatherapy such as Marguerite Maury explored the cosmetic benefits of essential oils combined with the whole aromatherapy experience, including massage. Today, work in the research and development departments of many leading cosmetic companies has led to the inclusion of essential oils in cosmetic products as active agents, and research exists to confirm the role of essential oils in skin care. Because of financial rivalry, results of cosmetic research conducted by leading companies are not widely diffused in the professional literature. What has been published confirms the valuable role of essential oils in dermatology (Denda et al, 2000; Hosoi et al, 2000; Monges et al, 1994; Mori et al, 2002), and one specialist aromatherapy text now exists for this field (Bensouilah et al, 2006).

The surge in popularity of the spa movement has also led to aromatherapy's being offered for well-being and cosmetic benefit. Many therapists training for the spa setting receive rudimentary instruction in aromatherapy along with other spa techniques and often use pre-blended commercial products rather than providing individualized care. It is also now common for basic aromatherapy training to be included in aesthetician's training programs.

Although the main styles of aromatherapy have been detailed earlier, there can be significant variations and, depending on the country in which each method has evolved, differences in technique and application. For example, while in the United Kingdom aromatherapy training and practice almost invariably include massage, in the United States (due to massage licensing laws, which can vary among states) often holistic aromatherapists are not massage practitioners, working instead with custom blends of essential oils that are then promoted for use in self-care. In addition, the various aromatherapy styles show significant interdependence, with holistic care usually at the core of all the styles (Figure 23-2).

It is also apparent from the earlier discussion that the main styles of aromatherapy may have different training requirements; however, the reality is that, although training provision is well structured for holistic aromatherapy, with minimum standards already established in a number of countries, training in clinical and medical styles is less well recognized and standards

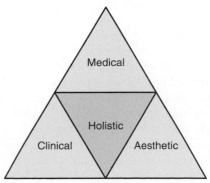

Figure 23-2 Interdependence of styles of aromatherapy.

are not consistent internationally. For example, in France, training in the medical aromatherapy style that is aimed at medical professionals is extremely variable in duration and content. A recent bold move in Australia is the establishment of national training standards and competencies for aromatic medicine as separate from aromatherapy (available through http://www. NTIS.gov.au); it is the first such move in the world, and it is anticipated that other countries will respond in a similar fashion in the future.

THERAPEUTIC POTENTIAL

There is a wealth of research to support the therapeutic value of essential oils, and in recent years this evidence has become increasingly disseminated and accessible in professional publications. The immense psychophysiological potential of essential oils is due to two or three factors.

1. Essential oils are fragrant substances. Thus they are able to impact the body-mind via the olfactory sense, with all its deep-seated limbic and higher brain connections that influence, among other things, emotions, memory, desire, basic drive, and hormonal response. The olfactory neurons travel directly to the frontal portions of the brain. For these reasons, inhalation of essential oil fragrance is considered a key aspect of an aromatherapy treatment.

The capacity of fragrant substances to influence emotions and behavior has led to the field of Aroma-Chology as defined by the Sense of Smell Institute (formerly the Olfactory Research Fund; http://www.senseofsmell.org) in 1989. This field is dedicated to the study of measurable effects of the interrelationships between psychology and fragrance technology and is not restricted to essential oils and naturally derived aromatics. However, there is a significant overlap between Aroma-Chology and aromatherapy, with aromatherapists going a step further to seek physiological benefits of essential oils, either indirectly via the olfactory sense or more directly through their absorption and pharmacological activity. A recent systematic review addressing the psychophysiological effects (on mood, cognition, behavior, performance, physiology) of fragrant substances (Herz, 2009) confirms that they can significantly impact the body-mind via inhalation.

Aromatherapists use these confirmed mood-enhancing benefits of fragrance to reduce stress and thereby improve general health and well-being. However, these effects are largely influenced by context, expectation, prior experience of the aroma, its concentration when presented, and perception of the fragrance as pleasant or unpleasant. Indeed, it may be possible that psychological effects can override the potential physiological properties of an essential oil (Moss et al, 2006; Robbins et al, 2007). This may explain the inconsistencies that are sometimes found when attempts are made to measure the effects of individual essential oils

on the body-mind (Neale et al, 2008). There is nevertheless supportive evidence for the positive and measurable effects of aromatherapy in relieving stress and anxiety and promoting well-being over a range of administration methods and evaluation tools (Atsumi et al, 2007; Cooke et al, 2000; Morris, 2008; Saeki, 2000).

2. Essential oils are pharmacologically active. Their chemical components are secondary metabolites produced by the plant predominantly for defensive purposes, and they are thus biologically active substances. Because of their lipophilic nature and small molecular size, many components of essential oils are able to penetrate the body irrespective of their route of administration and exert a pharmacological impact either locally (in the tissues surrounding their application site) or systemically (via the bloodstream). For these reasons, essential oils are often administered via different routes according to the needs of the individual. The capacity of essential oil components to enter the bloodstream via different routes has been studied, at least for inhalation (Buchbauer et al, 1991; Jager et al, 1996; Stimpfl et al, 1995) and topical administration (Fewell et al, 2007; Fuchs et al, 1997; Jager et al, 1992), and pharmacological effects are confirmed via ingestion for a range of pathologies (Goerg et al, 2003; Juergens et al, 2003; Kerhl et al, 2004). Because of the increased physical and metabolic barriers at the skin interface (stratum corneum, especially) compared with other routes of administration, this route is likely to result in extremely low (but nonnegligible) amounts of active components' reaching the bloodstream.

Assuming therefore that some essential oil components are able to enter the tissues locally and/or enter the bloodstream, there are a number of pharmacological possibilities. The main actions are listed in Table 23-1.

In addition to the aforementioned fragrance and pharmacological factors, many aromatherapists would add the following third dimension to essential oil therapeutics.

3. Essential oils are able to impact the individual at a subtle or vibrational level. Many therapists refer to essential oils as the "life force" of the plant and believe that their vibrational energetic qualities are able to influence the individual on a subtle level. Thus practitioners of different forms of energy medicine such as traditional Chinese and Ayurvedic medicines may use essential oils as part of their therapy and select these remedies according to energetic principles. A number of aromatherapy texts support these energetic approaches (Holmes, 2007, 2008; Miller et al, 1995; Mojay, 1996). While it is as yet hard to find credible and reproducible evidence for the energetic-vibrational impact of essential oils, as has been previously seen, the impact of fragrance on the body-mind as well as the pharmacological activity of essential oils has been well studied. The vibrational energies of different flowering plants have been developed to offer their own forms of therapy, as with the Bach flower remedies, for example.

TABLE 23-1
Main Pharmacological Actions of Essential Oils

Action	Research studies (not exhaustive)
Analgesic	Yip et al, 2008 (ginger and orange)
	Le Faou et al, 2005
	Greenway et al, 2003 (geranium)
Antibacterial	Cermelli et al, 2008
	Enshaieh et al, 2007
	Dryden et al, 2004
Antifungal	Soković et al, 2008
	Khosravi et al, 2008
	Jirovetz et al, 2007
Antiinflammatory	Chao et al, 2008 (cinnamaldehyde)
	Lee et al, 2007
	Ghazanfari et al, 2006
Antioxidant	Singh et al, 2008
	Chung et al, 2007
	Zhang et al, 2006
Antiparasitic	Navarro et al, 2008
	Scanni et al, 2006
	Oladimeji et al, 2005
Antispasmodic	Goornemann et al, 2008
	Grigoleit et al, 2005
	Jahromi et al, 2003
Antiviral	Schnitzler et al, 2008
	Schnitzler et al, 2007
	Giraud-Robert, 2005
Carminative	Alexandrovich et al, 2003
	Goerg et al, 2003
Cicatrisant	Amanlou et al, 2007
	Orafidiya et al, 2005
	Orafidiya et al, 2003
Deodorizing	Warnke et al, 2006
	Mercier et al, 2005
	Sherry et al, 2003
Immune stimulating	Nam et al, 2008
	Serafino et al, 2008
	Mikhaeil et al, 2003
Mucolytic and expectorant	Fenu et al, 2008
	Kehrl et al, 2004
	Mattys et al, 2000
Rubefacient	Xu et al, 2006
	Hong et al, 1991
	Green et al, 1989
Sedative	Moss et al, 2006
	Lim et al, 2005
	Koo et al, 2003

EVALUATION

How the effectiveness of aromatherapy is assessed and reported in the literature is highly variable, ranging from single case study reports and evidence-based articles in professional publications to surveys of service provision,

audits, and full-scale clinical trials. A review of the literature demonstrates that the last 10 years have witnessed an increase in both the number and quality of documented benefits of aromatherapy integration into the clinical environment. The challenge always remains of how to evaluate successfully the benefits of what is in fact a multifaceted therapy that typically combines fragrance (aroma) with touch (typically with massage), potential pharmacological activity (chemical components), individualized care, and positive client-therapist interaction. For these reasons it is not surprising that some still question the validity of many aromatherapy interventions (e.g., Cooke et al, 2000). Wherever possible, this chapter reports on recent work and research and focuses mainly on human studies.

CLINICAL APPLICATIONS

Aromatherapy is increasingly integrated into a wide range of health care settings. These are summarized (not in order of prevalence) in Box 23-1.

To provide concrete examples of where and how aromatherapy is increasingly integrated, the following sections outline five of these clinical areas in more detail:

- Midwifery
- Cancer and palliative care
- Elder care
- Special needs
- Psychiatry

BOX 23-1
Examples of Health Care Areas into Which Aromatherapy Is Being Integrated

Cancer care
Critical care
Drug rehabilitation
Elder care
HIV/AIDS care
Midwifery
Neurology
Pain management
Palliative care
Pediatrics
Pneumology/ears, nose, and throat
Postoperative care
Preprocedural care
Prison and young offender units
Psychiatry
Rheumatology
Special needs
Sports rehabilitation
Therapy for staff and caregivers
Wound care

AIDS, Acquired immunodeficiency syndrome; *HIV,* human immunodeficiency virus.

MIDWIFERY

The holistic and clinical styles of aromatherapy have been used in pregnancy care and midwifery for many years, assisting the mother-to-be predominantly in stress and anxiety management but also providing relief with common pregnancy-associated symptoms such as nausea, skin changes, altered sleep patterns, pain, and fatigue. In the labor environment, essential oils are most often administered by midwife-aromatherapists, whereas preconception, antenatal, and postnatal aromatherapy care is often provided by nonmidwife aromatherapists and doulas.

The accidental or deliberate misuse of essential oils can pose a risk to the unborn child (Anderson et al, 1996; Weiss, 1973); however, so far no reports have been published of pregnancy-related risk when the holistic style of aromatherapy is used, although some have labelled aromatherapy provision by nonmidwives as "an accident waiting to happen" (Tiran, 1996). This issue of safety is a hotly debated topic in the midwifery field, and opinions differ as to what dosages should be employed and which essential oils are safe or hazardous in pregnancy. These discrepancies are due to lack of reporting of adverse effects, and thus risk assessment is based on prediction, speculation, and each practitioner's individual experience in this field. A few essential oil components such as sabinyl acetate have been confirmed as potentially hazardous to fetal development in animal studies (Pages et al, 1996); however, these components are not found in the essential oils commonly used in holistic aromatherapy.

Providing stress reduction during labor has multiple benefits for both mother and baby. These include less need for mechanical intervention and opioid analgesia, reduced use of epidural anesthesia, improved mobility during labor, and generally increased control over the labor process, all of which may contribute to a safer birthing process and a more alert baby (Bastard et al, 2006; Burns, 2005; Burns et al, 2000, 2007; Fanner, 2005; Simkin et al, 2007).

In the postnatal period, benefits can also be seen, including improved psychological status, improved bonding, and increased coping skills (Antoniak, 2008; Imura et al, 2006; Meyer, 2005).

CANCER CARE AND PALLIATIVE CARE

Along with the favorable effects of aromatherapy in midwifery, its benefits in oncology and palliative care environments are increasingly well surveyed, documented, and researched. Aromatherapy is the most popular complementary therapy for persons with cancer in the United Kingdom. The predominant style used in this setting is holistic aromatherapy coupled with massage or light touch techniques, and the focus is mostly on anxiety reduction and promotion of well-being (Abel, 2000; Cawthorne et al, 2000; De Valois et al, 2001; Dyer, 2004; Imanishi et al, 2009; Peace et al, 2002; Stringer, 2000; Wilkinson et al, 1999). With regard to

improvement in well-being and reduction of anxiety and fatigue, research shows that aromatherapy can offer significant benefit, at least in the short term, to persons with cancer and to their families and/or caregivers (Curry et al, 2008; Wilkinson et al, 2007). In some countries such as the United Kingdom clear guidelines have been established for the use of complementary therapies like aromatherapy in palliative care (Tavares, 2003).

A more recent development in oncology and palliative care is the increasing use of non–massage-associated clinical aromatherapy interventions with positive results for challenges such as nausea, fatigue, malodor, breathlessness, pain relief, wound management, skin care, and oral care (Dyer et al, 2008; Knevitt, 2004; Kohara et al, 2004; Louis et al, 2002; Mercier et al, 2005; Schwan, 2004; Warnke et al, 2006). These clinical interventions include the use of essential oils in the following:

- Foot baths
- Inhaler devices
- Nasal gels
- Airborne diffusers
- Airborne spritzers
- Topical preparations
- Wound dressings
- Mouth rinses

ELDER CARE

Aromatherapy is a well-established treatment in elder care in various countries, particularly in residential care environments. Nursing home physicians are generally in favor of using nonpharmacological interventions for management of behavioral disturbances associated with dementia, but their level of knowledge is variable; this may restrict patient access to therapies such as aromatherapy (Cohen-Mansfield et al, 2008).

Benefits have been reported in working with individuals who have dementia/Alzheimer disease, including help in reducing agitation, modifying behavior, providing stimulation and social interaction, and assisting in orientation (Ballard et al, 2002; Holmes et al, 2002; MacMahon et al, 1998; Smallwood et al, 2001), although a recent Cochrane systematic review confirms that more sound research evidence is required in this area (Thorgrimsen et al, 2003). In some cases of severe dementia, aromatherapy massage interventions might actually lead to an increase in agitation (Brooker et al, 1997). *Lavandula angustifolia* (lavender) essential oil is one of the most commonly used essential oils for elderly populations (Bowles et al, 2005); the benefit of its inhalation in reducing dementia-related agitation in one Chinese crossover randomized trial has been confirmed (Lin et al, 2007). Another element of importance in this field is providing aromatherapy support for caregivers of persons with dementia, who themselves are subject to significant stress and decline in health (Henry, 2008).

Other benefits of aromatherapy in these settings include malodor control and potential reduction in need for medication (Berlie, 2008) as well as improvement in sleep patterns in the older patient (Cannard, 1996). A recent study demonstrates that odor stimuli such as those provided by essential oils—in this case *Piper nigrum* (black pepper) and *Lavandula angustifolia* (lavender)—may improve posture and balance in older persons (Freeman et al, 2009), who are more prone to falling, whereas odor stimuli such as black pepper and menthol can assist in improving the swallowing reflex (Ebihara, Ebihara, and Maruyama, 2006; Ebihara, Ebihara, and Watando, 2006).

Another aspect of aromatherapy care for this age group is the management of pain (especially chronic pain). Here there is evidence that aromatherapy can offer at least short-term assistance with pain management (Bensouilah, 2004; Bowles et al, 2005; Yip et al, 2008).

SPECIAL NEEDS

In the field of special needs, a number of aromatherapists work independently, and to the author's knowledge, few clinical trials have been conducted in this domain. Therapists work with a range of patients with special needs, such as deaf and deaf-blind individuals (Armstrong et al, 2000), individuals with autism (Ellwood, 2008), and those with other mental health and special needs (Durell, 2002; Greenwood, 2008). One specialist text exists on aromatherapy for people with learning difficulties (Sanderson et al, 1991). Case reports, articles, and therapists' experience in the special needs environment demonstrate real benefits of using essential oils, some of which are the following:

- Promoting relaxation and well-being
- Aiding communication
- Reinforcing positive acceptance of touch
- Empowering the individual
- Improving mobility and posture
- Encouraging trust and confidence
- Helping with orientation in time and space

In most cases, therapy is given coupled with massage or other touch techniques and incorporates the use of other sensory stimuli. However, one crossover study examining four interventions (Snoezelen therapy, relaxation therapy, aromatherapy hand massage, and physical activity) did not find that the aromatherapy intervention was beneficial for improving alertness in individuals with profound learning disabilities (Lindsay et al, 1997).

PSYCHIATRY

As has already been shown, the benefits of fragrance on mood, cognition, and behavior are well established, and thus it is not surprising to find that aromatherapy is used widely in the care of persons with affective disorders and mental health issues. Indeed, olfactory impairment is associated with depressive behavior and occurs in the early stages of several central nervous system and neuropsychiatric diseases, such as depression, Parkinson disease, schizophrenia, Alzheimer disease, and multiple sclerosis (Atanasova et al, 2008; Moscavitch et al, 2009).

Self-care with essential oils to improve mood and well-being is common in the general population, and persons with mild to moderate depression and anxiety disorders are more likely to seek complementary therapies such as aromatherapy than are those with severe depression (Hsu et al, 2008). In addition to benefiting from simple self-care measures such as lavender baths for reducing anxiety (Morris, 2008), residents in short-term psychiatric care facilities may also profit from aromatherapy under the guidance of a qualified therapist, as reported by Kyle (2008).

Aromatherapy offers many benefits to the individual with psychiatric illness, including the following:

- Establishing a sense of normalcy
- Improving self-esteem and well-being
- Encouraging self-care
- Increasing confidence and providing choice
- Raising mood
- Increasing social interaction
- Improving sleep

In psychiatry, the main benefits of essential oils come through their inhalation via diffusion or the use of scented products applied to the skin or added to baths, with massage conferring added psychophysiological benefit. Inhalation of a pleasantly perceived fragrance has confirmed benefits in humans in reducing symptoms of depression and improving general immune function (Komori et al, 1995).When coupled with other mind-oriented therapies such as counselling, relaxation therapy, or hypnotherapy, a form of "odor conditioning" can be used successfully to assist the person, particularly in the realm of stress and anxiety management. This application is well illustrated in the work of Spector et al (1993) on the use of odor cues to promote relaxation in the treatment of speech anxiety and in the work of Betts (2003) on reducing the incidence of epileptiform convulsions through association of fragrance with hypnosis.

In addition to the aforementioned benefits, which are largely due to the effects of a pleasant fragrance, there may also be pharmacological activity, which further increases sedative, anxiolytic, and mood-enhancing effects (Buchbauer et al, 1993). The degree of sedation achieved may be on a par with that produced by benzodiazepines or other hypnotic medications and indeed may assist with withdrawal from or reduction in dependence on these drugs (Hardy et al, 1995; Komori et al, 2006). Both traditional and scientific evidence exists supporting the use of *Lavandula angustifolia* (lavender) and *Melissa officinalis* (lemon balm) essential oils to benefit individuals with anxiety, depression, and psychotic disorders (Abuhamdah et al, 2008; Huang et al, 2008).

It can be seen from the foregoing discussion that aromatherapy is increasingly accepted and implemented alongside mainstream medical care for patients in a diverse range of settings. Many essential oils are used in therapy worldwide. The most common ones are listed in Box 23-2.

BOX 23-2

Twenty-Seven Essential Oils Commonly Used in Clinical Environments (Latin Name and Common Name)

Boswellia carterii, frankincense
Cananga odorata, ylang ylang
Chamaemelum nobile, Roman chamomile
Citrus aurantium var. *amara flos.,* neroli
Citrus aurantium var. *amara fol.,* petitgrain
Citrus bergamia, bergamot
Citrus paradisii, grapefruit
Citrus sinensis, sweet orange
Cupressus sempervirens, cypress
Cymbopogon citratus, lemongrass
Cymbopogon martinii, palmarosa
Eucalyptus radiata, eucalyptus
Lavandula angustifolia, lavender
Lavandula latifolia, spike lavender
Matricaria recutita, German chamomile
Melaleuca alternifolia, tea tree
Mentha citrata, bergamot mint
Mentha x piperita, peppermint
Origanum majorana, sweet marjoram
Pelargonium x asperum, geranium
Piper nigrum, black pepper
Rosa damascena, rose
Rosmarinus officinalis, rosemary
Sabinyl acetate, juniper
Santalum album, sandalwood
Vetiveria zizanioides, vetiver
Zingiber officinale, ginger

Potential benefits such as lowered perception of stress by staff and caregivers comprise another important area of aromatherapy provision (Curry et al, 2008; Pemberton et al, 2008; Tysoe, 2000). Because of the multifaceted nature of the therapy, it can be challenging to measure outcomes effectively, but there is now increasingly sound qualitative and quantitative evidence to encourage its continued use in specialty areas such as elder care and cancer and palliative care. It is always essential, however, to link efficacy with safety, and issues of safe practice are of paramount importance.

ISSUES CONCERNING SAFE PRACTICE

Essential oils, as concentrated active agents, have the capacity to cause harm if not used appropriately. Because of their widespread inclusion in foods, flavorings, fragrances, and cosmetics, many have been rigorously assessed for their potential hazards, and guidelines exist for safe levels of their inclusion in these products, such as the code of practice and guidelines established by the International Fragrance Association (http://www.ifraorg.org) and the "generally recognized as safe" (GRAS) status conferred by the Flavor and Extracts Manufacturers Association (http://www.femaflavor.org). However, these limits and guidelines are not always applicable or relevant to the way that essential oils are employed in aromatherapy, and thus further safety advice for this discipline is of utmost importance.

Given the main routes of administration of essential oils, the predominant potential hazards are dermatitic reactions (allergic, irritant, and photocontact) and mucous membrane irritation. The risk of toxicity is very low unless the essential oil is consumed or used in inappropriate concentrations on the skin.

RISK TO THE CLIENT

There have been very few documented cases of client harm as a result of essential oil use when the oils are administered or recommended by aromatherapists. However, reporting of adverse effects is not well coordinated. Some aromatherapy member associations are considering implementing a yellow card vigilance scheme such as the Adverse Reactions to Aromatherapy (ARIA) system recently adopted by the International Federation of Professional Aromatherapists (http://www.ifparoma.org) for its members, whereby practitioners and patients can report adverse reactions should they arise (Kayne, 2006). Thus far, reporting has been extremely low.

Accidental or deliberate misuse of essential oils in the home environment is more widely reported and often involves children, who are generally more vulnerable to adverse effects (Beccara, 1995; Darben et al, 1998; Tibballs, 1995). Consistent abuse of airborne aromatics in the home environment can also lead to airborne contact dermatitis (Schaller et al, 1995) as well as skin allergy (Weiss et al, 1997). Occupational exposure can also lead to contact dermatitis reactions (Ackerman et al, 2009; Wakelin et al, 1998).

Anecdotal negative reporting regarding the use of professional aromatherapy in clinical environments includes instances in which clients or care staff find some aromas too harsh or strong, provoking headaches, malaise, nausea, or coughing, although such cases are extremely rare.

Because it is exceptionally difficult to control for adverse incidents in the use of essential oils by the general public, who have easy access to these potent substances without the necessary safety information, support, and guidance, the role of the aromatherapist as educator is of paramount importance.

RISK TO THE THERAPIST

Considering the increased exposure that aromatherapists have to essential oils and related products, in terms of both dose and frequency of exposure, it is not surprising that there is more reporting of risk to the therapist than of risk to the client, especially with regard to skin reactions such as allergic contact dermatitis, although these, too, remain sparsely documented. There are a number of case reports of aromatherapists (usually those who have been in practice for a number of years) becoming sensitized or allergic to the products that they consistently use over time (Bleasel et al, 2002; Selvaag et al, 1995). Because many of these products have similar chemical composition, once sensitization is established the therapist often reacts to not just one but several essential oils, which in some cases necessitates a change in career.

ESSENTIAL OIL QUALITY AND RISK FACTORS

It has been known for a number of years that the presence of oxidized essential oil components increases the risk of contact allergy and skin irritation (Chang et al, 1997; Christensson et al, 2008, 2009; Wakelin et al, 1998). These include the oxidation products of very common and unstable components such as d-limonene and linalool. This fact makes the issue of quality control of utmost importance to the aromatherapist in terms of sourcing and storage of essential oils. An additional challenge for the therapist is to obtain fresh and high-quality essential oils that are fully identified with regard to their species, plant part origin, and precise chemical composition.

POTENTIAL CONFLICT WITH MEDICATIONS

Few documented drug–essential oil interactions have been reported in the literature, and most pertain to the internal consumption of essential oils rather than exposure via dermal application or inhalation. This situation is in contrast to the well-documented drug-herb interactions such as those involving *Hypericum perforatum, Panax ginseng, Gingko biloba,* and other herbs. As a result of lack of reporting, much of the information on risk of interactions between drugs and essential oils is speculative, with most research evidence coming from animal studies rather than actual reporting of interactions in humans.

Most potential for interaction lies in the fact that many essential oil components have been found to be inducers or inhibitors of enzyme systems such as members of the cytochrome P-450 family and glutathione *S*-transferase (Ganzera et al, 2006; Jori et al, 1969; Lam et al, 1991; Parke et al, 1974). However, because of pharmacokinetic differences as well as the relatively low concentrations of doses of essential oils when they are inhaled or topically applied, the likelihood of drug–essential oil interaction is greatly reduced if traditional holistic aromatherapy interventions are used (unless the drug is also administered topically or inhaled).

When essential oils are taken orally on a regular basis, however, given their concentrated nature, the risk of interaction is possibly equal to or greater than that with ingested herbal medicines. The fact that as yet there is little reporting of this risk may relate to the relatively recent upsurge in interest and use of ingestion as a means of administering essential oils. The aromatherapy profession needs to remain vigilant in this regard, because in some countries, ingestion of essential oils by the general public without support or professional supervision is increasingly promoted by companies, and the assumption is that natural products are without risk and are safe alternatives to medical care.

Even when essential oils are administered via inhalation, the therapist needs to be aware of possible conflicts, such as between essential oils that contain 1,8-cineole (e.g., niaouli, eucalyptus) and certain drugs like barbiturates (Jori et al, 1970). This component has been shown to induce enzyme systems and thus drug detoxification.

As with all potential drug interactions, the risk is raised when the patient is prescribed drugs that have a low therapeutic index, such as warfarin, barbiturates, and digoxin. With these medications, any small shift in serum levels can have profound consequences, and thus typically aromatherapists use lower doses of oils and work only with topical and inhaled formulations for patients taking these medications. They also need to be aware of the increased risk associated with certain essential oils containing potent components such as methyl salicylate (e.g., wintergreen) and eugenol (e.g., cloves), even when applied externally, because of the higher risk of bleeding if the patient is taking anticoagulant therapy or has a clotting disorder (Joss et al, 2000; Srivastava et al, 1990).

When essential oils are administered via the skin, the therapist needs to beware of potential conflict with topical drug preparations such as corticosteroids and transdermal drug delivery systems such as nicotine patches, hormone patches, and nausea medication patches.

INDIVIDUALS AT HIGHER RISK

As can be seen, the risk of harm from essential oils when used appropriately is extremely low. Certain individuals may be more at risk than others from essential oil hazards; these groups are listed in Box 23-3. Although aromatherapy is not contraindicated for these individuals, it is common for the aromatherapist to use extra caution with essential oil selection, dose, and route of administration to minimize risk.

FUTURE POTENTIAL FOR THE THERAPY

As can be seen, with the increase in research and publication of studies in professional journals that demonstrate the therapeutic benefits of essential oils in clinical settings, the future looks bright for continued integration

Individuals Most at Risk for Essential Oil Hazard

- Elderly
- Children and babies
- Pregnant women
- Individuals with skin diseases such as eczema
- Individuals with fragrance and cosmetic allergies
- Individuals with a history of allergy (including asthma, eczema)
- Individuals taking multiple medications, especially those with a low therapeutic index such as digoxin, warfarin, barbiturates
- Individuals with unstable medical conditions
- Individuals who have a history of an unstable psychiatric condition and who are taking psychotropic medications
- Individuals with significant renal or hepatic dysfunction

into a range of medical settings, especially as training standards improve and specialist courses are developed for certain areas such as elder care, psychiatry, oncology, palliative care, and midwifery.

A significant, as yet relatively unimplemented aspect of essential oil therapeutics is the role of essential oils in the realm of infection control (prevention and treatment). There is ever-increasing evidence that essential oils can exert significant antimicrobial effects via both direct contact (Jirovetz et al, 2007; Sherry et al, 2003) and airborne contact (Inouye, 2003; Inoue et al, 2001, 2003; Krist et al, 2006; Pibiri et al, 2006, Sato et al, 2007) and that they may offer antimicrobial solutions for multidrug-resistant organisms such as methicillin-resistant *Staphylococcus aureus* (Caelli et al, 2000; Dryden et al, 2004; Opalchenova et al, 2003). The natural presence of essential oils protects their host plants from microbial predation, and these oils may exert these same influences in clinical settings. This activity raises real possibilities for essential oils to offer direct solutions in clinical environments that typically have a high microbial load, in which patients are more likely to be prone to nosocomial infections that are resistant to antibiotic or antifungal therapy.

SUMMARY

With the increasing acceptance and efficacy of aromatherapy in the clinical setting, this discipline is also increasingly subject to scrutiny to ensure safety and cost effectiveness. Although ultimately these measures are beneficial in the long term, we may well see a reduction in aromatherapy service provision in the current health care climate until its efficacy, cost effectiveness, and safety can be further demonstrated. In a cost-driven society with the financial constraints that exist in medical settings, where departments of finance hold the purse strings and choose essential oil suppliers by cost alone, the result can be the sourcing of cheaper essential oils of poorer quality for therapy. This practice can ultimately be detrimental in terms of both reduced efficacy and increased risk to the client.

In addition, with the increase in the risk of litigation, certain constraints are put on the therapy that also can limit its potential use. One example is the use of airborne diffusion for effective disinfection in clinical environments. Despite clear evidence demonstrating the potential of these active agents to provide airborne disinfection, significantly reducing microbial load, including that of multiresistant strains, the diffusion of essential oils in public areas such as waiting rooms or hospital wards is not widely practiced for fear of complaint or adverse reactions that may result in legal claims.

One other limiting factor is the perceived rise in multiple chemical sensitivity syndrome and the development of "fragrance-free" environments. Because essential oils are viewed more as fragrances than as therapeutically active substances with potential benefit, their use in some hospitals has been withdrawn.

What is also needed is a clearer distinction between the main aromatherapy practice styles and greater public awareness of these styles. Currently public opinion of aromatherapy remains quite general, with little expectation as to its benefits other than providing a "feel good" therapy. Although the psychological benefits of aromatherapy can be readily appreciated through the well-being aspect of this pleasurable therapy, essential oils also offer demonstrated benefit in many other ways.

Chapter References can be found on the Evolve website at http://evolve.elsevier.com/Micozzi/complementary/

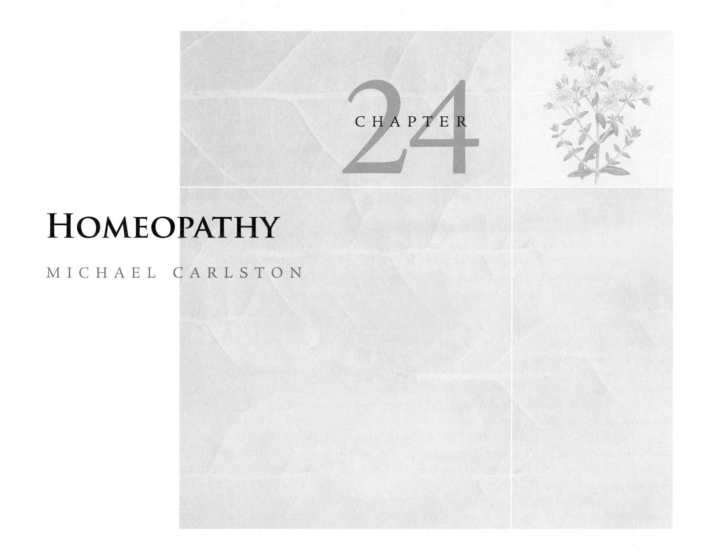

24

HOMEOPATHY

MICHAEL CARLSTON

omeopathy is a highly systematized method of heal-ing that follows the principle "use likes to treat likes" and is practiced by licensed physicians and other health care professionals throughout the world. In the United States, homeopathic medicines are protected by federal law, and most are available over the counter. Among the many challenges that homeopathy poses to conventional medicine and science, the greatest may be the common use of extremely diluted medicinal substances.

HISTORY

The homeopathic method was developed by Samuel Hahnemann, MD (1755-1843), a German physician, chemist, and author of a well-known textbook on the preparation and use of contemporary medicines (Figure 24-1). In a series of experiments conducted from 1790 to 1810, Hahnemann demonstrated that (1) medicinal substances each elicit a pattern of signs and symptoms in healthy people, and (2) the medicine whose symptom pattern most closely resembles that of the illness being treated is the one most likely to initiate a curative response for that patient (Hahnemann, 1833).

Hahnemann understood these experiments to mean that the outward manifestations of illness represent the concerted attempt of an organism to heal itself and that the corresponding remedy reinforces that attempt in some way. He coined the term *homeopathy* to describe his method of using remedies with the power to resonate with the illness as a whole, in contrast to the more conventional method of opposing symptoms with superior force.

The word *homeopathy* is derived from the Greek roots *omoios*, meaning "similar," and *pathos*, meaning "feeling." Hahnemann also began using *allopathy*, from the Greek *alloios*, meaning "other," to denote the standard practice of using medicines either to counteract symptoms or to produce an action unrelated to symptoms, such as purging, bloodletting, or blistering of the skin. ∾

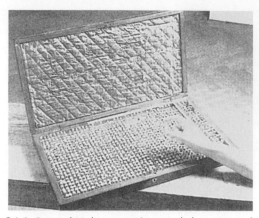

Figure 24-1 Samuel Hahnemann's remedy box. Many homeopaths kept their remedies in a similar box, but few had one that was so splendid. (From Richardson S: *Homeopathy: the illustrated guide.*)

Hippocrates, Celsus, Paracelsus, and others advocated treatment with "similars" for some patients. Hahnemann credited his teacher, Quarin, as the source of his own medical capabilities. Quarin's teacher, Stoerck, advocated testing drugs for their "like" effects: "If stramonium makes the healthy mentally sick through a confusion of the mind, why should one not determine whether it gives mental health in that it disturbs and alters the thoughts and sense in mental disease, and that if it gives health to those with spasms, to try and see if, on the other hand, they get spasms" (Stoerck, 1762).

Hahnemann was the first to base an entire therapeutic approach on the "likes cure likes" methodology. He believed that the detailed correspondence between the clinical symptoms of patients and the experimental pathogenesis of remedies reflected a universal law of healing with medicinal substances. His development of such a rigorous system integrating a medical philosophy, formalized drug testing, and protocols for clinical application is a unique achievement in medical history.

The Hahnemannian law of similars—*similia similibus curaentur,* or "Let likes be cured by likes"—never gained general acceptance in medicine and is considered implausible to most physicians. Even committed homeopaths regard it as a mystery not yet explained or proved. This tolerance of uncertainty is consistent with Hahnemann's commitment to the belief that theory must always be secondary to the patient's clinical benefit.

THEORETICAL BASIS

The physician's highest calling, his only calling, is to make sick people healthy—to heal, as it is termed.
—SAMUEL HAHNEMANN, *ORGANON OF MEDICINE*

In the opening line of the founding document of homeopathy Hahnemann forcefully establishes that the practical impact of any therapy on the patient's well-being is its sole importance. Although he goes on to elaborate the lesser significance of developing of theoretical systems, ironically many physicians and patients have been drawn to homeopathy precisely because of their attraction to the distinctive and internally consistent theoretical constructs of homeopathic medicine (Astin, 1998; Clark et al, 2008). The homeopathic view of the primacy of an inner world paralleling the common one is a familiar and appealing concept stretching across many religious and spiritual traditions, as well as more recent conceptualizations of an "energy" basis to biological organisms. Homeopathy's foundation is a radical innovation in the experimental investigation of medicinal substances. Its cardinal principles follow logically from the law of similars and the conceptual transformations required to accommodate this law.

The theory of like cures like is supported by the concept that a *symptom* represents the body's physiological response to an illness or disease in the effort to maintain homeostasis and to help heal or cure that illness or disease. For example, a fever is the physiological response to infection with pyrogenic bacteria. Elevated body temperature slows the rate of reproduction of bacteria (see Figure 1-1). Therefore, a fever is literally bacteriostatic. It was the bacteriostatic properties of early antibiotics that provided an elegant mechanism for treating infection, which resulted in the "miracle drugs" of the twentieth century.

With either fever or antibiotics, the immune system must still overcome the infection. These agents just give the body a chance to catch up by generating white blood cells faster than the bacteria can generate more bacterial cells. Thus a fever can be seen as nature's antibiotic. In the natural history of an infection, when a fever "breaks" it is a sign that the infection is being overcome. In a "healing crisis" the potentiation of a symptom like fever by a homeopathic remedy may be a means to cure.

PROVINGS

In 1790, while experimenting with cinchona (Peruvian bark), Hahnemann decided to ingest a therapeutic dose because he was frustrated by the conventional explanation of its medicinal action. Cinchona bark, also known as "Spanish bark" or "Jesuit bark," was brought back to Europe from South America, where it was used indigenously to treat remittent fevers.

It later became the source of quinine to treat malaria and quinidine to treat heart conditions. As a natural remedy with synergistic properties it remains effective against chloroquine-resistant malaria today (see Chapter 38). In Hahnemann's early experiments with cinchona, he soon experienced feelings of cold, numbness, drowsiness, thirst, and anxiety, as well as palpitations, prostration, and aching bones. He recognized these as the exact symptoms of *ague*, or intermittent fever, the syndrome that was then being treated with cinchona (Bradford, 1895). He allowed the effects of the dose to wear off before taking a second and a third dose, which confirmed his original observation that a natural substance that treated the disease also produced the same symptoms as the disease—or *like cures like.* The prevailing treatment of ague, familiar to modern readers as malaria, continued to be an extract of the cinchona tree (quinine) until recent times.

Hahnemann recognized this response as a confirmation of principles taught in Hippocratic writings and by Paracelsus. Excited by the possibilities of a fuller application of the approach, Hahnemann devoted the rest of his life to ascertaining the therapeutic properties of medicinal substances by administering them to healthy people: himself, his colleagues, and his students. His *Materia Medica Pura* records the detailed symptoms of more than 90 medicines, a monumental achievement that represents 20 years of painstaking labor (Hahnemann, 1833, 1880).

In these *provings,* as he called them, Hahnemann administered the substance in question to a group of reasonably healthy people in doses sufficient to elicit symptoms without provoking irreversible toxicity, anatomical changes, or organic damage. These experiments developed a unique composite portrait, or "symptom picture," for each substance. Therefore the homeopathic understanding of a medicinal substance, or "remedy," is a shorthand sum of the responses of all people who have taken that substance, a distinctive totality that must be studied as a whole and for its own sake, rather than simply as a weapon against a particular disease or a group of symptoms.

THE VITAL FORCE

Like acupuncture, herbalism, and other natural methods, homeopathy belongs to the vitalist tradition in medicine, based on the old *vis medicatrix naturae,* the natural healing capacity, and summarized in the aphorisms of Paracelsus, as follows:

> The art of healing comes from Nature, not the physician. . . . Every illness has its own remedy within itself. . . . A man could not be born alive and healthy were there not already a Physician hidden in him. (Jacobi, 1958)

Underlying these approaches is a coherent philosophy of ancient lineage (traced elsewhere in this book), the precepts of which still ring true despite modern efforts to ignore or surpass them (Box 24-1).

Within homeopathy, curative remedies imitate and therefore resonate with manifested signs and symptoms. Illness is viewed as the organism's attempt to heal itself. Hahnemann identified the life energy itself (the vital force) as the ultimate source of health and illness alike, ending only with the death of the organism. Hahnemann described his process of preparing remedies by sequentially diluting and shaking them (see later) as liberating the essence of the remedy from its material aspects and thereby increasing its potency. Whatever we choose to call it, some version of the vital force is required to refer to the bioenergetic integrity of living beings.

BOX 24-1

Precepts of Healing

- Healing is a concerted effort of the entire organism and cannot be achieved by any part in isolation from the whole.
- All healing is essentially self-healing, which is a basic property of all living beings.
- Healing applies only to individuals and therefore is inherently problematic, even risky, and never reducible to any technique or formula, however scientific its foundation.

THE HOMEOPATHIC MATERIA MEDICA

The Hahnemannian concept of medicinal action remains the most distinctive contribution of homeopathy to medical science, with implications for pharmacology, ethnobotany, and industrial medicine and toxicology. Without recourse to pathological models or unconsenting animal subjects, provings offer a purely experimental technique for investigating the medicinal action of any substance.

The homeopathic pharmacopeia currently recognizes more than 2000 remedies, with more added all the time. Most are of plant origin, including flowers, leaves, roots, barks, fruits, and resins. Although many are poisonous in their crude state (e.g., aconite, belladonna, digitalis, ergot, hellebore, nux vomica), others are common medicinal herbs (comfrey, eyebright, mullein, yellow dock); foods and spices (cayenne, garlic, mustard, onion); fragrances, resins, and residues (amber, petroleum, charcoal, creosote); and mushrooms, lichens, and mosses.

Mineral remedies include metals (copper, gold, lead, tin, zinc), metalloids (antimony, arsenic, selenium), salts (calcium sulfate, potassium carbonate, sodium chloride), alkalis, acids (hydrochloric, nitric, phosphoric, sulfuric), elemental substances (carbon, hydrogen, iodine, phosphorus, sulfur), and constituents of the earth's crust (silica, aluminum oxide, ores, rocks, lavas, mineral waters).

Remedies from the animal kingdom include venoms (from jellyfish, insects, spiders, molluscs, crustaceans, fish, amphibians, snakes); secretions (ambergris, cuttlefish ink, musk); milks, hormones, and glandular or tissue extracts (sarcodes); entire creatures (*Apis mellifera*, or honeybee; tarantula); and nosodes, or products of diseases (tuberculosis, gonorrhea, syphilis, abscesses) and vaccines.

The investigative method of provings is equally applicable to the study of conventional drugs, unproven folk remedies, toxic or laboratory chemicals, pollutants, and commercial or industrial products (dyes, insecticides, paints, solvents). Some homeopaths have extended the method to create and test remedies made from such surprising sources as the poles of the magnet and Coca-Cola (although today's formula is a secret, the original 1885 recipe created by Dr. John Pemberton, a physician in Atlanta, included extracts of coca leaf –including cocaine– and caffeine-rich kola nut [see Chapter 1]). The homeopathic materia medica is as boundless as the creation of the earth and as inexhaustible as its transformation by human or environmental forces.

Finally, the richness and diversity of the materia medica database increases the likelihood that some degree of medicinal help can be found for most people. At the same time, its basic principles are simple enough that even a novice can achieve some results with a small number of remedies. As long as a few commonsense guidelines are observed, the method is perfectly safe for laypeople of average intelligence to learn at their own pace and to use for first aid and for the treatment of common domestic ailments. Considerable study and experience are required, however, to take full advantage of the enormous body of homeopathic information collected over the past two centuries.

THE TOTALITY OF SYMPTOMS

Just as provings include the full range of symptoms elicited by each remedy, homeopathy teaches that illness is primarily a disturbance of the vital force and manifests itself as a totality of physical, mental, and emotional responses that is unique to each patient and cannot be adequately understood as a mere specimen of any disease process. The Hahnemannian totality of symptoms describes the entire complex of signs and symptoms as they appear in the patient.

To the practicing homeopath, this composite totality or psychophysical style—much more than any abstract disease category or printout of laboratory abnormalities—furnishes the truest picture of the health and illness of the individual patient as a whole.

In practice, determining the totality of the symptoms demands that the homeopathic prescriber take into account the living experience of the patient, including the full range of thoughts and feelings. This approach by no means rejects or ignores the technical expertise of the physician and does not hesitate to make use of pathological diagnosis or of conventional drugs or surgery. Homeopathy uses the technical language of abnormalities to educate the patient, allowing the patient to retain control and to participate at every step. The conventional diagnosis, particularly the disease severity and degree of tissue damage, can also be important in predicting patient response to homeopathic treatment.

The homeopathic principle of symptom totality also explains why mental and emotional symptoms that would sometimes seem irrelevant to a conventional physician on occasion weigh heavily in choosing the remedy. Whereas most physical symptoms relate to a certain part of the body (e.g., arm, nose, back, stomach), psychological states involve how patients feel as a whole (e.g., afraid, depressed, happy,

confused). The totality of symptoms gives special importance to describing the condition of the patient as a whole. Thus, homeopathy stands with all other therapeutic modalities labeled as complementary and alternative medicine (CAM) in that it is also a form of mind-body medicine.

Achieving a clear understanding of each individual's health is vital to a successful homeopathic prescription. Consequently, other approaches to analyzing the case may be necessary. Symptoms that are strange, rare, or peculiar help the homeopath understand the given patient's unique response to the illness. Symptoms affecting the person's emotions and mental abilities are more important, because they most deeply impact the person's well-being. Similarly, symptoms reflecting more serious disease must be given more attention, because a remedy without power to influence these problems cannot be the correct choice for a patient with such a condition. In some cases, modalities—factors that increase or diminish symptom severity—can help lead the homeopath to the correct remedy more than a specific symptom, because the modalities are more uniquely individual. Paying such close and careful attention to symptomatology requires listening intensively to the patient, as well as talking to the patient, to elicit responses. Listening and talking to the patient in itself is a powerful means of therapy, which in CAM modalities is not limited to the "talk therapies" of psychiatry, psychotherapy, and psychology in mainstream medicine today.

THE SINGLE REMEDY

Based on the materia medica, the Hahnemannian method uses one remedy at a time for the whole patient, comparing the symptoms of the individual with those associated with various remedies until the best possible match is found. The reason is that the homeopathic materia medica has been compiled by testing individual substances, and the effects of combining them are unpredictable. Although almost all homeopathic remedies are made from a complex mix of substances (e.g., plants, insects), they have been tested in toto, and the homeopathic materia medica establishes that even slight differences (e.g., the mineral *calcarea phosphorica* vs. *calcarea carbonica*) produce distinctly different symptom patterns.

The encyclopedic scale of the homeopathic materia medica ensures that it can never be grasped in its entirety. As a result, some have tried to abbreviate and simplify clinical use of homeopathic remedies. Over-the-counter combination remedies also are available in many pharmacies and health food stores and are safe and effective if used properly. Although the practice is controversial in some quarters, some respected physicians use two, three, or more remedies simultaneously.

Administering different remedies to affect each part of a patient makes it difficult to know which remedy has acted and, in the view of many homeopathic practitioners, is contrary to homeopathic tradition. For this reason, remedies would have to be selected according to the rough indications of folk medicine or the technical language of abnormalities, much as in conventional drug treatment. Although it is often disparaged as a general approach, even the staunchest supporters of classical homeopathic methods recognize that there are situations in which the best homeopathic remedy for a certain patient at a certain time can be indicated by a single very important symptom. This is most likely when the patient is extremely ill.

Studying the totality of symptoms enables the serious student to accumulate detailed personal experience with remedies and generates much of the excitement about learning how to use them. The revival of American homeopathy in recent years has been achieved largely on the strength of the single-remedy concept. Only the totality of symptoms can illuminate remedies, and patients are unique individuals worthy of study for their own sake.

THE MINIMUM DOSE

Because homeopathic remedies stimulate an ailing self-healing mechanism rather than correct a specific abnormality, large or prolonged doses are seldom required and might even have harmful effects. Homeopaths use the smallest possible doses and repeat them only as necessary, allowing remedies to complete their action without further interference. The remedy will not work unless it fits the illness so closely that it renders the patient uniquely susceptible to its action. The minuteness of the dose minimizes the likelihood of untoward or dangerous adverse effects.

Hahnemann's advocacy of infinitesimal doses remains one of the most controversial aspects of his work. No one has explained satisfactorily how medicines diluted beyond the molecular threshold of Avogadro's number could possibly have any effect, let alone a curative one. However, the standard argument that "the remedies are simply placebos" cuts both ways. People do heal themselves of serious illnesses without drugs or surgery. For 200 years, homeopathic patients have been spared the adverse effects of conventional treatments later derided by conventional practitioners. With a variety of basic scientific investigations ongoing and many showing evidence of physical change in homeopathic dilutions, homeopathy envisions a new bioenergetic science that is still in its infancy.

In the study of modern environmental sciences and toxicology the concept of *hormesis* has developed based on the observation that the behavior of biologically active substances at very low concentrations is very different from their activity at higher concentrations and that they do *not* demonstrate a simple dose-response curve across all concentrations. Highly dilute substances that are toxic at higher doses may demonstrate a trophic effect by stimulating physiological and metabolic processes. These observations from mainstream science may be useful in understanding the observed clinical benefits of homeopathy.

THE LAWS OF CURE

Consideration of the whole patient makes clear why drugs that successfully lower the blood pressure or kill bacteria may leave the patient feeling as bad or worse than before. Judgments about improvement, worsening, and the effectiveness of treatment are difficult to interpret apart from a more global perspective on how patients feel as a whole, and how they function according to their own individual standards. Perhaps the greatest shortcoming of the biomedical model is its failure to comprehend patients as integrated energy systems and to follow them throughout their lifetime.

Since the era of Hahnemann, classical homeopathy has addressed this critical issue by attempting to track the order in which symptoms and illnesses appear, the grouping of symptoms that appear and disappear together, and the relation of each group to the overall health and functioning of the patient. Constantine Hering (1865, 1875) proposed four general principles by which to evaluate the changes experienced by the patient during the recovery process (Box 24-2).

Like most attempts to succinctly define general principles, Hering's laws of cure can both confuse and elucidate. The fourth principle has proved most reliable for long-term case management. Although some health changes are obviously better or worse, more literal interpretations of Hering's law, particularly subtle distinctions about the relative importance of internal organs, are difficult and subjective. Some approximation of the totality of symptoms over time remains indispensable to the general assessment of the patient as a whole, for clinician and researcher alike.

These "laws of cure" provide clear standards by which to evaluate the actions of all therapies, including homeopathic medicine. When the intervention is followed by a lasting decline in the patient's condition as defined in this manner, the intervention was a poor choice. This pertains to homeopathy as well as to conventional medicine or other healing approaches.

BOX 24-2

Hering's Directions of Symptom Movement in the Cure and Recovery Process

1. From above downward, from the head toward the feet
2. From inside outward, from interior to peripheral parts
3. From more vital to less vital organs, from more visceral to less essential structures
4. From the most recent to the oldest, in the reverse order of their appearance in the life history of the patient

METHODOLOGY

PHARMACY

The Homeopathic Pharmacopoeia of the United States (American Institute of Homeopathy, 1989) is the official standard for the preparation of homeopathic medicines. Crude medicinal substances are transformed into remedies by serial dilution and succussion in a liquid or solid medium. First crushed and dissolved in a specified volume of 95% grain alcohol, crude plant materials are shaken and stored, and the supernatant liquid is kept as the "mother tincture." The same procedure is used for animal products, nosodes, and any other substances that are soluble in alcohol. Metals, ores, and other insoluble remedies are pulverized with mortar and pestle and diluted with lactose, undergoing succussion until they become soluble.

Tinctures are further diluted with alcohol or lactose, either 1:10 (the decimal scale, written "X") or 1:100 (the centesimal, written "C") and succussed vigorously, which yields the 1X or 1C dilution. The process is repeated for the 2X, 3X, 4X (or 2C, 3C, 4C) dilutions, and on up as desired.

In clinical practice any dilution may be used, but the most popular for self-care are the 6th, 12th, and 30th (X or C). Higher dilutions for professional work are in the centesimal scale, namely, the 200th, 1000th, 10,000th, and 50,000th, written 200C, 1M, 10M, and 50M, and representing dilutions of 10^{-400}, 10^{-2000}, $10^{-20,000}$, and $10^{-100,000}$, respectively.

The general skepticism about diluted remedies, as expressed by Oliver Wendell Holmes and modern critics, is readily understandable, because even the 12C and 30C remedies are well beyond the apparent limits imposed by Avogadro's number and therefore out of the realm of conventional chemistry entirely (Holmes, 1842). Because there is essentially no likelihood that any of the original substance remains in many homeopathic preparations, for 40 years researchers have been investigating changes in the solvents used in the transformation of a medicinal substance into a homeopathic remedy. (Holmes also expressed skepticism about regular medicine; for example, in an address to the Massachusetts Medical Society, publisher of the *New England Journal of Medicine,* in 1860 he stated, "If the entire materia medica as currently practiced could be sunk to the bottom of the sea, it would be all the better for mankind and all the worse for the fishes.")

CASE TAKING

As in general medicine, in homeopathy the evaluation requires more than simply taking down information or selecting remedies. Encouraging patients to tell their stories, in their entirety, relieves their burden of pain and suffering, which makes the homeopathic interview a powerful healing experience in its own right. It even might suggest a path of recovery, allowing remedies to continue the process.

Traditionally, patients are invited to speak and allowed to continue for as long as possible without interruption, while the homeopath asks, "What else?" as often as necessary to elicit more symptoms and to remind the patient that no one disease is being sought but rather the totality of symptoms. Symptoms are written down verbatim whenever possible, supplemented by the homeopath's own observations about the patient's temperament, behavioral patterns, and personality style.

After the patient finishes his or her story and the principal symptoms have been noted, the homeopath must investigate further to characterize symptoms in detail. Conventional diagnosis is based on common symptoms such as fever, pain, cough, and bleeding, whereas homeopaths look for unusual or idiosyncratic features that tend to be ignored or discarded by conventional physicians (Box 24-3).

Medical school faculty who learn about the process of homeopathic interviewing often comment that the careful attention to the patient's descriptions and nonjudgmental respect for the patient's experience would be useful skills for all medical students to learn.

The interview also includes physical examination and laboratory work as needed to establish a diagnosis, both homeopathic and conventional.

SELECTION OF THE REMEDY

Remedy selection, homeopathic "diagnosis" in a sense, is the product of the homeopath's understanding of the patient. Homeopathic prescribing is the clinical implementation of the correspondence between the database of the materia medica and the details of each patient's case record.

Because of the mass of information contained in the homeopathic materia medica, an encyclopedic memory or a computer with a similar capacity would be required to fully grasp the treatment options for each patient. Even experienced homeopathic specialists often use reference materials.

BOX 24-3

Fully Characterized Symptoms Described in a Homeopathic Interview

- Subjective sensations such as pain, vertigo, fatigue, and anger
- Localization of symptoms (one sided, wandering, radiating, circumscribed, or diffuse)
- Modalities, that is, factors by which symptoms are modified (intensified or relieved) according to changes in the time of day, the weather, diet, or emotional state
- Concomitants, or symptoms that appear simultaneously or in sequence (nausea with headache, fever after chill)

For professional homeopaths to consider as many remedies as possible, they need help in proceeding from the clinical totality to a menu of possible remedies that they can study and from which they can choose. This is the purpose of the *repertory*. Patients complain of problems and symptoms, but homeopathic materiae medicae are organized by the name of the medicinal substance. The repertory overcomes this problem by indexing the symptoms correlated with the remedies that have either elicited them in provings or cured them clinically. By finding the remedies that match the leading symptoms in a case, the search for a cure can be narrowed, and the homeopathic specialist can study most effectively.

Whether in the form of a book or computer software, the largest, most comprehensive repertories (Archibel, 2004; Kent Homeopathic Associates, 2008; Murphy, 2005; Schroyens, 2004; van Zandvoort, 2004) include all types of symptoms from every anatomical region and physiological system, as well as mental and emotional symptoms, "generalities" (physical symptoms or modalities attributable to the patient as a whole), and rare symptoms, the oddity of which may point directly to the remedy. The repertory is only a tool for locating remedies; these remedies must then be studied in the materia medica. The final selection is based more often on a total or qualitative fit than on any narrow, technical calculation.

REGIMEN AND PRECAUTIONS

Although they remain stable in the cold and across a wide range of temperatures, dilute remedies are inactivated by direct sunlight and should be stored in a dark, dry place, shielded from heat and radiation. Patients are instructed to put nothing in the mouth for at least 30 minutes before and after each dose, because competing tastes can interfere with the action of the remedy. Coffee and camphorated products might reverse the effects of the remedy, so patients should avoid them throughout the treatment period, even when no remedies are actually being taken. The use of medicinal herbs and exposure to mothballs and other aromatic substances also should be curtailed. Homeopaths may differ on how compulsive patients need to be about avoiding possible interferences.

Although conventional drugs often interfere and should be avoided when possible, severely ill patients should not stop taking medications. Because of their potentially synergistic effect, some homeopaths believe that acupuncture and chiropractic should not be started concurrently with homeopathic remedies. Relapse might also follow dental work that includes drilling and local anesthesia.

ADMINISTRATION AND DOSAGE

Remedies are dispensed in the form of tablets or pellets of sucrose or lactose that are taken dry on the tongue or dissolved in water. Lower dilutions are preferred in acute situations because they can be repeated as often as necessary and will be somewhat effective even if only broadly similar to the totality of the case. Higher dilutions are used mainly by professionals for long-term treatment. More care must be taken in the selection of higher dilutions, and administration should not be repeated while the remedy's action is in progress.

In homeopathy the term *dosage* refers primarily to the number and frequency of repetitions, which must be tailored to fit the patient, as with the choice of the remedy. In both acute and chronic cases, the rule is to stop the remedy once the reaction is apparent, repeating only when the reaction has subsided.

PROS AND CONS

There are few, if any, absolute contraindications to homeopathic treatment. Although patients with severely disabling illnesses or chronic drug dependence are difficult to help—by any method—homeopathy at least might be considered before resorting to more drastic measures or after conventional methods have failed. Homeopathic remedies are relatively safe, economical, simple to administer, and gentle in their action, with very few serious or prolonged adverse effects. Although subtle at first, the effects of treatment are prompt, thorough, and long lasting. Simple acute illnesses and injuries are easy for even untrained laypeople to treat homeopathically, because the amount of information required is minimal.

On the other hand, homeopathy is far from a panacea. It is a difficult and exacting art. Even after years of study and practice, a skilled prescriber might need to try several remedies before any benefit is obtained. Some patients might show little or no improvement, despite the most conscientious efforts. Remedies are rather delicate and easily inactivated, so certain precautions must be observed. Finally, how dilute remedies act is not understood, and how a patient will respond or which symptoms will change and in what order cannot be predicted with absolute certainty. As with all medicine, homeopathy is an art dependent on the living energy and variability of individual humans.

HISTORICAL DEVELOPMENT

EARLY CONTROVERSIES

Hahnemann's successful treatment and prophylaxis of scarlet fever during an epidemic brought wide fame to homeopathy throughout Europe. In America, successive waves of epidemics of yellow fever, cholera, influenza, typhus, and typhoid fever were successfully treated by homeopathy throughout the 1800s. With epidemics came converts—both physicians and patients—from regular medicine to homeopathy, discouraged at the failure of regular medicine and the poisoning that accompanied use of the materia medica as then practiced. One of the converts to homeopathy was Abraham Lincoln, who often resorted to "frontier medicine" where there was no physician; he referred to homeopathic remedies as a "soup made from the shadow of a pigeon's wing."

Nevertheless, Hahnemann was ridiculed and persecuted for his heresies until 1822, when he was awarded a stipend to publish his writings (Bradford, 1895). He fueled the controversy by his unflagging convictions and determination to speak out. Famously, he upset the local medical community when he published a letter in the paper decrying the care other physicians provided to the newly deceased emperor of Austria, claiming that instead of helping the patient, they hastened his demise. Similar claims were made that not only did the physicians hasten the demise of their patients but tortured them before death in the case of Charles II (1680s) and George III (1820s), as well as George Washington (December 1799).

In addition to his *Organon of Medicine* and *Materia Medica Pura,* Hahnemann wrote many technical and expository works, maintained a busy correspondence, and continued to practice and conduct experimental research. Hahnemann died secure in the knowledge that his students were practicing homeopathy throughout Europe and America. Fired by ambition and gifted with intellect, Hahnemann left a body of work and a method that have stood the test of time.

HOMEOPATHY IN AMERICA

In the latter half of the nineteenth century, the United States became the center of the homeopathy movement and produced some of its greatest masters, whose works still enjoy international use. Three major factors contributed to the rapid growth and development of American homeopathy.

The first was the absence of laws or bureaucracy to license the practice of medicine, a tolerant attitude born of the hope to break free from the oppressive social and economic constraints of Europe. When the first school of homeopathy opened in Pennsylvania during the 1830s, American physicians were organized on a voluntary basis, and state legislatures were reluctant to prevent uneducated or lay healers from helping anyone who wanted to use their services (Starr, 1982).

The second factor was the great migration of those seeking land and fortune in the West. The westward expansion of America into the wilderness stretched beyond the reach of established society, including medical care. Frontier mothers had to develop essential medical skills to enable the survival of their families. Hering's *Domestic Physician,* published in 1835, provided instructions in the lay use of homeopathic medicines. The book was so popular that the first homeopathic book to break its sales record was not published until 150 years had passed.

Third, the concept of the materia medica itself was easily adapted to Native American medicine. Introducing dozens of Native American herbs into the pharmacopeia,

American homeopathy was enriched by the botanical lore of midwives, medicine men, eclectics, and other herbalists whose recipes are still in use today (Hale, 1867).

Under these conditions, homeopathy flourished in the United States, inspiring the creation of hospitals, medical schools, and "insane asylums" that scored notable triumphs and attracted public attention (Coulter, 1973). Hahnemann was among the first European or American physicians to speak out against the violent treatment administered to mentally ill patients. Consequently, homeopathic asylums provided quite enlightened treatment compared with the prevailing standard of care (Gamwell, 1995). Published accounts indicate that, during epidemics of cholera, typhus, and scarlet fever, homeopathy proved its superiority over the often toxic conventional treatments then in vogue (Bradford, 1900).

Physicians practicing this new method quickly rose to social prominence, treating such rich and famous patients as members of President Lincoln's cabinet (Coulter, 1973). By the turn of the nineteenth century, 10% of all physicians used homeopathy in their practices (Ullman, 1991a, 1991b).

During and after the Civil War, however, the tremendous expansion of American industry transformed the nature of medicine. American homeopathy—with its use of minimal doses at rare intervals—never created a large or profitable industrial base capable of financing large educational or research institutions. Experimental medicine, based on rigorous physicochemical causality, generated such unprecedented technical achievements as anesthesia, antisepsis, surgery, microbiology, vaccines, and antibiotics (Bernard, 1957).

The American Medical Association (AMA) and its state societies forbade their members to consult or fraternize with homeopaths (Coulter, 1973). Such persecution had little effect until state legislatures began to license physicians and accredit medical schools, and the pharmaceutical industry won control of the process (Starr, 1982). Thereafter the AMA invited homeopaths and physicians of all schools to become members in exchange for licensing, creating a monopoly against lay healers, midwives, and herbalists. The Flexner Report, published in 1914, proposed a uniform standard of medical education for all physicians and used the power of accreditation to phase out homeopathic colleges that fell short of these standards (Starr, 1982). Philosophical disputes within the homeopathic community precluded unified action to maintain homeopathy's foothold in American medicine (Coulter, 1973).

The AMA strategy succeeded. By the 1920s, the homeopathic schools had closed or conformed to the new model, and homeopathy was reduced to a postgraduate specialty for the few physicians who were prepared to swim against the tide. Although some fine homeopathic physicians continued to practice, the movement declined rapidly over the next 40 years. By 1970, homeopathy appeared to be moribund, its teachers aged or dead (Kaufman, 1971).

American homeopathy has begun to flourish once more, largely because of the rebirth of the self-care movement, the health care crisis, and the overemphasis on technology that provoked these events (Illich, 1976; Lown, 1996; Ray, 2001). By eliminating lay healers and aspiring to control every abnormality by purely technical means, American medicine has become a colossus that thrives on great cost and great risk (Moskowitz, 1988), generating more iatrogenic illness (Steel, 1981), and consuming a greater share of the gross national product than anywhere else in the world. Facing crises in health insurance, malpractice litigation, and the physician-patient relationship (Moskowitz, 1988), the public—and now the medical profession itself—has turned to alternatives such as those described in this text.

Safe, effective, and inexpensive enough to sustain busy practices even without third-party reimbursement, homeopathy has become increasingly popular with young family physicians. As in frontier days, the renaissance of American homeopathy would not be occurring were it not for the devotion of laypeople—not only in performing self-care, but also in organizing study groups in their communities and teaching these methods to their friends and neighbors.

RESEARCH

Hahnemann's system of provings—using individuals to determine the symptoms that a medicine could produce—was the first research in homeopathy and some of the first systematic clinical research in medical history. Indeed, the whole field is based on this experimental work, which was unprecedented both in method and in scope. Provings are still conducted on many herbal medicines that have been used by traditional healers for centuries, particularly in Asia and in South America. The proving method also is being modernized; statistical methods are used to determine the significance of various symptoms. Some historians of medicine consider Hahnemann's system of provings to be the first phase 1 drug trials (Kaptchuk, 1998). Following Hahnemann's scientific bent, homeopaths have been conducting all types of research investigating the method since its inception. The proving methodology itself has been investigated as a means of demonstrating the effects of homeopathic dilutions with and without success (Brien et al, 2003; Dantas et al, 2007; Walach et al, 2001). The Samueli Institute for Information Biology published a very good overview of the field of homeopathic research as it stood in 2002 (Walach et al, 2002).

BASIC SCIENCE RESEARCH

Basic scientific research in homeopathy primarily has investigated the chemical and biological activity of highly diluted substances. As discussed previously, Hahnemann found that if the homeopathic remedies were highly diluted to concentrations as low as 10^{-30} to $10^{-20,000}$,

medicinal effect could be preserved while simultaneously minimizing adverse effects. Most scientists reject homeopathic theory because of the common usage of dilutions exceeding Avogadro's constant (1×10^{-23}), beyond which point no molecules of the original material should remain. Although some believe that conventional scientific knowledge already encompasses the most unlikely homeopathic principles (Eskinazi, 1999), that is a minority opinion. The general belief is that the purest scientific research is necessary to overcome entrenched intellectual resistance to this theory.

Toxicology

The model most often used for investigating biological effects of homeopathic dilutions is toxicological research. Generally these studies have used rats subjected to lethal doses of toxic metals (arsenic, mercury, lead). In a meta-analysis and critical review of published and unpublished work on this topic (Linde et al, 1994), the quality of the studies overall was found to be poor. Although this problem significantly impaired the ability to draw definitive conclusions, interestingly the best studies used dilutions exceeding Avogadro's number, and more than 70% of these studies reached findings in support of biological effects of the homeopathic dilutions.

Immunology

A number of studies on the effects of high dilutions have been conducted in the field of immunology (Bastide, 1994; Belon, 1987), including a study that prompted one of the most notorious controversies in recent scientific literature. This study of the effects of high dilutions showed degranulation of human basophils in response to immunoglobulin E antibodies diluted as much as 10^{-120} (Davenas et al, 1988). This article was highly criticized not only because the findings challenged the basic tenets of biomedicine, but also because of its handling by the *Nature* editors (Anderson, 1991; Benveniste, 1988; Coles, 1989; "When to believe the unbelievable," 1988), who published it conditional upon a subsequent investigation by a team that included a professional magician but no immunologist (Maddox et al, 1988). The controversy over this study continues, with attempts to repeat the experiment reporting both success and failure (Belon et al, 2004; Benveniste et al, 1991; Hirst et al, 1993).

Miscellaneous Life Sciences

A large number of research studies using animal, organ, tissue, plant, and cellular materials to evaluate aspects of homeopathic principles have been published in scientific journals. In fact, this line of inquiry has been followed for over 80 years; in 1927, researchers first published a study investigating the effects of a homeopathic dilution on developing tadpoles (Konig, 1927). To explore the foundations of these areas of homeopathic research further, refer to Bellavite and Signorini (1995, 2002) and Endler and Schulte (1994).

Fundamental Science

The two crucial aspects of homeopathic theory have frequently been investigated independently of each other. The similia principle ("likes cure likes") is often linked to well-established paradoxical effects of nearly all conventional medicines. Systematic study of the similia principle has mostly appeared under the guise of "hormesis" research (Calabrese et al, 2001; Jonas et al, 2008). However, others have performed investigations of this concept as a general physiological principle (van Vijk et al, 1994).

Investigations searching for evidence of physical changes created by the potentization process have a long and creative history. In the 1960s, researchers first assayed homeopathic dilutions using nuclear magnetic resonance imaging (Smith et al, 1966, 1968). As might be expected when attempts are made to apply new technology to an unconventional subject, these studies have generally been of very poor quality, and both cautious interpretation and excellent data are required (Aabel et al, 2001; Demangeat et al, 2001). More recently, as technology has advanced with finer instruments capable of measuring more subtle phenomena, scientists have begun to apply these tools to study homeopathic principles (Becker-Witt et al, 2003; Bellavite et al, 2002; Berezin, 1994; Lo et al, 1998; Poitevin et al, 2000).

CLINICAL RESEARCH

Before the mid-1980s, few reports of clinical research in homeopathy were published outside of homeopathic journals. The first double-blind experiment reported in a peer-reviewed medical journal showed statistically significant results in treating rheumatoid arthritis with individualized prescribing of remedies (Gibson et al, 1980). A later study on arthritis comparing response to a single homeopathic remedy with that to a conventional drug showed the homeopathic treatment to be inferior on almost every outcome measure (Shipley et al, 1983). This study provides an excellent example of the difficulties in adapting classical homeopathic practice to double-blind, randomized controlled trial protocols. Standard homeopathic practice calls for an individualized remedy selection and dosing scheme, as well as a long time frame for treatment of chronic conditions, but the Shipley study design violated all these essential components and led one of the experimenters later to recant the negative finding, as follows:

> One cannot logically extrapolate from this any conclusions about other potencies of Rhus tox., other homeopathic remedies, or homeopathic medicine in general. The most important lesson that we have learned from this study is that a double-blind crossover trial of short duration using a single potency of a remedy prescribed on local features is unlikely to be a fruitful method of seriously studying homeopathic medicine. (Lancet, 1983).

A study of recurrent respiratory illnesses in a pediatric population (de Lange de Klerk et al, 1995) recalls the Shipley study because of the problems in interpreting the data. Superficially, the pediatric study found no significant benefits of homeopathic medicine. However, good reasons exist to contest this conclusion. As one of the confounding factors, the "placebo" intervention included all the components typical of homeopathic clinical consultations (homeopathic interview, dietary and lifestyle advice, clinical management avoiding overuse of medication). Other studies have shown that these interventions appear to be effective in themselves, and the investigators found that both groups improved dramatically. Although the group who received the remedy improved even more, the difference between the groups was not statistically significant. Was the placebo group improvement in this case simply the course of natural history, or was it the effect of the homeopathic approach minus the remedy?

Other notable studies include work on pediatric diarrheal disease (Jacobs et al, 1993, 1994, 2000, 2003), fibrositis and fibromyalgia (Bell et al, 2004; Fisher et al, 1989), hay fever and pollinosis (Lüdtke et al, 1997), vertigo (Weiser et al, 1998), and otitis media (Jacobs et al, 2001), as well as use of the homeopathic standard arnica in surgery, trauma, and physical overexertion (Campbell, 1976; Hart et al, 1997; Ramelet et al, 2000; Stevinson et al, 2003; Tveiten et al, 1991, 1998, 2003; Vickers et al, 1998; Wolf et al, 2003).

Ferley et al's early positive findings (1989) for a homeopathic treatment for influenza have received equivocal support, best summarized in a recent meta-analysis (Vickers et al, 2004).

Probably the most impressive series of trials was conducted by Reilly's group investigating allergic rhinitis and asthma (Reilly et al, 1986, 1994; Taylor et al, 2000). For 15 years this group conducted research into these allergic diseases using homeopathically prepared allergens as an intervention in sensitive patients. They repeatedly achieved positive findings of such a degree that the pooled patient subjective data (visual analogue scale) resulted in a P value of .0007. This highly impressive finding was tarnished by a failed but admittedly imperfect attempt at replication (Lewith et al, 2002). A Cochrane review of trials of homeopathic treatment of asthma concluded that there was insufficient evidence to reach a determination of whether homeopathy was or was not effective (McCarney et al, 2004).

Systematic Reviews

In homeopathy, as in all areas of medicine, systematic reviews and meta-analyses have been in vogue as a means of refining our understanding of the research data. Some reviews were disease specific. Others were meta-analyses of general research, a few studies specifically considered quality issues, and one super meta-analysis even looked at the quality of the meta-analyses (Cucherat et al, 2000; Ernst, 2002; Jonas et al, 2001; Linde et al, 1997, 1998, 1999).

Among the conclusions were comments in every review regarding the poor quality of most of the studies. Each found results favoring homeopathy, which became more ambiguous as the quality of the studies improved. Unfortunately the quality of some of the meta-analyses themselves has become an issue, most notably that of Shang et al (2005). The strength of Shang et al's conclusions were at odds with important deficiencies in their design, which led to a volume of criticism that continues to this day (Lüdtke et al, 2008).

The *British Medical Journal* published the first meta-analysis of homeopathic clinical trials (Kleijnen et al, 1991). The authors' comments remain an interesting reflection on the intellectual and emotional milieu of the discussion as well as on homeopathic research:

> The amount of published evidence even among the best trials came as a surprise to us. Based on this evidence we would be ready to accept that homeopathy can be efficacious, if only the mechanism of action were more plausible. . . . The evidence presented in this review would probably be sufficient for establishing homeopathy as a regular treatment for certain indications. There is no reason to believe that the influence of publication bias, data massage, bad methodology, and so on is much less in conventional medicine and the financial interests for regular pharmaceutical companies are many times greater. Are the results of randomized double-blind trials convincing only if there is a plausible explanation? Are review articles of the clinical evidence only convincing if there is a plausible mechanism of action? Or is this a special case because the mechanisms are unknown or implausible?

GLOBAL MEASURES OF HOMEOPATHY: COST EFFECTIVENESS AND OUTCOMES

Another relevant area of research in homeopathy is cost effectiveness and outcomes. Many believe that outcomes research will prove to be the most important area of homeopathic research (Carlston, 2003; Jacobs et al, 1994). Like several other forms of CAM, homeopathic treatment is directed toward the patient's global well-being, not toward specific disease features. Therefore, general outcome measures such as overall health status (assessed using widely accepted scales), patient satisfaction, days missed from school or work, and the cost of treatment are most suitable for evaluating homeopathic treatment. Also, patients do not care if their treatment is merely statistically superior to placebo. They only want to get better, and thus many conventional medical researchers argue that measuring patient satisfaction is crucial. As Ian Chalmers, the founder of the Cochrane Collaboration, states, "The patient's opinion is the ultimate outcome measure."

A German study in which nearly 500 patients received either conventional or homeopathic care found that, although costs were similar, patients' clinical response to homeopathic treatment was significantly better as determined by both patient and physician ratings

(Witt, Keil et al, 2005). Another study of patient outcomes found a highly significant improvement in disease severity and quality of life among 3981 German and Swiss patients (Witt, Lüdtke et al, 2005). In France the annual cost to the social security system for a homeopathic physician is 15% less than that for a conventional physician, and the price of the average homeopathic medicine is one third that of standard drugs (Caisse Nationale des Assurances Maladie, 1991). Fisher found that expenditures for patients of the London Homeopathic Hospital were significantly lower than those for matched, conventionally treated patients. The reduction in expensive services documented in other studies also suggests a potential for cost effectiveness (Jacobs et al, 1998; Swayne, 1992; Van Wassenhoven et al, 2004).

HOMEOPATHY TODAY

The use of homeopathy is increasing rapidly throughout the world, particularly in Europe, Latin America, and Asia. In many European countries, homeopathy is the most popular form of alternative and integrative medicine. Developing countries have turned to homeopathy as the cost of conventional, Western medicine becomes too costly to afford. In both Argentina and Brazil, several thousand physicians use homeopathy, and Mexico has five medical colleges that provide homeopathic training. South Africa has homeopathic medical colleges in several major cities, and the health ministry in Israel has approved the importation of homeopathic preparations for sale in pharmacies (Kayne, 2003).

The use of homeopathy in the United States has increased tremendously in the last 20 years. A survey showed that 1% of the American population used homeopathy in 1989 (Eisenberg et al, 1993). Sales of homeopathic remedies increased by 1000% during the 1980s (U.S. Food and Drug Administration, 1985) and were reported to be $200 million in 1992, climbing at the rate of 25% per year (Swander, 1994). A 1999 survey found that 17% of Americans were using homeopathy for self-care (Roper Starch Worldwide, 1999).

Physician interest parallels patient enthusiasm. In Germany, 25% of all physicians use homeopathy (Ullman, 1991a, 1991b); in France, 32% of general practice physicians use it (Bouchayer, 1990); and in Great Britain, 42% of physicians refer patients to homeopaths (Wharton et al, 1986). In India, homeopathy is practiced in the national health service, at several hundred homeopathic medical schools, and by more than 100,000 homeopaths (Kishore, 1983). In 1995, about 10% of conventional U.S. medical schools offered elective instruction about homeopathy (Carlston et al, 1997). By 1998, almost 15% of U.S. medical schools required that students study homeopathy (Barzansky et al, 1998).

Because education in CAM has expanded dramatically, more recent numbers for homeopathy would likely be much higher. Data published in 2004 showed that almost 50% of American schools of osteopathic medicine include homeopathy in the required coursework (Saxon et al, 2004).

APPROPRIATE USE

Homeopathic remedies are most likely to be successful and to optimize overall health for the types of conditions listed in Box 24-4.

Homeopathy is less useful (1) for the treatment of chronic diseases involving advanced tissue damage, such as cirrhosis of the liver or severe cardiovascular disease; (2) for people with prolonged dependence on conventional medications such as corticosteroids, anticonvulsants, and antipsychotics; or (3) as a substitute for appropriate conventional treatments such as emergency surgery or reduction of fractures. Homeopathy is often used by homeopathic specialists as a treatment complementing conventional medicine in these circumstance or as a palliative measure when no other effective treatment exists.

BOX 24-4

Uses of Homeopathic Remedies

- Functional complaints with little or no tissue damage, such as headache, insomnia, chronic fatigue, and premenstrual syndrome
- Conditions for which conventional medicine has little to offer, such as viral illnesses, traumatic injuries, surgical wounds, and multiple sclerosis
- Chronic health conditions, such as allergies, recurring infections, arthritis, skin conditions, and digestive problems
- Conditions that have not been cured by conventional treatments because of the inappropriateness of the medication, determined nature of the disease, or patient noncompliance with the treatment regimen

PRACTICE PATTERNS

Surveys of American physicians document interesting differences between those using homeopathic medicines in their practices and those using more conventional remedies (Jacobs et al, 1998; Schappert, 1992). Physicians using homeopathy saw fewer patients and spent more than twice as much time with each patient than did conventional physicians, averaging 30 minutes per visit versus 12.5 minutes. In addition, homeopathic physicians ordered half as many diagnostic procedures and laboratory tests as conventional physicians and prescribed fewer standard medications.

Asthma, headaches, depression, allergies, psychological problems, and skin problems were among the top 10 conditions treated most frequently by homeopathic physicians (Jacobs et al, 1998). Schappert's contemporaneous survey (1992) found that conventional physicians, on the other hand, saw more patients with hypertension, upper respiratory tract infections, diabetes, sore throats, bronchitis, back disorders, and acute sprains and strains. These practice patterns suggest that patients were seeking homeopathic care mostly for chronic conditions not managed adequately by conventional medicine. The low number of acute problems treated by homeopaths may be the result of patients' treating these conditions on their own.

SUMMARY

Homeopathic medicine has persisted both in spite of and because of its dissident voice. Its theories usually contradict those of conventional medicine, and the intensive clinical interaction between patient and practitioner stands in opposition to the time pressures of managed care. Although its controversial aspects would seem to weaken homeopathic practice severely, in fact this distinction attracts interest, and in many ways this controversy serves to invigorate both conventional and homeopathic thought.

⊝ Chapter References can be found on the Evolve website at http://evolve.elsevier.com/Micozzi/complementary/

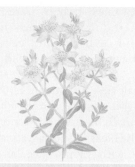

CHAPTER 25

NUTRITION AND HYDRATION

MARC S. MICOZZI

People eat food, not nutrients. When we rummage through the refrigerator for a snack or cruise the supermarket aisles trying to decide what to fix for dinner, our choices are much more likely to reflect cultural, social, and family patterns than to be based on the federal government's food pyramid and recommended daily allowances.

Food has powerful symbolic meaning and has played a key role in our religious and social rituals for thousands of years. From birthday cake to the bitter herbs of the Passover seder to Thanksgiving turkey to communion wafers, food helps form our social bonds, express our spirituality, and define who we are. Rituals remain powerful even when we no longer recall their origins. For example, Christians worldwide celebrate Easter by eating colored eggs, although few could explain the connection between hard-boiled eggs and Jesus' resurrection.

Substances can have radically different meanings for different groups. For Muslims, Christian Scientists, and members of Alcoholics Anonymous, wine is strictly "taboo," whereas for Catholics, wine is part of a sacrament that is by definition "an outward sign instituted by Christ to give grace." Individuals also bring very different perspectives to the table. For some vegetarians, chicken soup represents cruelty to animals, whereas for many other people, it recalls Mom's tender care during childhood illnesses.

An intellectual understanding of what constitutes good nutrition is no match for the powerful psychological, social, and spiritual forces that have been shaping human eating habits since the Stone Age.

EATING HABITS OF EARLY HUMANS

Humans are omnivores. We can eat almost everything found in nature, and with a few exceptions (e.g., wood, grass), we can extract nutrition from whatever we consume. For hundreds of thousands of years, our early ancestors roamed the forests and plains as hunter-gatherers. The hunters brought home very lean meat; wild game has only 4% to 6% body fat versus the 40% to 60% body fat found in modern domesticated animals. The gatherers collected plants that were high in fiber and

355

complex carbohydrates and provided many necessary vitamins. These early humans obtained calcium from animal bones and other minerals from the dirt that inevitably clung to wild plants and game.

Life was a constant struggle to obtain enough fat and calories, and our ancestors developed a decided preference for foods that tasted rich in these needed nutrients. In the small, hunter-gatherer tribes, food was often allocated on the basis of social status, gender, and age, which provided it with significance beyond the satisfaction of hunger. When agriculture was developed 10,500 years ago, diets became more stable. Seasonal crops led to seasonal feasts, which added another layer of cultural meaning to food consumption.

Although even the earliest farmers sought to improve their crops genetically—for example, selecting and sowing the seeds of wheat that had stronger stalks and quicker, more uniform germination—the quality of food did not change much. Humans learned to use yeast (made from microbes, which had been present on the planet for millions of years) to produce bread, beer, and wine; other microbes were used to make cheese and yogurt. These microbes made certain plants and dairy products easier (and more enjoyable) to consume and digest, but humans were still eating the diet for which their digestive system and metabolism were designed: low in fat and high in protein, complex carbohydrates, and fiber, with no refined sugar. Everything in the human diet remained completely natural—until modern times.

MODERN ERA: FOOLING MOTHER NATURE

Fast-forwarding to the twentieth century, we find a very different picture of food production and consumption. Early in the century, advances in biochemistry allowed scientists to isolate some of the active ingredients in food. In 1928, for example, it was discovered that limes, the British Navy's traditional method of preventing scurvy, worked by providing sailors with vitamin C. Unfortunately, although vitamin C supplements proved easier to store and dispense, they did not provide the full benefits of the fruit. Later research disclosed that lime pulp contains *bioflavonoids,* which are necessary for absorbing and processing vitamin C. Bioflavonoids also help maintain collagen and capillary walls and protect against infection and cancer. Scientists were discovering that replacing natural products with artificial ones did not always improve on the original.

This finding, however, did not stop scientists from trying to improve on nature. Currently, modern technology and agribusiness have "improved" crops by covering them with artificial chemicals, including pesticides, fungicides, ripening agents, and fumigants, all of which make them more efficient to grow, ship, and store. Genetic engineering

has changed the biological structure of many plants in ways not yet fully understood. Some plants are irradiated (flooded with "harmless" radiation) to lengthen their shelf life. Animals destined for the table are dosed with antibiotics to prevent disease and with hormones to make them fat and juicy.

Once vegetables, fruit, milk, meat, and eggs leave the farm, they are often "processed" into "food products," such as canned soup and frozen dinners. Processed foods are generally high in fat, salt, and sugar; are lower in nutrients than fresh foods; and contain a host of chemicals to boost flavor, color, texture, and shelf life. Consider the following:

- Pounds of sugar the average American consumed per year in the nineteenth century: less than 10
- Pounds of sugar the average American consumes per year today: 150

Among the many artificial substances used in processed foods are such synthetic sweeteners as aspartame, silicon dioxide, phenylalanine, tribasic calcium phosphate, benzosulfimide, and calcium silicate. The effects of all these chemicals on our bodies are not entirely known, but saccharin, the first widely used artificial sweetener, was shown to cause cancer in laboratory animals. Aspartame (NutraSweet) is now being studied for possible neurological effects. Large quantities of one of its ingredients, methanol, have been shown to cause blindness, brain swelling, and inflammation of the pancreas and heart muscle.

In addition to pseudosugars, we now have "fake fats." Partially hydrogenated oil does not occur in nature but in the laboratory, when liquid vegetable fats are turned into solids by pumping hydrogen into them. This makes them more like animal fats in taste and feel, as well as in their harmful effects on the cardiovascular system; in fact, partially hydrogenated fats have been associated with higher cancer rates than saturated fats. *Trans*-fatty acids (TFAs) are formed when unsaturated fatty acids (the building blocks of fat) are deformed by certain heat or chemical treatments. These deformed fats may be toxic. TFAs in the diet may damage the regulatory machinery of the body, significantly compromising health. Despite these concerns, partially hydrogenated oils and TFAs are found in a wide range of processed foods, including almost all margarines, mass-produced breads, convenience foods, and junk foods, as well as some baby foods.

For a variety of reasons, including productivity, efficiency, convenience, profit, arrogance, and curiosity, we have found abundant ways to change the nature of our diets and the nature of the animals and plants that feed us. As a group, the U.S. population eats high on the food chain, consuming unprecedented amounts of meat, chicken, fish, dairy products, fat, salt, and sugar. We cover our food with artificial chemicals while it is grown, processed, preserved, and genetically altered in ways that have only recently been introduced on this planet. After hundreds of thousands of years of evolution, during which our bodies became perfectly adapted to drawing nutrition from the natural environment, we have suddenly introduced large quantities of new, artificial substances into our diets, hoping to improve on nature.

How have these "advances" affected our health?

DISEASES OF AFFLUENCE

We have become a nation in which one third of the U.S. population is significantly overweight, and more than one quarter—24% of adult males, 27% of adult females, and 27% of children—are obese. Although this is caused by a variety of factors, ranging from genetics to the introduction of the car (reducing the necessity to move around) and television (reducing the desire to move around), a clear and direct correlation exists between food consumption and excess body weight.

Research has shown an equally clear and direct connection between excess body weight and illness, especially the leading killers in the United States: cardiovascular disease and cancer. Today, 60 million Americans have cardiovascular disease, including high blood pressure, heart disease, and stroke. This year, cardiovascular disease will kill about 1 million Americans, more than 2600 a day, or one death every 33 seconds. Another 1.2 million people will be diagnosed with cancer this year, and almost 600,000 will die of it. Thousands more will suffer from other diseases related to diet: diabetes, gallbladder disease, respiratory disease, sleep apnea, gout, osteoporosis, and a host of other conditions.

For more than a century, the U.S. Department of Agriculture (USDA) has been trying to improve our eating habits by issuing dietary recommendations. It currently spends $333.3 million per year educating the public about what we should and should not consume and in what quantities (USDA, 1997). That seems a great expenditure until we consider that America's food manufacturers spend that amount promoting snacks and nuts; their total annual advertising budget is more than $7 billion, most of which is spent promoting highly processed, packaged foods. The fast-paced American lifestyle relies on these convenience foods and on restaurant and take-out fare. We now spend 45% of our food dollars on away-from-home meals and snacks, most of which are higher in fat, salt, and sugar and lower in fiber and calcium than meals prepared at home.

According to the USDA's *Healthy Eating Index,* some small improvements have been made in the American diet. On a scale of 1 to 100, the average U.S. score rose from 61.5 in 1990 to 63.8 in 1995, but it still falls far short of the 80 or above that marks a good diet. Put another way, Americans are earning about a C− in healthy eating practices.

Box 25-1 lists trends in American eating habits in the twentieth century.

BOX 25-1

American Eating Habits: 1900 to 1980

Fresh fruit and vegetable consumption drops from 40% to 5% of the diet.
Sugar consumption rises 50%.
Beef consumption rises 50%.
Fat and oil consumption rises 150%.
Cheese consumption rises 400%.
Margarine consumption rises 800%.

WHAT SHOULD WE BE EATING?

Most Americans know (but don't necessarily act on) the basic facts: a healthy diet includes lots of fresh, unprocessed fruits, vegetables, and grains; modest amounts of protein and fat; and very little white sugar and salt. The question of precisely how much of each type of food we need, however, becomes more complicated.

All food provides energy, which is measured in units called *calories.* Nutritionists generally recommend daily intake of 1600 calories for older adults and sedentary women; 2200 calories for children, teenage girls, active women, and sedentary men; and 2800 calories for teenage boys, active men, and very active women. Calories are taken into our bodies as carbohydrates, proteins, and fats (which are known as *macronutrients,* or major constituents of diet). We also require vitamins and minerals (which are effective in small amounts and thus are known as *micronutrients*) to process these nutrients and maintain body functions.

Nutritionists, physicians, research scientists, alternative practitioners, food manufacturers, and consumers hold differing views about what percentage of calories we should obtain from each macronutrient. People favoring a largely vegetarian, low-fat diet tend to recommend that we receive about 15% of our calories from protein, 60% from carbohydrates, and 25% from fats. Proponents of high-protein diets often advocate 30% protein, 40% carbohydrates, and 30% fats. The food pyramid, developed by the U.S. Department of Health and Human Services and USDA, suggests that we use fat "sparingly" and that our daily fare include 2 to 3 servings of dairy products; 2 to 3 servings of meat, poultry, fish, eggs, beans, and nuts; 3 to 5 servings of vegetables; 2 to 4 servings of fruit; and 6 to 11 servings of bread, cereal, rice, and pasta (Box 25-2).

Although these numbers may provide useful guidelines, they do not address one crucial factor: the *quality* of nutrients in each category. The food pyramid, which recommends 6 to 11 servings of grain-based foods, fails to distinguish, for example, between the empty calories of frozen waffles, which are composed primarily of white sugar and white flour, and a bowl of whole-grain cereal. It encourages us to use fats "sparingly" but advocates 2 or 3 helpings of cheese and whole milk, which contain at least 8 g of fat per serving, plus up to 3 servings of meat, which

The Changing Shape of U.S. Government Guidelines

Over the years, the U.S. Department of Agriculture has revised its dietary recommendations in response to research findings and new concepts of nutrition.

1946 to 1958: The "Basic 7" Daily Food Guide
Leafy, green, and yellow vegetables: 1 or more servings
Citrus fruit, tomatoes, raw cabbage: 1 or more servings
Potatoes and other vegetables and fruits: 2 or more servings
Milk, cheese, ice cream: children, 1 to 4 cups of milk; adults, 2 or more cups
Meat, poultry, fish, eggs, dried peas, beans: 1 to 2 servings
Bread, cereal, flour: 2 or more servings
Butter and fortified margarine: 2 tablespoons

1958 to 1979: The Four Basic Food Groups (per day, for adults)
Milk group: 2 or more cups
Meat group: 2 or more servings
Vegetable and fruit group: 4 or more servings
Bread and cereal group: 4 or more servings

1979 to 2005 The Food Pyramid (per day)
Fats, oils, sweets: use sparingly
Milk, yogurt, cheese: 3 to 5 servings
Dried beans, nuts, seeds, eggs, meat: 2 to 3 servings
Vegetables: 3 to 5 servings
Fruits: 2 to 4 servings
Bread, cereal, rice, pasta: 6 to 11 servings

2005 MyPyramid
Customized based on personal characteristics
Personal plans available at http://www.mypyramid.gov

can contain up to 26 g of fat per serving. Is a Whopper (40 g of fat) part of a healthy diet? Are PopTarts (20 g of white sugar) giving us the right kind of energy to start the day?

Clearly the numbers alone do not tell the whole story. All carbohydrates are not created equal, nor does everyone need the same amount of them, or of any given nutrient. Our food needs are influenced by many factors, such as age, gender, body size, activity level, and reproductive status, and will change over time. To determine what type of diet is best for our bodies at different stages of our lives, we need some understanding of how the nutrients in food enable our bodies to function.

CARBOHYDRATES

Carbohydrates provide large amounts of quick energy. We obtain carbohydrates from fruits, vegetables, beans, grains, and other plant materials, as well as from dairy products.

Our bodies easily transform carbohydrates into *glucose* (blood sugar), which the body needs for fuel, and into *glycogen,* a form of sugar that can be stored in the liver and muscles until needed, then transformed into glucose.

There are two types of carbohydrates: simple and complex. *Simple* carbohydrates, or simple sugars, include white table sugar (sucrose), the sugar in fruit (fructose), and the sugar in milk (lactose). In *complex* carbohydrates, such as whole grains, beans, and vegetables, the sugar molecules are linked together in longer, more complicated chains.

Both types of carbohydrates become blood sugar, but the simple sugars are converted more quickly, elevating insulin levels and providing a "sugar rush" that quickly abates, often leading to feelings of tiredness. Complex carbohydrates are metabolized more slowly, providing a sustained supply of energy. One complex carbohydrate has a different role: fiber is not absorbed into the body at all but helps with digestive and bowel function. One of the disadvantages of an overprocessed, highly refined diet is that foods tend to linger in the body, which can allow carcinogens (cancer-causing substances) to be absorbed or produced by the body (see Chapter 21). Fiber in the diet has been shown to reduce constipation, which decreases the risk of colon, breast, and other cancers; it also shrinks intestinal polyps (growths), which can lead to cancers. About 25 g of fiber a day is usually sufficient and will occur naturally in a diet that includes a good supply of complex carbohydrates.

PROTEINS

Protein is essential for the growth, maintenance, and repair of every cell in the body and for the production of hormones, antibodies, and digestive enzymes. When we consume dietary protein, we break it down into amino acids, which are the building blocks we need to make our own proteins.

There are two types of dietary proteins: complete and incomplete. *Complete* proteins, which are found in meat, poultry, fish, eggs, dairy products, and soybeans, provide the full range of essential amino acids we need. *Incomplete* proteins, which include some but not all needed amino acids, are found in grains, beans, nuts, seeds, and leafy green vegetables. However, incomplete proteins can be combined to provide the full range of amino acids our bodies require. For example, brown rice served with beans, nuts, or seeds forms a whole protein.

Protein cannot be stored in the body for future use, so we need to replenish our supply every day. Most Americans consume twice the protein they need. When more protein is taken in than the body can use, the excess is either burned off as energy or stored in the body as fat.

FATS

Fat is the most concentrated form of energy available to us and is necessary for growth and healthy function. As babies and children, we needed fat for brain development.

As adults, many of us consume more than we need, which leads to weight gain and a national obsession about staying thin, especially for women. Conflicting cultural pressures make it difficult to obtain a realistic picture of the amount and types of fat we need.

Our body's fats are made up of fatty acids, which come in three major types: saturated, polyunsaturated, and monounsaturated.

Saturated fatty acids come from meats (e.g., beef, lamb, veal, pork), egg yolks, dairy products (e.g., cream, whole milk), and a few plant products, including coconut oil and vegetable shortening. The liver turns saturated fat into cholesterol, which is used to make cell membranes, hormones, and vitamin D.

Cholesterol travels through the body in the form of lipoproteins. *Low-density lipoproteins* (LDLs, or "bad cholesterol") contain large amounts of cholesterol, whereas *high-density lipoproteins* (HDLs, or "good cholesterol") carry relatively little cholesterol and help remove excess cholesterol from blood and tissues. If the LDL level is too high for the HDLs to clear away the excess cholesterol, it forms plaque on the artery walls, which can lead to heart disease.

Polyunsaturated fatty acids (PUFAs) are found in corn, soybean, safflower, and sunflower oils and some fish oils. PUFAs may actually lower "bad" cholesterol levels, but they have a tendency to lower HDL levels as well, leaving the body less capable of removing the amounts of cholesterol that are present. Although not as harmful as the saturated type, PUFAs can pose a health risk if too many are used in the diet.

Monounsaturated fatty acids are found in olive, peanut, canola, and other vegetable and nut oils. These fats actually reduce LDL level slightly and do not reduce HDL level, so they may benefit the body when taken in moderation.

Many oils are actually a combination of these different types of fatty acids, but in general, one type predominates, which is how the oil is described on the food label.

The Whole Truth About Whole Milk

Cow's milk is the ideal food—for calves. When it comes to human infants, children, and adults, the milk issue is cloudy. Cow's milk is three times higher in protein than is human breast milk. In fact, human breast milk has among the lowest levels of protein of any milk from mammals. Among different animal species, the higher the growth rate of infants of that species, the high the protein content of the species' milk. Survival among the young of most species requires rapid rates of growth and maturation. This is not the case for human infants, who grow more slowly and mature over a longer time period.

Not only does cow's milk have a higher total protein content, but the *type* of protein present is very different from that in human milk. Cow's milk is six times higher in casein protein (which has been shown to promote tumors in some laboratory animal experiments). Also, cow's milk is low in linoleic acid, which may be important for early human growth and health. For these reasons and more, cow's milk is not a good food for human infants. And there is no reason on earth to think that it should be.

Among adults around the world, it is rare in most populations to consume whole milk in the diet. However, in some parts of the world, dairy animal domestication represents a renewable resource for converting plants and grasses from the environment (which are inedible for humans) into usable human food sources. Humans can't digest or extract nutrients from many plants containing cellulose. And, in fact, neither can cows—by themselves. However, ruminants like cows have multiple stomachs, which allow bacteria present in them to ferment cellulose so that it can be digested. In the cow, it is converted to meat and milk. Even termites rely on bacteria in their digestive tracts to digest cellulose from the wood they eat. The use of domesticated animals to graze on grasses allows humans to survive in relatively harsh, dry environments where there may not be enough other food to eat. Dairy animal domestication can be traced back approximately 10,000 years to parts of the world now called the Middle East, where the use of these animals allowed humans to survive in areas where they otherwise might not.

Human digestive problems can also be caused by milk consumption, however. Milk contains *lactose,* or milk sugar, which can only be digested by a special enzyme called *lactase* that breaks down lactose. All infants have lactase to digest milk sugar. However, most adults in most populations lose the lactase enzyme when they get older (and no longer would normally be expected to drink milk). These adults are intolerant of milk because of the lactose, which they cannot digest. They experience indigestion, intestinal problems, and possible malnutrition from drinking milk. In the Middle East and the Mediterranean region, local cultures have developed processes that allow bacteria to break down lactose through fermentation. Thus, production of cheeses, yogurts, and other cultured dairy products allows people to eat dairy foods without getting the lactose in whole milk that causes digestive problems. In China and East Asia, there is no dairy production at all, and milk and milk products do not form any part of the diet. This raises a question: how do over 1 billion of the world's people get adequate calcium without dairy? (See later.)

Northern European adults generally have the lactase enzyme, which allows them to digest milk and its lactose sugar without digestive problems. But whole milk

(Continued)

The Whole Truth About Whole Milk—cont'd

remains an unnecessary source of fat in what should be a beverage. It is hard for Americans to avoid too much fat in their foods, but to drink it in our beverages is really making it difficult.

But what about calcium? Don't we need to drink milk to get calcium ?

Milk as a Source of Calcium

Milk is a good source of calcium, but there are ways of getting dietary calcium while bypassing the cow. There is much evidence to suggest that humans do not build bone by milk alone. Dairy-free diets are not necessarily low in calcium. Other good sources of calcium in the diet include fish, some vegetables, grains, and seeds. Over 1 billion people in China somehow get enough calcium in the diet, although, as noted earlier, there is absolutely no dairy industry or dairy consumption there. The Chinese refer to butter and cheese as "animal secretion" when they encounter it. There are no words in Chinese for products that do not exist there. The Chinese also have high rates of lactose intolerance, which perhaps explains why a dairy industry never developed there. Perhaps the Chinese get enough calcium from eating bits of bone and sinew left behind in traditional preparations of (lean) meat dishes. Bone is the best source of calcium of all, whether people eat the bones of sardines or whether normally herbivorous animals consume bone. When deprived of calcium even cows (and other ruminants) will eat the bones of other animals (although they are normally vegetarian).

Proper calcium nutrition is dependent on getting enough calcium in the diet and having adequate vitamin D to absorb it from the gastrointestinal (GI) tract. Vitamin D must be activated by sunlight on the bare skin to be effective (see the sidebar "The Light Cure and Vitamin D" in Chapter 11). So adequate calcium nutrition depends on the GI tract, liver, kidneys, bone, and skin cells. Vitamin D deficiency became a problem in many people when populations moved into dark urban centers during the Industrial Revolution in the last two centuries. People no longer got enough fresh vegetables (since they had left the farms) and they did not get enough sun because they were kept indoors. The result was high rates of rickets.

Plants naturally contain vitamin D sources, which normally are eaten but then must be activated by sunlight in the skin cells. This is the kind of vitamin D usually contained in cow's milk, which comes from plants eaten by the cow. Today, milk does contain artificially activated vitamin D that does not require conversion by sunlight in the skin. However, with enough consumption of vegetables and adequate exposure of the skin to sunlight, it should be possible for most people to get adequate amounts of vitamin D.

Other Problems with Milk—Nothing to Sneeze At

Beyond the nutritional consequences of milk, cow's milk proteins may produce allergies in infants and children, which may threaten proper growth and be present for life. These infant allergies may have long-lasting effects on the immune systems. Many have noted an increase in adult allergies, which have been blamed on all manner of modern pollutants and allergens. I have wondered whether a whole generation of infants raised on the "enlightened" practice of bottle feeding with cow's milk are now a generation of adults with lifelong allergies.

Certified raw milk has also been found to be contaminated with *Listeria,* a dangerous bacteria responsible for the deaths of infants and children and harm to pregnant women. Historically cows and cow's milk have been carriers of diseases, including tuberculosis. The reason milk requires pasteurization is that it can be contaminated with dangerous bacteria. Some of my own research into the history of diseases shows that human tuberculosis may have originated with contact between humans and cows beginning 10,000 years ago.

The health costs of cows are real (not to mention the environmental costs). Today the risks of chronic disease from excess consumption of fats and proteins, as present in whole milk, are becoming clear for adults. The risks to infants are obvious. Failure to breastfeed in infancy often leads to overnourished and overweight infants. Human infants given cow's milk are by definition overfed. This overfeeding during infancy may cause excess fat deposition and increase body mass. These problems may have long-lasting consequences.

Americans still drink much more whole milk than other low-fat varieties such as skim. Substitute skim milk for whole milk and learn to like it. Drinking liquid fat (whole milk) has got to be an acquired taste. Better yet, cast off cow's milk. And by all means, for infants, breast is best.

VITAMINS

In 1913, American biochemist Elmer McCollum became the first scientist to isolate a vitamin. Further research revealed that this substance, which became known as vitamin A, helps maintain skin, teeth, bones, hair, mucous membranes, and reproductive capacity. We can obtain vitamin A from cream, butter, egg yolks, cod liver oil, and some leafy green and yellow vegetables, or we can simply take a pill containing vitamin A. This is the great vitamin debate: for decades scientists have been arguing about whether supplements containing vitamins and minerals are a useful addition to the diet or whether we can and should obtain all the vitamins and minerals we need from the foods we eat.

No one disputes the need for vitamins, which enable us to make use of the energy stored in food to perform a variety of functions, ranging from maintaining the nervous system to forming red blood cells. There are two main categories of vitamins: fat soluble and water soluble. The *fat-soluble* vitamins, including A, D, E, and K, can be stored in the body's fat for days or weeks, whereas *water-soluble* vitamins dissolve quickly in the bloodstream and are removed in urine or sweat. Because water-soluble vitamins cannot be stored, these vitamins need to be resupplied on a daily basis. The most essential water-soluble vitamins are B_1, B_2, B_6, B_{12}, folic acid, C, niacin, pantothenic acid, and biotin.

There is some controversy about how much of each vitamin we need to stay healthy. The U.S. Food and Drug Administration has issued guidelines based on the National Academy of Science's recommended daily allowances (often listed on supplement labels as RDAs). Some consider these numbers the minimum needed to maintain health, whereas others maintain that these are maximum amounts that should not be exceeded.

Vitamin C, one of the most popular and widely debated vitamins, provides a good example of these divergent views. The RDA for vitamin C is 60 mg/day, the amount found in a single orange. Consuming less than this amount compromises the immune system, bones, and skin and even the ability to reproduce. Researchers at the University of California at Berkeley and the USDA's Western Human Nutritional Research Center determined that without 60 mg of vitamin C per day, waste products of metabolism known as *free radicals* can damage DNA. This can lead to cancer, heart disease, and other illnesses in all of us. For would-be fathers, this means sperm may contain genetic mutations that can result in birth defects, genetic disease, and cancer in future children.

Since the amount of vitamin C in a single orange can prevent all that, what can larger amounts do?

Linus Pauling, winner of Nobel prizes for chemistry and peace, would respond that megadoses of vitamin C can fight colds and boost the immune system. He consumed 300 times the recommended amount, about 18,000 mg, every day. Because vitamin C is water soluble, he pointed out, any excess will wash out harmlessly in the urine. Some scientists argue that our physiology and metabolism may not be equipped to handle micronutrients at levels higher than could be found in nature. Many complementary and alternative medicine practitioners take the middle path, advocating 300 to 3000 mg of vitamin C per day.

Then there is the real controversy: are you better off eating oranges or taking vitamin C tablets? To some extent, that depends on where you stand in the dosage debate; eating 1 orange a day is manageable, eating 300 is not. As we learned with limes, natural foods are complex arrangements of ingredients that tend to work best together rather than in isolation or synthesized form. We have identified a number of vitamins and their uses but may be far from understanding the full range of benefits we obtain from whole foods. Most physicians recommend receiving vitamins from a healthy diet. This is good advice, but in a nation earning a C− in nutrition, not very realistic. If your intake for the day consists of frozen waffles and coffee for breakfast, a hot dog with fries and cola for lunch, and pizza for dinner, you are probably going to miss a few nutrients. The most practical approach is to eat the best diet possible and take a multivitamin (without iron) as a "backstop," for those days when life is too hectic to squeeze in even a single orange.

Vitamin A

The medical world has been very vigilant about the possible toxicity of micronutrients (see later) while remaining reluctant to embrace the evidence that optimal levels of micronutrients to help prevent or treat diseases are higher than the well-established RDAs. Vitamin A is a particular example. Because it is a fat-soluble vitamin, excess intake is not readily eliminated, which leads to the possibility of toxicity. Today, although reports of hypervitaminosis A are rare, deficiency of vitamin A is common and can even be considered an epidemic in certain portions of the world population.

National data from the American Association of Poison Control Centers repeatedly fail to show even one death from vitamin A per year. Vitamin A is very safe. However, pregnancy is a special case in which prolonged intake of too much preformed oil-form vitamin A might be harmful to the fetus, even at relatively low levels (under 20,000 IU/day). Interestingly, you can get over 100,000 IU of vitamin A from eating only 7 oz of beef liver. Have you ever yet seen a pregnancy overdose warning on a supermarket package of liver?

In fact, lack of vitamin A, especially during pregnancy and in infancy, poses far greater risks. Deficiency of vitamin A in developing babies is known to cause birth defects, poor tooth enamel, a weakened immune system, and literally hundreds of thousands of cases of blindness per year worldwide. This is why developing countries safely give megadoses of vitamin A to newborns.

Vitamin A Metabolism
Vitamin A (retinol) functions as a constituent of visual pigments, allows for normal reproductive capacity in both males and females, and permits normal cellular growth and differentiation. Among micronutrients, only retinol and its chemical derivatives can serve all of these biological functions.

(Continued)

Vitamin A—cont'd

The fat-soluble substance essential for normal growth that we now call vitamin A was recognized in 1909 and named in 1920, of. Preformed vitamin A, or the aldehyde and alcohol forms and their esters, are found mainly in animal products, including milk, eggs, meat, and fish, and is not synthesized by plants. However, provitamin A, which includes β-carotene among several other carotenoids, is found in plant sources and cannot be synthesized either by humans or animals. Both forms are also commonly found in over-the-counter pharmaceutical compounds. For the most part, β-carotene is converted to vitamin A during absorption through the intestinal mucosa, where it and preformed vitamin A are transported in the plasma by lipoproteins. Vitamin A is then stored in the liver in fat cells.

Wolbach and Howe (1925) were the first investigators to discover a relation between vitamin A and neoplasia; that is, dietary deficiencies in rats led to "preneoplastic abnormalities," and restoration of vitamin A to their diet reversed the neoplastic process.

Many subsequent studies, including that in 1941 by Abels et al which associated vitamin A deficiency with human cancer, strongly supported the link between vitamin A and neoplastic disease. Recognition that vitamin A deficiency leads to abnormal growth of the skin and to preneoplastic changes spurred an initial rush to treat skin disorders with this new drug; however, early excitement was tempered because of toxic effects in many patients, especially liver toxicity.

Toxicity

A hominid or prehuman skeleton of *Homo erectus* (approximately 100,000 years ago) discovered in Kenya exhibited the earliest pathologically documented changes consistent with chronic excessive intake of vitamin A, or hypervitaminosis A. The clinical effects of excessive intake of vitamin A were first reported over 100 years ago, many years before vitamin A itself had even been positively identified. These reports involved the ingestion of polar bear and seal livers (5 to 8 mg retinal per gram of liver) by Eskimos and Arctic explorers. Their acute symptoms included severe headaches, drowsiness, irritability, nausea, and vomiting. Twelve to 24 hours after ingestion, redness and loss of the skin of the face, trunk, palms, and soles developed. Seven to 10 days later, all symptoms resolved.

Subsequent clinical observations verified these major acute symptoms of hypervitaminosis A, which occur when the intake of vitamin A exceeds the capacity of the liver to remove and store it, and after ingestion of a dose of at least 350,000 IU of vitamin A by infants and 1,000,000 IU by adults. Minor acute side effects are more frequent and better described. They include

dryness of skin and mucous membranes as well as ocular, gastrointestinal, and musculoskeletal complaints such as tenderness of long bones. Specific major chronic vitamin A toxicities include abnormalities of the following: embryological development, reproductive function, serum lipids, liver function, and the skeletal system. Minor chronic side effects resemble the minor acute toxicities described earlier but are more subtle. (See Table A.)

Micronutrient Interactions

The principal micronutrients shown to interact with vitamin A are selenium, zinc, vitamins E and C, and iron. Selenium is an effective cancer-preventive agent in its own right, and its mechanism of action may be similar to that of vitamin A

Several studies have indicated that interactions occur between zinc and vitamin A at many levels of cellular activity. Some human enzyme systems requiring zinc are directly and indirectly critical to vitamin A metabolism. Zinc reportedly influences the enzyme that catalyzes the conversion of retinaldehyde to retinoic acid. Indirectly, zinc may affect vitamin A through zinc-dependent enzymes, which may be involved in the synthesis of vitamin A carriers and cellular binding proteins.

Research suggests that interactions occur between both vitamins C and E and vitamin A. Some investigators believe that vitamin E has only a nonspecific, antioxidant role in its relationship with vitamin A. Vitamin E stabilizes cell membranes, and vitamin E deficiency shortens the survival time of red blood cells and accelerates the

TABLE A

Acute and Chronic, Major and Minor, Effects of Hypervitaminosis A

	Minor	Major
Acute	Dryness of skin and mucous membranes Eye, gastrointestinal, muscle complaints Tenderness of long bones	Headache, drowsiness, irritability, nausea and vomiting Redness and loss of skin on the face, trunk, palms, soles
Chronic		Reproductive and embryological abnormalities Liver toxicity Serum lipid abnormalities Skeletal abnormalities

Vitamin A—cont'd

depletion rate of liver stores of vitamin A. Vitamin E provides vitamin A and carotenoids with protection from oxidation in mixed diets. This protection results in higher levels of liver vitamin A and, under certain circumstances, higher circulating vitamin A levels. Studies of vitamin E-deficient rats fed vitamin A indicate that vitamin E protects vitamin A at a cellular level as well. Vitamin E may also reduce vitamin A toxicity.

Vitamin A deficiency and excess appear to influence the liver's synthesis of vitamin C (ascorbic acid), and vitamin C apparently acts as an antioxidant for vitamin A. Some reports claim to demonstrate a direct association between vitamin A deficiency and vitamin C synthesis.

High levels of iron in the intestine may contribute to destruction of vitamin A–active compounds. However, no data indicate that intake of high levels of inorganic iron causes vitamin A deficiency. Studies of human volunteers have revealed that vitamin A deficiency produces the gradual onset of anemia that responds to vitamin A but not to medicinal iron supplementation. Nutrition surveys commonly reveal an association between anemia and inadequate dietary vitamin A.

Epidemiological studies of children in developing countries showed a parallel increase in hemoglobin and serum iron levels with increasing blood levels of vitamin A. Experimental studies of the interaction between iron and vitamin A show that iron absorption is not altered by vitamin A deficiency and that vitamin A appears to help mobilize stored iron and incorporate it into red blood cells.

Vitamin A: Cancer Cure or Cancer Cause?

A few researchers have claimed that vitamin A, in test-tube experiments, will push stem cells to change into cells that can build blood vessels. They contend that this activity may increase cancer. When structures similar to blood vessels developed within the tumor masses grown in culture, the investigators concluded that vitamin A promotes carcinogenesis. However, an in vitro (test-tube) experiment is far from clinical proof. Even the study authors admit that vitamin A is known to be necessary for embryonic development precisely because it helps to differentiate stem cells, pushing them to become normal tissue—which is fundamentally an "anti-cancer" activity.

There is an anticancer drug that specifically acts by blocking the breakdown of retinoic acid, derived from vitamin A. This approach has been found to be effective in treating animal models of human prostate cancer. Daily injections of the agent VN/14-1 resulted in up to a 50 percent decrease in tumor volume in mice implanted with human prostate cancer cells. No further tumor growth was seen during the 5-week study. It seems that when cancerous tumors have more vitamin A available, they shrink. Keeping more retinoic acid available within cancer cells redirects these cells back into their normal growth patterns, which includes programmed cell death. This potent agent causes cancer cells to differentiate, forcing them to turn back to a noncancerous state. Vitamin A seems to induce positive, healthy, cell changes. Vitamin A derivatives are already in wide use to fight skin cancer.

Sensational warnings and outright misstatements that natural vitamin A may "incite" cancer actually serve to excite newspaper readers and television viewers. Upon closer examination, a "vitamin promotes cancer" study often has the appearance of being conducted to prove an intended point. As the authors fuel fears about vitamin A, they also give away their goal, stating that these findings open a new door to drug development. New marketing avenues for the development of patentable vitamin A–like drugs are a commercial opportunity that the pharmaceutical industry has not overlooked.

A vitamin A derivative could protect against lung cancer development in former smokers, says another report. Significantly, the vitamin A derivative is used in combination with α-tocopherol (vitamin E) to reduce toxicity known to be associated with 13-*cis*-retinoic acid (the vitamin A derivative) therapy. This point illustrates why nutritional physicians do not use high doses of vitamin A by itself, but rather give it in conjunction with other important, synergistic nutrients. All nutrients are needed in a living body.

The following is an example: A study published in the *Journal of Nutritional Biochemistry* found that administering both vitamin A and vitamin C to cultured human breast cancer cells was more than three times as effective as administering either compound alone. The combination of the two vitamins inhibited proliferation by over 75% compared with untreated cells. The ability of retinoic acid (vitamin A) to inhibit tumor cell proliferation is well known, although its mechanism has not been defined. The authors suggested that the synergistic effect observed in this study was due to ascorbic acid's ability to slow the degradation of retinoic acid, thereby increasing vitamin A's cell proliferation inhibitory effects. Vitamin C helps vitamin A work even better.

Doctors' experience and clinical evidence both show that vitamin A helps prevent cancer, which has been known for a long time. The association of vitamin A and cancer was initially reported in 1926 when rats, fed a vitamin A–deficient diet, developed gastric carcinomas. The first investigation showing a relationship between vitamin A and human cancer was performed in 1941 by Abels et al, mentioned earlier, who found low plasma vitamin A levels in patients with gastrointestinal cancer.

(Continued)

Vitamin A—cont'd

My colleague Tom Moon and his associates reported that daily supplemental doses of 25,000 IU of vitamin A prevented squamous cell carcinoma. And de Klerk et al reported findings of significantly lower rates of mesothelioma among subjects assigned to receive retinol. Studies in animal models have shown that retinoids (including vitamin A) can act in the promotion-progression phase of carcinogenesis and block the development of invasive carcinoma at several epithelial sites, including the head and neck and lung. The Linus Pauling Institute states that studies in cell culture and animal models have documented the capacity for natural and synthetic retinoids to reduce carcinogenesis significantly in the skin, breast, liver, colon, prostate, and other sites.

There will always be people bent on believing that vitamins must be harmful somehow. For them, it only remains to set up some test tubes to try to prove it. Such has been done with other vitamins, perhaps most notably a famous experiment that claimed that vitamin C promoted cancer. The study, reported in *New Scientist,* September 22, 2001, was a prime example of sketchy science carelessly reported. The article would have readers uncritically extend the questionable findings of a highly artificial, electrical-current-vibrated quartz crystal test tube study and conclude that 2000 mg of vitamin C can (somehow) do some sort of mischief to human DNA in real life. If 2000 mg of vitamin C was harmful, the entire animal kingdom would be dead. Our nearest primate relatives all eat well in excess of 2000 mg of vitamin C each day. And, pound for pound, most animals actually manufacture from 2000 to 10,000 mg of vitamin C daily, right inside their bodies. If such generous quantities of vitamin C were harmful, evolution would have had millions of years to select against it. The same is true for vitamin A. If it "promoted" cancer, every animal eating it would get cancer.

They don't, of course. And if we consume enough vitamin A, perhaps neither do we. The National Institutes of Health state that dietary intake studies suggest an association between diets rich in β-carotene and vitamin A and a lower risk of many types of cancer. A higher intake of green and yellow vegetables or other food sources of β-carotene and/or vitamin A may decrease the risk of lung cancer. A study of over 82,000 people showed that high intakes of vitamin A reduce the risk of stomach cancer by one half. Dr. Jennifer Brett comments that "vitamin A fights cancer by inhibiting the production of DNA in cancerous cells. It slows down tumor growth in established cancers and may keep leukemia cells from dividing." A derivative of the vitamin has been shown to kill CEM-C7 human T lymphoblastoid leukemia cells and P1798-C7 murine T lymphoma cells.

Vitamin A is very far from being a cancer "promoter." Rather, it may be very near to a cancer solution. ∾

 Vitamin D

The term *vitamin D* actually refers to a pair of biologically inactive precursors of a critical micronutrient. They are vitamin D_3, also known as cholecalciferol, and vitamin D_2, also known as ergocalciferol.

Cholecalciferol (D_3) is produced in the skin by a photoreaction on exposure to ultraviolet B light from the sun (wavelength 290 to 320 nm). Ergocalciferol (D_2) is produced in plants and enters the human diet through consumption of plant sources.

Once present in the circulation, both D_2 and D_3 enter the liver and kidneys, where they are hydroxylated to form both 25-hydroxyvitamin D and 1,25-dihydroxyvitamin D. The former, 25-hydroxyvitamin D, is relatively nonactive and represents the storage form of vitamin D. By contrast, 1,25-dihydroxyvitamin D is highly active metabolically, and its levels are tightly controlled. Vitamin D has many critical metabolic functions. There has been recent confusion in the literature regarding differences in relative abundance, availability and effects of vitamin D_2 and D_3, which have been reconciled by thoughtful investigation.

The major circulating form of vitamin D_3 in human blood is 25-hydroxyvitamin D_3, and therefore it is the form measured by physicians to evaluate vitamin D status in people worldwide. It takes a long time for this form to work on calcium absorption and mobilization, however, and it must be converted or metabolized to the more active 1,25-dihydroxyvitamin D for effectiveness in the body.

Knowledge of the role of vitamin D metabolic activity, its role in human health, and identification of the forms and metabolic pathways for vitamin D had been building for many decades but only became fully elucidated during the 1970s. Although nutrition is fundamental in human health, understanding of nutritional metabolism has generally lagged behind the pace of medical investigation and practice focusing on factors external to the host such as infectious microorganisms.

Versatility of Vitamin D

The first major functions of vitamin D to be recognized were (1) enhancement of calcium absorption from the diet through the intestine and (2) mobilization and reabsorption of calcium from bone, which represents the major store of calcium (or "calcium bank") in the body. (See figure.) Calcium in turn is critical for cellular metabolism and membrane actions, enzymatic reactions, muscle function, skeletal structure, and a host of activities needed to sustain life and maintain homeostasis. Because vitamin D has long been recognized for its role in calcium metabolism, it has long been used to treat patients with renal failure and bone diseases. It also has an important role in the treatment of postmenopausal

Vitamin D
Photoconversion and Hydroxylation, and Metabolic Actions

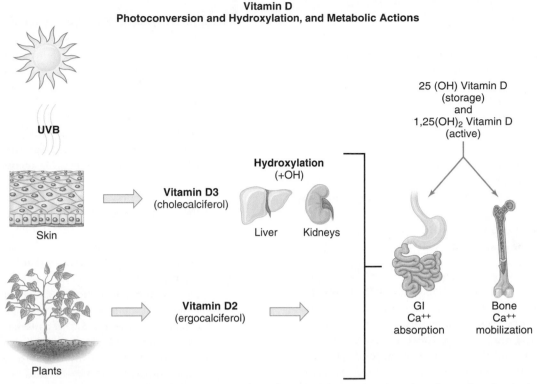

Sources and photoconversion of vitamin D. (Original artwork by Marc Micozzi, redrawn by Elsevier.)

Vitamin D—cont'd

osteoporosis and the current epidemic of bone fractures in the elderly.

In 1979, however, DeLuca found that vitamin D is actually recognized by every tissue in the body. Every cell has receptors for vitamin D. Since then vitamin D has been used to treat hyperproliferative skin diseases such as psoriasis.

In the immune system, the large white blood cell macrophages activate vitamin D. The activated vitamin D in turn causes macrophages to make a peptide that specifically kills infective agents such as tuberculosis mycobacteria. Vitamin D also has a role in helping prevent autoimmune diseases such as multiple sclerosis, rheumatoid arthritis, and diabetes type 1.

Vitamin D's activity in the kidney has long been recognized, and it has been found to affect the production of renin and angiotensin, the major regulators of blood pressure, in the kidney. There is a direct correlation between higher (further from the equator) latitudes (where both sunlight and vitamin D levels are lower) and higher blood pressure in both the northern and southern hemispheres of the earth. People at high latitudes with high blood pressure experience a return to normal blood pressure levels after exposure to ultraviolet B light in a tanning bed three times a week for 3 months

and restoration of active vitamin D levels (and you thought it only worked if the sunlight was captured on a beach in the Bahamas!).

Multiple sclerosis also shows a marked association with higher latitudes worldwide, and there may be a similar protective role for vitamin D for this disease.

Vitamin D is also thought to have an important role in cancer. As early as the 1940s it was noted that living at higher latitudes is associated with a higher incidence of several cancers (whereas only skin cancer specifically has a lower incidence at higher latitudes). Recent epidemiological observations have continued to bear out this association. A high frequency of sunbathing before age 20 was found to reduce the risk of non-Hodgkin lymphoma. And, although sun exposure is related to an increased incidence of malignant melanoma, it was also found to be associated with increased survival from melanoma in a recent study. In some of the sunniest spots on earth, both the Australian College of Dermatologists, the Cancer Council of Australia, and the New Zealand Bone and Mineral Society have concluded that a balance is required between avoiding an increased risk of skin cancer and achieving enough ultraviolet light exposure to maintain adequate vitamin D levels.

As in all things involving nutrition, achieving a balance is a good goal and guide for optimal health. It was

(Continued)

Vitamin D—cont'd

thought that a balanced approach to this problem could be achieved through thoughtful dermatological screening for skin cancers. Thus, most skin cancers should be detected and treated early, because they are by definition visible on the surface of the skin, unlike cancers of other tissues, which begin growing hidden and undetected deep inside the body.

Dermatological intervention also took another, different direction, however. Rather than just focusing on early detection and treatment of skin cancer, dermatologists began fighting against the sun. That, in turn, has had profound effects on vitamin D nutrition and deficiency over the past 40 years.

Global Dimensions of D-ficiency

Essentially little or no active vitamin D is available from regular dietary sources. It is principally found in fish oils, sun-dried mushrooms, and fortified foods like milk and orange juice. However, many countries worldwide forbid the fortification of foods. There is potentially plenty of vitamin D in the food chain, because both phytoplankton and zooplankton exposed to sunlight make vitamin D. Wild-caught salmon, which feeds on natural food sources, for example, has available vitamin D. However, farmed salmon fed food pellets with little nutritional value have only 10% of the vitamin D of wild fish. The "perfect storm" of photophobia, lack of exposure to sunlight, and insufficiency of available dietary vitamin D has led to a national and worldwide epidemic of vitamin D deficiency.

Estimates are that at least 30% and as much as 80% of the U.S. population is vitamin D deficient. In the United States, at latitudes north of Atlanta, the skin does not make (photoconvert) any vitamin D from November through March (i.e., essentially outside of daylight savings time; so although we shift the clock around, it does not salvage vitamin D synthesis). During this season the angle of the sun in the sky is too low to allow UVB light to penetrate the atmosphere, and it is absorbed by the ozone layer. Even in the late spring, summer, and early fall, most vitamin D is made between 10 am and 3 pm when UVB from the sun penetrates the atmosphere and reaches the earth's surface.

It might be expected that vitamin D deficiency would be a problem limited to northern latitudes.

In Bangor, Maine, among young girls 9 to 11 years old, nearly 50% were deficient at the end of winter and nearly 20% remained deficient at the end of summer. At Boston Children's Hospital, over 50% of adolescent girls and African American and Hispanic boys were found to be vitamin D deficient year round. In another study in Boston 34% of whites, 40% of Hispanics, and 84% of African American adults over age 50 were found to be deficient.

Vitamin D deficiency is also a national problem, however. The U.S. Centers for Disease Control and Prevention completed a national survey at the end of winter and found that nearly 50% of African American women aged 15 to 49 years were deficient. These are women in the critical childbearing years. A growing fetus must receive adequate vitamin D from the mother, especially because breast milk does not provide adequate vitamin D. A study of pregnant women in Boston found that in 40 mother-infant pairs at the time of labor and delivery, over 75% of mothers and 80% of newborns were deficient. This observation was made despite the fact that pregnant women were instructed to take a prenatal vitamin that included 400 IU of vitamin D and to drink two glasses of milk per day.

Further, vitamin D deficiency is a global problem. Even in India, home to 1 billion of the earth's people, where there is plenty of sun, 30% to 50% of children, 50% to 80% of adults, and 90% of physicians are deficient. In South Africa, vitamin D deficiency is also a problem even though Cape Town is situated at 34 degrees latitude.

Although there are many new bilateral and multilateral governmental and private efforts to export Western medical technology and pharmaceuticals to the Third World to combat infectious diseases such as acquired immunodeficiency syndrome (AIDS), there is no comparable effort to acknowledge and address the global dimensions of the vitamin D deficiency epidemic. The U.S. Congress and president just deemed it as a great achievement to give $40 billion in tax dollars to U.S. pharmaceutical companies to send expensive drug treatments for AIDS (a preventable disease) overseas. By contrast, addressing the vitamin D deficiency epidemic could be accomplished with much safer and less expensive nutritional supplements together with sunlight, the only source of energy that is still free.

Vitamin D Dose, Toxicity, and Formulation

It has been well established that giving 100 IU of vitamin D daily to children will prevent rickets (Table B).

As with most of established thinking about recommended daily allowances (RDAs), the dosages are those that prevent the development of frank nutritional deficiencies and associated pathology. The idea of levels for optimal health does not enter the picture. Even the capricious RDA process raised the recommendation from 200 IU to 400 IU/day in 1997 (although technically it is not an "RDA" but an "IA," or adequate intake).

Currently, those more knowledgeable about human nutrition than the group involved in the outdated RDA/IA process recommend 1000 IU daily for both children and adults to maintain blood levels of 25-hydroxyvitamin D above 30 ng/mL. It is now recognized that each 100 IU

TABLE B

The Evolving Picture of Vitamin D Daily Intake

Daily intake	Associated effects
100 IU	Prevents rickets, frank nutritional deficiency disease
	Amount in one glass of milk or fortified orange juice
200 IU	"Adequate intake" per RDA pre-1997
400 IU	"Adequate intake" per RDA post-1997
	Reduces risk of rheumatoid arthritis in women by 50%
1000 IU	Reduces risk of cancer (breast, colorectal, ovarian, prostate) by 50%
2000 IU	Reduces risk of diabetes by 80%
	Reduces incidence of upper respiratory tract infections in the elderly by 90%
	Reduces PSA levels in men by 50%
30,000 IU	Minimum to develop toxicity over several months or years

PSA, Prostate-specific antigen; *RDA*, recommended daily allowance.

TABLE C

Blood Levels of Vitamin D (25-Hydroxyvitamin D)

Level (ng/mL)	Associated intakes and effects
1	Amount blood level is raised by 100 IU intake
1-20	Deficiency
21-29	Insufficiency
30-150	Sufficiency, reached by 50,000 IU weekly for 8 weeks
50	Reduces risk of breast cancer by 50% (vs. 20 ng/mL)
150-200	Onset of toxicity

Vitamin D—cont'd

of vitamin D ingested raises blood levels by only 1 ng/mL (Table C).

Although a typical recommendation is in the range of 1000 to 2000 IU/day, it is reasonable to recommend up to 5000 IU/day.

It is not easy to become vitamin D intoxicated. Sunlight actually destroys any excess vitamin D that is made in the body, so it is not possible to become vitamin D intoxicated from too much sunlight alone. In a world in which dangerous and expensive drugs are doled out like candy, it is ironic to witness the degree of concern in the medical establishment over exposures to physiological levels of natural substances such as vitamins, and even sunlight!

Nonetheless, a medical lore has developed over the possible risks of excess vitamin D intake, although vitamin D intoxication is one of the most rare medical conditions in the world. If vitamin D were considered as a drug, it demonstrates a remarkably high therapeutic index of at least 300 for disease treatment (ratio of minimum toxic dose to dose given to treat rickets) and at least 20 for chronic disease prevention. If the patient has a chronic granulomatous disorder such as histoplasmosis, sarcoidosis, or tuberculosis, however, a vitamin D blood level above 30 ng/mL will cause hypercalcemia and hypercalciuria. Therefore, supplementation should be avoided in these cases.

Because the only pharmaceutical preparation of vitamin D is in 50,000-IU doses, one therapeutic regimen is 50,000 IU per *week* for 8 weeks to treat deficiency, with 50,000 IU *every 2 weeks* thereafter for maintenance of adequate vitamin D levels. Dietary supplements are also good choices for vitamin D.

Manufacturers often add 50% more vitamin D than is listed on the label to maintain potency during the shelf life of the product. Thus, a 1000-IU formulation that actually contains 1500 IU is still perfectly safe.

Despite the inadequacy of the RDA/IA process there is ample evidence and clinical experience indicating that vitamin D blood levels and daily intakes should be much higher than they are, not only for prevention of bone diseases but to provide optimal health and help reduce the risk of many common chronic diseases, disorders, and medical conditions. Together with healthy sun exposure, Vitamin D supplementation can be accomplished safely and effectively and should be a first-line consideration in any clinical practice and for the general population.

MINERALS

Minerals are everywhere in nature and range from beneficial (calcium) to poisonous (arsenic). The minerals essential to human function include calcium, phosphorus, potassium, sodium (salt), chloride, and magnesium. In addition, we need a number of trace elements, including iron, zinc, selenium, manganese, copper, iodine, molybdenum, cobalt, chromium, and fluorine. As with vitamins, most physicians recommend obtaining minerals from a healthy diet, whereas many complementary and alternative medicine practitioners advocate supplements to ensure a regular supply.

RDAs have been established for only six minerals—calcium, phosphorus, iron, magnesium, iodine, and zinc—and two of those guidelines have recently been questioned. Much recent publicity has surrounded the role of calcium in preventing osteoporosis, the brittle bones that come with age, especially for women. The National Academy of Science recently raised the RDA for calcium from 800 to 1000 mg for nonpregnant women and from 1200 to 1500 mg for pregnant women. Although this is a step in the right direction, compliance remains doubtful. The old RDAs were not met by 68% of the total population; more significantly, they were not met by 84% of women between ages 35 and 50 and 87% of girls between 15 and 18 years of age. With higher standards, these compliance percentages may slip still lower.

The one mineral that medical professionals have been successful in promoting, *iron,* has turned out to be potentially harmful. For many years, although expressing now-discredited concerns about potential dangers from most supplements, the medical profession advocated the use of iron supplements. Vital for the production of hemoglobin, which transports oxygen to the body's cells, iron is also necessary for many immune, growth, and enzyme functions. Lack of iron leads to anemia, especially in pregnant women, and to other conditions, including fatigue, fragile bones, and mental disorders. However, because iron is stored in the body, excesses can easily build up, causing the production of free radicals, which have been associated with cancer and heart disease. This author has conducted independent research showing that excess iron can cause cancer. More often, overuse of iron supplements causes digestive discomforts and disorders. Dietary guidelines for iron are now being revised downward, and many multivitamin supplements are now available without iron.

Exactly how much of any nutrient is needed depends largely on the physical condition of the individual. Pregnant women, athletes, smokers, people with chronic illnesses, and those of various ages and lifestyles all have different dietary requirements. The one dietary requirement that is relatively consistent for all of us is the need for water.

WATER AND FLUID AND ELECTROLYTES

The human body can survive up to 5 weeks without food but rarely lasts beyond a few days without water. Our bodies are almost 70% water, which is vital for every bodily process, including absorbing and digesting food, transporting nutrients throughout the body, and carrying out waste materials. Water is naturally lost through sweat and elimination. Caffeine, alcohol, and other constituents act as diuretics, which increase urination and further deplete the body's reserves of liquids. To replace all this lost fluid, we need to drink at least eight glasses of water a day. Dry mouth, headache, and fatigue are often signs we are dehydrated. Exercise, massage, and other activities increase our need for water. When we are ill, additional fluids help flush toxins from the body and restore well-being.

Fluid and electrolyte balance is critical for good health and physical performance. The salinity of the blood and tissues matches the salinity of the oceans at the time life is thought to have emerged from the sea into the terrestrial environment. Water itself has some unique properties that has enabled life to exist on earth. Liquids generally freeze from the bottom up; as liquids cool, the colder molecules of the liquid (with lower kinetic energy) fall toward the bottom because they become more dense—and thus the liquid will become solid (freeze) from the bottom up. Water, to the contrary, has a distinctive molecular configuration. As water cools the molecular configuration becomes more dense until it reaches approximately 40° F at which point a remarkable effect takes hold. The water molecules begin to lock into a molecular configuration that is less dense, and the molecules rise to the top as they freeze. In large bodies of water, the frozen layer at the top then tends to trap any heat energy in the lower reaches, thus preventing the entire body of water from freezing. Imagine the implications for life on earth if bodies of water froze from the bottom up.

Individual organisms rely on water to carry blood cells and nutrients to all parts of the body in the blood circulation, to bathe the tissue cells in extracellular fluid, to support the central nervous system through the cerebrospinal fluid, and to return excess body fluids to the circulation through the lymphatic vessels. It is one large, complex hydraulic system.

It is important to maintain both fluid and electrolyte levels. The formation of urine occurs at a relatively constant rate to filter the blood and remove metabolic by-products to eliminate them from the body. Although carbohydrate is broken down in the body to carbon dioxide (which is breathed out through the lungs) and water vapor (both breathed out and eliminated in urine), organic nutrients containing nitrogen must be eliminated as metabolic by-products and excreted through the urine. The fate of proteins, purines, and pyrimidines (nucleic acids) is ultimately to become urea and uric acid in the urine. Buildup of uric acid in the blood leads to gout with deposits of uric acid crystals in joints and cartilage (such as in the earlobes). In kidney failure, nitrogen-containing metabolites build up in the blood to the point that they cause central nervous toxicity (renal encephalopathy).

In addition to elimination of fluid and electrolytes in the urine, there are continual insensible losses of water through respiration (the exhaled air carries out water vapor) as well as losses of both water and electrolytes through sweating. Humans, who are less hirsute mammals, have sweat glands throughout the skin of the body. Cooling by evaporation of water allows the surface of the body to reduce surface temperature. Hairier animals covered with fur cannot use this mechanism and rely on hyperpnea, or rapid panting, which allows blood in the tongue to be cooled by contact with air (like the old air-cooled engines of the Volkswagen Beetle). When people sweat due to high ambient temperatures and/or high physical performance, it is important to replace both fluid and electrolytes.

Body water and electrolytes may also be lost by excretion of excessive fluids in the stool, as in diarrhea and dysentery (the latter implies loss of blood as well as water and electrolytes in the stool). In the case of cholera, the cholera bacteria produce a toxin that inhibits reabsorption of water from the intestinal contents by the cells lining the intestines. The result is massive fluid and electrolyte loss, which may result in death from dehydration within days. Diarrhea is still a very common cause of death in infants in third world countries, especially where nursing mothers are encouraged to use infant formula (made with contaminated water) instead of staying with the proven benefits of natural breastfeeding.

DIET AS THERAPY

Although most mainstream Western physicians receive little training in diet and rarely consider it as a therapy, many other health practitioners consider food a vital part of preventing and treating illness (see Chapters 21, 26, 29, and 32).

CHINESE MEDICINE

Since ancient times, the Chinese have used food for medicinal purposes, and many contemporary medical schools include a classroom kitchen to train students in preparing beneficial foods. Families and some restaurants routinely prepare special dishes to meet the needs of people who are ill, elderly, pregnant, or lactating. Beneficial foods are identified and selected on the basis of such traditional Chinese medical concepts as the five-phase theory and yin and yang, two models for the dynamic processes governing the universe and human bodies. *Yin* is associated with the female principle, and its properties include cold, slowness, darkness, the interior, and deficiency. *Yang* is associated with the male principle; its properties include heat, light, speed, the exterior, and excess. A disease characterized by too much cold would be associated with yin, and a practitioner might prescribe foods and herbs that stimulate yang by enhancing heat or "scattering the cold" (see Chapter 26 and later section on macrobiotics).

AYURVEDA

Developed in ancient India, Ayurveda (Sanskrit for "the knowledge of long life") has always incorporated food into its holistic approach to health. In Ayurveda, three *doshas* (vata, pitta, and kapha) define the three basic mind-body or constitutional types. Each dosha finds certain foods and flavors beneficial, whereas others may be harmful if taken in too large a quantity. For instance, people whose dominant dosha is *vata,* which is responsible for the body's kinetic energy and associated with the element of air, may suffer from nervous energy and will be soothed by warm, moist, sweet foods and aggravated by pungent, bitter, raw foods. Following an appropriate vata diet can help people avoid or recover from a wide range of vata disorders, such as insomnia, constipation, anxiety, high blood pressure, and arthritis (see Chapters 29 and 32).

NATUROPATHY

A synthesis and refinement of nineteenth-century nature cures, naturopathy considers a wholesome diet one of the cornerstones of good health, along with exercise, fresh air, adequate sleep, and low-stress lifestyle. Naturopaths believe that the body has an innate tendency to heal itself and that nourishing food is necessary for the body's self-maintenance and repairs. Practitioners recommend a diet of whole (unprocessed) foods, especially fresh fruits and vegetables, which should be organic (free of chemicals and other additives) if possible. Fasting, including juice fasts, may be prescribed to rid the body of toxins. Naturopaths started the first "health food stores" in America and developed many foods, such as graham crackers, that were revolutionary in their use of whole grains (see Chapter 21).

MACROBIOTICS

Loosely based on the traditional Chinese concepts of yin and yang, the macrobiotic diet was developed in the 1950s by George Osawa, a Japanese educator and philosopher. The name is derived from the Greek *makros* ("big" or "long") and *bios* ("life"), and its practitioners believe a long and healthy life can be achieved through a balanced diet and other beneficial practices. As do traditional Chinese physicians, macrobiotics advocates believe all foods have yin or yang properties. Yin foods, which are thought to be calming, include green vegetables, fruits, nuts, and honey. Yang foods, said to be strengthening, include meat, fish, eggs, and beans. Whole grains, which have balanced yin and yang, form the cornerstone of the diet. Too much yin food can leave a person feeling resentful and worried; an overly yang meal may generate feelings of aggressiveness. Eating the proper foods can help rebalance feelings and restore physical well-being.

REVERSAL OF HEART DISEASE

Heart disease was considered irreversible until the 1980s, when cardiologist Dean Ornish proved that heart patients could restore heart health through diet, exercise, and stress management. Based on the Pritikin diet, Ornish's diet is very low in fat (perhaps too low at 15% of calories) and cholesterol and is high (perhaps too high) in carbohydrates and fiber. It excludes almost all animal products except for skim milk and fat-free yogurt. An occasional glass of wine is permitted; smoking is not. In a rigorous week-long training session, participants are taught how to cook and eat according to Ornish's guidelines and are instructed in exercise, yoga, and meditation. When they go home, they are expected to continue the regimen indefinitely. This approach is not easy to maintain, but when the alternative is heart bypass surgery, possibly followed by another operation in 5 years, participants are motivated; in 99% of cases, those who followed the regimen successfully reversed the course of their heart disease. Many who question whether the Ornish diet itself is optimal point to the benefits of social support and stress reduction to help account for these results.

VEGETARIAN AND VEGAN DIETS

A *vegetarian* does not eat meat, poultry, or fish but does eat eggs and dairy products. Research has demonstrated that a vegetarian diet can reduce the risk of heart disease, high blood pressure, diabetes, osteoporosis, gallbladder disease, colon cancer, and other conditions. A *vegan* diet excludes all animal-based foods, including dairy products, eggs, and honey. Unless supplements are used, vegans risk deficiency of vitamin B_{12}. The vegan diet has been used to treat asthma, arthritis, high blood pressure, and angina.

RAW FOODS

In the late nineteenth century, Swiss physician Max Bircher-Benner developed a diet that is 70% uncooked vegetables and fruits; the balance of the diet can include meat, dairy products, grains, nuts, and seeds. He believed that raw foods (1) are more natural and appropriate for the human digestive system, (2) maintain their nutrients better than cooked food, and (3) prolong the life span.

DETOXIFICATION

Since ancient times, people have sought to eliminate toxins from the body by fasting and special diets, often in conjunction with other means, such as emetics and enemas. At present, many Americans are concerned about ridding their bodies of waste products that have accumulated because of poor digestion or sluggish elimination or that have resulted from environmental toxins. Practitioners recommend eating only raw fruits and vegetables and drinking large amounts of water; yogurt may also be included in the regimen (see also Chapter 21).

THE ATKINS DIET

In the 1970s, Robert Atkins developed a diet based on the principle that sugar and refined carbohydrates increase the body's production of insulin, a hormone necessary for the transformation of carbohydrates to blood sugar. Consumption of white bread, pasta, cereal, and other highly processed, low-fat foods causes insulin levels to spike. When the carbohydrates are absorbed and high amounts of insulin are no longer needed, insulin levels drop sharply, which reduces energy and encourages thoughts of a carbohydrate-laden snack. Atkins developed a diet that severely restricts the intake of processed and refined carbohydrates and promotes instead a diet focusing on "nutrient-dense" foods—proteins, fats, and complex carbohydrates—supported by multivitamins and other supplements (Atkins Center, n.d.). The Atkins diet has been demonstrated to be effective for short-term weight loss, but the long-term health effects are of concern to some.

THE "ZONE" DIET

Like Atkins, Barry Sears designed a diet that reduces the intake of processed foods and sugar to control insulin level. Sears's diet, which he calls "Zone Perfect" and most people know as "the Zone," uses food as a drug to keep insulin levels in the "therapeutic zone" 24 hours a day. According to Sears, every meal and snack should contain a set ratio of macronutrients: 30% protein, 40% carbohydrates, and 30% fats. Sears also suggests adding supplements, such as ω-3 fish oils and antioxidants, to enhance the Zone diet (Zone Perfect, n.d.).

FOOD OR DRUG?

Sears and Atkins are not the only people using food's druglike properties to affect the body. Scientists have long been aware that many fruits, vegetables, grains, and beans appear to reduce the risk of heart disease, cancer, and other conditions because they contain *antioxidants* (vitamins, minerals, and enzymes that protect cells from being damaged by oxidation). Now another group of disease-fighting nutrients has been identified: phytochemicals, also known as "nutraceuticals."

Phytochemicals are thought to fight cancer and other ailments by keeping disease-causing substances from latching onto healthy cells and by removing toxins before they can cause harm. There are many thousands of phytochemicals—tomatoes alone contain 10,000 different kinds—each with a slightly different function. Genistein, for example, which is found in soybeans, prevents the formation of the capillaries needed to nourish tumors. Indoles, which increase immune function, are found in members of the Brassica family such as broccoli and cauliflower. The bioflavonoids found in limes prevent certain cancer-causing hormones from attaching to the body's cells. Much as an earlier generation of scientists sought to identify and synthesize vitamins, today's researchers are working to isolate and manufacture phytochemicals. However, it is unlikely that they will be able to reproduce the rich mix of beneficial substances found in a single tomato or a handful of soybeans.

Sometimes we do not need to eat the plant to obtain the benefits of phytochemicals. For example, brewing teas such as green tea can provide a natural mixture of antioxidants to be drunk as a beverage. The antioxidant profile of green tea (from Asia) has been studied extensively in terms of its anticancer effects. A newly popular red tea (from South Africa) has a similar profile of antioxidants, but without the caffeine, and also shows anticancer properties.

FOOD ALLERGIES

Soybeans may be bristling with needed nutrients and phytochemicals, but they are among the common foods that trigger allergies. Other major offenders include nuts (especially peanuts), dairy products, fish, shellfish, wheat, eggs, and food additives, especially preservatives and coloring agents.

An *allergy* occurs when the immune system reacts to an ordinary food as if it were a hostile invader, producing an antibody known as immunoglobin E. This antibody attaches itself to specialized immune cells known as masts, and when the offending food is encountered again, the antibody causes the mast cell to release chemicals that produce the allergic reaction. The result may be skin disorders (e.g., hives, eczema), respiratory conditions (e.g., allergic rhinitis, asthma), stomach problems (e.g., cramps, diarrhea), or headaches. In severe cases, people may develop anaphylactic shock, which causes collapse and possibly even death.

No one knows for certain what causes allergies to arise, but it is common for them to run in families, although each family member may have a different type. Some theorize a possible psychological component; on some deep level, allergy sufferers may view the world as inherently hostile. "It is fairly common to be sensitive to one or two foods," notes physician Christiane Northrup. "But women with multiple food allergies that are resistant to simple dietary change often have a history of abuse of some type, or they are continuing to live in dysfunctional relationships or to stay in overly stressful jobs" (Northrup, 1994).

START WITH THE USUAL SUSPECTS

The offending substance (known as an *allergen*) can often be identified by a simple skin prick test, in which one after another of the "usual suspects" is injected under the skin to see how the body responds. Another investigative technique is the radioallergosorbent test, in which blood is drawn, serum containing antibodies is extracted, and possible allergens are added to test for a reaction. Naturopaths favor an *elimination diet,* in which various foods are systematically removed from the menu for 2 weeks. When symptoms disappear, foods are reintroduced one by one until a reaction takes place, indicating which one is causing the allergy.

Herbalists often recommend that the elimination diet be accompanied by intake of immune boosters such as echinacea and red clover, digestive aids (e.g., slippery elm, marshmallow, hops), and dandelion root to support liver function (see Chapter 22). Yoga practitioners can teach postures designed to aid digestion and overall well-being (see Chapter 31). Nutritionists with expertise in supplements advise taking vitamins and minerals, including zinc, selenium, vitamin C, magnesium, and manganese.

Homeopaths treat allergies with a form immunotherapy in which highly diluted amounts of the allergen are given with the aim of overcoming the reaction (see Chapter 24). This is similar to the controversial approach known as *desensitization,* in which people are exposed to minute but increasing amounts of the allergen until a higher level of tolerance is achieved. Enzymes have proved effective in treating some milk sugar allergies. For the majority of those with allergies, the most effective treatment is avoiding the allergen in question.

FUNCTIONAL FOODS

The American food industry is currently responding to the public's desire for healthier fare by creating a variety of products that, they claim, provide enhanced health benefits, such as lowering cholesterol and heightening mental abilities. Known as *functional foods,* these products include snacks, cereals, margarines, and salad dressings laced with calcium, vitamins, fiber, and such new constituents as DHA (docosahexaenoic acid), which is currently being used in Japanese schoolchildren and is said to improve concentration.

To achieve the benefits of functional foods, large quantities of them must be consumed. One margarine, for example, must be eaten three times a day for 2 weeks to lower cholesterol by 10%. To obtain their full allotment of vitamins from snack foods, toddlers must eat three and a half cookies a day. Often six times as expensive as standard fare (e.g., one margarine retails for $17.22 a pound), these functional foods require a level of commitment many families are not prepared to make.

The greatest drawback to many functional foods is the flavor. As *New York Times* food critic William Grimes noted, one cholesterol-controlling apricot and orange cereal bar has the "texture of a rubber eraser, enlivened by a hideously artificial fruit flavor." He noted that a "sugar controller" for diabetic patients, a fudge brownie flavor nutrition bar, "chews like a plug of tobacco, minus the flavor, except for a haylike aftertaste. The chocolate coating seems to be for color only. Nuts depicted on the wrapping fail to show up in the actual bar" (Grimes, 1999). In a taste test of 13 functional foods, five got a "thumb's up," including the bone-building Aviva Instant Hot Chocolate and Viactiv's caramel-flavored soft calcium chews; the majority of products received a "thumb's down." Grimes addressed the "pleasure principle" as follows:

> All food is functional. That's why humans eat three times a day. But unlike animals and insects, they do not eat for function's sake alone. Somewhere in the tortured mental software that governs eating behavior, the pleasure principle lives in more or less uneasy proximity to the efficiency principle. We eat to live, but we also live to eat.

NUTRITION VERSUS NOURISHMENT

Food and emotions are very deeply linked in human beings for reasons far older than our current obsession with thinness. For centuries the human race was able to survive because we ate the things our tribes said were okay to eat. We avoided the poisonous berries and ate what Mother said was safe. Food has always been an essential part of the daily ritual of living, and the foods we were fed in childhood have left a very deep impression on us. At an unconscious and conscious level, they help us feel safe and cared for (Northrup, 1994).

One of the reasons diets and food fads are so popular is that we are tribal beings who take our cues about what to eat from those around us. One of the reasons diets so often fail is that they conflict with much deeper cultural programming that comes from our family of origin. If generations of your relatives served beef brisket (or borscht, or macaroni and cheese) for dinner every Sunday, that dish will forever be equated with family gatherings and feelings of belonging. However flawed they may be, our families usually present our strongest links to our past and to others; in a profound way, they represent safety and the sense of being at home.

Unfortunately, the eating patterns of the past do not always work well in the twenty-first century. The rib roast with gravy and buttered potatoes that once nourished our great grandparents on the farm may lead to a heart attack in someone whose most strenuous daily activity is booting up the computer. On the other hand, the food products our contemporary culture urges us to consume—loaded with fat, salt, sugar, artificial ingredients, and chemical additives and stripped of nutrients during processing—are equally unlikely to sustain us into a healthy and advanced old age. Taking a scientific, reductionist approach is not the answer either. Obsessing about every calorie and gram of fat on our plates can turn food into an enemy. Eating is one of the most vital ways we connect with our environment and with each other. Treating food as a hostile force is not good for our bodies, our souls, or our relationship with the world.

So, what is the key to healthy eating? Moderation and common sense are a good starting point. Once we understand our basic nutritional needs and which foods we would be wise to avoid when possible, we can move gradually into patterns of eating that provide us with a sense of physical well-being. However, unless we have a medical condition such as diabetes that requires strict dietary controls, healthy eating does not mean abandoning favorite foods forever. On occasion a piece of grandmother's fried chicken at a family gathering, an ice cream cone on a summer afternoon, or a mug of sugary cocoa after sledding is a necessary reminder that being alive is sometimes supposed to be fun and that sharing food with the people we love can be healthy for our hearts in ways not yet recognized by biomedical science. Food is rich in cultural, social, and personal meaning as well as nutrients, and all these elements are necessary for a balanced diet.

⊕ Chapter References can be found on the Evolve website at http://evolve.elsevier.com/Micozzi/complementary/

CHAPTER

26

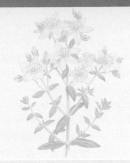

TRADITIONAL MEDICINE OF CHINA

KEVIN V. ERGIL

Sections Five and Six provide a survey of the fundamentals of global health traditions that form integrated systems of thought and practice, following from an explanation of their relevant world views. The sections are divided geographically into Asia (Section Five) and Africa and the Americas (Section Six). Although this book aims to present a unified body of the theories and practices of alternative medicines, many healing traditions throughout the world are marked by significant heterogeneity, consistent with their historical evolution and their underlying philosophies. Refer to the Evolve site at http://evolve.elsevier.com/Micozzi/complementary for the Tibetan Medicine chapter. ∾

CHINA'S TRADITIONAL MEDICINE IN CULTURAL PERSPECTIVE

Certain considerations are important to understanding ethnomedical systems in general and Chinese medicine in particular. Medicine is a human endeavor and as such is shaped by the considerations of the humans using and practicing it. These considerations sometimes have very little to do with curing disease in the most simple and efficient way and a great deal to do with economics, politics, and culture. Ideology, belief, and even simple ignorance have influenced the practice of medicine more than rationality. A medical historian or a physician might perceive medicine to be a steady march from ignorance to the light, but these are typically revisionist histories. Medicine is a human enterprise embedded in and intersected by myriad other human projects. Even the choice of how to conduct a medical procedure or what type of health care to choose may have more to do with habit or economics than with rationality or efficacy.

For example, American gynecologists position their patients for maximum visual exposure during routine examinations, whereas physicians in the United Kingdom allow the patient to lie on her side, assuming a more relaxed posture during the examination (Payer, 1988). An example more relevant to this chapter is the case of a Chinese patient who chose traditional herbal medicine to manage painful and debilitating kidney stones. Although the treatment was ultimately efficacious, the patient's choice was not motivated by a desire for efficacy. Undergoing surgery would have meant that the patient would have been classified as an "invalid" on the work papers and therefore barred from advancement. As a final example, a hospital in California closes its doors to the practice of acupuncture, even though acupuncturists in the state are licensed medical practitioners and their services are routinely requested by hospital patients. In each instance, considerations that are not directly linked to the rational and effective delivery of medical care influence medical choices.

Our own perspectives on medicine and our experience of our own medical systems provide us with ideas of what is normal or typical for medicine. We respond to aspects of a traditional system that correspond with our expectations. We imagine Chinese herbal medicine to be a gentle therapy using nontoxic ingredients. Its use of highly toxic substances or drastic purgative therapies is easily overlooked. It is unlikely, for example, that the traditional form of Tibetan therapeutic cautery applied with a hot iron will elicit substantial interest as a form of alternative therapy. Naturalistic and rational elements of systems intrigue us. Unfamiliar or magical diagnostic and therapeutic modes cause us concern.

It is easy to make intellectual errors when dealing with medical systems. We forget that our own perspectives may prevent us from understanding the meaning and use of practices that have been developed within another culture. That failure to account for our own needs and biases also can lead to the overenthusiastic acceptance of ideas whose genesis and application we really do not understand.

If we want to avoid these errors, we must think about medical systems as being embedded in their respective cultures. Each system's structure and elements are vital to their practice in a particular cultural context. "Culture," in this sense, does not imply an all-embracing system of meaning subscribed to by all members of a community, country, or ethnicity. Culture is a complex network of signification; some elements might resonate only in a local sense, whereas other aspects have almost global relevance. This does not mean that the medical ideas and practices of one society cannot or will not be successfully appropriated by another, but rather that aspects of a system that are meaningful to one group of people might not be meaningful at all to another.

For example, neurasthenia *(sheng jin shuai ruo)* is an important syndrome in traditional Chinese medicine and Chinese psychiatry, even though this diagnosis has fallen into disrepute among Western psychiatrists and the condition is no longer classified as a disease entity in diagnostic manuals. Neurasthenia was an exceptionally popular diagnosis in the nineteenth century during periods of extensive medical exchange between the United States and China and Japan. The diagnosis has continued to be clinically important in China because it fits well into certain traditional medical models and responds well to cultural and political concerns about mental illness (Kleinman, 1986). Americans and Europeans who encounter neurasthenia within the corpus of Chinese medicine

sometimes find it an unusual or obscure concept despite its relevance for Chinese medical practice.

Sometimes, on encountering a new idea, we choose to think about it in familiar terms. One example is the use of the word *energy* to express the idea of qi. An extension of this is the frequent translation of the term for the therapeutic method of draining evil influences from channels as "sedation." Neither energy nor sedation has much to do with the concepts that underlie qi and draining; however, these terms are more familiar to us and make Chinese medicine more accessible. Unfortunately, this practice can obscure the breadth of meaning in these terms (Wiseman et al, 1990).

We try to make sense of the world from our position in it, historically as well as culturally. We tend to view history as progressing, as if by design, to a specific end. Events of the past, viewed from the perspective of the present, offer tempting opportunities for reinterpretation in relation to current experience. For example, in the context of current perspectives on disease causation, Wu You Ke's statements that "miscellaneous qi" could cause epidemic disease and his concept of "one disease, one qi" (Wiseman, 1993) have led contemporary sources in China to suggest that, coming before the invention of the microscope, such an insight is quite remarkable (Wiseman et al, 1995). The idea that Wu You Ke's observation represented a precursor of germ theory is attractive to Chinese practitioners who are trying to find a place for traditional practices in an increasingly biomedicalized world. In fact, the concept of miscellaneous or pestilential qi has been used extensively in adapting traditional theory to the management of human immunodeficiency virus (HIV) infection. However, as Wiseman points out, it never was explored in relation to the causation of disease by microscopic organisms, nor was it ever conceived as a basis for such an exploration. Its relation to this concept is a retrospective interpretation.

The preceding points are generally relevant to almost any system or collection of medical practices. Some additional points are crucial to understanding the progression of medical thought in China. Although we tend to think that Chinese medicine has been practiced without significant change for millennia, this is simply not true. Chinese medicine has undergone significant change and development over the centuries. Ideas that once were important are now almost invisible, and ideas that were left by the wayside for centuries found favor in later times. Recent ideas have been relatively significant in the organization of the system. Changes in technology, for example, have broadened the clinical use of acupuncture and increased its safety. Ideas, substances, and medical practices have come to China from all over the world; some of them have become significant parts of traditional Chinese medicine, and some of them remain only as observations in ancient texts.

Within China itself, many competing ideas have existed side by side. Old theories have been rejected or discovered anew and accorded even more importance than they had at their conception. Some ideas found more fertile ground in other Asian countries, as with the transmission of acupuncture and Chinese herbal medicine to Japan, where particular aspects of the Chinese tradition were emphasized and adapted.

Historian and anthropologist Paul Unschuld (1985) critiques the perspective of Chinese medicine as a homogenous monolithic structure, as follows:

> Proponents of this view depict "Chinese Medicine" as an identifiable, coherent system, the contents of which they attempt to characterize. Such an approach is both ahistorical and selective. It focuses on but one of the many distinctly conceptualized systems of therapy in Chinese history, that is the medicine of systematic correspondence, and it neglects both the changing interpretations of basic paradigms offered by Chinese authors through the ages and the synchronic plurality of differing opinions and ideas that existed for twenty centuries concerning even fundamental aspects of this therapy system such as pulse-diagnosis.

This is a particularly important point, because it is extremely tempting to encounter medical systems with the expectation that they be possessed of an internal logic that reconciles all their aspects. Although many aspects of Chinese medicine can be applied with complete consistency, other aspects or concepts seem to be quite contradictory. This trait leads us to what has been probably the most important aspect of Chinese medicine throughout its history: it is a medical tradition that never threw anything away. Certain medical practices might have been relegated to the attic, but they were available if necessary. A striking example of this is the work of Zhang Zhong Jing, whose system of diagnosis and therapy did not attract much attention during his lifetime but who became highly influential centuries after his death. Later, authors believed his theory to be incomplete and broadened its perspective, but his theories and these new theories that emerged in response to them are still important to the contemporary clinician. In the West an incomplete theory is rejected and disappears. In the history of Chinese medicine, theories, practices, and concepts may fade, but they do not entirely disappear. A new theory can exist beside the one that it sought to correct. Clinicians can choose to apply the perspective that they believe is most relevant. In this way, conflicting concepts of cause, systems of diagnosis, and treatment have continued to exist side by side.

Unschuld considers this one of the basic characteristics distinguishing traditional Chinese thought from modern Western science (Unschuld, 1985). It also is the aspect of Chinese medicine that is most challenging to Western students. The extent to which deductive reasoning and its necessary condition of "either this or that but not both" are pervasive in our society have made it difficult to approach a medical tradition that dispenses with what we view as a necessary precondition of valid human knowledge. Even European or American advocates of

Chinese medical traditions sometimes err and insist that only certain theoretical perspectives or therapeutic methods are correct or authentic.

Years earlier, Lin Yutang (1942) wrote that systematic metaphysics or epistemology were alien to traditional Chinese thought, as follows:

> The temperament for systematic philosophy simply wasn't there, and will not be there so long as the Chinese remain Chinese. They have too much sense for that. The sea of human life forever laps upon the shores of Chinese thought, and the arrogance and absurdities of the logician, the assumption that "I am exclusively right and you are exclusively wrong," are not Chinese faults, whatever other faults they may have.

The history of Chinese medical thought also includes many individuals who thought that they were exclusively right. However, the breadth of traditional Chinese medical thought was sustained by an intellectual climate that retained all possible ideas for use and exploration. A given philosopher or clinician might reject an idea, but the idea itself would remain available for future use.

For example, during the Ming dynasty, Wu You Ke (ca. 1644) was the leading exponent of the "offensive precipitation sect" *(gong xia pai)* of physicians whose tenets included a distinctive set of ideas concerning the management of epidemic disease and a wholehearted rejection of many established ideas in Chinese medicine (Wong et al, 1985). He was subsequently viewed alternatively as a contributor to Chinese medical thought, a proponent of a divergent and uninformed theory, and finally (as noted previously) as the intellectual antecedent of Koch, the discoverer of the tuberculosis bacillus. At no point were his ideas discarded.

Interestingly, in modern China, where the sheer volume of information and the nation's health care needs makes it necessary to teach a standard curriculum to thousands of students each year, this tolerance for varying clinical perspectives continues. For example, certain herbal physicians are known as minor *Bupleurum* decoction *(xiao chai hu tang)* doctors because their prescriptions are organized around one formula from the *Treatise on Cold Damage (Shang Han Lun),* an early text on diagnosis and herbal therapy written during the Han dynasty (206 BC–AD 220). Also, some herbal physicians reject traditional formulas entirely and use contemporary perspectives on the Chinese pharmacopeia to organize their prescriptions.

Some acupuncturists may have a clinical focus dedicated almost entirely to six acupuncture points and may use computed tomographic scans to plan clinical interventions. At the same time, two floors down in the same hospital, physicians base their selection of acupuncture points on obscure and complex aspects of traditional calendrics and systems such as the "Magic Turtle."

Once it is understood that Chinese medicine is a large and varied tradition with many manifestations and philosophies, it is possible to begin its exploration.

HISTORY

Chinese medicine has an extensive history. As with most medical traditions, this history can be approached from several perspectives. There is the ancient mythology of Chinese medicine, which attributes the birth of medicine to the legendary emperors Fu Xi, Shen Nong, and Huang Di. There is the history that can be deduced from the careful study of available ancient texts and records, which indicate, for example, that there is no reference to acupuncture as a therapeutic method in any Chinese text before 90 BC, and that the oldest existing text to discuss medical practices resembling current Chinese medicine dates from the end of the third century BC (Unschuld, 1985). Finally, there are the more extravagant interpretations of archaeological evidence and textual materials that seek to establish the ancient character of certain Chinese medical practices. An example is the frequent assertion that the stone "needles" excavated at different times in various parts of China were remnants of ancient acupuncture (Chuang, 1982; Wang, 1986). This assertion is based on references to the ancient surgical application of sharp stones in texts from later periods and morphological similarities between the excavated stones and later metal needles.

LEGENDARY AND SEMI-MYTHICAL ORIGINS

The origins of Chinese medicine are mythically linked to three legendary emperors: Fu Xi, Shen Nong, and Huang Di. Fu Xi, or the Ox Tamer (ca. 2953 BC), taught people how to domesticate animals and divined the *Ba Gua,* eight symbols that became the basis for the *I Ching (Yi Jing),* or *Book of Changes.*

Shen Nong, or the Divine Husbandman, also known as the Fire Emperor, is said to have lived from 2838 to 2698 BC and is considered the founder of agriculture in China. He taught the Chinese people how to cultivate plants and raise livestock. He also is considered the originator of herbal medicine in China, having learned the therapeutic properties of herbs and substances by tasting them. Later authors would attribute their work to Shen Nong to indicate the antiquity and importance of their text. The *Divine Husbandman's Classic of the Materia Medica (Shen Nong Ben Cao Jing)* is a case in point. The text probably was written in AD 220 and reconstructed in AD 500 by Tao Hong Jing. Given that all historical evidence points to the ancient character of herbal medicine in China, it is appropriate that Shen Nong is considered its originator (Figure 26-1).

Huang Di, the Yellow Emperor (2698-2598 BC), is known as the originator of the traditional medicine of China. He also is seen as the "Father of the Chinese Nation." He is credited with teaching the Chinese how to make wooden houses, silk cloth, boats, carts, the bow and

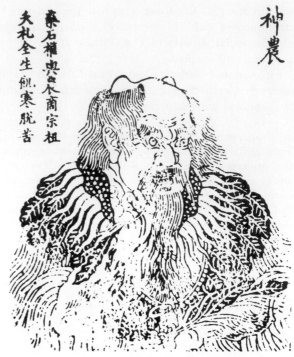

Figure 26-1 Image of Shen Nong.

arrow, and ceramics, and introducing the art of writing. Legend has it that he gained his knowledge from visiting the immortals. Most important to this discussion is his work the *Yellow Emperor's Inner Classic (Huang Di Nei Jing),* in which the traditional medicine of China is first expressed in a form that is familiar to us today. The text is divided into two books. *Simple Questions (Su Wen)* is concerned with medical theory, such as the principles of yin and yang, the five phases, and the effects of seasons. The *Spiritual Axis (Ling Shu)* deals predominantly with acupuncture and moxibustion. The texts are written as a series of dialogues between the emperor and his ministers. Qi Bo, the most famous among the ministers, is said to have tested the actions of drugs, cured people's sickness, and written books on medicine and therapeutics.

QI BO EXPLAINS THE ORDERLY LIFE OF TIMES PAST

The first book of *Simple Questions* begins with the Yellow Emperor asking Qi Bo why peoples' life spans are now so short when in the past they lived close to a hundred years. Qi Bo explains that in the past people maintained an orderly life. "In ancient times those people who understood Dao patterned themselves upon the yin and the yang and they lived in harmony with the arts of divination." (Veith, 1972)

It is generally agreed now that the *Yellow Emperor's Inner Classic* was first compiled around 200 to 100 BC. In terms of both legend and practice, it remains a text that is critical to Chinese medicine.

ANCIENT MEDICINE: 2205 TO 206 BC

Little is actually known about the practice of medicine in China before 200 BC. The Shang dynasty (1766-1121 BC) is the first dynasty of which there exists clear archaeological evidence. It appears likely that before the Shang, nomadic cultures were scattered across northern China. Interaction among these groups eventually led to the development of the Shang. This dynasty left the first traces of some form of therapeutic activity. In addition to developing the first Chinese scripts, the Shang had clearly defined social relations. There was a king and nobility, and perhaps most importantly, the people were no longer nomadic.

The Shang response to illness is documented by archaeological finds and writings from the succeeding Zhou dynasty (1122-221 BC). During this period, ideas developed that would be central to Chinese culture; specifically, a relationship between the living and the dead developed into a ritualized veneration of ancestors. Ancestors could be consulted concerning a variety of issues, including the cause of illness, through the use of oracle bones. Tortoise shells and the scapula of oxen were heated and rapidly cooled, which caused them to crack. The resulting patterns would be used for guidance in resolving questions. Often the question posed to the ancestors would be inscribed on the bone itself. Bones could be used for more than one divination. One tomb has yielded more than 100,000 oracle bones, displaying questions such as "Swelling of the abdomen. Is there a curse? Does the deceased Chin-wu desire something of the king?" (Unschuld, 1985). The ancestors were appropriately placated according to the response. Natural causes of illness also were encountered, but these appear to have been addressed through the intervention of ancestors as well.

The Zhou dynasty resulted from a political conflict with a group of Chinese-speaking descendants of the same Neolithic peoples who had settled to form the Shang. The defeat of the Shang established one of China's longest dynasties, as well as a pattern of governance that would characterize Chinese society—a central government working in relation to smaller principalities.

The Zhou continued the practices of the Shang rulers, consulting tortoise shell oracles with the aid of *wu*, or shamans. The wu acted as intermediaries between the living and the dead, played important ritual roles in court activities and with regard to the weather, and were called on to combat the demons who caused illness. During this period the shamanic activity of chasing evil spirits away from towns and homes with spears might have been transferred to the human body, and the practice of acupuncture emerged. Later accounts (eighth century AD) describe the needling techniques used by the physician Bian Qu (fifth century BC) to drive out demons. However, we have no clear evidence of this.

The Warring States period, toward the close of the Zhou, was marked by political strife and social upheaval. This era saw the emergence of two philosophers, Kong Fu Zi (Confucius) and Lao Zi (Lao Tzu), whose ideas about social and natural order were to have a lasting impact on Chinese culture. A similar trend occurred within medicine: the human body no longer was seen as subject only to the whims of spirits and demons, but as a part of nature and subject to discernible natural relationships. Those ideas were elaborated on during the Han dynasty.

FLOWERING OF CHINESE MEDICINE: 206 BC TO AD 907

In 206 BC the empire was reunited under the Han. The Han (206 BC–AD 220) created a stable aristocratic social order, expanded geographically and economically, and spread Chinese political influence throughout Vietnam and Korea. The Chinese people currently refer to themselves as the Han. This dynasty presided over a period of great development for the Chinese, including the integration of the Confucian doctrine, elements of yin and yang, and the five-phase theory into the political picture. Textual evidence reveals the emergence of a medicine that is similar to current Chinese medicine.

The earliest texts available were recovered from three tombs dating to 168 BC that were excavated at Ma Wang Dui in Hunan province (Unschuld, 1985). These texts discuss magical and demonological concepts, as well as some ideas about yin and yang in relation to the body. The texts present an early concept of channels in the body, but in a less developed fashion than the later *Yellow Emperor's Inner Classic*. Ma Wang Dui texts mention moxibustion and the use of heated stones, but they do not speak about acupuncture or specific points on the body, which implies that the idea of acupuncture had not yet emerged.

A biography written by a contemporary in 90 BC describes Chun Yu Yi, the first physician known to record personal observations of clinical cases. Interestingly, he also was tried for malpractice because of his use of the apparently unfamiliar method of acupuncture to change the flow of qi (Unschuld, 1985).

The *Divine Husbandman's Classic of the Materia Medica*, mentioned earlier, appears during this era as well. This text is the first known formal presentation of individual medicinal substances, the first in a long line of such texts.

 Sun Si Miao Explains the Incurable Nature of Physicians

Finally, it is inappropriate to emphasize one's reputation, to belittle the rest of the physicians and to praise only one's own virtue. Indeed, in actual life someone who has accidentally healed a disease, then stalks around with his head raised, shows conceit and announces that no one in the entire world could measure up to him. In this respect all physicians are evidently incurable. ❧

Quoted in Unschuld P: *Medical ethics in Imperial China: a study in historical anthropology*, Berkeley, Calif, 1979, University of California Press.

The *Classic of Difficult Issues (Nan Jing)* was compiled sometime during the first or second century AD, although its authorship is attributed to the legendary physician Bian Qu. This text has had and continues to have a marked influence on the practice of Chinese medicine and, to an even greater extent, on the practice of Chinese medicine in Japan. It marks a drastic shift in medical thinking, systematically organizing the theory and practice of therapeutic acupuncture in terms of body structure, illness, diagnosis, and treatment. It is almost entirely devoid of magical elements. The author(s) of the *Classic of Difficult Issues* reconciled the contradictions of the *Inner Classic,* in addition to providing many new observations. Although it is thought to have been written as an independent text, the *Classic of Difficult Issues* met with so much resistance because of its radical organization that it became known as a commentary on the *Inner Classic.*

The *Treatise on Cold Damage* and the *Survey of Important Elements from the Golden Cabinet and Jade Container (Jin Gui Yao Lue)* were written in the second century AD by Zhang Zhong Jing, also known as Zhang Ji (AD 142-220). Chinese medical texts of this period were primarily philosophical, but as with the authors of the *Classic of Difficult Issues,* Zhang studied disease from a clinical standpoint, emphasizing the physical signs, symptoms, and course of disease; the method of treatment; and the action of the substances used. He was interested especially in fevers, because most of the people in his village died from fever epidemics (possibly typhoid). Although published during the Han dynasty, these texts remained relatively obscure until the Sung dynasty (after AD 960), when medical thinkers realized that the concepts of diagnosis and therapy presented reflected their own concerns. These texts enormously influenced the practice of herbal medicine in Japan. We examine an herbal formula derived from the *Treatise on Cold Damage* later in this chapter.

Hua Tou (AD 110-207), acupuncturist, herbalist, and surgeon, is a near-legendary figure in Chinese medicine. Not only did he reportedly use acupuncture and herbs, his adaptation of animal postures is one of the early forms of qigong. He is said to have used the anesthetic properties of plants to render a patient insensible to pain, which enabled him to practice surgery successfully.

Despite Hua Tou's reputation, his surgical innovations seem to have departed with him. Chinese medical history reveals the practice of a variety of minor surgical interventions for growths, hemorrhoids, and wound healing, but none of the significant abdominal surgeries attributed to Hua Tou. The surgical castration used to produce eunuchs for the imperial court was medically significant, and there is textual evidence of Chinese exposure to the surgical practices developed in India for the treatment of cataracts, but these did not form surgical traditions per se.

Huang Pu Mi (AD 215-286) wrote the *Systematic Classic of Acupuncture (and Moxibustion) (Zhen Jiu Jia Yi Jing),* which exercised substantial influence over the acupuncture traditions of China, Korea, and Japan. This text presented

and reorganized material from the *Inner Classic* and earlier texts.

It is important to realize that the histories of individual physicians and the texts that have come down to us reflect the medicine of the literate elite of China more than the medical traditions of that nation as a whole. About 80% of the total population consisted of farmers, peasants, and farming villages. These people lived at a level of bare subsistence and worked extremely hard to stay there, entirely dependent on the soil and the weather. They were not exposed to formal education and typically were illiterate. Very little is known of what these people knew or thought at any particular time. Their traditions were regionally oriented and full of folk superstition, historical legend, and aspirations dominated by the hope of survival.

Some authors, especially compilers of materia medica texts, did explore the nonliterate traditions of the Chinese people, but the first systematic publication of this material did not occur until late in the Qing dynasty (Unschuld, 1985). Folk herbal and medical traditions were most systematically explored under the guidance of the postrevolutionary government of China. Texts such as *The Barefoot Doctor's Manual* reflect the inclusion of this type of material.

In AD 220, after approximately 30 years of strife and religious rebellion by Daoist sects, the Han dynasty fell. After the Han there was another long period of division in China, although not as violent or as divisive as the Warring States period after the Zhou dynasty. In AD 589 the Sui dynasty reunified China and soon was succeeded by the Tang dynasty, considered by many to be the height of China's cultural development. The Tang dynasty spread China's influence as far as Mongolia, Vietnam, Central Asia, Korea, and Japan. During this period, both Buddhism and Daoism strongly influenced medical thought.

Sun Si Miao (AD 581-682), a famous physician of the period, was a prolific author and a productive scholar who was well versed in both Daoist and Buddhist practice. His works include *Thousand Ducat Prescriptions (Qian Jin Yao Fang),* a text on eye disorders, and the *Classic of Spells,* a guide to magic in medicine. The *Thousand Ducat Prescriptions* contains a section titled "On the Absolute Sincerity of Great Physicians" that established him as China's first medical ethicist. He addresses the need for diligent scholarship, compassion toward the patient, and high moral standards in the physician, which remain pertinent and seem to speak directly to current medical issues.

ACADEMIC MEDICINE AND SYSTEMATIC THERAPEUTICS: AD 960 TO 1368

By the time of the Sung dynasty the practice of medicine had become more specialized, and efforts were made to integrate past insights systematically. The number of texts published during the period of this dynasty may have exceeded the number written during all the previous dynasties. In 1027, Wang Wei Yi oversaw the casting of two bronze figures that he designed to illustrate the location of acupuncture points. One of these was used in the Imperial Medical College. The bronzes were pierced at the location of the acupuncture points, covered with wax, and filled with water. When a student found the hole under the wax with a needle, water would drip out, indicating it to be the correct spot.

During the Sung dynasty, great advances occurred in herbal therapeutics, and several complete herbal texts with illustrations were published under imperial decree. Tastes and properties were assigned to herbs according to their yin or yang nature, and functions were assigned based on the herb's nature and its ability to treat specific symptoms. Efforts were made to systematize herbal therapeutics. The writings of Zhang Zhong Jing received great interest because of his systematic application of traditional theoretical principles to the use of herbal medicine. The revival of the *Treatise on Cold Damage* influenced medicine for the next several hundred years, because it sparked the development of warm-induced disease theory *(wen bing xue)* during the Ming dynasty.

During the Sung dynasty the education of physicians became more formal. The Imperial College, which had provided for the training of the emperor's physicians, was expanded. In 1076 the Imperial Medical College was founded, with an enrollment of 300 students. There were regional schools as well.

The Jin and Yuan dynasties saw the continuation of specialized medical thought and independent inquiry. Much of what we recognize as Chinese medicine today—and what we discuss in the section on fundamental concepts—stems from the Sung, Jin, and Yuan dynasties. Physicians of this period developed ideas involving the elaboration of therapeutic approaches on the basis of early theory. They espoused the application of five-phase theory in relation to seasonal influences, supplementing the body, purging the body to eliminate evil influences, and supplementing the yin.

MEDICINE IN THE MING AND QING DYNASTIES: AD 1368 TO 1911

During the Ming and Qing dynasties physicians continued to pursue lines of inquiry explored in preceding dynasties, such as the far-reaching naturalistic explorations of Li Shi Zhen (1518-1593). His *Grand Materia Medica (Ben Cao Gang Mu)* included discussions of 1892 substances and, among its topics, described the use of kelp and deer thyroid to treat goiter.

The exploration of more precise linkages between factors in disease causation and therapeutics continued, and a number of medical sects emerged. During a virulent epidemic that struck from 1641 to 1644, Wu You Ke (Xing) (1592-1672) used an unorthodox treatment method that was highly successful. His text, *Discussion of Warm Epidemics (Wen Yi Lun)*, explored the theoretical basis for his treatment.

Some authors consider the Ming dynasty to be the peak of the cultural expression of acupuncture and moxibustion in China (Qiu, 1993). This period saw the production of numerous texts on the subject. One of the most influential acupuncture texts, the *Great Compendium of Acupuncture and Moxibustion (Zhen Jiu Da Cheng)*, was written by Yang Ji Zhou toward the end of the Ming dynasty.

Intellectual trends of the Ming continued into the Qing dynasty. The *Discussion of Warm Disease (Wen Re Lun)* by Ye Tian Shi complemented Zhang Zhong Jing's method of diagnosing and treating diseases caused by cold with an equally systematic method of diagnosing and treating those caused by heat.

Political, economic, and social trends during the Qing dynasty exacerbated the isolation of the Manchu rulers of the time and exposed the Chinese to the power of Western knowledge, technology, and science. The broadening of cultural horizons and the broadening of medical inquiry combined to shake the classical underpinnings of Chinese medical thought. In 1822, acupuncture was formally eliminated from the Imperial Medical College (Qiu, 1993).

By the close of the Qing dynasty in 1911, political and cultural institutions were in a state of decline. The scattered practitioners of traditional Chinese medicine found themselves increasingly under fire from the advocates of a new and modern China and a new and modern medicine.

The collapse of the Qing and the formation of the Republic laid traditional medicine open to the conquering influence of Western medicine. The Imperial College of Physicians was eliminated (Wong et al, 1985), and the Western-educated proponents of reform began to work toward the elimination of the traditional medicine of China and the establishment of Western medicine as the dominant medical system.

From 1914 through 1936 a series of encounters and clashes occurred over the regulation, establishment, or elimination of practitioners of Chinese medicine (Wong et al, 1985). The traditional medicine of China, or "medicine" *(yi)* as it had been known, came to be termed "Chinese medicine" *(zhong yi)*. Both nationalist and Marxist reformers intensely disliked Chinese medicine.

SO-CALLED CHINESE MEDICINE

Initially the external threat reduced the internal spectrum of competing Chinese interpretations of the classics. The great diversity of individual efforts to reconcile insights from personal experience with the ancient theories of yin yang and the five phases, as well as with other older views about the structure of the body, disappeared behind the illusion of a so-called Chinese medicine *(chung-I [zhong yi])*, supposedly well defined and with theory easily converted into practice. This situation, in turn, has given rise to the historically misleading impression that these diverse elements, like the concepts and practices of Western medicine, constituted a unified, coherent system. (Unschuld, 1985)

A critical feature of this new Chinese medicine was its rejection of practices that were manifestly "unscientific," represented in the creation of zhong yi. This disciplined form of medicine has emerged today as traditional Chinese medicine.

The aspects of the traditional medicine of China that were secured in zhong yi were later appropriated by the Chinese Marxists in an effort to build a strong medical infrastructure for substantial populations in the face of economic and technical limitations. Chairman Mao's declaration in 1958 that "Chinese medicine is a great treasure house! We must uncover it and raise its standards!" (Unschuld, 1985) inspired efforts to rehabilitate the traditional medicine of China and to "discover" a primitive dialectic within the theoretical underpinnings of the system. The *Revised Outline of Chinese Medicine* stated that "yin-yang and the five phases *(wu-hsing [wu xing])* are ancient Chinese philosophical ideas. They are spontaneous, naive materialist theories that also contain elementary dialectic ideas" (Sivin, 1987).

The development of Chinese medicine as a system parallel to Western medicine was under way by the time of Mao's declaration. In 1956, four colleges of Chinese medicine were created, with many more to follow. At present, zhong yi exists as a parallel medical system, integrating necessary biomedical elements while retaining fidelity to the traditional concepts of Chinese medicine. Educational programs emphasize acupuncture and herbal medicine and range from an undergraduate technical certificate to doctoral programs. Most independent practitioners enter the field with a 5-year medical baccalaureate degree (MB/BS) that is earned after high school (Ergil, 1994). In this system, both inpatient and outpatient medical care is delivered from large, well-equipped hospitals, as well as private clinics and pharmacies.

FUNDAMENTAL CONCEPTS

YIN AND YANG

The philosophy of Chinese medicine begins with yin and yang. These two terms can be used to express the broadest philosophical concepts as well as the most focused perceptions of the natural world. Yin and yang express the idea of opposing but complementary phenomena that exist in a state of dynamic equilibrium. The most ancient expression of this idea seems to have been that of the shady and sunny sides of a hill (Unschuld, 1985, p. 55; Wilhelm, 1967, p. 297). The sunlit southern side was the yang, and the shaded northern side was the yin. The contrast between the bright and dark sides of a single hill portrayed the yang and the yin, respectively. If you imagine, for a moment, the different environments that exist on either side of this one hill, you can begin to get an idea of yin and yang. On the bright, sunny side, plants and animals that enjoy light are more prevalent, the air is

drier, and the rocks are warm; on the dim, shaded side, the air seems moist and cool.

Yin and yang are always present simultaneously. The paired opposites observed in the world gave tangible expression to the otherwise uncontemplatable Dao of ancient Chinese thought (Box 26-1).

The *Book of Changes*, which sought to explore the myriad manifestations of yin and yang, expressed the idea as follows: "That which lets now the dark, now the light appear is tao" (Wilhelm, 1967).

The *Yellow Emperor's Inner Classic*, the oldest text to discuss the medical application of yin and yang in a comprehensive way (Unschuld, 1985, p. 56), states that "yin and yang are the way of heaven and earth" (Wiseman et al, 1985). This text showed how yin and yang were to be used to correlate the body and other phenomena to the human experience of health and disease.

The Inner Classic on Yin and Yang

> As to the yin and yang of the human body, the outer part is yang and the inner part is yin. As to the trunk, the back is yang and the abdomen is yin. As to the organs, the viscera are yin whereas the bowels are yang. The liver, heart, spleen, lung, and kidney are yin; the gallbladder, stomach, intestines, bladder, and triple burner are yang. (Wiseman et al, 1993)

It is important to note that the preceding quote is taken from the translation of an important contemporary textbook of Chinese medicine. Many ideas expressed in the *Yellow Emperor's Inner Classic* are taught and applied routinely in the contemporary clinical practice of Chinese medicine.

Yin and yang were used to express ideas about both normal physiology and pathological processes. They were applied to the organization of phenomena in many ways, for example, to organize phenomena in terms of the emergence of its dominant yin or yang character. Summer was yang within yang, fall was yin within yang, winter was yin within yin, and spring was yang within yin. Thus the coldest, darkest, and most yin period was yin within yin,

---

BOX 26-1

Origins of Yin and Yang

Out of Tao, One is born;
Out of One, Two;
Out of Two, Three;
Out of Three, the created universe.
The created universe carries the yin at its back and the yang in front;
Through the union of the pervading principles it reaches harmony.

—LAO ZI

Quoted in Lin Y: Laotse, the book of Tao. In Lin Y, editor: *The wisdom of China and India*, New York, 1942, Modern Library.

whereas spring, when the yang began to emerge from the yin, was yang within yin.

There is a distinctly ecological orientation to the worldview that is supported by yin and yang; each phenomenon is seen in relation to its surroundings, and it is expected that each phenomenon will exert an influence on its surroundings that is balanced by an equal but opposing influence (Table 26-1). Just as the language of ecology is the language of interrelation and interdependence, the language of Chinese medicine is a language of interrelation and interdependence. The external landscape, or human environment, is understood to be in profound and dynamic relationship with the internal landscape, or human organism. This idea becomes clearer when we explore disease causation later (see Chapter 4).

The ancient Chinese understood humans to have a nature and structure inseparable from yin and yang and, as such, inseparable from the world around them—a structure that is to be understood by the same rules that guide us in understanding the world in which we live. Life on the shaded side of a mountain has characteristics that differ from those on the sunny side. Finally, the comprehension and adjustment of life in relation to yin and yang would support life itself. Thus it was said, "To follow (the laws of) yin and yang means life; to act contrary to (the laws of yin and yang) means death" (Unschuld, 1985).

Within the traditional medical community of contemporary China, there is debate over the actual nature of yin and yang. Some exponents of a more scientific, less traditional perspective on Chinese medicine want yin and yang to be used as concepts to organize phenomena. Others who express a less modern perspective emphatically state that yin and yang are actually tangible phenomena (Farquhar, 1987). Although it is probably easiest to think about yin and yang as descriptive terms that help the Chinese physician organize information, it should be remembered (especially in traditional pharmaceutics) that the yin and yang constituents of the body are actual things that can be reinforced by specific substances or actions.

A useful analogy for thinking about yin and yang in this way is that of a candle. If one considers the yin aspect of the candle to be the wax and the yang aspect to be the flame, one can see how the yin nourishes and supports the yang and how the yang consumes the yin and thus burns brightly. When the wax is gone, so is the flame. Yin and yang exist in dependence on each other.

THE FIVE PHASES

Another idea that has played a significant part in the development of some aspects of Chinese medicine is that of the five phases (wu xing). The five phases are earth, metal, water, wood, and fire. In Chinese wu means "five" and xing expresses the idea of movement, "to go." For a time the wu xing were translated as "the five elements." This translation conveys little of the dynamism of the Chinese concept, instead focusing on the apparent similarities between the wu xing and the elements of medieval alchemy. This is an example of the translation problem in which we use the familiar to understand the new. However useful this method may be at first, it can lead to some confusion in the long run. Wu xing may include the implication of material elements, but in general, the five phases refer to a set of dynamic relations occurring among phenomena that are organized in terms of the five phases. This philosophy can cover almost every aspect of phenomena, from seasons to odors (Table 26-2).

QI AND THE ESSENTIAL SUBSTANCES OF THE BODY

Apart from the ideas of yin and yang and the five phases, no concept is more crucial to Chinese medicine than qi—the idea that the body is pervaded by subtle material and mobile influences that cause most physiological functions and maintain the health and vitality of the individual. This idea is not typical of biomedical thinking about the body. It is not unusual to see the concept of qi translated using the term energy, but this translation conceals its distinctly material attributes. Furthermore, although energy is defined as the capacity of a system to do work, the character of qi extends considerably further.

The Chinese character for qi is traditionally composed of two radicals; the radical that symbolizes breath or rising vapor is placed above the radical for rice (Figure 26-2). Qi is linked with the concept of "vapors arising from food" (Unschuld, 1985). Over time this concept broadened but never lost its distinctively material aspect. Unschuld favors the use of the phrase "finest matter influences" or "influences" to translate this concept. Some phenomena labeled as qi do not fit conventional definitions of substance or matter, which further confused the

---

TABLE 26-1

Yang and Yin Correspondences

Yang	Yin
Light	Dark
Heaven	Earth
Sun	Moon
Day	Night
Spring	Autumn
Summer	Winter
Hot	Cold
Male	Female
Fast	Slow
Up	Down
Outside	Inside
Fire	Water
Wood	Metal

TABLE 26-2

Correspondences of the Five Phases

Category	Wood	Fire	Earth	Metal	Water
Viscus	Liver	Heart	Spleen	Lungs	Kidney
Bowel	Gallbladder	Small intestine	Stomach	Large intestine	Urinary bladder
Season	Spring	Summer	Late summer	Autumn	Winter
Time of day	Before sunrise	Forenoon	Afternoon	Late afternoon	Midnight
Climate	Wind	Heat	Damp	Dryness	Cold
Direction	East	South	Center	West	North
Development	Birth	Growth	Maturity	Withdrawal	Dormancy
Color	Cyan	Red	Yellow	White	Black
Taste	Sour	Bitter	Sweet	Pungent	Salty
Sense organ	Eyes	Tongue	Mouth	Nose	Ears
Odor	Goatish	Scorched	Fragrant	Raw fish	Putrid
Vocalization	Shouting	Laughing	Singing	Weeping	Sighing
Tissue	Sinews	Vessels	Flesh	Body hair	Bones
Mind	Anger	Joy	Thought	Sorrow	Fear

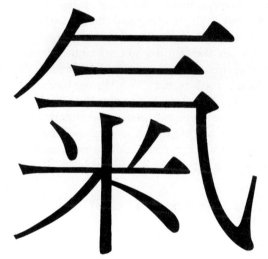

Figure 26-2 The character qi.

TABLE 26-3

Types of Qi

Type	Category	Function
Ying qi	Construction qi	Supports and nourishes the body
Wei qi	Defense qi	Protects and warms the body
Jing qi	Channel qi	Flows in the channels (felt during acupuncture)
Zang qi	Organ qi	Flows in the organs (physiological function of organs)
Zong qi	Ancestral qi	Responsible for respiration and circulation

issue (Wiseman et al, 1995). For this reason, many authors prefer to leave the term *qi* untranslated.

The idea of qi is extremely broad, encompassing almost every variety of natural phenomena. Many different types of qi are in the body. In general, the features that distinguish each type derive from its source, location, and function. There is considerable room for debate in this area, and exploration of a wide range of materials can suggest different ideas about categories of qi. In general, qi has the functions of activation, warming, defense, transformation, and containment (Table 26-3).

The qi concept is important to many aspects of Chinese medicine. Organ qi and channel qi are influenced by acupuncture. In fact, one characteristic feature of acupuncture treatment is the sensation of obtaining the qi, or *de qi. Qigong* is a general term for the many systems of meditation, exercise, and therapeutics that

are rooted in the concept of mobilizing and regulating the movement of qi in the body. Qi is sometimes compared with wind captured in a sail; we cannot observe the wind directly, but we can infer its presence as it fills the sail. In a similar fashion, the movements of the body and the movement of substances within the body are all signs of the action of qi.

In relation to qi, blood and fluids constitute the yin aspects of the body. *Blood* is produced by the construction qi, which in turn is derived from food and water. Blood nourishes the body. Blood is understood to have a slightly broader and less definite range of actions in Chinese medicine than it does in biomedicine. Within the body, qi and blood are closely linked, because blood is considered to flow with qi and to be conveyed by it. This relationship often is expressed by the Chinese saying "Qi is the commander of blood and blood is the mother of qi," and some suggest that qi and blood are linked as a person and his or her shadow are linked.

Fluids are a general category of thin and viscous substances that serve to moisten and lubricate the body. Fluids can be conceptually separated into humor and liquid. *Humor* is thick and related to the body's organs; its functions include lubrication of the joints. *Liquid* is thin and is responsible for moistening the surface areas of the body, including the skin, eyes, and mouth.

ESSENCE AND SPIRIT

Qi, essence, and spirit make up the *three treasures* in Chinese medicine. In brief, essence is the gift of one's parents, and spirit is the gift of heaven. *Essence* is the most fundamental source of human physiological processes, the bodily reserves that support human life and that must be replenished by food and rest, and the actual reproductive substances of the body. *Spirit* is the alert and radiant aspect of human life. We encounter spirit in the luster of the eyes and face in healthy persons, as well as in their ability to think and respond appropriately to the world around them. The idea expressed by spirit, or *shen* in Chinese, encompasses consciousness and healthy mental and physical function.

The relation of the mind to the body in Chinese medicine does not include the notion of a distinct separation. It is understood that the psyche and soma interact with each other and that aspects of mental and emotional experience can have an impact on the body, and vice versa. In this sense, spirit is linked both to the health of the body and to the health of the mind. Similarly, aspects of human experience that are understood as predominantly mental in a biomedical frame of reference are linked to specific organs in Chinese medicine. For example, anger is related to the liver, obsessive thought to the spleen, and joy to the heart.

VISCERA AND BOWELS (*ZANG* AND *FU*)

The ancient Chinese understood human anatomy in ways not dissimilar from those of their European contemporaries, up to the seventeenth century. Chinese history includes cases of systematic dissection, but none of these reached the extensive explorations into the structure of the body that characterized European medicine by the fifteenth century. Instead, the Chinese medical perspective of the body, although rooted in familiar anatomical structures, represented a system in which organs serve as markers of associated physiological functions rather than actual physical structures.

The physician of Chinese medicine encounters a body in which 12 organs function. These organs are divided into the "viscera," which include six *zang* or solid organs, and the "bowels," which include six *fu* or hollow organs.

These organs often are related to the physical structures that we associate with conventional biomedical anatomy. The six viscera are heart, lungs, liver, spleen, kidneys, and pericardium. The six bowels are the small intestine, large intestine, gallbladder, stomach, urinary bladder, and "triple burner" *(san jiao)*. These organs have physiological functions that often are similar to those associated with them in biomedicine, but that also might be very different. The liver is said to store blood and to distribute it to the extremities as needed. The spleen is viewed as an organ of digestion. The Chinese understood the physical structure and location of most of the organs, but because systematic dissection was not extensively pursued, the close observation of physiological function was more often the basis of medical thought.

For example, circulation and elimination of fluids were observed and attributed to an organ that was said to have a name, but no form was established. This organ, the triple burner, is considered either the combined expression of the activity of other organs in the body or a group of spaces in the body. This example clearly expresses the idea that physiological function, rather than substance, establishes an organ in Chinese medicine. At the same time, the triple burner has always been surrounded by debate, because it does not have a clear anatomical structure.

The organs of viscera and bowel are paired in the yin and yang, or *interior-exterior relationship*. The heart is linked with the small intestine, the spleen with the stomach, and so on. Each viscus and each bowel has an associated channel that runs through the organ, through the organ with which it is paired, within the body, and across the body's surface, then connects with the channel of the related organ.

Historical evidence suggests that the idea of channels is more ancient than the idea of specific acupuncture points. Although disagreement surrounds the location of specific points, research in the People's Republic of China recently led to the publication of a number of texts dedicated to resolving historical, philological, and anatomical questions about acupuncture points. At this time, 12 primary channels and 8 extraordinary vessels are understood to exist. The 12 channels are classically organized in terms of a sixfold yin-and-yang organizational scheme, although they can also be organized in terms of five-phase theory. Qi is understood to flow in these channels, making a rhythmical circuit.

Along the pathways of 14 of these channels (the 12 regular channels and 2 of the extraordinary channels) lie 361 specific points. In addition, a large number of "extra" points have been derived from clinical experience but are not traditionally considered part of the major channel systems. Beyond this, various individual elaborations of acupuncture theory suggest new points. There are also local microsystems of acupuncture points that have postulated numerous points on the ear, scalp, hand, foot, and other areas of the body.

Acupuncture points appear at many locations on the body. Most often they are located where a gentle and sensitive hand can detect a declivity (slope) with slight pressure on the skin surface. Points are located at the margins or bellies of muscles, between bones, and over distinctive bony features that can be detected through the skin. Methods used to locate points vary. In general, points are found by seeking anatomical landmarks, by proportionally measuring the body, and by using finger measurements; the first method is considered the most reliable. With time and clinical experience, some practitioners can be less formal in their approach to locating acupuncture points, but this topic interests even advanced practitioners. In Japan, clinicians gather regularly to hone their point location skills. In China, point location in relation to classical sources, anatomical study, and empirical evidence is an area of advanced study.

As with qi, the actual term and use of the Chinese expression that we translate as "point" is important. The character *xue*, which has been translated as "point," actually means "hole" in Chinese. A hole often is part of the clinician's subjective experience of the acupuncture point. Xue are holes in which the qi of the channels can be influenced by inserting a needle or by other means. Imagining the channel system as a vast subcutaneous waterway, with caves and springs punctuating its course as it flows to the surface, provides a concept of the holes similar to the way the Chinese thought of them for many centuries (Box 26-2).

Holes, or points along the channels, have been categorized and organized in myriad ways. One of the oldest and most well known is a system of categories based on the idea of *shu*, or transport points. This system of point categories applies exclusively to points on the forearm and lower leg, which embody the image of qi welling gently from a mountainous source at the fingertips and gradually gaining strength and depth as it reaches the seas located at the elbow and knee joints.

In reading the preceding brief discussion of the essential anatomy and physiology of Chinese medicine, it is important to remember that this anatomy forms a general reference for physiological function rather than an anatomy of direct links between discrete categories of tissue and specific physiological processes. A strength of

Chinese medicine is that its theory allows for generalizations about complex physical processes, in addition to responding to signs and symptoms whose origins are obscure. Also, the distinction between mind and body is not present in Chinese medicine. Although Chinese physicians may display a disconcerting lack of interest in contemporary psychotherapy or its patients, they are quick to posit a link between affect and physiological process, in a manner that might intrigue a contemporary psychobiologist. On this basis, we can proceed to examine how illness manifests in the body.

CAUSES OF DISEASE

Ultimately, all illness is a disturbance of qi within the body. Its expression as a pathological process displaying specific signs and symptoms depends on the location of the disturbance. Contemporary formal discussions on disease causation use the ideas of Chen Yen (1161-1174), who wrote *Prescriptions Elucidated on the Premise that All Pathological Symptoms Have Only Three Primary Causes (San Yin Qi Yi Bing Cheng Fang Lun)*, and an additional idea of Wu You Ke that each disease has its own qi.

The three categories of disease are organized in terms of external causes of disease, internal causes, and causes that are neither external nor internal (Wiseman et al, 1995) (Box 26-3). The first category includes six influences that are distinctly environmental: wind, cold, fire, dampness, summer heat, and dryness. When they cause disease, these six influences are known as *evils*. If the defense qi is not robust or the correct qi is not strong, or if the evil is powerful, the evil may enter the surface of the body and, under certain conditions, penetrate to the interior.

The nature of the evil and its impact on the body were understood through the observation of nature and the observation of the body in illness. The clinical meaning of the causes of disease does not lie, for the most part, in the expression of a distinct etiology, but in the manifestation of a specific set of clinical signs. In this sense, the biomedical distinction between etiology and diagnosis is somewhat blurred in Chinese medical theory.

For example, the evils of wind and cold often are implicated in the sudden onset of symptoms associated with the common cold: headache, pronounced aversion to

---

BOX 26-2

Set Acupuncture Points: Leg Three Li

- *Location:* 3 cun (body inch) below the depression below the patella, one fingerbreadth from the anterior crest of the tibia
- *Indications:* Stomach pain, vomiting, abdominal distention, indigestion, diarrhea, constipation, dizziness, mastitis, mental disorders, hemiplegia, pain in knee joint and leg
- *Depth of needle insertion:* 0.5 to 1.3 inches

BOX 26-3

The Three Causes of Disease (San Yin)

- *External causes*, or "the six evils": Wind, cold, fire, dampness, summer heat, and dryness
- *Internal causes*, or internal damage by the "seven affects": Joy, anger, anxiety, thought, sorrow, fear, and fright
- *Nonexternal, noninternal causes:* Dietary irregularities, excessive sexual activity, taxation fatigue, trauma, and parasites

cold, aching muscles and bones, fever, and a scratchy throat. Wind is expressed in the sudden onset of the symptoms and in their manifestation in the upper part of the body, and cold is displayed in the pronounced aversion to cold and the aching muscles and bones. Whether the patient had a specific encounter with a cold wind shortly before the onset of the symptoms is not particularly relevant. Although a patient may mention being outside on a chilly and windy day before the onset of a cold, such exposure could easily result in signs of wind heat as well; that is, a less marked aversion to cold, a distinctly sore throat, and a dry mouth. The six evils are not agents of specific etiology but agents of specific symptomatology. These ideas developed in a setting in which the possibility of investigating a bacterial or viral cause was nonexistent. Rather, careful observation of the body's response to disease provided the information necessary for treatment.

Each of the evils affects the body in a manner similar to its behavior in the environment. Images of these processes observed in nature and society were inscribed on the body to permit its processes to be readily understood. The human body stood between heaven and earth and was subject to all their influences in a relationship of continuity with its environment. Although these six evils are identified as environmental influences that attack the body's surface, it also is clearly understood they may occur within the body, causing internal disruption.

In the second category of disease causation, "internal damage by the seven affects" refers to the way in which mental states can influence body processes. However, such a statement expresses a separation not implied in Chinese medicine. Each of the seven affects, or internal causes, can disturb the body if it is strongly or frequently expressed. As discussed earlier, each of the mental states—joy, anger, anxiety, thought, sorrow, fear, and fright—is related to a specific organ.

In the third category, nonexternal, noninternal causes encompass the causes of disease that do not result specifically from environmental influences or mental states. These include dietary irregularities, excessive sexual activity, taxation fatigue, trauma, and parasites. "Excessive sexual activity" suggests the possibility that too frequent emission of semen by the male can cause illness. This can occur because semen is directly related to the concept of essence, which is considered vital to the body's function and difficult to replace. This category also includes possible damage to the essence through excessive childbearing or bearing a child when the mother is too young or too old.

"Taxation fatigue" expresses the dangers of engaging in a variety of activities for a prolonged period. This category includes both the idea of overexertion and the idea of inactivity as possible causes of disease. All the concepts included within taxation fatigue reflect the essential thought of Chinese medicine that moderation is the key to health. Lying down for prolonged periods damages the

qi, and prolonged standing damages the bones. From the moment that the Yellow Emperor asked Qi Bo why people now die before their time and received his answer, the images of balance, harmony, and moderation have informed Chinese medicine.

Each of the causes of disease, from prosaic causes such as dietary irregularities to exotic notions such as wind evil, disrupts the balance of yang and yin within the body and disrupts the free movement of qi. The next step is to determine the precise pattern of imbalance.

Diagnosis

Diagnostics in Chinese medicine is traditionally expressed within four categories: inspection, listening and smelling, inquiry, and palpation. The fundamental goal is to collect information that reflects the status of physiological processes, then analyze this information to determine which impact a disorder has on that process.

The first of the four diagnostic methods, *inspection (wang)*, refers to the visual assessment of the patient, particularly the spirit, form and bearing, head and face, and substances excreted by the body. Inspection uses a large body of empirically derived information and theoretical considerations. The color, shape, markings, and coating of the tongue are inspected. For the patient attacked by wind and cold, the examiner would expect to see a moist tongue with a thin white coating, signaling the presence of cold. If heat were present, the examiner might expect a dry mouth and a red tongue. The observation of the spirit, which is considered very important in assessing the patient's prognosis, relies on assessing the overall appearance of the patient, especially the eyes, the complexion, and the quality of the patient's voice. Good spirit, even in the presence of serious illness, is thought to bode well for the patient.

The second aspect of diagnosis, *listening and smelling*, refers to listening to the quality of speech, breath, and other sounds, as well as being aware of the odors of breath, body, and excreta. As with each aspect of diagnosis, the five-phase theory can be incorporated into the assessment of the patient's condition. Each phase and each pair of viscus and bowel have a corresponding vocalization and smell.

The third aspect of diagnosis, *inquiry*, is the process of taking a comprehensive medical history. This process has been presented in many ways, but perhaps best known is the system of 10 questions described by Zhang Jie Bin in the Ming dynasty. The questions were presented as an outline of diagnostic inquiry and included querying the patient about sensations of hot and cold, perspiration, head and body, excreta, diet, chest, hearing, thirst, previous illnesses, and previous medications and their effects. For example, the examiner might expect the patient who has wind and cold symptoms to report an aversion to exposure to cold, headache, body aches, and an absence of thirst.

This step is considered critical to a good diagnosis. Although pulse diagnosis is sometimes regarded as a central feature of Chinese medicine and is rightly regarded as an art, it should not form the sole basis of a complete diagnosis, as follows:

> The *simple questions* expresses the following idea: If, in conducting the examination, the practitioner neither inquires as to how and when the condition arose nor asks about the nature of the patient's complaint, about dietary irregularities, excesses of sleeping and waking, and poisoning, but instead proceeds immediately to take the pulse, he will not succeed in identifying the disease. (Wiseman et al, 1995)

Contemporaries of Li Shi Zhen, the author of the *Pulse Studies of Bin Hu (Bin Hu Mai Xue),* placed great emphasis on the pulse. Although considered an expert, he rejected the idea that one would place an unequal emphasis on any aspect of the diagnostic process.

Palpation (qie), the fourth diagnostic method, includes pulse examination, general palpation of the body, and palpation of the acupuncture points. *Pulse diagnosis* offers a range of approaches and can provide a remarkable amount of information about the patient's condition. The process of pulse diagnosis is carried out on the radial arteries of the left and right wrists. The patient may be seated or lying down and should be calm. The pulse is divided into three parts. The middle part is adjacent to the styloid process of the radius and is called the "bar" position; the "inch" is distal to it, and the "cubit" is proximal. The *inch position,* which is nearest the wrist, can indicate the status of the body above the diaphragm; the *bar position* indicates the status of the body between the diaphragm and the navel; and the *cubit position* indicates the area below the navel. Beyond this simple conceptual structure, each pulse position can be interpreted to determine the status of the organs and the channels.

Table 26-4 summarizes two models of what can be felt at each pulse position. The first chart is derived from the *Classic of Difficult Issues,* which first presented this type of pulse diagnosis in a systematic way, and the second chart shows a less elaborate, contemporary pattern. Some authors suggest that the pattern associated with the *Classic of Difficult Issues* is related more to the use of pulse diagnosis in the practice of acupuncture, whereas the later pattern is more relevant to the herbalist (Maciocia, 1989). Not all herbalists or acupuncturists make use of the pulse, but certain styles of acupuncture rely quite heavily on it. There are many possible approaches to the pulse, which makes it a rich area for the clinician and a vexing area for the biomedically oriented researcher (Birch, 1994).

The pulse allows the clinician to feel the quality of the qi and blood at different locations in the body. Table 26-5 provides a list of 29 pulse qualities and possible associations (Wiseman, 1993). Pulse qualities are organized on the basis of the size, rate, depth, force, and volume of the pulse. The overall quality of the pulse and the variations in quality at certain positions can become quite meaningful to the clinician after several years of close attention. The patient afflicted with a wind cold evil might display a floating and tight pulse, signaling the presence of a cold evil on the surface of the body.

After carrying out the diagnostic process, the practitioner of Chinese medicine must make sense of the information derived. The practitioner constructs an appropriate image of the configuration of the disease so that it can be addressed by effective therapy. Central to this process is the concept of *pattern identification (bian zheng),* which involves gathering signs and symptoms through the diagnostic process and using traditional theory to understand their impact on the fundamental substances of the body, the organs, and the channels. Many intellectual aspects of the diagnostic processes of Chinese medicine, especially when applied to the practice of herbal medicine, are as analytical as a biomedical clinical encounter. The physician must elicit signs and symptoms from the patient and then use them to understand the disruption of underlying physiological processes.

The first step of pattern identification is the localization of the disorder and the assessment of its essential nature, using the eight principles that are an expansion of

TABLE 26-4

Pulse Positions

Position	Left		Right	
	Deep	Superficial	Deep	Superficial
Nan Jing				
Inch	Heart	Small intestine	Lung	Large intestine
Bar	Liver	Gallbladder	Spleen	Stomach
Cubit	Kidney	Urinary bladder	Pericardium	Triple warmer
Contemporary Chinese Sources				
Inch	Heart		Lung	
Bar	Liver	Gallbladder	Spleen	Stomach
Cubit	Kidney	Urinary bladder	Kidney	Urinary bladder

TABLE 26-5

Pulse Types

	English	Chinese	General Association
1	Normal	zheng chang mai	Normal pulse
2	Floating	fu mai	Exterior condition
3	Deep	chen mai	Interior condition
4	Slow	chi mai	Cold and yang vacuity
5	Rapid	shuo mai	Heat
6	Surging	hong mai	Exuberant heat, hemorrhage
7	Faint	wei mai	Qi and blood vacuity desertion
8	Fine	xi mai	Blood and yin vacuity
9	Scattered	san mai	Dissipation of qi and blood, critical
10	Vacuous	xu mai	Vacuity
11	Replete	shi mai	Exuberant evil with right qi strong
12	Slippery	hua mai	Pregnancy, phlegm, abundant qi and blood
13	Rough	se mai	Blood stasis, vacuity of qi and blood
14	Long	chang mai	Often normal
15	Short	duan mai	Vacuity of qi and blood
16	Stringlike	xian mai	Liver disorders, severe pain
17	Hollow	kou mai	Blood loss
18	Tight	jin mai	Cold, pain
19	Moderate	huan mai	Slower than normal, not pathological
20	Drum skin	ge mai	Blood loss
21	Confined	lao mai	Cold, pain
22	Weak	ruo mai	Vacuity of qi and blood
23	Soggy	ru mai	Vacuity of qi and blood with dampness
24	Hidden	fu mai	Deep-lying internal cold
25	Stirred	dong mai	High fever, pregnancy
26	Rapid, irregular	cu mai	Debility of visceral qi or emotional distress
27	Slow, irregular	jie mai	Debility of visceral qi or emotional distress
28	Regularly intermittent	dai mai	Debility of visceral qi or emotional distress
29	Racing	ji mai	Heat, possible vacuity

Data from Wiseman N, Ellis A, Zmiewski P, et al: *Fundamentals of Chinese medicine,* Brookline, Mass, 1995, Paradigm.

yin and yang correspondences: yin, yang, cold, hot, interior, exterior, vacuity, and repletion.*

As with many other aspects of contemporary Chinese medicine, the *eight principles* originated in the Sung dynasty. Kou Zong Shi proposed a structure that organized disease into eight essentials: cold, hot, interior, exterior, vacuity, repletion, evil qi, and right qi (Bensky et al, 1990). These were improved on in 1732, in the text *Awakening the Mind in Medical Studies (Yi Xue Xin Wu)* (Sivin, 1987). The original source was written, in the spirit of the times, to create a formal diagnostic structure for herbs that could be conceptually integrated with the ideas already in use for acupuncture. Today this formal structure is applied to both acupuncture and herbal medicine.

The patient with a wind cold evil had these symptoms: marked aversion to exposure to cold, headache, body aches, absence of thirst, a moist tongue with a thin white coating, and a floating and tight pulse. In terms of the eight principles, this would be an exterior, cold, repletion pattern. The principles of yin and yang would not directly apply.

What does this mean? The eight principles serve fundamentally to localize a condition. When Chinese physicians say that a condition is "external," they mean that it has not yet penetrated beyond the skin and channels to the deeper parts of the body. In this case, a cold condition betrays itself through the body's expression of cold signs. To say a condition is "replete" is to say that the evil attacking the body is strong, or that the body itself is strong.

Assessment according to the eight principles is typically the first step in developing a clear pattern identification,

*Although many authors continue to use the terms *excess* and *deficiency* to express the Chinese expressions *shi* and *xu,* I prefer Wiseman's "repletion" and "vacuity" as a translation. The use of "excess" simply is incorrect because of the existence of other Chinese terms that convey this idea exactly. "Deficiency" is problematic because it implies measurable quantity, which is not a consideration in the Chinese concept (Wiseman et al, 1990). Unschuld uses "depletion" and "repletion" instead.

especially if the patient has organ involvement. The eight principles are the application of a yin and yang–based theoretical structure.

A single biomedical disease entity can be associated with several Chinese diagnostic patterns (Box 26-4). For example, viral hepatitis is associated with at least six distinct diagnostic patterns, and lower urinary tract infection might be related to one of four patterns (Ergil, 1995a, 1995b). Each of these patterns would be treated in different ways, according to the saying "One disease, different treatments." The patient whose clinical pattern is wind cold has the common cold and a headache, but the same disease could manifest in other patterns.

Also, many different diseases may be captured within one pattern, thus the saying "Different diseases, one treatment." One contemporary text lists such diverse entities as nephritis, dysfunctional uterine bleeding, pyelonephritis, and rheumatic heart disease under the diagnostic pattern of "disharmony between the heart and kidney" (Huang et al, 1993, p. 79).

This comparatively precise diagnostic linkage begins to be broadly appreciated in the historical trends of the Sung, Jin, and Yuan dynasties. The six-channel pattern identification proposed by Zhang Zhong Jing is one of many patterns currently used. The patient who has encountered a wind cold evil would, under Zhang Jong Jing's system, be categorized as having *tai yang* disease. There is considerable room for overlap within the available methods of pattern identification.

THERAPEUTIC CONCEPTS

Once a diagnosis has been determined and, when relevant, a pattern has been differentiated, therapy begins. Therapeutics in Chinese medicine is fundamentally allopathic; that is, it addresses the pathological condition with opposing measures, as follows:

> Cold is treated with heat, heat is treated with cold, vacuity is treated by supplementation, and repletion is treated by drainage (*Inner Classic* in Wiseman et al, 1985).

Within the realm of acupuncture, moxibustion, and herbal medicine, three fundamental principles of

therapy are understood: (1) treating disease from its root, (2) eliminating evil influences and supporting the right, and (3) restoring the balance of yin and yang. These refer to approaches that are appropriate to the patient's condition. It would be appropriate to eliminate the cold evil and support the right qi of the patient with a wind cold pattern. In a patient with symptoms that reflect a complex underlying pattern, the physician might attempt to treat the root of the patient's condition. For example, functional uterine bleeding caused by a disharmony of the heart and kidney would be addressed primarily by harmonizing the heart and kidney; treating the root of the condition would adjust its symptoms. Treatment methods vary widely; Box 26-5 provides the simplest expression of their organization.

THERAPEUTIC METHODS

This section introduces the therapeutic methods of acupuncture and moxibustion, and discusses cupping and bleeding, Chinese massage, qi cultivation, Chinese herbal medicine, and dietetics.

ACUPUNCTURE AND MOXIBUSTION

Although acupuncture and moxibustion can be used independently, they are so deeply interrelated in Chinese medicine that the term for this therapy is *zhen jiu*, meaning "needle moxibustion." To capture the distinctively composite character of this phrase, some authors translate the expression as "acumoxa therapy." This close linkage is based on the ancient origins of these methods, and moxibustion apparently was the form of therapy first applied to the channels and holes to treat problems on or within the body. Both acupuncture and moxibustion are used to provide a discrete stimulus to points that lie along channel pathways or to other appropriate sites.

Points may be chosen on the basis of the actual trajectory of the channel on which the points lie. For example, *Union Valley* is considered an important point for the head

---

BOX 26-4

Types of Diagnostic Patterns

- Eight principles
- Six evils
- Qi and blood and fluids
- Five phases
- Channel patterns
- Viscera and bowels
- Triple burner
- Six channels
- Four levels

BOX 26-5

Methods of Treatment

- Diaphoresis
- Clearing
- Ejection
- Precipitation
- Harmonization
- Warming
- Supplementation
- Dispersion
- Orifice opening
- Securing astriction
- Settling and absorption

and face because it lies on the pathway of the large intestine channel, which traverses that area of the body. Similarly, points on the lower extremity that lie on the urinary bladder channel, which traverses the entire back, often are used for treatment of back pain (Figure 26-3).

Points also are often selected entirely on the basis of their sensitivity to palpation or based on a variation in texture perceived by the practitioner. Often a number of suitable acupuncture points in a specific area may be assessed to determine which would be most suitable for needling. In some cases, points that do not lie on specific channels or form part of the collection of recognized extra points can be identified by their tenderness. These points are known as *ah shi*, or "Ouch, that's it," points and are an important part of clinical acupuncture's traditional history and contemporary practice.

With many acupuncture points from which to choose, and multiple methods on which to base that choice, it is not surprising that many clinicians focus on a few specific methods or a particular collection of points. Some clinicians restrict their approach so that they can focus on adjusting the application of treatment.

A detailed discussion of acupuncture as a therapeutic method can be found in Chapter 27.

MOXIBUSTION (*JIU FA*)

Moxibustion (*jiu*) refers to the burning of the dried and powdered leaves of *Artemisia vulgaris (ai ye)*, either on or in proximity to the skin, to affect the movement of qi in the channel, locally or at a distance. *A. vulgaris* is said to be acrid and bitter and, when used as moxa, to have the ability to warm and enter the channels. References to moxa appear in early materials, such as the texts recovered from the excavated tombs at Ma Wang Dui (Unschuld, 1985). These texts discuss a number of therapeutic methods, including moxibustion, but do not mention acupuncture. The *Treatise on Moxibustion of the Eleven Vessels of Yin and Yang (Yin Yang Shi Yi Mai Jiu Jing)* describes the application of moxa to treat illness by performing moxibustion on the channels (Auteroche et al, 1992).

Moxibustion can be applied to the body in many ways: directly, indirectly, using the pole method, and using the warm needle method. *Direct moxibustion* involves burning a small amount of moxa, about the size of a grain of rice, directly on the skin. Depending on the desired effect, larger or smaller pieces of moxa can be used, and the moxa fluff can be allowed to burn directly to the skin, causing a blister or a scar, or it can be removed before it has burnt down to the skin. Such techniques are used to stimulate acupuncture points in cases in which the action of moxibustion is traditionally indicated or in which warming the point seems to be the most appropriate response. Older texts described the use of direct moxibustion on Leg Three Li and other acupuncture points as a method of health maintenance and prevention.

Indirect moxibustion involves the insertion of a mediating substance between the moxa fluff and the patient's skin. This gives the practitioner greater control over the amount of heat applied to the patient's body and offers the patient increased protection from burning, which allows for the treatment of delicate areas such as the face and back. Popular substances include ginger slices, garlic slices, and salt. The mediating substance is often chosen on the basis of its own medicinal properties and the way these combine with the properties of moxa. Ginger might be selected in patients with vacuity cold, whereas garlic is considered useful for treating hot and toxic conditions. Figure 26-4 shows a patient being treated for facial paralysis with indirect moxibustion using ginger slices.

During *pole moxibustion* a cigar-shaped roll of moxa wrapped in paper is used to warm the acupuncture points gently without touching the skin. This is a safe method of moxibustion that can be taught to patients for self-application.

The *warm needle method* is accomplished by first inserting an acupuncture needle into the point and then placing

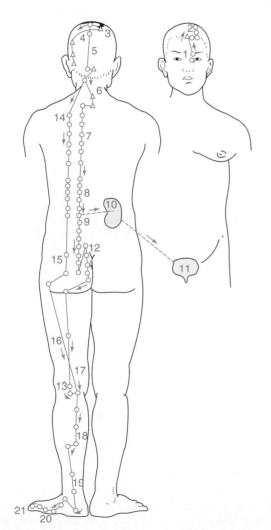

Figure 26-3 The course of the urinary bladder channel of the foot tai yang. (Modified from Qiu ML: Chinese acupuncture and moxibustion, Edinburgh, 1993, Churchill Livingstone, p 103.)

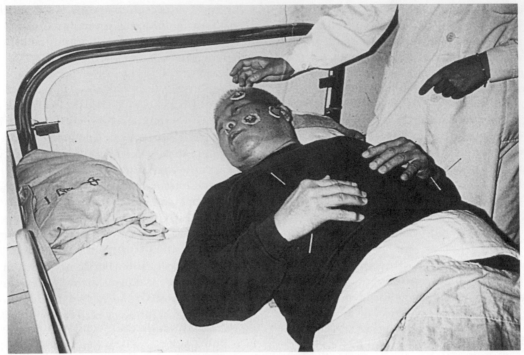

Figure 26-4 Patient receiving indirect moxa. (Courtesy Wind Horse, Marnae Ergil.)

moxa fluff on its handle. After the moxa is ignited, it burns gradually, imparting a sensation of gentle warmth to the acupuncture point and channel. This method is especially useful for patients with arthritic joint pain.

Combined Therapy with Acupuncture

Together, moxibustion and acupuncture are used to treat, or at least ameliorate, a wide range of conditions and symptoms. On the basis of the simple premise that all disease involves the disruption of the flow of qi and that acupuncture and moxibustion regulate the movement of qi, all disease theoretically can benefit from these methods. A brief review of acupuncture texts provides ample evidence of the range of conditions for which acupuncture is considered appropriate. Over the years, efforts have been made outside of China to parse the range of conditions treatable by acupuncture, including that by a World Health Organization (WHO) interregional seminar in the late 1970s (Bannerman, 1979). More recently the WHO established selection criteria for evaluating reports of controlled clinical trials of acupuncture as a basis for reporting on the use of acupuncture in the treatment of various diseases and disorders; Boxes 26-6 and 26-7 list partial results (WHO, 2002). Although these lists are comparatively short compared with the disorders enumerated in a clinical manual or acupuncture textbook, they are informative in terms of the routine application of acupuncture in China and elsewhere. It is also instructive to compare these two lists with the report of the National Institutes of Health (NIH) Consensus Conference discussed later.

For further discussion of acupuncture and the adjunctive use of moxibustion, see Chapter 27.

CUPPING AND BLEEDING

Two methods important to the practice of Chinese medicine are cupping and bleeding. These may be used separately or together and are often used with other methods, such as moxibustion and acupuncture. *Cupping* involves inducing a vacuum in a small glass or bamboo cup and promptly applying it to the skin surface. This therapy brings blood and lymph to the skin surface under the cup, which increases local circulation. Cupping is often used to drain or remove cold and damp evils from the body or to assist blood circulation. *Bleeding* is done to drain a channel or to remove heat from the body at a specific location. Unlike the bloodletting practiced by Western physicians throughout the nineteenth century, this method expresses comparatively small amounts of blood, from a drop to a few centiliters. Figure 26-5 shows a patient receiving cupping and bleeding at an acupuncture point on the urinary bladder channel associated with the lungs.

CHINESE MASSAGE (*TUI NA*)

Literally "pushing and pulling," *tui na* refers to a system of massage, manual acupuncture point stimulation, and manipulation that is vast enough to warrant its own chapter. These methods have been practiced at least as long as moxibustion, but the first massage training class was instituted in Shanghai in 1956 (Wang et al, 1990, p. 16). At present, this field of study can serve as a minor component of a traditional medical education or an area of extensive clinical specialization.

Diseases and Disorders Effectively Treated with Acupuncture*

Adverse reactions to radiotherapy and/or chemotherapy
Allergic rhinitis (including hay fever)
Biliary colic
Depression (including depressive neurosis and depression following stroke)
Dysentery, acute bacillary
Dysmenorrhea, primary
Epigastralgia, acute (in peptic ulcer, acute and chronic gastritis, and gastrospasm)
Facial pain (including craniomandibular disorders)
Headache
Hypertension, essential
Hypotension, primary
Induction of labor
Knee pain
Leukopenia
Low back pain
Malposition of fetus, correction of
Morning sickness
Nausea and vomiting
Neck pain
Pain in dentistry (including dental pain and temporomandibular dysfunction)
Periarthritis of shoulder
Postoperative pain
Renal colic
Rheumatoid arthritis
Sciatica
Sprain
Stroke
Tennis elbow

*Diseases, symptoms, or conditions for which acupuncture has been proved—through controlled trials—to be an effective treatment.

A distinct aspect of tui na is the extensive training of the hands necessary for clinical practice. The practitioner's hands are trained to accomplish focused and forceful movements that can be applied to various areas of the body. Techniques such as pushing, rolling, kneading, rubbing, and grasping are practiced repetitively until they become second nature (Figure 26-6). Students practice on a small bag of rice until their hands develop the necessary strength and dexterity.

Tui na often is applied to limited areas of the body, and the techniques can be quite forceful and intense. Tui na is applied routinely for orthopedic and neurological conditions. It also is applied for conditions not usually viewed as susceptible to treatment through manipulation, such as asthma, dysmenorrhea, and chronic gastritis. Tui na is used as an adjunct to acupuncture to increase the range of motion of a joint or instead of acupuncture when

needles are uncomfortable or inappropriate, such as in pediatric applications.

As with all aspects of Chinese medicine, regional styles and family lineages of massage practice abound. The formal tui na curriculum available in Chinese programs is extensive, but probably not a complete expression of the range of possibilities.

QI CULTIVATION (QIGONG)

Qigong is a term that literally embraces almost every aspect of the manipulation of qi by means of exercise, breathing, and the influence of the mind, as discussed later and in Chapter 28. Qigong includes practices ranging from the meditative systems of Daoist and Buddhist practitioners to the martial arts traditions of China. Qigong is relevant to medicine in three specific areas. First, it allows the practitioner to cultivate demeanor and stamina to perform the strenuous activities of tui na, to sustain the constant demands of clinical practice, and to quiet the mind to facilitate diagnostic perception. Second, qigong cultivates the practitioner's ability to transmit qi safely to the patient. Practitioners may direct qi to the patient either through the needles or directly through their hands. This activity may be the main focus of treatment or an adjunctive aspect, in which case the qi paradigm is expanded to include direct interaction between the patient's qi and the clinician's qi. Third, the patient may be taught to engage in specific qigong practices that are useful for the patient's illness.

Qi cultivation makes extensive use of the principles of traditional Chinese medicine, and its history is intertwined with that of famous physicians. The history of qi cultivation practices is considered to extend back into antiquity and to indicate the early recognition of the importance of exercise to the health of the body. In Lu's *Spring and Autumn* annals, the following famous aphorism relates the importance of movement to the maintenance of health and function (Engelhardt, 1989):

> Flowing water will never turn stale, the hinge of the door will never be eaten by worms. They never rest in their activity: that's why.

In this text, Lu described the role of dance and movement in correcting the movement of qi and yin within the body and benefiting the muscles (Zhang, 1990).

Descriptions of qi cultivation practices and exercises are attributed to the early Daoist masters. Zhuang Zi, writing in the fourth century BC, reveals the role of breathing and physical exercise in promoting longevity and describes a sage intent on extending his life (Despeux, 1989), as follows:

> To pant, to puff, to hail, to sip, to spit out the old breath and draw in the new, practicing bear hangings and bird-stretches, longevity his only concern (Watson, 1968).

BOX 26-7

Diseases and Disorders for Which Acupuncture Shows Therapeutic Effects*

Abdominal pain (in acute gastroenteritis or due to gastro-intestinal spasm)	Neuralgia, postherpetic
Acne vulgaris	Neurodermatitis
Alcohol dependence and detoxification	Obesity
Bell palsy	Opium, cocaine, and heroin dependence
Bronchial asthma	Osteoarthritis
Cancer pain	Pain due to endoscopic examination
Cardiac neurosis	Pain in thromboangiitis obliterans
Cholecystitis, chronic, with acute exacerbation	Polycystic ovary syndrome (Stein-Leventhal syndrome)
Cholelithiasis	Postextubation in children
Competition stress syndrome	Postoperative convalescence
Craniocerebral injury, closed	Premenstrual syndrome
Diabetes mellitus, non–insulin dependent	Prostatitis, chronic
Earache	Pruritus
Epidemic hemorrhagic fever	Radicular and pseudoradicular pain syndrome
Epistaxis, simple (without generalized or local disease)	Raynaud syndrome, primary
Eye pain due to subconjunctival injection	Recurrent lower urinary tract infection
Facial spasm	Reflex sympathetic dystrophy
Female infertility	Retention of urine, traumatic
Female urethral syndrome	Schizophrenia
Fibromyalgia and fasciitis	Sialism, drug induced
Gastrokinetic disturbance	Sjögren syndrome
Gouty arthritis	Sore throat (including tonsillitis)
Hepatitis B virus carrier status	Spine pain, acute
Herpes zoster (human [alpha] herpesvirus 3)	Stiff neck
Hyperlipemia	Temporomandibular joint dysfunction
Hypo-ovarianism	Tietze syndrome
Insomnia	Tobacco dependence
Labor pain	Tourette syndrome
Lactation deficiency	Ulcerative colitis, chronic
Male sexual dysfunction, nonorganic	Urolithiasis
Ménière disease	Vascular dementia
	Whooping cough (pertussis)

*Diseases, symptoms, or conditions for which the therapeutic effect of acupuncture has been shown but for which further proof of its effect is needed.

Among the texts recovered at Ma Huang Dui are a series of illustrated guides to the practice of conduction (dao yin) that provide guidance to the physical postures and therapeutic properties of this form of qi cultivation (Despeux, 1989, p. 226).

The famous physician of second-century China, Hua Tou, is credited with the creation of a series of exercises. These were based on the movements of the tiger, the deer, the bear, the monkey, and a bird and were to be practiced to ward off disease.

Zhang Zhong Jing, in his Golden Cabinet Prescriptions, recommended the practices of dao yin or conduction and tui na or exhalation and inhalation to treat disease.

A wide variety of forms of qi cultivation were developed over the centuries, and many have achieved great popularity. Since the 1950s, qigong training programs have been implemented and sanatoria built, specializing in the therapeutic application of qigong to the treatment of disease (see Chapter 28).

Fundamental Concepts

Qi cultivation rests on several fundamental principles intended to support activity to enhance the movement of qi and to increase health. Most discussions of qi cultivation address the relaxation of the body, the regulation or control of breathing, and the calming of the mind. Qi cultivation generally is performed in a relaxed standing, sitting, or lying posture. Once the correct position is achieved, the practitioner begins to regulate breathing in concert with specific mental and physical exercises.

For example, one form of qigong involves the action of visualizing the internal and external pathways of the channels and imagining the movement of the qi along these channels in concert with the breath. As the practice develops, the practitioner begins to experience the sensation of qi traveling along the channel pathways. Traditionally, it is considered that the mind guides the qi to a specific area of the body and that the qi then guides the

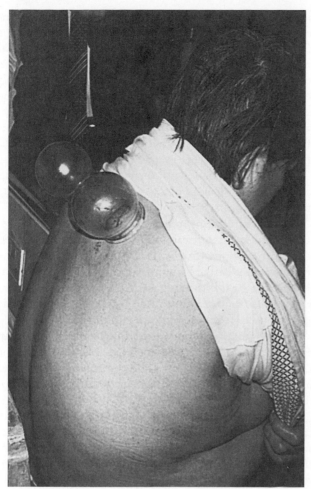

Figure 26-5 Cupping and bleeding. (Courtesy Wind Horse, Marnae Ergil.)

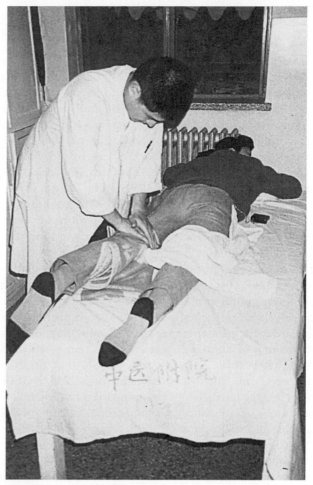

Figure 26-6 Tui na in clinical practice. (Courtesy Wind Horse, Marnae Ergil.)

blood there as well, which improves circulation in the area. From this point of view, this particular exercise trains the qi and blood to move freely along the channel pathways, which leads to good health.

Another exercise involves the use of breath, visualization, and simple physical exercises to benefit the qi of the lungs. This therapeutic exercise is recommended for bronchitis, emphysema, and bronchial asthma. It is begun by assuming a relaxed posture, whether sitting, lying, or standing. The exercise is begun by breathing naturally and allowing the mind to become calm. The upper and lower teeth are then clicked together by closing the mouth gently 36 times. As saliva is produced, it is retained in the mouth, swirled with the tongue, and then swallowed in three parts while one imagines that it is flowing into the middle of the chest and then to an area about three fingerbreadths below the navel (the *dan tian,* or cinnabar field). At this point, one imagines that one is sitting in front of a reservoir of white qi that enters the mouth on inhalation and is transmitted through the body as one exhales, first to the lungs, then to the dan tian, and finally out to the skin and body hair. This process of visualization is repeated 18 times.

This process makes use of the relationship between the mind and qi to strengthen the function of the lungs and to pattern regions of the body associated with the area where the qi governing the lungs and respiration is stored. This area is associated with the acupuncture point *dan zhong,* or chest center (ren 17), which is located in the middle of the chest. Next the qi is directed to the cinnabar field, which is associated with another location on the ren channel *qi hai,* or sea of qi (ren 6), just below the umbilicus. This area is considered to be important to the production and storage of the body's qi and to the lungs on exhalation.

This exercise typifies the three aspects of a qigong exercise described previously: relaxation, mental tranquility, and breath control. It induces relaxation through mental concentration, because the exercise of focusing on breathing and the visualized process help remove distracting thoughts from the mind, and the patterning of the breath with visualization controls and regulates the breathing.

It should be stressed that although many forms of qigong exist, they share general principles of application and a relationship to Chinese medicine concepts.

CHINESE HERBAL MEDICINE (ZHONG YAO)

Since the legendary emperor Shen Nong tasted herbs and guided the Chinese people in herbal use, diet, and therapeutics, herbal medicine has been an integral part of Chinese culture and medical practice. The traditional Chinese materia medica includes much more than herbs; minerals and animal parts are listed as well. The number of substances currently identified is 5767, as recorded in the *Encyclopedia of Traditional Chinese Medicinal Substances (Zhong Yao Da Ci Dian)* published in 1977 by the Jiangsu College of New Medicine (Bensky et al, 1986). This publication is the latest in a long line of definitive discussions of materia medica that have been produced in China over the millennia. The earliest known is the *Divine Husbandman's Classic of the Materia Medica,* reconstructed by Tao Hong Jing (AD 452-536). This text classified herbs into upper, middle, and lower grades and discussed the tastes, temperatures, toxicities, and medicinal properties of 364 substances.

Currently, substances are categorized systematically as expansions of the eight methods of therapy discussed earlier (Box 26-8). Subcategories exist within the basic categories into which substances are organized. Prescribing rules take into account the compatibilities and incompatibilities of substances, the traditional pairings of substances, and their combination for treatment of specific symptoms.

Both the Ma Wan Dui texts and the *Inner Classic* provide recommendations for the therapeutic combination of substances. Zhang Zhong Jing's work in systematizing herbal prescriptions as therapeutic approaches for specific diagnostic patterns based on yin and yang correspondences was unusual for its time. It was not until physicians of the Sung dynasty became interested in relating herbal practice to a systematic theory and organizing diagnostics accordingly that interest was renewed in the *Treatise on Cold Damage*. This book remains a significant resource for the current practitioner of Chinese herbal medicine. One of the most comprehensive English-language compilations of Chinese herbal prescriptions derives approximately 20% of its formulas from this source (Bensky et al, 1990).

Not all herbal prescriptions or texts discussing application followed the lead of Zhang Zhong Jing. Many texts offered herbs or prescriptions for specific symptoms without reference to distinct theoretical structures or diagnostic principles. The general population probably applied herbs in exactly this manner. Even today, although the prescription of herbal formulas is primarily driven by traditional diagnostic theory and pattern diagnosis, extensive compilations of empirically derived herbal formulas with symptomatic indications are published.

Contemporary compilations of formulas follow an organization similar to that used for substances. The result is that both substances and formulas are organized in a manner that makes them accessible in terms of traditional theories (Box 26-9).

Let us examine the formula and its constituent substances that might be provided to our patient who has encountered a wind cold evil or who, in the pattern identification system described in the *Treatise on Cold Damage,* would be said to have a "tai yang stage pattern." In either case, ephedra decoction *(ma huang tang)* would be an appropriate choice, particularly if the patient had a

---

BOX 26-8

Fundamental Categories of Chinese Materia Medica

- Exterior resolving
- Heat clearing
- Ejection producing
- Precipitant
- Wind dispelling
- Water disinhibiting dampness percolating
- Interior warming
- Qi rectifying
- Food dispersing
- Worm expelling
- Blood rectifying
- Phlegm transforming, cough suppressing, panting-calming
- Spirit quieting
- Liver calming, wind extinguishing
- Orifice opening
- Supplementing
- Securing and astringing
- External use

BOX 26-9

Fundamental Categories for Chinese Herbal Medicine

- Exterior resolving
- Heat clearing
- Ejection producing
- Precipitant
- Harmonizing
- Dampness dispelling
- Interior warming
- Qi rectifying
- Dispersing
- Blood rectifying
- Phlegm transforming, cough suppressing, panting-calming
- Spirit quieting
- Tetany settling
- Orifice opening
- Supplementing
- Securing and astringing
- Oral formulas for sores
- External use

slight cough as well. The constituents and dosage of the formula are 9 g of ephedra *(ma huang)*, 6 g of cinnamon twig *(gui zhi)*, 9 g of apricot kernel *(xing ren)*, and 3 g of licorice *(gan cao)*. These ingredients are cooked together in water to make a slightly concentrated tea, which is drunk in successive doses. The tea is taken warm to induce sweating, a sign that the qi of the surface of the body that had been impeded by the cold evil is free to move and throw off the evil. The patient stops drinking the tea once sweat arrives.

A traditional system of organizing a formula is to identify ingredients as the ruler, minister, adjutant, and emissary. In this case the *ruler* of the formula is ephedra. The ruler sets the therapeutic direction of the formula. Acrid and warm, ephedra promotes sweating, dispels cold, and resolves the surface. (We examine ephedra again in the discussion of herbal research.) Cinnamon twig is the *minister,* working to assist the ruler in carrying out its objectives. As with ephedra, it too is said to warm the body. Apricot kernel is the *adjutant,* so it addresses the possible involvement of the lung and moderates the acrid flavor of the other two substances. Because the lung is the organ most immediately affected by wind cold or wind heat, the formula addresses the organ. Finally, licorice is the *emissary,* serving both to render the action of the other herbs harmonious and to distribute this action through the body.

The previous example is brief and simple but illustrates fundamental concepts. Chinese herbal therapeutics can be complex. Its practice is broad, and the range of conditions addressed is more extensive than with acupuncture. In terms of complexity and the diagnostic acumen required of the practitioner, it resembles the practice of internal medicine. Herbal therapy also encompasses the external applications of herbs and a variety of methods of preparation. Besides being prepared as the traditional water decoction, or tea, substances may be powdered or rendered into pills, pastes, or tinctures.

DIETETICS

Traditional dietetics encompasses the practice of herbal therapy but also addresses traditional Chinese foods in terms of the theoretical constructs of Chinese medicine. Five-phase theory has been applied to foods since the time of the *Inner Classic.* It is not unusual to see a classroom in a college of Chinese medicine equipped as a kitchen. In larger cities, special restaurants prepare meals with specific medicinal purposes. The practices of this field are deeply rooted in the cultural practices of China and cultural beliefs about diet. Many of the foods organized for use in therapy also are routinely prepared by families to promote health when the seasons change and when illness strikes, as well as to strengthen a woman after birth, to cause milk to fill the breasts of a new mother, or to nourish elderly persons in their declining years.

CHINESE MEDICINE OVERSEAS

China's traditional medicine is practiced in various forms all over the world. Sometimes its practice follows the contemporary patterns of *traditional Chinese medicine* (zhong yi). Sometimes its practice is deeply informed by local custom, preference, or regional elaborations.

CHINESE MEDICINE IN KOREA

A close relationship exists between China and Korea. Chinese medicine arrived in Korea during the Qin dynasty (221-207 BC). However, the textual basis of Korean medicine in the literary tradition of Chinese medicine seems to have been established during the Han and Tang dynasties (Hsu et al, 1977), during a period of political domination by the Chinese. The closeness between China and Korea during the Kingdom of Silla (AD 400-700) facilitated this exchange of ideas. Formal medical instruction by government-appointed physicians began in AD 693. Texts such as the *Systematic Classic of Acupuncture (and Moxibustion)* were important to the development of the tradition. With the formation of the Liao dynasty (AD 907-1168), Korea established its independence from Chinese rule, but cultural and medical exchange continued. During the Li dynasty (1392-1910), many texts, including the *Illustrated Classic of Acupuncture Points as Found on the Bronze Model,* reached Korea (Chuang, 1982). Widely used techniques of acupuncture point selection based on five-phase theory have emerged from Korea, including those of the Buddhist priest Sa-am (1544-1610).

At least two comparatively recent innovations based on Chinese medicine have been developed in Korea and have become well known in other parts of the world. Korean *constitutional diagnosis* was developed initially by Jhema Lee (1836-1900) and based a system of herbal therapeutics on a system of diagnostic patterning that used the four divisions of yin and yang. In 1965, Dowon Kuan expanded the system to an eightfold classification and applied it to acupuncture (Hirsch, 1985). *Koryo sooji chim,* the system of Korean *hand and finger acupuncture,* was developed by Yoo Tae Woo and published in 1971. The system maps the channel pathways and acupuncture points of the entire body onto the hands, where they are stimulated using very short, fine needles and magnets. This system has gained a significant level of international exposure.

CHINESE MEDICINE IN JAPAN

The history of cultural exchange between China and Japan dates to at least AD 57. Kon Mu was the first physician to go to Japan and use Chinese methods; he was sent in AD 414 by the king of Silla, in southeast Korea, to treat the emperor Inkyo Tenno. This interaction continued; in 552 a Korean delegation brought a selection of Chinese medical texts to Japan (Bowers, 1970). In 562, Zhi Cong came from southern China with more than 100 books on the practice of Chinese medicine (Huard et al, 1968), including the *Systematic Classic of Acupuncture (and Moxibustion)* (Chuang, 1982). By the early eighth century the influence of Chinese medicine was well established. With the adoption of the Taiho code in 702, provision was made for a ministry of health composed of specialists, physicians, students, and researchers (Lock, 1980). In 754 a Buddhist priest, Chien Chen, brought many medical texts from China to Japan. His influence was memorialized in a shrine in Nishinokyo (Chuang, 1982).

Chinese influences on Japanese medicine were derived primarily from the *Classic of Difficult Issues* and *Systematic Classic of Acupuncture (and Moxibustion)*. A revisionist movement in the late seventeenth century established the *Treatise on Cold Damage* (*Shokanron*) as the core text of herbal medicine, or *kanpo* (Chinese method), in Japan (Lock, 1980).

Several factors have influenced the development of Chinese medicine in Japan, giving it a somewhat unique appearance. The scarcity of ingredients for the preparation of Chinese herbal formulas led to an emphasis on lower dosages in herbal prescriptions than are typical in China. An emphasis on palpatory diagnosis involving channel pathways and the abdomen also became well established. The use of finer-gauge needles and shallow insertion became typical of Japanese acupuncture.

In the mid-seventeenth century, Waichi Sugiyama, a blind man, began to train the blind in acupuncture using very fine needles and guide tubes. Because it had become customary in the earlier part of the Edo period for blind persons to do massage, both massage and acupuncture now became associated with blind practitioners. This contributed to a lower social position for acupuncture practitioners and to specialization in medical practice. Kanpo physicians became primarily practitioners of herbal medicine (Lock, 1980).

This trend toward specialization has continued to the present, with the division of acupuncture, moxibustion, and massage into separately licensed practices (although many individuals hold all three licenses) and the actual practice of herbal medicine being retained in the hands of medical physicians. Interestingly, many Chinese herbal prescriptions are recognized as appropriate therapy for certain medical conditions according to regulations governing health care in Japan.

Japan has seen both focused specialization in and the innovative exploration and expansion of traditional acupuncture. The *Classic of Difficult Issues* often has been the focus for movements to revive the practices of traditional acupuncture. Its influence has contributed heavily to the comparatively recent development of groups of acupuncturists advocating *meridian therapy (keiraku chiryo)* based on the application of concepts in the *Classic of Difficult Issues* and their subsequent interpretation by later Chinese authors. A distinctive feature of meridian therapy is the application of five-phase theory to the transport points, a practice that has influenced the perception and adoption of five-phase theory by European practitioners (Kaptchuk, 1983).

The pioneering work of Yoshio Manaka also has contributed dramatically to the practice of acupuncture. Manaka, a physician who experimented with acupuncture principles when medical supplies were lacking during World War II, became convinced of the efficacy and physiological relevance of traditional theories and continued to experiment and develop them throughout his life.

Japanese acupuncture practitioners have a broad range of practices and interests. Although some are particular partisans of specific schools of thought, including some based on contemporary Chinese medicine perspectives, many practitioners have adopted a comparatively eclectic approach.

CHINESE MEDICINE IN EUROPE

The history of Chinese medicine in Europe, particularly acupuncture, is both long-standing and broadly developed. The medical use of acupuncture in Europe dates from the middle of the sixteenth century (Peacher, 1975). The work of Willem Ten Rhyne (1647-1690) in this area culminated in the publication in 1683 of *Dissertatio de Arthritide: Mantissa Schematica: de Acupunctura: et Orationes Tres*, based on information gathered during his service in Japan as a physician for the Dutch East India Company. The German physician Kampfer, who also traveled with the Dutch East India Company and spent time in Japan, contributed his observations.

In France the Jesuit Du Halde published a text in 1735 that included a detailed discussion of Chinese medicine (Hsu, 1989). Soulié de Morant's publication of *L'Acupuncture Chinoise* was an extensive discussion of the practice of acupuncture based on direct translation, observation, and actual practice by the author. Published in 1939, the text was rooted in Soulié de Morant's exposure to the medicine of China in that country from 1901 to 1917.

England saw the publication of J.M. Churchill's *A Description of Surgical Operations Peculiar to Japanese and Chinese* in 1825. Among early notable English acupuncturists were Drs. Felix Mann and Sidney Rose-Neil, both of whom began their explorations of acupuncture in the late 1950s and have influenced its development substantially in English-speaking countries. J.R. Worsley, a physical therapist, began his studies of acupuncture in 1962 and had a substantial impact on the perceptions of many English and U.S. practitioners. He visited Hong Kong and Taiwan for a brief period and then became a part of the study group established by Rose-Neil (Hsu et al, 1977). Worsley went on to create the British College of Traditional Chinese Acupuncture and two U.S. schools.

CHINESE MEDICINE IN THE UNITED STATES

In 1826, Bache became one of the first American physicians to use acupuncture in his practice (Haller, 1973). Ten Rhyne's text was a part of Sir William Osler's library (Peacher, 1975), and in his *Principles and Practice of Medicine,* Osler prescribes acupuncture for lumbago (Osler, 1913).

Although only occasionally explored by the conventional U.S. medical community, the traditional medicine of China has been practiced in the United States since the middle of the nineteenth century. Herbal merchants, entrepreneurs, and physicians accompanied the Chinese who sold their labor in the United States. The practice of the China doctor of John Day, Oregon, Doc Ing Hay, is one of the most famous (Barlow et al, 1979). Ah Fong Chuck, who came to the United States in 1866, became the first licensed practitioner of traditional Chinese medicine in the United States in 1901, when he successfully won a medical license through legal action in Idaho (Muench, 1984). With the strengthening of medical practice acts throughout the United States, the interruption of the herb supply from China, and the advent of World War II, these practices disappeared or retreated into Chinatowns nationwide.

Substantial attention was focused on acupuncture, the traditional medicine of China, and its regional variants, as a result of James Reston's highly publicized appendectomy and postoperative care in 1971 and the subsequent opening of China by Nixon. As a result, medical practices largely confined to Asia and the Chinatowns of America gained visibility throughout the United States. Increased visibility led to substantial public interest in acupuncture and gradually to licensure and the development of training programs in many states. Currently, 41 states (including the District of Columbia) license, certify, or register the practice of acupuncture and a range of other activities, including the practice of herbal medicine, by nonphysicians. More than 57 U.S. programs offer training in acupuncture and Oriental medicine.

Americans have a clear interest in the available range of expressions of Chinese medical tradition. In the United States, European interpretations of the application of five-phase theory, Korean constitutional acupuncture, traditional chinese medicine (acupuncture, herbs, qigong, tui na), Japanese meridian therapy, and the approaches of special family lineages within the Chinese tradition all are taught and practiced. This willingness to accept and explore the traditional and contemporary interpretations of traditional Chinese medicine has led to the emergence of the concept of "Oriental medicine" as an umbrella term for the global domain of practice in this area.

The extent to which the practice of Chinese medicine has come to be viewed as an established therapeutic practice in the United States was recently illustrated by a regulatory action taken by the U.S. Food and Drug Administration (FDA). After a series of reports of adverse events surrounding the use of ephedra-containing supplements in support of weight loss regimens and athletic training, neither of which can be considered to constitute the practice of Chinese medicine, the FDA was compelled to act. In February 2004 the FDA issued a final rule prohibiting the sale of dietary supplements containing ephedrine alkaloids (ephedra), "because such supplements present an unreasonable risk of illness or injury" (U.S. FDA, 2004). Intriguingly, it was specifically stated that the "scope of the rule does not pertain to traditional Chinese herbal remedies." Although the logistics of honoring this exemption have yet to be worked out, it is a definite acknowledgment of the professional practice of Chinese herbal medicine in the United States.

PRACTICE SETTINGS

In general, traditional Chinese medicine is practiced in a range of clinical settings. Large hospitals entirely devoted to its practice are common in China. In this setting, acupuncture, herbal medicine, and tui na are provided on both an inpatient and an outpatient basis. It is not unusual to see a large outpatient facility treating 20 patients simultaneously in the same space. Other settings include smaller practices and even roadside stands. Herbal prescriptions can be obtained from a Chinese herb store in most countries with a significant Chinese population. In Japan, small hospitals, large clinics, and private offices are typical settings.

Wherever traditional Chinese medicine is practiced, the delivery settings are not significantly different from the environment in which biomedical services are provided, unless the practitioner wants to emphasize the distinctive character of the practice or the practice is marginalized through lack of regulation. In the United States, record-keeping processes, insurance billing, biomedical screening, and concerns about office hygiene often produce a setting that—except for such peculiarities as acupuncture needles, moxa fluff, and herbs—looks very much like a typical physician's office.

RESEARCH AND EVALUATION

Aspects of Chinese medicine have been the focus of concerted research efforts in China and Japan since the mid-twentieth century, or earlier if one considers research into Chinese herbal medicine in Japan. Recently, substantial research initiatives in this area have been undertaken in the United States and Europe as well, developing rapidly in terms of quality and quantity in the last 20 years. The actual and perceived quality of such research, in both the East and the West, can vary widely. As is the case with medical systems, research standards—and even scientific research—are subject to cultural influences. The randomized, placebo-controlled, and double-blind clinical trial is the definitive standard for an unambiguous biomedical recognition of efficacy, but not all societies require or encourage their medical communities to secure knowledge in this manner. In addition, the simple accessibility of research data is influenced by the language and location of publication. These problems can pose obstacles to the availability and use of research information. Therefore, research that is meaningful to the scientific communities of China, Japan, Europe, or the United States can vary in its relevance to and impact on other communities.

Study design is another problem that emerges with clinical research in Chinese medicine. Problems with research methods have arisen as the Chinese medicine community in the United States and Europe has participated more in research and as the biomedical community has become better educated about various modalities of Chinese medicine.

Efforts by the Office of Alternative Medicine (OAM), created in 1991 under the NIH, substantially contributed to this process within the United States. The OAM hosted several conferences dealing with methodological considerations in the field of alternative medicine, and each event addressed aspects of traditional Chinese medicine. Other OAM-supported projects included funding of numerous small research grants, many in the area of Chinese or Oriental medicine.

The OAM also sponsored a workshop on acupuncture in cooperation with the FDA. In April 1994, members of the acupuncture medical and scientific community gave presentations detailing the safety and the apparent clinical efficacy of acupuncture needles. These presentations became the core of a petition that led, in March 1996, to the reclassification of acupuncture needles by the FDA from a class III, or experimental, device to a class II, or medical, device for use by qualified practitioners with special controls (sterility and single use).

In November 1997 the NIH convened a consensus development conference on the safety and efficacy of acupuncture for the treatment of specific conditions. Acupuncture experts presented evidence to a scientific panel, who reached the following formal conclusion:

> Acupuncture as a therapeutic intervention is widely practiced in the United States. While there have been many studies of its potential usefulness, many of these studies provide equivocal results because of design, sample size, and other factors. The issue is further complicated by inherent difficulties in the use of appropriate controls, such as placebos and sham acupuncture groups. However, promising results have emerged, for example, showing efficacy of acupuncture in adult postoperative and chemotherapy nausea and vomiting and in postoperative dental pain. There are other situations such as addiction, stroke rehabilitation, headache, menstrual cramps, tennis elbow, fibromyalgia, myofascial pain, osteoarthritis, low back pain, carpal tunnel syndrome, and asthma, in which acupuncture may be useful as an adjunct treatment or an acceptable alternative or be included in a comprehensive management program. Further research is likely to uncover additional areas where acupuncture interventions will be useful. (NIH, 1997)

Considering that less than 2 years earlier, acupuncture needles were still considered an experimental device in the United States, this finding marked significant progress.

In late 1998 the OAM was established as the National Center for Complementary and Alternative Medicine (NCCAM) and was provided with a significant increase in funding (Box 26-10). Since its inception, OAM/NCCAM has continued to refine and develop its approach to fostering research into complementary and alternative medicine (CAM). One strategy is the funding of CAM research centers with developed institutional resources. At present, these specialty centers number 22; many have developed or proposed research that includes aspects of traditional Chinese medicine (Boxes 26-11 and 26-12). Some centers, such as the Center for Alternative Medicine Pain Research

---

BOX 26-10

Acupuncture Studies Sponsored by NCCAM

Acupuncture and Hypertension

Acupuncture and Moxa: A RCT for Chronic Diarrhea in HIV Patients

Acupuncture for Shortness of Breath in Cancer Patients

Acupuncture for the Treatment of Chronic Daily Headaches

Acupuncture for the Treatment of Hot Flashes in Breast Cancer Patients

Acupuncture for the Treatment of Posttraumatic Stress Disorder (PTSD)

Acupuncture in Cardiovascular Disease

Acupuncture in Fibromyalgia

Acupuncture in the Treatment of Depression

Acupuncture Needling on Connective Tissue by Ultrasound

Acupuncture Safety/Efficacy in Knee Osteoarthritis

Acupuncture to Prevent Postoperative Bowel Paralysis (Paralytic Ileus)

Acupuncture to Reduce Symptoms of Advanced Colorectal Cancer

Acupuncture vs. Placebo in Irritable Bowel Syndrome

Efficacy of Acupuncture for Chronic Low Back Pain

Efficacy of Acupuncture in the Treatment of Fibromyalgia

Efficacy of Acupuncture with Physical Therapy for Knee Osteo-Arthritis

Interaction Between Patient and Healthcare Provider: Response to Acupuncture in Knee Osteoarthritis

A Randomized Study of Electroacupuncture Treatment for Delayed Chemotherapy-Induced Nausea and Vomiting in Patients with Pediatric Sarcomas

Use of Acupuncture for Dental Pain: Testing a Model

HIV, Human immunodeficiency virus (infection); *NCCAM*, National Center for Complementary and Alternative Medicine; *RCT*, randomized controlled trial.

BOX 26-11

NCCAM Research Centers Examining Aspects of Chinese Medicine

Center of Excellence for the Neuroimaging of Acupuncture Effects on Human Brain Activity
Specialty: Acupuncture
Massachusetts General Hospital
Charlestown, MA
Investigating the neural basis for the effects of acupuncture through the use of functional magnetic resonance imaging.

New England School of Acupuncture–Harvard Acupuncture Research Collaborative
Specialty: Acupuncture
New England School of Acupuncture
Watertown, MA
This developmental center for research will bring together leaders from the Oriental medicine and conventional medicine communities to critically evaluate the efficacy and safety of acupuncture and to develop sound methodologies for acupuncture research.

Center for CAM Research in Aging and Women's Health
Specialty: Aging and women's health
Columbia University
College of Physicians and Surgeons
New York, NY
Studies include a basic science evaluation of various biological activities of a Chinese herbal preparation to help assess its safety for women with or at risk for breast cancer.

Center for Alternative Medicine Research on Arthritis
Specialty: Arthritis
University of Maryland School of Medicine
Baltimore, MD
The center will investigate the cost effectiveness of and long-term outcomes following acupuncture treatment for osteoarthritis of the knee; the mechanism of action and effects of electroacupuncture on persistent pain and inflammation; and the mechanism of action of an herbal combination with immunomodulatory properties.

CAM Research Center for Cardiovascular Diseases
Specialty: Cardiovascular diseases
University of Michigan Taubman Health Care Center
Ann Arbor, MI
The center will assess the impact of traditional Chinese medicine techniques of qigong on post–coronary artery bypass grafting pain, healing, and outcome.

Center for CAM in Neurodegenerative Diseases
Specialty: Neurodegenerative diseases
Emory University School of Medicine
Atlanta, GA
Current projects include the investigation of the effect of the Chinese mind-body modalities of t'ai chi ch'uan and qigong on motor disabilities associated with Parkinson's disease.

CAM, Complementary and alternative medicine; NCCAM, National Center for Complementary and Alternative Medicine.

on Arthritis at the University of Maryland School of Medicine, have built their centers around long-term and sustained research efforts in specific areas. This has allowed them to make substantial strides as increased funding became available because of interest in CAM therapies. Recently, traditional acupuncture and Oriental medicine programs have begun to emerge as visible partners in research initiatives. The New England School of Acupuncture has partnered with Harvard in a research collaboration.

Other organizations, such as the Society for Acupuncture Research (SAR), have emerged from the broad-based community of acupuncturists, physicians, and researchers interested in the range of research issues posed by this field. The SAR holds annual meetings and publishes its proceedings. Among its objectives are scholarly exchange between researchers in acupuncture and other modalities related to Oriental medicine, encouragement of research activities by acupuncturists, and clarification of methodological issues related to research in these areas. In 1996, two SAR officers, Stephen Birch and Richard Hammerschlag, compiled a definitive summary of the most successful, well-designed, controlled clinical trials produced to date.

RESEARCH INTO SPECIFIC AREAS OF CHINESE MEDICINE

Research on fundamental concepts, or what might be called *fundamental theory*, includes the exploration of whether concepts such as qi, the channels, acupuncture points, the diagnostic aspects of the pulse, and aspects of pattern diagnosis actually can refer to reproducibly identifiable and quantifiable phenomena. All these areas have been or are being actively pursued in a number of countries. This research resembles basic research in physiology and relies on the development of sophisticated models and the design of instrumentation to test these models.

Research questions derived from the search for the physiological basis of Chinese medical concepts have been pursued for some time in China. One such study investigated the nature of kidney yang and concluded that patients displaying a diagnostic pattern associated with kidney yang vacuity showed low levels of 17-hydroxy corticosteroids in their urine, which ultimately suggests a relationship between the concept of kidney yang and the adrenocortical system (Hao, 1983).

NCCAM-Sponsored Studies in Chinese Medicine Modalities

Chinese Herbal Medicine
Alternative Medicine Approaches for Women with Temporomandibular Disorders
Consistency of Traditional Chinese Medicine Diagnoses and Herbal Prescriptions for Rheumatoid Arthritis
Herbal Treatment of Hepatitis C in Methadone Maintained Patients

T'ai Chi Ch'uan
Alternative Stress Management Approaches in HIV Disease
Complementary/Alternative Medicine for Abnormality in the Vestibular (Balance) System
Tai Chi Chih and Varicella Zoster Immunity

Qigong
Qigong Therapy for Heart Device Patients
Chinese Exercise Modalities in Parkinson's Disease

HIV, Human immunodeficiency virus; *NCCAM,* National Center for Complementary and Alternative Medicine.

Research on the correlation between the force and waveforms of the radial artery and the diagnostic perceptions of clinicians and physical status of patients has long been pursued in China, the United States, Japan, and Korea (Broffman et al, 1986; Takashima, 1995; Zhu, 1991). Typically, this research depends on the use of pressure sensors that are pressed against the skin overlying the radial artery in a manner and location that replicates that of the finger position of the traditional clinician. Pulse patterns are recorded and correlated to observations made by the clinician in an effort to determine the physical features that must be present for a diagnostic perception. Preliminary results are intriguing, but methodological questions concerning population size and standardization of measurement remain.

Research concerning channels and acupuncture points has relied on a variety of techniques, including the measurement of electrical resistance, thermography, tracing of the pathways of injected radioisotopes, and dissection. Dissection has not produced particularly interesting results; the so-called Bong Han corpuscles, identified on dissection by Kim Bong Han in Korea, once were proposed as the anatomical basis of acupuncture points. These research findings have not been replicated, and although occasionally referred to in contemporary materials (Burton Goldberg Group, 1993), it generally is not perceived as credible.

More interesting are the discussions that propose or demonstrate an archaic or cellularly mediated signaling system that uses the bioelectrical properties of the body to propagate information. Early contributors in this area include Robert O. Becker, an orthopedist whose interest in the body's bioelectric properties and bone healing led him to explore the electrical properties of acupuncture points and channel pathways (Becker, 1985; Reichmanis et al, 1975). A component of this hypothesis is the measurable lowered electrical resistance of the skin at acupuncture points. This unusual electrical property is characteristic of many acupuncture points (Pomeranz, 1988).

Yoshio Manaka, a Japanese surgeon and acupuncturist, hypothesized the presence of an archaic signaling system he called the "X-signal system," based on information theory concepts of biological systems, texts such as the *Inner Classic* and *Classic of Difficult Issues,* and experimental observations in his acupuncture clinic (Manaka et al, 1994). Manaka's perspective grew out of exploration of both Chinese and Japanese needling methods and the use of the gentler needling techniques associated with the school of meridian therapy that arose in Japan.

In his extensive discussion of the biophysical basis of acupuncture phenomena, James Oschman observes that the solid-state phenomena and the piezoelectric properties of the body's connective tissues provide a potential structure and mechanism that would allow for the existence of a signaling system similar in role to the channels and points described in traditional literature (Oschman, 1993). Oschman goes on to explore a rich range of topics, including the measurable emission of electromagnetic fields from the hands of qigong practitioners (Seto et al, 1992). Recently, Helene Langevin's work on the relationship between connective tissue and acupuncture phenomena such as *de qi* has demonstrated a mechanism that may support some of the hypotheses advanced by Oschman (Langevin et al, 2002).

All these explorations are preliminary. Even when research has been carried out and replicated, as in the case of lowered electrical resistance over acupuncture points, continued exploration is needed. We are not likely to see a precise validation of the concepts of Chinese medicine in these areas, but rather to see a validation of the physiological basis for the existence of such concepts. The genius of Chinese medicine in these areas may lie in its ability to generalize about the manifestations of incredibly complex biological phenomena in an articulate and useful fashion. Given the preliminary findings on the possible nature of acupuncture points and channels, or on the variety of mechanisms that seem to be involved in acupuncture as a therapeutic phenomena, it seems increasingly likely that a concept such as "qi," or the therapeutic effects of an acupuncture point, must represent the action of many discrete and identifiable physiological processes. The likelihood is that aspects of these processes, observed as a whole, are the basis of the traditional concept.

MATERIA MEDICA AND TRADITIONAL PHARMACOLOGY

Investigations of materia medica and traditional pharmacology have been ongoing since the early part of the twentieth century, in both China and Japan. The quality of research work is generally high, and the availability of translated literature is comparatively extensive. This research can be divided into two areas of examination: the pharmacological properties of traditional materia medica and the clinical efficacy of traditional pharmacology. The first area does not differ from the typical concerns of pharmacological research. In vitro studies and exploration of traditional use can suggest the potential usefulness of certain substances. If one becomes aware of a substance that is alleged to have pharmacological properties, it is comparatively easy to conduct studies to assess the presence of these properties and to isolate apparently active compounds.

A famous case in point is the first herb listed in the Chinese materia medica: *herba ephedra,* known botanically as *Ephedra sinica* Stapf (ma huang). Herba ephedra is recorded in the *Divine Husbandman's Classic of Materia Medica.* Its chief active component was isolated in 1887 in Japan but remained largely unexplored for 35 years, until C.F. Schmidt and K.K. Chen began to explore its pharmacological effects at the Peking Union Medical College, where the department of pharmacology was beginning a systematic exploration of the Chinese materia medica (Chen, 1977).

These explorations revealed that ephedrine was a sympathomimetic with properties of epinephrine, causing an increase in blood pressure, vasoconstriction, and bronchodilation. Clinically, ephedrine had several distinct advantages over epinephrine; ephedrine could be used orally, had a long duration of action, and was less toxic. It also was found to be useful in the management of bronchial asthma and hay fever and to support the patient's vital signs during the administration of spinal anesthesia. In subsequent years it became possible to synthesize ephedrine. This product of the Chinese materia medica currently is found in a number of pharmaceuticals, including over-the-counter products such as Sudafed and Actifed.

Historically and clinically, herba ephedra has been applied in a similar fashion in Chinese medicine, except for spinal anesthesia. As mentioned earlier, it is a principal ingredient in the herbal formula ephedra decoction. This herb also figures prominently in formulas used to address presentations that relate to asthma and allergy. The study of herba ephedra represents an early and impressive example of pharmacological research in the Chinese materia medica. Other single herbs for which the traditional clinical applications are supported in recent clinical experimentation include *herba artemisiae* (*yin chen hao*) for hepatitis and *caulis mu tong* (*mu tong*) for urinary tract infections. Extensive compilations discussing identified active constituents, clinical studies, and toxicity of large numbers of substances have been prepared (Chang, 1986).

Explorations of traditional pharmacology are somewhat more complex, although they too are amenable to the methods of double blinding and placebo control that are critical to recognition in the biomedical world. However, given the breadth of possible substances that may be applied clinically (more than 5000) and the number of possible permutations for their combination in formulas, the scope of the inquiry becomes quite large. In addition, there is the question of whether to include the traditional considerations that surround diagnosis and pattern identification in the process of prescription and selection of herbal formulas for investigation. Some contemporary studies are designed to take this into account, with the traditional clinician being able to assign individuals to specific treatment groups on the basis of symptoms while still being blinded with regard to the actual constituents of the substances administered to the patients. A recent example of this approach can be seen in a randomized clinical trial of the use of Chinese herbal medicine for the treatment of irritable bowel syndrome conducted by Alan Bensoussan under the auspices of the Research Unit for Complementary Medicine at the University of Western Sydney. This study, in which patients were randomly assigned to one of three treatment groups—placebo, standard formula, and individualized formula—showed that Chinese herbal medicine provided significant reduction in the symptoms of irritable bowel syndrome (Bensoussan et al, 1998). Research in this area has been extensive in both China and Japan and is emerging in the United States.

ACUPUNCTURE

Research into the theoretical basis, safety, and therapeutic effects of acupuncture is discussed in Chapter 27.

QI CULTIVATION

Considerable numbers of intriguing studies of qi cultivation have been conducted in China, and the subject is beginning to be explored in the United States. Qi cultivation has been examined in relationship to an increase in immunocompetence, as measured by lymphocyte profiles (Ryu et al, 1995) and by changes in electroencephalographic patterns. Qi cultivation has been explored as a tool for managing gastritis, and numerous Chinese studies have suggested that it might be a promising method for treating hypertension.

Unfortunately, many of the problems that have confronted acupuncture research also surround research into qi cultivation. In addition, although there is great interest in qi cultivation in the West, there has not been the equivalent enthusiasm for resolving methodological problems and beginning to establish strong research initiatives.

Research into qi cultivation that investigates the role of the practice of qi cultivation exercises in the beneficial alteration of physiological processes is similar, in many respects, to the investigation of the effects of meditation, yoga, guided imagery, and what Benson termed the *relaxation response*. The challenge here is developing an effective control and ruling out other variables that may influence the results.

Attempts to examine the effects of externally transmitted qi have led to special problems. In some cases, as discussed earlier, it is believed that this phenomenon involves measurable portions of the electromagnetic spectrum. In cases in which investigators hypothesize qi as an existent, but presently unmeasurable, phenomenon, they seek to establish the presence and effect of externally transmitted qi by examining its apparent effects on other systems that can be directly observed.

Given the extensive range of phenomena under investigation and the range of claims for the healing potential of qi cultivation, there is a certain amount of skepticism about the field as a whole. Even in China there is some question as to whether qi cultivation should be established as a standard method of treatment within the corpus of Chinese medicine. There is also the belief that some of the practices associated with qi cultivation have the potential for abuse and charlatanism (Tang, 1994).

Qi cultivation remains a challenging part of the broad fabric of China's traditional medicine. Researchers within the field hope that over time it will be possible to increase the availability of well-designed and accessible studies in the field (Sancier, 1996).

Acknowledgments

As is apparent from the text, this presentation owes a heavy debt to the work of Paul Unschuld and Nigel Wiseman. The scholarship and enterprise of these two individuals is reflected in their work and the help that they have provided to students of Chinese medicine such as myself. Marnae Ergil, my wife and colleague, contributed enormously by reviewing text, answering questions, and being willing to check technical points in Chinese language materials at any hour of the day or night. This project would not have been possible without the institutional commitment to scholarship and the support provided by the Pacific College of Oriental Medicine, and later by Touro College.

⊖ Chapter References can be found on the Evolve website at http://evolve.elsevier.com/Micozzi/complementary/

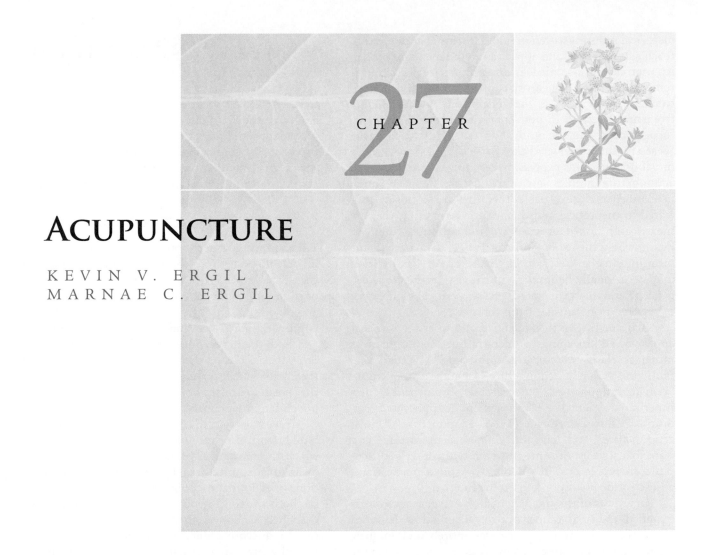

CHAPTER 27

ACUPUNCTURE

KEVIN V. ERGIL
MARNAE C. ERGIL

THE IDEA OF ACUPUNCTURE

Acupuncture, literally "sharp puncture," simultaneously invokes impressions of simplicity and complexity. A sharp object, a needle, is simple, whereas the body, its object, is complex. The surface of the body, when compared in area with the point of the needle, provides an almost limitless number of locations in which the needle might be inserted. The needle is "yang" in its sharp, metallic, focused, and intrusive form. The body is "yin," comparatively soft, organic, expansive, and complex.

Acupuncture, however, is not just about the yang and yin of a needle and a body, but rather the system of ideas, understood relationships, and practices that inform the clinician about where that needle, or needles, might be placed. How many, of what diameter and length, for how long, at what angle, with what movements, and with what intentions and intentionality? What other interventions might be applied to warm and/or stimulate the surface of the body? All these aspects, then, are part of acupuncture.

This chapter gives a detailed overview of acupuncture theory to provide the reader with a strong conceptual understanding of the fundamental ideas and practices from which acupuncture emerges. Particular attention is paid to the acupuncture channels and networks (meridians) themselves, the significance of which frequently goes unexplored even in many of the popular contemporary acupuncture texts. Models for acupuncture point selection and the use of associated techniques are discussed. The way in which these models inform the diverse traditions in acupuncture is explored, and, finally, acupuncture research and the relationship (or the lack of one) between this research and acupuncture theory are examined.

This chapter is designed to be read after finishing Chapter 26, Chinese Medicine. Many of the ideas developed in the following discussion rely on or refer to concepts already presented in that chapter. Although certain points are amplified here, the reader should be familiar with the basic concepts discussed in that chapter, such as historical developments in Chinese medicine, important text sources, the idea of yin and yang, the five phases, the six evils, the viscera and bowels, and disease causation.

The word *acupuncture* has attained a meaning in the West that allows the term to float free of its cultural and historical moorings, even in popular texts that purport to teach acupuncture, and appear as an independent modality that can be qualified in any number of ways and is removed from its obligatory context. The first decontextualizing movement is the separation of acupuncture from moxibustion. In both ancient and modern China, "acupuncture," in the sense that the term is used in the West, is actually known as *zhen jiu* (针灸), meaning "needle moxibustion." This expression recognizes that, although acupuncture needles and moxibustion floss are often used independently of each other, they are so closely associated in theoretical and therapeutic terms that they are inextricably linked. A similar construction is found in Japan, where the expression *shin kyu* (针灸) has the same meaning. In the West, although the use of moxibustion may occasionally be implicit in the use of the term *acupuncture,* it remains unstated, and so a critical component of the tradition vanishes from view.

"Acupuncture" is then qualified in a variety of ways that appear to add meaning to the term but often obscure as much as clarify. "Medical acupuncture," "Western acupuncture," "Chinese acupuncture," Japanese acupuncture," "Korean acupuncture," "Vietnamese acupuncture," "new American acupuncture," "five-element acupuncture," "traditional Chinese medicine (TCM) acupuncture," "Taoist acupuncture," and "classical Chinese acupuncture" is a nonexhaustive list of some common types or styles of acupuncture represented in schools, workshops, publications, and scientific literature, and on the Internet.

Regardless of the way in which the term *acupuncture* is qualified, the basic framework for all practices described under these varying rubrics derives entirely and uniquely from acupuncture principles and concepts described in the great classics of Chinese medicine— the *Yellow Emperor's Inner Classic (Huang Di Nei Jing)* comprising the *Spiritual Axis (Ling Shu)* and *Simple Questions (Su Wen),* ca. 200 to 100 BC; the *Classic of Difficult Issues (Nan Jing)* ca. AD 200; and the *Systematic Classic of Acupuncture and Moxibustion (Zhen Jiu Jia Yi Jing),* AD 282—and from later books based on these, such as the *Great Compendium of Acupuncture and Moxibustion (Zhen Jiu Da Cheng).*

This chapter expands the exploration of acupuncture concepts begun in Chapter 26 to provide a detailed foundation of the core acupuncture concepts that form the basis for all contemporary acupuncture traditions or practice styles. Later in this chapter these various types or traditions of acupuncture are examined in greater detail. At this point, however, it is important to establish what might be termed the common conceptual sources of acupuncture (or acupuncture and moxibustion) theory and practice. These are ideas that, except for minor refinements, represent the core of acupuncture theory that was well established in China by the third century AD and have continued to provide the basis of theoretical elaboration and incremental development through to modern times. Although there are many innovative approaches to acupuncture therapeutics, all innovation and all traditions, as we shall see, can be and ideally should be understood in reference to this conceptual core.

CORE ACUPUNCTURE THEORY AND PRACTICE

Core acupuncture theory is based on the principles of yin and yang; the five phases; the vital substances of the body (qi, blood, and fluids); the viscera and bowels, which act to produce, distribute, and store these vital substances; and the channels and networks that permit the flow and distribution of these substances throughout the body.

CHANNEL AND NETWORK THEORY

The channels and networks are the pathways that carry qi, blood, and body fluids throughout the body, including to the surface and to the internal organs. They are the paths of communication between all parts of the body. When qi and blood flow through the channels smoothly, the body is properly nourished and healthy. The organs, the skin and body hair, the sinews and flesh, the bones, and all other tissues rely on the free flow of qi and blood through the channels. Ultimately, it is the channels and networks that create a unified body in which all parts are interacting and interdependent.

As we have seen in Chapter 26, the channels appear to have historical primacy over the points or holes through which the movement of qi and blood is manipulated by means of acupuncture and other techniques. Clear descriptions of acupuncture points appear well after the ancient methods of stimulating channels with heat or stones are described. Channels, then, are equivalent in importance to acupuncture points in acupuncture theory and are typically presented first in standard acupuncture texts. Although acupuncture points often seem to be the primary object of therapy (and can be the subject of intense care in the process of point location in which palpation, anatomical location, and measurement are used to establish a point for treatment), the channels are the basis for all relations among points and body regions.

Functions of the Channel and Network System

There are five major functions of the channel and network system: transporting, regulating, protective and diagnostic, therapeutic, and integrating (Table 27-1). These functions inform clinical practice. For example, when an evil invades the exterior of the body, it first enters the skin and body hair. If not expelled it may enter various levels of the channels or network vessels. Eventually it may even reach the internal organs. Understanding the path that an evil may take into the body helps the clinician to assess where the evil is and how best to treat it. Similarly, the channels can reflect the relative vacuity of the body's correct qi or the replete condition of an organ or body region due to illness. By observing changes to the channels and their nature and location, by palpating the channels, and by understanding channel relationships the clinician can choose appropriate points to use to treat the condition.

TABLE 27-1

Functions of the Channel System

Function	Clinical relevance of channel system function
Transportation	The channel system encompasses all of the pathways for the circulation of qi and blood throughout the body, thus providing qi and blood to all of the organs and tissues for nourishment and moistening.
Regulation	The channel system maintains the flow of qi and blood through the pathways, which then maintains the balance of yin and yang to regulate the functions of the organs.
Protection and diagnosis	The channel system protects the body against the invasion of evils. If evils invade or are internally generated, then the channel system reflects the signs and symptoms of the disease. This might include observable signs such as color change, rashes, and so forth; palpable signs such as changes in resistance, lumps, and so forth; or subjective changes such as pain, numbness, and so forth, along a pathway.
Therapy	The signs and symptoms of disease are reflected in the channel (diagnosis), and then treatment is based on the selection of points along the channels that have a direct impact on the affected organ systems.
Integration	The channel system connects the viscera and bowels with each other and with the limbs and body surface. It also connects the internal and external parts of the body, including the organs of the five senses, tissues, bone, sinew, muscle, and orifices.

Structure of the Channel and Network System

The pathways through which qi and blood flow are divided into two types: the channels and the networks. The channels are bilateral and symmetrical; they travel vertically through the body and are relatively deep within the body. The networks are branches of the channels. They connect interiorly-exteriorly related organs, and they connect channels. The networks are also bilateral and symmetrical, but they travel in all directions, and relative to the channels, they are more superficial.

The Twelve Regular Channels

The 12 regular channels are the most well-known and frequently discussed channels. They contain the preponderance of acupuncture points that are located on channels, and each corresponds to one of the 12 organs of Chinese medicine. They are best known by their surface pathways.

Distribution and nomenclature. There are six yang and six yin channels, which are distributed bilaterally on the body. The yin channels run along the inner surface of the limbs (three on the arms and three on the legs) and across the chest and abdomen. Each yin channel is associated with specific viscera. With the exception of the stomach channel, the yang channels run along the outer surfaces of the limbs (three on the arms and three on the legs) and along the buttocks and back. Each yang channel is associated with a specific bowel.

Within the classification of yin and yang, the channels are further divided based on their relative location on the anterior, midline, or posterior aspect of the limb. The yin channels include the greater yin, located on the anterior, medial aspect of the limbs; the lesser yin, located on the posterior, medial aspect of the limbs; and the reverting yin, located on the midline of the medial aspect of the

limbs. The yang channels include the yang brightness, located on the anterior lateral aspect of the limbs; the greater yang, located on the posterior lateral aspect of the limbs; and the lesser yang, located on the midline of the lateral aspect of the limbs.

The name of each of the channels is based on three features: (1) the distribution of the channel along either the upper limbs (the hand channels) or the lower limbs (the foot channels), (2) the yin-yang classification of the channel, and (3) the organ with which the channel is directly associated. Thus, the channel associated with the lung is referred to as the hand greater yin lung channel, because it runs from the interior of the abdomen out to the tip of the thumb, it runs along the anterior medial aspect of the arm, and it is directly associated with the lung.

The flow of qi in the twelve regular channels. In addition to being directly associated with one of the internal organs, each of the six yin channels is paired with its interiorly-exteriorly related yang channel. This pairing expresses an important physiological connection between the associated viscera and bowel and an anatomical relation between the channels. In addition, each hand channel is associated with a foot channel based on its yin-yang classification and location.

These two ways of pairing the channels are expressed in three circuits of the flow of qi through the 12 regular channels. The flow of qi in each circuit begins in a yin channel on the chest and passes to the interiorly-exteriorly related yang channel at the hand. It then ascends along the yang channel to the face, where it passes into the hand yang channel's paired foot yang channel. It then descends to the foot, where it passes to the interiorly-exteriorly related yin channel and ascends back to the chest to begin a new circuit. Thus, the qi passes from the chest to the hand to the face to the foot and back to the chest three times, traversing a complete circuit through the body and covering both the yin (anterior) and yang (posterior) aspects of the body before it completes its circuit of the 12 channels (Figure 27-1).

The directionality of qi flow is often exploited by means of specialized needling techniques. To drain qi and so to reduce activity in a channel, the direction of the flow is opposed. To strengthen or supplement the qi in a channel or organ, the needle can be oriented in the direction of flow (Table 27-2).

The three hand yang and three foot yang channels all meet in the head. The head is the most yang aspect of the body. Many of the diseases that manifest in the head, certain types of headache, acne, and so on, are caused by repletion yang qi. Because yang is active and upbearing, the repletion will often rise via the yang channels to the head. Treatment entails downbearing the yang qi and draining the repletion. Often

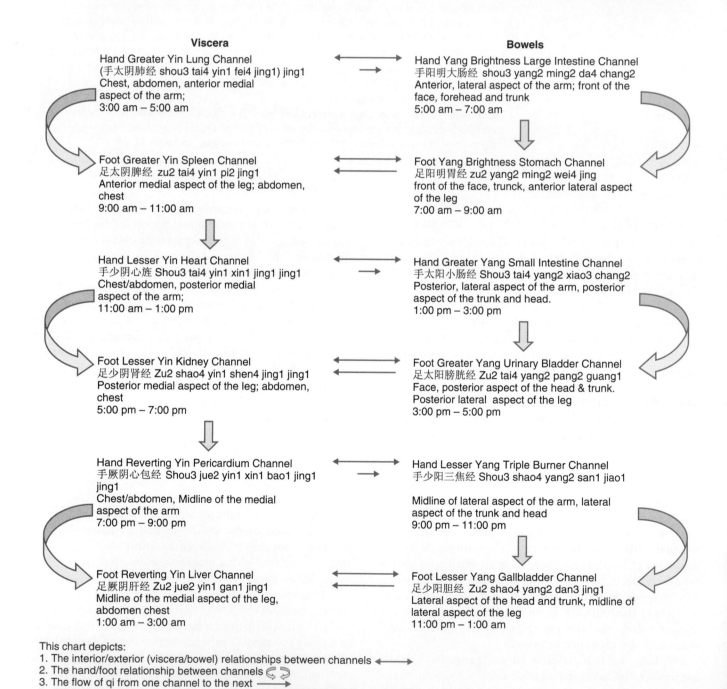

Viscera

Hand Greater Yin Lung Channel
(手太阴肺经) (shou3 tai4 yin1 fei4 jing1) jing1
Chest, abdomen, anterior medial
aspect of the arm;
3:00 am – 5:00 am

Foot Greater Yin Spleen Channel
足太阴脾经 zu2 tai4 yin1 pi2 jing1
Anterior medial aspect of the leg; abdomen,
chest
9:00 am – 11:00 am

Hand Lesser Yin Heart Channel
手少阴心旌 Shou3 tai4 yin1 xin1 jing1 jing1
Chest/abdomen, posterior medial
aspect of the arm;
11:00 am – 1:00 pm

Foot Lesser Yin Kidney Channel
足少阴肾经 Zu2 shao4 yin1 shen4 jing1 jing1
Posterior medial aspect of the leg; abdomen,
chest
5:00 pm – 7:00 pm

Hand Reverting Yin Pericardium Channel
手厥阴心包经 Shou3 jue2 yin1 xin1 bao1 jing1
jing1
Chest/abdomen, Midline of the medial
aspect of the arm
7:00 pm – 9:00 pm

Foot Reverting Yin Liver Channel
足厥阴肝经 Zu2 jue2 yin1 gan1 jing1
Midline of the medial aspect of the leg,
abdomen chest
1:00 am – 3:00 am

Bowels

Hand Yang Brightness Large Intestine Channel
手阳明大肠经 shou3 yang2 ming2 da4 chang2
Anterior, lateral aspect of the arm; front of the
face, forehead and trunk
5:00 am – 7:00 am

Foot Yang Brightness Stomach Channel
足阳明胃经 zu2 yang2 ming2 wei4 jing
front of the face, trunck, anterior lateral aspect
of the leg
7:00 am – 9:00 am

Hand Greater Yang Small Intestine Channel
手太阳小肠经 Shou3 tai4 yang2 xiao3 chang2
Posterior, lateral aspect of the arm, posterior
aspect of the trunk and head.
1:00 pm – 3:00 pm

Foot Greater Yang Urinary Bladder Channel
足太阳膀胱经 Zu2 tai4 yang2 pang2 guang1
Face, posterior aspect of the head & trunk.
Posterior lateral aspect of the leg
3:00 pm – 5:00 pm

Hand Lesser Yang Triple Burner Channel
手少阳三焦经 Shou3 shao4 yang2 san1 jiao1

Midline of lateral aspect of the arm, lateral
aspect of the trunk and head
9:00 pm – 11:00 pm

Foot Lesser Yang Gallbladder Channel
足少阳胆经 Zu2 shao4 yang2 dan3 jing1
Lateral aspect of the head and trunk, midline of
lateral aspect of the leg
11:00 pm – 1:00 am

This chart depicts:
1. The interior/exterior (viscera/bowel) relationships between channels ⟷
2. The hand/foot relationship between channels ⟳⟲
3. The flow of qi from one channel to the next ⟶
4. The 3 loops of the body (chest – hand – face – abdomen) that the qi completes in one day
5. The relative location of each channel on the limbs of the body
6. The time of day during which the qi is said to pass through each channel

Figure 27-1 Flow in channels and organs. (Courtesy Marnae Ergil.)

TABLE 27-2

Direction of Qi Flow in the Twelve Regular Channels

The three yin channels of the hand (LU, HT, PC) start in the chest and run along the medial aspect of the arms to the hands, where they meet and join their internally-externally paired yang channel. For example, the hand greater yin lung channel meets the hand yang brightness large intestine channel on the hand.

The three yang channels of the hand (LI, SI, SJ) start on the hands and run along the lateral aspect of the arms to the head and face, where they meet their paired foot yang channel. For example, the hand yang brightness large intestine channel meets the foot yang brightness stomach channel on the face.

The three yang channels of the feet (ST, BL, GB) start from the head and face and descend to the feet to meet their internally-externally paired yin channels. For example, the foot greater yang stomach channel meets the foot greater yin spleen channel on the foot.

The three yin channels of the feet (SP, KI, LR) start at the toes and ascend to the abdomen or chest to meet the three yin channels of the of the hands. For example, the foot greater yin spleen channel ascends to the abdomen, where it meets the hand lesser yin heart channel.

In each channel, the qi is said to flow in a particular direction.

BL, Bladder; GB, gallbladder; HT, heart; KI, kidney; LI, large intestine; LR, liver; LU, lung; PC, pericardium; SI, small intestine; SJ, triple burner (san jiao); SP, spleen; ST, stomach.

points located on the ends of the hands and feet will be used to drain the repletion down and out of the head.

The three hand yin and the three foot yin channels all meet in the chest and abdomen. The chest and abdomen are the place where all of the organs of the body reside.

The yin and yang channels of the hand meet on the hands.

The yin and yang channels of the feet meet on the feet. ∾

Qi and blood circulate through the body via the channels ceaselessly, from one channel to the next. Before returning to the beginning of the circuit, the qi and blood passes through the body in three loops. Over the course of one 24-hour period, the qi and blood in the channels pass through the entire body in the following sequence:

$$LU \rightarrow LI \rightarrow ST \rightarrow SP \rightarrow HT \rightarrow SI \rightarrow UB \rightarrow KI$$
$$\rightarrow PC \rightarrow SJ \rightarrow GB \rightarrow LR$$

where *LU* = lung; *LI* = large intestine; *ST* = stomach; *SP* = spleen; *HT* = heart; *SI* = small intestine; *UB* = urinary bladder; *KI* = kidney; *PC* = pericardium; *SJ* = triple burner (san jiao); *GB* = gallbladder; and *LR* = liver.

The flow of qi is cyclic. At any given time of day, as determined by ancient Chinese time-measuring methods of 2-hour increments, the flow of qi will be strongest in one specific organ. This idea can be used in both diagnosis and treatment. In the course of 1 day, the strength of qi will pass one time through each of the 12 channels. When the qi is passing through a given channel, the organ associated with that channel is considered to be at its strongest. The qi of the organ associated with the channel on the opposite side of the diurnal clock is considered to be

at its weakest. Thus, from 3:00 AM to 5:00 AM, the qi of the lung is at its strongest and the qi of the urinary bladder is at its weakest.

Clinically, this information might be applied in several ways. For example, if an asthmatic patient consistently wakes between 3:00 and 5:00 in the morning with an asthmatic attack, one might think that the qi of the lung, which should be especially strong at this time, is instead exceptionally weak, which creates a circumstance in which the patient cannot breathe easily and other organs, the liver in particular, take advantage of this weakness and overwhelm the lung, causing an asthmatic attack. Or, if an elderly person wakes between 5:00 and 7:00 in the morning with an immediate need to move the bowels, one might suspect that the qi of the large intestine (5:00 to 7:00 AM) is weak and the qi of the kidney (5:00 to 7:00 PM), which is responsible for securing the loss of substances from the body, is also weak and unable to restrain the large intestine.

Pathology and treatment of the twelve regular channels. Each of the channels has its own pathological symptoms and signs that guide the practitioner in determining a diagnosis and in choosing points for treatment. Pathology that is specific to the channel may present as pain, tension, rashes, and so on that manifest along a specific channel pathway. For example, a patient who has shoulder and arm pain that covers the posterior portion of the shoulder, crosses over the scapula and trapezius muscle, and goes down the posterior aspect of the arm might be diagnosed with stagnation of qi and blood in the small intestine channel, which engenders pain.

Because the internal pathways of the channels connect directly to the associated organs, channel pathology may also be a reflection of organ pathology. For example, a patient who experiences constipation might also experience shoulder and neck pain along the pathway of the large intestine. Although the patient may not make the connection, through inquiry, a good diagnostician might learn that when the bowels move, the pain diminishes and both the pain and the constipation improve when there is less stress. Often, the patient will complain only of the shoulder pain and then be pleasantly surprised when both the shoulder pain and the constipation clear up. Thus, when discussing channel pathology we refer not only to what is visible or what is manifesting along the exterior portion of the pathway, but also to the internal pathway and its organ connections (Table 27-3).

The internal branches always need to be considered when inquiring about symptomatology and when coming to a diagnostic conclusion. For example, an internal branch of the foot greater yin spleen channel travels to the bottom of the tongue and spreads over the bottom of the

TABLE 27-3

Signs of the External and Internal Pathways of the Channels

Channel	External channel pathway signs	Internal channel pathway signs
Lung	Heat effusion and aversion to cold, nasal congestion, headache, pain along the channel pathway	Cough, panting, wheezing, rapid breathing, fullness in the chest, expectoration of phlegm, dry throat, change in urine color
Large intestine	Heat effusion, parched mouth, thirst, sore throat, nosebleed, toothache, swelling of the neck, pain along the channel pathway	Lower abdominal pain, wandering abdominal pain, rumbling intestines, sloppy stool, and excretion of thick, slimy yellow matter
Stomach	High fever, red face, sweating, delirium, manic agitation, pain in the eyes, dry nose, nosebleed, lip and mouth sores, deviated mouth, pain along the channel pathway	Abdominal distention and fullness, water swelling, vexation and discomfort while active or recumbent, mania and withdrawal, swift digestion and rapid hungering, yellow urine
Spleen	Heaviness in the head or body, weak limbs, motor impairment of the tongue, cold along the inside of the thigh and knee, swelling of the legs and feet	Pain in the stomach duct, sloppy diarrhea, stool containing untransformed food, rumbling intestines, nausea, reduced foot intake, jaundice
Heart	Headache, eye pain, pain in the chest and back muscles, dry throat, thirst with desire to drink, hot or painful palms, pain in the scapular region and/or the medial aspect of the forearm	Heart pain, fullness and pain in the chest, pain in the hypochondriac region, heat vexation, rapid breathing, discomfort in the lying posture, dizziness with fainting spells, mental diseases
Small intestine	Erosion of the glossal and oral mucosa, pain in the cheeks, tearing, pain along the channel pathway	Lower abdominal pain and distention with the pain stretching around to the lumbus or into the testicles, diarrhea, stomach pain with dry feces
Urinary bladder	Heat effusion and aversion to cold, headache, stiff neck, pain in the lumbar spine, eye pain and tearing, pain along the channel pathway	Lower abdominal pain and distention, inhibited urination, urinary block, enuresis, mental disorders, arched-back rigidity
Kidney	Lumbar pain, weak legs, dry mouth, pain along the channel pathway	Dizziness, facial swelling, blurred vision, gray facial complexion, shortness of breath, enduring diarrhea, sloppy stool, dry stool, impotence
Pericardium	Stiffness of the neck, spasm in the limbs, red complexion, pain in the eyes, pain along the channel pathway	Delirious speech, heat vexation, fullness and oppression in the chest and rib-side, heart palpitations, heart pain, constant laughing
Triple burner	Sore throat, pain in the cheeks, red painful eyes, deafness, pain behind the ears and along the channel pathway	Abdominal distention and fullness, hardness and fullness in the lower abdomen, urinary frequency, enuresis, edema
Gallbladder	Alternating heat effusion and aversion to cold, headache, malaria, eye pain, deafness, pain along the channel pathway	Rib-side pain, vomiting, bitter taste in the mouth, chest pain
Liver	Headache, dizziness, blurred vision, tinnitus, heat effusion	Fullness, distention, and pain in the rib side; fullness and oppression in the chest; abdominal pain; vomiting; jaundice; mounting qi; enuresis; urinary block; yellow urine

tongue. Thus, when the tongue is examined, if the bottom is especially pale, one might consider the possibility of blood vacuity as a result of dysfunction of the spleen in producing blood. An internal branch of the liver channel travels up to the tissues surrounding the eyes and to the vertex of the head. Clinically, symptoms such as vertex headaches might be indicative of repletion of yang qi in the liver channel. All of the 12 regular channels have several of these internal pathways, along which there are no specific points that can be accessed but which must be considered in relation to diagnosis and treatment.

In addition to the 12 regular channel pathways, there are four additional types of channels that are directly associated with the 12 regular channels and similarly named. These are the 12 cutaneous regions, the 12 sinew channels, and the 12 divergent channels.

The Twelve Cutaneous Regions

The 12 cutaneous regions are the most superficial of the channel pathways and divide the surface of the body into 12 segments. Their distribution follows the course of the regular channels; however, their pathway is distributed entirely over the body surface. They do not distribute interiorly, and they have no starting or terminating points and no directional flow. These are very broad pathways that cover a much larger area than any of the other channel pathways.

The cutaneous regions function to circulate defense qi and blood to the body surface, regulate the function of the skin and pores, and strengthen the body's resistance to disease and injury. All of these functions are related to the functions of the lung system. Thus, if the lung system is functioning well, then the cutaneous regions are well nourished, and there is sufficient defense qi on the surface of the body to keep the pores regulated and prevent the loss of qi through sweat or the invasion of an evil into the body.

Although specific descriptions of pathology of the 12 cutaneous regions do not exist, clinically skin disorders (rashes, discolorations, growths) may indicate a disorder of the related regular channel or organ. Channel obstruction manifesting as specific pain conditions can also show signs in the cutaneous regions. In addition, a patient who is susceptible to colds or who feels easily chilled on the exterior of the body might be showing signs of an insufficiency of defense qi circulating in the cutaneous regions.

The cutaneous regions also remind us that, although there is better or worse channel stimulation and more and less accurate point location, no place exists on the body at which a needle is not providing some degree of stimulation to associated organs or channels. Acupuncture points may be very specific in their locations, but the body as described by classical acupuncture theory is not a switchboard or a wiring diagram. Specificity in location of points is necessary when needling so as to obtain qi in the regular channel. But a stimulus can still be provided to the channel even when the site of stimulation is not exact. Thus, several techniques have been developed to treat the cutaneous channels and to stimulate broader areas. Some of these are gua sha, plum blossom or seven-star needling, moxibustion, cupping, shiatsu, and tui na. In addition, opinions about point location may vary.

The Twelve Sinew Channels

The sinew channels are also relatively superficial channels, although somewhat deeper than the cutaneous regions. They follow approximately the same pathways as the regular channels with which they share their names; however, they do not travel internally at all. They are called "sinew channels" because they travel across the sinews, which include what we refer to as muscles, tendons, and ligaments. The sinew channels all branch off from the regular channels at the tips of the fingers or toes, then travel upward and inward across the body.

As surface channels, the sinew channels are said to contain only defense qi, and thus, like the cutaneous regions, they defend the body against the invasion of evils. If the defense qi in the sinew channels is overcome by the invasion of evil qi from the exterior, it may travel down the sinew channel to the tips of the fingers, where the sinew channels meet the regular channels, and from there enter the regular channels and travel internally.

For example, often when one is first catching a cold, one might experience pain, stiffness, or discomfort in the neck and shoulders. This muscular discomfort is indicative of the presence of a cold evil lodged in the sinew channels of the urinary bladder and small intestine channels. The presence of this evil may simply lead to a common cold. However, if the evil is able to invade into the urinary bladder or small intestine regular channel, and from there progress to the organ, then, in addition to the cold, the patient may develop signs such as scanty, dark urine and short or even painful urination: signs of a urinary tract infection. Thus, it is always best to treat signs of dysfunction in the sinew channels early, before the dysfunction progresses to more serious or complicated conditions.

In addition, the sinew channels supplement the regular channels by emphasizing the circulation of qi and blood to the muscles, tissues, joints, and body surface. They connect the muscles, tendons, and ligaments to the joints; link the structures of the body; and facilitate articulation and normal movement as well as protecting the bones.

The 12 sinew channels may reflect symptomatology of their associated organs, but in general, pathology in these channels will manifest as impediment patterns (associated with pain from obstruction of qi and blood and seen in conditions such as osteoarthritis), trauma, muscle strain due to overuse, or muscle tension and contraction, which may be caused by long-standing emotional or physical stressors. The primary symptom of all of these pathologies is pain. Whether the condition is replete or vacuous is determined by the presentation. Repletion conditions present with muscle spasms or contracture, edema, inflammation, and relatively sharp or severe pain, especially with light pressure. Vacuity conditions manifest with atony, dull pain or numbness that is often very deep and elicited with deep pressure, a lack of skin tone, poor motor control, and paleness or coldness of the skin.

Because the 12 sinew channels do not have their own points, it is necessary to use points on the associated regular channel or to think about other types of points. *Ah shi* ("That's it!") points are frequently needled to release the stagnation of qi and blood in the sinew channels. Ah shi points are essentially points that are tender and painful to the touch and are located by palpation. In addition to being clearly sensitive to the patient when palpated, these points are also identifiable to the practitioner by their distinct qualities (tension, stiffness, contraction) on palpation. Ah shi points may be located on or off the regular channels and are frequently found some distance from established acupuncture points. The concept of a "trigger point" used in the West since the 1960s has a great deal of similarity to the ah shi point, which formally emerged in Chinese medical thought around the seventh century AD. Cutaneous stimulation is also useful. The points located on the tips of the fingers and toes (the well points) as well as other points that are local, adjacent, and distal to the site of pain may be used. To effectively course a sinew channel, one might choose to use the first and last points on the associated regular channel pathways along with other points.

The Twelve Channel Divergences

Channel divergences is a general term for 12 major branches of the 12 regular channels. These channels are distributed inside the body and have no points of their own. They are called "divergences" because they break off or diverge from the regular pathway and conduct qi and blood to different areas of the body. These channels make important internal linkages that may not be made by the primary channels and so serve to explain the actions and indications of many of the channel points.

The 12 divergent channels separate from the regular channel at a relatively superficial level of the body, usually at a spot near the elbow or knee joints. The yin and yang internally-externally related pair then merge together and enter the chest and abdomen to travel to the viscera and bowels. Together, they emerge from the body cavity at the neck or head, and finally merge with the regular yang channel of a yin-yang pair.

Like the sinew channels, the divergent channels run from the extremities to the trunk, face, and head, with the exception of the triple burner divergent channel, which runs from the vertex of the head down the body to the middle burner. Like the cutaneous and sinew channels, the 12 divergent channels contain only defense qi.

The divergent channels have three major functions: (1) they supply defense qi to the viscera and bowels, and act as a secondary line of defense against the invasion of evil; (2) they strengthen the connection between organs and channels; and (3) they integrate areas of the body that are not covered by the main pathways.

Although the divergent channels are mentioned in the *Inner Classic,* there is no clear description of divergent channel pathology. Generally, the divergent channels are thought to share the same pathologies as the regular channels. However, when disease has entered the divergent channels, the symptoms produced are often intermittent or cyclic and one-sided. Divergent channel symptoms are produced by the pathogen's encounter with the defense qi, and thus as the defense qi waxes and wanes in flow, there will be an exacerbation or amelioration of symptoms. The point where the divergent channels separate from the regular channel and the point where they merge with the regular yang channel are the most important points for treatment of divergent channel pathology (Table 27-4).

The Eight Extraordinary Vessels

Although often discussed as an entirely different category of channels, the eight extraordinary vessels actually are a part of the general channel system. They are "extraordinary" because they do not fit the pattern of the other major channels. There are two primary differences between the eight extraordinary vessels and the 12 regular channels:

1. The eight extraordinary vessels do not have a continuous, interlinking pattern of circulation. In other words, although they have connections with each other and with the 12 major channels, they do not link one to the next as do the 12 regular channels.
2. The eight extraordinary vessels are not each associated with a specific organ system as are the 12 regular channels. Rather, the eight extraordinary vessels are associated with specific types of disorders based on their location and functions.

The eight extraordinary vessels function as reservoirs of qi and blood. They fill and empty in response to changing conditions and pathologies of the regular channels or of the organ systems, and they exert a regulating effect on the regular channels. All of the eight extraordinary vessels are considered to be very closely related to the functions of the liver and kidney systems and also to the functioning of the uterus and the brain (Table 27-5).

The basic functions of the eight extraordinary vessels are as follows:

To provide additional interconnections among the major channels and the organ systems.

To regulate the flow of qi and blood in the regular channels. Surplus qi or blood from the regular channels may be stored in the eight extraordinary vessels and released when required.

TABLE 27-4

Comparison of the Various Parts of the Channel System

	12 Regular channels	12 Cutaneous regions	12 Sinew channels	12 Divergent channels
Pathways	Bilateral Internal and external pathways Have points to access qi	Bilateral Mostly superficial Divide the body into 12 broad regions	Bilateral Superficial, follow the regular channels but broader, cover muscle areas	Bilateral Travel from the limbs to the interior of the body and the head
Flow of qi	From chest to hand, hand to head, head to foot, foot to abdomen/chest	Nondirectional	From tips of fingers/toes inward along regular channel pathway	From elbows/knees, internally and then up to head
Functions	Transport Regulate Protect and aid diagnosis Treat Integrate	Circulate defense qi and blood to the body surface Regulate the function of the skin and pores Strengthen immunity	Defend the body against evils Supplement the regular channels' circulation of qi and blood to the muscles, tissues, joints, and body surface	Supply defense qi to the viscera and bowels Act as a secondary line of defense against the invasion of evil Strengthen the connection channels and organs Integrate areas of the body that are not covered by the main pathways
Pathology	Varied	Skin disorders (rashes, discolorations, growths	Pain Symptoms reflecting symptomatology of associated organ	No clear description of pathology; symptoms are often intermittent or cyclic and one-sided
Treatment	Acupuncture points	Gua sha, plum blossom or seven-star needling, moxibustion, cupping, shiatsu, tui na	Ah shi ("That's It!") points Cutaneous stimulation First and last channel points	Regular channel points Diverging and merging points

Like the regular channels, each of the eight extraordinary vessels has its own distinct pathway. However, only two of the eight extraordinary vessels (the controlling vessel and the governing vessel) have acupuncture points. These two channels traverse the midline of the body, and the functions of their points are often associated with the functions of the organs lying in proximity to them.

Not only are specific points located on the controlling and governing vessels, but all of the eight extraordinary vessels are closely associated with a specific point on one of the 12 regular channels. This point, called a "confluent point," is used to access the qi and blood of the extraordinary vessel and make it available for use by the organ systems. Clinically, each of the eight extraordinary vessels is paired with another, which makes four couplets. Typically, when the confluent point on one channel is used, the confluent point of its paired channel is also used.

The Network Vessels

As discussed earlier, there are two types of major pathways in the body. All of the various types of channels have already been reviewed. The other major pathways are the network vessels. These are branches of the channels; however, they also have their own functions and pathologies. They connect interiorly-exteriorly related organs and they connect channels. Like the regular channels, the network vessels are bilateral and symmetrical, but they travel in all directions and are relatively superficial. As a general function, with the rest of the channel system, the network vessels form a network of pathways that integrate the entire body and distribute qi and blood, especially to the surface of the body.

There are two types of network vessels: (1) the network divergences, and (2) the superficial network vessels, also called the "grandchild network vessels" or the "blood network vessels." The network divergences can also be divided into two subcategories, the transverse network vessels,

TABLE 27-5

Eight Extraordinary Vessels

Extraordinary vessel	Functions of the extraordinary vessel	Common clinical conditions indicating disharmony of the extraordinary vessel
Governing Vessel Confluent point: SI3 Paired vessel: yang springing	Sea of the yang channels Regulates all yang channels Sea of marrow Homes to the brain Reflects physiology and pathology of the brain and the spinal fluid	Pain and stiffness in the back, heavy-headedness, hemorrhoids, infertility, malaria, mental disorders Points along the channel influence areas and organs of the body located near the point.
Controlling Vessel Confluent point: LU7 Paired vessel: yin springing	Sea of yin channels Regulates all yin channels Regulates menstruation and nurtures the fetus	Menstrual irregularities, menstrual block, miscarriage, infertility, enuresis, abdominal masses Points along the channel influence areas and organs of the body located near the point.
Penetrating Vessel Confluent point: SP4 Paired vessel: yin linking	Sea of the regular channels Regulates the 12 regular channels Sea of blood Regulates menstruation	Women: Uterine bleeding, miscarriage, menstrual block, menstrual irregularities, scant breast milk, lower abdominal pain, facial hair Men: seminal emission, impotence, prostatitis, urethritis, orchitis
Girdling Vessel Confluent point: GB41 Paired vessel: yang linking	Binds all the channels running up and down the trunk Regulates the balance between upward and downward flow of qi Wraps around the body; the only channel to not travel vertically up and down the body	Vaginal discharge, prolapse of the uterus, abdominal distention and fullness, limpness, weakness or pain in the low back
Yang Springing Vessel Confluent point: UB62 Paired vessel: governing	Control opening and closing of the eyes Control the ascent of fluids and the descent of qi Balance the yin and yang qi of the body Balance gait and movement of the legs	Eye problems, insomnia, muscle spasms along the lateral aspect of the lower leg with flaccidity on the medial aspect
Yin Springing Vessel Confluent point: KI6 Paired channel: controlling	Control opening and closing of the eyes Control the ascent of fluids and the descent of qi Balance the yin and yang qi of the body Balance gait and movement of the legs	Eye problems, somnolence, lower abdominal or genital pain, muscle spasms along the medial aspect of the lower leg with flaccidity on the lateral aspect
Yang Linking Vessel Confluent point: SJ5 Paired channel: girdling	Unites all the major yang channels Compensates for superabundance or insufficiency in channel circulation Regulates yang channel activity Governs the exterior of the body	Exterior invasion, especially of heat
Yin Linking Vessel Confluent point: PC6 Paired channel: penetrating/chong	Unites all the major yin channels Regulates yin channel activity Governs the interior of the body Balances the emotions	Used for many different internal conditions

GB, Gallbladder; *KI*, kidney; *LU*, lung; *PC*, pericardium; *SI*, small intestine; *SJ*, triple burner (san jiao); *SP*, spleen; *UB*, urinary bladder.
Adapted from Ellis A, Wiseman N, Boss, K: *Fundamentals of Chinese acupuncture*, Brookline, Mass, 1991, Paradigm; Wiseman 1998; Ni 1996.

which connect an interiorly-exteriorly related channel pair, and the longitudinal network vessels, which separate from the regular channels and have their own specific symptomatology.

Network divergences. According to the *Inner Classic,* the transverse and longitudinal network vessels are one vessel with multiple pathways. However, their pathways are sufficiently distinct, and the functions and related symptomatologies different enough, that it is useful to separate them for discussion.

There are 12 transverse network vessels. These pathways are not definitively mapped, but they run from the connecting point on each channel to its interiorly-exteriorly related channel. Thus, the lung transverse network vessel breaks off from the lung connecting point and travels to the large intestine channel, and the large intestine transverse network point breaks off from the large intestine connecting point and travels to the lung channel. Clinically, through the use of these network vessels and the associated connecting and source points of the channels, the qi in a channel can be balanced or harmonized. Essentially, these rather short pathways serve as a direct connection between the yin and yang channels of an internally-externally related pair. This direct connection through the transverse network vessel strengthens the relationship between internally-externally related channels. Through a "source-connecting point" treatment, replete qi in one channel of a pair can be drained into the other, or a vacuity of qi in one channel of a pair can be supplemented through the use of the qi of its pair.

There are 16 longitudinal network divergences, one for each of the 12 regular channels, one for the governing vessel, and one for the controlling vessel, as well as the great network of the spleen and the great network of the stomach. As with the transverse network vessels, these vessels break off from the connecting points of their named channels. Often, acupuncturists will forget about or be unaware of the pathways or symptomatology of the longitudinal network divergences. However, awareness of these pathways and their associated symptoms can aid the acupuncturist is determining appropriate treatment. The longitudinal network divergences are treated using the connecting point of the affected channel.

Grandchild network vessels. The grandchild network vessels, also called the "superficial network vessels," are the small branches of the network divergences that appear on the surface of the skin. These are closely associated with minute blood vessels. Should these superficial network vessels change in color and become dark or stagnant, or should there be another need to treat them, a technique called "network vessel pricking" is used. In this method, a three-edged needle is used to prick the superficial network vessels and release blood.

Summing Up Channel Theory

If there is any single major misconception concerning acupuncture theory in the West, it is that acupuncture is primarily about the points, the location where a needle or other therapeutic tool is applied. Perhaps because they are the locus of therapeutic action, they figure prominently in the mind of the Westerner encountering acupuncture. Channels and networks are, however, the complex substrate that organizes and provides meaning to acupuncture points. As we have seen, channel theory is rich and complex, although very often completely ignored when the West encounters acupuncture. It may be that the early translation of the terms *channels* and *networks* as "meridians" and *holes* as "points" provided the sense that both were imaginary constructs inscribed on the surface of the body and, as such, only vague and imaginary markings engraved on an anatomically established body. However, channels and holes are tangible entities and the objects of vivid experience as documented in the classical texts of acupuncture. Although there is no reason to privilege them as a form of distinct or alternate anatomy, it is unwise, if we wish to understand acupuncture as an object of clinical and scientific inquiry, to ignore them as abstract fantasies.

The acupuncture point or hole is where the classics tell us we can touch the qi, blood, and spirit of the patient. Why and where we would wish to do this is guided entirely by channel theory and the characteristics of the holes themselves.

ACUPUNCTURE POINT CATEGORIES, GROUPINGS, AND ASSOCIATIONS

Just as the specific pathway of each of the channels and networks discussed earlier is well beyond the scope of this chapter, so is an exhaustive discussion of individual acupuncture points. There are some 361 acupuncture points associated with the 12 regular channels and the governing and controlling vessels. In addition there are numerous extra points, special reflex system points, and ah shi points. As we have discussed, an acupuncture point can best be considered as a hole where qi and blood can be manipulated in relation to a channel, organ, or body region. Historically the locations of acupuncture points have been described with varying degrees of precision and accuracy depending on the ease of fixing their locations by means of anatomical landmarks or measurement methods. Opinions about these have varied to some extent in the classics. Over the last half-century, efforts of the State Administration of Traditional Chinese Medicine in China, the World Health Organization (WHO), and other bodies have been devoted to determining standard reference locations. However, the existence of standard locations should not negate the opinions of various traditions of practice or clinicians, because, in the end, the location of an acupuncture point is established by its ability to summon qi, to influence the body, and to cure illness. In some instances, precise location of acupuncture points in terms of anatomy and measurement is critical; in others, the dynamics of the response of the point to touch, the presence of qi, is the determining factor in establishing location.

> Altogether, the points or holes on the 12 regular channels and on the governing and controlling vessels of the eight extraordinary vessels total 361. ∾

12 Regular Channels (listed in order of the flow of qi)

Lung channel	11 points
Large intestine channel	20 points
Stomach channel	45 points
Spleen channel	21 points
Heart channel	9 points
Small intestine channel	19 points
Urinary bladder channel	67 points
Kidney channel	27 points
Pericardium channel	9 points
Triple burner channel	23 points
Gallbladder channel	44 points
Liver channel	14 points
Extraordinary Vessels	
Governing vessel	28 points
Controlling vessel	24 points

As we shall see later, many points belong to special point groupings that help to define their clinical efficacy. However, generalizations can also be made about points on specific channels or groups of channels. So, for example, points on the three hand yin channels all treat disorders of the chest, but on each individual channel the points treat signs and symptoms associated with the organ for which the channel is named (Table 27-6).

Special Point Categories and Groups

One of the most important parts of the acupuncture treatment planning process is to understand the clinical significance of special group points. Every point has specific functions and is able to help treat specific symptoms or conditions. Many points belong to special groups. Membership in a special group helps to define the functions of a given point. A summary of the more commonly used special groups can be found in Table 27-7. Points that belong to special groups tend to be used more commonly than many other points. A good working knowledge of what these special groups are, what points belong in each group, and how that group affects a point's function is essential to designing clear, well-delineated point prescriptions. In the following sections a few of the special groups are described in detail to help the reader to understand their importance.

Five transport points (five-phase points). Perhaps the most powerful and certainly the most commonly used points on the body are the transport points. These points, located on the arms and legs below the elbow or knee, are associated with the five phases. Beginning at the tip of the finger or toe and moving up to the elbow or knee are five points on each channel that are associated with the five phases, for a total of 80 points. The five points are the jing-well, ying-spring, shu-stream, jing-river, and he-uniting

(sea) points. The category name for each of these points is associated with the flow of water, which is used as a metaphor for the flow of qi through the body and for the depth of the qi at these points. The qi flows from the well points, on the tips of the fingers and toes (the tip of the mountains), where the qi is said to be "shallow and meek," to the next proximal point, the spring, where the qi has a "gushing quality." From the spring, the qi travels to the stream points, where the flow pours from shallow to deep. From the stream, flow continues to the river, where the force becomes more powerful and the qi is found at a deeper level. Finally, the qi reaches the uniting (sea) points at the knees and elbows. At the uniting points, the qi unites with its home organ, just as a river reaches its final destination, the sea. The names of the points describe the nature of the qi at each of the points. This description of the nature of the qi is not the same as the directional flow of qi through the channels.

There are two major ways in which these points are used clinically and which inform point selection.

In the *Classic of Difficult Issues,* the points that held membership in each of these point categories were identified as being especially effective in treating certain types of conditions (Table 27-8). Thus, the appropriate point on a given channel might be selected to treat the corresponding condition manifesting in a particular organ.

These points are also frequently selected according to their five-phase correspondences (see Table 27-8). Each of the transport points is related to a specific phase (as is the organ of the channel on which the points lie). These relationships are used in theory-based treatment models that, when taken to their fullest extreme, can become quite complex.

Using the five-phase organizational scheme, on a basic level vacuity conditions are treated by supplementing the mother of the affected channel/organ and repletion conditions are addressed by draining the child of the affected channel/organ. Thus, if there is a vacuity in the fire phase, then the mother point on the fire channel might be supplemented (the wood point on the heart channel). In addition, one can supplement the same-phase points on the mother channel (wood point on the liver channel).

Alternatively, if there is a repletion condition in the fire phase, then one could drain the child point on the fire channel (the earth point on the heart channel) or the same-phase point on the child channel (the earth point on the spleen channel).

Some classic point selection texts discuss variants of these techniques, originally suggested by the theoretical discussions in the *Classic of Difficult Issues.* These approaches became very popular in the 1930s and again in the 1950s when there was a revival of interest, especially in Japan, in the acupuncture theories of the *Classic of Difficult Issues.* Contemporary schools of clinical thought in Japan, such as "meridian therapy," use transport points extensively based on a five-phase paradigm. This approach to acupuncture point selection is also practiced in Korea

TABLE 27-6

Clinical Applications of Major Points on the Four Limbs

Channel categorization	Channel/organ name	General clinical applications	Specific system clinical applications
Three hand yin channels	Lung	Chest disorders	Respiratory conditions, throat, nose, exterior patterns
	Pericardium		Mental-emotional conditions, heart conditions, stomach distress (nausea, vomiting)
	Heart		Mental-emotional conditions, heart conditions (angina, palpitations, etc.), eye conditions
Three hand yang channels	Large intestine	Face, head, sense organs, febrile diseases	Front of the face and head, including frontal headaches, nasal congestion, tooth pain, sores on the gums
	Small intestine		Occipital headaches, neck soreness, stiffness and pain, scapular pain
	Triple burner		Temporal headaches, earaches, ear congestion, pain, swelling or discomfort on the sides of the head or face, pain in the hypochondriac region
Three foot yin channels	Spleen	Urogenital, abdomen, and chest disorders	Digestive disorders such as nausea, poor appetite, loose stools
	Kidney		Urinary disorders such as incontinence, infertility conditions
	Liver		Liver and gallbladder conditions such as insomnia, anger, menstrual irregularities, genital sores or itching
Three foot yang channels	Stomach	Mental disorders, febrile diseases, eye problems	Pain on the frontal aspect of the face or head, acne, acid reflux, mania
	Urinary bladder		Pain in the occipital area or nape, back, and lumbus; urinary problems such as incontinence, dysuria
	Gallbladder		Temporal headaches, migraine headaches; pain or discomfort of the side of the head and face, hypochondriac region, or hip

Adapted from Ellis A, Wiseman N, Boss, K: *Fundamentals of Chinese acupuncture*, Brookline, Mass, 1991, Paradigm, p 57.

(notably in the Korean four-point method) and elaborated in China with the six-point method. Essentially, the theory is that if a particular phase is vacuous or replete, then the relationships of the engendering and restraining cycles can be used to supplement or drain the affected phase as needed.

For example, a patient comes for treatment with loose stools and nausea that are exacerbated by stress. One might diagnosis this as spleen qi vacuity with the liver overacting on the spleen. First, one would focus on supplementing the spleen by supplementing the mother point on the affected channel, the spleen channel. The spleen is associated with earth, thus its mother would be fire. This means that the fire point (the ying-spring point) on the spleen channel would be supplemented. In addition, the fire point on the fire channel would be supplemented. This would be the ying-spring point on the heart channel. Taken further, one would drain the controlling phase on the affected channel, which in this case would be the wood point (the jing-well point) on the spleen channel and drain the wood point on the controlling channel or

the jing-well point on the liver channel. (See Table 27-9 for a summary of the Korean four-point and Chinese six-point treatments.)

Five-phase approaches to treatment have had a substantial influence on some portions of the English and American acupuncture communities through the work of J.R. Worsley. Worsley's studies with exponents of meridian therapy led him to develop an approach to acupuncture diagnosis and treatment based almost exclusively on five-phase correspondences and the use of phase-associated transport points.

The use of the five-phase points in point selection entails a much more complex theoretical structure and understanding than is needed for use of most of the other point categories. The *Classic of Difficult Issues* discusses the alarm mu points and the back transport points together in the sixty-seventh difficult issue. Frequently the alarm mu and the back transport points will be used together in treatment or they will be used in alternate treatments.

Alarm mu points. Alarm mu points are points on the chest and abdomen where qi collects. There is one alarm

TABLE 27-7

Point Categories

Category	Description of point category
Source points	Called "source points" because these are points at which the source qi of the associated organ collects. There is one source point for each channel. The source qi is stored by the kidneys and spread throughout the body by the triple burner. Used to promote the flow of source qi and regulate the function of the internal organs. Often used in a treatment that entails the appropriate draining or supplementing of the source and the network point to treat simultaneously affected internally-externally related channels.
Network (luo) points	The site on a channel where the network vessel splits from the regular channel. There are 16 of these points: one for each regular channel, one on the controlling vessel, one on the governing vessel, and one each for the great luo of the spleen and the great luo of the stomach. Used to treat interiorly-exteriorly related organs and the specific symptomatology of the longitudinal network vessel. Frequently, these points are combined with source points to treat internally-externally related channels.
Eight meeting (influential) points	Each of the eight points is associated with a specific substance or tissue. The substances with which the points are associated include qi, blood, viscera, bowels, sinews, marrow, bones, and vessels. These are very general points and can treat any aspect of disharmony in their related tissue or substance. They are generally combined with other points to increase their specificity.
Four command points	These points are especially effective in treating disorders located in a particular anatomical area of the body. Each point is associated with a specific area of the body. The areas covered are the abdomen, the back, the head and back of the neck, and the face and mouth. Whenever one of these areas is involved in a patient's complaint, it would be appropriate to use the command point for that area.
Eight confluent points	Each of the eight extraordinary channels has a single point on one of the 12 regular channels that is said to be confluent with the associated extraordinary channel and to open or access that channel (see discussion in The Eight Extraordinary Vessels).
Cleft points	As qi and blood circulate through the channels they accumulate in the cleft points. Palpation and observation of these points can indicate repletion or vacuity in the channel. Sharp or intense pain on pressure or redness and swelling indicates repletion, and dull or mild pain or a depression indicates vacuity. They are used for both stubborn and acute conditions. They are also thought to be good for the treatment of bleeding conditions associated with the organ.
Ma Dan Yang's 12 heavenly star points	These are 12 points that Song dynasty physician Ma Dan Yang considered to be extremely useful. The points were compiled into song form by his students to be passed down through the generations. The 12 points are not used together. Among the 12 points are many that that belong to other point categories and so are generally recognized as very useful.
Window of heaven points	A list of 10 points first mentioned in the *Inner Classic (Nei Jing)*. They were never well explicated, and all but two of the points are located on the neck. Analysis of the points and their actions indicates that they seem to be useful for treating conditions that manifest primarily in the head or the sense organs but are the result of a disharmony of the movement of qi between the head and the body.
Nine needles for returning yang	A set of nine points that, when needled together, are indicated for yang desertion manifesting as loss of consciousness, generalized cold, counterflow cold of the limbs, cyanosis, etc.
13 Ghost points	Thirteen points compiled by the seventh-century physician and ethicist Sun Si Miao for the treatment of mental conditions. The original names of the points all contained the character *gui* (鬼), which means ghost or demon.
Points of the four seas	The four seas, first described in the *Inner Classic,* are the sea of qi, the sea of blood, the sea of water and grain, and the sea of marrow. There are several points that are directly associated with one of the four seas and are thought to be especially useful for treatment of disorders of the particular sea.
Extra points	Extra points, also called "new" points, are points that have specific locations but are not a part of the channel and network system. This category of points continues to grow as more points are found with specific uses.
Crossing points or intersection points	These are points where two or three channels meet. Because channels meet here, these points have a strong therapeutic effect on any of the channels that cross. Use of these points can eliminate the need to use multiple points when more than one channel is affected.
Ah shi ("That's it!") points	These are nonspecific points on the body that are particularly sensitive to palpation. There is no defined location for these points, they are simply tender spots that are most often used to treat disorders in their immediate vicinity.

TABLE 27-8

Nature and Location of the Transport Points and Their Classical Clinical Actions

Point location	Point category	Phase relationship on a yin channel	Phase relationship on a yang channel	Representation of qi	Classical clinical actions
Near the end of finger or toe	Jing-well	Wood	Metal	Shallow and meek	Revive clouded spirit Clear heat
Second most distal point on the channel	Ying-spring	Fire	Water	Like a small spring with somewhat more force	Treat externally contracted heat conditions
Usually the third most distal point on the channel	Shu-stream	Earth	Wood	Pouring down from a shallow place to a deeper one	Treat pain in the joints
On the wrists or ankles	Jing-river	Metal	Fire	Free flowing like the water in a river	Treat cough and panting
At the elbow or knee	He-uniting (sea)	Water	Earth	Large and deep as it unites with the organ of the home channel	Correct bowel patterns

TABLE 27-9

Korean Four-Point and Chinese Six-Point Treatment Strategy

Vacuity Conditions

Korean four point — Supplement the mother point on the channel of the affected organ
Supplement the phase point on the mother channel
Drain the controlling phase point (the grandmother point) on the affected organ's channel
Drain the phase point on the controlling phase (the grandmother) channel

Chinese six point — Drain the phase controlled by the affected phase (the grandchild point) on the channel of the affected organ
Drain the phase point on the channel controlled by the affected phase (the grandchild channel)

Repletion Conditions

Korean four point — Drain the child of the affected phase on the channel of the affected organ
Drain the phase point on the child channel of the affected organ
Supplement the phase point on the channel that controls the affected organ (the grandmother channel)
Supplement the control point (the grandmother point) on the channel of the affected organ

Chinese six point — Supplement the phase controlled by the affected phase (the grandchild point) on the channel of the affected organ
Supplement the phase point on the channel controlled by the affected phase (the grandchild channel)

point associated with and named for each of the 12 organs. These points may be palpated for tenderness, lumps, gatherings, depressions, and so forth, and also used to treat their associated organs. If, for example, a patient were to have either diarrhea or constipation, the practitioner would be likely to palpate and probably use the alarm point of the large intestine, which is located on the stomach channel, just lateral to the umbilicus. All of the alarm points are located in close proximity to the organ with which they are associated, but generally not on the channel associated with that organ. In fact, many of the alarm points are located on the controlling vessel, because that channel crosses over the entire abdomen and chest, passing through many of the organs.

Back transport points. Back transport points are points that are all located on the urinary bladder channel, lateral to the spine. There is one back transport point for each organ, and the qi of that organ runs through the point. In addition, there are back transport points for the governing vessel, for the diaphragm, for the sea of qi, and for other concepts in Chinese medicine. These points are regulating points, so they can be used to treat vacuity or repletion in the associated organ. Back transport points are frequently combined with alarm mu points to treat diseases of the viscera and bowels.

As noted earlier, a good working knowledge of what the point categories are, what points belong in each category, and how that category influences a point's function is essential to designing clear, well-delineated point prescriptions. Without this knowledge it is difficult to design a point prescription that will effectively and efficiently treat the presenting condition. This underscores the importance of a thorough understanding of the channel and network theory and of point theory for the practitioner. Without it, one begins to practice acupuncture as simply a technique that is not associated with a specific medical paradigm rather than as a part of a larger medical system that works best when used within its defined paradigm.

ACUPUNCTURE TREATMENT PLANNING

The classical Chinese therapeutic goal of acupuncture is to regulate qi and blood. Qi and blood flow through the body, its organs, and the channel pathways. When they flow freely, the body is healthy. When some cause, such as an evil, an emotion, trauma, and so on, disrupts the flow of qi or blood, illness or pain can result. Or, if the body does not have enough qi or blood, then symptoms such as fatigue, poor appetite, and so on, may appear. Acupuncture may be used to remove evils, to direct qi to where it is insufficient, to move obstructions and allow qi to flow, or to boost the functions of organs to produce more qi or blood.

Today, stimulation of acupuncture points is accomplished using a wide variety of tools and methods, but the most common is the filiform needle. The needle itself can vary significantly in structure, diameter, and length.

A typical acupuncture needle has a shaft that is 1 to 1.5 inches (25.4 to 38.1 mm) long and a handle of approximately 1 inch. The distinctive part of the needle is the tip, which is round and moderately sharp, much like the tip of a pine needle. The acupuncture needle is solid and gently tapered; it does not have the lumen or cutting edge of the hypodermic needle. The length of an acupuncture needle can vary from as little as 0.25 inch (6.4 mm) for very specialized applications to as much as 7 inches (17.8 cm). The shortest typical length is 0.5 inch (12.7 mm) for use in auricular acupuncture. Needles may be as long as 7 inches

or more for transverse or very deep needle insertion. Typical long needles are about 5 inches (12.7 cm) for deep insertion at points in the gluteal region.

The diameter of the acupuncture needle can range from as little as 0.12 mm to as much as 0.46 mm. Typically needles used for medium (0.25 to 1 inch), deep, and very deep insertive techniques range from about 0.22 mm to 0.46 mm, whereas needles used for shallow and minimally insertive techniques (often seen in certain Japanese styles) are in the 0.12- to 0.20-mm range. The diameter most commonly used by American practitioners of medium and deep insertion is 0.25 mm (Figures 27-2 and 27-3).

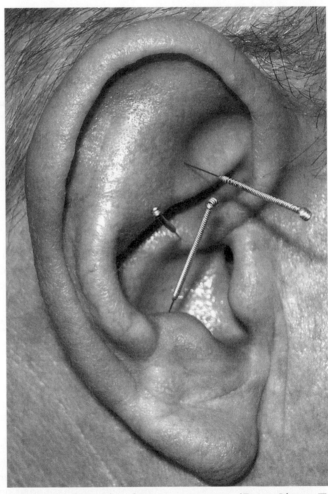

Figure 27-2 Example of Ear Acupuncture. (From Oleson T: *Auriculotherapy manual: Chinese and western systems of ear acupuncture,* ed. 3, Edinburgh, 2003, Churchill Livingstone.)

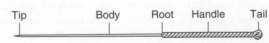

Figure 27-3 The structure of the filiform needle. (From Qiu ML: *Chinese acupuncture and moxibustion,* Edinburgh, 1993, Churchill Livingstone.)

From a classical and modern Chinese acupuncture point of view, the aim of the acupuncturist is to obtain qi at the site of insertion. The obtaining of qi may be seen or felt by the practitioner, the patient, or both parties. The practitioner seeks either an objective or subjective indication that the qi has arrived. The arrival of qi may be experienced by the practitioner as sensations felt by the hands as the needle is manipulated or through observation of color changes or of skin appearance at the site of insertion. The sensation of the arrival of qi often is felt by the practitioner as a gentle grasping of the needle at the site, as if one is fishing and one's line has suddenly been seized by the fish. The patient may feel the arrival of qi as a sensation of itching, numbness, soreness, or a swollen or distended feeling, or the patient might experience local temperature changes or an "electrical" sensation. Sometimes, the patient may not have any sensation, but the practitioner will be aware that qi has arrived, or the patient may be aware of the arrival of qi before the practitioner. Although the sensation or observation of the arrival of qi is not absolutely necessary for a successful treatment, it is considered to be one of the goals of traditional needling styles.

Perspectives on qi arrival, its signs and significance, and detection of qi by the practitioner, patient, or both can vary with the tradition of practice. In some styles of practice emerging out of the Japanese tradition, insertion of the needle is very minimal (or nonexistent) and the arrival of qi is to be detected by the clinician and not experienced by the patient, at least not as a distinct local sensation.

For the purposes of this section acupuncture techniques are presented from a primarily Chinese perspective. Although many of the concepts and practices described apply to other traditions, schools, or styles, there may be variations from what is presented here.

When a site for insertion has been determined, the needle is rapidly inserted and then adjusted to an appropriate depth. Many considerations will alter the angle and depth of insertion, methods of manipulation, and length of retention. A twelfth-century text, *Ode of the Subtleties of Flow*, states, "Insert the needle with noble speed then proceed (to the point) slowly, withdraw the needle with noble slowness as haste will cause injury" (Shanghai College of Traditional Chinese Medicine, 1981).

Once a point has been needled and qi obtained, the practitioner may manipulate the needle to achieve a specific therapeutic effect. Methods of manipulation range from simply inserting the needle and leaving it, to using techniques that involve slow or rapid insertion, to performing deeper or shallower insertions. Rotation of the needle will influence the therapeutic effect, as will other, more complex manipulations. The needle may be withdrawn immediately after qi arrives or may be retained for 20 to 30 minutes, or a very short, fine needle (known as an *intradermal*) may be retained for several days. In all cases, the goal of the clinician is to influence the flow or production of qi.

Practitioners use different methods to select acupuncture points for a particular patient or condition. Points may be chosen on the basis of the trajectory of the channel on which they lie, on the basis of membership in a particular traditional point category, or through an empirical understanding of what points work best for a given condition, based on the experience of generations of practitioners. Points may also be selected based on sensitivity to palpation or changes in texture that are perceived by the practitioner. Each of these methods gives the practitioner information about a particular point and should be considered when creating a treatment plan (Table 27-10).

To correctly determine the appropriate points to be used in treatment, a correct Chinese medicine diagnosis must be reached. Often, points will be chosen to treat the presenting symptoms of a specific biomedical condition. Although these points may give some symptomatic relief of the condition, they generally will not treat the root cause of the symptoms, and thus the condition will not be

TABLE 27-10

Acupuncture Treatment Planning in Chinese Medicine

A. Point matching: determining a large set of potentially appropriate points
  1. Diagnosis
  2. Treatment principle and method
  3. Matching of points to fulfill the treatment principle based on:
     a. Channel theory and channel pathways
     b. Areas of effect
     c. Special group points
     d. Pathology-condition points
B. Point selection: creating specific treatment plans
  1. Address tip and root
  2. Ensure balance
     a. Yin and yang channels
     b. Front and back of the body
     c. Top and bottom of the body
     d. Left and right sides of the body
  3. Include local, adjacent, and distal points
  4. Determine the overall purpose of each point prescription
  5. Determine the appropriate size of a point prescription
  6. Choose appropriate adjunctive techniques
     a. Moxibustion
     b. Cupping
     c. Bleeding
     d. Plum blossom (seven-star) needling
     e. Gua sha
     f. Electroacupuncture
     g. Laser
     h. Magnets
     i. Bodywork/tui na
     j. Microsystems

resolved. For example, if a patient comes for treatment of chronic low back pain, there are many points that might be chosen to treat the pain. However, there are several different possible Chinese medicine diagnoses for low back pain. If the practitioner does not concern himself or herself with the diagnosis, the techniques employed and even some of the points used to "treat" the low back pain at best might be inappropriate and at worst might worsen the condition.

Once a Chinese medicine diagnosis has been determined, the practitioner begins the process of choosing a set of points to treat the condition. The process begins with point matching. Point matching entails creating a large set of points (usually 20 to 40 points) that might possibly be appropriate for the given diagnosis. These points should address both the root cause of the condition and the presenting symptoms. This large set of points is chosen based on an understanding of channel theory and knowledge of the areas that different channels affect, on a clear knowledge of point categories and how points in specific categories affect areas of the body or substances in the body, on knowledge of specific channel points and how they differ, and on knowledge about empirical points that might be appropriate for a given diagnosis or condition.

Point Selection

Once the large set of points has been created, from this set two to five smaller acupuncture prescriptions are developed. This is a process called *point selection*. When creating the smaller prescriptions, the practitioner must be mindful of additional considerations.

First, a point prescription must address both the tip and the root of the problem. For example, if a patient arrives with a chief complaint of loose stools, the practitioner must develop a point prescription that will treat the root cause of the loose stools, which might be spleen qi vacuity, kidney yang vacuity, damp heat, and so forth. The prescription should also address the presenting symptom of the loose stools. If the focus is entirely on the root, it may be that for several weeks there will be no improvement in the stools. But if the focus is entirely on the tip, the loose stools, then although there may be temporary improvement, the condition will not be fully resolved.

Second, a point prescription must be balanced. Achieving balance includes balancing points between the upper and lower portions of the body, balancing points between the left and right sides of the body, balancing points between the front and the back of the body, and balancing points between yin and yang channels. Frequently students of acupuncture will, for example, create a point prescription that consists of only yin channel points or only points on the legs with no arm points, and so on. This type of treatment may leave the patient feeling unbalanced or as if the treatment were incomplete.

Third, point selection is based on choice of local, adjacent, and distal points. For low back pain, one might choose several local points on the lower back. In addition, one would choose points near the site of the pain (e.g., in the hip, the sacrum). Finally, one would choose appropriate distal points on the four limbs. For loose stools, one might choose several local points directly over the large intestine on the abdomen, adjacent points on the upper abdomen associated with the spleen and stomach, and, again, distal points on the leg to address the root of the loose stools. This process gives a balance to the prescription and allows the qi to move or be acted upon so that it will address both the clinical problem or symptom (the tip) and its cause (the root).

Finally, the elements of function and size of the treatment must be considered. Each individual point chosen has its own functions and indications; however, the overall point prescription should also have a general function or purpose. If the cause of the low back pain is qi and blood stagnation due to trauma, then the points chosen should act together to move the qi and blood to reduce the pain and improve healing. If the cause is a kidney vacuity, then the points chosen should still move the qi, albeit more gently; however, points should also be chosen to boost the kidneys, and adjunctive techniques such as moxibustion might be appropriate. Essentially, the function of the point prescription should match the treatment principle that is determined by the diagnosis.

The number of needles being inserted is an important consideration. Some practitioners say that no more than eight needles should be inserted. Others say that about eight bilateral points (16 needles) should be used. There is no absolute rule about the number of needles used, but choosing points that might work on several aspects of treatment is often more effective than choosing points that act only on one symptom. The age, constitution, and gender of the patient should also be considered when determining the number of needles. Some treatments might require a higher number of needles, but if, for example, the patient is elderly or debilitated, use of a large number of needles could cause the patient to become extremely tired or uncomfortable. On children, as few needles as possible should be used, and on menstruating women, fewer needles are generally desirable.

The frequency of treatment, as well as the various techniques to be used, are also addressed when thinking about point selection. In China, a typical course of treatment is 10 treatments, which are usually given every day or every other day for 10 to 20 days followed by a break for 10 days. Then, if necessary, treatment recommences. In the West, although 10 treatments may be considered an appropriate course of treatment, practitioners tend to treat once a week for 10 weeks. This method is probably not as effective for treating pain conditions as more frequent sessions would be. Techniques vary widely depending on the style in which the practitioner is trained, whether it be TCM, one of the many systems coming out of Japan or Korea, or one of the schools or styles developed outside of Asia.

Adjunctive Techniques

All of the techniques described in what follows are important elements of the training of an acupuncturist. Although they may or may not involve the insertion of a needle, they are all forms of stimulation that can be used over large areas of the body, over channel pathways, or over specific points to achieve a therapeutic effect. They might be used by themselves or in conjunction with acupuncture. In some traditions or schools they have been very highly developed as specialized and independently utilized stimulation techniques, whereas in others they are used as adjunctive techniques to complement and support the acupuncture needle treatment. The discussion here is provided primarily from the point of view of the Chinese tradition and is necessarily very cursory.

Moxibustion. Moxibustion refers to the burning of dried, powdered leaves of *Artemisia vulgaris* (*ai ye* or mugwort), either on or close to the skin, to affect the flow of qi in the channel. Artemisia is acrid and bitter, and it warms and enters the channels. References to warming techniques appear in very early materials, including the Ma Wang tomb texts (Unschuld, 1985). As mentioned at the beginning of this chapter, the term *zhen jiu* literally means "needle moxibustion," although in the West we typically use simply the term *acupuncture* when referring to these techniques.

Moxibustion can be applied to the body in many ways. *Direct moxibustion* involves burning a small amount of moxa (about the size of a small grain of rice) directly on the skin. The moxa can be allowed to burn down to the skin, causing a blister or scar, or it can be removed before it has burned down to the skin. This technique is used less frequently in the West than other techniques because of the scarring.

Indirect moxibustion involves putting a substance between the moxa and the patient's skin. This gives the practitioner greater control over the amount of heat and helps to protect the patient from burns. Some frequently used substances are ginger slices, garlic slices, and salt. The overall action of the technique changes slightly depending on the medium used. For example, moxa on salt is more astringent and is used to help stop diarrhea, whereas moxa on ginger is more warming.

Other techniques include pole moxa and warm needle moxa. In *pole moxa* a cigar-shaped roll of moxa wrapped in paper is used to gently warm an area without touching the skin. This is a very safe method of moxibustion that can be taught to patients for self-application. The *warm needle method* is accomplished by inserting an acupuncture needle and then placing moxa on its handle. After the moxa is ignited, it burns slowly, giving a gentle sensation of warmth to the acupuncture point and to the channel.

Any of these techniques might be used to stimulate acupuncture points or areas of the body, especially when warming is appropriate. For example, if a patient is suffering from joint pain that worsens in cold, damp weather, applying moxa either directly or indirectly to the affected area will help to relieve the pain by warming the area and allowing the qi to flow more smoothly. In some places, most notably Japan, moxibustion techniques are highly developed, and specialized training is required to become a moxibustion practitioner (Figure 27-4).

Cupping. In *cupping*, once known as "horning" because animal horns were traditionally employed, a flame is used to induce a vacuum in a small glass or bamboo cup, which is then applied to the skin. The subsequent suction on the skin helps to drain or remove cold and damp evils from the body or to assist blood circulation. For example, if a patient arrives with a common cold accompanied by cough and sore muscles on the upper back, cupping might be performed on the upper back to move the qi and dispel the evil. The cups may remain static on the area to which they are applied or a medium may be applied to the body and the cups then drawn over the medium to cover a larger area. When the cups are removed, the patient is usually left with discoloration at the site of the vacuum. Today, some practitioners use small glass or plastic cups with a suction valve and then attach a hand-held vacuum to remove the air.

Gua sha. Usually thought of as a folk technique, *gua sha*, literally "sand scraping," is used throughout Asia. It entails applying an oily medium to the skin and then using a spoon, a horn, or some other smooth utensil to scrape along the surface of the skin. Although the resulting marks on the skin look quite painful, patients describe the sensation as like having a very deep itch that they have been unable to scratch scratched. The release of the sha from the muscles releases evils from the muscle layer of the body, allows qi and blood to flow more freely, and often reduces muscular pain and stiffness. The technique is primarily used to release external evils or to relieve muscular pain, stiffness, and tension.

Bleeding. *Bleeding* is done to drain a channel or to remove heat from the body. In this method small amounts of blood are expressed, from a drop to a few centiliters. It is commonly used on points that are located on the tips of the fingers or toes or over areas where there is a large

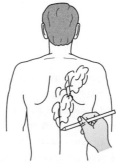

Figure 27-4 Moxibustion. (From Wang Y: *Microacupuncture in practice*, St. Louis, 2009, Churchill Livingstone.)

vessel. On the tips of the fingers or toes, it is used to release acute heat that might be causing a sore throat or a severe headache. On the back of the knee, or in the crease of the elbow, it might be used to release heat that is causing a skin condition such as eczema or acne. Bleeding the tip of the ear can cause a rapid drop in blood pressure and is an emergency technique for preventing stroke.

Electroacupuncture. A relatively modern acupuncture technique involves the application of a small electrical current to needles that have been inserted into the body. The intensity of the stimulus provided is determined by the patient and the patient's condition. The purpose of the technique is to apply continual stimulation to the needle throughout treatment. Electroacupuncture is particularly useful in the treatment of pain conditions and is frequently used for wind stroke. The electrical stimulus may be applied to regular body points as well as to auricular points, facial points, or the head. The technique is also frequently used in acupuncture anesthesia.

Plum blossom needling (seven-star needling). A plum blossom or seven-star needle was traditionally made by binding five or seven sewing needles to a bamboo stick. Today, five or seven very small needles are attached to a metal or plastic hammer. The hammer is used to lightly tap the skin. The technique may be used on a particular area of the body, on a specific point, or over the pathway of a channel. It is used to treat areas of numbness or paralysis, and even to treat balding. It is also used as a treatment for children or individuals who are hesitant about being needled.

Tui na. Bodywork is an important part of many health care systems. The technique developed in China is called *tui na,* literally "pushing and pulling." In China, many practitioners specialize in tui na and become practitioners of tui na alone. The techniques are varied. They include rubbing pressing, pinching, pulling, rolling, and so on. Like the other techniques described here, tui na may be used over large areas of the body, over channel pathways, or simply at a specific point. In some cases, a patient may receive a full-body tui na treatment. Traditionally, the art of bone setting was also a part of the practice of a tui na practitioner. In fact, many of the tui na techniques bear a close resemblance to some of the techniques used today by chiropractors or osteopaths (see Chapters 17 and 18).

MICROSYSTEMS

All of the various microsystems that are used in the context of acupuncture treatment are comparatively modern developments. Almost all claim roots in classical Chinese acupuncture theory; however, in most cases there is little evidence of anything in the classics supporting the degree of elaboration seen in contemporary systems. Almost all of the microsystems can be considered as reflex zones, specific and bounded areas of the body that can be stimulated to influence all regions of the body itself. They are essentially maps of the body and its organ systems drawn on various specific areas of the body, which can then be used to treat the entire system.

The theoretical rationale for the reflex zones that comprise most microsystems is typically based on interpreted neurology or developmental biology, and thus they are usually connected with contemporary ideas about neurology, development, and anatomy. However, the idea that a bounded region of the body can relate directly to all body regions is seen in the diagnostic principles described in classical texts (particularly face and tongue diagnosis), and thus the principle of reflex zones is not without its classical antecedents.

The reflex zones are typically used in one of three ways: (1) Chinese medicine theory may be applied to the choice of points (i.e., for a diagnosis of kidney qi vacuity, the kidney points in a given system might be chosen); (2) biomedical concepts may be applied to choose the points (i.e., if there is a problem with the pancreas, then the pancreas region in a given system might be chosen); or (3) the points in the reflex zone might be used symptomatically (i.e., if there is pain in the back and knees, then the back and knee region in a given system might be chosen for stimulation).

A number of different microsystems have been developed. The ear and scalp microsystems are particularly biomedicalized, whereas hand, foot, nose, face, and abdomen systems are perhaps a little less so. Although some microsystems are relatively obscure and the province of specialists with expertise in their application, the use of others is comparatively common in clinical settings. Almost all require some degree of specialized training to use effectively. In general the microsystems are used in conjunction with conventional acupuncture points, but some, such as the Korean hand acupuncture system, are intended to be used as independent acupuncture systems. Two common systems, auricular acupuncture and scalp acupuncture, are discussed here.

Auricular Acupuncture

Auricular or ear acupuncture is a widely used acupuncture microsystem. In 1951, Dr. Paul Nogier, a French physician, encountered patients who had been treated for sciatica by the application of cautery to specific areas of the ear as part of a folk tradition. These patients claimed reduction of their symptoms (Nogier, 1976, 1983). Nogier became interested and began a deep exploration of the therapeutic stimulation of the ear to treat medical conditions. He used a number of stimulus methods, including acupuncture, which was well known to French physicians. Nogier's work led him to describe a pattern of reflex areas that corresponded with an inverted homunculus mapped onto the human ear.

Subsequent to the initial publication of his ideas in 1957, his work was translated into Chinese and republished in 1958. Based on Nogier's publications and subsequent work in China, the academy of TCM in Beijing published its version of an auricular acupuncture chart in 1977, blending Nogier's model with Chinese additions. It is from this point that auricular therapy can be said to be an important aspect of Chinese acupuncture. It has become so integrated with Chinese acupuncture practice that both Chinese and Western practitioners are often surprised to learn of its European roots.

Ear acupuncture is used as an adjunct to group and behavioral therapies in supporting patients who are addressing substance abuse issues. Typically, in what is known as the National Acupuncture Detoxification Association (NADA) protocol, the shenmen, liver, kidney, lung, and sympathetic ear points are needled bilaterally on a daily basis for several weeks. The NADA protocol is also used to address posttraumatic stress disorder.

Scalp Acupuncture

Standard acupuncture theory posits that all of the qi of the organs rises to the head via the various channel pathways; thus the flourishing of qi and blood is reflected in the head. In the 1950s and 1960s, based on knowledge gained from cerebral cortex mapping, a system of acupuncture was developed to treat central nervous system (CNS) conditions. Over the past 50+ years, other scalp systems have also been developed, but all are based on the areas of the brain associated with specific functions. Some use very carefully defined and measured lines as the locations for needle insertion, whereas others use more general zones to identify needling locations.

The earliest system identified lines on the scalp that corresponded with areas of the brain associated with motor skills and sensory perceptions. In addition, there are lines for tremors, for vertigo and hearing, for speech, for vision, and for balance, as well as several others. Based on the understanding of the crossing of the spinal nerves, contralateral needling is done for conditions affecting one limb. Bilateral needling is done for conditions affecting both limbs or for systemic conditions. Relatively thick (0.30- or 0.28-mm) needles are inserted horizontally into the scalp and then manipulated with strong continuous stimulation for 3 to 4 minutes. After manipulation, the needles are retained for several more minutes.

Scalp acupuncture appears to be quite useful for treatment of conditions such as poststroke paralysis, Parkinson disease, and other conditions related to balance and movement, and is frequently used when acupuncture is focused on rehabilitation.

TRADITIONS, SCHOOLS, STYLES, AND SYSTEMS

The idea that *acupuncture* is a term that floats freely and that may be distinguished by the addition of various qualifiers was introduced earlier. This section examines a range of approaches to acupuncture that are bound together through their common engagement with elements of the core traditions of Chinese medicine and are, at the same time, distinctive with regard to specific aspects of their approaches to therapy. Although it is tempting simply to refer to all of these approaches as particular "styles" of acupuncture, as does Ahn (2008), it may be helpful to draw a distinction of scale regarding what constitutes a tradition, a school, a style, and a system to clarify some of what is seen in the field of acupuncture.

When this scalar approach is used (see Chapter 5) an acupuncture *tradition* can be said to be organized so broadly that it has only a limited degree of central focus and may, in fact, contain diverse schools and systems within it. At the same time any distinct elements of the tradition will still have characteristics in common. Very often traditions will have regional associations and characteristics (like regional styles of cooking within Chinese cuisine). From this point of view, what is termed "traditional Chinese medicine" or "Chinese medicine," as well as "Japanese acupuncture," can be said to be acupuncture traditions in their own right.

Acupuncture *schools* are approaches to practice that are organized around a central figure or organization. A school promulgates a distinctive doctrine that guides practice and insists on some degree of conformity to its methods, although it may exist within a larger tradition. Toyohari and keiraku chiryo within the Japanese tradition represent schools in that sense, as does five-element acupuncture.

A *style* involves the appropriation, or rejection, of the elements of a tradition or school and the assertion of a kind of distinctiveness, without the requirement for a great deal of clarity about the antecedents or basis for its assertions. "Western acupuncture" or "medical acupuncture" exemplifies an acupuncture style from this point of view.

Finally, *systems* involve specific and highly structured approaches to treatment that do not require a commitment to any specific school or tradition and can be easily incorporated into different styles of practice. Ryodaraku, Yoshio Manaka's five-step treatment protocol, auricular acupuncture, and Master Dong's points are examples of acupuncture systems (Table 27-11).

The ideas presented in the sections addressing channels, networks, and points represent the common core of the East Asian acupuncture traditions that have developed in China, Japan, Korea, and Vietnam, as well as most of those to be found in the West. This core pertains even to those systems that overtly eschew any engagement with core theory (such as Western acupuncture) and simply use acupuncture points removed from any traditional context, because the points themselves would not exist as objects of knowledge without the centuries of exploration contributed by the ancient Chinese. In this sense, then, there is no acupuncture tradition that is not, in essence, based on the originating contributions of the Chinese.

TABLE 27-11

Scalars in Acupuncture Practice

Tradition	A regionally distinct approach or set of approaches that can be characterized by regional developments
School	Approach to practice organized around a central figure or organization, e.g., meridian therapy, toyohari, five-element acupuncture
Style	Appropriation or rejection of a school or tradition, with the assertion of distinctiveness but with limited development of a distinctive theory of application, e.g., Western acupuncture, medical acupuncture, Japanese-style acupuncture
System	Specific highly structured approaches to treatment not requiring adherence to a specific school or tradition and easily incorporated into different practice styles, e.g., five-step treatment protocol, auricular acupuncture, Korean hand acupuncture, abdominal needling

Even within China, however, and certainly in Japan, Korea, Vietnam, Europe, and the United States, there have been shifts of emphasis, theoretical elaborations, clinical developments, and refinements in technique that have produced approaches to acupuncture that seem so distinctive to their developers or their adherents that they have come to be identified as specific schools or systems of acupuncture. This is definitely the case with the wide range of practices that are subsumed under the general heading of "Japanese acupuncture," in which myriad distinctive schools of practice show both a strong relationship to the acupuncture traditions and texts of China, and regional innovation and development.

Intriguingly, many of these systems that have developed outside China and East Asia often seek to contrast their practice methodologies with what is seen as the dominant, even hegemonic, paradigm of TCM. In China, however, divergent or distinctive practice styles are always understood to be part of the greater "Chinese medicine" or "acupuncture and moxibustion" paradigms, even when they break truly new ground or diverge significantly from traditional approaches to practice. There are many possible reasons for this contrast in attitudes between those within China and those without. The two most apparent are the following: In some cases a degree of national pride suggests that it is important to demonstrate that the distinctive practice was developed outside of China, whereas exponents of the Chinese tradition may wish to point clearly to the Chinese origins of every acupuncture practice. In other instances an attempt to brand acupuncture is occurring, and the acupuncture style in question may make an effort to distinguish itself

from standard professional acupuncture by asserting engagement with more authentic practices, development of areas said to be neglected by TCM, or rejection of practices attributed to TCM.

This section proposes no evaluation of the merits of competing claims, nor will we pronounce on the validity of differing practice styles. The goal here is to provide the reader with some guidance to the significance of some of the common qualifiers applied to the term *acupuncture*. We make no claim to providing an exhaustive list of traditions, schools, systems, and styles of acupuncture practice, but rather offer a window into the diversity of approaches to clinical practice by presenting some of the commonly encountered models for delivering acupuncture therapy.

CHINESE ACUPUNCTURE STYLES AND SYSTEMS

Readers of Chapter 26 recall that there is exceptional conceptual flexibility in theoretical approaches to Chinese medical practice. Even today in China, during one of the comparatively most standardized periods of acupuncture practice in Chinese history, the diversity of practice styles and schools as one departs from the standard curricula of academic institutions and enters private and institutional practice settings is immense. However, the persistence of the Chinese cultural tendency to integrate, incorporate, and retain tends to cause even proponents of the most radical departures from "standard" Chinese medicine to find that their distinctive school or system has been absorbed into the greater paradigm of the Chinese tradition.

For all intents and purposes *Chinese acupuncture, traditional Chinese acupuncture,* and *TCM acupuncture* can be considered virtually synonymous terms that convey the acupuncture practiced in the dominant paradigm of modern China. "Classical Chinese acupuncture" is an expression that tries to assert a distinction between itself and the modern practice traditions of China, but that in actuality conveys nothing, because it refers to the same classical texts and traditions as the predominant paradigm.

"Daoist acupuncture" is an expression that has emerged over the years. What seems to be meant is a repertoire of acupuncture point selection strategies associated with Daoist physicians or traditions of Daoist ritual practice. There are also texts that assert a "Daoist" lineage for their acupuncture practices (Liu, 1999) and even training programs in the United States that claim a privileged connection between the traditions of Daoism and their instructional content. The problem is that a great number of physicians in China were, in fact, Daoists (and often Buddhists and Confucians as well), and so a great deal of "standard"— that is, classically derived and widely disseminated— acupuncture theory can be attributed to texts that are associated with Daoist traditions. Many of the most notable "Daoist" components are systems of acupuncture point selection based on the *I Ching (Yi Jing)* or on the stems and branches (traditional calendrics). However, all these methods are practiced in the context of standard acupuncture theory and so distinguish themselves mainly in the details.

JAPANESE ACUPUNCTURE SCHOOLS AND SYSTEMS

As discussed in Chapter 26, the recorded history of cultural exchange between China and Japan dates back to at least AD 57 (obviously there were important contacts in prehistory as well), and the exchange has been a long and productive one, especially in the field of medicine. Today acupuncture in Japan encompasses a wide range of schools and systems. The typical Japanese acupuncturist draws from the many different schools and systems of practice in an eclectic fashion. Alternatively, some practitioners adhere closely to the tenets of a particular school. For this reason it is not entirely accurate to generalize about Japanese acupuncture except, perhaps, as a tradition of practice. Rather, it is more useful to speak of the schools and systems that have emerged from Japan. Japan has seen both focused specialization in, and the innovative exploration and expansion of, acupuncture practice.

Meridian Therapy

The *Classic of Difficult Issues* has historically been the focus for movements to revive the practices of "traditional" acupuncture in Japan. The text was an important influence in the development of meridian therapy (keiraku chiryo), a school of acupuncture developed in the 1930s based on the application of concepts in the *Classic of Difficult Issues* and their subsequent interpretation by later Chinese authors. A distinctive feature of meridian therapy is the application of five-phase theory to the transport points, a practice that has influenced the perception and adoption of five-phase theory by European practitioners (Kaptchuk, 1983).

Toyohari

Toyohari is a distinctive school of acupuncture practice that grew out of meridian therapy. Like meridian therapy it is built on the foundations of the *Classic of Difficult Issues* and uses the approach of pulse and abdominal diagnoses to select acupuncture points based on five-phase concepts. It is distinguished by an exceptionally gentle needling technique that can range from minimally insertive to entirely noninsertive (the effectiveness of noninsertive acupuncture fundamentally calls into question the mechanisms of action that have been proposed by Western biomedicine, which essentially relate to the physiology of skin puncture). Many of Japan's toyohari practitioners are blind, which links them closely with the historical tradition of

acupuncture as a field of practice for the blind, as with shiatsu (see Chapter 20). In the mid-seventeenth century, Waichi Sugiyama, a blind man, began to train the blind in acupuncture using very fine needles and guide tubes. Practitioners of toyohari cultivate special sensitivity to the sensations felt by the practitioner with the arrival of qi, which is summoned to the acupuncture points with little if any needle insertion.

An interesting system of acupuncture therapy is the pioneering work of Yoshio Manaka. Manaka, a physician who experimented with acupuncture principles during a period when medical supplies were unavailable during World War II, became convinced of the efficacy and physiological relevance of traditional theories and continued to experiment and develop them throughout his life. His work, specifically his five-step protocol and the use of ion pumping cords, has contributed dramatically to the practice of acupuncture.

The variety of systems emerging from Japan also include systems such as shoni shin (literally "pediatric needles"), akabane and many others. Each of these systems is quite unique, and yet the term *Japanese acupuncture* has been used to cover all of them. This misnomer leads one to believe that a specific tradition developed in Japan, when in fact all of the systems emerging from Japan are grounded in the core texts of the Chinese tradition and the core acupuncture theory of China.

KOREAN SCHOOLS AND SYSTEMS

Widely used techniques of acupuncture point selection based on five-phase theory have emerged from Korea, including those of the Buddhist priest Sa-am (1544-1610). Although these are known as Korean four-point (eight-needle) techniques, however, the method has been established for so long that it has become integrated into many other acupuncture traditions and schools.

Two comparatively recent acupuncture systems developed in Korea have become relatively well known in other parts of the world. Korean constitutional diagnosis was developed initially by Jhema Lee (1836-1900). It based a system of herbal therapeutics on a set of diagnostic patterns using the four divisions of yin and yang. In 1965, Dowon Kuan expanded Jhema Lee's system to an eightfold classification and applied it to acupuncture (Hirsch, 1985). This system became known as *Korean constitutional acupuncture*.

Another influential contemporary system is *koryo sooji chim*, the system of Korean hand and finger acupuncture developed by Yoo Tae Woo and published in 1971. This system has gained a significant level of international exposure. Koryo sooji chim maps the channel pathways and acupuncture points of the entire body onto the hands, where they are stimulated using very short, fine needles and magnets. Specialized tools are required to insert the small needles into very specific areas on the hands and fingers.

WESTERN EUROPEAN TRADITIONS AND STYLES

"Medical acupuncture" is an expression with a wide and slightly contrasting range of uses. Its primary meaning is any form of acupuncture (tradition, school, style, or system) practiced by an individual who is a licensed physician.

The American Association of Medical Acupuncture (n.d.) defines medical acupuncture as "the clinical discipline of acupuncture as practiced by a physician who is also trained and licensed in Western biomedicine. Founded on medical texts of ancient China, the interpretation and application of acupuncture within the context of contemporary medicine is an extension of the physician's biomedical training. The medical acupuncture physician uniquely offers a comprehensive approach to healthcare, which combines classic and modern forms of acupuncture with conventional biomedicine."

In this context the term *medical acupuncture* distinguishes only the professional status of the person performing the acupuncture, and this form of acupuncture relies substantially on a wide range of practice traditions and schools.

A somewhat less frequently encountered meaning of "medical acupuncture" is that of a system of acupuncture that typically (but not always) retains the acupuncture points derived from the Chinese tradition but seeks to describe a bioscience-based paradigm for their application (Filshie et al, 1998; Jin et al, 2006). In some cases acupuncture points are renamed and reorganized to provide a less traditional, more "scientific" appearance (Ma, et al, 2005).

Western acupuncture and *Western-style acupuncture* are terms that appears periodically in the literature, typically in descriptions of research in which the acupuncture to be provided is "Western," which seems to mean that it involves acupuncture stimulation of both standard acupuncture points and "trigger points" in the presence of a Western medical diagnosis but without, in some instances, any described process for determining the points selected for treatment.

Occasionally the term *dry needling* is used in association with the concept of Western acupuncture. Strictly speaking, dry needling is done with a hypodermic needle, not an acupuncture needle. The needle is different in that it has a lumen and a cutting edge. The technique emerged from Travell's approach to the treatment of myofascial trigger points (MTrPs) by injection (of lidocaine, saline, etc.), using a "wet needle" containing a substance to be injected. Some clinicians concluded that the use of a needle without injection of any substance was sufficient, hence "dry" needling. The term *dry needling* then implies (1) the use of a hypodermic needle inserted into (2) a trigger point. In the sense that a needle and a type of acupuncture point (the ah shi point) are involved this could be said to be acupuncture, but the acupuncture paradigm is otherwise entirely absent from the method, and the use of the cutting needle creates different effects as well.

French Energetic Acupuncture

Several distinct influences shaped what might best be termed a collection of acupuncture styles rooted in classical Chinese acupuncture theory and early-twentieth-century Chinese acupuncture practice. The French diplomat George Soulié de Morant, who studied acupuncture in China from 1901 through 1917 and was recognized as a physician by the Chinese, produced several very influential texts in France during the 1930s and 1950s. His work substantially influenced the development of acupuncture in France and provided the basis for the engagement of French acupuncture with post–World War II Japanese and Vietnamese perspectives on acupuncture practice. The fact that Soulié de Morant chose to translate *qi* as energy and that his collaborator (and later nemesis) Niboyet chose to integrate acupuncture closely with homeopathy seems to have contributed substantially to the "energetic" orientation of this style.

Five-Element Acupuncture

J.R. Worsley, a physical therapist who began his studies of acupuncture in 1962, came to have a substantial impact on the perceptions of many practitioners in England and the United States. He visited Hong Kong and Taiwan for a brief period and then became a part of the study group established by Rose-Neil (Hsu et al, 1977). Worsley went on to create the College of Traditional Chinese Acupuncture in the United Kingdom and two institutions in the United States. Worsley's five-element acupuncture constitutes a school of practice blending elements of Japanese acupuncture traditions, notably meridian therapy and akabane, with a very broadly developed interpretation of five-element theory based on ideas expressed in the *Yellow Emperor's Inner Classic*. Since the death of its founder and the appropriation of Worsley's five-element model of practice by others, there can also be said to be five-element styles.

What we hope to have made clear in this section is that throughout Asia and Europe a variety of schools, systems, and styles of acupuncture have developed. And yet, with few exceptions, all of them refer back to the classical texts that emerged out of the Han dynasty in China. The basic core acupuncture theory that we have discussed in this chapter continues to be the core of almost all of the traditions, schools, systems, and styles, for without that core theory, there is no structure for understanding the actions of individual points or for developing different methods of point selection.

ACUPUNCTURE RESEARCH

What we might term the "modern" history of acupuncture research in the West has a scope of just under 40 years (and perhaps 60 years in East Asia). This is not to say that there are not earlier instances of research activities in both East Asia and the West. However, these are distinct, isolated, and comparatively limited and certainly not part of the system of internationalized research communication that constitutes what we term "modern."

Ongoing lines of scientific inquiry into acupuncture have focused primarily on three specific types of questions: (1) Are there physiological processes that can, at least partially, explain acupuncture effects such as pain control? (2) Is acupuncture safe? (3) Can acupuncture be shown to treat specific clinical conditions effectively?

The answer to questions 1 and 2 is yes, and the answer to question 3 is a qualified yes for many clinical conditions. This section reviews work done on each of these questions to give the reader an understanding of the complexity of the questions and the amount of research that has been done over the last 40+ years.

ANATOMY AND PHYSIOLOGY OF ACUPUNCTURE EFFECTS

One of the advantages of acupuncture, as its practitioners and advocates seek to increase its acceptance into mainstream health care, is that its primary therapeutic tools and methods are not abstract in any sense. The acupuncture needle is a tangible object that is introduced into or adjacent to tissue. That simple physicality has formed the basis for many intriguing investigations into the basic physiology of acupuncture. When Kaptchuk (1983, 2002) stated that acupuncture is the most credible of complementary therapies in terms of acceptance by the medical community, he proposes that this greater acceptance may be the result of the existence of a substantial body of data showing that acupuncture in the laboratory has measurable and replicable physiological effects that can begin to offer plausible mechanisms for the presumed actions. This point is echoed by Filshie and White (1998) when they tell us, "Acupuncture owes much of its respectability to the discovery that it releases opiate peptides" (pp. 3-4). The fact that acupuncture can point to a body of basic research that provides a number of scientifically derived hypotheses for many of its clinically observed effects has been helpful in supporting its acceptance in a variety of medical settings.

The contrast between ancient and traditional models of acupuncture and contemporary biomechanistic models is quite distinct. As we have seen, the classical constructs of acupuncture theory model a system that has been described through the observation of the body in health and disease and the body's response to stimulus. Although these models are explanatory, they were not developed in the context of the linearity and reductionism of the currently popular positivist, reductionist scientific enterprise. Instead they were developed on the basis of observation and an effort to describe observed relations systematically. They capture a diverse range of information in very broad and general terms (Table 27-12).

TABLE 27-12

Comparison of Biomechanistic Model and Acupuncture Model

Reductionist science-based model	Acupuncture theory model
Events attributed to observed or hypothe-sized physiological processes	Events attributed to described system (based on observations of results of physiological processes)
Narrowly described	Broadly described
Incomplete	Comprehensive
Implicit reductionism	Implicit holism
Developing model	Static model

Contemporary biomechanistic models are constructed on the basis of currently established understandings of anatomy and physiology. The most prevalent models apply concepts derived from studying the neurophysiology of pain and, because of this, seek to explain acupuncture in terms of what is already "known" about the body. Newer models have actually used traditional descriptions of physical responses to acupuncture stimulation to develop experiments that have led to new understanding of the way the body, particularly connective tissue, responds to acupuncture. From an acupuncturist's perspective, 30 years of basic science research into acupuncture using a biomechanistic model has furnished valid and valuable insight into many acupuncture phenomena, but cannot yet fully explain the range of observed acupuncture phenomena. There is, in fact, no reason that it should be expected to do so. Science consists of a rigorous process of investigation and explanation that relies on careful descriptions of observable processes. The methodology of science derives its power from the strict limitations placed on its methods. Scientific knowledge is continually developing, and so we should expect two things from proposed scientific models of acupuncture: (1) that they will be limited or incomplete because the current state of our knowledge about the body is incomplete, and (2) that they will continue to develop as our understanding develops.

Acupuncture theories, on the other hand, are based on observations of the results of processes that are then organized in very general terms and in terms that make sense of observable results, but not the underlying processes (see Table 27-12). It should not surprise us at all when acupuncture theories are not entirely captured by current scientific models or, to put it another way, when scientific models fail to capture all aspects of acupuncture theory.

What we can see when we investigate some of the basic science underlying our understanding of acupuncture is that acupuncture exploits a wide range of bodily responses to stimulation in a systematic fashion. No single physiological process fully explains all of acupuncture's effects, and at this time, acupuncture theory may offer a more coherent model for organizing and using (while not describing the causes of) acupuncture effects.

For instance, there are now two very suggestive theories concerning the significance of channels from a scientific point of view. One theory suggests that there is a detectable difference in the electrical impedance of channels compared with that of surrounding tissue. Another suggests that described channels may correspond to the distribution and spatial organization of fascia (connective tissue) and that the network formed by interstitial connective tissue throughout the body may form the basis of the communicating channels and networks described by acupuncture (Langevin and Yandow, 2002, p. 263). Although both theories are highly suggestive, neither of these theories has been completely demonstrated to be correct, nor would they fully explain all of acupuncture's observed effects.

This situation should not surprise us. Acupuncturists have been thinking about acupuncture for over 2000 years, whereas scientists have been thinking about it for perhaps 100 years. This is not to say that all acupuncture theory is "true" in scientific terms, but that a rush to reduce its meaning to a few very basic physiological processes may ultimately limit our understanding of both acupuncture and physiology.

Are Channels and Points Real?

The contrast between scientific understanding and the traditional forms of knowledge associated with acupuncture becomes vividly clear when we contemplate the two most well-known acupuncture concepts: points and the external pathways of the regular channels. Depending on the approach guiding the research—and, perhaps, the disposition of the researcher or the interpreter of the data—it can be concluded that either there is no such thing as an acupuncture point or channel at all, or that channel theory represents a reasonably accurate description of a collection of interacting structures and processes.

From a reductionistic point of view the impulse is to clearly establish an absolute physical structure that correlates precisely to all aspects of the acupuncture model. It was this impulse that led to the tragedy and travesty of the Korean researcher Bong Han, who became a virtual cultural hero in Korea during the 1960s because of his reported discovery of Bong Han corpuscles, distinct tissue structures that were found only at acupuncture points and along channels. These were later shown to be artifacts of microscopic slide preparation, and Bong Han committed suicide. Of course, the entire modern practice of pathology, for example, is based on the systematic artifacts introduced when devitalized tissues removed from the living body are manipulated by chemical and mechanical processes and rendered in a two-dimensional plane of microscopic slide preparations.

Although there is research suggesting that the areas defined as acupuncture points and external channels may have features associated with them that are distinctive (and that distinguish them from other areas of the body's surface), there is nothing to suggest that there are any specific physical structures corresponding precisely to points and channels. Instead there is research indicating that the regions described by acupuncture points are particularly rich in nerve bundles and small blood vessels, that the tissues specified by channels and points may have different electrical characteristics than surrounding tissues, and that the organization of fascia shows distinctive characteristics underneath many acupuncture points and along channel pathways (Langevin et al , 2001; 2002) The idea that there are differentials in the electrical resistance of acupuncture points and channels is a comparatively old one, dating to research efforts as far back as 1950 (Macphearson et al, 2007). The work of Becker (1985) and Tiller (1997) has been very influential in suggesting that the activity of acupuncture channels and points may be closely related to their electrical properties. It is hypothesized by clinicians applying these ideas that variations in the electrical activity of acupuncture points and channels in disease states may aid in diagnosis of disease states, or that variations among acupuncture points, channels, and surrounding skin surface can be detected by measuring differences in electrical resistance. Although these concepts have given rise to the production, sale, and use of a vast array of electrodiagnostic devices and "point detectors," the present state of the science does not support their clinical use. This situation represents a general challenge in complementary and alternative medicine (CAM), in which many "alternative" therapies have robust data, but alternative diagnostics remain problematic.

All of these devices work by measuring galvanic current, the standing current produced by the normal skin surface. The measurement of galvanic current is achieved with what is essentially an ohmmeter. The subject holds an electrode in one hand and a probe is applied to a desired area of the skin surface. Typically direct current is supplied through the probe and measured by the meter. However, even slight variation in the pressure with which the probe is applied can cause significant fluctuations in current flow (resistance), which essentially causes a point to be detected wherever the probe is pressed firmly against the skin. For this reason, although the few well-designed studies of these phenomena are very suggestive, conclusive statements about the electrodermal properties of acupuncture channels and points remain elusive.

The idea that fascia might have a distinctive role in acupuncture phenomena has become very well established as a consequence of the work of Helene Langevin and her research team at the University of Vermont Medical School. Langevin began with a question concerning the physical basis of *de qi,* the sensation of the needle's being "grabbed" on insertion that is associated in many acupuncture traditions with the arrival of qi. She asked if there could be an actual anatomical event associated with the sensation reported by practitioners for centuries of acupuncture practice. Her initial hypotheses were that the "needle grasp," or the gripping associated with de qi phenomenon, was caused by the winding of connective tissue around the needle during rotation and that the manipulation of the needle, now coupled with connective tissue, "transmits a mechanical signal to connective tissue cells via mechanotransduction" (Langevin, Churchill, and Cipolla, 2001, p. 2275). She was able to demonstrate that the increased pull-out force associated with rotated needles was 18% greater at acupuncture points than at control points (Langevin, Churchill, Fox et al, 2001). She simultaneously proposed a mechanism through which the physical stimulation of connective tissue at the needling site might produce a variety of "downstream" changes in interstitial connective tissue that might be implicated in acupuncture effects. A later paper demonstrated a close relation between channel pathways and connective tissue and between acupuncture points and areas where intermuscular and intramuscular connective tissue was particularly dense (Langevin and Yandow, 2002).

Her work demonstrates the potential existence of a nonneural signaling system, the course and structure of which parallels ancient observations concerning channels and networks. At present the data are only suggestive. Langevin's work substantially supports the ideas of other authors who have proposed that acupuncture effects not attributable to neural events may be related to connective tissue signaling systems (Oschman, 1993).

Intriguingly, the concept of MTrPs is often presented as a science-based and medically established version of the idea of acupuncture points. MTrPs have a long history of conceptual development based on the palpation of tender regions in the musculature of patients with pain. Travell and Simons substantially organized the concept and coined the term, which is applied to points that are located on palpation and are exquisitely tender on palpation (and are typically found in areas where the patient is experiencing pain). Unlike the locations of channel and extra points, which are substantially fixed, the described locations of MTrPs are areas where MTrPs may be found if they are present. The presence of an MTrP is evidenced by acute tenderness on palpation and, in the case of an active MTrP, by local pain as well.

As is the case with acupuncture points, there is no clear evidence of any distinctive anatomical features specific to MTrPs; however, because they are conceptualized within the biomedical model, and because there are bioscience-based hypotheses concerning their production and action, MTrPs are considered to be a scientifically developed idea. The publication in 1977 by Melzack (of the Melzack-Wall gate theory of pain) of a paper claiming a 71% correlation between acupuncture points and these "trigger points" seemed to suggest that acupuncture points formed part of a well-described domain in the neurobiology of pain (Melzack et al, 1977). Since publication

of this paper, MTrPs originally described in relation to the diagnosis and treatment of myofascial pain are frequently invoked to explain or dismiss effects or models described in traditional acupuncture theory (Baldrey, 1993, 1998; Bowsher, 1998).

Ironically, as Steve Birch has been careful (2008) to point out, some 6 years after the publication of Melzack's article, Travell and Simons's textbook on trigger points contained an analysis of the Melzack et al study. Their conclusion: "Acupuncture points and trigger points are derived from vastly different concepts. The fact that a number of pain points overlap does not change that basic difference. The two terms should not be used interchangeably" (Travell et al, 1983, p. 21, quoted in Birch, 2008, p. 343).

Although it is clear from our earlier discussion that a region that is tender on palpation, or an ah shi point, is an important category of point in acupuncture therapy, it is not so clear that many, or even a majority, of acupuncture points used in the treatment of pain are equivalent to trigger points. This issue has been well demonstrated. A careful analysis of Melzack's assertions (Birch, 1999, 2003), suggests that the actual correlation between trigger points and the acupuncture points examined by Melzack that are actually used for the treatment of pain is approximately 18%.

As suggested by Birch, however, the desire to establish that acupuncture points fall fully within the domain described by MTrPs seems to be deeply compelling to segments of the medical community. The unsuccessful attempt of Dorsher (2008) to rebut Birch's analysis of Melzack et al by insisting that the majority of acupuncture points are directly equivalent to trigger points is an example of this determination.

In the end it is important to remember that acupuncture points may be channels points, extra points, or ah shi points. It is clear that the ah shi point and the MTrP are almost exactly equivalent in concept. They both are present when they elicit pain on palpation and are not present when they do not. Channel points or extra points may be painful on palpation and may even act as ah shi points, but their clinical application is not limited to pain, nor are they present only when painful. From this point of view, acupuncture and trigger point therapy exploit similar physical observations with regard to exceptionally tender myofascial points. The close agreement of the trigger point theory and the theory of ah shi points suggests that an equivalent physiological phenomena has been independently observed by two very different traditions of clinical practice. However, the conceptualization of acupuncture points as purely MTrPs limits the complete understanding of acupuncture channels, channel points, and extra points.

Although it is very clear that acupuncture channels and points as traditionally described do not define new or distinct structures unknown to science, it is quite likely that they describe relations among existing tissue and processes that may cooperate and interact in ways that are not presently completely understood.

How Does Acupuncture Work?

Acupuncture, like any therapy, must interact with existing anatomy and physiology to produce its effects. There are a number of well-described and scientifically demonstrated models of the way in which acupuncture might achieve its effects. What is very clear is that acupuncture effects are the consequence not of a single physiological process, but rather of a complex dynamic of local tissue, vascular, and CNS-mediated neuroendocrine events.

Birch's description of the "splinter effect"(Birch et al, 1999, p. 163) illustrates the complex range of vascular events that occur when the body encounters a common injury. This model suggests that many of the physiological responses to acupuncture are quite common to the body's response to injury with any sharp object, hence the splinter effect. The splinter effect captures the potential complexity surrounding such an obviously "simple" event as insertion of an acupuncture needle. Birch presents his concept of the splinter effect to illustrate a range of local and regional vascular effects that can occur with acupuncture (Table 27-13). The splinter effect involves a series of vascular responses to acupuncture that are equivalent to the changes provoked by any tissue damage with a sharp object. Local vascular effects are one of the many changes provoked by acupuncture.

Based on his interpretation of the research data, Ma has created a useful description of seven specific events or "chain reactions" that acupuncture activates in both local tissue and the CNS (Ma et al, 2005, p. 26). Although most of these are local, central responses are also described, because Ma correctly considers local and central responses to be "physiologically inseparable" (Table 27-14). Ma's

TABLE 27-13

The "Splinter" Effect

Splinter or needle pierces skin.
Vasoconstriction commences to halt blood loss and prevent circulation of any microorganisms carried on the object (duration 20 minutes).
Slightly later vasodilation increases local circulation to allow white blood cells and other cells to enter the area to assist in infection control and tissue repair (duration 2 to 3 hours).
Vasomotion begins after 1 hour. This is the pumping of microscopic vessels to allow flushing away of damaged cells and blood (duration 1 hour).
Birch's splinter effect (Birch et al, 1999) describes a series of vascular changes that support defensive, tissue repair, and metabolic processes that are typical of the body's response to a wound and illustrate the immediate vascular changes associated with acupuncture.

TABLE 27-14

Seven Local and Central Reactions to Needling an Acupuncture Point

Skin and tissue reactions at needle site, including induction of "current of injury"
Interaction between needle shaft and connective tissue
Relaxation of contracted muscle, increased circulation to site
Nociception and motor neuronal activation, neuroendocrine activation via central nervous system, segmental, and nonsegmental pathways
Blood coagulation, lymphatic circulation
Local immune response
Tissue repair (DNA synthesis) at site of injury (needling)

outline captures the elements of Birch's splinter effect and points out some additional interesting features of the physiological events provoked by acupuncture. His observations capture complex local effects such as "current of injury," which refers to the creation of a current flow produced by any lesion in tissue. In this case the acupuncture needle produces a very focused lesion with a small current (10 mA) that supports tissue growth and healing (Ma et al, 2005, p. 27).

Ma's inclusion of nociception and motorneuronal activation and neuroendocrine activation via CNS, segmental, and nonsegmental pathways captures the idea that acupuncture needling which provides a detectable level of stimulus (some styles do not) invokes a complex of neurophysiological responses that diminish pain. In particular, acupuncture is considered to invoke descending pain regulation by stimulating the production of the body's own chemical messengers for pain control.

The comparatively recent discovery in 1975 by Solomon Snyder and Candace Pert of opiate neuropeptides, which have come to be known as endorphins, shed a great deal of light on certain aspects of the process of pain control. This discovery occurred coincident with recently emergent medical interest in acupuncture and acupuncture effects in pain control. By 1977 published studies strongly suggested that acupuncture effects in pain control or acupuncture analgesia might be linked to the activity of endorphins (Mayer et al, 1977; Pomeranz et al, 1976). These studies showed that the effects of acupuncture analgesia, induced both by manual stimulation of acupuncture needles and by electrical stimulation, could be blocked by the administration of the opiate antagonist naloxone. This finding suggested that acupuncture's ability to control pain relied, at least in part, on its ability to trigger the release of endogenous opiates. Responding later to criticism that the reversal of acupuncture analgesia by the administration of naloxone was insufficient to validate the hypothesis that acupuncture analgesia was produced by endorphins, Pomeranz (1988) provided a list of 17 distinct lines of experimental evidence that support the acupuncture analgesia–endorphin hypothesis. Six examples of these lines of experimentation are provided in Table 27-15.

Based on these data, it is conventionally accepted that many of acupuncture's perceived effects in the direct reduction of pain are likely mediated by the production of endogenous opiates. This conclusion may be overly general in light of the specific nature of the evidence that supports it; however, the assertion that endorphin secretion lies at the root of acupuncture effects is still a popular one.

Functional magnetic resonance imaging (fMRI) has been applied to the investigation of acupuncture since the late 1990s. Within the limitations of the technology, which includes limited access to the body and the need for the subject to remain immobile during data collection, fMRI studies of acupuncture have produced intriguing results. One of the earliest studies presented the dramatic conclusion that there might be a direct correlation between the stimulation of an acupuncture point and cortical activation (Cho, 1998). What appeared initially to be evidence of the specificity of the action of acupuncture points, as demonstrated by regional neural activation, was later seen to be a comparatively typical response to needling. Over the years, the preponderance of evidence has suggested that acupuncture effects revealed by fMRI need to be understood in terms of the role of the CNS in processing the signals produced by the acupuncture stimulus.

TABLE 27-15

Examples of Experimental Evidence Supporting the Endorphin Hypothesis for Acupuncture Analgesia

- Different opiate antagonists block acupuncture analgesia.
- Rats with endorphin deficiency show poor acupuncture analgesia.
- Mice with genetic deficiency in opiate receptors show poor acupuncture analgesia.
- When endorphins are protected from enzymatic degradation acupuncture analgesia is enhanced.
- Transference or cross circulation of cerebral spinal fluid from an animal with induced acupuncture analgesia to a second animal will produce acupuncture analgesia, and this effect is blocked by naloxone.
- Lesions of the periaqueductal gray, an important endorphin site, eliminates acupuncture analgesia.

Adapted from Pomeranz B, Stux G: Basics of acupuncture, Springer-Verlag, 1998; Pomeranz 2000.

Other research has suggested that traditional Chinese needling techniques that elicit "de qi" can create neural deactivation of the limbic system in a way that can benefit patients with chronic pain (Hui et al, 2000, 2006).

This line of inquiry has produced research showing that patients with carpal tunnel syndrome respond to acupuncture very differently than healthy subjects. Patients experiencing the pain of carpal tunnel syndrome have been shown to respond to acupuncture stimulation with neural deactivation of the limbic system, which can be hyperactivated in chronic pain conditions (Napadow et al, 2007). Concurrent activation of the lateral hypothalamic area, a region critical to the release of endogenous opiates, which are the body's pain control system, also occurs. This information has been interpreted to suggest that patients with pain respond differently to acupuncture than do healthy individuals.

SAFETY OF ACUPUNCTURE

In a clinical setting patient safety is of critical importance. Although substantial work remains to be done to demonstrate the efficacy of acupuncture treatment in all areas to the degree that it has been demonstrated in the treatment of postextraction dental pain or the nausea and vomiting associated with cancer chemotherapy, the data on the clinical safety of acupuncture are exceptionally strong. A recent analysis (Birch, 2004a, 2004b) of published reviews of acupuncture safety conducted between 1993 and 2003 indicates that acupuncture is a comparatively safe therapy. This is not to suggest that serious adverse events cannot occur with acupuncture, but these are quite rare. Pneumothorax, for example, was found to have occurred twice in the course of almost a quarter million treatments (Ernst et al, 2001).

Although a comprehensive review of findings in relation to acupuncture safety lies beyond the scope of this chapter, it is important to point out that emerging data continue to confirm the safety of clinical acupuncture. A recent study presented to the Society for Integrative Oncology at its 2006 Boston meetings demonstrated the safety of acupuncture in patient populations with exceptionally low platelet counts (well below 50 μMol/mL), a population typically excluded from acupuncture based on surgical guidelines applied to acupuncture without clinical evidence (Taormina, 2006). (Table 27-16).

Considering the number of patients treated (estimated 9-12 million treatments per year [in the United States]) and the number of needles used per treatment (estimated average of 6-8), "there are ... remarkably few serious complications" (American Medical Association, 1981).

From Lytle, 1993, quoted in Birch, 2004a.

TABLE 27-16

Acupuncture Adverse Events

Minor	Serious
Bleeding or bruising	Organ puncture (pneumothorax)
Pain	Infection (*Staphylococcus*, hepatitis B virus)
Transient nerve damage	Spinal lesions
Feelings of tiredness	Syncope

One of the advantages of acupuncture is that the incidence of adverse effects is substantially lower than that of many drugs or other accepted medical procedures used for the same conditions. As an example, musculoskeletal conditions, such as fibromyalgia, myofascial pain, and tennis elbow, or epicondylitis, are conditions for which acupuncture may be beneficial. These painful conditions are often treated with, among other things, anti-inflammatory medications (aspirin, ibuprofen, etc.) or with steroid injections. Both medical interventions have a potential for deleterious side effects but are still widely used and are considered acceptable treatments. The evidence supporting these therapies is no better than that for acupuncture. ◌

From National Institutes of Health: Acupuncture, *NIH Consens Statement* 15(5):9, 1997.

CLINICAL EFFICACY OF ACUPUNCTURE

The clinical application of acupuncture has been an object of concerted research efforts in China and Japan since the mid-twentieth century. More recently substantial research initiatives in this area have been undertaken in the United States and Europe as well, and these have developed rapidly in terms of quality and quantity in the last 25 years.

There has been a corresponding increase in the volume of publication on acupuncture research. Since 1970 reports of 1077 clinical trials of acupuncture have been published in indexed journals. Of these, 756 have been randomized controlled trials. Two hundred of these were published between 1970 and 1995, 89 were published between 1995 and 2001, and 467 have been published since 2001. Although the creation of new CAM journals accommodated the publication of scientifically correct, but not politically correct, studies during the 1990s and first part of this decade, the era of an "alternative medical literature" is ending with the growing acceptance of CAM and acupuncture studies in the regular medical literature.

The actual and perceived quality of such research can vary widely. As is the case for medical systems, research standards—even for scientific research—are subject to cultural influences. Whereas the randomized,

placebo-controlled, double-blind clinical trial is the definitive standard for an unambiguous biomedical recognition of pharmaceutical efficacy, not all societies require or encourage their medical communities to secure knowledge in this fashion. In addition, the simple matter of the accessibility of research data, and the more complex issue of the acceptability of such data, are both deeply influenced by the language and location of data publication. All of these factors can present challenges and obstacles to the effective design, availability, and use of research.

There is a history of productive acupuncture research in the United States dating from the early 1970s as the diplomatic and cultural exchange was restored with President Nixon's visit to China. Acupuncture piqued the imaginations of American physicians and researchers, especially in relation to pain control, and basic science research and small clinical studies were carried out. The establishment in the United States of the Office of Alternative Medicine (OAM) in 1991 under the National Institutes of Health (NIH) led to a distinct increase in the quality and scope of acupuncture research, particularly clinical research, in the United States and, to some extent, abroad.

The OAM hosted conferences dealing with methodological considerations in the field of alternative medicine, and at each of these, acupuncture research occupied an important place. The Workshop on Acupuncture sponsored by the OAM in cooperation with the U.S. Food and Drug Administration (FDA) in 1994 was crucial to the continued development of acupuncture in the United States. The event was research based, and members of the acupuncture medical and scientific community gave presentations detailing the safety of acupuncture needles and the apparent clinical efficacy of acupuncture. These presentations formed the core of a petition that led, in March 1996, to the reclassification of acupuncture needles by the FDA from a class III or experimental device to a class II or medical device for use by qualified practitioners with special controls (sterility and single use).

In November 1997 the NIH convened a Consensus Development Conference on Acupuncture that included 2 days of presentations of the evidence for the safety and efficacy of acupuncture for the treatment of specific conditions. This evidence was presented by experts in the field to a panel that reviewed reports of research on the use of acupuncture in the treatment of a wide variety of conditions. The panel reached the following formal conclusion:

> Acupuncture as a therapeutic intervention is widely practiced in the United States. Although there have been many studies of its potential usefulness, many of these studies provide equivocal results because of design, sample size, and other factors. The issue is further complicated by inherent difficulties in the use of appropriate controls, such as placebos and sham acupuncture groups. However, promising results have emerged, for example, showing efficacy of acupuncture in adult postoperative and chemotherapy nausea and vomiting and in postoperative dental pain. There

are other situations such as addiction, stroke rehabilitation, headache, menstrual cramps, tennis elbow, fibromyalgia, myofascial pain, osteoarthritis, low back pain, carpal tunnel syndrome, and asthma, in which acupuncture may be useful as an adjunct treatment or an acceptable alternative or be included in a comprehensive management program. Further research is likely to uncover additional areas where acupuncture interventions will be useful. (NIH, 1997)

Given that less than 2 years previously acupuncture needles had still been considered an experimental device in the eyes of the federal government, this marked a significant degree of progress for acupuncture in the West.

Many of the studies presented at the Workshop on Acupuncture sponsored by the OAM in 1994 were also presented at the consensus development workshop in 1997. For the most part the best clinical research could be clustered into five specific areas that seemed to represent the best and most positive research related to acupuncture. These areas were (1) antiemesis treatment, (2) the management of acute and chronic pain, (3) substance abuse treatment, (4) the treatment of paralysis caused by stroke, and (5) the treatment of respiratory disease. In addition, there are areas such as female infertility, breech presentation, menopause, depression, and urinary dysfunction in which acupuncture was able to show good clinical results (Birch et al, 1996) (Table 27-17).

A review of the list of clinical conditions presented in the consensus statement reveals that all but four are pain conditions. Pain control is the one application of acupuncture that has been well accepted by the conventional medical community in Europe and the United States for many years. This area became very visible in the United States in the 1970s as a result of Chinese reports on acupuncture anesthesia (more correctly termed *acupuncture analgesia*) that were coincident with the restoration of diplomatic relations with China. The fact that the effects of acupuncture on pain appeared to be readily explainable in terms of familiar Western constructs already associated with the understanding of pain (e.g., gate-control theory, counterirritation, trigger points, and the actions of endorphins) provided an acceptable mechanism for acupuncture's effects on pain and further legitimized this area of exploration. As a result, this is one of the most widely researched applications of acupuncture. However, it has been not without problems.

Some of the problems that are typical of research on acupuncture treatments for pain, as well as acupuncture therapy in general, are exemplified by the results of two early meta-analyses of studies that examined the use of acupuncture in the management of chronic pain. The first was conducted by pooling data from 14 studies that carried out randomized controlled trials of acupuncture to treat chronic pain and that measured their outcomes in terms of the number of patients whose condition was improved (Patel et al, 1989). This meta-analysis reached a number of conclusions concerning the relationship of study design to research outcomes and concluded that acupuncture compared favorably with placebo and conventional treatment.

A second meta-analysis reviewed 51 studies and compared the quality of published controlled clinical trials in terms of research design and other specific factors, including randomization, single and double blinding, and numbers of subjects. This meta-analysis concluded that, of the studies reviewed, those with results favorable to acupuncture were more poorly designed than those that found negative results for acupuncture. The evidence suggested that the efficacy of acupuncture as a treatment for chronic pain is doubtful (ter Riet et al, 1990).

A careful review of the ter Reit et al meta-analysis by Delis and Morris (1993) suggested that its authors had "included studies which did not meet their criteria," such as a study that was not controlled and a study in which laser light was used instead of acupuncture needles. This finding prompted Delis and Morris to conduct their own analysis and to reanalyze the studies examined by ter Riet et al in relation to a number of factors, including investigator training and the appropriateness of treatment. Their meta-analysis showed a trend toward improvement in study design over time, which suggested that many poorly designed acupuncture studies might best be viewed as preliminary efforts by investigators who were insufficiently familiar with the modality to design effective studies.

All three of these meta-analyses pointed out significant issues in relation to acupuncture study design. Besides questions concerning randomization, blinding, placebo control, and sample size, a variety of questions

---

TABLE 27-17

Conditions for which Acupuncture is Proven Effective

1. Adult postoperative and chemotherapy-induced nausea and vomiting
2. Postoperative dental pain
3. Addiction
4. Stroke rehabilitation
5. Headache
6. Menstrual cramps
7. Tennis elbow
8. Fibromyalgia
9. Myofascial pain
10. Osteoarthritis
11. Low back pain
12. Carpal tunnel syndrome
13. Asthma

The consensus statement developed at the 1997 Consensus Development Conference on Acupuncture mentioned 13 clinical conditions for which acupuncture showed either efficacy or usefulness as an adjunctive or alternative treatment. Of these, only three—addiction, postoperative dental pain, and osteoarthritis—had been targets of National Institutes of Health–funded research. By 2007 an additional seven areas had been examined by NIH-funded studies: carpal tunnel syndrome, fibromyalgia, headache, low back pain, menstrual cramps, myofascial pain, and nausea and vomiting (MacPherson et al, 2008).

emerged pertinent to the practice of acupuncture as a distinct modality. Is the investigator trained in acupuncture? Is the acupuncture treatment appropriate for the condition? Does the study allow for adjusting the treatment to the individual patient's needs according to traditional diagnostics? Are outcome measures clear? Is placebo or sham acupuncture used, and how is it administered?

Of all the debated areas in acupuncture research, this last has received the most attention. The problem of how to provide a sham treatment in acupuncture is a vexing one. In herbal studies a capsule of inert material that appears similar to the capsule of the medication being investigated can be provided to the patient. Because the patient cannot tell the difference between the two capsules, he or she is effectively blind to the use of a placebo. In acupuncture the problem becomes rather more complex. This is because the patient may be able to observe and feel all the sensations associated with either a true or a false treatment.

Proposed solutions vary from comparing real acupuncture with other modalities to carefully selecting a treatment with few effects (Vincent, 1993) or selecting acupuncture points that are entirely irrelevant (BRITS method) to the conditions being treated. In addition, methods of providing simulated acupuncture have been used successfully (Lao et al, 1999).

If a clinical trial compares acupuncture to an inactive treatment that does not involve the insertion of needles, the trial may be criticized because the act of simply inserting needles into a subject may have a greater placebo effect than other inactive interventions. Thus the study might not be able to determine whether the observed effects of acupuncture were greater than those of a placebo because the effects observed in the study might only be the result of acupuncture's being a better placebo. A second criticism leveled at failure to test acupuncture against a control that involves an insertive sham is that hypothesized effects such as diffuse noxious inhibitory control (an aspect of descending pain regulation systems) might be the actual cause of the observed effects rather than any specific acupuncture treatment.

The level of sophistication at which the problem of designing studies with appropriate inactive treatments, shams, or placebo acupuncture has been addressed has increased dramatically over the years. However, the essential characteristics of the problem remain. Some studies have produced results that show the selected form of "sham" acupuncture to have clinical effects that are essentially equivalent to those of "real" acupuncture, and these will be discussed later.

Understanding of the criteria for study design has improved substantially. The publication of Birch's paper (2004b) presenting 64 critical points that must be assessed in the design or review of controlled trials of acupuncture, the routine application of standards such as the Jadad score to published studies in meta-analyses, and the improvement of the quality of meta-analyses (and the resultant improvement of study design) as a consequence of the work of the Cochrane Collaboration have all produced improvements in the quality of acupuncture research.

Acupuncture and Pain

The control of pain is considered to be a major area for the clinical application of acupuncture, and although some of the research in this area has been problematic, a number of studies strongly indicate the importance of acupuncture in pain management. As we have seen, one of the conclusions of the Consensus Development Conference on Acupuncture was that acupuncture could be demonstrated to be efficacious for reduction of postoperative dental pain. One study showed that patients receiving acupuncture required less postoperative analgesia after oral surgery than a group receiving a sham acupuncture treatment (Lao et al, 1995).

Although patients frequently seek out acupuncture for low back pain and acupuncturists regard low back pain as an area in which they provide effective treatment, the research evidence produced over the years remains equivocal. A systematic review of randomized controlled trials determined that "acupuncture for acute back pain has not been well studied" and that the value of acupuncture in treating chronic back pain "remains in question" (Cherkin et al, 2003, p. 905). Birch's review of reviews (2004a) found that only two out of the seven reviews examined indicated that acupuncture had been shown to be effective for low back pain. The remaining reviews found promising or contradictory results.

A 2005 meta-analysis (Manheimer et al) concluded that acupuncture provided short-term relief of chronic low back pain. In addition it was concluded that true acupuncture worked better than sham acupuncture. The authors also stated that they could not reach a conclusion about the effectiveness of acupuncture compared with other active treatments.

It is against this background that published results of the findings of the German acupuncture trials are particularly striking (Haake et al, 2007). These trials were conducted from 2001 through 2005 and involved 340 outpatient practices. In all, 1162 patients were treated for low back pain and received ten 30-minute sessions of acupuncture each week. The study offered acupuncture delivered according to TCM principles (administered by physicians trained in acupuncture) and two control treatments. One of the control treatments was sham acupuncture, which was provided by needling areas that were identified as "nonacupuncture points" (Molsberger et al, 2006), and the other was conventional therapy consisting of drugs, physical therapy, or exercise. At the end of the study when patients were assessed 6 months after concluding treatment, the response rate for acupuncture was 48%, whereas the response rate for conventional therapy was 27%. These statistically significant results demonstrated unequivocally that acupuncture could be more effective than conventional therapy in the treatment of low back pain. The greatest surprise lay in the patient response to sham acupuncture, which was 44%, almost as high as the response to true acupuncture treatment. These results, while substantiating acupuncture's claim to therapeutic effectiveness, have raised significant questions about the importance of specific point location in effective acupuncture treatment.

Because the points chosen for sham acupuncture were typically 5 cm away from any described acupuncture points and were needled shallowly (3 mm), the results of this study strongly suggest that there may be little importance to needling at traditionally described needling sites or that, at least, the degree of specificity implied by traditional locations is not relevant to this acupuncture effect. These are provocative findings.

Over the years, a number of studies have suggested that the pain of osteoarthritis seems to respond well to acupuncture (Dickens et al, 1989; Junnila, 1982; Thomas et al, 1991), and one study suggested a significant cost benefit when the use of acupuncture removed the need for surgical intervention (Christensen et al, 1992). The implications of these studies have led to the increased commitment of resources to the investigation of the potential role of acupuncture in the management of osteoarthritis and the production of promising clinical data (Berman et al, 1999). This work culminated in 2004 with publication of the results of a large-scale trial of acupuncture involving 570 subjects who received either acupuncture, sham acupuncture, or patient education. The study's authors concluded that acupuncture provided improvement in function and pain relief when used as an adjunctive therapy for osteoarthritis (Berman et al, 2004).

Headache pain is often treated with acupuncture. Twenty years ago a controlled trial of the use of acupuncture in the management of migraines was conducted that enrolled 30 patients who had chronic migraine headaches. Acupuncture was significantly effective in controlling the pain of migraine headaches (Vincent, 1989). A recent pragmatic trial of acupuncture for chronic headache and migraine demonstrated clinical benefits for patients and low costs (Vickers et al, 2004).

Acupuncture in Other Clinical Areas

The 1997 Consensus Development Conference concluded that acupuncture has been demonstrated to be efficacious for the treatment of adult postoperative and chemotherapy-related nausea and vomiting. Research in the area of antiemesis revolves around the use of the acupuncture point "inner gate" (neiguan, P6) to control nausea and vomiting. The use of this point in acupressure to control nausea and vomiting is well known, and its use to control the nausea of pregnancy with pressure bands has been determined to be effective as well (Aloysio et al, 1992). Consumer products are even available that

exploit this effect by applying light pressure to the acupuncture point in question, although their clinical usefulness remains in question. The inner gate point also has been investigated in relation to its use to control perioperative emesis resulting from premedication and anesthetic agents (Ghaly et al, 1987) and nausea and vomiting induced by cancer chemotherapy (Dundee et al, 1989, Ezzo et al, 2006). Today, the inner gate point forms the basis of many clinical acupuncture interventions to provide relief to patients receiving chemotherapy in hospital-based oncology services. The application of acupuncture in this context is so routine that in at least one metropolitan area biomedical clinicians refer to P6 as "the Sloane point," using the name of a hospital with a pioneering application of acupuncture in its oncology service.

On the basis of clinical experiences in China, acupuncture is used extensively in the United States for the management of symptoms associated with withdrawal from a variety of substances, including alcohol and cocaine. The summary conclusion reached by presenters at the 1994 OAM Workshop on Acupuncture panel on substance abuse was that early trials and empirical findings suggested positive treatment effects (Kiresuk et al, 1994). Although acupuncture continues to be widely used in this area, the research evidence remains equivocal.

Asthma continues to be a complex area in which to assess acupuncture's effectiveness. An early extensive review of acupuncture in the treatment of pulmonary disease led its author to conclude that acupuncture produced favorable effects in the management of patients with bronchial asthma, chronic bronchitis, and chronic disabling breathlessness (Jobst, 1995). Since 1996 only 12 randomized controlled trials examining acupuncture in the treatment of asthma have been conducted. Although earlier trials focused on lung function as a primary outcome measure, more recent randomized controlled trials have also evaluated acupuncture's effects on the patient's quality of life and inflammatory response. These randomized controlled trials have demonstrated significant reduction in irritability and anxiety (Mehl-Madrona et al, 2007), which may trigger asthma; reduction in days of "acute febrile disease" (Stockert et al, 2007); and reduced medication use (Bernacki, 1998; Mehl-Madrona et al, 2007). The use of acupuncture for asthma management still fares somewhat poorly in systematic reviews (McCarney et al, 2007; Passalacqua et al, 2005). McCarney et al declared that "more pilot data" should be acquired before investigators proceed to any large-scale randomized trials in this clinical area and spoke to the difficulty of developing "objective comparisons between different acupuncture types" on the basis of existing data.

A study conducted at a private fertility center in Denmark examined the timing of acupuncture treatment in in vitro fertilization to maximize the likelihood of pregnancy. The study showed that pregnancy rates were significantly higher when acupuncture was received on the day of embryo transfer. Although the control group had an ongoing pregnancy rate of 22%, the acupuncture group had a rate of 36% (Westergaard et al, 2006). Acupuncture also has shown promise in reducing the pain associated with in vitro fertilization (Sator-Katzenschlager et al, 2006) and improving its clinical outcomes.

What Acupuncture Can Treat

Although the preceding discussion reviews recent developments in clinical research into acupuncture, it may be helpful to explore the question of what conditions acupuncture can be said to treat. The answer to this question may be very broad or a very narrow depending on who provides the response. From the perspective of the acupuncturist there are very few clinical conditions that acupuncture cannot at least palliate or make more tolerable for the patient. Based on the strictest standard of clinical efficacy perhaps only conditions such as postextraction dental pain or chemotherapy-associated nausea and vomiting can be said, unequivocally, to be well treated by acupuncture. The middle ground can be captured based on an examination of two wide-ranging systematic reviews. One was completed by the WHO (2002) and included Chinese-language sources, and the other was completed by Birch et al (2004a, 2004b). Neither of these can be considered complete. The WHO document is a systematic review of controlled clinical trials for which results were published through early 1999. The Birch et al review is essentially a review of reviews and thus consolidates the data from several very rigorous reviews of acupuncture trials from the English-language literature. Both reviews assessed the research in similar ways and described acupuncture as either "effective" or "promising" in treating a given condition. Table 27-18 summarizes the findings of the two reviews. WHO reviewers evaluated 30 of 46 specific conditions examined as ones in which acupuncture had a proven or demonstrated therapeutic effect. Birch et al's stringent assessment of the evidence gleaned by other reviewers entirely omits Chinese-language publications and is purely a review of systematic reviews of randomized controlled trials. Their more stringent criteria rated acupuncture as "effective" for 4 of the 46 conditions and as "promising" for 8.

This analysis is limited, and it could appropriately be criticized on the basis of either what it has included or what it has failed to include. There are numerous promising studies, some of which have been examined here, that would support arguments for a broader and more inclusive list. The clinical experience of many acupuncturists would also support broadening this list. On the other hand, it is likely that rigorously constructed meta-analyses could fail to find compelling evidence for the usefulness of acupuncture in the management of many of these conditions. On this basis, then, the list in Table 27-18 provides a roster of the clinical domains for which comparatively robust clinical research data exist to support the use of acupuncture.

TABLE 27-18

What Acupuncture Treats

	WHO*	Birch†
Acute and Chronic Pain		
Abdominal pain	2	
Back pain (chronic low back pain)	1	1
Neck pain	1	
Biliary colic	1	
Bursitis, tendonitis	1	
Cancer pain	2	
Carpal tunnel syndrome		2
Facial pain	1	
Fibromyalgia	2	2
Joint pain related to bursitis, tendonitis, or arthritis	1, 2	2
Neuralgias (trigeminal, herpes zoster, postherpetic)	1, 2	
Pain associated with sprains, contusions, fractures	1	
Posttraumatic or postoperative pain	1	
Acute postoperative dental pain	1	1
Sciatica	1	
Tennis elbow	1	2
Other Conditions		
Allergic rhinitis	1	
Asthma	2	2
Bell palsy	2	
Dysmenorrhea	1	2
Functional gastrointestinal disorders	1, 2	
Headache	1	1
Hypertension	1	
Insomnia	2	
Mild depression	1	
Muscle spasms, tremors, tics, and contractures	2	
Nausea and/or vomiting	1	
Premenstrual syndrome	1	
Sequelae of cerebrovascular accidents (aphasia, hemiplegia)		2
Substance abuse	2	2
Temporomandibular joint dysfunction, bruxism	2	1
Overweight	2	

Acupuncture is considered to be effective in treating or ameliorating those conditions marked 1 and to show promise of clinical effectiveness in treating those marked 2.

LOOKING FORWARD

The way forward in acupuncture research includes an emergent effort to examine acupuncture in pragmatic terms. Many clinical trials of acupuncture, in order to isolate its effects, reduce variables, and control for placebo effects, apply a clinical research model—the randomized controlled trial—that is designed to establish the "efficacy" of a pharmaceutical agent. Although such trials can help us learn more about what aspects or components of acupuncture treatment do or do not have specific effects, they do not offer much guidance to the clinician or the patient, because the acupuncture treatments they examine are often different from the acupuncture therapy that occurs in normal practice.

Hammerschlag (2003) speaks to the heart of this matter when he asserts the need to reassess the importance of a central tenet of evidence based medicine: that acupuncture should outperform placebo and suggests that it is time to think about research that considers whole systems of care rather than modalities.

Many researchers see pragmatic trials as a potential solution that addresses this issue. These trials examine interventions that are very close to normal treatment approaches and typically involve comparisons with conventional therapy. This type of trial provides information that is valuable to patients and clinicians. The findings of German acupuncture trials, which compared acupuncture with conventional care, resulted in acupuncture's becoming a covered therapy for chronic low back pain in Germany, based on the clear demonstration of acupuncture's superiority to conventional care. This occurred even though the trials problematized the question of the specific location of acupuncture points, which suggests that shallow needling might be as effective as deeper needling, and failed to control for nonspecific effects.

What is striking as we observe the past several decades of acupuncture research is that the insights afforded us by technological advances offer greater knowledge of human anatomy and physiology and also broaden our appreciation of the complex models advanced by acupuncture theory. Although it is far too early to say whether all propositions of the systems described in the first section of this chapter are based on "real" anatomical or physiological processes, recent discoveries emerging out of research into the properties of fascia or into neural activation based on MRI suggest the existence of complex and interacting systems and may ultimately validate many of the insights provided by acupuncture theory.

The challenge we confront is simultaneously to pursue scientific inquiry and a comprehensive engagement with traditions of acupuncture theory and practice.

⊖ Please refer to the Evolve website at http://evolve.elsevier.com/Micozzi/complementary for a chapter on Tibetan Medicine by Kevin V. Ergil.

⊖ Chapter References can be found on the Evolve website at http://evolve.elsevier.com/Micozzi/complementary/

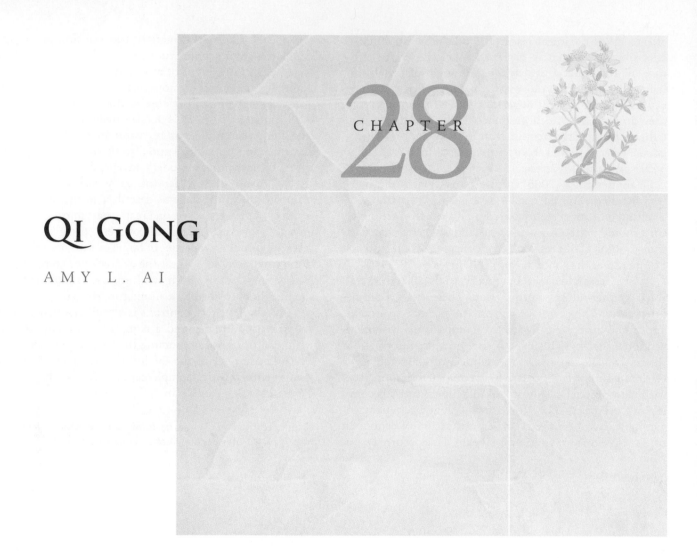

CHAPTER

28

QI GONG

AMY L. AI

This chapter provides an introduction to *qi gong* or *qigong* (QG; also Qi Gong, QiGong), a type of energy-based health practice anchored in an energy-centered worldview (Ai et al, 2001). Along with herbs, acupuncture, and other therapeutic approaches, QG is one aspect of traditional Chinese medicine (TCM), with a rich history spanning thousands of years. The primary goal of this chapter is to summarize its important components and to help the reader better understand this ancient healing art.

It is impossible to understand the rationale for QG without a knowledge of its primary guiding philosophy, *Daoism* (Taoism). In its Chinese character, *dao* refers to the way, or the universal order, to be followed in life and in nature (Ai, 2003). In a cosmic sense, dao refers to the ultimate, indefinable principle underlying all movements—the process involving every aspect in the universe. This chapter therefore begins with a discussion of the concepts and basics of QG, then introduces the philosophical foundation, Daoism, and next presents its influence on TCM and QG. Finally, the contemporary scientific investigation of QG is summarized.

DEFINITION

Qi gong is the phonetic juxtaposition of two Chinese characters: *qi*, meaning "flow of air" in a more literal sense or "vital energy" in a more symbolic sense, and *gong*, meaning "perseverant practice" (Ai, 2003). The translation of the concept of QG has been influenced by different perspectives. American QG master Cohen (1997), trained by Chinese teachers, referred to it as "working with the life energy, learning how to control the flow and distribution of qi to improve the health and harmony of mind and body." Shen (1986) considered QG as an ancient therapeutic martial art. Qian (1982), an advocate of the scientific study of QG in China and the American-trained leading physicist there, defined QG as an ancient system for self-development that involves movement, breathing exercises, and conscious control of body energy. Integrating these perspectives, I consider QG as an energy-based health practice and healing process involving deep breath and meditation with movement (internal or external) that may provide potential medical benefits.

Notably, the idea of the flowing vital energy is shared by many non-Western legacies, as well as the shamanic tradition in Western culture, which is traced back to ancient Egypt (Graham, 1990). Some indigenous people in Africa call it "num," whereas Native American tribes speak of the "Holy Wind" (Cohen, 1997). Indians term it "prana," and Russians name it "bioplasma" in contemporary technical terms (Willis, 1991). The uniqueness of the Chinese concept of qi lies in (1) its focus on holistic health in terms of multilevel energy patterns rather than solely on the physical body or on an external divinity or ghost-like spirit, (2) its pathway of qi circulation (i.e., the acupuncture channel system consisting of several hundred points) (Shen, 1986), and (3) its rationale, which resembles an accepted tenet of quantum theory in modern physics (Capra, 1991). In this view, relations and activities of energy patterns are seen as fundamental in both human nature and the universe. The term *qi* refers not only to the essence of all material objects, but also to their interactions in terms of the rhythmic alternation of two fundamental forces, *yin* and *yang*, similar to positive and negative charges in modern chemistry. This ying-yang relation is elaborated further in the next section.

HISTORY

The inclusion of the qi system in health and healing was documented 4000 to 5000 years ago in the classic book of TCM, the *Yellow Emperor's Inner Classic (Hung De Nei Jing Su Wen)* (Liao, 1992). The *Inner Classic* system viewed the human in both cosmic and geographical terms. It explicitly rejected earlier supernatural and magical healing and instead described illness and therapies in terms of pernicious and emotional disturbances. This system is based on principles describing the movement of qi in the human body and its relationships to physical and mental health. The *Inner Classic* recommended the earliest documented form of QG, Dao Yi, as a healing exercise to cure chills and fevers and to achieve the state of a tranquilly content, sagelike person who is full of vital spirit (Cohen, 1997).

In many early forms of QG, slow-moving dance reproducing animal postures was used to promote animal-like vitality, balance, grace, and strength. The founder of Daoist philosophy, Lao Zi (Lao Tzu), first described basic QG principles that had been followed by practitioners for centuries, such as concentration, emptiness of desire, quiescence, flexibility, and infantlike breath. In the fourth century BC, Zhuang Zi, Lao Zi's follower, wrote about the role of infantlike breathing and physical exercise in promoting longevity and described a sage intent on extending his life (Despeux, 1989). In the second century AD the TCM doctor Hua Tuo was known for both his famous anesthetic herb formula, Ma Fu San, and his QG practice, Five Animal Plays, based on the movements of the tiger, deer, bear, monkey, and bird. Throughout Chinese history, many forms of QG have been developed

among Daoists, Buddhists, TCM practitioners, and martial artists (Shen, 1986).

According to Cohen (1997), QG first reached Europe in the late eighteenth and early nineteenth centuries. In 1779 the Jesuit P.M. Cibot translated Daoist QG exercise and respiratory techniques in terms of cong-fou (kung fu, kong-fu, gongfu) into French with illustrations. His translated text later became influential for Per Henrik Ling (1776-1839), who founded medical gymnastics on the basis of a vital energy theory to promote health. Described by Dally as "a sort of photographic image of Taoist kung-fu" (Cohen, 1997), Ling's theory and practice laid the foundation for contemporary physical education. The idea of vital energy was dropped, however, in the clash with modern materialistic science.

In the East, in contrast, the culturally rooted legacy of qi has never been abandoned, despite the rapid changes in political regimes in China during the twentieth century. The initial use of QG in the formal medical profession began in the 1950s, when some QG rehabilitation institutes established by the Chinese government demonstrated the therapeutic effects of internal QG in treating hypertension and neurasthenia. The late 1970s witnessed a true renaissance in the practice of medical QG or QG therapy for the purpose of medical care and rehabilitation. An influential advocate was an elderly master, Guo Lin, who had persistently practiced Daoist QG after she developed advanced uterine cancer in her thirties (Shen, 1986). She and her students used QG to heal diseases with diagnoses in Western medicine, especially cancer. Since then, numerous styles of QG therapy have been invented, all of which share the essential principles of ancient Daoism and its expression in TCM.

CURRENT CLASSIFICATION AND DEVELOPMENT OF QI GONG

In practice, QG consists of two foundational forms: (1) *dynamic* or *active* QG, which involves visible movement of the body, typically through a set of slowly enacted exercises, and (2) *meditative* or *passive* QG, which entails still positions with inner movement of the diaphragm. Essential to both are precise control of abdominal breathing, alert concentration, and a tranquil state of mind. The most well-known dynamic QG in the Western world is *t'ai chi* (tai ji). Dynamic QG also includes varied forms of martial QG (kung fu), which focus on the development of physical capacity. In contrast to Western exercise, however, dynamic QG centers on flexibility and inner strength rather than masculinity and body size. Based on different philosophical foundations, affiliated intentionality, and spiritual goals, QG can also be classified intellectually and spiritually into Daoist, Buddhist, and Confucianist forms (Dao Jia Gong, Fa Jia Gong, and Ru Jia Gong).

From a clinical perspective, QG therapy can be classified into two systems (Sancier, 1996). *Internal* QG aims to control internal qi flow, to promote one's own health, or to self-heal illness through an individual's own practice. *External* QG attempts to achieve healing by manipulating or transmitting another's qi, based on the idea that energy can be led outside or travel through a therapist's body and be conducted to other living and nonliving systems. This form of therapy is performed by a QG master whose practice has reached an advanced level or who has an inherent talent in this respect (Qian, 1982). A healer can provide qi through projection without direct contact or through other methods with contact, such as touching of acupoints, massage, and osteopathic adjustments. Diseases treated by internal QG in China include cardiovascular diseases such as essential hypertension, coronary heart disease, heart arrhythmia, rheumatic heart disease, and stroke as well as other functional and organic diseases (Cohen, 1997; Eisenberg, 1985; Sancier, 1996; Shen, 1986).

Public interest in QG spurred basic and clinical research in China during the 1980s and some international interest in its role and mechanisms in the 1990s (Cohen, 1997; Hisamitsu et al, 1996; Sancier, 1996; Shen, 1986; Tiller et al, 1995). However, relatively few clinical studies on QG's efficacy have been conducted outside China. Moreover, less documentation has been found, even in China, regarding the clinical research of external QG, except for a single case report on its experimental use as anesthesia. Heise (1993) discussed the effectiveness of t'ai chi and QG in the treatment of psychosomatic disorders in Germany. McGarry (1996) advocated the integration of Eastern perceptions of the bioenergy field into Western belief systems and approaches to therapeutic interventions in Australia.

The practice of QG became known in the United States during the 1990s. *New York Magazine* reported Dr. Mehmet Oz's experiments using American therapists during open heart surgery at Columbia-Presbyterian Medical Center (Brown, 1995). An acupoint known as yongquan (bubbling spring or KI1), at the beginning part of the kidney meridian located on the soles of the feet, was used in the application of "energy medicine." At the dawn of the new millennium, the National Institutes of Health began to fund scientific investigations of QG efficacy (Ai et al, 2001; Wu et al, 1999). Since then, dozens of randomized controlled trials (RCTs) investigating the effect of internal and external QG on health and mental health conditions have been published worldwide, alongside new systematic reviews.

PHILOSOPHICAL DIFFERENCES UNDERLYING WESTERN AND EASTERN MEDICINE

Because of the different worldviews (cosmologies; see Chapter 5) underlying Chinese medicine and modern biomedical sciences, conducting RCTs is not an easy task. The fundamental difference stems from a philosophical perspective that distinguishes aspects of Eastern and Western cultures. For the most part, the operative philosophy of science is embodied in Aristotelian empirical materialism, in which knowledge in antiquity was systematically organized into the scheme that underlies much of the Western view of the universe. The formulation of a Cartesian mind/matter *(res cogitans/res extensa)* dualism in the seventeenth century also helped bring about the birth of modern science (Ai, 1996). In this paradigm, matter as the observed object is completely separated from the scientist as an observer. Biomedicine, as the offspring of this outlook, focuses primarily on the material structure of the body, which is further broken down into systems, organs, tissues, cells, chromosomes, genes, and molecules. In this biomedical model the heart, for example, is treated as a pump, a mechanical organ with regular outputs. The diagnosis and treatment of heart disease are centered on aspects of the material organ or other levels of structure: physical, physiological, biochemical, and genetic.

In Chinese medicine, however, the heart signifies more than an anatomical organ. Strangely, the energetic concept of heart, often referred to as "heart qi" in China, also contains some function of the mind (Ai, 1996). In a modern view, this involves the brain-heart relationship, which is more explainable in terms of the heart-related functions involving neuroendocrinology, immunology, and the pituitary-hypothalamic-adrenal axis. Without these scientific concepts, the ancient Chinese perspective organized all these phenomena in a system of vital energy movement. The circulation of qi within the human body and its interactions thus became essential to theory. Accordingly, the QG modality was built on an energy-centered worldview, a Daoist view that differs remarkably from that supporting contemporary Western medicine, both ontologically and epistemologically.

DAOIST DIALECTIC VIEW OF THE WORLD AND HUMANS

ENERGY-CENTERED OUTLOOK

More than 2000 years ago, Daoism crystallized one of many ancient intellectual legacies of the Chinese culture. The emergence of Daoism echoes the historical environment of its founder, Lao Zi, who is believed to have lived between 571 and 471 BC during the Spring and Autumn Period of the late Zhou dynasty, which lasted for 242 years. This historical period was marked by chaotic and ceaseless battles among hundreds of warring dukes and by schools of varied philosophies. Reality was perceived by Daoists in complex relations; the truth in human nature and in universal phenomena was nothing short of ambiguity, paradox, and contradiction. Ancient Daoists sought to achieve a conscious awareness and philosophical understanding of universal principles, or the manner and process of change that underlies all cosmological processes. By embodying the invisible but perceivable image of "flow of air," the word *qi* was used as a vivid metaphor to illustrate the changing energy patterns in universal processes.

In ancient Greece, Aristotle described the world as a systematic structure, and Democritus pioneered the concept of atoms as the basic unit of natural substances. These philosophical perspectives established the fundamental materialistic worldview underlying all modern sciences, in particular classic physical theory. Ancient Daoists, however, were more interested in mastering the order of ever-changing patterns that explained the interactive phenomena at multiple levels in nature, including humans (Ai, 2003). Concurrently, they observed that the transformation of energy is the unifying principle or force among all beings. The ontological difference between the outlooks of the Greek and Chinese traditions was noted by a modern physicist, Fritjof Capra. In *The Tao of Physics,* he suggests that the Daoist ontology resembles that of quantum physics (Capra, 1991). Both traditions propose that all forms of substance are nothing but the materialization of energy. Both view the dynamic patterns of energy as the primary and continual forces in nature, whereas substantive aspects are secondary.

Nonbeing as the Fundamental

Without scientific terminology, Lao Zi used *nonbeing,* or *wu* in Chinese, and *being,* or *yu,* to summarize the energetic and substantive aspects of all things. An original energy in the pure form of nonbeing was considered as the primary force that generated the materialistic universe, the sum of all being. In his world-famous *Dao De Jing (Tao Te Ching),* Lao Zi wrote: "All things are born of being; *being is born of nonbeing.* All living things are formed by being, and shaped by their environment, growing if nourished well by virtue, the being from nonbeing" (emphasis added). In other words, an invisible energetic force as the origin of the world existed before all material substances emerged. Accordingly, the Daoist worldview considers invisible energy movements as constant, ultimate reality, whereas visible materialistic aspects of the world are transit phenomena in a cosmos sense. For example, each human body has its circle between life and death, but the energetic movement of its particles would continue at different levels beyond this circle.

The Chinese character *yu* can be translated as *something exists.* In contrast, *wu* can be translated or interpreted as *nothing exists* or *nothingness.* The latter interpretation is somewhat similar to the Buddhist *nothingness* or *emptiness.* Both concepts refer to images of reality, mean that "nothing exists," and are perceived through intuition rather than empirical observation. However, the Daoist nonbeing tends to differ from the Buddhist emptiness in both perspective and content. The Daoist concept concerns the nature of ultimate reality itself. It conceptualizes the origin of the universe or all objective being in the form of energetic nonbeing, or *wu,* or in modern terms, a void field filled with energetic movement. The Buddhism concept *emptiness* involves subjective reflection to that ultimate reality. It offers a cognitive solution as detachment to human suffering through the emptiness of the mind. Taking Lao Zi's dialectic view, therefore, *nothingness* could imply something within, such as moving energy, or Daoist qi, or the awareness of spiritual truth through Buddhist liberation, or *Nirvana,* and enlightenment. This ontological difference shapes the different focus of meditative QG, as described later.

Daoist Dialectical Epistemology

The *being* versus *nonbeing* relation in the Lao Zi excerpt implies not only the Daoist ontology concerning the nature of the universe, including humans, but its dialectical epistemology as well. Capra (1991) noted that the Eastern tradition appreciates intuitive thinking above rational thinking more than its Western counterpart. Despite their basic outlook shared with modern physicists, Daoists do not employ *form* logical thinking, empirical observation, and deductive reasoning. Rather, their way of knowing is based on dialectical thinking, intuitive imagery, and cyclical patterning. Because of their puzzling dialectics and multiplicity of meanings, some Daoist passages seem to be logically incomprehensible. As Lao Zi said in *Dao De Jing:* "When living by the Tao, awareness of self is not required, for in this way of life, the self exists, and is also non-existent, being conceived of, not as existentiality, nor as non-existent." Stated abstractly, in this passage, fact *A* holds with both *B* and *non-B.* Seemingly contradictory arguments such as this are expressed throughout his book, because paradox and mutuality are a part of truth in the Daoist philosophy.

The Daoist dialectic way of circular reasoning presents a stark contrast to the laws of *form logic* tracing back to ancient Greek, and particularly Aristotelian, reasoning (Peng et al, 1999). Central to the latter are three laws: *identity, noncontradiction,* and *the excluded middle.* The first law claims that everything must be identical with itself. The second law insists that no statement can be both true and false. The third law declares that *A* is either *B* or *non-B.* For example, in *The Republic,* Plato recorded a conversation about beauty and ugliness with Socrates that clearly differs from the previous Lao Zi passage: "Since fair is the opposite of ugly, they are two." "Of course." "Since they are two, isn't each also one?" "That is so as well." "The same argument also applies then to justice and injustice, good and bad, and all the forms" (Bloom, 1968). Accordingly, at least until recently, the order of the world in the Western perspective has tended to follow a path of *certainty, specification,* and *a linear logic that links cause to effect.* (For example, if *A* leads to *B* and *B* leads to *C,* then *A* also leads to *C.*) Form logic defines the relative truth concerning the contingent reality in structures, which allows natural law to be comprehensible within specified domains. It eventually paved a way to the emergence of modern science that nourished current medical science.

Central to Daoist dialectics, by contrast, are three different but interrelated principles: *change, contradiction,* and *holism* (Peng et al, 1999). The first principle claims that reality is *in constant flux*. The second principle states that reality is full of paradoxes. The last principle declares that all things are interdependent and interactive. The order of the world, including human health, therefore tends to follow a path of *uncertainty, mutuality,* and *the circling logic that links an individual part to the whole.* This last principle is the essence of dialectical thinking as the consequence of the first two. The truth thus is often presented in a liquid sense in reference to its context, or as opposite but related aspects, rather than in an isolated and absolute stage. As Lao Zi said, "We cannot know the Tao itself, nor see its qualities directly, but only see by differentiation, which it manifests. Thus, that which is seen as beautiful is beautiful compared with that which is seen as lacking beauty."

THREE BASIC PRINCIPLES

Corresponding to this last principle, *holism,* Daoists believe that all things in the world are interrelated and affect every other thing in mutually interactive and cyclical ways. The parts become meaningful only in relation to the whole context. Accordingly, ancient Daoists summarized the absolute truth concerning the ultimate reality in a mysterious web of complex energy systems, which appears to be incomprehensible as the whole. However, its manifestation in the form of changing patterns, such as health, is perceivable in comparison to and in connection with opposing and multiple aspects within all phenomena. Daoist dialectics did not lead to classic science or its structurally detailed modern medical diagnosis and intervention, but it can be a helpful lens in comprehending the dynamic energetic totality, such as with TCM and modern physics. Daoists, however, present natural law through different paths than those of scientists. Their energy system was shown in interactive images, symbols, and metaphors. To demonstrate the universal part-whole dynamics of energetic patterns, the Daoist tai ji symbol is shown in a half-black and half-white round pattern, a sign of two interactive cosmic forces, *yin* and *yang,* or a dynamic union of two forces generating the vital energy, qi.

Corresponding to the second principle, *contradiction,* the polarized yin and yang aspects define each other in all paradoxical relations, such as being and nonbeing, energy and substance, spirit and matter, or mind and body. The S curve dividing line between the yin-yang halves in the tai ji symbol implies the constant cyclical movement in contradictive pairs, mutually creating, controlling, and penetrating. Both sides can influence and transform into each other in certain ways, such as in the relationship between health and illness. From this relativist perspective, the metaphor of the qi and the yin-yang relation can be used to describe the energetic and functional relationship of both physical nature and human phenomena. Metaphorically, at an atomic level, this relation can be understood as one between positive and negative particles. At a physical and physiological level, each person has both yin and yang sides at multiple levels, such as the relation of invisible functions to solid organs. At the basic neuropsychological level, all humans have both a rational left hemisphere and an intuitive right hemisphere (Ai, 2003).

Daoism respects nature and emphasizes a harmonic relationship with nature, as do many ancient traditions such as Buddhism, Hinduism, and Native American thought (Ai, 2003). Yet, in keeping with the first principle, *change,* Daoists were uniquely interested more in the constant movements in the *nonbeing* aspect of nature than in the visible (e.g., physical landscape) or invisible (e.g., the spirit) properties in its *being* aspects. The universal principle of all change is presented by a single word, *dao,* the law inherent in nature rather than that created by a creator. The law of nature is not perceived in a fixed order but in a continuous flow in the constant movement of both *nonbeing* and *being* aspects within a hierarchical system, for example, from a higher level of the universe to a lower level of humans. This basic idea is stated by Lao Zi in *Dao De Jing:* "When the consistency of the Tao is known, the mind is receptive to its states of change. Man's laws should follow natural laws, just as nature gives rise to physical laws, whilst following from universal law, which follows the Tao." The law of the universe, not of human logic, is what Daoism intends to comprehend philosophically, to appreciate aesthetically, or to worship spiritually (Crosby, 2002).

I CHING: A CODING SYSTEM FOR UNIVERSAL CHANGES

Daoism uniquely employs mathematics to predict changing patterns in nature and humans. Unlike for scientists, however, even the mathematical patterns of such principles are displayed in symbolic ways. This manner can be traced back 5000 years to an ancient book, *I Ching* (*Yi Jing*), or the *Book of Changes,* which has had profound influence on the Eastern tradition, including TCM and QG. The book is entirely devoted to the basic ordering principles and was used to calculate predictable changing patterns in ancient times. The 64 hexagrams of the *I Ching* are considered an oracle (Capra, 1991). Each of these 64 figures is composed of six lines, as shown in Figure 28-1. A line disconnected in the middle, "– –," represents yin and a complete line, "——," represents yang. The 64 hexagrams register the maximum possible combinations of yin and yang in six lines. Yin and yang, therefore, are the two basic codes in this complex patterning system, including human health. This dichotomized coding system resembles, but emerged thousands of years before, the zero-one language used in computer science. Capra (1991) praises the *I Ching* in *The Tao of Physics:* "Because of its notion of dynamic patterns, the *I Ching* is perhaps the closest analogy to S-matrix theory in Eastern thought. In both systems, the emphasis is on the process rather than object."

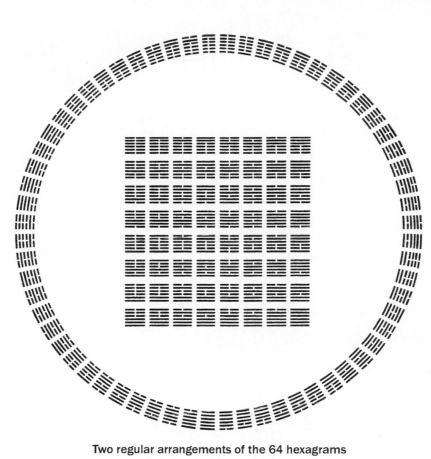

Two regular arrangements of the 64 hexagrams

Figure 28-1 The 64 hexagrams of the *I Ching*.

DAOIST INFLUENCES ON QI GONG PRACTICE

ENERGETIC FUNCTION–CENTERED ORGAN SYSTEM

Throughout Chinese history, Daoism has been the most influential intellectual tradition underlying the development of QG. Like Daoist ontology, QG in theory becomes a function and health-centered rather than a structure- and disease-oriented system. Each person is considered as an energetic cosmos in miniature. Health phenomena are viewed in light of a complex hierarchical web of qi, rather than as merely isolated physical matters. One's energy movement manifests the same pattern as does the universe. As shown in Figure 28-2, the physical parts and major acupoints of an ancient figure in practice was illustrated and described in accordance with moon images and other symbols, which indicates that qi patterns in humans correspond to those in seasonal changes and cosmic movements.

Because the energetic *nonbeing* is more fundamental than the substantive *being*, QG focus primarily on the holistic processes of multilevel energy patterns and their interrelations rather than on the material structure of body parts, as does Western medicine. Even organs *(zhang fu)* are primarily described in terms of qi, with reference to interactive functions within each one and among all, rather than in terms of their exact anatomical structures, because organs are the reservoir of qi in TCM. Likewise, QG exercise places more emphasis on the internal movement via breath technology to cultivate essential qi, rather than on external movement via muscular training to build up body size, as do Western physical exercises. However, Daoist healing systems do not deny physical aspects of human health. Instead, these phenomena are integrated into the primary energetic process.

Identified in their physical structures, the 12 organs are not too distant from their placement by European contemporaries in biomedical anatomy. These organs are divided into the viscera, including six *zang* or solid organs, and the bowels, including six *fu* or hollow organs. The organs of the viscera (heart, lungs, liver, spleen, kidneys, pericardium) and bowel (small intestine, large intestine, gallbladder, stomach, urinary bladder, "triple burner" [*san jiao*]) are paired in terms of their *interior-exterior* (yin-yang) relationship. Aside from the triple burner, in TCM the major physiological functions of these organs are close to those associated with organs similarly named in biomedicine.

Unique to this system, however, are two energy-oriented concepts essential to QG practice. One is san jiao, which has no corresponding anatomical structure. This concept refers to the three energetic locations at the middle of the chest, diaphragm, and abdomen, which

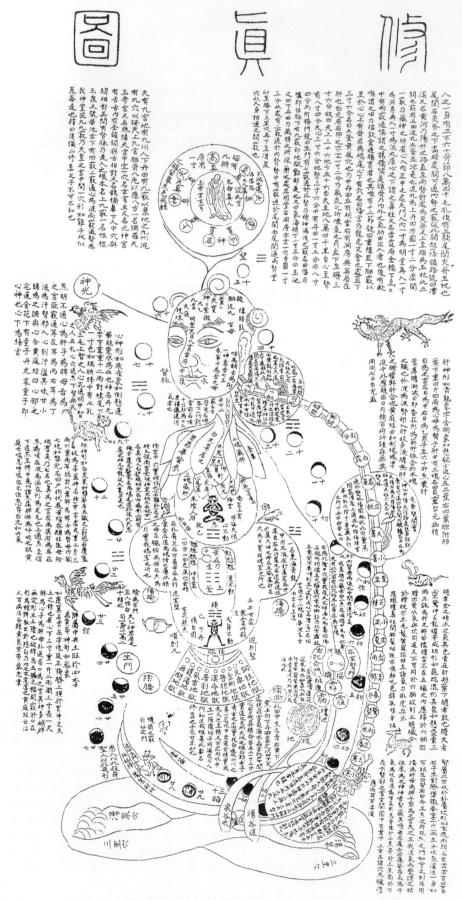

Figure 28-2 An ancient figure in practice.

express the functional connection and interaction among paired organs. Another concept relates to acupuncture *meridians* (or channels), a circulation system of qi, which also has no identifiable anatomical structure. It consists of 12 primary channels corresponding to the six pairs of yin-yang organs and an additional set of eight extraordinary vessels. Along the pathways of 14 of these channels (the 12 regular channels and two of the extra channels) lie 361 specific acupuncture points. Qi flows along these channels, making a rhythmic circuit over 24 hours daily. Each channel has its own peak energetic time in a daily circle, which can be explained by the fluctuation of the immune and neuroendocrinology systems over 24 hours. To cultivate vital energy, some Daoist QG styles emphasize meditation on certain acupoints and qi pathways at certain times every day according to the temporal order of daily qi flow *(zi wu liu zu)*.

In principle, health and illness conditions in QG theories follow the coding system in the *I Ching* by matching multilevel energetic components of each individual. Ancient Greeks used four elements—*water, fire, earth,* and *air*—to represent the basic qualities of natural phenomena. Similarly, in the Han dynasty about 2000 years ago, a five-element system—*wood, fire, earth, metal,* and *water*- was introduced (Maciocia, 1989). The energetic interaction among the five elements follows the mutual generating and controlling processes. The five-element theory was combined with the yin-yang system in the *I Ching* to register the complex energetic interplay among multilevel phenomena that are associated with health (Ai, 2003). Paired organs, tissues, meridians, some acupuncture points, pulse, tongue status, sounds, tastes, colors, time, seasons, directions, planets, temperament, herbs, food, and external pathogens are all coded by these integrated categories along with interconnected relations (Maciocia, 1989; Unschuld, 1985). Organized by the five-element theory, seven emotions or psychic elements (joy, anger, anxiety, concentration, grief, fear, fright) are also linked with the energetic patterns of all functional organs.

Based on this system, the "qi flow of the human" becomes a relatively predictable phenomenon, corresponding to the similarly ordered energetic phenomena in the universe.

HEALTH: HOLISTIC BALANCE IN EVER-CHANGING QI PROCESSES

Consistent with Daoist epistemology, QG theory is literally a systematic elaboration on the changing patterns of qi with respect to the intrarelationship and interrelationship of body, mind, and spirit, as well as their interactions with the energetic environment, in terms of nature, society, and cosmos. Health is maintained only in the internal and external energetic qi contexts of each individual and is perceived with constant changes, contradictions, and holism. Because of the principle of *holism,* illness conditions are often individually assessed and addressed using

multiple principles concerning the whole energy system rather than using a standardized diagnosis and assessment for structural abnormality. Because of the principle of *contradiction,* health is not viewed as the state of opposition to or absence of disease but rather as an uncertain process of constantly balancing normal and abnormal qi patterns. Because of the principle of *change,* health and illness can be transformed into each other, depending on the interaction between the ailment stage and health practice by an individual. Accordingly, QG practice should be integrated into one's lifestyle, which then can boost overall energy, balance the effect of illness, and allow the natural healing capacities to prevail constantly and to transform an ill state into a healthy process.

Such Daoist essence is reflected in the Chinese character *zhong yi. Yi* means "medicine," and *zhong* usually means "middle," but it also refers to the internally balanced "golden medium." According to an expert on the *I Ching,* zhong yi does not mean the "medicine of middle kingdom," or of China, but refers to the "medicine for inner balance" (Yuan, 1997). Inner balance lies in the harmonic pattern of ever-changing qi in relation to the interplay between ying and yang at all levels of human function, as well as in one's habits and environment. This perspective enables QG practice to focus on the prevention of illness conditions through sensitive recognition and management of qi and to emphasize the treatment of preillness stages (e.g., *functional disorders*) before ailments are manifest. A classic text of Chinese medicine, the *Classic of Difficult Issues (Nan Jing),* compiled over 2000 years ago, presented many therapeutic principles for becoming an excellent doctor who can prevent substantive illnesses from progressing to a state of pathology and mortality (Wang et al, 1988).

Each individual therefore must take the responsibility for his or her own healthy lifestyle, harmonic attitude, and energy exercise, QG. In keeping with its preventive orientation, QG as an energy-oriented practice becomes an art of health, healing, and holistic life, integrating body, mind, and spirit, not a "magic bullet" for treatment of specific diseases.

BREATHING MEDITATIVE PRACTICE: BALANCED ENERGY AND MIND-BODY CONNECTION

The spirit of Daoism also guides QG practice with a heavy emphasis on breathing technique as one approach to holistic health. Lao Zi stated in *Dao De Jing,*

> Maintaining unity is virtuous, for the inner world of thought is one with the external world of action and of things. The sage avoids their separation, by breathing as the sleeping babe, and thus maintaining harmony.... From constancy, there develops harmony, and from harmony, enlightenment. It is unwise to rush from here to there. To hold one's breathe causes the body strain; exhaustion follows when too much energy is used, for this is not the natural way."

Held in the posture of standing, sitting, or lying, the meditative Daoist QG practice appears to be similar to the Zen Buddhist approach. Both emphasize deep breathing, concentration, and relaxation. However, these two approaches differ from each other in terms of goals and techniques. Buddhism stresses the experience of awakening from the illusion of life (enlightenment), whereas Daoism emphasizes a more muscular practice (literally, in the example of QG) cultivating energy and spirit *(shen)* as well as promoting health and longevity. Buddhist practice tends to center on the emptiness of mind (detachment), whereas some Daoist practices guide consciousness to follow the flow of qi passively along a certain meridian system, such as "heavenly circulation" *(zhou tian)* around the middle line in front and back of the body. Daoist QG practice also tends to concentrate on the most important energy center, the cinnabar field *(dan tian)*, at about three finger widths below the navel. This area is considered to be the "ocean of qi," where the root of vital energy and longevity reside.

In modern terms, QG is essentially a mind-body practice and also a spiritual cultivation. As with early Hippocratic medicine, the approach of QG is psychosomatic and does not follow a soma and psyche dualism (Hammer, 1990; Temkin, 1991). Physical health and ailments are seen not only as inseparable from, but also as internal responses to, emotional stimuli and environmental stress. From a perspective that joined QG theories and psychiatric diagnoses, Hammer (1990), an American psychiatrist, devoted an entire book to an explanation of the nature of the movement of qi in relation to emotion and illness. When any type of affect becomes overwhelming, emotions become internal agents of illness. Conversely, the dysfunction of organs will be manifested not only in somatic symptoms but also in certain types of emotional distress. For example, the heart is classified as the "fire" element—an "emperor" organ that houses the individual's spirit (shen) and mental energy, with a tendency to be excessive. It is related to the color red and the emotion of joy. Indeed, in light of modern neuroendocrinology, the heart beats faster because of the increased secretion of adrenal hormones in an ecstatic emotional state, and many patients with cardiovascular disease also experience depression and anxiety (Ai, 1996). Interestingly, some American physicians also speak of this mind-body aspect of the heart in terms of "dual heats" in a human: first a pulsating of muscle in the chest and a then a precious second cable of communicating neurons that create feeling, longing, and love (Lewis et al, 2001). This view recognizes the important role of neuroendocrinology and the immune system in organ-brain or body-mind communication, an ancient idea essentially expressed in the concept of qi and QG practice.

QG practice thus emphasizes the guidance of mind for the qi flow through constant meditative breathing exercise, which in turn spontaneously affects the bodily function. Following Daoist dialectics, no type of emotion is seen as absolutely positive or completely negative. For example, excessive joy is believed to cause harm to one's energetic balance, as do negative emotions such as anger. This situation can be understood in modern terms. For example, a person with coronary heart disease can experience sudden cardiac arrest when attending holiday festivities, a family gathering, or a birthday party. This heart attack may result from excessive joy or excitement that in turn leads to extra stress. To protect well-being, the TCM emphasis is on zhong (i.e., balancing mood, in relation to organs' health) rather than positivity per se (i.e., pursing happiness at its extreme end). The key to health in this QG perspective lies in the integration and balancing of overall energetic functions rather than in the pursuit of extremity.

Likewise, Daoist QG practice does not deny sexuality as a sinful desire, nor does it encourage extreme sexual play in the spirit of hedonism. Rather, sexual energy and behaviors are inseparable parts of health, emotion, and longevity, but they may also be associated with certain illness in malpractice. Some QG support techniques promote healthy sexuality in relation to physical and emotional heath. Returning to the fire organ example, the qi of the pericardium, a parallel fire organ to the heart, acts to facilitate sexual functioning. A defective pericardium function is believed to affect human activity in varied ways, ranging from hyposexuality to hypersexuality, as well as impacted joy. Currently, this conception may also be explainable by neuroendocrinology and psychology. QG practice helps maintain the tranquil qi balance in these fire organs, readjust dysfunction of both organs and emotions, and restore healthy energetic patterns in related sexuality.

CLINICAL STUDIES ON THE EFFICACY OF INTERNAL QI GONG

Despite the public interest in and theories behind QG, whether QG practice can "cure" medically diagnosed diseases remains an underinvestigated subject by Western standards (Ai et al, 2001). The primary reason may lie in the role of this millennia-old practice, one that has primarily been used for promoting health-related well-being, rather than for curing diseases of modern diagnoses in century-young Western biomedicine. A second reason may be the lack of close contact between QG practice and modern clinical research methodology until the late twentieth century, when the People's Republic of China reopened its doors to the world. Before 1997, Sancier (1996) and Cohen (1997) reported on some studies from Chinese sources with limited information about research designs. Clearly, most studies were not conducted using the RCT design, which limits conclusions on causality with regard to treatment efficacy. Over the past decade, however, a growing number of RCTs on QG with better designs have been conducted and results published around world, including in China. These studies have offered more solid evidence on certain health benefits of QG and on the underlying mechanisms as well, despite the limits in both the number of trials and their sample sizes.

STUDIES ON QI GONG IN CHINA BEFORE 1997

As mentioned earlier, studies conducted in China during the 1980s dealt mostly with internal QG. Of these, most were descriptive, and very few were reported in peer-reviewed journals in English. The most noteworthy studies reviewed by Sancier (1996) and Cohen (1997) are described in the first part of this section and serve as a sampling of earlier investigation on QG. Those investigating the effect of QG on cardiovascular diseases had better designs than those looking at other chronic conditions.

Hypertension and Cardiac Function

Sancier (1996) gathered more than 10 reports from China about the effects of QG on hypertension, whereas Cohen (1997) mentioned one large-sample study investigating the combined use of QG practice and biofeedback devices in treating hypertension. Both reviewers highlighted prevention of stroke and mortality, but most studies did not use a control group. One study investigated the effects of QG practice on the blood chemistry of hypertensive patients (Kuang et al, 1991a, 1991b; Sancier et al, 1991). Improvement was found in plasma coagulation and fibrinolysis indices, blood viscosity, erythrocyte deformation index, and plasma levels of tissue-type plasminogen activator, plasminogen activator inhibitor, factor VIII–related antigen, and antithrombin III. Changes in the activities of two messenger nucleotides (cyclic adenosine monophosphate and cyclic guanosine monophosphate) were also reported.

One identified RCT followed 204 hypertensive patients (Kuang et al, 1991a, 1991b; Sancier et al, 1991). At the 6-month follow-up, the combination of QG and antihypertension medication was found to be 19% more effective than medication alone. The QG group showed reduced plasma dopamine-β-hydroxylase activity, increased plasma high-density lipoprotein (HDL) levels, and improvement in blood viscosity and platelet aggregation abnormalities. Hyperresponse of blood pressure to stress was also decreased. The clinical effectiveness was 87% ± 3% and 68% ± 1% for the QG and control groups, respectively. Total and stroke mortality rates were 17.3% and 11.5% in the QG group, compared with 32.0% and 23.0% in the control group. The most interesting controlled trial tracked 242 patients for 30 years (Cohen, 1997). Both the QG and control groups took standardized antihypertension medication. Significant differences were found in mortality rates (25.41% in the QG group, 47.76% in the control group), stroke rate (20.49% in the QG group, 40.83% in the control group),

and stroke-related mortality rate (15.57% in the QG group, 32.50% in the control group).

Some studies of healthy subjects showed beneficial QG effects on cardiac function, microcirculation, and cardiovascular diseases (Chu et al, 1988; Ma, 1983; Mo, Xu et al, 1993; Mo, Wan et al, 1993; Qin, 1988; Wang et al, 1990, 1993). In one study a group of 66 young men were divided into two groups (QG exercise vs. regular exercise). Both groups practiced their exercises for 4 weeks before suddenly entering a highland area. Symptoms of altitude sickness and physiological changes were measured for both groups before and after the experiment. The QG group showed less altitude stress than did the controls, as indicated by blood pressure, heart rate, oxygen consumption, microcirculation on the apex of the tongue and nail fold, and temperature at the lao gong acupoint (P8) in the palm of the left hand (Mo, Xu et al, 1993). Another study compared microcirculation disorders in 22 air force pilots practicing QG for 8 weeks and in 18 pilots in a control group performing regular physical exercise (Mo, Wan et al, 1993). The abnormalities (before and after entering a highland area) were significantly less in the QG group than in the control group.

Other Chronic Conditions and Aging-Related Indices

As reported by Cohen (1997), a study using a pretest-posttest design and involving 14 elderly patients with cardiac or pulmonary diseases observed improvements in lung function after 18 months of QG practice, including the following: (1) the volume of air exhaled after a full inhalation increased by 3.31+%, (2) the volume of air in the lungs after the deepest inhalation increased by 7.34+%, and (3) the volume of air exhaled with maximum effort and speed increased by 16.11% ($P < .001$). In another study patients with bronchial asthma received 2 to 3 months of standardized training in the practice of tranquil breathing for 20 to 30 minutes twice per day, concentration on certain acupoints, and self-massage (Cohen, 1997). The 4-year follow-up of 93 patients (out of an initial sample of 99) found a significantly lower frequency, severity, and duration of asthma attacks; less medication use; and better capacity for physical labor among program participants.

Several large-sample studies of patients with gastric and duodenal ulcers reviewed by Cohen (1997) provided only reports of high percentages of cure rates after QG practice without including any information on research design or medication use. Another study involving patients with advanced cancers compared 97 patients who underwent chemotherapy and practiced QG for 2 hours per day for 3 months with 30 patients who underwent chemotherapy only (Cohen, 1997). Favorable outcomes were observed in terms of symptoms, body weight, and standard immunological indices for those who practiced QG in addition to receiving chemotherapy. Despite reports of similar results in replicated samples, no information was available about the details of control design and assessment of outcome measures.

With regard to the potential antiaging effects of QG, Kuang et al (1991a, 1991b) compared the impact of QG exercise and a control condition on bone density. After 1 year of practice, 18 middle-aged subjects (50 to 59 years) increased their bone density from 0.627 ± 0.040 to 0.696 ± 0.069 g/cm^3. Among 12 older subjects (60 to 69 years), bone density increased to a lesser degree. But the increases in bone density in both subgroups exceeded the increases in the control subgroups of the same age ranges. A better-designed study examined the levels of active superoxide dismutase (SOD), an enzyme that protects cells against damage from superoxide (Cohen, 1997). Two hundred subjects were evenly divided into a QG group (which performed QG exercise for about 30 minutes per day) and a control group, with 50 males and 50 females in each group. After subjects practiced QG, relaxation, and self-massage for 1 year, the level of active SOD was higher in the QG exercisers than in the controls ($P < .001$). This outcome was replicated by Ye et al in a study in which 116 subjects practiced QG for 2 months, but no control group was mentioned (Cohen, 1997).

Kuang et al (1991a, 1991b) also differentiated the effects of QG exercise on the levels of sex hormone (estradiol) in 70 men (aged 40 to 69) and women (aged 51 to 67). After 1 year of QG practice, the plasma levels decreased among men but increased among women. An auxiliary study observed a decrease in both 24-hour urine estradiol levels and the estradiol/testosterone ratio in 30 men (aged 50 to 69) after 1 year of exercise, accompanied by changes in symptoms of kidney deficiency as defined by TCM theory (e.g., soreness, dizziness, insomnia, hair loss, impotence, incontinence) (Xu et al, 1994). Ye et al (1990) reported similar changes in plasma levels of estradiol but not of testosterone in 77 QG exercisers, compared with 27 controls, after 2 months of practice. Still, questions could arise concerning the conclusions on causality drawn by these studies because of the expectations of the researchers regarding outcomes, based on their potential cultural bias.

Electroencephalographic Patterns and Mental Health

Chinese researchers identified a unique electroencephalographic (EEG) pattern present in healthy QG practitioners, especially long-term practitioners, involving four types of brain waves (Cohen, 1997). The first, slowest type, *delta* waves (0.5 to 4 Hz), tends to be prevalent during infancy or during deep sleep in adults. Yet delta waves were recorded when QG healers were awake, a phenomenon that seems to concur with Lao Zi's reference to "breathing like a sleeping babe." The second, next slowest type, *theta* waves (4 to 8 Hz), is normally present during drowsy, barely conscious states and is likely accompanied by dreamlike images. However, theta waves were present in trained practitioners in a fully awake but relaxed state. The third, faster type, *alpha* waves (8 to 13 Hz), can be produced in most people by closing the eyes and during relaxation. It is most frequently produced during meditative QG. The final one, the fastest type, *beta* waves (13 to 26 Hz or higher), is mostly associated with waking consciousness in adults. During the practice of QG, brain waves slow down from beta to alpha, theta, or a combination of alpha and theta. In particular, alpha waves change from the appearance of ripples on a pond on the EEG to a preponderance of high-amplitude, high-crested "ocean waves." This indicates that more brain tissues are acting in the same way simultaneously. More powerful alpha waves in the left hemisphere of the brain characterize the practitioner's attentive meditation on an object. Those in the right hemisphere occur during silent awareness with no object of attention in meditation. Increased alpha and theta waves tend to be recorded in the frontal portions of the brain during QG practice. The coherence among these types of waves produced by various parts of the brain also increases, which appears to support the yin-yang balance theory in TCM and QG.

Wang (1993) examined the effect of duration of QG practice on mental health. Among 155 QG practitioners, 119 individuals with more than 2 years of experience demonstrated considerably better mental health than did those with less than 2 years of experience. Outcome measures included scores on standardized instruments for assessing obsessive-compulsive traits, anxiety or phobic anxiety, depression or psychosis, general mental health, and interpersonal sensitivity. Wang (1993) also assessed type A behaviors in 89 individuals who practiced QG and 144 individuals who did not. Type A traits were shown by 22.43% of the QG group and 51.39% of the control group. Nevertheless, the lack of RCT designs has made conclusions regarding causality somewhat questionable.

Chinese researchers also investigated a rare side effect of inadequate QG practice, called *qi gong deviation* (QD) (Ai, 2003). QD manifested at a functional level in some aspect of mental health, but its clinical characteristics did not allow it to be clearly classified into existing psychiatric disease diagnoses. In 1994 the term *qi gong psychotic reaction,* the U.S. term for QD, was included in the Glossary of Culture-Bound Syndromes in the *Diagnostic and Statistical Manual of Mental Disorders* (fourth edition) of the American Psychiatric Association.

Using standardized psychiatric rating scales (Brief Psychiatric Scale, Hamilton Depression and Anxiety Scales, Improved Minnesota Multiphasic Personality Inventory), Shan et al (1989) assessed 109 patients (aged 18 to 69, 89% males) who had mental disorders attributed to QG. Of these, 74 were self-taught learners of QG, who practiced QG mostly for self-healing. Patients who experienced QD presented abnormalities in perception, thinking, and behavior to varying degrees. Most of them also experienced specific QD physical symptoms. Patients with QD were categorized into two groups: the schizophrenic type (47 cases) and the neurotic type (62 cases). Most of the QD patients, however, recovered in a short time with no recurrence of attention disorder, delusion, hallucination, depression, anxiety, or behavior disturbances. Although QD is considered a temporary condition, its existence suggests the need for appropriate guidance in practice.

STUDIES ON QI GONG AROUND THE WORLD AFTER 1997

The popularity of complementary and alternative medicine (CAM) over the past two decades has led to the spread of QG practice and research around the world. This section focuses on the evidence for the beneficial effects of QG in various areas, mostly from reports of RCTs published since 1997. My own online search identified over a dozen RCTs on QG between 1997 and 2008; results of all were published in English. In addition, there are two current systematic review articles of QG trials. Ng and Tsang (2009) conducted the first review, focusing on the health areas showing benefit from QG and the underlying psychophysiological mechanism of QG. They identified around two dozen trials conducted between 1997 and 2006, involving a total of 750+ subjects (aged 52.5±) (Note that of the original 26 reports, 4 publications appeared to have been generated from two samples in Korea.) Some of the articles were published in Chinese. Of these RCTs, 12 used a comparable control group (e.g., conventional therapy or attention placebo), whereas the rest used a no-treatment control group. In the selected programs participants received instruction from a QG master or followed audiovisual training materials. All studies used individual and/or group-based QG practice as the main intervention, although in some QG was integrated with other interventions (e.g., mindfulness). Ng and Tsang concluded that QG had some clinical effects in reducing blood pressure, total cholesterol level, and depressive symptoms and posited that the explanatory pathways or underlying mechanisms were related to *stress reduction* via the QG regulation of neuroendocrine and immune functions.

A second review by Rogers et al (2009) selected 36 reports of research on both QG and t'ai chi conducted between 1993 and 2007 with a total of 3700 participants (aged 55 or older). Identified categories of study outcomes included falls and balance, physical function, cardiovascular diseases, and psychological and additional disease-specific responses. The reviewers concluded that QG and t'ai chi interventions may help improve physical function, reduce blood pressure, decrease fall risk, and mitigate depression and anxiety. Major trials identified in my own literature search and in Ng and Tsang's review (2009), including a few overlapping studies, are summarized in the following sections, which correspond roughly to the categories for studies conducted before 1997. Because the principle of QG has not always been integrated in the popular practice of

t'ai chi, to be conservative this chapter discusses only the four trials from Rogers et al's review (2009) that clearly identified QG as the primary intervention.

Hypertension, Metabolic Syndrome, and Cardiac Function

Consistent with earlier hypertension studies performed by Chinese researchers before 1997, the reviews by both Ng and Tsang (2009) and Rogers et al (2009) found support for an effect of QG on lowering systolic blood pressure (SBP) and diastolic blood pressure (DBP). Lee and various colleagues in Korea randomly assigned study participants (Lee, Lee et al, 2004; Lee, Lim et al, 2004; Lee, Lee, Choi et al, 2003; Lee, Lee, Kim et al, 2003) to one of two groups: a Shuxinpingxue QG group, or a wait-list, no-treatment control group. After 8 to 10 weeks of QG practice (30 minutes per session and twice per week), the QG group showed a significant decrease in both SBP and DBP compared with the control group (P <.001). For the QG group, the average reduction in both SBP and DBP appeared to be more than 10 mm Hg as judged from a data figure, but actual values were not reported. However, Cheung et al (2005) did not find a significant difference between the practice of Goulin QG (60 minutes in the morning and 15 minutes in the evening for 16 weeks) and conventional exercise in the treatment of mild hypertension, although blood pressure was significantly reduced in both the QG group and the regular exercise group. In Australia, Liu et al (2008) used a quasi-experimental, pretest-posttest design to assess the effect of QG (three times per week for 12 weeks) on blood pressure. SBP decreased by 11.64± mm Hg and DBP decreased by 9.73 mm Hg (P <.001) in patients who practiced QG. Because there was no adequate control, however, such numbers may serve only as references for others' trials. Unfortunately, all the studies just described had a small sample size.

Besides showing an effect of QG on blood pressure, the majority of these trials also demonstrated its impact on the physical and/or hematological indicators of metabolic syndrome. In the study by Lee, Lee et al (2004), levels of total cholesterol, HDL cholesterol, triglycerides, and apolipoprotein A-I were significantly reduced in hypertensive patients who engaged in QG exercise compared with the no-treatment control group. Cheung et al (2005) reported a similar significant reduction in triglyceride level, body mass index (BMI), and waist circumference in both the group practicing QG and the group engaging in regular exercise. Liu et al (2008), using a pretest-posttest design to study the effects of QG in adults with elevated blood glucose levels, did not find changes in triglyceride level, HDL level, or fasting blood glucose level, but a significant improvement was seen in insulin resistance (as measured with the Homeostatic Model Assessment), hemoglobin A1c (HbA1c) level, BMI, and waist circumference. In addition, Liu et al (2006) in China compared a 3-month regimen of Eight Brocade QG with a control regimen of walking and attention in patients with hyperlipidemia. They reported significant improvement in the levels of total cholesterol, high- and low-density lipoprotein cholesterol, and triglycerides in the QG group but not in the control group.

In Japan, Iwao et al (1999) found no difference in the effect of QG walking and conventional walking (30 minutes after lunch) on plasma glucose levels in 10 patients with diabetes mellitus and associated complications. Participants in both types of walking showed significantly lower plasma glucose levels than those who did not walk. However, the pulse rate was significantly higher in patients who practiced conventional walking than in those who practiced QG walking or did not walk after lunch, which may suggest a calming effect associated with the QG walking exercise. Also, Tsujiuchi et al (2002) employed dietary advice and exercise treatment as the control to test the effect of QG on glucose metabolism in patients with type 2 diabetes. Significantly reduced levels of HbA1c and C peptide were observed in those who practiced QG over 4 months, especially in patients with higher preintervention levels of HbA1c levels.

A few studies investigated cardiac function in participants with or without cardiac disease. In Italy, Pippa et al (2007) compared QG training with a wait-list control condition in older patients with chronic atrial fibrillation. Results on the 6-minute walk test improved in the QG group but declined in the control group, although no significant changes were found in ejection fraction, BMI, and lipid levels. In Sweden, Stenlund et al (2006) studied 109 older patients with coronary artery disease (aged 77.5±). After 3 months, the group engaging in QG practice showed considerable improvements in self-estimated level of physical activity and performance on the one-leg stance test and the coordination and box-climbing test, compared with the group receiving usual care. In China Du et al (2006), in a study involving 69 patients (aged 60.6±), and Wang et al (2006), in a trial encompassing 220 patients (aged 50 to 70), used echocardiogram findings to compare the effect of Yi Jin Jing QG exercise (five times per week for 6 months) and a no-treatment control condition on cardiac function indices. Both studies reported significant differences in stroke volume, peak early transmitral filling velocity (VE), and peak late transmitral filling velocity (VA) across time and between groups. These authors attributed the observed improvement in cardiac function to regular QG practice.

Other Chronic Conditions, Aging-Related Indices, and Stress Biomarkers

Xu (2000) in China randomly assigned older patients with chronic obstructive pulmonary disease to practice respiration QG (20 minutes twice per day) and self-massage or to receive external diaphragm pacer (EDP) therapy. After 20 days, both groups exhibited improvement in lung function (forced vital capacity, forced expiratory volume in 1 second, peak expiratory flow rate), blood gas values

(arterial partial pressure of oxygen and carbon dioxide, arterial oxygen saturation), and descending and ascending excursion of the diaphragm. However, QG was superior to EDP in enhancing lung functioning. Mannerkorpi and Arndorw (2004) in Sweden noted that practicing dynamic QG for 3 months appeared to improve movement harmony in patients with fibromyalgia compared with a no-treatment control group, but no improvement was seen in fibromyalgia symptoms or physical function. However, they also reported an adverse event related to the practice of standing QG. Astin et al (2003) in the United States found comparable improvement (as measured by pain and disability scores on the Fibromyalgia Impact Questionnaire) in patients with fibromyalgia who practiced either mindfulness meditation and Phoenix QG or exercise for the same length of time. Likewise, Tsang et al (2003) in Hong Kong found a similar effect for both Eight Brocade QG and conventional rehabilitation activities relying on physical therapy and occupational therapy in improving physical health, ability to perform activities of daily living, and social function in 50 adults (aged 74.7±) with chronic disabilities. These findings, along with those of others trials on the effect of QG on mild hypertension (Cheung, 2005) and diabetes (Iwao et al, 1999), suggest that QG can be an alternative to regular exercise for management of certain chronic conditions.

To examine the effect of QG on the physical status of 71 women (aged 45 to 55), Tsai et al (2008) in Hong Kong compared Muscle-Tendon Change Classic (MTCC) QG with a no-treatment control condition. After 8 weeks of practice, the MMCC QG group had improved significantly in muscular endurance, body fat, waist-to-hip ratio, and BMI. Wenneberg et al (2004) in Sweden explored the benefit of QG in 31 patients (aged 51.4±) with muscular dystrophy. After 30 months of practice, those in the QG group reported better status with regard to perceived health (Medical Outcome Study Short Form Health Survey) and coping skills (Ways of Coping Questionnaire), but not in physical ability (Berg Balance Scale), compared with those in a no-treatment control group. In the United States, Yang et al (2007a) examined the effect of QG and t'ai chi on falls and balance in 82 healthy adults older than age 65. The group practicing QG demonstrated significantly better scores than the wait-list control group on vestibular ratios of the Sensory Organization Test and on Base of Support measures but not on visual ratios of the Sensory Organization Test and on feet opening angle. German researchers Schmitz-Hubsch et al (2006) compared the effects of integrated Crane and Eight Brocade QG with no treatment in 56 patients (aged 63.8±) with Parkinson disease. More patients in the QG group than in the no-treatment control group showed improvement in motor symptoms (as assessed by the Unified Parkinson's Disease Rating Scale, motor part) at the 3-month and 6-month follow-up, but not at 12-month follow-up. These results indicate the need for a long-term commitment to practicing QG.

Many age-related health conditions can interact with perceived stress. Quite a few RCTs investigating the benefits of QG have assessed neuroendocrine and immune biomarkers that tend to be associated with both chronic diseases and stress. Testing 87 women (aged 45.2±) Chen et al (2006) in China found a significant reduction in interlukin-6 levels and maintenance of bone mineral density in those who practiced Eight Brocade QG for 12 weeks. By contrast, those in the control group (who followed their usual lifestyle) showed a significant reduction in bone mineral density. Manzaneque et al (2004) in Spain assigned 29 naive subjects to either QG training or a control condition. After 30 minutes of daily practice for 1 month, the QG group showed significantly decreased numbers of total leukocytes and eosinophils, decreased number and percentage of monocytes, and lower complement C3 concentrations compared with the control group. Lee, Huh et al (2003) in Korea compared Chun Do Sun Bup (CDSB) QG with similar motion without breathing and mental technique in 60 subjects (aged 36±). After a 2-hour practice, levels of peripheral blood white blood cells and lymphocytes increased in CDSB QG participants, but not in those in the control group. In another sample of 18 subjects (aged 26.5±), Lee's group found that NK cell cytotoxicity, but not NK cell numbers, significantly increased in the CDSB QG group compared with the no-treatment control (Lee et al, 2005). The results of these RCTs indicate that QG has certain effects in modulating immune functions. Further, in Lee et al's trials of QG in patients with hypertension, a significant decrease in plasma levels of norepinephrine and epinephrine (Lee, Huh et al, 2003) and a decrease in urinary levels of catecholamines (norepinephrine, epinephrine, and metanephrine) (Lee, Lee, Choi et al, 2003) were shown in the group practicing QG. These findings suggest the stabilizing influence of QG on the sympathetic nervous system. In 50 older adults (aged 77.2±) with a history of flu immunization and sedentary lifestyle, Yang et al (2007b) reported higher immune function in the group practicing QG (hemagglutination inhibition assay [HIA] increased 109%) than in the wait-list no-treatment group (HIA increased about 10%).

Mental Health and Addiction

Some previously mentioned post-1997 research also assessed certain aspects of mental health and psychological conditions. Astin et al (2003) found that QG practice reduced depression (as measured by the Beck Depression Inventory) in patients with fibromyalgia. Lee's group reported increased levels of general and exercise self-efficacy (Lee, Lim et al, 2004) and decreased levels of stress (Lee, Lee, Kim et al, 2003) in hypertensive patients. Tsang et al (2006) compared Eight Brocade QG with newspaper reading as the attention control in 72 older adults (older than age 65) with a history of depression and chronic illness. Those who practiced QG experienced significantly decreased depression (as measured using the Geriatric Depression Scale),

as well as increased well-being, perceived benefits, and self-efficacy, compared with those in the control group. Further, Zhang et al (2006) and Zhong and Zhang (2006) demonstrated the beneficial effect of Yi Jin Jing QG in older adults in improving cognitive performance (e.g., reaction time, digit memory) after 6 months of QG practice and in improving psychological health (e.g., depression, obsession, and anxiety, as measured using the Symptoms Checklist 90) after 1 year of practice, compared with a no-treatment control condition (124 to 214 subjects, aged 61±; unclear whether the two samples overlapped).

Finally, in a study of detoxification treatment involving 60 subjects (aged 32.4±) Li et al (2002) found that the group practicing Pan Gu Giong QG showed negative urine test results (for morphine) by day 5, whereas the usual-care control group had negative results by day 9. The QG group also experienced more rapid reduction of withdrawal symptoms (e.g., hallucinations, behavioral deviation, nausea, vomiting) and had significantly lower anxiety scores (on the Hamilton Anxiety Scale).

In sum, the enthusiasm about QG studies in China a decade ago certainly generated both interesting data and some doubts about certain results because of weak research design, and future investigation is merited. The pioneering work conducted there provided valuable hypotheses for further testing of QG effects and underlying mechanisms, and opened opportunities for international collaboration in a new wave of QG research around world. As the extension of this early work, the clinical studies performed over the past decade in many parts of the world, including China, have advanced research design and methodology in this area. The new evidence obtained lends support for beneficial effects of QG in improving health and function, especially in some chronic conditions associated with aging and related physical and psychological well-being, as noted by Ng and Tsang (2009) as well as by Rogers et al (2009). New RCTs have also offered a balanced view of QG, including its limitations in treating certain heritable and highly debilitating disease that have yet to be offered a definitive pharmaceutical cure. The international trials have also helped ease some of the concerns about cultural bias in drawing conclusions regarding the healing effects of QG that would have arisen had such studies been conducted only in its homeland, China. However, gaps still remain in this research area. Most of the existing RCTs have used small samples, and not all of them have employed an adequate control. In fact, just what is the appropriate sham QG to use a control will remain a question, as does the use of sham needles in acupuncture research. Korean scholars' use of a motion similar to QG but without breathing and mental technique can be seen as a creative attempt to address this issue (Lee, Huh et al, 2003). Further, because there are numerous forms of QG, it will be interesting to test which form may especially benefit which chronic conditions. As noted by Mannerkorpi and Arndorw (2004), certain forms of practice may be harmful for certain diseases. Likewise, the QD phenomena observed in China also calls for more investigation of the interplay between forms of QG and personality types. When the use of internal QG spreads in the West, evidence-based regulations on training and practice may also be established, as was the case with acupuncture. At present, perhaps one thing can be said to be certain. QG is one type of mind-body, healthy lifestyle exercise, and its long-term benefits can be realized only with committed and appropriate practice.

CLINICAL STUDIES ON THE EFFICACY OF EXTERNAL QI GONG

At the dawn of the new millennium, the surging public interest in complementary, alternative, and integrative medicine in the United States prompted the initiation of several RCTs funded by the National Institutes of Health (NIH). These trials investigated the role of external QG in the treatment of medically diagnosed conditions and conformed to a higher standard of clinical research design. Often, such investigation has to involve interdisciplinary collaborations and multiple standardized assessments of physical and mental health outcomes (Ai et al, 2001; Chen et al, 2008; Wu et al, 1999). Yet this type of investigation can raise more design questions than studies of internal QG practice.

QUESTIONS ABOUT "PLACEBO" CONTROL IN QI GONG TRIALS

One important question about external QG concerns the placebo effect. In designing the second large-sample QG trial funded by the National Center for Complementary and Alternative Medicine (NCCAM), Ai et al (2001) argued that there are limitations in using the classic RCT design, based on a materialistic scientific philosophy, to assess the role of qi or other forms of invisible bioenergy. A unique question arises about both the adequate placebo and the appropriate comparison. Unlike in pharmaceutical trials, in which a placebo tablet looks identical to the medicine but does not contain the active ingredient, a placebo treatment for energy healing trials cannot be so well defined. A basic difference between drug and energy-healing trials is that the former does not involve a living person as the tool of intervention, so researchers do not need to worry about the type of interpersonal influence that occurs, as in the latter. Although neither clinicians nor patients can distinguish a placebo from a real drug, QG masters cannot be blind as to whether or not they are conducting real therapy. From a conventional perspective, the very notion of energy healing appears to fall into the category of what allopathic medicine terms the *placebo effect*, which seems to be created from nothing other than the expectations of physicians and/or patients.

To address this interpersonal influence in assessing external QG, the *first* solution is simply to make the placebo aspect of healing invisible (Ai et al, 2001). The investigated therapy can take place on unconscious individuals (those asleep or anesthetized) or with the therapist behind a wall or a screen, or even at a considerable distance. The *second* solution, when this invisible form is implausible, is to conduct the assessment with two control groups, such as by comparing a "treatment" group with both a "no treatment" group and a "sham" (mimic) therapy group. Comparison groups must be designed so that expectations on the part of the research participants can be held constant. If benefits still occur for participants in the actual treatment group, the researcher can conclude that effects were not simply caused by expectations. The *third* solution is to reconsider the effective role of the placebo or expectations in the design rather than ignore or eliminate it. As in psychotherapy, confidence in or hope for the efficacy of a therapist-involved treatment may be more important than any particular technique. QG researchers should heed the historical lesson of Franz Anton Mesmer's claims of the miraculous cure brought about by his redistribution of animal magnetism in people's bodies in eighteenth-century Europe (Wyckoff, 1975). Despite the court's intent to trivialize the cures as resulting from patients' expectations, techniques of mesmerism have survived as hypnotism and are considered legitimate for medical use today (see Chapters 6 and 9). Thus the so-called placebo effect in QG healing and similar therapies, such as other types of energy healing, can still be seen as part of a real cure and should be examined in its own right. A few RCTs examining the effects of external QG are summarized in the following sections.

OUTCOMES OF RANDOMIZED CONTROLLED TRIALS ON EXTERNAL QI GONG

First NIH-Funded Small-Scale Randomized Controlled Trial

The first study funded by the NIH through NCCAM was an interdisciplinary effort involving multiple-session assessments of 26 patients (aged 18 to 65) with treatment-resistant late-stage complex regional pain syndrome type I (Wu et al, 1999). The trial included one QG experimental group and one placebo control (sham QG) group, with six 40-minute sessions of either QG or sham treatment over 3 weeks. Comprehensive evaluation was performed at baseline and at 6- and 10-month follow-up. All 22 patients who completed the trial underwent several mental health and domestic functioning assessments using the Symptoms Checklist 90, Sickness Impact Profile, Beck Depression Inventory, and Cognitive-Somatic Anxiety Questionnaire. Eighty-two percent of QG patients reported less pain by the end of the first session, compared with 45% of control patients. By the last session, 91% of QG patients reported analgesia compared with 36% of control patients.

The results demonstrate that external QG led to transient pain reduction and long-term reduction of anxiety in the experimental group, even in such a small sample. This report suggests that by using a sound research design, it may be possible to provide valid scientific evidence of QG effects on mental health and quality of life.

Second NIH-Funded Large-Scale Randomized Controlled Trial

A second NIH/NCCAM-funded, large-sample trial was designed to examine the efficacy of QG for in-hospital rehabilitation of middle-aged and older patients after open-heart surgery (Ai et al, 2001). The study design combined the methodology of an RCT in clinical medicine with that of a multiwave survey to achieve multiple interrelated objectives. The RCT part had three layered goals. The first goal was to design a conventional efficacy trial for QG. The second goal was to test the mechanisms of action of QG, such as the energy alteration that occurs in physiological functions. This potential energy alteration may mediate the effect of QG on postoperative wound healing and pain control in this study. The third goal was to test the placebo effect. Researchers randomly assigned 400 cardiac surgery patients into three groups that received either (1) no treatment, (2) sham QG by trained actors, or (3) real QG by a master. Patients, surgeons, and evaluating research assistants and physicians were all blinded to the intervention assignment. The efficacy of QG was assessed by measures of wound healing, pain relief, use of pain medication, and length of hospitalization. To address the placebo effect further, patients were asked after their participation in the trial if they believed they had received the effective (real) treatment. It was hypothesized that there would be no improvement in the no treatment group, some minimal improvement in the sham QG group, and more improvement in the real QG group. End point measurements and assessments were made at multiple points (2 weeks before hospitalization, day before surgery, during postoperative 4 days in the hospital, and 2 months, 6 months, and 2 years after surgery).

As with the first study, however, a limitation in this second trial was the need to collect complicated measures on some difficult conditions immediately after severe surgical trauma. Namely, QG healers had only 3 to 4 days to deliver their treatment during the hospitalization. Both conditions (wound healing and pain relief) tend not to be within the norm of regular treatment using complementary, alternative, and integrative medicine, including QG, which primarily focuses on the prevention of disease and maintenance of health rather than on the treatment of medical diseases. Clearly, this limitation means that the short-term efficacy of QG in this study may be affected by the "dosage" (treatment length or intensity) required by these difficult conditions, as well as by the level of the QG healers' "energy power." The original principal investigator and designer of this trial left the University of Michigan Integrative Medicine Program immediately after the NCCAM funding became available. The RCT trial data from 400 patients were collected, cleaned, and analyzed but have never been written up. Through personal contact, it was learned that, unsurprisingly, the trial found only a placebo effect. Several factors may help explain this finding. First, there may be no QG effect on these difficult conditions occurring during a severe medical crisis. Second, the "dosage," with respect to the length or times of the QG treatment, may be insufficient. Third, the energy power of the QG healers in this trial may not have been at the appropriate level. The original QG master who was to be tested in this trial did not participate in the RCT, rather his students did. One of these healers was later tested by a biophysicist expert researcher in the University of California system, who indicated that the tested level of the healer was "B+."

Third NIH-Funded Medium-Scale Randomized Controlled Trial

The third NIH-funded trial was designed to assess the efficacy of QG in reducing pain and improving functionality in patients with knee osteoarthritis. Chen et al (2008) randomly assigned 112 patients (older than age 50) to receive either genuine QG from one of two QG masters or sham QG from one sham master for five to six sessions over 3 weeks. Both the patients and the examining physician were blinded to the assignment. Of the 106 patients who completed the trial, those in both treatment groups reported significant reduction in pain scores (on the Western Ontario and MacMaster University Osteoarthritis Index) after QG intervention. Results for the patients treated by the two healers were then analyzed separately. Compared with those in the sham control group, patients treated by healer 2 reported greater reduction in pain (mean improvement -25.7 ± 6.6 vs. -13.1 ± 3.0; $P < .01$) and more improvement in functionality (-28.1 ± 9.7 vs. -13.2 ± 3.4; $P < .01$), as well as a reduction in negative mood but not in anxiety or depression. Patients treated by healer 1 experienced improvement similar to that of the control group. The results of therapy persisted at 3-month follow-up for all groups. Mixed-effect models confirmed these findings with control for possible confounders (e.g., gender, BMI, belief in CAM therapies, and duration of osteoarthritis pain). The results of this study are consistent with the third possibility raised for the second NIH-funded RCT, which suggests that the efficacy of external QG may depend on the unknown energy power of the QG healer. The apparent difference between healers calls for more scientific investigation on the measurable capacity in both QG and other forms of energy healing.

Another Small-Scale Randomized Controlled Trial and Other Laboratory Experiments

Jang and Lee (2004) in Korea assigned 36 naive female subjects (college students) with premenstrual syndrome (PMS) to receive either real QG treatment or a sham QG placebo. Each treatment was performed eight times during the second and third cycles with subjects completing a treatment diary. Significant improvements were reported by the QG group in terms of negative feeling, pain, water retention, and total PMS symptoms, compared with the control group. Finally, Mo et al (2003) in China and Chen et al (2002) in the United States have use RCTs to investigate the effect of QG on morphine-abstinent mice and rats and on the in vivo growth of transplantable murine lymphoma cells in mice, respectively, and have obtained some preliminary findings. These types of studies are not the primary focus of this chapter, nor is information concerning the historical documentation of QG, practical instructions for practice, or the more scientific exploration of the nature of qi and other biofield phenomena, which is addressed elsewhere in this book or in specialized sources.

SUMMARY

At the end of their research article, Ai et al (2001) described the implications of these new investigations of QG for clinical sciences as follows:

> Inquiry into controversial issues surrounding QG does not arise only from the need to improve the quality of research design on energy healing trials. It is also a call for continuing innovation of research methodology to address the unique challenge of evaluating the complicated frameworks of CAM modalities. Through close cooperation between researchers and CAM practitioners, standardized approaches to valid research protocols can be developed. By scientific testing of plural pathway models, the blossoming of research on energy healing may eventually enrich methodologies used in clinical research on other types of health care.

Acknowledgments

The author has been supported by National Institute on Aging training grant T32-AG0017, National Institute on Aging grant R03-AGO-15686-01, National Center for Complementary and Alternative Medicine grant P50-AT00011, a grant from the John Templeton Foundation, and the John Hartford Faculty Scholars Program. Amy L. Ai, PhD, is professor at the University of Pittsburgh and an affiliated researcher at the University of Michigan Health System Integrative Medicine Program.

⊖ Chapter References can be found on the Evolve website at http://evolve.elsevier.com/Micozzi/complementary/

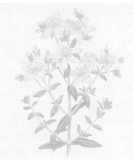

CHAPTER

29

TRADITIONAL MEDICINE OF INDIA: AYURVEDA AND SIDDHA

KENNETH G. ZYSK

As the health care professions look seriously at complementary and alternative modalities of medicine, a growing interest in Ayurveda and Siddha medicine, the traditional Indian medicine, is also emerging. Three traditional medicinal systems predominate in modern India: Ayurveda, Siddha, and Unani. Ayurveda is found mostly in northern India and in Kerala in the south. Siddha medicine occurs in Tamil Nadu and parts of Kerala. Unani, which derives from Arabic medicine, is found throughout India, mainly in the urban areas. This chapter focuses on Ayurveda and Siddha medicine (Tamil, *Citta vaittiyam*) and its history and practice in South India, with an eye toward the similarities and differences between Siddha medicine and Ayurveda.

Thus, in addition to being a highly developed and complex form of "ethnomedicine," both Ayurveda and Siddha remain living systems in current use as available forms of primary health care in India. Ayurveda, in particular, is becoming increasingly available as a complementary and alternative medical system through the practice of integrative medicine in the West, which actively is bringing complementary and alternative medical modalities into current practice.

AYURVEDIC MEDICINE

Ayurveda is literally the "science of life," or of longevity. As with any popular development, aspects of the Indian medical system and its cures have sometimes been appropriated by individuals not wholly familiar with the basics of Ayurveda or the science of longevity. As a result inaccurate information or even misinformation circulates in various publications about Ayurveda. Fortunately, well-trained scholars have undertaken serious study of this ancient healing tradition, and this chapter aims to present the fundamental principles and practices of traditional Ayurveda as they may be understood from scholarly study of classical Sanskrit sources and according to accounts by traditional Indian practitioners.

HISTORY

Available literary sources indicate that the history of Indian medicine can be divided into four main phases (Zysk, 1991, 1993a, 1993b). The first, or Vedic, phase dates from about 1200 to 800 BC. Information about medicine during this period is obtained from numerous curative incantations and references to healing that are found in the *Atharvaveda* and the *Rigveda,* two religious scriptures that reveal a "magicoreligious" approach to healing (Zysk, 1993a, 1993b). The second, or classical, phase is marked by the advent of the first Sanskrit medical treatises, the *Caraka* (Sharma, 1981-1994) and *Sushruta Samhita* (Bhishagratana, 1983), which probably date from a few centuries before to several centuries after the start of the common (Christian) era. This period includes all subsequent medical treatises dating from before the Muslim invasions of India at the beginning of the eleventh century, because these works tend to follow the earlier classical compilations closely and provide the basis of traditional Ayurveda. The third, or syncretic, phase is marked by clear influences on the classical medicine from Islamic or Unani, South Indian Siddha, and other nonclassical medical systems. Bhavamishra's sixteenth century *Bhavaprakasha* is one text that reveals the results of these influences, which included diagnosis by examination of pulse or urine (Upadhyay, 1986). This phase extends from the Muslim incursions to the present era. I would term the final phase "New Age Ayurveda," in which the classical paradigm is being adapted to the world of modern science and technology, including quantum physics, mind-body science, and advanced biomedical science. This recent manifestation of Ayurveda is most visible in the Western world, although there are indications that it has already taken hold in India. These four phases of Indian medical history provide a chronological grid for understanding the development of this ancient system of medicine.

THEORY

From its beginnings during the Vedic era Indian medicine always has adhered closely to the principle of a fundamental connection between the microcosm and macrocosm. Human beings are minute representations of the universe and contain within them everything that makes up the surrounding world. Comprehending the world is crucial to comprehending the human being, and conversely, understanding the world is necessary to understanding the human.

The Human Body

According to Ayurveda the cosmos consists of five basic elements: earth, air, fire, water, and space. Certain forces cause these to interact, giving rise to all that exists. In human beings these five elements occur in the form of the three *doshas,* forces that, along with the seven *dhatus* (tissues) and three *malas* (waste products), make up the human body.

The three doshas. When in equilibrium the three doshas maintain health, but when an imbalance occurs among them, they defile the normal functioning of the body, leading to the manifestation of disease. An imbalance indicates an increase or decrease in one, two, or all

three of the doshas. The three doshas are *vata, pitta,* and *kapha* (Svoboda, 1984).

Vata or *vayu,* meaning "wind," is composed of the elements air and space. It is the principle of kinetic energy and is responsible for all bodily movement and nervous functions. It is located below the navel and in the bladder, large intestines, nervous system, pelvic region, thighs, bone marrow, and legs; its principal seat is the colon. When disrupted, its primary manifestation is gas and muscular or nervous energy, which leads to pain.

Pitta, or bile, is made up of the elements of fire and water or, according to some, just fire. It governs enzymes and hormones and is responsible for digestion, pigmentation, body temperature, hunger, thirst, sight, courage, and mental activity. It is located between the navel and the chest and in the stomach, small intestines, liver, spleen, skin, and blood; its principal seat is the stomach. When disrupted, its primary manifestation is acid and bile, which leads to inflammation.

Kapha or *shleshman,* meaning "phlegm," is made up of the elements of earth and water. It connotes the principle of cohesion and stability. It regulates vata and pitta and is responsible for keeping the body lubricated and maintaining its solid nature, tissues, sexual power, and strength. It also controls patience. Its normal locations are the upper part of the body, thorax, head, neck, upper portion of the stomach, pleural cavity, fat tissues, and areas between joints; its principal seat is the lungs. When it is disrupted, its primary manifestation is liquid and mucus, which leads to swelling, with or without discharge.

The attributes of each dosha help determine the individual's basic bodily and mental makeup and to isolate which dosha is responsible for a disease. The qualities of vata are dryness, cold, light, irregularity, mobility, roughness, and abundance. Dryness occurs when vata is disturbed and is a side effect of motion. Too much dryness produces irregularity in the body and mind. Pitta is hot, light, intense, fluid, liquid, putrid, pungent, and sour. Heat appears when pitta is disturbed, resulting from change caused by pitta. The intensity of excessive heat produces irritability in the body and mind. Kapha is heavy, unctuous, cold, stable, dense, soft, and smooth. Heaviness occurs when kapha is disturbed and results from firmness caused by kapha. The viscosity of excessive heaviness and stability produces slowness in body and mind.

Prakriti. There are seven normal body constitutions (*prakriti*) based on the three doshas: *vata, pitta, kapha, vata-pitta, pitta-kapha, vata-kapha,* and *sama.* The last is triple balanced, which is best, but extremely rare. Most people are a combination of doshas, in which one dosha predominates. In general, vata-type people tend to be anxious and fearful, exhibit light and "airy" characteristics, and are prone to vata diseases. Pitta-type people are aggressive and impatient, exhibit fiery and hot-headed characteristics, and are prone to pitta diseases. Kapha-type people are stable and entrenched; exhibit heavy, wet, and earthy characteristics;

and are prone to kapha diseases (Svoboda, 1984). A person's balanced condition, therefore, is the same as his or her prakriti, so that every individual's state of balanced doshas is unique.

The seven dhatus. The seven dhatus or tissues are responsible for sustaining the body. Each dhatu is responsible for the one that comes next in the following order:

1. *Rasa,* meaning sap or juice, includes the tissue fluids, bile, lymph, and plasma, and functions as nourishment. It comes from digested food.
2. *Blood* includes the red blood cells and functions to invigorate the body.
3. *Flesh* includes muscle tissue and functions as stabilization.
4. *Fat* includes adipose tissue and functions as lubrication.
5. *Bone* includes bone and cartilage and functions as support.
6. *Marrow* includes red and yellow bone marrow and functions as filling for the bones.
7. *Shukra* includes male and female sexual fluids and functions in reproduction and immunity.

The three malas. The malas are the waste products of digested food and drink. Ayurveda delineates three principal malas: *urine, feces,* and *sweat.* A fourth category of other waste products includes fatty excretions from the skin and intestines, sebum (earwax), mucus of the nose, saliva, tears, hair, and nails. According to Ayurveda an individual should evacuate the bowels once a day and eliminate urine six times a day.

Ayurveda considers digestion to be the most important function that takes place in the human body. It provides all that is required to sustain the organism and is the principal cause for all maladies from which an individual suffers. The process of digestion and assimilation of nutrients is discussed under the topics of the *agnis* (enzymes), *ama* (improperly digested food and drink), and the *srotas* (channels of circulation).

The three agnis. The agnis, or enzymes, assist in the digestion and assimilation of food and are divided into three types.

Jatharagni is active in the mouth, stomach, and gastrointestinal tract and helps break down food. The waste product of feces results from this activity.

Bhutagnis are five enzymes located in the liver. They adapt the broken-down food into a homologous chyle according to the five elements and assist the chyle to assimilate with the corresponding five elements in the body. The homologous chyle circulates in the blood channels as rasa, nourishing the body and supplying the seven dhatus.

Dhatvagnis are seven enzymes that synthesize the seven dhatus from the assimilated chyle homologized with the five elements. The remaining waste products result from this activity.

Ama. Ama, the chief cause of disease, is formed when there is a decrease in enzyme activity. As a product of improperly digested food and drink, it takes the form of a liquid sludge that travels through the same channels as the chyle. Because of its density, however, it lodges in different parts of the body, blocking the channels. It often mixes with the doshas that circulate through the same pathways and gravitates to a weak or stressed organ or to a site of a disease manifestation. Because all diseases invariably derive from ama, the word *amaya,* meaning "coming from ama," is a synonym for disease. Internal diseases begin with ama, and external diseases produce ama. In general, ama can be detected by a coating on the tongue; turbid urine with foul odor; and feces that are passed with undigested food, an offensive odor, and abundant gas. The principal course of treatment in Ayurveda involves the elimination of ama and the restoration of the balance of the doshas.

The thirteen kinds of srotas. The srotas are the vessels or channels of the body through which all substances circulate. They are either large, such as the large and small intestines and the uterus; medium sized, such as arteries and veins; or small, such as the capillaries. A healthy body has open and free-flowing channels. Blockage of the channels, usually by ama, results in disease. Following are the names, functions, and locations of the thirteen srotas:

1. *Pranavahasrotas* convey vitality and vital breath *(prana)* and originate in the heart and alimentary tract.
2. *Udakavahasrotas* convey water and fluids and originate in the palate and pancreas.
3. *Annavahasrotas* convey food from the outside and originate in the stomach.
4. *Rasavahasrotas* convey chyle, lymph, and plasma and originate in the heart and in the 10 vessels connected with the heart. Ama primarily accumulates within them.
5. *Raktavahasrotas* convey red blood cells and originate in the liver and spleen.
6. *Mamsavahasrotas* convey ingredients for muscle tissue and originate in the tendons, ligaments, and skin.
7. *Medovahasrotas* convey ingredients for fat tissue and originate in the kidneys and fat tissues of the abdomen.
8. *Asthavahasrotas* convey ingredients for bone tissue and originate in hip bone.
9. *Majjavahasrotas* convey ingredients for marrow and originate in the bones and joints.
10. *Shukravahasrotas* convey ingredients for the male and female reproductive tissues and originate in the testicles and ovary.
11. *Mutravahasrotas* convey urine and originate in the kidney and bladder.
12. *Purishavahasrotas* convey feces and originate in the colon and rectum.
13. *Svedavahasrotas* convey sweat and originate in the fat tissues and hair follicles.

This broad outline exhibits the Ayurvedic view that the human body's anatomical parts are composed of the five basic elements, which have undergone a process of metabolism and assimilation in the body. Human beings differ depending on their normal bodily constitution (prakriti), which is determined at the moment of conception and remains until death. The four factors that influence constitutional type include the father, the mother (particularly her food intake), the womb, and the season of the year. A large imbalance of the doshas in the mother will affect the growth of the embryo and fetus, and a moderate excess of one or two of the doshas will affect the constitution of the child.

These are the principal factors that help the Ayurvedic physician determine the correct course of treatment to be administered to a patient for a particular ailment.

Three mental states. In addition to physical constitution, Ayurveda understands that an individual is influenced by three mental states, based on the three qualities (gunas) of balance (sattva), energy (rajas), and inertia (tamas). In the state of balance the mind is in equilibrium and can discriminate correctly. In the state of energy the mind is excessively active, which causes weakness in discrimination. In the state of inertia the mind is excessively inactive, which also creates weak discrimination.

Ayurveda always has recognized that the body and the mind interact to create a healthy, normal (prakriti) or unhealthy, abnormal (vikriti) condition. A good Ayurvedic physician will determine both the mental and physical condition of the patient before proceeding with any form of diagnosis and treatment.

DISEASE

Aspects of the Ayurvedic understanding of disease have been mentioned in the previous section. Here the focus is specifically on the Ayurvedic classification of disease, the naming of disease, and the manifestations of disease (Dash, 1980; Dash et al, 1980).

Classification of Disease

Ayurveda identifies three broad categories of disease on the basis of causative factors.

Adhyatmika diseases originate within the body and may be subdivided into hereditary diseases, congenital diseases, and diseases caused by one or a combination of the doshas.

Adhibhautika diseases originate outside the body and include injuries from accidents or mishaps and, in the terminology of the modern era, from germs, viruses, and bacteria.

Adhidaivika diseases originate from supernatural sources and include diseases that are otherwise inexplicable, such as maladies stemming from providential causes, planetary influences, curses, and seasonal changes.

Disease Names

In Ayurveda diseases receive their names in one of six ways. A disease is named for the condition it produces (fever, or jvara), its chief symptom (diarrhea, or atisara), its chief physical sign (jaundice, or pandu), its principal nature (piles, or arshas), the chief dosha(s) involved (wind disease, or vata-roga), or the chief organ involved (disease of the duodenum, or grahani). Regardless of its given name, most diseases involve one or more of the doshas.

Manifestation of Disease

During the course of a disease an Ayurvedic physician seeks to identify its site of origin, its path of transportation, and its site of manifestation. The site of manifestation of a disease usually differs from its site of origin. Recognizing this distinction enables the physician to determine the correct course of treatment.

Ayurveda describes the manifestation of all diseases in the same fundamental way. Causative factors (e.g., food, drink, regimen, season, mental state) suppress digestive (enzyme) activity in the body, which leads to the formation of ama. The circulating ama blocks the channels. The site of the disease's origin is where the blockage occurs. The circulating ama, often combining with one or more of the doshas, then takes a divergent course, referred to as the path of transportation. Finally, the dosha(s) and ama mixture comes to rest in and afflicts a certain body part, which is known as the site of disease manifestation. Treatment entails correction of all the steps in the process resulting in disease manifestation, which thus restores the entire person to his or her particular balanced state.

TREATMENT

In Ayurveda restoring a person to health is not viewed simply as the eradication of disease. It entails a complete process of diagnosis and therapeutics that takes into account both mental and physical components integrated with the social and physical worlds in which the patient lives. It begins with Ayurvedic diagnosis, examination of the disease, and determination of types of therapeutics (Jolly, 1977; Lad, 1990; Sen Gupta, 1984).

Ayurvedic Diagnosis

Ayurveda established a detailed system of diagnosis, involving examination of pulse, urine, and physical features.

After a preliminary examination by means of visual observation, touch, and interrogation, the Ayurvedic physician undertakes an eightfold method of detailed examination to determine the patient's type of physical constitution and mental status and to get an indication of any abnormality.

Pulse examination. Pulse examination is first mentioned in a medical treatise from the late thirteenth or early fourteenth century AD. It is a highly specialized art. Not every Ayurvedic physician uses pulse examination.

The diagnostic process involves evenly placing the index, middle, and ring fingers of the right hand on the radial artery of the right hand of men and the left hand of women, just at the base of the thumb. A pulse resembling the movement of a snake at the index finger indicates a predominance of vata; a pulse resembling the movement of a frog at the middle finger indicates a predominance of pitta; a pulse resembling the movement of a swan or peacock at the ring finger indicates a predominance of kapha; and a pulse resembling the movement of a woodpecker indicates a predominance of all three doshas. To get an accurate reading, the physician must keep in mind the times when each of the doshas is normally excited and should take the pulse at least three times early in the morning when the stomach is empty, or 3 hours after eating in the afternoon, making sure to wash his or her hands after each reading (Upadhyay, 1986).

Urine examination. Like pulse examination, urine examination probably was formalized during the syncretic phase. After collecting the morning's midstream evacuation in a clear glass container, the physician submits the urine to two kinds of examination after sunrise. First, the physician studies it in the container to determine its color and degree of transparency. Pale yellow and oily urine indicates vata; intense yellow, reddish, or blue urine indicates pitta; white, foamy, and muddy urine indicates kapha; urine with a blackish tinge indicates a combination of doshas; and urine resembling lime juice or vinegar indicates ama. The physician also puts a few drops of sesame oil in the urine and examines it in sunlight. The shape, movement, and diffusion of the oil in the urine indicate the prognosis of the disease. The shape of the drops also reveals the specific dosha(s) involved. A snakelike shape indicates vata; an umbrella shape, pitta; and a earl shape, kapha.

Examination of bodily parts. The physician concludes the diagnostic examination with careful scrutiny of the tongue, skin, nails, and physical features to determine the particular dosha(s) affected. Using the basic characteristics of each of the doshas, the physician will examine the different parts of the body. Coldness, dryness, roughness, and cracking indicate vata; hotness and redness indicate pitta; and wetness, whiteness, and coldness indicate kapha.

Having completed this phase of the diagnosis, the Ayurvedic physician proceeds to examine any malady present.

Examination of the Disease

A detailed examination of the disease involves a five-step process, which leads to a complete understanding of the abnormality.

Cause. A disease results from one or several of the following factors: mental imbalances arising from the effects of past actions *(karma);* unbalanced contact between the senses and the objects of the senses affecting the body and the mind; effects of the seasons on the mental and doshic balance; the immediate causes of diet, regimen, and microorganisms; doshas and ama; and the combination or interaction of individual components, such as doshas and tissues, or doshas and microorganisms.

Early signs and symptoms. Early signs and symptoms that appear before the onset of disease provide clues to the diagnosis. Proper diet and administration of medicine can avert disease if it is recognized early enough.

Manifest signs and symptoms. The most crucial step in the diagnostic process is evaluation of manifest signs and symptoms. It involves determining the site of origin and of manifestation, and the path of transportation of the Ama and dosha(s). Most signs and symptoms are associated with the site of disease manifestation, from which the physician must work his or her way back to the site of the origin of disease to effect a complete cure. Although symptomatic treatment was largely absent in traditional Ayurveda, modern medicine in India has introduced Ayurvedic physicians to techniques of symptomatic treatment in cases of acute disease.

Exploratory therapy. Exploratory therapy involves 18 different experiments that use herbs, diet, and regimens to determine the precise nature of the malady and suitable therapy by allopathic and homeopathic means.

Pathogenesis. Pathogenesis is determined through a six-step process that identifies the manner by which a dosha becomes aggravated and moves through the different channels to produce disease. An accumulation of a dosha leads to its aggravation, which causes it to spread through the channels until it lodges in a particular organ of the body, bringing about a manifestation of disease. Once a general form of the disease appears, it progressively splits into specific varieties. As in systems of medicine the world over, many patients consult the Ayurvedic physician only after the disease appears.

Ayurveda delineates seven basic varieties of disease on the basis of the doshas: diseases involving a single dosha, diseases involving two doshas, and diseases involving all three doshas together.

Prognosis is the final step in the Ayurvedic diagnostic process. Because Ayurvedic physicians traditionally did not treat persons with incurable diseases, it was important for the physician to know precisely the patient's chances of full recovery. Therefore disease is one of three types. It is easily curable, it can be palliated, or it is incurable or difficult to cure. (By comparison, the Edwin Smith Papyrus on ancient Egyptian Medicine, from 3000 BC, on diseases of the head and neck—the rest of the papyrus on the lower body is missing—also categorizes "diseases I will treat," "diseases with which I will contend," and essentially "untreatable" from the standpoint of the physician). In general, if the disease type (vata, pitta, kapha) is different from the person's normal physical constitution, the disease is easy to cure. If the disease and constitution are the same, the disease is difficult to cure. If the disease, constitution, and season correspond to doshic type, the disease is nearly impossible to cure (Singhal, 1972-1993).

Having determined the patient's normal constitution, diagnosed his or her illness, and established a prognosis for recovery, the Ayurvedic physician can begin a proper course of treatment.

Prevention and Treatment

Ayurveda recognizes two courses of treatment on the basis of the condition of the patient. The first is *prevention,* for the healthy person who wants to maintain a normal condition based on his or her physical constitution and to prevent disease. The second is *therapy,* for an ill person who requires health to be restored. Once healthy, Ayurveda recommends continuous prophylaxis based on diet, regimen, medicines, and regular therapeutic purification procedures.

When a person is diagnosed with a doshic imbalance, either purification therapy, alleviation therapy, or a combination of these is prescribed.

Purification therapy. Purification therapy involves the fundamental *Pañchakarma,* or Five Action treatment. The fivefold process varies slightly in different traditions and regions of India, but a standard regimen generally is followed. All five procedures can be performed, or a selection of procedures can be chosen on the basis of different factors such as the physical constitution of the patient, his or her condition, the season, and the nature of the disease. Before any action is taken, the patient is given oil internally and externally (with massage) and is sweated to loosen and soften the dosha(s) and ama. An appropriate diet of food and drink is prescribed. After this twofold preparatory treatment, called *Purvakarma,* the five therapies are administered in sequence over the period of about a week. Because of the profound effects on the mind and body, the patient is advised to set aside time for treatment. First, the patient might be given an emetic and vomits until bilious matter is produced, thus removing kapha. Second, a purgative is given until mucus material appears, thus removing pitta. Third, an enema, either of oil or decocted medicines, is administered to remove excess vata. Fourth, head purgation is given in the form of smoke inhalation or nasal drops to eradicate the dosha(s) that have accumulated in the head and sinuses. Fifth, leeches may be applied and bloodletting performed to purify the blood. Some physicians do not consider bloodletting as one of the five therapies of Pañchakarma, instead counting oily and dry (decocted medicine) enemas as two separate forms (Singh, 1992).

Alleviation therapy. Alleviation therapy uses the basic condiments honey, butter or ghee, and sesame oil or castor oil to eliminate kapha, pitta, and vata, respectively. This therapy and Pañchakarma often are used in conjunction with one another.

Herbal medicine. Ayurveda prescribes a rich store of natural medicines that have been collected, tested, and recorded in medical treatises from ancient times. The tradition of collecting and preserving information about medicines in recipe books called *Nighantus* continued to the twentieth century (Nadkarni, 1908). The most traditional source of Ayurvedic medicine is the kitchen. It is likely that, at an early stage of its development, Indian medical and culinary traditions worked hand in hand with each other.

Because of the close association between food and medicine, Ayurveda classifies foods and drugs (usually vegetal) by the tongue, potency, and taste after digestion.

Rasa, taste by the tongue, is categorized into six separate tastes, with their individual elemental composition and doshic effect as follows:

1. *Sweet,* composed of earth and water, increases kapha and decreases pitta and vata.
2. *Sour,* composed of earth and fire, increases kapha and pitta and decreases vata.
3. *Saline,* composed of water and fire, increases kapha and pitta and decreases vata.
4. *Pungent,* composed of wind and fire, increases pitta and vata and decreases kapha.
5. *Bitter,* composed of wind and space, increases vata and decreases pitta and kapha.
6. *Astringent,* composed of wind and earth, increases vata and decreases pitta and kapha.

Virya, potency, comprises eight types that are divided into four pairs: hot-cold, unctuous-dry, heavy-light, and dull-sharp.

Vipaka, postdigestive taste, identifies three kinds of aftertaste: sweet, sour, and pungent.

Contrary foods and drugs are to be avoided always. For instance, clarified butter and honey should not be taken in equal quantities, alkalies and salt must not be taken for a long period, milk and fish should not be consumed together, and honey should not be put in hot drinks.

Four important criteria are considered when compounding plant substances and other ingredients into medical recipes. The substances that make up the recipe should have many attributes that enable it to cure several diseases. They should be usable in many pharmaceutical preparations, they should be suitable for the recipe and not cause unwanted side effects, and they should be culturally appropriate to the patients and their customs. Every medicine should be able to treat the disease's site of origin, site of manifestation, and its spread simultaneously.

A brief survey of the different kinds of medical preparations indicates the depth and content of Ayurvedic pharmaceuticals. The botanically based medicines derive largely from the Ayurvedic medical tradition, whereas the drugs based on minerals and inorganic substances derive from the Indian alchemical traditions, called *Rasashastra.*

1. *Juices* are cold presses and extractions made from plants.
2. *Powders* are prepared from parts of plants that have been dried in the shade and other dried ingredients.
3. *Infusions* are parts of plants and herbs that have been steeped in water and strained.

4. *Cold infusions* are parts of plants and herbs that were soaked in water overnight and filtered the next morning.
5. *Decoctions* are vegetal products boiled in a quantity of water proportionate to the hardness of the plant part and then reduced by a fourth. The decoction is then filtered and often used with butter, honey, or oils.
6. *Medicated pastes and oils.* Often the plant and herbal extracts are combined with other ingredients and formed into pastes, plasters, and oils. Used externally, pastes and plasters are applied for joint, muscular, and skin conditions, and oil is used for hair and head problems. Medicated oils also are used for massages and enemas.
7. *Large and small pills and suppositories.* Plant and herbal extracts are also formed into pills and suppositories to be used internally.
8. *Alcoholic preparations* are made by fermentation or distillation. Two preparations are delineated: one requires the drug to be boiled before it is fermented or distilled, and in the other, the drug is simply added to the preparation. Fifteen percent is the maximum allowable amount of alcohol content in a drug. Several Ayurvedic medicines are prepared from minerals and metals, especially mercury, and reflect the tradition of Indian alchemy.
9. *Sublimates* are prepared by an elaborate method leading to the sublimation of sulfur in a glass container. They are found in recipes *(rasayanas)* used in rejuvenation therapies.
10. *Bhasmas* are ash residues produced from the calcination of metals, gems, plants, and animal products. Most are metals and minerals that are first detoxified and then purified. An important bhasma is prepared from mercury, which undergoes an 18-stage detoxification and purification process. Ayurveda maintains that bhasmas are quickly absorbed in the blood and increase the number of red blood cells.
11. *Pishtis* are fine powders made by trituration of gems with juices and extracts.
12. *Collyrium* is made from antimony powder, lead oxide, or the soot from lamps burned with castor oil. Collyrium is used especially to improve vision.

Space does not allow a discussion of the individual plants used in Ayurvedic recipes. It is safe to say, however, that of the hundreds of plants mentioned in various Ayurvedic treatises, only a small portion are commonly used by most Ayurvedic physicians.

SIDDHA MEDICINE

Research into Siddha medicine in Tamil Nadu has revealed certain difficulties that must be overcome to understand properly this medical system and its history. The central problem lies in the reliability of the secondary sources, which are written primarily by Tamil Siddha doctors. Little scholarly research on the subject has been carried out by Western students and scholars of India and Indian medicine.

Due to the increased awareness of Tamil's Dravidian linguistic roots over the past decades, a strong nationalist movement has grown up in Tamil Nadu. Tamilians consider their cultural and linguistic heritage to be older and more important than that of the Indo-Aryans of northern India; some even claim that their ancestors comprised the first civilization on the planet. The fire of this controversy has recently been kindled by a debate centering on the still-to-be-deciphered script of the so-called Indus Valley civilization. This ancient urban culture, which extended along the Indus River and its tributaries in what is now Pakistan, resembled the great civilizations of ancient Egypt and Mesopotamia in size, development, and age. One side of the debate maintains that the script represents a language probably of Dravidian origin, whereas the other side claims that it does not represent a language at all. Tamilians, whose language is Dravidian, are anxiously following the debate, for if the former side prevails, it would confirm their antiquity on the Indian subcontinent. The lens through which Tamilians look at their own history will always distort the image in favor of Tamil superiority and antiquity.

HISTORY

References to Ayurveda occur early in Tamil literature. Already in the mid-fifth century AD text, *Cilappatikara,* there is reference to Ayurveda (Tamil, *āyulvetar*). Mention of the three humors (Tamil, *tiritocam;* Sanskrit, *tridosha*) occurs in the *Tirukural,* a collection of poems that dates from around AD 450 to 550.

The first Tamil Siddha text is the *Tirumandiram* written by Tirumular and dated probably to around the sixth or seventh century AD. In it there is mention of alchemy used to transform iron into gold, but no specific references to Tamil medicinal doctrines are found. The major sources of Siddha medicine are those belonging to religious groups who called themselves Kayasiddhas. They emphasized the "perfection of the body" by means of yoga, alchemy, medicine, and certain types of Tantric religious rituals. These works date from about the thirteenth to the fourteenth century AD and are attributed to numerous authors, including Akattiyar (Sanskrit, *Agastya*), the traditional founder of Siddha medicine, and Teraiyar (ca. late seventeenth century), who is said to have written 12 works on medicine, and whose famous disciple Iramatevar travelled to Mecca in the late seventeenth or early eighteenth century, where he studied, converted to Islam, and took on the name Yakkopu (Jacob). Most critical scholars of Siddha agree that on the basis of their language, the numerous texts on Siddha medicine, which present it as a system of healing, cannot be older than the sixteenth century.

We must, therefore, acknowledge that Tamil Siddha medicine, as it is now exists in both theory and practice, began in Tamil Nadu around the sixteenth century, but elements of healing practices that became part of Siddha medicine, including those held in common with Ayurveda, came from an earlier period.

Tamil folklore surrounding healing shares a common origin with Buddhism from northern India. To trace the origin of the name Teraiyar, legend says that Akattiyar performed a trephination on a sage to remove a toad *(terai)* from inside his skull. However, it was Akattiyar's disciple who, with an instrument, made the frog jump into a bowl of water. Because of his skill in removing the toad, Akattiyar gave the disciple the name Teraiyar; the latter is, however, a different person from the late-seventeenth-century medical author of the same name.

This is a particularly interesting legend because there is a similar account in Buddhist literature. In its earliest version found in the Pali texts of the Buddhist canon, a skilled physician, Jivaka Komarabhacca, opened up the skull of a merchant from Rajagriha and removed two centipedes by touching them with a hot poker. The merchant made a full recovery. Versions of this folk story occur in the Sanskrit literature of later Mahayana Buddhism and were translated into Tibetan and Chinese. The uniqueness of the story as a remarkable medical accomplishment and its spread throughout Buddhist Asia testifies to the influence of Buddhism in the dissemination of medical knowledge in premodern India.

Like all systems of Hindu knowledge, Siddha medicine attributes its origin to a divine source; hence its knowledge is sacred and eternal, passed down to humans for the benefit of all humanity. According to Hindu tradition, the god Shiva transmitted the knowledge of medicine to his wife Parvati, who in turn passed it on to Nandi, from whom it was given to the first practitioners of Siddha medicine, the Siddhars. Tradition lists a total number of 18 Siddhars, beginning with Nandi and the semilegendary Agattiyar through to the final Siddhar, Kudhambai. They are the acknowledged transmitters of Siddha medical doctrines and practices. By attributing a divine or extrahuman origin to its medicine, the Tamil Siddhars assured Siddha medicine a legitimate place in the corpus of Hindu knowledge. Although the transmission begins with Nandi, who in the form of a bull is Shiva's mode of transportation, tradition attributes the origin of medicine as well as of the Tamil language to Agattiyar.

PRINCIPLES

According to Siddha cosmology, all matter is composed of two primal forces of matter *(shiva)* and energy *(shakti)*. These two principles of existence operate in humans as well as nature and connect the microcosm with the macrocosm. This connection is expressed by the association between the human body and the signs of the zodiac in Indian astrology. The formulation of the sequence of body parts is interesting, because it follows a Babylonian and Greco-Roman system of head-to-toe rather than an Indian one, which begins at the toes and ends at the head. This formulation is illustrated in the following list, using Latin-based zodiac names.

1. ♈ Áries (0°) = the neck
2. ♉ Taurus (30°) = the shoulders
3. ♊ Gémini (60°) = the arms and hands
4. ♋ Cancer (90°) = the chest
5. ♌ Leo (120°) = the heart and the stomach
6. ♍ Virgo (150°) = the intestines
7. ♎ Libra (180°) = the kidneys
8. ♏ Scórpio (210°) = the genitals
9. ♐ Sagittárius (240°) = the hips
10. ♑ Capricornus (270°) = the knees
11. ♒ Aquárius (300°) = the legs
12. ♓ Pisces (330°) = the feet

In addition to this cosmic connection, which occurred in all traditions of Indian astrology, Siddha medicine relied entirely on Ayurveda for the medical doctrines that bridge the natural world and the human body. In modern-day Siddha practice, evidence of the following epistemology is not always noticed.

First, there are the five gross elements *(pañcamahabhutam)*, which make up the entire natural world: solid/earth, fluid/water, radiance/fire, gas/wind, and ether/space. These combine in certain ways to yield the three bodily humors, called *muppini* in modern Tamil. They are said to be in the proportion of 1 wind to ½ bile to ¼ phlegm, which is opposite to that found in Ayurveda:

1. *Wind* (Tamil, *vatham;* Sanskrit, *vata*) is a combination of space and wind, and is responsible for nervous actions, movement, activity, sensations, and so on. It is found in the form of the five bodily winds.
2. *Bile* (Tamil, *pittam;* Sanskrit, *pitta*) is made up of fire alone and takes care of metabolism, digestion, assimilation, warmth, and so forth. Its principal seat is in the alimentary canal from the cardiac region to small intestines. Some Ayurvedic formulations state that bile is a combination of the elements fire and water.
3. *Phlegm* (Tamil, *siletuman;* Sanskrit, *shleshman, kapha*) is a combination of earth and water and is responsible for stability in the body. Its principal seats are in the chest, throat, head, and joints.

Next, there is the shared doctrine of the seven tissues (Tamil, *dhatu*) of the body: lymph/chyle, blood, muscle, fat, bone, marrow, and sperm and ovum. Finally, there are the five winds (Tamil, *vatham;* Sanskrit, *prana*) that circulate in the body and initiate and carry out bodily functions: *pranam* is the inhaled breath and brings about swallowing; *apanam* is the exhaled breath and is responsible for expulsion, ejection, and excretion; *samanam* helps digestion; *vyanam* aids circulation of blood and nutrients; and *udanam* functions in the upper respiratory passages. There are also five secondary winds: *nagam,* the air of higher intellectual functions; *kurmam*, the air of yawning; *kirukaram*, the air of salivation; *devadhattham*, the air of laziness; and *dhananjayam*, the air that acts on death.

Like Ayurveda, Siddha medicine maintains that the three humors predominate in humans in accordance with their nature and stage of life, and that they vary with the seasons. Every individual is born with a unique configuration of the three humors, which is called the individual's "basic nature" (Sanskrit, *prakriti*). It is fixed at birth and forms the basis of his or her normal, healthy state. During the three different stages of life and during the different seasons, one humor usually predominates, which is normal, but such a domination of a humor must be understood in relation to the person's fundamental nature to maintain the balance that is the individual's basic state. The classification of the humors according to stages of life and seasons in Siddha differs from that found in Ayurveda. In the case of the seasons, the variation is attributed simply to the different climatic conditions that occur in the different parts of the year in the northern inland areas and the southern Tamil coastal and inland environments.

According to Siddha, wind predominates in the first third of life, bile in the second third, and phlegm in the last third of life, whereas in Ayurveda phlegm dominates the first third and wind the last third of life. In terms of climate the north is colder in the winter (December and January) than is the south, and the west coast has rain in June and July, when the east coast is extremely hot. A dry, cold climate is rare in the south, but it is precisely that climate which increases wind. Bile and phlegm, on the other hand, are increased when it is hot and wet.

DIAGNOSIS

The diagnosis of disease in Siddha medicine relies on the examination of eight anatomical features *(envagi thaervu)*, which are evaluated in terms of the three humors:

1. *Tongue:* Black indicates wind, yellow or red bile, and white phlegm; an ulcerated tongue points to anemia.
2. *Complexion:* Dark indicates wind, yellow or red bile, and pale phlegm.
3. *Voice:* Normal indicates wind, high-pitched bile, and low-pitched phlegm.
4. *Eyes:* Muddy colored indicates wind, yellowish or red bile, and pale phlegm.
5. *Touch:* Dryness indicates wind, warmness bile, and cold, clammy phlegm.
6. *Stool:* Black indicates wind, yellow bile, and pale phlegm.
7. *Pulse* (See later.)
8. *Urine* (See later.)

Most modern Siddha doctors place the greatest emphasis on the examination of the pulse, whereby both diagnosis and prognosis can be obtained through one process. These methods of diagnosis also occur in Ayurveda, but only after the fourteenth century. Before this time and in the Ayurvedic classical literature, diagnosis of disease was determined by a vitiation of one or more of the humors based on observation, touch, and interrogation.

Siddha pulse diagnosis (Tamil, *natiparitchai;* Sanskrit, *nadipariksha*), like that found in Ayurveda, in all probability owes it origins to Unani medicine. Moreover, it requires a highly developed sense of touch and a refined subjective awareness. According to Siddha, the following four conditions must not be present in the patient when a reading of the pulse is taken:

1. Oily hands
2. A full stomach or hunger
3. Physical exhaustion
4. Emotional distress

Moreover, if a reading cannot be taken on the hand, other arterial points may be used, such as the ankle, neck, or earlobes. It is also advisable to read the pulse at different times of the day and during different seasons of the year, because the body and the mind change during the course of the day and climatic conditions affect the person's psychological and physiological states.

The pulse is felt on the female's left and the male's right hand by the doctor's opposite hand, a few centimeters below the wrist joint using the index, middle, and ring fingers of the hand. Pressure should be applied by one finger after the other, beginning with the index finger. Each finger detects a particular humor, which in normal conditions has a movement representative of certain animals. The index finger feels the windy humor, which should have the movement of a swan, a cock, or a peacock; the middle finger feels the bilious humor, which should have the movement of a tortoise or a leach; and ring finger feels the phlegmatic humor, which should have the movement of a frog or a snake. Any deviation from these normal movements indicates which humor or humors are disturbed. If all humors are affected, the pulse is usually rapid with a good deal more volume than normal. After long periods of practice under the guidance of a skilled teacher, a student can begin to detect subtle differences in the flow, volume, and speed of the pulse at the point of each of the three fingers. These changes correspond to abnormalities in particular parts of the body, which the skilled Siddha doctor can pinpoint and for which the appropriate cure can be prescribed.

The examination of the urine *(muthira paritchai)* is another form of diagnosis in which Siddha medicine has demonstrated particular expertise. Not an original part of Ayurveda, urine examination probably derived from Unani medicine, in which this form of diagnosis can be noticed in early Arabic and Persian medical literature. In addition to examining the urine for its color, smell, and texture, Siddha medicine has developed a technique for determining the vitiated humor by reading the distribution of a drop of gingili (sesame) oil added to the urine. The meaning of the drop's configuration is as follows: longitudinal dispersal indicates windy humor; dispersal in a ring signals bilious humor; and lack of dispersal points to phlegmatic humor. Moreover, a combination of two types of dispersal means that two humors are involved. Slow dispersal in a circular form and a drop that forms the shape of an umbrella, a wheel, or a jasmine or lotus blossom indicate a favorable prognosis. If, however, the drop sinks, spreads rapidly with froth, splits into smaller drops and spreads rapidly, mixes with the urine, or spreads so that its pattern is that of an arrow, a sword, a spear, a pestle, a bull, or an elephant, the prognosis is unfavorable.

Finally, as in Ayurveda and Unani, the conditions of the eyes show which of the humors is vitiated as well as the patient's mental and emotional state: shifty, dry eyes point to wind; yellow eyes with photophobia indicates bile; watery, oily, eyes devoid of brightness reveals that phlegm is affected; and red, inflamed eyes show that all three humors are vitiated.

TREATMENT

According to traditional Siddha thinking, a physician must be knowledgeable in alchemy, astrology, and philosophy; he must be able to apply intuition and imagination; he must not seek fame or fortune from healing; he must not treat a patient before a proper diagnosis has been reached; and he must use only medicines that he has prepared himself.

Treatment and pharmaceutics are the two areas in which Siddha differs considerably from Ayurveda. As in Siddha Yoga, the principle aim of Siddha medicine is to make the body perfect and not vulnerable to decay, so that the maximum term of life can be achieved. Like Ayurveda, Siddha places emphasis on positive health, so that the object of the medicine is disease prevention. Beyond this fundamental agreement between the two systems, Siddha differs considerably from Ayurveda.

Siddha has developed expertise in five particular branches of medicine—general medicine, pediatrics, toxicology, ophthalmology, and rejuvenation—whereas traditional Ayurveda lists the following eight branches of medicine: general medicine, pediatrics, surgery, treatment of ailments above the neck, toxicology, treatment of mental disorders caused by seizure by evil spirits, rejuvenation therapy, and potency therapy. Whereas Ayurveda prescribes a therapeutic regimen involving treatments that produce the "five purifying actions"—emetics, purgatives, enemas, bloodletting, and errhines—Siddha employs only purgation.

Siddha medicine has excelled in ophthalmology. It has two separate treatises devoted to the treatment of 96 different eye diseases. This focus may be related to the strength of Arabic optics from the Unani tradition. Toxicology has formed a separate part of Siddha medicine and seems to be closely linked to indigenous systems of treating snakebites and other forms of poisoning. It may have some affinity to the Visha Vaidya (poison-doctor) tradition followed by certain Nambudiri Brahmins of

Kerala. As in this Keralan toxicological tradition, Siddha has adopted the Ayurvedic system of the three humors to explain the different effects of poisons, but it remains fundamentally an indigenous and local toxicological tradition. It classifies the severity and cure by means of the number of teeth or fang marks left on the victim. Four marks indicate the most severe condition, which is incurable; one mark indicates the least severe condition, which is cured by cold water baths and fomentation on the site of the bite.

Unlike Ayurveda, in which surgery forms a separate school of medicine, surgery per se is not a significant part of Siddha medicine. Medicated oils and pastes are applied to treat wounds and ulcers, but the use of a knife is hardly found in Siddha medicine.

Closely connected with the tradition of the martial arts in South India there developed a type of acupressure treatment based on the vital points in the human body, known as *varmam* (Sanskrit, *marman*). There are 108 points mentioned in the Ayurvedic classics, which identify them and explain that if they are injured, death can ensue. In Siddha medicine the number of important varmam points is also 108 (some say 107) out of a total of 400. Siddha doctors developed techniques of applying pressure to special points, called *varmakkalai,* to remove certain ailments and of massaging the points to cure diseases. They also specialized in bone setting and often practiced an Indian form of the martial arts, called *cilampam* or *silambattam,* that involved a kind of dueling with staffs.

According to Dr. Brigitte Sébastia of the French Institute in Pondicherry, India, the art of varmam is particularly widespread among the hereditary Siddha practitioners belonging to the Natar caste in the district of Kanyakumari in Tamil Nadu. The development of this special form of healing appears to have evolved naturally from the fact that the men of this caste, while carrying out their task of climbing coconut and *Borassus* trees to collect the fruits and sap for toddy, occasionally fell from great heights. To repair the injury or save the life of a fall victim, skills of bone setting and reviving an unconscious patient by massage developed among certain families within the caste, who have passed down their secret art from generation to generation by word of mouth. In the past, rulers employed members of this caste to cure injuries incurred in battle and to overpower their enemies by their knowledge of the Indian martial arts.

Closely connected with Siddha Yoga, the Siddha system of rejuvenation therapy, known as *Kayakalpa* (from Sanskrit, meaning "making the body competent for long life"), marks the most distinctive feature of Siddha medicine. It involves a five-step process for rejuvenating the body and prolonging life:

1. Preservation of vital energy via breath control (Tamil, *vasiyogam;* Sanskrit, *pranayama*) and yoga
2. Conservation of male semen and female secretions
3. Use of *muppu* earth salts

4. Use of calcinated powders (Tamil, *chunnam;* Sanskrit, *bhasma*) prepared from metals and minerals
5. Use of drugs prepared from plants special to each Siddha doctor

The esoteric substance called *muppu* is particular to Siddha medicine and may be considered as Siddha's equivalent of the "philosopher's stone." Its preparation is hidden in secrecy, known only by the guru and taught only when the student is deemed qualified to accept it. It is generally thought to consist of three salts *(mu-uppu)* called *puniru, kallupu,* and *vediyuppu,* which correspond respectively to the sun, moon, and fire. Puniru is said to be a certain kind of limestone composed of globules that are found underneath a type of clay known as fuller's earth. It is collected only on the night of the full moon in April, when it is said to bubble out from the limestone, and is then purified with the use of a special herb. Kallupu is hard salt or stone salt, (i.e., rock salt), which is dug up from mines under the earth or is obtained from saline deposits under the sea, or it can be gathered from the froth of seawater, which carries the undersea saline. It is considered to be useful in the consolidation of mercury and other metals. Finally, vediyuppu is potassium nitrate, which is cleaned seven times and purified with alum.

This religiomedical form of therapy is the cornerstone of the Siddha medical practice and provides the basis for the rich variety of alchemical preparations that make up the pharmacopoeia of Siddha medicine.

PHARMACOPOEIA

The precise origin of the system of Siddha pharmacology is not known, but it seems to have been closely linked to the Tantric religious movement, which can be traced back to the sixth century AD in North India and influenced both Buddhism and Hinduism. It was strongly anti-Brahminical and stressed ascetic practices and religious rituals that involved "forbidden" foods and sexual practices and often included the use of alchemical preparations.

The alchemical part of Siddha is present from at least the time of Tirumular's *Tirumandiram* (sixth or seventh century AD), in which various alchemical preparations are mentioned. Alchemy is also found in Sanskrit texts from North India, but only from about the sixth or seventh century AD, and later became the integral part of Ayurvedic medicine called *Rasashastra,* "traditional knowledge about mercury." In the classical treatises of Ayurveda, however, mention of alchemy is wanting, and only certain metals and minerals are mentioned in late classical texts from the seventh century AD by the author Vagbhata. Because alchemy had reached a far greater level of development in Siddha medicine than in Ayurveda, it is believed that medical alchemy may well have begun in South India among the Siddha yogis and ascetics and was later assimilated into Ayurveda.

There are three groups of drugs in Siddha medicine: plant products *(mulavargam),* inorganic substances *(thatuvargam),* and animal products *(jivavargam),* which are characterized by means of taste *(rasa),* quality *(guna),* potency *(virya),* postdigestive taste *(vipaka),* and specific action *(prabhava),* of which Ayurveda recognizes all but quality as the principal characteristics of a drug. Siddha has further classified the inorganic substances into six types:

1. *Uppu:* 25 or 31 varieties of salts and alkalis, which are water soluble and give out vapor when heated.
2. *Pashanam:* 64 varieties (32 natural, 32 artificial) of non–water soluble substances that emit vapor when heated.
3. *Uparasam:* seven types of non–water soluble substances that emit vapor when heated. They include mica, magnetic iron, antimony, zinc sulfate, iron pyrites, ferrous sulfate, and asafetida (hingu).
4. *Loham:* six varieties of metals and metallic alloys that are insoluble, but melt when heated and solidify when cooled. They include gold, silver, copper, iron, tin, and lead.
5. *Rasam:* drugs that are soft and sublime when heated, transforming into small crystals or amorphous powders, such as mercury, amalgams and compounds of mercury, and arsenic.
6. *Gandhakam:* sulfur, which is insoluble in water and burns off when heated. Rasam and gandhakam combine to make kattu, which is a "bound" substance, that is, a substance whose ingredients are united by a process of heating.

In addition there are 13 varieties of gems and minerals, 16 varieties of mud and siliceous earth, 35 varieties of animals, and 24 varieties of rocks.

Mercury and sulfur, combined to make mercuric sulfide, are the cornerstones of Siddha pharmacology and have been equated to the deity Shiva and his consort Parvati. The crucial ingredient in almost every Siddha alchemical preparation is mercury or quicksilver, which is used in five forms *(panchasthuta):* pure mercury *(rasam),* red sulfide of mercury *(lingam),* mercuric perchloride *(viram),* mercurous chloride *(puram),* and red oxide of mercury *(rasacheduram).* Although mercury plays a key role in both the Ayurvedic and Siddha forms of medical alchemy, mercury in its pure form is not found in India and therefore must be imported, often from Italy. If mercury never existed in its pure form in India, from where did alchemy come and how did it develop in India? Could it have come from trade with the Roman and Byzantine empires and subsequently the Italian city-states of the Middle Ages?

When combining drugs, Siddha has considered substances that have a natural affinity for each other, such as borax and ammonium sulfate, to be greater than the sum of their individual parts. Such a substance is called *nadabindu,* where *nada* is acidic and *bindu* is alkaline or, in the Siddha cosmology, female Shakti mated with male Shiva. The most important mixture of this kind is alkaline mercury with acidic sulfur. Similarly, Siddha has devised a classification of drugs as "friends" and "foes." The former increases the curative effect, whereas the latter reduces it.

Six pharmaceutical preparations are common to both Siddha and Ayurveda. They can be administered internally or on the skin and include calcinated metals and minerals (chunnam), powders (churanam), decoctions (kudinir), pastes (karkam), medicated clarified butter (nei), and medicated oils (ennai). Particular to Siddha medicine, however, are three special formulations: chunnam, metallic preparations that become alkaline, yielding calcium hydroxide, which must always be taken with another more palatable substance (anupana, "after drink"); mezhugu, waxy preparations that combine both metals and minerals; and kattu, inextricably bound preparations, which are impervious to water and flame. Sulfur and mercury or mercuric salts are combined to make them resistant to heat. While on the fire, certain juices are added by drops to empower the substance. The drug can be kept for long periods and given in small doses once a day. It should not, however, be completely turned into a powder, but should be rubbed on a sandal stone so as to yield only a few grains of the powerful substance.

Both Ayurveda's Rasashastra and Siddha's alchemy have devised slightly different methods for purifying or detoxifying metals and minerals, called suddhi murai in Tamil and shodhana in Sanskrit, before they are reduced to ash (Tamil, chunnam; Sanskrit, bhasman). Purification is done by one of two methods. In one, sheets of metal are repeatedly heated and plunged into various vegetable juices and decoctions. In the other method, called "killing" (marana), the metal or mineral is destroyed by the use of power herbs, so that it loses its identity and becomes converted into a fine powders, having the nature of oxides or sulfides, which can be processed by the intestinal juices. After this purification procedure, the metal or mineral is combined with its appropriate acid or alkaline and is prepared for its final transformation into an ash or bhasman by incineration in special furnaces fueled by cow dung cakes, which are often replaced by electric ovens in more modern establishments.

After the purification of the metals and minerals, they are then turned into ash or calcinated powders and are ready to be used as medicines. There are nine principles that must be followed in the calcination of metals and minerals:

1. There is no alchemical process without mercury.
2. There is no fixation without alkali.
3. There is no coloring without sulfur.
4. There is no quintessence without copper sulfate.
5. There is no animation without conflagration.
6. There is no calcination without corrosive lime.
7. There is no compound without correct blowing.
8. There is no fusion without suitable flux.
9. There is no strong fluid without sal ammoniac.

The traditional incineration process may vary slightly among the different Siddha doctors, but all procedures require repeated heating in a fire fueled by dung cakes.

The number of burnings can reach 100 for certain preparations. In traditional Ayurveda, the duration and intensity of the heat is regulated by the size of the pile of dung cakes, called a puta in Sanskrit. Siddha medicine has devised a method with a special substance made of inorganic salts, in Tamil called jayani, which reduces the number of burnings to only three or four. To increase the potency of the ash (chunnam), Siddha practitioners add the esoteric substance muppu, which seems to vary in individual composition from one Siddha doctor to the other. Other ingredients added to increase a chunnam's potency are healthy human urine (amuri) or urine salts (amuriuppu) obtained from the evaporation of large quantities of urine. Neither of these additives is found in Ayurveda's Rasashastra.

According to modern Siddha medicine different metals have different healing effects. Mercury is antibacterial and antisyphilitic; sulfur is used against scabies and skin diseases, rheumatoid arthritis, spasmodic asthma, jaundice, and blood poisoning, and is taken internally as a stool softener; gold is effective against rheumatoid arthritis and as a nervine tonic, an antidote, and a sexual stimulant; arsenic cures all fevers, asthma, and anemia; copper is used to treat leprosy and skin diseases, and to improve the blood; and iron is effective against anemia and jaundice, and as a general tonic for toning the body.

In terms of herbal drugs, the Siddha practitioners have a materia medica of at least 108 plants and plant products, some of which are imported from as far away as the Himalayas. These vegetal drugs are used in three ways in Siddha medicine. As mentioned earlier, certain drugs purify the minerals and metals before they are transformed into ash. Many plant and plant substances are used to eliminate waste products from the body through a process of body purification involving purgation of the nose and throat, enemas, and laxatives, and the removal of toxins from the skin by the application of medicated pastes. This procedure resembles the process of the five methods of purification (Sanskrit, pañcakarman) in Ayurveda. Finally, plants are employed in treating specific ailments and in the general toning of the body. Siddha doctors also used animal products, such as human and canine skulls, in the preparation of a special "ash" or chunnam (Tamil, peranda chunnam), which is said to be effective against mental disorders.

Despite the irrefutable scientific evidence that shows most of these minerals and metals to be toxic to the human body, both Ayurvedic and Siddha practitioners continue to use them in their everyday treatment of patients. They claim that their respective traditions have provided special techniques to detoxify the metals and minerals and to render them safe and extremely potent.

To make their products more accessible to a Western clientele, Ayurvedic pharmaceutical manufacturers in India have begun to adopt the Western system of "good manufacturing practices" and to resort to Ayurveda's rich pharmacopoeia of plant-based medicines. Such is not the case with

Siddha medicine, which has yet to experience the financial rewards that come from serving a Western clientele.

SUMMARY

Ayurveda is a sophisticated system of medicine that has been practiced in India for more than 2500 years. It focuses on the whole organism and its relation to the external world to reestablish and maintain the harmonious balance that exists within the body and between the body and its environment. Only a glimpse of this ancient form of medicine has been presented; there is much to be learned from a deeper exploration of Ayurveda. Studies of Ayurveda and related traditions in Tibetan medicine are being undertaken in India, Europe, and North America. Very few reliable sources for traditional Ayurveda are available in English. Most of the sound works are by and for specialists and are virtually inaccessible to the reader without knowledge of Sanskrit (e.g., Meulenbeld, 1974; Srikanta Murthy, 1984). A selective list of trustworthy and available books in English on traditional Ayurveda has been referenced as shown.

Unlike Ayurveda, which has a long and detailed textual tradition in Sanskrit from around the beginning of the common (Christian) era, Siddha medicine's textual history in Tamil is vague and uncertain until about the thirteenth century AD, when there is evidence of medical treatises. Most of the knowledge about Siddha medicine comes from modern-day practitioners, who often maintain a historically unverified development of their own tradition and who, because of the upsurge of Tamil pride, tend to make fantastic claims about the age and importance of Siddha medicine vis-à-vis its closest rival in India, Ayurveda.

Based on the evidence thus far marshalled by means of written secondary sources and the reports of fieldworkers in Siddha medicine, it would appear that Siddha and Ayurveda share a common theoretic foundation, but differ most strikingly in their respective forms of therapeutics. This would tend to suggest that the original form of Siddha medicine consisted principally in a series of treatments for specific ailments. To these therapeutic measures

was added a theoretical component based on, among others, Ayurveda and perhaps also Unani in the form of diagnosis by means of pulse and urine; Unani could well have been Ayurveda's source for these same means of diagnosis. The same pattern of medical development, which involves practice followed by theory, may also apply to other forms of Indian medicine, beginning with Ayurveda itself and including the more recent Visha Vaidya tradition of Kerala. The core of Siddha medicine is its alchemy, the fundamental principles of which conform to the alchemical traditions of ancient Greece and China as well as Arabic alchemy. It would, therefore, seem possible that both Siddha and Ayurvedic alchemy might well have derived from one or a combination of these older traditions. Further investigation into each system in relationship to Indian alchemy could reveal important connections between Indian and other systems of alchemy and medicine.

Ayurveda has left the soil of India and has found fertile ground in the West, where alternative and complementary forms of healing have become popular in recent decades. There are clear signs on the horizon that Siddha medicine is likely to follow the same course. These Indian systems of medicine must undergo changes and adaptations to be accommodated in a foreign environment. Some of these modifications have found and will continue to find their way back to India, where they become integrated into the indigenous system. Such has been the pattern of medicine in most parts of the world, so that the final chapter on a particular medical history can never be written. In fact, Siddha's medical history can only be truly understood when viewed in terms of Siddha's change and adaptation over time.

From a practice standpoint, the Indian Medicine Central Council Act of 1970 gave an official place in national health programs to the Ayurvedic and Unani medical systems of India. India now has more than 200,000 registered traditional medical practitioners, the majority of whom have received their training in government colleges of Ayurvedic or Unani medicine.

Chapter References can be found on the Evolve website at http://evolve.elsevier.com/Micozzi/complementary/

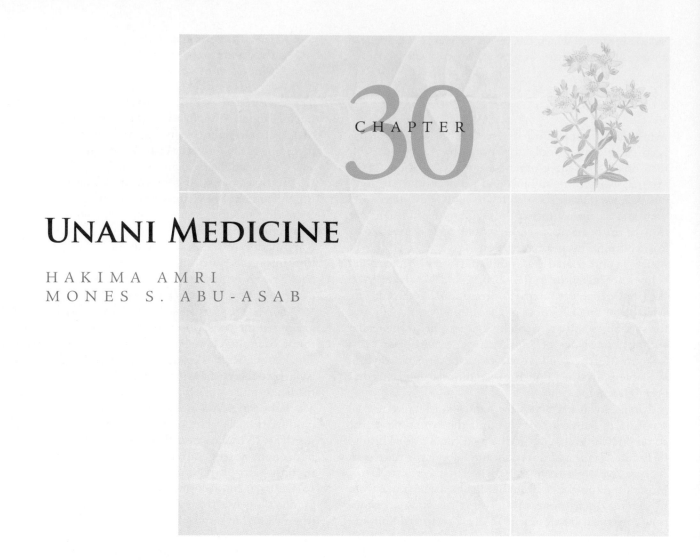

UNANI MEDICINE

HAKIMA AMRI
MONES S. ABU-ASAB

Looking back we may say that Islamic medicine and science reflected the light of the Hellenic sun, when its day had fled, and that they shone like a moon, illuminating the darkest night of the European Middle Ages; that some bright stars lent their own light, and that moon and stars alike faded at the dawn of a new day—the Renaissance. Since they had their share in the direction and introduction of that great movement, it may reasonably be claimed that they are with us yet.
—ARNOLD AND GUILLAUME (1931)

The Eastern Mediterranean region, known as the Levant, was the site of several milestones in the history of humanity. It is where early crops and animals were first domesticated, alphabetical letters were invented and used, and many sciences and religions were developed and studied. It is likewise the home of an ancient system of Greco-Arabic medicine known worldwide today as Unani medicine. This medical system may be seen at once as a bridge between East and West, and between ancient and modern. The word *Unani* is an Arabic adjective that means "Greek," referring mainly to the medical works of Hippocrates and Galen, which Arab and Muslim scholars translated from the Greek. However, as

documented, the roots of the practice go back to Egypt and Mesopotamia (Nunn, 2002).

In the West, modern writers have always thought of Greece as part of European civilization and not as an integral part of Africa, Middle Eastern, and Arabic regions—the Levant. Perhaps the European Renaissance was instigated by ancient Greek knowledge with no realization of its contemporary connections to the rest of the Levant. However, culturally, ethnically, and historically, Greece is part of the Eastern Mediterranean continuum (Bernal, 1987). When one studies Unani medical traditions, one can trace the continuity of medical knowledge from ancient Egypt to Greece and Turkey, to Syria and Iraq, and back to Egypt. This comprehensive traditional medical system that developed over thousands of years is now known by the name Unani medicine, or by its Arabic common name, *Tibb*. It is practiced in several parts of the world with a continued strong presence in India and Pakistan.

Unani medicine is recognized by the World Health Organization as one of the alternative systems of medicines (Bannerman et al, 1983; World Health Organization, 2002, n.d.). As a medical system, Unani practices can be traced back a few thousand years to their roots in Egypt and Mesopotamia, where the great Greek physician Hippocrates (ca. 460-370 BC) probably traveled at a young age and where Galen (ca. AD 129-199) studied and practiced medicine (King, 2001). Aside from some fragmented records from the walls of the Egyptian temples and burial sites and Egyptian papyri (such as the Edwin Smith papyrus), as well as some Sumerian clay tablets, the works of Hippocrates and Galen remain the most extensive ancient medical writings that have survived, mainly through the translations of Arab and Muslim scholars during the Middle Ages. Their works were further expanded by Arab and Muslim physicians such as Rhazes* and Avicenna,† who made additions from their own experience and pertinent observation. They corrected misconceptions and recorded their own discoveries, such as (1) the alcohol extraction of medicinal plants and distillation of rose oil, described for the first time in the greatest detail; (2) the distinctions between diseases such as smallpox and measles; and (3) explanations for the first time of meningitis and pleurisy. Rhazes focused on infectious diseases, whereas Avicenna identified over 750 drugs and emphasized preventive medicine, exercise, diet, and mental health. Rhazes and Avicenna authored Al-Hawi (Razi, 1955) and Al-Qanoon (Avicenna, 1993), respectively. The former is considered the largest medical encyclopedia to date, and the latter became the standard medical textbook for hundreds of years throughout most of the Old World until the development of chemistry and the rise of modern medicine. Unani medicine can be considered as the catalyst for the revival, modernization, and systematization of ancient Egypto-Greco-Roman medicine that laid the foundation for modern medicine (Porter, 1999).

Unani medicine has profoundly influenced medicine in the West. The allopathic Western medical system in Europe evolved from the Unani tradition, and during the eighteenth and nineteenth centuries, Unani medicine provided a source for other natural, holistic, and alternative practices such as homeopathy, naturopathy, and chiropractic in Europe and the United States.

The Unani medical system is also distinguished by including mental evaluation in patient examination (an early approach to mind-body medicine). In addition to physical signs, Unani physicians also use both mental and emotional characteristics to determine the temperament of the patient. They also attribute certain symptoms to mental causes and treat them as such.

The technically rudimentary methods of diagnosis of traditional medical systems do not imply that their medical knowledge and practice are primitive and unsophisticated. To the contrary, they represent an excellent understanding of biological systems and states of health and disease. These traditional systems with their simple methods of patient examination offer the most cost-effective real-time evaluation of patient status of any known method, one in which the caregiver does not have to rely on calibrated machines and delayed test results to treat an illness.

THEORETICAL BASIS OF UNANI MEDICINE

All traditional medical systems seek to harmonize the health of the individual with the universal elements of nature and the cosmos; they all aim for a balance between opposite, but complementary, elements of the human system. Similar to other traditional medical systems such as Chinese medicine and Ayurveda, Unani adheres to a holistic and balanced approach to health maintenance, diagnosis of illness, and restoration of health. As a holistic medical system, it aims to assist the natural recuperative power of the body; it recognizes all factors that contribute to human health status; and it avoids harming sound parts of the body when pursuing treatment options for a disease (Osborn, 2008).

Unani's theoretical basis encompasses the theory of naturals (tabie'iat), which is a unifying explanation of humans and nature. It explains the shared natural building elements of the universe and humans, and classifies normal constituents and functions of a healthy individual. Unani practice is based on the theory of causes (mousabibat), which identifies the elements underlying illness, and the theory of signs ('alamat), which identifies diagnostic symptoms (Chishti, 1991).

THE NATURALS OF UNANI (TABIE'IAT)

Avicenna defined Unani medicine as a branch of knowledge that is based on physical laws, the naturals, and not on dogma or superstition. There are seven main sets of naturals that form the essential constituents and the working principles of the body: the elements or phases (arkan), temperaments (mizaj), humors (akhlat), organs (a'dha'), spirits (arwah), faculties (quwa), and functions (af'al).

The Elements or Phases (Arkan)
The elements are also known in Arabic as the basics, or origins (ousoul). The four elements are earth, water, air, and fire. A fifth energetic element, the ether, is considered the source of the other four but is not used in Unani medicine (Figure 30-1). The ancient philosophers of the Levant attempted to formulate a unifying theory that explains all natural phenomena; however, because in their time they lacked the tools for molecular and atomic

*Abū Bakr Muhammad ibn Zakariyā Rāzī was a chemist, physician, philosopher, and scholar. Razi was born in Rayy, Iran, in the year AD 865 (251 AH) and died there in AD 925 (313 AH).
†Abū 'Alī al-Ḥusayn ibn 'Abd Allāh ibn Sīnā was born ca. AD 980 near Bukhara, Khorasan, and died in 1037 in Hamedan. He is also known as Ibn Seena.

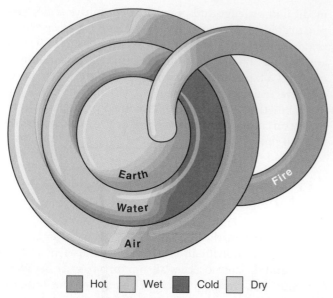

Hot □   Wet □   Cold ■   Dry □

Figure 30-1 The four elements and their relation to each other as described by Avicenna and illustrated by the authors. The earth element is surrounded by water, which is enveloped by air, whereas fire connects all of them. The shades are indicative of the two natures (temperaments) characterizing each element: earth is dry and cold, water is cold and wet-moist, air is wet-moist and hot, and fire is hot and dry. (Copyright © Hakima Amri and Abu-Asab Mones.)

investigations, they used symbolism to hypothesize, predict, and substitute for the unknown, and referred to things by their characteristics rather than their constitutions. For example, the elements also represent all physical phases of matter: solid, liquid, gas, and energy. These physical phases were considered to be the elements that form the ingredients of everything in the universe, including humans; their usage in medicine means that they confer their characteristics to the body, its organs, and its energies.

Avicenna described the earth element as "a simple motionless heavy object that occupies the center in a group of elements. It helps life forms attain cohesiveness, shape, and stability" (anticipating the Newtonian concept of gravity). He also described the physical relationships among the elements: "the water element engulfs the earth, and the two are surrounded by air." He placed the fire element as the connector between the other three elements (see Figure 30-1) and attributed to it the ability to bring earth and water from their elemental states into compounds by reducing their inertia. His characterization of the fire element is similar to a modern description of free energy. Furthermore, he pointed out that the air and fire are constituents of the life energies or spirits (see section on the spirits later).

Each element is associated with fixed qualitative characteristics (nature or temperament) called the "elemental

powers": these are hot, cold, wet or moist, and dry. Each element possesses two natures. Earth is cold and dry, water is cold and wet-moist, air is hot and wet-moist, and fire is hot and dry (Bakar, 1990). In addition, earth and water are associated with heaviness, and fire and air with lightness. Heavy elements are thought of as strong, negative, passive, and female, whereas light elements as weak, positive, active, heavenly, and male.

The four elements are dynamic, interacting and resulting in a continuous change within the human body. This change is either cyclical or directional. The food and water cycles are examples of cyclical change, whereas an abnormal growth of a tumor represents a directional change. Because the elements must exist in equilibrium to maintain health, any change in the elements is monitored to assess the health status of each part of the body. This necessitated the development of a monitoring classification called the "temperaments" (*mizaj*).

The Temperaments (*Mizaj*)

The literal meaning of *mizaj* is the quality or qualities of a mixture; its classic use means that it is a product of the opposite physical qualities of the four elements (hot, cold, wet, and dry). Temperament, as it is called in most literature, is the sum quality of the body, or any of its organs, resulting from the actions and reactions of the elements. Its definition can encompass the metabolic, behavioral, and mental profile of the individual; it can also be thought of as a physical state or phenotype. In modern interpretation, we have established that the individual acquires a temperamental phenotype during his or her life based on genotype, environmental effects, and lifestyle choices. The individual's genetic predisposition plays a role in the type of temperamental phenotype acquired. As explained in the section on Unani diagnosis, it is important to understand the theory of the temperaments, because certain conditions are associated with one temperament, signs that are normal for one temperament are abnormal for others, and the temperamental phenotype determines the suitability of a treatment and dosage of medication.

There are four basic temperaments: hot, cold, wet, and dry. Because these four can also occur in combination, however, the total number of temperaments is nine, although other sources like Al-Antaki* mention 17 (Antaki, 1982). These are classified into eight imbalanced and one balanced temperament. The eight imbalanced temperaments result from the unequal presence of opposing qualities. These include four single temperaments—hot, cold, wet, and dry—and four composite temperaments—hot and dry, hot and wet, cold and dry, and cold and wet. Because the elements are constantly interacting, the normal balanced state has a range and is not a strict point.

---

*Anṭākī, Dā'ūd ibn 'Umar, died in Mecca in AD 1599 (1008 AH).

Humans have a body temperament range that differs from that of animals; age groups and geographically based populations have their own ranges; and healthy ranges are different from ranges during illness. In addition, each organ has its own temperament with ranges of heat and cold, as well as wetness and dryness. For example, the hottest are breath, blood, liver, flesh, and muscles; the coldest are phlegm humor, hair, bones, cartilage, and ligaments; the wettest are phlegm humor, blood, oil, fat, and brain; and the driest are hair, bone, cartilage, ligaments, and tendons.

The Humors (*Akhlat*)

The term *humor* is derived from the Greek *chymos* (χυμός, juice or sap); however, the humoral theory is ancient and cannot be attributed to a single person. Most of the humoral descriptions reference Hippocrates, whose writing on the subject has survived to our day. The four humors are present in the bloodstream in different quantities and are considered the essential components of the body that occupy the vascular system. Later, Avicenna concurred with Hippocrates and added the tissue fluids (intercellular and intracellular) as the secondary humors.

Balanced humors are considered the source of health, and restoring the humoral balance is the *modus operandi* of Unani treatment to restore the health of sick individuals. Unani adheres to the humoral theory with four humors in the body: blood (*dam*), phlegm (*balgham*), yellow bile (*safra'*), and black bile (*sauda*). Ancient Greek medicine used only three humors, blood, phlegm, and bile, until Thales of Miletus (ca. 640–546 BC), who had been educated in ancient Egypt, suggested bringing Greek traditions in line with Egyptian medical concepts by adding the fourth humor, black bile (Osborn, 2008). Like the elements, each humor has two natures: blood is hot and humid, phlegm is cold and humid, yellow bile is hot and dry, and black bile is cold and dry. Thus, there is a parallelism between the natures of the human body and the natures of objects in physical world.

The temperament of the individual is the net result of the proportions of the four humors. There are four types of temperaments that are named after the predominant humor: sanguine (blood humor predominates; *damawi*), phlegmatic (phlegm humor predominates; *balghami*), bilious or choleric (yellow bile humor predominates; *safrawi*), and melancholic (black bile humor predominates; *saudawi*).

In the healthy state, each individual has a unique equilibrium of the humors that is maintained by the vital forces or powers called *quwa*, which may be considered as the metabolic strength and functions of organs (see section on the faculties later). Although strong emphasis is placed on diet and digestion for the restoration of humoral balance and health, the restorative power of quwa is considered very important, and quwa is usually fortified by the prescribed medications.

The Organs (*A'dha'*)

Based on structure, organs are classified into two types: simple and compound. The simple organs are homogeneous in structure, such as bones, nerves, tendons, veins, and arteries; the compound ones are heterogeneous and are composed of several other organs, such as the head. Unani medicine assigns four organs primary importance; these are the heart, brain, liver, and gonads. The heart is the essential distributor of the two vital energies (*pneuma* and *ignis,* see next section). The brain controls the mental faculties, senses, and movement. The liver carries out the nutritive and cleansing processes. The gonads give the masculine and feminine characteristics and temperaments, and form the reproductive elements.

The Spirits: Life Energies (*Arwah*)

The spirits here differ from the theological and mystical ones; they are purely physical and refer to the "energies of life." The term is used in Unani medicine to signify the driving forces or energies that help the faculties carry out their functions and also connect between them (see next paragraph). Arab-Muslim and Greek physicians divided spirits into two types: (1) *pneuma* (breath; *nafas*), which is homologous to the oxygen needed for cellular aerobic respiration; and (2) *ignis* (fire; *hararah*), the thermal energy produced by physiological respiration needed for digestion and metabolism. Pneuma was described as "pure, warm, light, and mobile air," whereas ignis was described as being responsible for providing the heat or energy needed to carry out metabolic processes.

Lungs take out pneuma from the air, mix it with blood, and send it to the heart, from which it is distributed throughout the body organs and facilitates various functions by these organs. Unani physicians attributed various physiologic functions to pneuma, not different organs, and divided pneuma into three forms in the human body on the basis of source and function: the natural, the psychic, and the vital. The vital or animalistic spirit (Greek, *pneuma zoticon;* Arabic, *hayawaniyyah*) stems from the heart and functions to preserve life by preparing suitable conditions for the other two spirits. The psychic spirit (*pneuma psychicon; nafsaniyyah*) originates in the brain, stimulating sensation and perception through cognitive faculty and triggering movement through motivation faculty. The natural spirit (*pneuma physicon; tab'iyyah*) derives from the liver and is associated with the nutritional and reproductive processes that are performed by the natural faculties.

Ignis is the fire or energy produced in the presence of air, pneuma; therefore, it does not exist without pneuma. It is the energy that drives all metabolic processes within the body and is also responsible for the body's innate heat emanated during these metabolic processes. Ignis occurs within the same major organs as pneuma and assumes similar names.

There is a striking similarity between this ancient explanation of the body's energies and our current knowledge of respiration physiology. In a modern scientific interpretation, the pneuma and ignis are equivalent to oxygen intake and the important functional role of oxygen as the electron acceptor in the mitochondria without which respiration-generated free heat and chemical energy in the form of adenosine triphosphate, the cell's energy currency, will not occur.

The Faculties (*Quwa*): Psychophysical Drives

A faculty is an ability or a potentiality. The faculties constitute the biological systems of organs and their physiological processes. There are three major faculties: the vital or animalistic (*hayawaniyyah*), the psychic (*nafsaniyyah*), and natural or physical (*tab'iyyah*) (Figure 30-2). Each of these faculties carries out its functions under its corresponding spirit (see previous section), and the locations of the faculties are also identical with those of their spirits.

Vital faculties are the source of the motive energy (the life force that is referred to as *thymos* by Classical Greeks). They are either the active type that is involuntary, such as heartbeat, or are acted upon (voluntary), such as the emotions of anger, happiness, and contempt.

Psychic faculties represent the conscious and unconscious mind. The psychic faculties perform three functions:

they underlie behavior, they stimulate voluntary movement, and they generate sensation.

The natural faculties have a hierarchical relationship, because they fall into those that serve other faculties and those that are served by others. For example, as the chart of faculties show (see Figure 30-2), the nutritive faculty is served by four others: the attractive, the retentive, the digestive, and the expulsive. These four serving faculties serve the nutritive faculty by attracting, retaining, digesting, and expelling. The nutritive faculty serves the growth faculty, which in turn, with the forming faculty, serve the generative faculty.

The Functions (*Af'al*)

The functions complement the faculties, and each faculty has its specific functions based on in its specific organ. Avicenna classifies functions into single (such as digestion) and compound (such as eating, which requires the desire for food, taste, and swallowing).

UNANI VIEW OF DISEASE

Causes (*Mousabibat/Alasbab*)

For the human to maintain good health, six essential factors have to be present: (1) fresh clean air, (2) food and drink, (3) movement and rest, (4) sleep and wakefulness, (5) eating and excreting, and (6) healthy mental state.

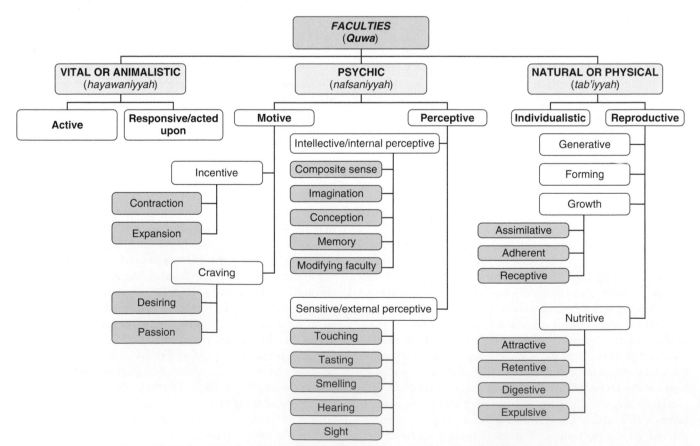

Figure 30-2 The three faculties and their characteristics as described by Unani physicians.

A long-term disruption of these essential factors results in illness. Illness is a state that affects the functions of the vital, psychic, or natural faculties because of an imbalance or obstruction of a temperament (dystemperament) or a combination of functions and temperaments. Unani physicians state that the body has three health conditions: (1) healthy (i.e., disease-free), (2) ill or diseased, and (3) a continuum between the two—situations in which the disease is still in its asymptomatic phase (which may manifest as a functional complaint or disorder before the detection of pathology) or the body is recuperating from a disease. The third state may manifest in three forms: (1) disease affects only one organ but the rest of the body is healthy; (2) the healthy state is not optimal, as in aging individuals; and (3) health and illness alternate in a temporal fashion, as in individuals with a hot temperament who are ill in the summer but well during the winter, or vice versa.

Dystemperament is either local or systemic and involves one or more of the four basic qualities of hot, cold, wet, or dry. The effect is usually caused by an outside and often unexpected source. On the other hand, humoral illness involves metabolic disorder, which results in imbalances in and/or corruptions of one or more of the four humors. The disorder is either quantitative (excess or deficiency), qualitative, or both simultaneously. Most humoral disorders originate internally due to metabolic errors that result in either excess (anabolism), such as high levels of triglycerides, or wasting (catabolism), such as degenerative diseases.

According to Al-Antaki there are four states in which the disease condition is not the result of an imbalance or a dystemperament (Antaki, 1982). Such diseases are of the following types: (1) congenital malformations and defects; (2) accidents (internal: poisoning; external: burn, fracture, wounds, etc.); (3) quantitative abnormality, organ enlargement or atrophy; and (4) dislocation, displaced organs.

Unani medicine (like Ayurveda) considers the origin of most illnesses to be the corruption of the *pepsis*: the digestive and metabolic processes (generation and distribution of the humors). Arab-Muslim medical literature is full of famous quotations that emphasize this point. According to Alkindi* "the stomach is the house of all illness," and he also advised not to eat when angry and not to bathe on a full stomach. The conditions under which digestion occur are as important as the diets that are consumed.

On a daily basis, the individual encounters potentially pathogenic stresses; however, most of these fail to cause illness. They succeed only when the individual's resistance and adaptive responses have been weakened or compromised and the virulence of the pathogen overwhelms the host's defenses, or the pathogen is able to establish itself through a weakness in the host systems.

*Abū Yūsuf Ya'qūb ibn Isḥāq al-Kindī, ca. AD 801-873, known in the West as Alkindus.

Signs of Imbalance (*'Alamat*)

Evaluation of an individual's health should take into consideration some innate traits (*lawazem*) such as age, gender, race, skin complexion, and geographic adaptations. Traits attributable to the long-term multigenerational adaptation to living in a particular geographic area should not be confused with signs of temperamental imbalance. For example, people from the warm equatorial parts of the world have hot temperaments, as well as dark complexions, eyes, and hair, whereas those from temperate zones have cold temperament, as well as light skin, eyes, and hair. Thus the cold temperament of the northerners is not an indication of a phlegmatic state.

Age also dictates different assessments depending on its phase. Four phases of life are recognized: youth (from birth to 28 years of age), adulthood (ends at 40), maturity (ends at 60), and elderliness (ends at death). Because bodily functions vary in their efficiency during each phase, each is also associated with its own innate temperament: youth is hot and wet; adulthood is hot and dry; maturity is cold and dry; and elderliness is cold and strangely wet. Therefore, *age temperament* should be considered before considering an *organ's temperament*, and the prescribed diet and herbal treatments should be suitable for the age group. There are also some traits that develop in association with age progression that should not be confused with symptoms of illness. For example, hair thinning and a desire for naps are associated with the phases of maturity and elderliness and are not indicative of an imbalance. These are life changes that should be accepted as normal with aging, rather than considered to require medical intervention.

Avicenna described a set of traits to be examined by the *hakim*, or Unani physician, to determine the temperamental status (Avicenna, 1993). These included the quality of skin texture and complexion (should be slightly moist, warm, smooth, elastic, and between white and red), the balance of muscle and fat, hair characteristics (should be full, thick, between straight and curly, with balanced growth in location and length), organ configuration, reaction time of the faculties, dreams, and the balance of sleep and waking. Also, the hakim looks for signs of humoral excesses in which all the humors are overabundant or one is in excess at the expense of another humor. Other focuses of observation are characteristics of stool and urine, stomach growling, mouth odor, shape of the nails, cheek color, involuntary movements (e.g., cough, spasm, shivering), congestion and blockage, gas formation and blockage, and tumors. Special attention is given to fevers, tongue color and texture, pain, pulse, and the eyes.

Imbalance of temperaments (dystemperament). The first diagnostic feature for which a hakim looks is a dystemperament of the ailing organ or system. There are four main dystemperaments: hot (hotter than usual, but not moister or drier); cold (colder than usual, but not moister or drier); dry (drier than usual, but not hotter or colder); and moist (more moist than usual, but not hotter or colder). These are dynamic, never static dystemperaments that are constantly changing and interacting. In addition, there are four possible compound dystemperaments that develop when a simple dystemperament persists long enough to effect a second one. For example, a hotter dystemperament expels moisture, which leads to a dry dystemperament; this produces a compound dystemperament. The four possible compound dystemperaments are hotter and moister, hotter and drier, colder and moister, and colder and drier.

Dystemperament can affect an organ, tissue, or system, and may include any of the humors or a combination of them. A dystemperament of a humor differs from a humoral disorder, because the humoral essence is not affected in this case and the humor or humors remain balanced. On the other hand, a humoral disorder progresses, ripens, and reveals itself after a period of time.

Dystemperaments are determined by the signs of the body or an organ. They are either qualitative (indicative of a disease) or material-spatial (indicative of the location). A dystemperament is qualitative if it is not located within an organ directly (as with a fever) and material if it is within an organ and causing changes there (e.g., a cold liver will produce pale urine and light stool).

It is only after gathering as much information as possible about the patient that the hakim tries to identify the form of humoral imbalance.

Imbalance of humors. Humoral disorders result from the corruption of the pepsis processes (digestion and metabolism within the body), which fall under the natural faculty. It is also important to add that nowadays industrial chemical pollutants can cause humoral disorders if they enter and persist in the body. When the metabolic process is weak, the humors are undersupplied and underperforming, which leads to problems in the functions of the systems and organs. Underperforming humors tend to generate more phlegm and less blood. On the other hand, an overactive metabolic process corrupts the humors with an unbalanced oversupply of metabolites, which is toxic to the system. This toxic accumulation loads the body with black and yellow biles.

Although humoral disorders are metabolic in nature, the humors may be affected by dystemperament like any other part or organ of the body. Coldness, dryness, and wetness slow them down, whereas heat puts them into overdrive.

The symptoms and diseases that are usually associated with each of the humors are summarized in Box 30-1 (Chishti, 1991; Osborn, 2008).

PRACTICAL BASIS OF UNANI MEDICINE

UNANI DIAGNOSIS (*TASHKHEES*)

Accurate diagnosis is the path to a successful treatment. The hakim relies on his or her senses, knowledge, reasoning, and experience to gather all signs of imbalance and

BOX 30-1

Signs of Humoral Imbalance

Blood Humor
Angina, bleeding disorders, canker sores, constant erection and spasm of penis, coughing, cracked nails, delirium, diphtheria, enlarged tongue, excessive menstrual flow, gout, headache, heart disease, hemorrhoids, lethargy, high blood pressure, loose teeth, migraine, nosebleed, nose itching, pleurisy, poor vision, slackness of uvula, swelling of liver, swollen palate, swollen testicles, tooth spaces, trembling lips, uremia, weak limbs

Phlegm Humor
Acne, arthritis, atonic dyspepsia, asthma, backache, bad breath, bad taste in mouth, baldness, boils, canker sores, chronic bronchitis, colic, conjunctivitis, constipation, constriction of throat, continuous trembling, convulsion of stomach, convulsions, corrupt appetite, cough, dandruff, dandruff of eyelids, deficient appetite, dilation of pupils, diphtheria, dull feeling in teeth, enlarged tongue, forgetfulness, foul odor from nose, grippe, headache, heart feels as if being pulled downward, erectile dysfunction, insomnia, itching of anus, joint ache, lethargy, madness, melancholy, muscular tension, weak nail growth, obstruction of liver, paralysis, pimples, pleurisy, respiratory allergies, retention of urine, ringing in ears, scabs, sebaceous cysts, severe perspiration, severe thirst, shedding eyelashes, sour mother's milk, styes, swelling of bladder, swelling of lips, swelling of lymph nodes, swelling of liver, swelling of spleen, swelling of testicles, swelling of uvula, swelling of womb, swollen eyelids, swollen palate, trembling limbs, ulcers of gums, ulcers of kidneys, upset stomach, vomiting, weak limbs, whiteness of lips

Yellow Bile Humor
Anal ulcer, biliousness and biliary congestion, boils on eyelid, burning urination, canker sores, cough, delirium, discolored teeth, dull teeth, excessive appetite, excessive menstrual flow, feeling of "smoke" in chest, gallstones, gastric and duodenal ulcers, gastritis, grippe, hard eyelids, headache, heart attack, hemorrhoids, hyperacidity and acid reflux, insomnia, jaundice, migraine, nose itching, photophobia, pleurisy, rheumatoid arthritis, swelling of liver, swelling of testicles, tendonitis, vomiting, yellowed nails

Black Bile Humor
Abnormal growths and hard tumors, arthritis, cancer, canker sores, clots and embolisms, colic, constipation, delirium, diphtheria, excessive appetite, excessive libido, flatulence, grippe, hallucinations, headache, heartburn, insomnia, insufficient mother's milk, intestinal obstruction, irritable bowel, neuralgia, seizures and convulsions, skin cancer, stiffness, swelling of bladder, swelling of liver, swelling of spleen, swelling of womb, swelling of stomach, thickened nails, varicose veins, vomiting

reach a diagnosis. In addition to taking the medical history of the patient, the hakim, through observation and physical examination, gathers the physical and mental signs of imbalance. The examination encompasses the tongue, nails, pulse, urine, and feces, and notes the presence of pain and fever.

Determination of the Patient's Temperament

As mentioned earlier, there are four types of temperaments in humans. The hakim determines the patient's temperament from three sets of characteristics: (1) appearance (complexion, build, touch, and hair), (2) physiological features (movement, diet preferences, seasonal preferences, sleep, and pulse), and (3) emotions (calm, angry, nervous, etc.).

The patient's humoral imbalance manifests itself in the patient's mental status, behavior, and mannerisms. Characteristics related to these aspects can be attributed to one of the four humors. A sanguine personality is usually balanced, stylish, refined, passionate, positive, genial, inquisitive, playful, sensual, and indulgent. A phlegmatic personality is calm, good natured, trusting, sluggish, inactive, sentimental, sensitive, loving, subjective, self-absorbed, and steady. A choleric personality is forceful, energetic, flamboyant, expressive, dramatic, bold, fidgety, short-tempered, angry, and argumentative. A melancholic personality is quiet, cool, aloof, detached, objective, withdrawn, cautious, prudent, frugal, stoic, stiff, inflexible, lonely, unhappy, thoughtful, and grumpy. A patient showing signs of mental fatigue or compulsiveness should be considered for examination. The hakim is usually on the lookout for behavioral signs that may provide a clue to the patient's illness.

Examination of Bodily Functions

Major traditional medical systems of the Old World use the same techniques to detect the signs of deviation from the normal range in order to determine the malfunctioning organ(s). Examinations of the pulse, tongue, urine, and feces are employed as diagnostic tools. Their usage is described briefly in the following sections.

Pulse (*nabd*). The heart is the distributor of pneuma to the rest of the body and directly determines the vitality of the system (the production of free energy and chemical energy); therefore, its health is of prime importance in Unani medicine. The current system of pulse diagnosis used in Unani medicine was developed by Avicenna. He studied all the available pulse information of his time and then integrated all in his synthesis. Galen and Avicenna understood the challenging nature of pulse diagnosis, as evident in their writings. Practicing hakims admit that it is the hardest part of Tibb to master.

A pulse is composed of two movements (systole and diastole), and two rests following each of the movements (Box 30-2). The pulse is felt at the radial artery near the wrist, where it is closer to the skin surface and easily

---

BOX 30-2

Ten Characteristics of Pulse Evaluation

Avicenna listed 10 characteristics of pulse evaluation. The first seven determine whether the pulse of an individual is regular. These are as follows:

The First Seven
1. Dimensions of expansion (length, width, and depth)
2. Strength as a force felt against the finger (strong, moderate, weak)
3. Speed (fast, moderate, slow)
4. Compressibility (soft, hard, and in between)
5. Turgor: tension of the artery between pulses—fullness (full, empty, and in between)
6. Temperature of the pulse (hot, cold, and in between)
7. Duration of diastole (short, long, and in between)

The Next Three
8. Regularity (regular in all preceding characteristics) or irregular
9. Order and disorder in irregularity
10. Rhythm, specific to the individual and usually measured as the ratio between the two movements and the two rests

He further classified the irregular pulse into *seven compound pulse types:*
a. Gazelle
b. Wavy
c. Wormy/cordlike/twisting
d. Antlike
e. Sawlike
f. Mouse tail
g. Snake tongue, needlelike/flickering

---

accessible. To examine the pulse, the hakim places the middle finger on the radial artery, directly between the carpus and the prominence of the radius, with the two adjoining fingers next to it in their natural positions and the index finger proximal to the heart. It is recommended that the pulse be examined on the right hand for a female and on the left hand for a male, with the palm turned upward for both.

Avicenna's description of pulse variation is very detailed and comprehensive. For example, he explained the underlying reasons for the natural heterogeneity of the pulse, the variation between male and female pulses, and pulse characteristics related to age, temperaments, seasons, geographical adaptations, food, sleep, sports, bathing, pain, tumors, and female gender.

A hot temperament, in a state of health, is associated with "great pulse," the best type of pulse, whereas a cold temperament is associated with a weaker pulse. A wet temperament produces a wavy and wide pulse, and a dry one is associated with tightness and stiffness and produces a spasmodic and shaky pulse. Furthermore, a sanguine temperament (hot and moist) is characterized by a moderate to slightly rapid pulse that is moderately soft and relaxed; a phlegmatic temperament (cold and wet) is associated with a deep, slow, and soft pulse; a melancholic temperament (cold and dry) produces a slow to weak, tense or constricted, thin, and well-defined pulse; and a choleric temperament (hot and dry) is associated with a strong, rapid, and well-defined pulse.

Tongue (*lisan*). There are two areas of interest with regard to the tongue: the body and the coat. The tongue body reflects the temperament and blood supply in the body in general, whereas the tongue coat reveals the health of digestive and metabolic processes, and humoral imbalances.

The tongue body texture is indicative of systemic or chronic conditions that are severe. The texture can be dry or rough, cracked, raw, rumpled, or wet and glossy. These characteristics may indicate lack of body moisture, nervousness, advanced sickness, inefficient digestion, and excess moisture, respectively.

The color, size, and texture of the tongue's coat are all taken into consideration in diagnosis. The coat reflects the health status of digestion, the digestive tract, and metabolism, and the surface location of the coat reflects the affected part of the system (e.g., pancreas, intestine, stomach, liver). An absent or thin coat denotes good digestive and metabolic health, whereas an increase in coat thickness reflects poor digestion, and the thickness is proportional to the accumulation of metabolic toxins in the body. Coat color indicates the nature of the buildup (e.g., phlegmatic, choleric), and its texture reflects moisture content.

Urine (*boul*). The urine provides a window on the metabolic status of the individual. Avicenna stated that the urine is indicative of the health of the liver, urinary tracts, and blood vessels. He stressed several specifics for urine collection to ensure accurate assessment. For example, the sample should be the first collection of the day before the individual eats any food, and the patient should have had no food the night before that may color the urine, should not have had intercourse, and should have been resting for a while before urination. Hakims assess the urine within the first hour of its collection by evaluating its quantity, color, foaminess, texture, clarity, and sediment. Avicenna eliminated touching and tasting the urine as part of the evaluation.

Urine may have one of several colors depending on the individual's state of health, ingested food, water intake, and use of drugs. It can be yellow, red, green, black, or white. Shades of yellow, for example, may range from straw yellow to lemon yellow to blond yellow to orange yellow to fiery yellow (saturated yellow) to saffron yellow with a tinge of red. The first two indicate a normal heat temperament, whereas the rest indicate increased heat or may be generated by extreme exercise, pain, hunger, or thirst.

The thick part of the urine is present as floats at the surface, particles suspended in the liquid, or sediment at the bottom. Foamy floats in urine are attributed to moisture and gases, especially in individuals with gaseous bloating. Abundance, persistence, and large bubble size of floats indicate an increase in viscosity caused by bad humor and cold. Thick elements of the other two type are referred to as sediment. Normal sediment is white, uniform, cohesive, and smooth, and readily precipitates. Suspended turbid sediment, however, denotes immature intermediates of metabolism.

It is axiomatic among hakims that the urine odor of an ill patient differs from that of healthy individuals. However, odorless urine signifies cold humor, immature digestion, acute sickness, and diminished metabolic vitality. A foul odor of the urine is caused mostly by infections and ulcers in the urinary tract. Acidic urine is produced by cold temperament that is affected by abnormal metabolism, but extreme acidity is a sign of death due to diminished innate heat. A sweet odor of the urine indicates the dominance of sanguine temperament, an extremely foul odor is produced by choleric temperament, and an acidic foul odor is caused by melancholic temperament.

Feces or Stool (*bouraz*). Feces, also called "alvine discharge," have characteristics that are indicative of the individual's pepsis and health. Normal feces are yellowish and cohesive with uniform softness similar in consistency to unfiltered honey. They come out easily without burning sensation, air sounds, or foam. The quantity of feces is compared with the amount of food ingested. A reduced amount is thought to be due to retention in the intestinal tract, and an increase points to the presence of humors. Wet feces (as in diarrhea) indicate weak digestion, weak absorption, or blockage, whereas hard feces (as in dehydration) may point to excessive urination, ingestion of dry food, prolonged retention, or fiery heat within the system. The color of the feces specifies the affecting humor; for example, a dark or black color is a sign of maturation of a melancholic disease, but only if one can exclude excessive heat or consumption of colored foods or a drink that produces black bile.

Pain (*waja'*). Pain is an unnatural transitory condition for the human body. It is usually caused by a dystemperament or an injury—loss of continuity (Box 30-3). Pain weakens the organ and halts its function. It warms the organ initially but later cools it down and saps its energy. Removal of the cause will halt the pain and is the preferred method of treatment (e.g., by applying a poultice of linseed *[Linum usitatissimum]* or dill *[Anethum graveolens]*, or by applying wet sedatives [alcohols] or cold anesthetics [all narcotics]).

Fever (*homa* [sing.], *homiat* [pl.]). In the fourth volume of his Al-Qanoon, Avicenna wrote a detailed study of fever types, symptoms, causes, and treatments. Fever is an unnatural heat "centered within the heart and spirits" (i.e., involving pneuma and ignis energies) and carried throughout the body by blood and the vascular system; it

BOX 30-3

The Fifteen Types of Pains and Their Causes

Avicenna listed 15 types of *pains* and their causes:
1. Itching (*hakak*), caused by a humor that is bitter or salty
2. Rough (*khashin*), caused by a rough humor
3. Stabbing (*nakhes*), caused by a humor that extends the muscle membrane and separates it
4. Flattening or extended (*moumaded*), caused by a humor or gas that pulls the nerve or muscle from two opposite ends
5. Pressing (*daghet*), caused by a substance that engulfs the organ and presses on it
6. Splitting (*moufasekh*), caused by a substance that seeps out of the muscle or its membrane and separates the two
7. Breaking (*moukaser*), caused by a substance, gas, or coldness in between the bone and its membrane
8. Softening (*rakhou*), caused by extension of only the muscle without the tendon
9. Boring (*thaqeb*), caused by the trapping of gas or a substance between the tissues of a hard organ such as the colon
10. Piercing (*masalee*), caused by the boring of a hard organ by a gas or substance
11. Dull (*khader*), caused by a cold temperament or obstruction of blood supply
12. Throbbing (*dharabani*), caused by hot inflammation next to an organ
13. Heavy (*thaqeel*), a sense of heaviness in an insensitive organ such as the lung, kidney, or spleen caused by inflammation or tumor, or by the tumor's disabling of the pain sensation, such as in cancer in the mouth of the stomach
14. Tiring (*a`ya`i*), could be caused by fatigue, or by an extending humor, gas, or ulcerative humor
15. Biting or incisive (*lathe'*), caused by a sour humor

is a disquieting sign of corruption and imbalance that requires attention. On the basis of origin, there are two main classes of fevers: (1) fevers associated with infections (*waba'yah*), and (2) transient fevers associated with warming effects, foul humor, hyperplasia, and blockage. Based on their causes and locations, the second class has three subtypes of fevers: (1) ephemeral fevers (*homa youm*), (2) humoral fevers/putrefactive fevers (*homa khalt/'ofounah*), and (3) organ fevers/hectic fevers (*homa daq*).

Avicenna attributed infection and its associated fever to the contamination of air and water with "malevolent soil objects" that are taken into the body. These "objects" corrupt the body's "spirit" and produce unnatural heat that spreads throughout the body. However, he ascribed the infection's success to the presence of corrupt humors that permits the infection to take place.

All of the *ephemeral fevers* are caused by external warming effects: the sun's heat, exhaustion, hot food and medications, sports, and emotional tension. These fevers usually last 1 day (hence the name *youm*, which means "a day" in Arabic) and rarely up to 3 days. The persistence of a fever beyond 3 days, however, signifies that it has spread to an organ or a humor and could turn into a putrefactive or hectic type.

Putrefactive fevers are caused by corruption of the humors. They arise in the body due to the ingestion of contaminated food and the effects of its by-products, consumption of high-moisture fruits, incomplete digestion, and lack of oxygen and proper breathing. Putrefaction may affect the whole body, or an organ, or a humor. Because putrefactive fevers are associated with humors, they are classified according to the affected humor: (1) *alghibb* fever is alternating fever, day on/day off, caused by the putrefaction of yellow bile humor; (2) *mutbiqah* fever is consistent and caused by the putrefaction of blood humor; (3) *na'bbah* fever is caused by the putrefaction of phlegm humor; (4) *alroub'* fever recurs in cycles of 1 day on and 2 days off and is caused by the putrefaction of black bile humor.

Organ fever (or *hectic fever*) may follow after the other fever types mentioned previously. It is considered difficult to diagnose but easy to treat at its incipience, easy to diagnose but difficult to treat at its end, and untreatable if the patient withers. Organ fever affects the moisture at three stages: at the first stage it reduces moisture in the vessels; at the second stage it reduces moisture between the tissues and produces wilting (*thoubool*); and at the third stage it is decomposing (*moufatit*) and reduces moisture within the tissues.

HEALTH MAINTENANCE, PREVENTION, AND TREATMENT OF DISEASE

Unani medicine emphasizes healthy practices of exercise and diet for health maintenance and prevention of sickness. Avicenna divided medicine into theoretical and practical, and further subdivided the practical into two sections: (1) management of healthy bodies, which he also called the "science of health preservation"; and (2) management of sick bodies (Figure 30-3).

Health is maintained by the proper internal balance of heat and moisture that allows the innate heat to be generated and participate in the proper functioning of the body. The body uses food to generate its needed energy and to provide building blocks to maintain structural integrity of the body.

Exercise (*Riyadhah*)

Avicenna placed exercise at the forefront as the most effective means for health maintenance. He claimed that regular exercise prevents dregs from accumulating in the body. In addition, exercise increases the innate heat, lightens the body, and strengthens muscles and tendons.

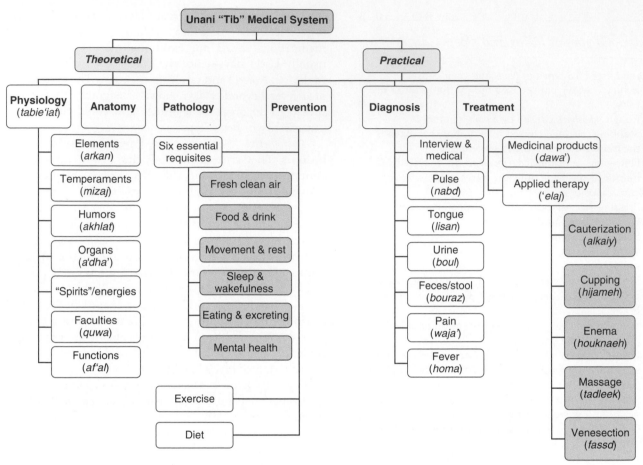

Figure 30-3 Organization of the Unani Tibb medical system.

It also prepares the organs to take in nutrients, reduces their stiffness, and prevents their weakness.

The Al-Qanoon section on exercise is extensive and lists a large number of general physical exercises such as running, archery, speed walking, jumping, horseback riding, wrestling, and rowing, as well as specific organ exercises such as exercises for the eye and ear. It also instructs on the time of exercise and on preparation for it, and goes on to describe the types of fatigue and other conditions that results from exercise and the methods to treat them. This section also encompasses the use of massage and steam baths.

Diet for Health and Healing (*Alghitha'*)

Health is also maintained by food that is balanced in quality and quantity. However, excretion does not get rid of all unutilized food material; there are residues that remain in the body that keep accumulating over time. These dregs have bad effects on the body: their by-products will harm the body, their accumulation in larger quantity leads to dystemperament, and their overload will produce the diseases of excesses. Accumulation of dregs in an organ produces tissue enlargement, and their spread throughout the tissues corrupts the ignis. Expulsion of dregs is accomplished with poisonous drugs most of the time or by

detoxification. When humoral imbalance is addressed, a ripening of the humoral substances is performed first, usually with laxatives, followed by purging.

The process of detoxification is carried out to rid the body of the accumulated dregs (toxins, superfluous matter). Over a period of a few days, the individual deviates from the regular daily diet and takes in food and drink that will induce detoxification. The process culminates in a "healing crisis" or catharsis of elimination in which the elimination may occur as diarrhea, nosebleed, perspiration, urination, or vomiting. There are many recipes for detoxification by food ingestion or administration of enemas; however, detoxification should not be carried out more than once a year.

Recognizing that humans have different needs at their various life stages, Avicenna described the types of diets that should be followed for infants, pregnant and breast-feeding women, adults, and elderly individuals. He also described and treated the various conditions that may arise from the diet because of excesses or imbalances for each age group.

The therapeutic diet of Unani medicine is used to restore balance by providing the proper food that suits the individual's temperament and that of his or her digestive system. Such a diet entails the elimination of unsuitable food, low-quality or contaminated food, excesses of one type of food and unhealthful mixtures; reduction in the number of meals; and the introduction of foods stimulating digestion, breathing, circulation, and innate heat such as spices, vegetables, and oils.

Medicinal products (*Dawa'*)

Treating with medications (botanical, zoological, and metallic substances) is the second choice for treatment after diet. Unani use of herbs is extensive and is well documented in many old texts that are still in current use (Antaki, 1982; Avicenna, 1993; Levey et al, 1967). These treatments cover almost all known diseases. Unani hakims use single and compound formulas as well as internal and external applications.

There are three rules to treating with medications: the first is to know the temperament of the medication (hot, cold, moist, dry); the second, to determine the quantity to be given to the patient and its effect (warming/cooling, drying/wetting); and the third, to determine the most effective time of its administration. Selection of the medication follows the diagnosis of illness, and as a rule, the medication is opposite in its temperament to that of the disease. The characteristics of the diseased organ, however, determine the quantity of the medication. These include its temperament, architecture, position, and strength. For example, the quantity of the medication should correspond to the amount of deviation from the normal temperament. Additional factors are also considered in calculating the quantity, such as the patient's strength, gender, and age, as well as time of the year (season), and geographic location.

Food and medications are ranked according to their power to affect the human body into eight classes: four degrees for hot food and medications and four degrees for cold ones. Unani formularies always give the power degree; for example, a medication may be followed by "hot in the second degree" or "cold in the third degree." Table 30-1 summarizes the various degrees of action.

Use of aromatic oil and alcohol extracts is featured prominently in Unani treatments. Avicenna invented steam distillation of rose oil; alcohol extraction and preservation of active ingredients of botanicals was earlier discovered by Arab chemists and put to use by hakims. Herbal treatments can be delivered in a number of ways, including capsules, conserve, decoction, essence, fomentation, infusion, ointment, oxymel, plaster, poultice, salve, suppository, syrup, and tincture (Avicenna, 1993; Chishti, 1991).

Applied and Manual Therapy (*'elaj*)

Cupping (*hijameh*) is the external application of vacuum suction to the skin to draw humors to the surface away from an organ or an area. It is used for treatment of an inflammation and for detoxification. The type of disease determines the location of cupping; for example, cupping on the heels is beneficial for amenorrhea, varicose veins, and gout, whereas cupping on the sides of the neck affects the organs of the head. Cupping is not advised for people over 60 years of age.

Enema (*houknaeh*) is an effective method for emptying the intestines (especially after vomiting), reducing kidney and bladder pain and enlargement, and detoxifying the upper organs. A harsh enema, however, may weaken the liver and produce fever.

TABLE 30-1

Summary of the Degrees of Action of Food and Drugs on the Metabolism

Hot food and medications (increase metabolism)	Cold food and medications (decrease metabolism)
First Degree Mostly neutral in its effect, but has a light stimulative action on the body if applied in large amount or repeated, e.g., hot water, chamomile (*Anthemis nobilis*).	*First Degree* Mostly neutral in its effect, but has a light suppressive action on the body if applied in large amount or repeated, e.g., cold water, cistus (*Cistus landaniferus*).
Second Degree Stimulates metabolism without adverse effects, e.g., ginger.	*Second Degree* Suppresses metabolism without adverse effects, e.g., Syrian rhubarb (*Rheum ribes*).
Third Degree Overwhelming in its action and effects but does not cause death except in overdose or repeated use. Most medications fall within this category, e.g., senna.	*Third Degree* Downregulates metabolism in a substantial manner but does not cause death except in overdose or repeated use, e.g., resin of cypress (*Cupressus sempervirens*).
Fourth Degree Hot poisons. Corrupt the metabolic process and bring death, e.g., hemlock and belladonna. Used only in small amounts by a hakim.	*Fourth Degree* Cold poisons. Bring metabolism to a halt and cause death, e.g., narcotics such as opium or heavy metals like arsenic. Administered by a hakim only in measured quantity.

Massage (*tadleek*) and bathing (*istihmam*) are ancient traditions in the Old World that can be considered one integral activity. It takes place in a warm bathhouse, the *hammam*, which is usually built on a freshwater source, and starts with a vigorous cleansing rub with a soapy loofa (*leefeh*), usually from a dried fruit of the *Luffa* plant, or a linen mitt. After a good rinse, an oil massage is performed with the fingers and palm using various pressures depending on the treatment goals.

Blood humor is purged through a procedure of bloodletting from a vein called *venesection* (*fassd*). There are two main conditions that require venesection: (1) excess of blood, and (2) low quality of blood. However, venesection also should be carried out at the early signs of some diseases such as varicose vein, gout, joint pain, high blood pressure, epilepsy, and melancholy. Use of leeches (*al'alaq*) is another method of bloodletting. Leeches are placed on the skin of the patient. They attach to the skin by their oral suckers, remain there until they are full, and then fall off to digest the blood. This method is still in use today in both Eastern and Western countries (Munshi et al, 2008).

Cauterization (*alkaiy*) is the application of heated metal or a corrosive directly to the skin surface. It is considered a treatment of last resort because of its harsh effects. One of the main purposes of its use is to prevent disease from spreading to healthy parts of the body. However, it is also applied to infected areas and unhealthy flesh, and is used to strengthen weak parts.

UNANI VIEW ON TUMORS (*AWRAM*) AND CANCER (*SARATAN*)

Avicenna placed tumors, both benign and malignant, into the category of the compound diseases that are multicausal and emphasized that they are rarely homogenous. He declared that, developmentally, tumors recapitulate all known disease types: dystemperament due to corrupting substance; disfigurement of histology and shape; and discontinuity. He also stated that there is no clear cause of cancer, but he speculated that it may be caused by a harmful humor that is usually kept in check by good humors and then carries out its harmful action when humors become imbalanced, or it may be caused by the movement of a substance from one organ to another.

There are six types of tumor based on origin: tumors originating from the four humors as well as aqueous (*ma'yeh*) tumors and gaseous (*reehia*) tumors. Hot tumors originate from a sanguine or choleric humor and are named after their humors. The purely sanguine tumors are called *phalghamonia*, the purely choleric tumors *jamra*, and the combination of the two *kharaj*. The last type, if it occurs in soft tissues such as under the axilla or behind the ears, is termed *ta'oon*.

There are four origins for cold tumors: melancholic, phlegmatic, aqueous, and gaseous. Avicenna attributed cold melancholic tumor formation to a corrupt black bile that originated from yellow bile, or a substance containing yellow bile, and its fast growth to the abundance of nutrients. There are three types of melancholic tumors: solid, cancerous, and glandular. The latter are tumors that have glandular secretory contents at their inception, such as those of the neck lymph nodes, termed *khanazeer*, and cutaneous glands, termed *sal'*. Solid tumors begin as localized, painless, and slowly developing solid growths, whereas cancers are mobile, fast growing, and begin within the organs, thus destroying sensation and eventually the organ itself. Phlegmatic tumors are of two types: soft tumors (*rakhu*) that are mixed and indistinct, and soft encapsulated glandular tumors (*sal' layen*).

Cancerous tumors separate from the organ and develop their own vascular supply. Avicenna concurred with Hippocrates that it is best not to disturb an internal tumor because it may lead eventually to death, and suggested that a cold and moist diet of barley water, ground fish, and hard-boiled egg yolk may prolong the life of the patient. For a tumor that is accompanied by fever, however, he advised the intake of filtered cow's buttermilk, legumes, and cucurbits. Small tumors can be cut out; however, the best treatment for them is an aggressive surgery. Surgery was developed and practiced by several hakims for virtually all parts of the body, including brain and nerves (Rahimi et al, 2007).

Aqueous tumors develop due to the accumulation of liquids in cysts or within the tissues. Gaseous tumors result from the accumulation of gas in the organ's cavity or within the organ's tissue.

SUMMARY

It is important to emphasize that the contributions of Arab and Muslim scholars to modern medicine originally involved translation of the Greco-Roman medical texts but evolved to encompass development of methodical approaches to disease etiology, prognosis, and diagnosis; systematization of medical practice; construction of organized hospitals and clinics; expansion of the repertoires of drugs and catalogues of surgical instruments; and establishment of a professional ethical code. Unani medicine thus represents a vital link, fertile ground, and prerequisite to the modern medicine that developed later in the West during the decline of the Arab-Muslim Empire.

Despite the comprehensive compendia and encyclopedic books transcribed by Unani Tibb physicians and the widespread practice and teaching of Unani medicine in the West as well as other parts of the world for centuries, the Unani medical system today is restricted to South Asia, where it survives alongside Ayurveda and Siddha. The recognition of Unani Tibb as a traditional medical system by the West today is lagging, probably because of the lack of scholarly endeavors and the interest in South Asian countries in developing and exporting Ayurveda (perhaps with mention that Unani is so close as to be almost an identical system). These two systems do have a few similarities, but they also have fundamental differences. Although the practical side of Unani medicine shows similarities, the theoretical as well as some philosophical aspects are different from those of Ayurveda. A synthesis by the reader of the chapters on the subject matter offered in this book will delineate the commonalities and differences of the two systems. The reader's view could also be influenced by a general perception that Unani is a Greco-Muslim rather than a Greco-Arabic medical system. It is important to emphasize that Unani physicians were not all Muslims but also included Jews (Rabbi Moses ben Maimon, 1134-1204, known as Maimonides), Christians (Hunayn Ibn Ishaq, 808-873, known as Johannitus), and Persians who wrote and practiced in Arabic because it was the language of the political elite and of the sciences in the golden age of the Arab-Muslim civilization that extended from Spain to Central Asia for over 700 years. Arabic was also the language of the religion that highly praised knowledge and tolerance. Among traditional medical systems, Unani represents a complete system of practice with a highly developed system of physical diagnosis.

⊖ Chapter References can be found on the Evolve website at http://evolve.elsevier.com/Micozzi/complementary/

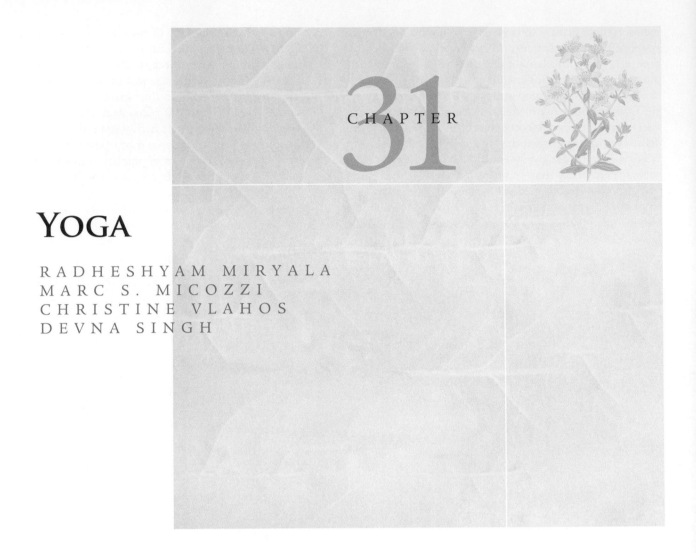

31

YOGA

RADHESHYAM MIRYALA
MARC S. MICOZZI
CHRISTINE VLAHOS
DEVNA SINGH

The practice of yoga has spread from India and become popularized throughout the world. Over time, many different schools of thought and styles of practice of yoga have flourished. Although a few schools focus on the original deep spiritual aspects of yoga, many people understand yoga to be a posturing and breathing technique to induce relaxation. This is a preliminary aspect of it; however, the true practice of yoga goes deep into mysticism and occultism. The philosophy of yoga addresses some of the greatest mysteries of life and the universe as it deals with the obscure astral and spiritual planes of human existence. Yogic literature is replete with statements attesting that true yogic knowledge is "revealed" wisdom and that it cannot be learned by reading books, listening to lectures, performing postural exercises, or using breathing techniques. It is regarded as a secret knowledge that cannot be imparted by words, but only experienced through sincere and dedicated practice. This revealed wisdom is beyond the limits of the individual intellect and imagination. It is a knowledge that describes methods to achieve direct consciousness of Divinity and Reality through meditation and intuition. Although yoga viewed as a physical culture involving postural exercises and breathing techniques has provided tremendous benefit to the world as a means of relaxation, it is important for a holistic practitioner to have a preliminary understanding of the deeper spiritual aspects of the science of yoga. A review of the complementary and alternative medicine (CAM) literature reveals a scant amount of modern rigorous research on the benefits of the postural exercises and breathing techniques; but research into the mystical aspects of yoga using contemporary methodology is nonexistent. This chapter briefly discusses the history and philosophies of yoga.

Let us start with the definition of the word *yoga*. *Yoga* is a Sanskrit word that is derived from the root *yuj*, which means "union" or "to join." This union is understood by the popular mind-body-spirit movement that has flourished recently to mean that the mind, body, and spirit are harmoniously joined together. Although this is partially correct, the real meaning is a union of the *Jivatma* (human soul) with the *Paramatma* (Divine Soul), or the merging of human consciousness with that of Divine Consciousness. The spiritual journey involves expanding the human consciousness until it is one with Divine Consciousness. To achieve this state of unification is considered to be the highest goal of human life, and this is the meaning of yoga. The mental process and discipline through which this union is attained is also called yoga. Thus, in essence, yoga is the ways and means of achieving the goal and it is also the goal itself. In ancient India, yogic scholars have experimented and developed methods of training and practice to efficiently help the interested seeker to achieve this goal. This experimental nature of the techniques is what makes yoga a true science of spirituality.

A problem that exists when discussing yogic philosophy is that it was originally written in Sanskrit. Many Sanskrit words and yogic philosophies do not translate perfectly into English. Some concepts in yogic literature do not have an equivalent in Western belief systems. Yogic science is a very specific and complex science. The difficulty in translating the concepts has led to many oversimplifications that have been detrimental to the true understanding of yoga. As yoga has spread throughout the world, various different schools of practice have evolved. Different techniques and methods have been developed over the years. Some schools continue to stress the importance of the true goal of yoga, whereas others have oversimplified the practice to focus on physical aspects of yogic techniques to improve balance and flexibility, induce relaxation, and so on. An in-depth evaluation of yogic science and the various different schools and styles of practice is beyond the scope of this chapter. Rather, this chapter focuses on explaining the fundamentals in a simple and succinct manner.

BACKGROUND AND HISTORY

The history of yoga starts around 1500 BC in the Indus Valley civilization that is now present-day India and Pakistan. Evidence of yogic beliefs and practices may be observed in the ancient *Vedas,* a collection of Sanskrit texts regarding "knowledge" of humanity, God, and the universe. According to Indian tradition, the Vedas were revealed through a vibrational medium *(shruta)* to seers *(rishis)* in the form of poems or hymns based on their mystical insights and are regarded as "revealed wisdom." This wisdom was not heard and perceived by the intellect as is commonly understood, but was intuitionally felt at a subtle vibrational level. The yogic truths are based on the experiences of mystics, saints, and sages who have experienced them throughout the ages. In India, these individuals were referred to as *rishis.* Swami Vivekananda, an influential spiritual leader of the early twentieth century and authoritative expert on Vedantic knowledge, describes rishis as follows: "They who having attained the supreme soul in knowledge were filled with wisdom, and having found him in union with the soul were in perfect harmony with the inner self, they having realized him in the heart were free from all selfish desires, and having

experienced him in all the activities of the world had attained calmness, . . . having reached the supreme God from all sides, had found abiding peace, had become united with all, had entered into the life of the Universe." (Vivekananda, n.d.) (see also Chapter 7).

This mystical tradition continued to flourish in India, and in the period between 600 BC and about 300 BC, the Upanishads were composed, which further described philosophies pertaining to yoga such as *paramatman* (Divine Soul), *atman* (human soul), *moksha* (liberation), and *dhyana* (meditation). It was also around this time that the *Bhagavad Gita* (Song of the Lord) was written. The Bhagavad Gita discusses three key elements of yogic philosophy: *karma* (action), *bhakti* (devotion), and *jyana* (knowledge from introspection). The Bhagavad Gita illustrates the divine relationship between humans and Divinity. In 200 BC, the sage Patanjali compiled a history of oral tradition regarding yoga into the *Yoga Darshan* or *Yoga Sutras,* which give specific details of classic yogic practices.

FUNDAMENTAL CONCEPTS

To understand how yoga is a science of spirituality, it is important to understand the fundamental concepts that are a part of this system of beliefs. Yogic philosophy addresses the basic questions of human life: (1) Who am I? (2) Why am I here? (3) What is the nature of suffering? (4) What is the method of escaping suffering? Yogic philosophy basically deals with the nature of humanity, God, and the manifest universe and the relationship among the three. It also deals with the way our thoughts and actions influence our spiritual journey and details ways and means of bringing our thoughts and actions into a regulated state. Yogic philosophy asserts that this spiritual journey is germane to all human beings independent of race, class, intelligence, and so on, but exists as a latent phenomenon. The preliminary aspect of the journey begins when we begin to question the nature of our existence. The awakening of this dormant phenomenon occurs when we choose to undergo the quest to understand the nature of our existence, and the journey ends when we merge our conscious ness with the Divine Consciousness.

A fundamental aspect of yogic philosophy is the belief that the cosmos is composed of two principal elements, *purusha* and *prakriti.* Purusha is composed of the Divine Soul and all souls of living things, including the human soul. Prakriti is the cosmic substance in the form of the physical world and the manifest universe. Human beings are composed of both purusha and prakriti, because their souls are a part of the Divine Soul and their outer selves are a manifestation of the cosmic substance in the form of the physical body. Prakriti does not have any conscious energy and exists in an inanimate state. The purusha is the Divine Soul, which is the animator of prakriti. The purusha is the source or base of everything in the manifest universe. Prakriti is the outer physical world and universe and our outer physical selves, including the body, mind, thoughts, and perceptions. The purusha is the substratum of all these things. All manifestations in the cosmos exist as a combination of both purusha and prakriti. Yogic philosophy states that essentially the human soul and the Divine Soul are the same. Through the process of human birth, the human soul becomes subjectively separated from the Divine Soul and must spend time in the manifest universe to make an attempt to become united with the Divine Soul again in consciousness. Yogic philosophy states that individuals are "bound" when they only identify themselves with prakriti, the outer self and the manifest universe, and are "freed" when they identify themselves with the purusha, the true inner self. In essence, yogic philosophy deals with the nature of God, humanity, and the manifest universe and the relationship between the three.

THE NATURE OF DIVINITY

Although yogic philosophy deals with God and soul, it is not considered to be a religious doctrine. It emphasizes that divinity is inside everyone and proposes scientific methods for achieving this realization. God is referred to by many different names, including *Brahman, Purusha, Isvara, Paramatma, Nirguna Brahma,* and *Saguna Brahma,* and there are subtle differences in the exact meanings of these terms. God is sometimes referred to as the Divine Soul who is without attributes. Different authors use the various terms interchangeably depending on the nature of the topic of discussion. At times God is referred to as a divine being with attributes, and the many names of gods of the Hindu pantheon are used as representations of God. However, the fundamentals of yoga refer to a divinity that is without attributes.

Many different schools of thought developed in yogic philosophy to describe the nature of God, either as a divinity without attributes or as a divinity with attributes. The two popular beliefs regarding the nature of God are embodied in the nondualistic and dualistic schools of thought. Adi Shankaracharya was a yogic scholar of the eighth century who expounded on the concepts of nondualism. The nondualistic philosophy states that the human soul and the Divine Soul are equal and the same. In the nondualistic school of thought, God is the Divine Soul that exists without attributes. The Divine Soul is said to be infinite, incorporeal, impersonal, unchanging, eternal, and absolute. The Divine Soul is the divine ground of all matter and sentient beings in the universe. Although the Divine Soul is the origin of all existence, forces, and substances in the material world, it is beyond the perception of the senses. It is this aspect of being beyond the perception of the senses that creates a difficulty in comprehending the experience of the Divine Soul. Because the Divine Soul is beyond the senses, it becomes difficult for the imagination to envision what this experience might be.

The experience of the Divine Soul cannot be described, but is often termed *Sat-Chit-Anandam* (Infinite Truth, Infinite Consciousness, Infinite Bliss).

The Divine Soul is formless and attributeless and cannot be described to be this or that. The problem arises when humans try to offer devotion or attempt to surrender to a God without attributes. Yogic methods attempt to achieve conscious awareness of this Divine Soul without attributes, but to wrap the human mind around an entity that is without form and function is quite difficult. This difficulty led to the birth of the dualistic school of thought. Because an attributeless God is difficult to fathom, the dualistic school of thought describes God to be with attributes. The purpose is to create an object of devotion that the human mind can perceive. The various gods of the Hindu pantheon represent different deities with godly attributes used by yoga followers to offer devotion and practice self-surrender. Over time, different sects and schools developed, each with its own personal deity. Also, certain schools have chosen a guru or spiritual teacher to be their object of devotion. This technique has been said to be a very efficient method of progressing on the spiritual journey, provided that the guru is one of the highest caliber who is merged with Divine Consciousness.

As noted, the nondualistic school of thought states that God is the substratum that courses through all souls and substances in the cosmos, and that there is no difference between the Divine Soul and the human soul. The dualistic school interprets the relationship between God, humans, and the universe differently. The dualistic school of thought states that differences exist between God, the human soul, and the manifest universe. Regardless, both schools of thought hold that even if a God with attributes in the form of a deity or guru is used as an object of devotion, the real ultimate God is an absolute divinity without attributes. In the end, the differences in the two schools of thought may be only a matter of semantics, because both claim that the goal of life is to merge the individual human soul with the Divine Soul.

THE NATURE OF THE MANIFEST UNIVERSE (PRAKRITI)

Yogic philosophy describes the origin of matter and the different phenomenon inherent to matter that make up the manifest universe. It states that in the beginning there was nothingness. Then a primordial stir occurred that sent out a wave of creation. This primordial stir is said to have been the awakening of the dormant will of God. From this primordial stir came the existence of prakriti (the manifest universe). When matter at its most primal subatomic state came into existence, so did its sense of individual identity apart from other forms of matter and apart from the Divine Consciousness. This is the basis of ego, or the "I-am-ness" of matter. As the complexity of physical matter evolved, so did the complexity of the individuating principle. Matter evolved to become the various objects and beings in the universe. The individuating principle evolved to include not only ego, but also intellect, mind, and consciousness.

Yogic philosophy details the creation of the manifest universe. It evolved from the basic subatomic particles to grosser and denser entities. Further complexities of the manifest universe include the five subtle potential energies of nature: sound potential, touch potential, sight potential, taste potential, and smell potential. These subtle potential energies correspond to the five fundamental elements of nature: ether/space, air/force, fire/energy, water/liquid, and earth/solid. This phenomenon of the five elements is also seen in other spiritual movements of the East and in Ayurvedic medicine and Chinese medicine. These five elements are related to the five "organs" of sense: hearing, feeling, seeing, tasting, smelling. To interact with the physical world, the five "organs" of action came into being: expressing, performing tasks, moving, excreting, and procreating. As matter evolved to denser and denser forms, it became the manifest universe with all matter and living beings. The variety of objects and creatures of the world are all composed of different proportions of the five potential energies and the five elements of nature.

Humans, including their organs of sense and organs of action, are also a combination of the subtle potential energies and elements of nature. The human being, in essence, is a microcosm of the macrocosm of the universe. Human beings interact with the phenomenal world through the organs of sense and organs of action. When humans attach themselves to the phenomenal world that they perceive with the senses and manipulate by action, they subjectively experience the pleasures and pains associated with this attachment. So in one sense, it seems that nature serves to keep humans hidden from their real selves by keeping them involved in the complexities of the material world. However, yogic literature says that the true purpose of nature is to provide the necessary experiences for the unfolding of the human being's higher consciousness. It is humans' ignorance (avidya) of their inner selves that binds them to the material world and its objects. This perception is referred to as maya, the illusory manifest universe. Taking the inner journey and gaining conscious awareness of the inner divinity in themselves, humans break free of the complex illusory power of the manifest universe. When the association with maya is removed, the condition of spiritual liberation (moksha) can take place.

THE NATURE OF HUMANITY

Humans are composed of both purusha and prakriti. As purusha, humans contain a portion of the Divine Soul in the form of the human soul. As prakriti, they contain a portion of the manifest universe in the form of the physical outer coverings of the body. In a simplistic sense, it appears that the physical body is the only covering to the human soul, but in reality the human soul is hidden under innumerable coverings. The spiritual journey of human beings involves increasing the consciousness to move from the outer physical body through these innumerable coverings to get to the divinity of the inner self. As these layers are traversed, an intuitional knowledge "reveals" itself, and the individual gets an opportunity to experience the soul. An essential element of the mystical practice of yoga is to remove these coverings layer by layer. Although there are innumerable layers or coverings to the soul, the human being is said to be composed of three bodies: the physical body, the astral body, and the causal body. This is similar to the traditional Chinese medicine view that the human being is composed of the physical body and the ethereal body.

The outer body is the physical body, which is a component of the manifest universe and is made up of the five basic elements of nature. The outward aspects of the physical body result from the mixture of the genetic components of the mother and the father. The physical body goes through the changes of life as it is born, grows, decays, and then dies. At death, it is meant to return to nature to reenter the food cycle. The physical body contains the five organs of sense and the five organs of expression that interact with the material world. Yoga states that there is a fundamental unity among all living creatures and all that exists in the universe. Yoga stresses the importance of the physical body's living in cosmic equilibrium and harmony, because we affect our surroundings and our surroundings affect us. The steps recommended for achieving this equilibrium include eating a simple natural diet, avoiding indulgences, and taking only the minimum from nature to maintain our existence. The practice of yoga attempts to bring about this harmony by bringing the physical body under the conscious control of the mind. When this is achieved, the body can enable higher spiritual pursuits. The physical body is the grossest part of the human body, and each successive layer has a greater subtlety to it.

The middle body is the astral body composed of prana (life force), manas (mind), buddhi (intellect), chit (consciousness) and ahankar (ego). Every living being has an astral body. The astral body is connected to the physical body through the layer of prana from which vital energies flow to the physical body. The layer of prana of the astral body has a shape similar to that of the physical body, but is more subtle than the physical body. Prana is the subtle life force that courses through the astral body. It is similar to the qi or chi of ancient Chinese beliefs. Prana exists in every form of matter in the manifest universe. As has already been said, prakriti or matter is inanimate and needs purusha to activate it. Prana activates matter by linking matter to energy on the physical level. The physical body is inanimate without the currents of prana. Prana is often referred to as "breath," but it is actually the force or energy that keeps up the activities of the physical body. The currents of prana flow along well-marked channels into every organ and part of the body. There are over 72,000 *nadis* (subtle energy channels) through which prana flows. These should not be confused with the nervous system, which is part of the physical body. The channels of prana have a very close similarity to the meridians of acupuncture. All matter in the manifest universe has a layer of prana, and the physical world is dependent on this flow of energy. Similarly, the physical body is also dependent on the flow of energy from the layer of prana. When prana ceases to function, the physical body dies.

Beyond the layer of prana is the layer of the mind. The mind should not be construed to be the brain. The brain is part of the physical body, whereas the mind is part of the astral or ethereal body. In an unregulated state, the mind produces spurious thoughts, both positive and negative. The input from the five senses also influences the quality and wandering nature of the mind. The mind does not involve reflexive reaction, such as moving one's hand away from a hot object. Such reflexive actions are part of the brain and nervous system, which exist in the physical body. The mind's activity moves in an unregulated manner when the individual associates himself or herself with the outer physical body and the feelings of comfort, joy, misery, and sorrow that accompany this association. As this association becomes stronger and stronger, the power of the mind keeps the individual's consciousness unaware of the inner human soul. Through sincere and dedicated spiritual practice the mind can be regulated. In a regulated state, the mind can be trained to look inward to ascertain the nature of the soul. When the mind is regulated, it becomes the most powerful vehicle for the spiritual journey. As the process of creation of the manifest universe occurred, the individuating principle of the mind also spread throughout this universe. Yogic theory states that the human mind is related to this Universal Mind and has latent functions and powers similar to those of the Universal Mind.

Beyond the layer of the mind is the region of consciousness, intellect, and ego. Although the words *mind* and *intellect* are used, these words are not perfect translations from the Sanskrit words *manas* and *buddhi*. In yogic knowledge, the mind and intellect are not part of the brain. The brain is part of the physical body. The mind and intellect are part of the astral body, and they are more subtle than the prana. Beyond the mind and the intellect is the ego. The term *ego* does not correlate with the traditional usage of the word in Western psychology. It is not the ego of Freud's id, ego, and superego theory, nor is it the part of the human mind from which conscious urges and desires arise, nor an inflated feeling of self-pride or superiority to others. The ego in yogic theory refers to the sense of "I-am-ness." In the densest form of ego, it is the

"I-am-ness" of the material world in which we associate ourselves with our professions, our hobbies, our likes and dislikes, our ties to others, and so on. In the subtlest form of ego, it is the "I-am-ness" of the human soul feeling separated from the Divine Soul.

The third body is the causal body, which houses the human soul. Yogic theory states that all our actions and thoughts create a causal effect on the outside world and also on our causal body. These subtle impressions produced by all our thoughts and actions create coverings around the soul. They control the formation and growth of the other two bodies and determine every aspect of our lives. Beyond these coverings is the soul, which is indestructible and unchangeable. The soul remains a passive onlooker to all the activities of life. At the time of death, both the causal and astral bodies (which remain together) separate from the physical body. The physical body disintegrates into the five elements to reenter the food cycle. If in this lifetime the human soul does not achieve merger with the Divine Soul, the causal body and astral body become reincarnated.

Yogic theory discusses the phenomenon of reincarnation. At the time of death the physical body dies and returns to the basic five elements of nature. The soul, which is trapped in the causal and astral bodies, takes another journey. Liberation (moksha) is the condition in which the individual's consciousness has evolved to an extent that the individual is freed from the cycle of birth and death. If the condition of liberation is achieved in this lifetime, the soul is spared from the cycle of birth and death. If the individual does not achieve liberation, the soul along with the causal body, astral body, and all the impressions from past thoughts and actions come back to the manifest universe to take up another life. A belief in the theory of reincarnation is not required to practice yoga, because the goal of yoga is meant to be achieved in one's current life.

PATANJALI'S YOGA SUTRAS

Sage Patanjali is credited with compiling the philosophy of yoga into the Yoga Sutras. This book deals with the definition of yoga, the goals of yoga, the obstacles on the path of yoga, and the ways and means of achieving the goals. Patanjali also describes the different stages of progress and the different stages of consciousness that are achieved with steady progress. According to I.K. Taimini (1961), Patanjali describes the obstacles that distract the mind as being disease, languor, doubt, carelessness, laziness, worldly-mindedness, delusion, nonachievement of a stage, and instability.

Patanjali defines the goal of yoga as *chitta-vritta-nirodha*, which translates as "inhibition of the fluctuating states of mind" or "whirlpools" of the mind. When the mind is regulated and exists in a state of stillness, the individual experiences his or her consciousness in its essential and fundamental nature. When the mind is unregulated, the individual's consciousness is assimilated into the various fluctuating states of the mind. The five fluctuating states of the mind are described as (1) knowledge from direct cognition, (2) knowledge from a false conception, (3) experience based on fancy or imagination, (4) sleep, and (5) experience based on memory. To achieve a state of stillness in the mind, the fluctuating states of the mind need to be regulated. Suppression of the fluctuating nature of the mind is the goal of yoga.

You can try a brief exercise to illustrate the difficulty of achieving a stillness of the mind. Try to examine the contents of your mind without making any particular effort for 5 minutes. Try to catalogue the varying fluctuations of the mind. For most, it will be difficult to go even a few seconds without the mind's being involved in one of its five states. The rapidly changing mental images that present themselves are derived from the ever-changing impressions produced by the outer world through the vibrations impinging on the sense organs, memories of past experiences floating in the mind, and mental images connected with anticipations of the future. Meditation is the vehicle that allows one to develop the ability to suppress the modifications of the mind, so that one can experience one's true inner self.

Patanjali also details the afflictions *(kleshas)*, obstacles on the path to attaining the goal of yoga, that must be overcome for the spiritual aspirant to progress on his or her spiritual journey. Yogic philosophy also states that these afflictions or obstacles are the root cause of human suffering. The five obstacles are ignorance, egoism, attraction to specific people or objects, repulsion toward specific people or objects, and the strong desire to continue living or a fear of death. Ignorance refers to a lack of awareness of the inner divinity and is the root cause of all of the other afflictions. Ignorance is not lack of knowledge, but refers to a spiritual ignorance in which the individual takes the material world to be Reality and remains ignorant of his or her true inner divinity. This leads to egoism or "I-am-ness," in which the individual's consciousness associates itself with the physical body and its sense organs, which experience the manifest universe (prakriti). This is when the individual becomes "bound" to prakriti. As this involution progresses, the association of the consciousness with the physical body and the illusory objects surrounding it becomes strengthened. Then, the individual starts to associate the pleasures and pain the individual experiences with the illusory objects of the manifest universe. This leads to a sense of attraction or repulsion toward objects and persons that cause pleasure and pain. This attraction and repulsion to innumerable persons and things in the manifest universe condition the individual's life, and the individual begins to think, feel, and act according to the biases produced by these bonds. Yogic philosophy states that when the individual is bound to these attractions and repulsions, the person curtails his or her

individual freedom. This binding is considered to be the cause of most of human misery. The last obstacle is a strong desire for mortal life or fear of death, which results from the compounding effects of the first four obstacles. A sincere and dedicated practice of yoga is the means for attenuation of these obstacles on the path to realization. As one progresses on the spiritual journey through yoga, there is a reduction of the obstacles, which leads to a reduction of the detrimental effects these obstacles have on meditation and progress on the spiritual path.

As one progresses and evolves along the spiritual path, the subtle essence of one's inner nature slowly reveals itself. Yogic literature states that with some spiritual progress, the mind becomes regulated, and its capacity for higher functions and greater levels of consciousness grows. The sincere spiritual aspirant can use this regulated mind and turn its attention inward to understand the nature of the manifest universe, the Divine Soul, and his or her true inner self. As this understanding of the relationship between prakriti and purusha unfolds, the individual mind begins to understand the functions of the Universal Mind. When this occurs the mind can become harnessed to develop certain powers *(siddhis)*. The powers described by Patanjali include clairvoyance, knowledge of past and future, telepathy, communication with previously liberated souls, extraordinary strength, and so on. Patanjali stresses that although one may acquire these powers, the sincere spiritual aspirant should shy away from these powers. They serve as temptations and distractions along the journey, and the aspirant should remain focused on the true goal of yoga. Patanjali states that these powers become manifest as consciousness expands, but the spiritually adept aspirant also gains the wisdom not to misuse these powers.

PATANJALI'S RAJA YOGA

Raja Yoga, or "kingly yoga," was detailed by Patanjali in his Yoga Sutras. He describes Raja Yoga as an efficient means of achieving the goal of yoga. Raja Yoga is a systematic method used to achieve a state of stillness in the mind. It consists of eight steps or limbs and is sometimes referred to as *Ashtanga Yoga.* The eight steps are progressive stages of practice to enable successful meditation and realization of the goal. The steps systematically reduce the obstacles on the path to self-realization. In Raja Yoga, the method adopted for bringing about changes in consciousness is based essentially on regulation of the mind by the will of the individual. This leads to a gradual suppression of the fluctuating and wandering nature of the mind. The techniques of Raja Yoga enable the gradual elimination of all sources of disturbance to the mind, both external and internal. With progress, the mind becomes regulated and is able to achieve the stillness that is required for further progress. The eight steps of Raja Yoga are as follows:

1. *Yama* (forbearance). This initial step details the way in which the spiritual aspirant should interact with the outside world. Because human beings are a part of the manifest universe, the aspirant should live his or her life in a regulated manner in balance with the laws of nature. The aspirant should avoid killing or causing pain, be truthful, refrain from taking what belongs to others, develop self-restraint rather than yielding to impulse or desire, and not covet means of enjoyment.

2. *Niyama* (self-discipline). The second step deals with mental and physical purity, introspection, and development of a profound devotion to God. The social and personal codes of conduct (yama and niyama) prepare the mind and body for the higher stages of meditation by reducing attachment and inducing tranquility.

3. *Asana* (yogic posture). The asana refers to a pose to be used to sit for meditation. The pose recommended is one that is comfortable and allows the aspirant to remain steady for a period of time. The aspirant should be able to remain stationary without feeling cramped and restless. The pose should be natural without strain or discomfort. The aspirant should be able to sit comfortably and go deep into meditation where he or she may experience a loss of body consciousness. The complicated poses that are taught as yoga in the West were not described by Patanjali. These complicated poses represent a later addition to yoga known as *Hatha Yoga* and are deemed by many to be nonessential for the true practice of yoga.

4. *Pranayama*. Pranayama refers to the regulation of the currents of prana that flow in the astral body discussed earlier. Pranayama is generally misconstrued to mean either regulation of breath or a deep breathing exercise. Pranayama is the regulation of prana (life force) and not the breath. Breathing, however, is one manifestation of prana as an action in the physical body. This close connection between prana and breathing enables the spiritual aspirant to manipulate currents of prana by manipulating breathing. With practice, the prana becomes purified, and this promotes the harmonious flow of prana in the body. Regulation of prana promotes serenity and steadiness in the body and stills the fluctuation of the mind.

5. *Pratyahara*. The mind is inundated by the impressions registered by the sense organs and the experiences produced by the outside world. This step aims to turn the mind inward so that it withdraws itself from the impressions of the sense organs. In this stage, the aspirant exercises his or her will so that the mind is able to restrain itself from influences from the outside world.

6. *Dharana*. This stage deals with development of concentration. The main focus of this stage is to train the mind to stay continuously concentrated on a chosen object. When concentration breaks, the spiritual aspirant is to bring the mind back to engaging on the chosen object. With practice, the wandering of the mind and disturbances regarding memories of the past, fantasies of future events, and so on, become curtailed and the aspirant is able to maintain prolonged concentration on the object. This stage prepares the aspirant for meditation.

7. *Dhyana*. All of the previous stages are to prepare the aspirant for this stage, which is meditation. In this stage, the mind is engaged in an uninterrupted flow toward the object of meditation. When the spiritual aspirant succeeds in completely eliminating all distractions and is able to concentrate on the object uninterruptedly for as long as desired, the aspirant masters the stage of dhyana. The difference between dharana and dhyana is that in the stage of dharana, the aspirant experiences occasional distractions from concentration. In dhyana, the mind has been regulated and is totally and continually absorbed on the object of meditation.

8. *Samadhi*. Samadhi is attained when dhyana reaches a state in which only the awareness of the object of meditation remains, and not awareness of the mind itself. Samadhi is the state of complete absorption in meditation. In this stage, only consciousness of the object exists without concurrent consciousness of the mind. The stages from dharana to samadhi represent different degrees of attainment of concentration and consciousness, with one leading to the next.

OTHER YOGIC PRACTICES

Patanjali's Raja Yoga is the oldest practice of yoga that has been documented. Over time, different practices have come into existence. The Bhagavad Gita describes three other paths of yoga: *Karma Yoga* (yoga of action), *Bhakthi Yoga* (yoga of devotion), and *Jnana Yoga* (yoga of knowledge from introspection). Patanjali's original Raja Yoga incorporated these elements of yoga, but did not recommend practicing them exclusively. *Hatha Yoga* is the other yogic movement that has become popularized over the years. It deals mostly with the postural aspects of yoga. Today, there are innumerable schools of yoga, each emphasizing different aspects of practice. However, the key elements of universal love and tolerance, surrendering to the will of the Divine, and devotion to the Divine are germane to all paths. Interested individuals should take caution in picking a path that suits their stage in life and fits their spiritual goals. At the same time, individuals should note that the true goal of yoga is to merge the inner self with the Divine Self. As the Bhagavad Gita says, "A person is said to have achieved yoga, the union with the self, when the perfectly disciplined mind gets freedom from all desires, and becomes absorbed in the self alone."

KARMA YOGA

Karma Yoga describes the performance of actions (karma) in a selfless service to God as a means of achieving merger with the Divine Consciousness. Actions should be performed in remembrance of God without anticipation of reward or failure. This should become a continuous process and include all activities of daily life, such as eating, caring for children, and so on. When this practice becomes established as a continuous process, it becomes like meditation in which the individual is continually absorbed in the remembrance of God. The individual begins to think of himself or herself only as an instrument of the Divine Consciousness, and no longer considers himself or herself the doer of actions. As this stage progresses, the individual loses attachment to the work and the antecedent joys and sorrows associated with the work. As the individual surrenders to the will of the Divine Consciousness, his or her will strengthens, and the individual is able to achieve things beyond his or her self-imposed limitations. In Karma Yoga, the individual lives and works in a harmonious manner with the outside world. The person performs his or her duty in such a way that this work becomes a spiritual practice.

JNANA (GYANA) YOGA

Jnana Yoga is the path of knowledge. This path aims at attaining Divine Consciousness through studying sacred books and engaging in deep inquiry and contemplation of the eternal truths. It involves recognizing God as the Creator of the Universe; the Almighty, Omnipotent, Omnipresent, and Omniscient One; and the Source of all spiritual knowledge. The knowledge obtained through this yoga helps a person understand the true nature of God, soul, and prakriti. This enlightenment enables the individual to break attachments to material things and allows the soul to become awakened so that it may merge with the Divine.

BHAKTHI YOGA

Bhakthi means "devotion," and Bhakthi Yoga is based on complete love of and devotion to God or Divine Consciousness. The object of devotion can be any deity or divine incarnation, or one's guru (spiritual teacher). Through constant devotion, the aspirant discovers Divinity reflected in every aspect of living and in every part of the universe. As the individual sees Divinity in everything, his or her capacity for love grows, and the individual is able to develop universal love and tolerance. Through love and devotion, the aspirant's ego or "I-am-ness" becomes subjugated, and the aspirant feels everything to be a part of the Divine.

HATHA YOGA

Hatha Yoga was developed in the fifteenth century by Yogi Swatmarama. He compiled his teachings into the *Hatha Yoga Pradipika*. Hatha Yoga uses physical purification as a means to purify the mind. Compared with the seated asanas of Patanjali's Raja Yoga, which were a means of preparing for meditation, the asanas of Hatha Yoga were developed as full body postures. Hatha Yoga also describes the various nadis and chakras of the astral body and details methods used to awaken these centers. Hatha Yoga in its many modern variations is the style that most people actually associate with the word *yoga* today. Unfortunately, many of these branches have ignored the deeper spiritual planes of this yoga and are satisfied with the physical health and vitality that its practice brings. In some schools, Hatha Yoga has been reduced to another form of fitness training.

MEDITATION

All of the yogic practices do eventually include meditation, which is the point at which all paths seem to converge. Yogic philosophy has influenced other spiritual movements, including Sufism, Buddhism, Sikhism, and Kaballah. Even these different movements also include meditation as an important part of the practice. Interestingly, the Chinese word *chan* and the Japanese word *zen* are derived from the Sanskrit word *dhyan,* and all these words refer to meditation. Meditation is said to be the vehicle used to travel on the spiritual journey. It is through meditation that higher states of consciousness unfold. It is also said that through meditation the various supernatural powers become manifest in the individual. Yogic literature states that the effects of meditation do not last just during the time spent meditating. The effects start to permeate throughout the day and influence all aspects of life. The goal of meditation is not just to experience the effects of meditation, but through it to achieve a condition in which the individual feels connected to the Divine throughout the day. Consider, for example, a quote from the Great Master Shri Ram Chandra Maharaj of Shahjahanpur, who founded the Sahaj Marg system of spiritual practice: "The real state of samadhi is that in which we remain attached with Reality, pure and simple, every moment—no matter how busy we may be all the time with worldly work and duties. It is known as sahaj samadhi—one of the highest achievements, and the very basis of nirvana. Its merits cannot be described by words, but can be realized by one who abides in it."

Yogic literature describes many different techniques for meditation. Some schools of yoga advocate a visualization technique using the form of their deity or their guru as the object of meditation. An effective yogic method is described in which the aspirant chooses to use a capable guru as the object of meditation, provided that the individual has developed love and devotion for the guru and surrenders himself or herself to the will of the guru. Patanjali describes several different techniques of meditation, including meditation on the heart, which is said to be an effective method for understanding the nature of the mind and for developing a sense of universal love. Patanjali also describes meditative techniques to improve intuitional capacity as well as methods to develop some supernatural powers such as clairvoyance. Another common method for meditation is the use of sacred sounds or *mantras*. The primordial stir or vibration of the universe is said to be articulated as "OM (A-U-M)," which is a very popular mantra used in meditation. One mantra technique is to meditate on the sacred sound OM by mentally repeating the sound in the mind. With time and practice, the mind becomes naturally integrated with the mantra and reverberates with the sound of the mantra. This renders the mind still and enables deeper states of meditation.

STAGES OF THE SPIRITUAL JOURNEY

Regardless of which path an individual chooses, the goal of yoga remains the same. Although the outer trappings of the paths may be different, there are certain stages common to all paths. After some preliminary progress, there exist four stages of which the aspirant must gain understanding and which must be incorporated into the aspirant's life. These four stages must be attained by every individual regardless of the chosen path. These are compulsory if the aspirant is genuinely interested in achieving the true goal of yoga. The four stages or conditions to be achieved are *viveka, vairagya, shat sampat,* and *mumukshutva*.

The first step is the acquisition of *viveka*. Viveka is the power of discrimination, which means the ability to discriminate between the real and the unreal, between the permanent and the impermanent, between that which is the inner self and that which is not of the inner self. As the individual progresses on the spiritual journey, the power of discrimination grows stronger, and the individual gains inner strength and mental peace. The state of viveka becomes more and more a permanent condition. This allows the individual to deal efficiently with the material world, because the individual always remains alert and does not become entangled in the trappings of the world.

The second step is the acquisition of *vairagya*, dispassion or nonattachment. An individual without vairagya is a slave to the attractions and repulsions of worldly life. When the aspirant gains the state of vairagya, the aspirant is not bothered by the attractions and repulsions of the

material world. This aids concentration of the mind and generates a strong yearning for liberation. Vairagya does not imply that the spiritual aspirant should abandon the social duties and responsibilities of life. Rather, the individual is to attend to them as a service to the Divine. Theoretically, it is easy to talk of viveka and vairagya, but the practical application of the two on a continuous basis can be difficult. With continuous sincere, dedicated effort, the condition of viveka and vairagya can exist as a natural part of the individual.

The third requisite is *shat sampat*, or sixfold virtue, which brings about tranquility and regulation of the functions of the mind. The six virtues are as follows:

1. *Shama* is tranquility of mind brought about by fixing the mind's attention on the Divine. In this stage, the mind is unaffected by the impressions created by the sense organs and action organs.
2. *Dama* is control of the sense organs and action organs. The mind regulates these organs, instead of being controlled by them. This does not imply austerity. The individual offers himself or herself and the organs of action to the service of the Divine.
3. *Uparati* is the condition in which the function of the mind ceases to be influenced by external objects. In this stage the individual develops a contentment with regard to objects, tolerance with regard to persons, and acceptance of his or her role in life.
4. *Titiksha* is power of endurance. In this stage, the aspirant patiently bears all afflictions and trying conditions without anxiety or lament.
5. *Shraddha* is the condition in which the individual develops intense faith in the words of the guru or the spiritual scriptures. But above all, it is the intense faith that the individual has in himself or herself and in his or her ability to reach the goal.
6. *Samadhana* is a state of perfect concentration of mind. In this condition, the mind is permanently fixed on the inner self. The individual in this stage performs all actions while the mind dwells in union with the Divine.

The fourth necessary stage is *mumukshutva*, which is an intense desire for liberation. In this condition, the aspirant's attention is permanently fixed on the goal of achieving union with the Divine. To attain this stage, the spiritual aspirant must have equipped himself or herself by progressing through the first three stages. The order of achieving these stages is important, because one leads to the other and they culminate in the development of an intense desire for liberation.

INNER AWAKENINGS

The goal of yoga is to merge the human soul with the Divine Soul. The journey to this goal involves progressing through various stages of consciousness. The four stages described earlier are also part of this journey. As the consciousness expands, there is also another journey that takes place. This is the journey of the currents of prana in the astral body. Yogic literature describes the journey of the consciousness and the journey of the currents of the astral body in great detail. The journey of the currents of the astral body involves the nadis and chakras.

NADIS AND CHAKRAS

Nadis are the channels through which the prana (life force) of the astral or ethereal body are said to flow (Figure 31-1). Prana is related to the qi or chi in Chinese-based systems, and the nadis seem to correspond to the meridians of traditional Chinese medicine. As noted earlier, there are over 72,000 nadis (subtle energy channels), and the places where multiple nadis merge form chakras. A chakra is defined as a center of activity that receives, assimilates, and expresses the prana (life force). The human body is said to contain seven chakras that are aligned in an ascending column from the base of the spine to the top of the head.

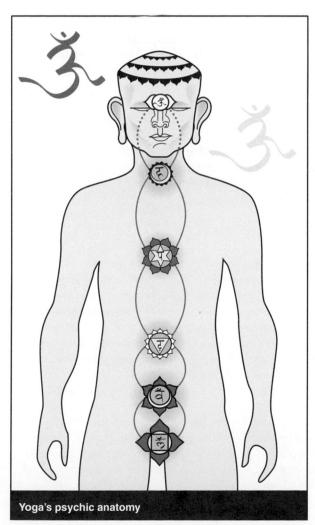

Yoga's psychic anatomy

Figure 31-1 Symbolic representation of the yogic nadi model.

Although they appear to be in the spinal column, the nadis and chakras exist only in the astral body and are not actually part of the spinal column, which is a part of the physical body. The seven chakras represent various aspects of consciousness. They are described as having different colors and are visualized as lotuses or flowers. As the spiritual journey progresses, the different chakras begin to become awakened as deeper levels of spiritual subtlety are achieved.

Although there are over 72,000 nadis, the three main ones are the *ida, pingala,* and *sushumna* nadis. The sushumna nadi starts at the base of the spinal column, moves straight up the body, and terminates at the top of the head. The ida and pingala nadis also start at the base of the spinal column, but they crisscross, forming semicircular curves. The journey of the chakras starts with the awakening of the *kundalini shakthi,* which lies dormant at the base of the ida, pingala, and sushumna nadis at the base chakra, the *muladhara* chakra. The kundalini is likened to a sleeping serpent coiled at the base of the spine. As the spiritual journey marches forward, the kundalini becomes awakened and starts to move up the ida, pingala, and sushumna nadis. As it travels up these nadis, it awakens the chakras along its path. As successive chakras are awakened, they correspond to higher states of consciousness, culminating at the top, which represents the Divine Consciousness. The seven chakras are the following:

1. *Muladhara:* symbolized by a lotus with four petals, located in the perineum, corresponds to the sacro-coccygeal nerve plexus, associated with the earth element. This is the resting place of the dormant kundalini shakthi (serpent power).
2. *Svadhishthana:* symbolized by a lotus with six petals, located in the sacrum, corresponds to the sacral plexus at the fourth lumbar vertebra, associated with the water element.
3. *Manipura:* symbolized by a lotus with 10 petals, located at the navel, corresponds to the solar plexus, associated with the fire element.
4. *Anahata:* symbolized by a lotus with 12 petals, located at the heart, corresponds to the cardiac plexus, associated with the air element. It is said that meditation on this region generates qualities of universal love and tolerance in the spiritual aspirant.
5. *Vishuddhi:* symbolized by a lotus with 16 petals, located at the base of the throat, corresponds to communication and sound vibrations, associated with the ether element.
6. *Ajna:* symbolized by a lotus with two petals, located in the middle of the forehead, considered to correspond with the vestigial third eye, associated with awareness, time, and light.
7. *Sahasrara dal kamal:* translates as "a lotus with 1000 petals," located at the crown of the head, associated with Divine Consciousness.

Many different texts offer different descriptions of the chakras. Some declare that each chakra has its own color, and some state that each chakra has its own vibrational sound. The chakras are also described as relating to different emotions. For example, awakening of the anahata (heart) chakra is associated with increased capacity for love and tolerance. We can get a very preliminary understanding of the chakras by reading about them, but yogic literature asserts that true knowledge of a chakra can be achieved only by the awakening of the chakra in the individual. Although many yogic practices focus on awakening the kundalini and taking the journey from the muladhara chakra to the sahasrara dal kamal, there are other inner journeys described in the yogic literature. For example, the Sahaj Marg system of spiritual training starts with the heart chakra and describes levels of spiritual attainment that goes far beyond the sahasrara dal kamal chakra.

IMPORTANCE OF THE GURU

I am the way, and the truth, and the life; no one comes to the Father but through Me.

—JESUS CHRIST

Adi Shankaracharya, who expounded on the philosophy of nondualism, states, "These three things are hard to achieve, and are attained only by the grace of God: human birth, the desire for liberation, and finding refuge with a great sage." In fact yogic literature is replete with statements attesting to the importance of finding a capable guru in undergoing the spiritual journey. Guru Nanak, who founded the Sikh movement, says on the importance of a guru, "Let no man in the world live in delusion. Without a guru none can cross over to the other shore."

The word *guru* comes from Sanskrit, and its roots are *gu*, meaning "darkness," and *ru*, signifying "dispeller." A guru is an awakened being who has merged his or her consciousness with that of the Divine. By an application of will, the guru is able to transmit this higher consciousness to the aspirant, thereby removing the darkness enveloping the aspirant's awareness. The spiritual path is long and fraught with obstacles of desire and ego, along with the individual's own delusions, fears, prejudices, fixations, and stagnant tendencies. A guru is a spiritual teacher who guides the aspirant on the spiritual path and helps to remove these obstacles. The guru devotes his or her life to guiding the aspirant along the spiritual path, the summation of which is the realization of the inner self and merging of the inner self with the Divine Self. Just as the nature of spirituality is one of mysticism and esotericism, so is the nature of the guru. As Shri Ram Chandra (Babuji Maharaj) states, "A guru is a mystery that solves another mystery—that of God."

In a world that is engrossed in satisfying the whims and desires of the physical body, it is easy to see why this spiritual journey to the inner self is not popular with the general public. And for the few who might have a casual interest in the matter, choosing a guru might be unpleasant to the ego. Dr. Georg Feuerstein, a German-American Indologist, echoes this sentiment in the following statement: "The traditional role of the guru, or spiritual teacher, is not widely understood in the West, even by those professing to practice yoga or some other Eastern tradition entailing discipleship. . . . Spiritual teachers, by their very nature, swim against the stream of conventional values and pursuits. They are not interested in acquiring and accumulating material wealth or in competing in the marketplace, or in pleasing egos. They are not even about morality. Typically, their message is of a radical nature, asking that we live consciously, inspect our motives, transcend our egoist passions, overcome our intellectual blindness, live peacefully with our fellow humans, and, finally, realize the deepest core of human nature, the Spirit. For those wishing to devote their time and energy to the pursuit of conventional life, this kind of message is revolutionary, subversive, and profoundly disturbing."

As with all things in life, there are organizations and people who are sincere and those who are fraudulent. The same holds true for spiritual organizations and spiritual teachers. In some countries, such as India, the guru-disciple tradition is an integral part of the culture. There have, however, been self-proclaimed gurus and spiritual organizations that have duped and defrauded the naive and misguided spiritual aspirant. This has made the general public wary of joining any spiritual organization. This has done great harm to the sincere spiritual movements. The interested spiritual aspirant is encouraged to take great care in making decisions regarding joining a spiritual organization or choosing a guru.

APPLICATION OF YOGA

Perverted, negative, and excessive use of sense objects, time, and the power of discrimination is the threefold cause of both psychic and somatic disorders. Both body and mind are the locations of disorders as well as pleasure. [The inner self] is devoid of disorders; it is the cause of consciousness in conjunction with the mind, and the five elements (the senses—sound, touch, appearance, flavor, odor) and the sense organs (hearing, feeling, seeing, tasting, smelling); it is eternal—the seer who sees all the actions.

—AYURVEDIC LITERATURE

It is important for holistic practitioners to have an understanding of the fundamental aspects of yogic philosophy. When yogic philosophies and practices are understood, CAM practitioners can find ways to incorporate them into Western medicine. These philosophies have already been incorporated into Ayurvedic medicine. In fact, they are a large part of Ayurvedic practice. Ayurvedic medicine's goals are also said to be aligned with the goals of yoga. Ayurveda suggests that overindulgence of the senses is implicated in certain disease processes, and yoga offers a way to curtail the indulgence of the senses. In Western medicine, spiritual practices such as meditation are recommended for the health benefits that they provide. Ayurvedic medicine also attests to this, but in Ayurveda the focus is on keeping the body healthy to pursue spiritual goals. Yogic philosophy views the body as a vehicle for the soul in the journey toward enlightenment. In yogic philosophy, meditation is not practiced to improve the health of the physical body; rather, health is maintained so that one can meditate and make progress on the spiritual journey. This is a radically different paradigm from that of Western medicine.

In the Western medical climate, our patients suffer from many chronic conditions such as depression and back pain. Traditional Western medicine has not found sustainable long-term cures for many of these chronic conditions. The role that CAM and holistic practitioners play in finding solutions to these chronic problems is an important one, and vital to the health of the public. Yogic philosophies and practices can become an important tool used to bring solutions for these chronic conditions. The fundamental yogic belief that all human suffering stems from the individual's unawareness of his or her inner divinity is a powerful paradigm shift to be introduced into modern medicine. This would radically alter our approach to treatment of chronic maladies such as depression, anxiety, fibromyalgia, and chronic pain syndromes.

There is little rigorous research on the use of yoga to treat various conditions; however, there is an abundance of anecdotal information on the benefits of yoga. Yoga teachers and practitioners claim that yoga relieves stress; enhances physical strength, stamina, and flexibility; facilitates impulse control; boosts immune function; improves blood circulation; increases memory and concentration; enables positive thinking; and bestows peace of mind. There are claims that yoga provides therapeutic relief for many ailments, including heartburn, asthma, arthritis, anxiety, depression, and hypertension. Research into the field of yoga is slowly gaining momentum; however, there are no studies focusing on the deeper spiritual aspects of yoga. It is this field of knowledge that could greatly influence modern medicine.

At the core of yogic practice is meditation. Yogic literature offers many techniques to enable effective meditation. The effects of meditation have been studied, and meditation has been proven to have many benefits, including reduction in stress and blood pressure. Modern medicine is making great discoveries regarding the benefits of meditation, but little research is being done on the relative effectiveness of different meditative practices. This is one area in which the field of yoga could be naturally integrated into modern medicine. Yoga offers various meditative techniques, but more importantly it has an abundant store of knowledge on ways to curtail distractions during meditation. Given that meditation has a positive effect, it

becomes important for the holistic practitioner to learn the ways and means to enable deep meditative states. This is perhaps one of the most important contributions yoga can make to modern medicine.

The application of yogic principles to the fields of preventive medicine and whole person wellness is another area in which modern Western medicine might garner great benefit. Yogic philosophy recommends that the practice of yoga be incorporated into one's existence as a way of life. Yogic literature claims that the dedicated practice of yoga leads to a cleansing of the subtle energy channels. These energy channels are said to course through all organs and parts of the body. This leads to a purification of the body and enables proper functioning of the organs. Further research is needed to validate these claims and to ascertain any benefit at the physical level. The dedicated practice of yoga is also said to lead to the condition in which the individual is grounded in the true inner self and is not afflicted by the transient phenomenal world. In our present culture, a large percentage of patients have mental disorders such as depression, anxiety, and a variety of psychosomatic conditions. When patients are taught methods that allow them to regulate their minds to understand their spiritual selves, they will develop the mental equipoise that can keep such mental disorders at bay. If the practice of yoga is started before individuals develop psychiatric disorders, it might work as prophylaxis against such disorders. Yogic literature recommends living in balance with nature. It also provides means for the individual's faculties of body, mind, and spirit to exist in union with nature, which could lead to an increased sense of whole person wellness.

The application of yoga in modern Western medicine involves many radical paradigm shifts. This should not discourage the scientific community from pursuing a deeper understanding of yogic knowledge in order to apply it to modern medical practice. Yogic theories, at a minimum, reinforce the belief that the human is a physical, mental, and spiritual being. Yoga also supports theories of bioenergies with its detailed explanation of the various subtle energy channels in the astral body. At a simple level, it offers methods for achieving physical and mental well-being. At a deeper level, it offers methods for enlivening the inner spirit. However, yogic literature declares that higher spiritual states cannot be measured, they can only be experienced. Modern medicine, along with the mind-body-spirit movement in CAM fields, has made great strides in understanding the spirit and applying it to health, but the "unknown" aspects of this spiritual science have not been explored. The unmeasurableness of the unknown is perhaps one of the reasons that these mystical aspects have not been explored in depth. Modern science is dedicated to providing measurable and tangible results, but this is not possible for the deep mystical aspects of yoga. This arena is beyond the region of the intellect and can only be experienced by intuition. The surrogate markers of cortisol levels and brain waves do not tell the whole story. Relying on such measures is like trying to appreciate a Picasso painting by looking at a chart that details the percentage of each color used in the painting. To harvest the higher fruits of yoga for application in modern medicine will require the concerted, dedicated, and creative efforts of the professionals involved in CAM research. This will make possible a higher level of wellness and improved well-being for the individual and for society in general.

THE HEART OF THE MATTER

Beyond the senses are the objects; beyond the objects is the mind; beyond the mind, the intellect; beyond the intellect, the Great Atman; beyond the Great Atman, the Unmanifest; beyond the Unmanifest, the Purusha. Beyond the Purusha there is nothing: this is the end, the Supreme Goal.

—KATHA UPANISHAD

In a world culture that promotes the indulgence of our senses and the cultivation of our ego, it is easy to understand why this journey to the inner self is not so popular. Our societies are defined by the flavors of cuisine, fashions of dress, and styles of music and various other instruments designed to satisfy the senses. Our cultures judge individuals based on wealth, professions, power, social status, and a myriad of other mechanisms designed to keep the individual's ego attached to the material world. It would appear that the world as the manifest universe exists to keep humans occupied so that they ignore the inner self. However, yogic literature declares that the world exists to provide experiences for the individual so that the individual's higher consciousness may unfold. This journey from the association with the outside world to the inner divinity is long and fraught with many obstacles. At a minimum, the individual should have an earnest desire to undergo the journey. Although only a small percentage of people fit into this category, yogic literature holds that the desire for knowledge of self exists in all individuals, although it is a latent phenomenon in most.

Yoga in essence is concerned with the expansion of human awareness or consciousness until it is merged with Divine Consciousness. Although the journey toward this expanded consciousness involves concepts of renunciation, this should not be interpreted to mean escapism or austerity. The human being exists as a part of the manifest universe, and the "awakened" individual is meant to live and function in the material world. When the individual experiences an expansion of consciousness, the person is meant to use this for the betterment of his or her surroundings. As a sentient being who is part of the manifest universe, the individual has a responsibility to care for the manifest universe. This responsibility includes existing in a state of balance with nature, and extends to assisting one's fellow humans on the spiritual journey. The expanded awareness is not meant to be an escapism that occurs during meditation, but a general state of being that stays with the individual while the individual is performing his or her duties in the world.

Yoga is a complex science that has evolved over thousands of years. As yoga has evolved through the ages, many different movements and branches have been established. Some have attempted to simplify the methods to suit modern times. The innumerable organizations have adopted different methods and different goals. Some have abandoned the goal of merging with the Divine Consciousness and have chosen instead to focus on techniques to promote physical fitness and mental relaxation. The serious spiritual aspirant is encouraged to consider the true goal of yoga when choosing a path. Yogic literature repeatedly states the importance of having a capable spiritual master to gain knowledge of the deeper spiritual aspects of yoga. Regardless of the path chosen, Yoga is a lifelong dedicated practice, and the aspirant should be wary of any weekend courses that promise profound changes. The benefits of yoga are commensurate with the dedication, sincerity, and discipline that the spiritual aspirant brings to the practice.

Acknowledgments

All gratitude to Puya Shri Parthasarathi Rajagopalachari, for all that he has given and for all that he is waiting to give.

⊖ Chapter References can be found on the Evolve website at http://evolve.elsevier.com/Micozzi/complementary/

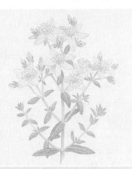

CHAPTER

32

CONTEMPORARY AYURVEDA

HARI M. SHARMA

HISTORY

Ayurveda is a holistic system of natural health care that originated in the ancient Vedic civilization of India. During centuries of foreign rule in India, beginning in the fifteenth century, Ayurvedic institutions declined or were suppressed, and much of the Ayurvedic knowledge was fragmented, misunderstood, and not used in its totality. Ayurveda has been revived in its completeness, in accordance with the classical texts, by Maharishi Mahesh Yogi in collaboration with leading Ayurvedic scholars and physicians, known as *vaidyas*. This specific reformulation of Ayurveda is known as *Maharishi Ayurveda (MAV)*.

The Sanskrit name *Ayurveda* is a compound of two words: *Ayus,* which means "life" or "life span," and *Veda,* which means "knowledge," with a connotation of completeness or wholeness of knowledge. The element of "wholeness" in Ayurvedic knowledge has profound clinical significance: the MAV clinician uses more than 20 treatment approaches that deal with the full range of the

patient's life: the body, mind, behavior, environment, and, most importantly, the patient's consciousness, his or her "innermost life." MAV considers consciousness to be of primary importance in maintaining optimal health and emphasizes meditation techniques to develop integrated holistic functioning of the nervous system.

MAV includes a sophisticated theoretical framework that provides clinical insight into the functioning of both mind and body. Understanding of the patient's mind-body type is essential to diagnosis and treatment, and special emphasis is placed on the therapeutic effects of diet and healthy digestion, as well as techniques to balance behavior and emotions. An extensive materia medica describes the therapeutic use of medicinal plants, and there is a detailed understanding of biological rhythms, which form the basis for daily and seasonal behavioral routines to strengthen the immune system and homeostatic mechanisms.

Ancient Ayurvedic texts typically begin with a thorough description of strategies of prevention before discussing modalities for treatment.

495

The Ayurvedic classics include three major texts (*Brihat Trayi*), the *Charaka Samhita*, *Sushruta Samhita*, and *Ashtanga Hridaya* of Vagbhata, and three minor texts (*Laghu Trayi*), the *Sarngadhara Samhita*, *Bhavaprakash Samhita*, and *Madhava Nidanam*. Most of these texts have been translated into English (*Charaka Samhita*, 1977; Madhavakava, 1986; Sarngadhara, 1984; *Sushruta Samhita*, 1963; Vagbhata, 1982). These texts address eight main sections of Ayurveda: *Shalya*—surgery in general; *Shalakya*—head and neck surgery for supraclavicular diseases; *Kaya Chikitsa*—treatment, diagnosis, and internal medicine; *Kaumarya Birtya*—pediatrics, obstetrics, and gynecology; *Agad Tantra*—toxicology and medical jurisprudence; *Bhut Vidya*—psychosomatic medicine; *Rasayana*—materia medica to promote vitality, stamina, resistance to disease, and longevity; and *Vajikarana*—fertility and potency. (See also Chapter 29.)

In addition to preventive techniques, MAV offers a holistic theory of prevention. Western medical attempts to develop preventive medical strategies, although laudable, conspicuously lack such a theory. As for the fields of diagnosis and treatment, MAV offers a large body of procedures and protocols, including a set of noninvasive diagnostic techniques, and addresses certain deficiencies of Western allopathic medicine. For example, functional diseases, such as irritable bowel syndrome and poor digestion, account for approximately one third of patient visits to family practitioners. Western medicine, however, lacks well-developed theories or methods of treatment for these disorders.

Another area of concern is iatrogenic (physician-caused) diseases, which are estimated to be the third leading cause of death in the United States (Starfield, 2000). A study of hospitalized patients found that 36% had iatrogenic illnesses (Steel et al, 1981). At least one serious "adverse event" (another term for iatrogenic occurrence) resulting from inappropriate care lengthened the hospital stay of 17.7% of hospital patients (Andrews et al, 1997), and nearly 14% of the adverse events led to death (Berwick et al, 1999). A large percentage of iatrogenic illnesses are the result of side effects from drugs. Adverse drug reactions have now become the fourth leading cause of death in the United States (Lazarou et al, 1998). To consider one example, Western approaches to cancer treatment can have severe side effects, and some antitumor drugs contribute to the development of new cancers. MAV modalities have been effective in reducing the side effects of several of these treatments (Dwivedi et al, 2005; Misra et al, 1994; Sharma et al, 1994; Srivastava et al, 2000), and laboratory research has shown that some MAV herbal preparations reduce cancer growth directly (Patel et al, 1992; Penza et al, 2007; Prasad et al, 1992, 1993; Sharma et al, 1990, 1991).

MAV is being practiced in clinics worldwide in India, Europe, Japan, Africa, Russia, Australia, and South and North America by specially trained physicians, many of whom also practice privately. In various ways, MAV directs its objectives not only to individual patients, but also to the life of society as a whole.

THEORETICAL BASIS: A "CONSCIOUSNESS MODEL" OF MEDICINE

MAV's contribution to patient care and clinical practice results from the model of health and disease on which it is based. Whereas Western medicine bases its model for understanding health and disease on the *material* of the body, the MAV model is based on the body's *nonmaterial* substrate, which is conceived as a field of pure intelligence. Western medicine's paradigm may seem more scientific, but in certain respects, Ayurveda's may be seen to presage today's advanced theories of physics.

From the time of Newton until the early twentieth century, the field of physics was based on a materialist approach to the natural world (see Chapter 1). The allopathic medical paradigm, developed in the nineteenth century, is based on this theory of materialism; it views the body as a complex machine. However, discoveries by twentieth-century physicists have undermined this materialist worldview and uncovered a fundamental role for consciousness in the physical world. Because the nature and importance of consciousness are not usually considered in allopathic medicine, twentieth-century physics provides a useful background for understanding MAV.

According to the materialist theory that dominated physics until the 1900s, the universe is made up of solid, discrete bits of matter. These particles affect each other only through direct interactions. Four basic principles support this "common sense" view of reality, as follows:

1. *Solid matter.* The world is fundamentally made up of solid material objects, the building blocks of nature.
2. *Strict causality.* Change in motion of one object can be caused only by direct interaction with another object.
3. *Locality.* Interactions between particles can occur only through collisions or through influences radiated through the electromagnetic or gravitational fields at the speed of light, or less. No nonlocal interaction can occur.
4. *Reductionism.* Large systems in nature—including, in principle, the human body and even the entire universe—can be understood completely by understanding the properties and local, causal interactions of their smallest discrete components.

In the materialist theory the consciousness of the scientist is considered separate from the material objects being studied. The knower (consciousness) and the known (object) are thought to exist in completely distinct domains. This separation is thought to be the basis of "objective" science. Throughout the history of science, however, the separation of consciousness from the apparently material world has led to theoretical difficulties. For example, if consciousness is completely separate from matter, it is difficult to explain how consciousness could arise from the purely mechanical interactions of solid matter within the brain.

In the twentieth century the terms of this discussion were changed by the fundamental discoveries of quantum physics. Experiments performed in the first quarter of the twentieth century indicated that subatomic particles, the supposed building blocks of nature, did not appear to be composed of solid matter. In some of these experiments, particles behaved as if they were waves. In others, electrons took instantaneous, discontinuous quantum jumps from one atomic orbit to another, with no intervening time and no journey through space—an impossible act for a classic particle. It also was shown that an individual subatomic particle cannot have both a precise position and a precise momentum simultaneously (the "uncertainty" principle), another situation that would not apply to a solid material particle. Finally, it was found that electrons can, with predictable regularity, tunnel through a solid barrier that, classically, would be impenetrable.

On the basis of these findings, the basic principles of quantum mechanics (often known as the *Copenhagen interpretation*) challenge the materialist worldview, as follows:

1. *No solid matter.* This interpretation accepted the scientific findings (wave/particle, quantum jumps, uncertainty, tunneling) that contradict the notion of solid matter.
2. *No strict causality.* Precise predictions for individual subatomic particles are impossible. Quantum mechanics thus loses the ability to trace causal relations among individual particles.
3. *No locality.* Quantum mechanical equations indicate that two particles, once they have interacted, are instantaneously connected, even across astronomical distances. This defies the strictly local connections allowed in classic materialism.
4. *No reductionism.* If apparently separate particles actually are connected nonlocally, a reductionist view based on isolated particles is untenable.

The Copenhagen interpretation was not put to experimental test for decades, which left some physicists unconvinced that solidity, causality, locality, and reductionism had to be abandoned. In the 1980s, however, a number of different experiments produced results that consistently contradicted the theories of materialism (often called *local realism*) and consistently confirmed the predictions of quantum mechanics (Aspect et al, 1981; Rarity et al, 1990). These studies found that once two particles have interacted, they are instantaneously

correlated nonlocally, over arbitrarily vast distances—an impossibility in materialism.

These results do not invalidate materialism altogether. In the everyday world of "large" objects, the mechanistic causation of Newtonian physics is approximately correct, which is why much of medicine has been able to rely on it without apparently ill consequences. However, at the fundamental, subatomic level, materialism conflicts both with theory and with frequently replicated experimental evidence. This gives rise to a fundamentally different worldview. Many physicists now argue that nature is composed of *probability waves* that are a function of *intelligence alone*, not of discrete physical particles. The equations of quantum mechanics thus describe a world made of abstract patterns of intelligence.

> In view of these uniformly idea-like characteristics of the quantum-physical world, the proper answer to our question, "What sort of world do we live in?" would seem to be this: "We live in an idea-like world, not a matter-like world." There is, in fact, in the quantum universe no natural place for matter. This conclusion, curiously, is the exact reverse of the circumstance that in the classic physical universe there was not a natural place for mind. (Stapp, 1994)

Quantum field theory, the most accurate version of quantum mechanics, can be related to the core tenet of MAV's paradigm. In quantum field theory the probability wave for a particle is described as a fluctuation in an underlying, nonmaterial field (known as a *force field* or *matter field*). Furthermore, in the most recent superunified theories, physicists have described all the force and matter fields that make up the universe as modes of vibration of one underlying, unified field, sometimes called the *superfield* or *superstring field*. All the order and intelligence of the laws of nature arise from this one fundamental, nonmaterial field, as does all matter. Not only are particles really just waves, but those waves ultimately are made of an underlying field, as ocean waves are made of ocean water. This field is one of pure intelligence, having the attributes that we associate with consciousness. This lends support to the statement of the quantum mechanical pioneer Max Planck, who said, "I regard consciousness as primary. I regard matter as derivative from consciousness," and of Sir Arthur Eddington, the physicist who first provided evidence in support of Einstein's general theory of relativity, who said, "The stuff of the world is mind-stuff" (Eddington, 1974).

Unified field theory may seem worlds away from the concerns of a clinician. The current allopathic approach assumes that the body can be explained by material reductionism, as if it were machinery. MAV, by contrast, has viewed it as an abstract pattern of intelligence. Because this latter view appears to be consistent with fundamental science, it is not unreasonable to consider that it might contribute to the clinician's capacity to promote health. Let us examine how MAV's "consciousness model" is applied in clinical practice.

APPLICATION OF THE CONSCIOUSNESS MODEL IN MAHARISHI AYURVEDA

TRANSCENDENTAL MEDITATION

To understand the most basic application of the consciousness model, we must briefly touch on physics again. Vedic thought discusses a unified field of pure, nonmaterial intelligence and consciousness whose modes of vibration manifest as the material universe. These modes of vibration are called *Veda*. The Vedic description is strikingly similar to that of physics but emphasizes an idea less often discussed in physics: that the unified field is the field of pure consciousness. The differentiation between consciousness and matter, between knower and known, loses its significance at the level of the unified field.

> These various modes of vibration known as *Veda* are described and written down in the voluminous Vedic literature. The different aspects of Vedic literature have been found to correspond with specific areas of the human physiology (Nader, 1993). ◦

In MAV the ultimate basis of disease is losing one's connection to (or, to use a central Vedic description, one's memory of) the unified field, which is the innermost core of one's own being and experience. This loss is known technically as *pragya-aparadh*. The ultimate basis of prevention and cure is restoring one's conscious connection to (or memory of) this innermost core of one's being and experience. This reconnection is the basis of an integrated approach to health care; integration of the different layers of life begins with reconnecting one's life to the substrate on which all its layers are based. The innermost core of one's experience is considered identical to the home of all the laws of nature that operate throughout the universe. The body contains, at its basis, the total potential of natural law, and all of MAV's modalities aim to enable the full expression of the body's inner intelligence.

The foremost means for accomplishing this are the Vedic techniques for developing consciousness, the most important of which is *Transcendental Meditation (TM)*. The term *transcendental* indicates that the mind *transcends* even the subtlest impulses of thought and settles down to the simplest state of awareness (in MAV terms, identical to the unified field). This state of awareness is known technically as *Transcendental Consciousness (TC)*.

Interestingly, a large body of published research has demonstrated that, during the subjective experience of TC, the body's metabolism and electroencephalogram (EEG) tracings take on a unique pattern of profound physiological rest and balance, with a metabolic reduction significantly deeper than that experienced during sleep or eyes-closed rest (Gallois, 1984; Wallace, 1970). Periods of clear experience of TC have been characterized by suspension of respiration without oxygen deprivation (Badawi et al, 1984; Farrow et al, 1982), stabilization of the autonomic nervous system (Orme-Johnson, 1973), and a decrease in plasma levels of lactate, a chemical marker of metabolic activity (Jevning et al, 1983) and cortisol levels (Jevning et al, 1978). Simultaneous with this metabolic rest, blood flow to the brain increases markedly (Jevning et al, 1978), and the brain displays a state of "restful alertness," characterized by greatly increased coherence between the EEG patterns of different areas of the brain, that is, stable phase relations between two EEG signals as measured by Fourier analyses that attain correlations of more than 0.95 (Badawi et al, 1984; Levine, 1976).

The state of TC can thus be defined physiologically and experientially. This corroborates MAV's view of TC as the fourth major state of human consciousness, in the sense that the three common states of waking, sleeping, and dreaming can be defined physiologically as well. MAV also discusses three higher states of consciousness in which the full potential of consciousness progressively unfolds. Long-term TM practitioners have reported that the experience of TC, which first occurred only during their practice of the TM technique, now subjectively coexists with waking and sleeping states. Several studies have investigated this integrated state, and results show that the increased EEG coherence that is characteristic of the TM practice appears to become a stable EEG trait during computer tasks (Travis et al, 2002). Long-term TM practitioners have significantly higher levels of frontal EEG coherence during performance of computer tasks than subjects who do not practice TM (Travis et al, 2006).

MAV views unfolding consciousness as the most important strategy of both disease prevention and cure. Consistent with this theory, data suggest that regular experience of TC has significant health benefits. Such research supports the MAV concept that "remembering" the unified field enlivens the orderly patterns that prevail in a healthy body. For example, TM has been found in several studies to retard biological aging (Glaser et al, 1992; Wallace et al, 1982). In a Harvard study of elderly nursing home residents that compared TM with two other types of meditation and relaxation techniques over 3 years, the TM group had the lowest mortality rate and the greatest reductions in stress and blood pressure (Alexander et al, 1989). A follow-up study that evaluated the long-term effects of TM on mortality in patients with systemic hypertension showed that TM practice was associated with a 23% decrease in all-cause mortality and a 30% decrease in the rate of cardiovascular mortality compared with other behavioral interventions and usual care (Schneider et al, 2005a). Several studies have found that TM significantly reduces high blood pressure (Cooper et al, 1978; Schneider et al, 1992, 2005b; Wallace et al, 1983). In a randomized controlled trial Schneider et al (1995) found TM to be approximately twice as effective as progressive muscle relaxation in reducing hypertension in older African Americans. Barnes et al (2004) studied the effect of TM on African American adolescents with high normal blood pressure and found that the TM group had greater decreases in daytime systolic and diastolic blood pressure than a control group who received health education. A recent meta-analysis of nine randomized controlled trials indicated that the regular practice of TM is associated with a significant reduction in systolic and diastolic blood pressure (Anderson et al, 2008). A previous meta-analysis of 17 randomized controlled trials indicated that practice of TM was associated with significant reductions in blood pressure, whereas simple biofeedback, relaxation-assisted biofeedback, progressive muscle relaxation, and stress management training did not result in statistically significant reductions (Rainforth et al, 2007).

A study of adolescents by Barnes et al (2001) found that TM had a beneficial effect on cardiovascular functioning, as measured by blood pressure, heart rate, and cardiac output. Studies of TM have shown that it significantly reduces cholesterol level (Cooper et al, 1978, 1979) and levels of lipid peroxide, fat that has been damaged by free radicals and can in turn cause damage of its own (Schneider et al, 1998). A noninvasive method of detecting free radical activity is the measurement of human ultra-weak photon emission, with lower emission intensities indicating lower levels of free radical activity. A study of long-term TM practitioners showed lower emission intensities in the TM group than in controls who did not meditate (Van Wijk et al, 2006). A follow-up study showed that TM practitioners had significantly lower emission intensities than practitioners of other meditation techniques and controls who did not practice meditation (Van Wijk et al, 2008). A study measuring catecholamine levels in TM practitioners showed that epinephrine and norepinephrine levels were significantly lower in the TM group than in the control group, although anxiety levels were similar in both groups (Infante et al, 2001). This indicates that the regular practice of TM results in a low hormonal response to daily stress. Because TM has been shown to reduce several important risk factors for heart disease (TM decreases high blood pressure, cholesterol level, and lipid peroxide level, and modulates the body's response to stress), TM should be helpful in the treatment of heart disease (Barnes et al, 2006). Research has borne this out—patients with heart disease were challenged by exercising on a bicycle, and those who practiced TM showed better results on several heart-related parameters (Zamarra et al, 1996). A randomized controlled clinical trial showed that practice of TM is associated with a reduction in atherosclerosis—hardening of the blood vessels that can lead to heart attack or stroke (Castillo-Richmond et al, 2000). A randomized controlled study of African Americans with congestive heart failure showed that those practicing TM had significantly improved functional capacity as measured by a 6-minute walk test, compared

with the health education control group. The TM group showed a significant decrease in depression compared with controls and had fewer rehospitalizations during the 6-month follow-up period (Jayadevappa et al, 2007).

The metabolic syndrome is regarded as a risk factor for coronary heart disease. Insulin resistance is considered a key component of the metabolic syndrome and is associated with hypertension. A randomized controlled trial of TM in patients with coronary heart disease showed that blood pressure and insulin resistance was significantly improved in the TM group compared with a health education control group (Paul-Labrador et al, 2006). A pilot study of postmenopausal women showed that TM reduced cortisol response to a metabolic stressor (Walton et al, 2004). This may play a role in the preventive effects of TM on cardiovascular disease and coronary heart disease, because elevated cortisol levels may be involved in producing the metabolic syndrome.

A meta-analysis of research on meditation and trait anxiety conducted at the Stanford Research Institute found that TM is approximately twice as effective as other meditation techniques in reducing trait anxiety (Eppley et al, 1989). Orme-Johnson and Walton (1998) conducted an analysis of meditation and relaxation techniques that showed TM to be more effective than other approaches in reducing anxiety, improving psychological health, and reducing tobacco, alcohol, and drug use. These and similar studies and meta-analyses (Alexander, Robinson, Orme-Johnson et al, 1994; Alexander, Robinson, Rainforth, 1994; Alexander et al, 1991) seem to corroborate MAV's theory, in that relaxation and other types of meditation appeared to be a less significant variable compared with experiencing the fourth state of consciousness (i.e., TC) via TM. Hundreds of other published studies of TM have documented a wide range of benefits in such areas as intellectual development and rehabilitation (many of these studies are reprinted in Chalmers et al, 1989a, 1989b, 1989c; Orme-Johnson et al, 1977; and Wallace et al, 1989).

Regular practice of TM has also been found to reduce health care costs significantly, as measured by insurance statistics; TM practitioners needed hospitalization for illness or surgery 80% less often than a matched control group (Orme-Johnson, 1987). A study of Canadian citizens enrolled in the government health insurance program showed that over a 6-year period, practice of the TM technique reduced government payments to physicians by 13% each year (Herron et al, 2000). A subsequent study of Canadian citizens over the age of 65 showed even greater reductions in medical expenditures. Mean physician payments for the TM group decreased 24% annually compared with those for controls. There was a 5-year cumulative decline of 70% in physician payments compared with those for controls (Herron et al, 2005). This suggests that a TM program would be a valuable component of any comprehensive health care cost containment strategy or health care system reform effort.

PREVENTION, PATHOGENESIS, AND BALANCE

Viewing the body as a pattern of intelligence is the basis of a central tenet of MAV: for optimal health, it is necessary to maintain the body's natural state of internal balance. This tenet has applications for strengthening immunity, as well as for prevention, diagnosis, and treatment. The natural state of balance is understood in terms of another important Ayurvedic concept: three principles known as *doshas* govern the functioning of the body. The three doshas are *vata, pitta,* and *kapha.* Each has specific qualities and governs certain physiological activities. The doshas are not thought of as specifically physiological but as subtle principles that emerge early in the manifestation of the unified field. Therefore they are understood to operate throughout nature.

The doshas are considered to be derived from combinations of still subtler expressions, the five *mahabhutas,* or "great elements." The physicist John Hagelin, a major contributor to grand unification theory, has pointed out that physics also identifies five basic "elements," known as spin types. All the force and particle fields of physics belong to one of these five categories, and the characteristics of the five spin types correspond closely to those of the five mahabhutas.

Vata governs flow and motion in the body. It is at the basis of the activity of the locomotor system. Vata controls functions such as blood circulation, the expansion and contraction of the lungs and heart, intestinal peristalsis and elimination, activities of the nervous system, the contractile process in muscle, ionic transport across membranes (e.g., the sodium pump), cell division, and the unwinding of DNA during the process of transcription or replication. Vata is of prime importance in all homeostatic mechanisms and controls the other two principles, pitta and kapha.

Pitta governs bodily functions concerned with heat and metabolism, and directs all biochemical reactions and the process of energy exchange. For example, it regulates digestion, functions of the exocrine glands and endocrine hormones, and intracellular metabolic pathways such as glycolysis, the tricarboxylic acid cycle, and the respiratory chain.

Kapha governs the structure and cohesion of the organism. It is responsible for biological strength, natural tissue resistance, and proper body structure. Microscopically, it is related to anatomical connections in the cell, such as the intracellular matrix, cell membrane, membranes of organelles, and synapses. On a biochemical level, kapha structures receptors and the various forms of chemical binding.

When the doshas are balanced in their natural states and bodily locations, they produce health; when aggravated or imbalanced, they produce disease. A balanced pitta dosha, for example, ensures healthy digestion, but an aggravated pitta can cause ulcers and acid indigestion. MAV holds that all disease results from disruption of the natural balance of the doshas, and immune strength results from maintaining balance of the doshas. As Table 32-1 shows, the natural dosha balance can be thrown off by a wide variety of factors, such as unhealthy diet, poor digestion, unnatural daily routine, pollutants, and certain behaviors. The balance is restored by a variety of dietary and behavioral modalities, as well as other modalities discussed in this chapter, such as TM and herbal mixtures.

Each dosha has five subdivisions that govern different aspects of the body. For example, *bhrajaka pitta,* one of the subdivisions of pitta, relates to the skin. When balanced, it gives luster to the skin; when aggravated, bhrajaka pitta results in acne, boils, and rashes.

The concept of doshas—underlying metabolic principles—simplifies the practitioner's tasks and increases his or her effectiveness. The tridosha concept can help in clarifying the possible side effects of any treatment, customizing treatments for a specific patient, predicting risk factors and tendencies toward specific diseases, and noticing clusters of apparently unrelated syndromes that may have a similar underlying cause.

Some of these aspects result from the doshas' ability to provide the basis for a more precise description of the individual's natural state of balance. An individual may have a natural predominance of one or more doshas. These doshas need not be present in equal proportion to ensure physiological balance, but they need to be functioning in harmony with one another. This state is called *prakriti.* When the doshas are out of balance, they create *vikriti,* which results in disorder and disease. Box 32-1 describes the classic characteristics of vata, pitta, and kapha prakritis. More common than these are mixed prakritis, which involve various combinations of the three classic types, such as vata-pitta, or pitta-kapha. These also describe the normal state of balance for individuals who possess them. Treatment in MAV is tailored to the individual patient through careful evaluation of both prakriti and vikriti.

Because MAV views disease as resulting from disruption of the natural balance of the doshas, the doshas play a key role in MAV's approach to understanding pathogenesis. In Western medicine a disease is detected as a result of its symptoms. The emergence of symptoms, however, must be preceded by earlier stages of imbalance. MAV identifies six stages of pathogenesis, the first three of which have highly subtle symptoms with which allopathic medicine is not familiar. These first three stages involve aggravation of the normal functioning of the doshas. A skilled MAV diagnostician can detect these early pathogenic stages before overt

TABLE 32-1

The Three Doshas

Dosha	Effect of balanced dosha	Effect of imbalanced dosha	Factors aggravating dosha
Vata	Exhilaration	Rough skin	Excessive exercise
	Clear and alert mind	Weight loss	Wakefulness
	Perfect functioning of bowels and urinary tract	Anxiety, worry	Falling, bone fractures
	Proper formation of all bodily tissues	Restlessness	Tuberculosis
	Sound sleep	Constipation	Suppression of natural urges
	Excellent vitality and immunity	Decreased strength	Cold
		Arthritis	Fear or grief
		Hypertension	Agitation or anger
		Rheumatic disorder	Fasting
		Cardiac arrhythmia	Pungent, astringent, or bitter foods
		Insomnia	In USA: Late autumn and winter
		Irritable bowel syndrome	In India: Summer and rainy season
Pitta	Lustrous complexion	Yellowish complexion	Anger
	Contentment	Excessive body heat	Strong sunshine
	Perfect digestion	Insufficient sleep	Burning sensations
	Softness of body	Weak digestion	Fasting
	Perfectly balanced heat and thirst mechanisms	Inflammation	Sesame products, linseed
	Balanced intellect	Inflammatory bowel diseases	Yogurt
		Skin diseases	Wine, vinegar
		Heartburn	Pungent, sour, or salty foods
		Peptic ulcer	In USA: Summer and early autumn
		Anger	In India: Rainy season and autumn
Kapha	Strength	Pale complexion	Sleeping during daytime
	Normal joints	Coldness	Heavy food
	Stability of mind	Laziness, dullness	Sweet, sour, or salty foods
	Dignity	Excessive sleep	Milk products
	Affectionate, forgiving nature	Sinusitis	Sugar
	Strong and properly proportioned body	Respiratory diseases, asthma	In USA: Spring
	Courage	Excessive weight gain	In India: Late winter and spring
	Vitality	Loose joints	
		Depression	

symptoms emerge, using the techniques discussed in the next section.

DIAGNOSIS

MAV adds a number of diagnostic techniques to the clinician's repertoire. All of them are noninvasive and reveal much information about underlying imbalances and about specific illnesses. Chief among these techniques is *nadi vigyan* (pulse diagnosis), which allows one to retrieve detailed information about the internal functioning of the body and its organs through signals present in the radial pulse. This information involves not only the cardiovascular system but other bodily systems as well. From the pulse, the diagnostician gains information about the functioning of the bodily tissues, the state of the doshas, and much more. Pulse diagnosis reveals early stages of imbalance that precede full-blown symptoms. In this and other MAV diagnostic modalities, perceiving the body as a pattern of intelligence enables physicians to retrieve enormous amounts of information in a noninvasive manner.

PHARMACOLOGY

Perception of the body in terms of patterns of intelligence is also demonstrated in MAV's approach to pharmacology, which makes sophisticated use of thousands of herbs and other plants.

Western pharmacology, applying the mechanistic model of the body, isolates and then synthesizes single

Classic Characteristics of Vata, Pitta, and Kapha Prakritis

Vata Prakriti
Light, thin build
Performs activity quickly
Tendency to dry skin
Aversion to cold weather
Irregular hunger and digestion
Quick to grasp new information, also quick to forget
Tendency toward worry
Tendency toward constipation
Tendency toward light and interrupted sleep

Pitta Prakriti
Moderate build
Performs activity with medium speed
Aversion to hot weather
Sharp hunger and digestion
Medium time to grasp new information
Medium memory
Tendency toward irritability and temper
Enterprising and sharp in character
Prefers cold foods and drinks
Cannot skip meals
Good speaker
Tendency toward reddish complexion and hair, moles, and freckles

Kapha Prakriti
Solid, heavier build
Greater strength and endurance
Slow, methodical in activity
Oily, smooth skin
Tranquil, steady personality
Slow to grasp new information, slow to forget
Slow to become excited or irritated
Sleeps heavily and for long periods
Plentiful hair that tends to be dark in color
Slow digestion, mild hunger

active ingredients from herbs and plants. For example, the Ayurvedic remedy willow bark was the source of acetylsalicylic acid, and the Ayurvedic remedy rauwolfia was the source of reserpine. The active ingredient model reflects a weakness of the scientific method: its inability to deal with complex systems and its requirement that the researcher radically simplify a process to evaluate it (Sharma, 1997). In contrast, Ayurvedic pharmacology, called *dravyaguna,* uses the synergistic cooperation of substances as they coexist in natural sources. It uses single plants or, more often, mixtures of plants whose effects are complementary. Such synergistic effects are gaining consideration in Western medical research, which is finding, for example, that *combinations* of antioxidants may halt oxidative damage and cancer cell growth more effectively than the single substances acting alone.

In terms of MAV's consciousness model, the effectiveness of herbal mixtures relative to active ingredients can be explained by the idea that plants, especially herbs, are concentrated repositories of nature's intelligence that, when used properly, can increase the expression of that intelligence in the body. Research and experience with MAV herbal mixtures known as *rasayanas* shows that synergism enhances the free radical–scavenging properties of herbs and mitigates the harmful side effects that often accompany Western drugs (Sharma, 2002).

According to MAV, rasayanas promote longevity, stamina, immunity, and overall well-being (Sharma, 1993). Research has shown several rasayanas to have significant antioxidant properties (Bondy et al, 1994; Cullen et al, 1997; Dwivedi et al, 1991, 2005; Engineer et al, 1992; Hanna et al, 1994; Niwa, 1991; Sharma et al, 1995). The rasayana known as *Maharishi Amrit Kalash (MAK)* is approximately 1000 times more effective at scavenging free radicals than vitamin C, vitamin E, and a pharmaceutical antioxidant (Sharma et al, 1992).

MAK has been researched extensively in laboratory, animal, and clinical settings, and has been found to have a wide range of significant beneficial properties. MAK prevented and treated breast cancer (Sharma et al, 1990; Sharma et al, 1991); prevented metastasis of lung cancer (Patel et al, 1992); caused nervous system tumor cells (neuroblastoma) to regain normal cell functioning (Prasad et al, 1992); enhanced the effect of nerve growth factor in causing morphological differentiation of nervous system tumor cells (pheochromocytoma) (Rodella et al, 2004); inhibited the growth of skin cancer cells (melanoma) (Prasad et al, 1993); and inhibited liver cancer (Penza et al, 2007). In clinical studies, MAK has been shown to reduce the side effects of chemotherapy without reducing the efficacy of the cancer treatment (Misra et al, 1994; Srivastava et al, 2000).

MAK also reduces several risk factors for heart disease. It prevented human platelet aggregation (Sharma et al, 1989) and reduced atherosclerosis in laboratory animals by 53% (Lee et al, 1996). In clinical studies of patients with heart disease, MAK reduced the frequency of angina, improved exercise tolerance, and lowered systolic blood pressure and lipid peroxide levels (Dogra et al, 1994, 2005). A study of hyperlipidemic patients showed that MAK increases the resistance of low-density lipoprotein to oxidation, which is important for the prevention of atherosclerosis (Sundaram et al, 1997).

A strong immune system is vital to the maintenance of health. Several studies have shown that MAK significantly enhances immune functioning (Dileepan et al, 1990, 1993; Inaba et al, 1995, 1996, 1997, 2005). MAK has also demonstrated antiaging effects. It improved age-related visual discrimination in older men (Gelderloos et al, 1990) and has been shown to rejuvenate the antioxidant defense system and protect against mitochondrial deterioration in the aging central nervous system (Vohra et al, 1999, 2001a). In the aging brain, MAK reduced lipid peroxidation and lipofuscin pigment accumulation, restored normal oxygen consumption, and enhanced cholinergic enzymes (Vohra et al, 2001b, 2001c). It has also been shown to decrease the number of dark neurons in the brain, which indicates that MAK protects the neurons from injury (Vohra et al, 2002).

A modified form of MAK, known as Amrit Nectar tablets, has powerful antioxidant properties. In a study of the inhibition of lipid peroxidation, an aqueous extract of Amrit Nectar tablets was 16 times more potent and an alcoholic extract was 166 times more potent than vitamin E, a well-known antioxidant. Amrit Nectar tablets also protected against the toxic side effects of the chemotherapeutic drugs doxorubicin (Adriamycin) and cisplatin (Dwivedi et al, 2005).

DIET

Western medical research is accumulating increasing evidence that diet plays a critical role in the development of heart disease and cancer. The American Cancer Society reports that about one third of the cancer deaths that occur each year in the United States are from cancers for which diet is a significant risk factor (*Cancer Facts and Figures*, 2008). Scientists estimate that 60% to 70% of cancers could be prevented by simple changes in diet and lifestyle (Sharma et al, 2002). It is known that a diet rich in the wrong types of fat creates a higher risk of heart disease, the number one killer in the United States today (American Heart Association, 2007; Sharma et al, 1998). Ayurveda has long considered problems of diet and digestion to be among the central causes of all disease and has considered improvement of diet and digestion to be crucial to almost any therapeutic regimen. Ayurveda views faulty diet as not only contributing to specific degenerative diseases, but also throwing off the body's natural balance, thus weakening immunity.

MAV's approach to diet rests on the consciousness model. Food is viewed as providing not only matter and energy to the body but also intelligence, order, and balance. This brings to mind the observation of the Nobel laureate physicist Erwin Schrödinger that food helps the body resist the second law of thermodynamics, which normally leads any complex system into chaos (Schrödinger, 1967). In this view, when we eat, we are eating not only nutrients but also "orderliness." MAV dietetics considers not only the nutritional value and caloric content of food but also the food's impact on the body's underlying state of balance. Food affects the doshas, and diet must be suited to the individual's vikriti and prakriti. It must also reflect the climate and season, as well as specific health conditions.

The influence of food on the doshas is specific to the food, but can usually be determined by knowing to which generic categories of taste and qualities the food belongs. According to MAV, the six categories of taste are sweet, sour, salty, pungent, bitter, and astringent. The six major categories of qualities are heavy, light, oily, dry, hot, and cold. Box 32-2 summarizes how taste and food qualities affect the doshas, and Box 32-3 gives examples of foods that possess these various qualities and tastes.

As an example of how this information would be applied clinically, a patient with kapha syndromes (e.g., sinusitis, certain types of obesity) would be advised to minimize consumption of heavy, oily, and cold foods, as well as foods with sweet, sour, and salty tastes. It would be recommended that the patient give predominance to foods exhibiting the remaining qualities and tastes.

MAV recommends a lactovegetarian diet for optimal health. Meat is more difficult to digest and has been linked to numerous diseases, including heart disease, cancer, and diabetes. MAV also recommends eating fresh fruits and vegetables. These emphases map well with emerging Western findings on diet, which have shown significant health benefits from a meatless diet and from increased consumption of fruits and vegetables ("Vegetarianism: addition by subtraction," 2004). A long-term study of vegetarians revealed that eating fresh fruit daily results in a significant reduction in mortality from ischemic heart disease, cerebrovascular disease, and all causes combined

---

BOX 32-2

Tastes and Food Qualities: Effects on the Doshas

Tastes	
Decrease Vata	*Increase Vata*
Sweet	Pungent
Sour	Bitter
Salty	Astringent
Decrease Pitta	*Increase Pitta*
Sweet	Pungent
Bitter	Sour
Astringent	Salty
Decrease Kapha	*Increase Kapha*
Pungent	Sweet
Bitter	Sour
Astringent	Salty

Major Food Qualities	
Decrease Vata	*Increase Vata*
Heavy	Light
Oily	Dry
Hot	Cold
Decrease Pitta	*Increase Pitta*
Cold	Hot
Heavy	Light
Oily	Dry
Decrease Kapha	*Increase Kapha*
Light	Heavy
Dry	Oily
Hot	Cold

BOX 32-3

Common Examples of the Six Tastes and Major Food Qualities

Six Tastes and Common Examples
Sweet: sugar, milk, butter, rice, breads
Sour: yogurt, lemon, cheese
Salty: salt
Pungent: spicy foods, peppers, ginger, cumin
Bitter: spinach, other green leafy vegetables
Astringent: beans, pomegranate

Six Major Food Qualities and Common Examples
Heavy: cheese, yogurt, wheat products
Light: barley, corn, spinach, apples
Oily: dairy products, fatty foods, oils
Dry: barley, corn, potato, beans
Hot: hot (temperature) foods and drinks
Cold: cold (temperature) foods and drinks

(Key et al, 1996). Higher consumption of fruits has also been associated with lower risks of lung, prostate, and pancreatic cancers. Vegetarians have lower risks of obesity, hypertension, diabetes, arthritis, colon cancer, prostate cancer, fatal ischemic heart disease, and death from all causes (Fraser, 1999; Kwok et al, 2000). A long-term study of male Seventh-Day Adventists found that meat eating correlated positively with all forms of mortality measured (Snowdon, 1988).

Multiple studies have demonstrated that eating meat increases the risk of heart disease, whereas a vegetarian diet affords protection against heart disease. A study of Seventh-Day Adventists showed a significant association between beef consumption and fatal ischemic heart disease in men, compared with vegetarians. The lifetime risk of ischemic heart disease was decreased by 37% in male vegetarians compared with nonvegetarians (Fraser, 1999). The risk of developing ischemic heart disease is also significantly lower in older vegetarian women than in older nonvegetarian women (Kwok et al, 2000). The Health Professionals Follow-up Study found consumption of red meat to be associated with coronary artery disease in men (Ascherio et al, 1994). Other studies also indicate that vegetarians have a significantly lower incidence of coronary heart disease (Claude-Chang et al, 1992; Dwyer, 1988; Slattery et al, 1991). Patients on a vegetarian diet show reduced frequency, duration, and severity of angina; regression of atherosclerosis; and improvement in coronary perfusion (Segasothy et al, 1999). Long-term vegetarians have a reduced risk of lipid peroxidation (Krajcovicova-Kudlackova, Simoncic, Babinska et al, 1995; Krajcovicova-Kudlackova, Simoncic, Bederova et al, 1995) and lower levels of cholesterol (Key et al, 1999; Kwok et al, 2000).

A vegetarian diet has shown protective effects against cancer, whereas eating meat has been correlated with the development of various types of cancer. Nonvegetarians have a significantly higher risk of developing colon cancer and prostate cancer (Fraser, 1999). Women who eat red meat daily are at twice the risk of developing colon cancer compared with women who eat red meat less than once a month (Willett et al, 1990). The association between red meat and colon cancer was elucidated in a clinical study that showed increased levels of endogenous N-nitrosation due to increased nitrogenous residues from red meat (Bingham et al, 2002). A large prospective study, the National Institutes of Health–AARP Diet and Health Study, found that eating red meat was associated with a significantly elevated risk of colorectal cancer, lung cancer, esophageal cancer, and liver cancer. Eating processed meats resulted in a significantly elevated risk of colorectal cancer and lung cancer (Cross et al, 2007). A study of vegetarian diet found a 40% reduction in cancer mortality in non–meat eaters compared with meat eaters (Thorogood et al, 1994). Increased consumption of fruit has been associated with lower risks of lung, prostate, and pancreatic cancers (Fraser, 1999).

Type 2 diabetes mellitus is another chronic disease that has been associated with meat intake. In a 17-year prospective study of Adventists, subjects who ate meat at least weekly had a 74% increase in diabetes risk compared with those who did not eat meat (Vang et al, 2008). The Nurses' Health Study showed that consumption of red meat and processed meats were both associated with an increased risk of diabetes in women (Fung et al, 2004). Processed meats were also implicated in diabetes in the Nurses' Health Study II, in which increased processed meat consumption was strongly associated with a progressively higher risk for diabetes in women. This study was also found that consumption of bacon, hot dogs, sausage, salami, and bologna were all individually associated with a higher risk of diabetes (Schulze et al, 2003). Similar results were seen in the Women's Health Study: higher consumption of total red meat, higher consumption of processed meat, and higher consumption individually of bacon and hot dogs were all significantly associated with increased risk of diabetes in women (Song et al, 2004). Findings are comparable for men: the Health Professionals Follow-up Study showed that frequent consumption of processed meat was significantly associated with a higher risk of diabetes (van Dam et al, 2002). Eating fruits and vegetables provides protection against diabetes. A 12-year prospective study showed that higher fruit and vegetable intake is associated with a substantially decreased risk of diabetes (Harding et al, 2008).

A vegetarian diet has proven beneficial in other chronic disorders as well. The prevalence of hypertension was shown to be lower among long-term vegetarians than among nonvegetarians in a study of Seventh-Day Adventists (Brathwaite et al, 2003). Diets rich in fruits and vegetables significantly reduced blood pressure in the Dietary Approaches to Stop Hypertension (DASH) clinical trial (Appel et al, 1997). This study also found that increasing fruit and vegetable consumption decreases urinary calcium excretion, which has positive implications for bone health

(Appel et al, 1997). Several population-based studies have shown that eating fruits and vegetables is beneficial for axial and peripheral bone mass and bone metabolism in men and women of all ages (New, 2003). Considering all the benefits of a vegetarian diet, it is not surprising that studies have shown vegetarians to have a longer life span (Fraser, 1999; Fraser et al, 2001; Singh et al, 2003). A long-term study found that vegetarians have a mortality rate that is half that of the general population (Key et al, 1996).

The hazards of a meat-based diet may be due to characteristics of the meat itself as well as multiple aspects involved in the production, preservation, processing, and cooking of meat and meat products (Cross et al, 2007; Singh et al, 2003). Saturated fat in meat contributes to atherogenesis and carcinogenesis. Heme iron in meat contributes to higher oxidative stress, which is linked to both heart disease and cancer. Meat increases the endogenous formation of N-nitroso compounds, which are carcinogenic. Processed meats containing nitrite preservatives are an exogenous source of N-nitroso compounds. Smoked and salted meats containing N-nitrosodimethylamine are a carcinogenic risk. Heterocyclic amines and polycyclic aromatic hydrocarbons are known mutagens that are formed during high-temperature cooking of meat (e.g., grilling). Other hazards of ingesting meat relate to what the animals themselves have eaten, for example, feed containing herbicides and pesticides that become concentrated in the fatty tissues and membranes of the meat. Cattle feed supplemented with rendered cattle carcasses has been implicated in the development of the transmissible prion disease known as "mad cow disease." Antibiotics administered to livestock may contribute to antibiotic resistance in those who consume their meat.

The benefits of a vegetarian diet relate to lower intake of saturated fat, cholesterol, and animal protein and increased intake of complex carbohydrates, dietary fiber, trace minerals, vitamins, and a myriad of biologically active phytochemicals (Lampe, 1999; Leitzmann, 2005). Clinical dietary studies of plant foods and their constituents have shown that fruits and vegetables affect the human biological system in many beneficial ways. They have antioxidant properties, stimulate the immune system, modulate detoxification enzymes, and alter cholesterol synthesis and hormone metabolism. Many phytochemicals have overlapping mechanisms of action and can have synergistic or additive effects. It is noteworthy that the protective effects of fruit and vegetable consumption observed in the epidemiologic studies are not seen with pharmacological doses of the plant foods or their constituents. The benefits were observed when these foods were eaten as part of the subjects' diet (Lampe, 1999).

DIGESTION

MAV focuses not only on what one eats but also on how one digests it. The emphasis on digestion contrasts with Western allopathic medicine, which deals with digestion only when it is significantly disrupted. In MAV, excellent digestion is considered critical to robust health. MAV contains a number of techniques for improving digestion and treating digestive disorders. They center on the concept of *agni*, which literally means "fire" and refers to metabolic and digestive activities that convert foodstuff into bodily substances. Ayurveda describes 13 types of agni in the body. Their importance in Ayurvedic health care is suggested by the fact that one of the eight branches of Ayurveda, *Kaya Chikitsa* (internal medicine), focuses on the strength or weakness of the agnis. This emphasis on digestion becomes clearer when we consider the end product of poor digestion, which Ayurveda calls *ama*. Ama plays a key role in pathogenesis, interacting with aggravated doshas and causing them to "stick" to areas where they do not belong. Healthy digestion reduces the amount of ama produced.

The central role of food and digestion is demonstrated particularly well by consideration of another central MAV concept: the importance of a substance called *ojas*. Ojas is said to be the finest manifestation of the unified field, which serves as a sort of glue to link consciousness and matter. Ojas maintains the integrity of the seven bodily tissues (*dhatus*), which are plasma (*rasa*), blood (*rakta*), muscle (*mamsa*), fat (*meda*), bone (*asthi*), bone marrow and nervous system (*majja*), and sperm and ovum (*sukra*). The end product of truly healthy diet and digestion is said to contain significant amounts of ojas. According to an MAV expression, "Like a bee that gets honey from the flowers, we get ojas from our food." Most MAV therapies and behavioral advice are designed to maximize the presence of ojas, and almost all MAV proscriptions are designed to minimize the depletion of ojas.

The manner in which food is eaten is considered to have an effect on healthy digestion. Food should be eaten in a warm, congenial, and uplifting atmosphere. Arguing or any other negativity at meals interferes with digestion, producing ama instead of ojas. Positive, loving emotions enhance digestion and increase the abundance of ojas.

PAÑCHAKARMA (PURIFICATION THERAPIES)

To rid the body of accumulated ama, pollutants, and other pathogenic impurities that disrupt or block the natural expression of the body's inner intelligence, MAV emphasizes the importance of purification therapies. Foremost among these is *Pañchakarma* (or *Panchakarma*; see Chapter 29), which literally means "five activities." Pañchakarma includes five main treatment modalities:

1. Whole-body massage with herbalized oil (*abhyanga*)
2. Continuous flow of warm herbalized oil on the forehead (*shirodhara*)
3. Fomentation of the body with herbalized heat (*swedana*)

4. Special herbalized oil head massage and nasal administration of herbs *(nasya)*
5. Sesame oil retention or herbalized eliminative enemas *(basti)*

Daily treatments, administered for 2 to 14 days or longer, are recommended with each change of the seasons. Certain aspects of Pañchakarma can also fit easily into a patient's daily preventive regimen. Preliminary research has shown that regular Pañchakarma reduces several cardiovascular risk factors, including cholesterol (Sharma et al, 1993; Waldschütz, 1988). Sesame oil, which is used topically and for colonic irrigation in Pañchakarma, has been shown to inhibit in vitro malignant melanoma growth (Smith et al, 1992) and human colon adenocarcinoma cell line growth (Salerno et al, 1991). Preliminary research on Pañchakarma has shown that it reduces levels of fat-soluble toxicants in humans. Levels of polychlorinated biphenyls (PCBs) and agrochemicals were reduced by 50% in subjects who received Pañchakarma. PCBs have been banned for years, but previous exposure can result in a lingering accumulation of the toxicant in fat tissue. Lipophilic toxicants have been associated with hormonal disorders, suppression of the immune system, reproductive disorders, cancer, and other diseases (Herron et al, 2002).

BEHAVIOR, EMOTIONS, AND THE SENSES

MAV regards behavior, speech, and emotions as having a significant impact on health. This concept springs naturally from the model that places consciousness at the basis of the body. Emotions can be understood as fine fluctuations of consciousness (or the unified field); as such, their impact on the more expressed physical levels of the body is immense. Recently, Western medicine has begun to investigate the effect of emotions on health, with interesting findings; Ayurveda has discussed this field for millennia. Ayurvedic texts include detailed discussions of lifestyle and behavior and their impact on health. Interestingly, traditional virtues—such as respect for elders, teachers, loved ones, and family members; pardoning those who wrong you; practicing nonviolence; and not speaking ill of others—are understood to promote the health of the individual's mind and body, as well as of the community and society.

According to Ayurveda, information entering through the five senses (sight, sound, taste, touch, and smell) is digested and metabolized in its own specific ways, and the by-products influence physiology. Thus, sensory input is considered to have an impact on health. This idea is applied clinically, not only in terms of behavioral advice but also in the form of sensory therapies such as aromatherapy and sound therapy. The use of sound therapy includes music (called *Gandharva Veda*) and primordial sounds used for their healing qualities. A study of MAV primordial sound therapy (specifically, Vedic sounds known as *Sama Veda*) found that it reduces human tumor

cell growth significantly, whereas hard rock music tends to increase growth significantly (Sharma et al, 1996) (see Chapter 31).

BIOLOGICAL RHYTHMS

In MAV, attuning the patient's lifestyle to natural biorhythms is considered a crucial element of prevention and treatment. MAV gives a detailed analysis of circadian and circannual rhythms, with recommendations for daily and seasonal routines. These include advice such as rising and retiring early, and eating one's main meal at lunchtime when the digestive "fires" are strongest. Many other recommendations are also given; as always, this advice must be tailored to the individual. Emerging Western data on biorhythms correlate well with the ancient Ayurvedic knowledge. Again, the idea of a connection between patterns of order in nature and in the human body was obvious to Ayurveda millennia ago.

The three-dosha concept plays a key role in understanding these connections. Different times of the day are associated with different doshas, as are different seasons and the different stages of the human life cycle (Box 32-4). For example, the summer is dominated by pitta (the dosha that governs heat and metabolism), whereas the spring is dominated by kapha (which has qualities of coolness and moisture). Childhood is dominated by kapha (which governs structure, substance, and growth) and old age by vata. In fact, physicians see a preponderance of kapha-based disorders, such as colds and respiratory illnesses, in children and an ever-increasing number of vata disorders, such as constipation and lighter, shorter, and more frequently interrupted sleep, in elderly patients. They also see more kapha-type disorders in spring and

---

BOX 32-4

Times of Day, Seasons, and Life Cycle Classified According to the Doshas

Kapha time: Approximately 6 AM (sunrise) to 10 AM and 6 PM to 10 PM
Kapha season: In USA, spring; in India, late winter and spring
Kapha period in life cycle: Childhood

Pitta time: Approximately 10 AM to 2 PM and 10 PM to 2 AM
Pitta season: In USA, summer and early autumn; in India, rainy season and autumn
Pitta period in life cycle: Adulthood

Vata time: Approximately 2 AM to 6 AM (sunrise) and 2 PM to 6 PM
Vata season: In USA, late autumn and winter; in India, summer and rainy season
Vata period in life cycle: Old age

pitta disorders in summer. Understanding the concept of doshas is helpful in treating these ailments.

COLLECTIVE HEALTH AND THE ENVIRONMENT

MAV holds great promise in several areas of collective health. In terms of infectious disease and epidemics, the Western approach of using antibiotics has an inherent limitation and risk caused by the process of natural selection, which produces new, resistant strains of microbes. As a result, overreliance on antibiotics can foster the development of serious new infectious diseases. MAV's focus on strengthening immunity and its techniques for dealing directly with epidemics offer a more effective and safer means of ensuring collective health.

In terms of chronic disease, Western medicine has long recognized that preventing and treating these disorders requires changes in lifestyle, diet, and behavior. However, allopathic medicine has been at a loss as to how to effect these changes in patients for a prolonged time. Research has shown that those who practice TM are better able to give up harmful habits such as cigarette smoking, alcohol consumption, and illegal drug use, and incorporate healthy dietary and lifestyle changes (Alexander et al, 1994b; Gelderloos et al, 1991; Monahan, 1977). MAV offers other time-tested modalities that benefit individual patients, such as daily routine and purification procedures, which could be useful in large-scale applications. MAV also offers an overall theory of prevention involving elements such as the three-dosha concept that could be of value for research on preventive medicine.

The most significant public health approach of MAV deals with larger social disorders and the dangers they pose. War, crime, and violence are rarely considered subjects of public health policy, but their implications for health are obvious. As with individual disease, MAV understands these as originating not in material factors but ultimately in consciousness—in this case, both individual and collective consciousness. Just as an abstract field of consciousness underlies the individual's mind and body, such a field underlies societal trends. Society reflects the influence of its members not only in a linear, additive way—in the sense that a green forest is made of green trees—but also through a field effect—in the sense that a gravitational field's influences are not localized. If the individual consciousness of a sufficient number of members of a society is coherent, harmonious, and life supporting, those influences spread through the "field" of the collective consciousness of the society, influencing the society as a whole.

This idea has been tested in a number of different settings. A study conducted in 1983 during the Lebanon War found that when a sufficiently large group of practitioners of the TM and advanced TM-Sidhi techniques meditated together as a group in Israel, war deaths in Lebanon

were significantly reduced compared with casualty rates on days when the number of practitioners meditating together decreased below a certain threshold (Orme-Johnson, Alexander et al, 1988). This study was replicated and extended; the results showed that the group practice of meditation techniques in a series of seven assemblies occurring over a 2.25-year period of the Lebanon War had a significant beneficial impact, including an estimated 48% reduction in conflict, 71% reduction in war fatalities, and 68% reduction in war injuries during the assemblies (Davies et al, 2005). Studies in other localities have also shown beneficial effects, usually involving reductions in the rate of violent crime (Dillbeck et al, 1981, 1988; Orme-Johnson and Gelderloos, 1988). For example, a 1993 study in Washington, DC, showed that when a large group of practitioners of the TM and TM-Sidhi programs assembled to meditate during the summer, there was an 18% reduction in violent crime compared with levels that had been predicted on the basis of previous years' crime levels and weather trends (Hagelin et al, 1999).

There has been much discussion and debate regarding these observations and the validity of what has been called the *Maharishi effect*. A psychoneuroendocrine mechanism for the observed societal effects has been investigated in a prospective time series study. It was found that day-to-day increases in the size of a group practicing the TM program were predictive of biochemical changes in nonpractitioners living and working up to 20 miles away from the TM group. There were changes in the levels of cortisol, a major stress hormone, and 5-hydroxyindoleacetic acid (5-HIAA), the main metabolite of serotonin, a widely distributed neurotransmitter in the brain that is associated with a sense of well-being. As the size of the TM group increased, excretion of cortisol decreased, excretion of 5-HIAA increased, and the ratio of excretion rates of 5-HIAA to cortisol increased. This preliminary study supports the hypothesis that group practice of the TM technique reduces stress and increases well-being on a biochemical level in individuals who are not in physical contact or in communication with the meditators (Orme-Johnson, 2005; Walton et al, 2005).

FUTURE DIRECTIONS

Many central elements of Ayurveda, such as the ideas that diet and emotions play a crucial role in disease and prevention, were not taken seriously by Western medicine a generation ago but are now major themes of research. Other areas of Ayurveda might prove to be of value in both clinical work and research. Already, study of the TM technique and herbal preparations have produced bodies of significant research findings whose implications have yet to be fully explored. Other areas in which research is just beginning include using a biostatistical approach to quantify the three doshas (Joshi, 2004); using the scientific framework of systems analysis to establish the three doshas as universal properties of all living organisms (Hankey, 2001, 2005); and identifying a genetic basis for prakriti (Patwardhan et al, 2005, 2008).

The clinical use of Ayurveda appears to be most dramatic when applied to diseases that Western medicine finds it difficult to treat, such as poor digestion, heart disease, cancer, and other chronic diseases (Janssen, 1989; Orme-Johnson, 1987). Its clinical value extends to other areas not discussed previously, including pediatrics, in which it has been found to reduce significantly the incidence of childhood ailments such as frequent colds, and gynecology, in which it has been shown to reduce the severity of menstrual and premenstrual disorders. Ayurveda is a comprehensive system of health care that uses multiple modalities for the treatment of disorders. Clinical research trials are generally designed to investigate single treatments for ease of interpretation and characterization of the results; however, this type of investigation fragments Ayurvedic treatment. A randomized trial of a whole-system Ayurvedic protocol was conducted in patients who were newly diagnosed with type 2 diabetes. The experimental group received instruction in TM and yoga stretches, dietary instructions in accordance with Ayurvedic principles, recommendations for daily routine and exercise, and an Ayurvedic herbal supplement. This preliminary study found statistically significant improvements in those patients in the Ayurvedic group who had higher baseline values of glycosylated hemoglobin (Elder et al, 2006).

Several medical institutions have incorporated Ayurveda into their teaching curricula. In the future it is likely that Ayurveda will gain further recognition as an effective system of natural health care. Its comprehensive modalities can be used to create health and well-being in the individual and in society as a whole.

Ⓔ Chapter References can be found on the Evolve website at http://evolve.elsevier.com/Micozzi/complementary/

CHAPTER

33

SUFISM AND RAPID HEALING

HOWARD HALL

HISTORICAL BACKGROUND

The history of Sufism is rooted back about 15 centuries, or around 600 years after Jesus, to the time of the Prophet Muhammad and the birth of Islam. The Prophet Muhammad lived from AD 570 to 632 and was born in the city of Mecca, which today is in Saudi Arabia. He was an orphan by age 6 years and was taken in by his uncle Abu Talib. At age 25, he worked as a merchant for a widow, Khadija, transporting goods to Syria. Khadija was 15 years older than Muhammad but was so impressed with his character that she later proposed marriage to him. They were married for about a quarter of a century until her death, during which time he never took any other wives, even though polygamy was common practice (Fatoohi, 2002).

Muhammad would frequently retire for meditation to a cave, later known as Hira, on top of a mountain north of Mecca called Nur, or "Light." At age 40 in the year AD 610, while meditating in that cave, it is said that Muhammad received the first of a series of revelations though the Angel Gabriel. These revelations to this "unlettered"

prophet continued over about 23 years; they were memorized and written down by Muhammad's followers and became the *Quran,* the holy text of Islam. The Quran (or Qur'an) consists of 114 chapters and has not been modified since it was written down; thus it is the same text today as was revealed to Muhammad during his lifetime (Fatoohi, 2002). Tradition also holds that the Quran is divinely protected from being corrupted (Quran 15:9). The Quran is also remarkable for its internal consistency, its external agreement with historical and archaeological evidence, as well as its inclusion of new information and scientific findings that did not come to light until the nineteenth and twentieth centuries (Fatoohi et al, 1999). For example, human fetal development was vividly described well before the dawn of scientific knowledge of embryology (Quran 22:5, 23:12-14, and 40:67). Furthermore, unlike the personages in some other religious traditions, Muhammad is not worshipped or seen as divine, but rather is credited with the revelation of a literary masterpiece, along with the founding of a major religion and a new world power (Armstrong, 1993).

509

The terms *Islam* and *Muslim* were never meant to represent an elusive religion. Rather, Islam refers to the universal concept of peace through "surrendering oneself to the will of *Allah*" (the Arabic word for "the God"). Likewise, a Muslim is one who surrenders his or her whole self to the one God. Thus, all living creatures, including animals and insects, are natural Muslims following God's divine design by their instinctual behaviors (Armstrong, 1993). However, it is only humans who can choose to surrender to the will of Allah or rebel and follow selfish desires. This struggle between surrender and rebellion represents the history of human spiritual evolution, with Allah sending prophets to lead people back to the creator. Also, Islam is represented as the religion of peace, as expressed in the letters that form the word *Islam* from *salam,* which means "peace." In addition, one of the names of Allah as described in the Quran is "Al-Salam." Further, the greeting of the believers is "Peace," or "Asalamualaikum." Finally, believers are ordered by Muhammad to spread "salam."

The Quran teaches that Allah sent the same basic religion and revelation to humans, including Judaism, Christianity, and Islam, without holding one of the earlier religions above the later ones. This universal religion was revealed to the Biblical first human, Adam, and to all the earlier prophets: Noah, Abraham, Ishmael, Isaac, Jacob, Joseph, Moses, Aaron, David, Solomon, Zachariah, John, and Jesus. As stated in the Quran, "The same religion has He established for you as that which He enjoined on Noah—that which We have sent by inspiration to thee—and that which We enjoined on Abraham, Moses, and Jesus; Namely, that ye should remain steadfast in Religion, and make no divisions therein" (42:13).

Contrary to popular belief, Islam is not anti-Judaism or anti-Christianity but commands that all Muslims respect and revere all the previous messengers and the books and messages revealed to them. Because Jews and Christians received earlier revelations, they are referred to as "People or family of the Book" in the Quran (Fatoohi, 2002). Thus the Quran holds that Allah's universal message has come to people across the ages through appointed messengers as a type of "progressive revelation" (2:106). The form of this message may change according to the needs of the people and their circumstances, but it is the same basic message of surrender. Thus, the true Islamic view is acceptance of these other religions as noted in the Quran: "The Messenger believeth in what hath been revealed to him from his Lord, as do the men of faith. Each one (of them) believeth in Allah, His angels, His books, and His Messengers. 'We make no distinction between one and another of His Messengers'" (2:285).

Islam also sees people as equals, distinguished only by their righteousness: "O mankind! We created you from a single (pair) of a male and a female, and made you into nations and tribes, that ye may know each other (Not that ye may despise each other). Verily the most honoured of

you in the sight of Allah is (he who is) the most righteous of you" (49:13).

In addition to a belief in prior messengers and scriptures, the central belief of Islam is the oneness of God (Allah). Not only is there just one God, but God (Allah) is in control of everything in the universe, regardless of whether we humans judge outcomes in the world as positive or negative. Islam also accepts the existence of angels and the Day of Judgment and holds that Muhammad is the last prophet and that the Quran is the last of Allah's holy books (Fatoohi, 2002).

Sufism is the mystical spiritual tradition within Islam, which directs humans toward a "nearness" to the God (Allah) so that they can become agents for Allah. As noted in the introduction of the Quran (Abdullah Yusuf Ali edition, C:1):

> Glory to Allah Most High, full of Grace and Mercy; He created All, including Man. To Man He gave a special place in His Creation. He honoured man to be His Agent, and to that end, endued him with understanding, purified his affections, and gave him spiritual insight; so that man should understand Nature, understand himself, and know Allah through His wondrous Signs, and glorify Him in Truth, reverence, and unity.

The commentator then discusses how humans were given a "will" so that they may choose to follow the will of Allah (i.e., submission or Islam) (C:2) and how humans became distant from Allah when their lower self rebelled against Allah's will (C:3):

> For the fulfillment of this great trust man was further given a Will, so that his acts should reflect Allah's universal Law, and his mind, freely choosing, should experience the sublime joy of being in harmony with the Infinite, and with the great drama of the world around him, and with his own spiritual growth.
>
> But, created though he was in the best of moulds, man fell from Unity when his Will was warped, and he chose the crooked path of Discord. And sorrow and pain, selfishness and degradation, ignorance and hatred, despair and unbelief poisoned his life, and he saw shapes of evil in the physical, moral, and spiritual world, and in himself.

Thus the spiritual tradition of Sufism represents the direct path back to Allah or, as noted in the Quran's "Opening" (first surah or chapter), "the straight way" (1:6).

The Sufi musician Hazrat Inayat Khan (1983) provides the following description of spiritual development: "The word 'spiritual' does not apply to goodness or to wonder-working, the power of producing miracles, or to great intellectual power. The whole of life in all its aspects is one single music; and the real spiritual attainment is to tune oneself to the harmony of this perfect music" (p. 129).

The foundation of Sufism is belief in the mystical aspects of the spirituality of the Muhammad (Hussein et al, 1997). During his lifetime, pious individuals from different nations learned under his guidance the spiritual laws of Islam, because these laws led toward direct experience of the divine or nearness to Allah (Ansha, 1991).

The spiritual leader of a Sufi school is known as a *shaikh.* The spiritual knowledge of the shaikh can be traced back to Muhammad, who later converted his cousin and son-in-law Ali bin abi Talib. Ali is considered a spiritual heir to the Prophet and the one who inherited his spiritual knowledge and power. Thus, all Sufi masters are his students, directly or indirectly, and this hierarchy is the origin of the title "Shaikh of the Shaikhs." Through a line of succession, each shaikh initiates a successor based on revelations from Allah, maintaining a direct spiritual link or attachment with Muhammad to the present spiritual leader (Chishti, 1991). This chain from Muhammad down to the present master of a Sufi school is known as a *silsila* (Hussein et al, 1997). At present, there are more than 150 orders or schools of Sufism.

A shaikh is a *mediator* or guide to Allah in Sufism to help the student draw near to Allah, battle the lower self (jihad), and channel the spiritual power from Allah to perform paranormal acts (discussed in the section on the metapsychology of Sufism). As noted in the teaching of Shaikh Gaylani,

> the mediator is essential. Ask your Lord for a physician who can treat the diseases of your hearts, a healer who can heal you, a guide who can guide you and take you by the hand. Draw near to those whom He has brought near to him, His elite, the ushers of His nearness, the keepers of His door. You have consented to serving your lower selves and pursuing your passions and natural inclinations. You work hard to satisfy and satiate your lower selves in this world, although this is something that you will never achieve. You keep to this state hour after hour, day after day, month after month and year after year, until you find that death has suddenly come to you and you cannot release yourselves from its grip. (Al-Casnaszani al-Husseini, 1999, p. 15)

If Allah did not reveal someone with the attributes that qualify a person to be a shaikh, the shaikh would not name a successor, and the silsila of that particular *tariqa* (way) would discontinue. In this case the dervishes would have to join another tariqa after the departure of their shaikh to maintain the spiritual link necessary for the attainment of their spiritual goal.

The unifying factor and ultimate aim of the Sufi way is the attainment of nearness to Allah by following a chain of masters who have already attained nearness to Allah and by following the path of the Prophet. This process of drawing near also is related to purifying one's lower self through personal internal struggle, or *jihad*. The process of drawing near to Allah may include the acquisition of paranormal powers, such as rapid wound healing, and paranormal knowledge, including Quranic knowledge. One of the great Sufi masters, Shaikh Abd al-Qadir al-Gaylani, used to describe what the dervish would obtain

as being "something that no eye has ever seen, no ear has ever heard, and has never occurred to any human heart." In Sufi terms, the attainment of nearness to Allah means the transformation into light by becoming absorbed or extinct in the Light (i.e., Allah). Allah describes himself in the Quran as being "nur" (light): "Allah is the Light of the heavens and the earth" (24:35). The nearer one draws to Allah, the more of Allah's attributes one acquires. When one achieves the ultimate goal of total "extinction" (Arabic, *fana*) in Allah, one will lose one's own will and become an instrument in the hands of Allah, thus experiencing the ultimate submission of one's will to Allah. With this nearness to Allah, one can reach the high stage of being an agent (vicegerent) for Allah, with spiritual guidance, vision, and power to help transform the world and people. The broad implication for society is having an *umma*, or community, united by following the will of Allah rather than clinging to the traditional tribal, blood, and kinship allegiances with accompanying blood feuds that were so prevalent during the time of the Prophet and remain so today (Armstrong, 1993).

Sufism is not associated with terrorism or fundamentalism. The Sufi spiritual viewpoint may not be generally accepted by traditional Muslims; it has even been met with hostility by some Muslim schools of thought (Hussein et al, 1997). Of course, traditional Muslims accept that righteous living in this life will lead them to Allah in the next life, but Sufi, like other mystical traditions, believes that one can gain direct experience of Allah in this life by following the spiritual path.

THE WAY

An integral part of Sufism is the notion of a "path" or "way" toward Allah through self-understanding, certain practices, and discipline (Ansha, 1991). Thus, Sufism is the straight path, or one of the shortest paths, to God. Many great spiritual traditions use the concept of a path or way toward the experience of the divine. For example, Buddhism is known as a path toward *nirvana* or enlightenment (Clarke, 1993). In the Bible, Psalm 25:4 states, "Show me thy ways, O Lord; teach me thy paths." Continuing with verses 9-10, "The meek will he guide in judgment: and the meek will he teach his way. All the paths of the Lord are mercy and truth unto such as keep his covenant and his testimonies." In the New Testament, Jesus said, "I am the way, the truth, and the life; no man cometh unto the Father, but by me" (John 14:6). Similarly, in the beginning chapter of the Quran, Al Fatihah ("The Opening") 1:6-7, Allah teaches the people how to pray to him in these verses: "Show us the straight way, The way of those on whom Thou hast bestowed Thy Grace, Those whose portion is not wrath, and who go not astray."

The idea of a spiritual path has a corollary in the Western philosophical concept of "means" versus "end."

John Dewey (1922) noted the following when discussing means and end concerning an activity:

> The distinction of means and end arise[s] in surveying the course of a proposed line of action, a connected series in time. The "end" is the last act thought of; the means are the acts to be performed prior to it in time. To reach an end we must take our mind off from it and attend to the act that is next to be performed. We must make that the end.

Dewey's concept of means and end were greatly influenced by the mind-body movement therapy work of F. Matthias Alexander (1910). Alexander observed that many postural problems people encountered were caused by unconscious movements to gain some end, such as sitting or standing, without much thought as to the means, way, or path of accomplishing this goal. Alexander taught individuals to focus on the "means whereby" of doing a simple act such as the process of moving from sitting to standing rather than focusing on the end results or "end gaining," as he termed it. The process of attending to the "means" or "way" resulted in increased conscious guidance and control of the self. Alexander (1910) noted the following:

> This triumph is not to be won in sleep, in trance, in submission, in paralysis, or in anaesthesia, but in a clear, open-eyed, reasoning, deliberate consciousness and apprehension of the wonderful potentialities possessed by mankind, the transcendent inheritance of a conscious mind.

From this perspective, following a path or way or attending to a means may be associated with increased awareness or consciousness, or perhaps even a higher consciousness. This mindfulness is comparable to the increased consciousness or awareness of one's body movements found by following instructions in the Alexander method (Alexander, 1910) (see Chapters 7 and 15).

ISLAMIC TRADITIONS AND HEALTH

As a spiritual tradition within Islam, Sufism follows the five pillars of Islam: (1) the statement of belief or *Shahada* ("There is no God, but the God [Allah] and Muhammad is the messenger of Allah"), (2) prayer, (3) fasting, (4) charity, and (5) *hajj* (pilgrimage). Traditional Islam includes spiritually based and healthy practices, such as prayer five times a day (early morning, noon, midafternoon, sunset, and evening), fasting, and prohibition against the consumption of pork products and intoxicating liquors. There are also prohibitions against gambling, sexual relations outside of marriage, and behavior or dress that is indecent (Abdalati, 1996).

There are obvious health benefits to avoiding high-risk behaviors such as those proscribed by Islamic tradition. Avoiding alcohol intoxication also helps prevent its disinhibiting effects and the accompanying social problems. "It has been said that the super-ego is the alcohol-soluble portion of the personality" (Friend, 1957, p. 84). Avoiding pork would also provide protection against swine-related foodborne diseases, such as *Salmonella typhimurium* gastroenteritis (Gessner et al, 1994), *Yersinia* enterocolitis (Tauxe, 1997), and viral illnesses from pork or pork products, including foot-and-mouth disease, classic swine fever (hog cholera), African swine fever, trichinosis, and swine vesicular viral disease (Farez et al, 1997; McKercher et al, 1978). Jewish laws in the Old Testament earlier forbade consuming pork or touching the dead carcasses of swine because they are "unclean to you" (Leviticus 11:7-8; Deuteronomy 14:8). This description of pigs as unclean is consistent with their habit of eating dirt, urine and fecal matter, decaying animals and vegetables, maggots, and cancerous growths on other animals. Pigs are also helpful in clearing an area of rattlesnakes, because they will eat the snakes and not be harmed by their venomous bites. Within a few days after being butchered a pig's flesh quickly fills with worms. Also, because of pigs' unclean diet and their inability to sweat or perspire, the meat and fat of pork can be 30 times more toxic than beef or venison. Pork is also digested more rapidly than beef or venison (4 hours versus 8 or 9 hours), which results in a much higher level of toxins when it is consumed. Even the use of modern microwave ovens may fail to protect against pork-related illnesses such as salmonellosis (Gessner et al, 1994). There may be no safe cooking temperature to ensure the killing of the dozens of parasites in pork, such as flukes, tapeworms, trichinae, and other worms. Pork is not the only source of foodborne diseases, and foodborne pathogens in general are emerging as a major public health challenge (Tauxe, 1997).

FASTING

Being hungry is better than the maladies that come with satiety. Subtlety and lightness and being true to your devotion are some of the advantages of fasting.

—RUMI (1991)

During the lunar holy month of Ramadan, Muslims all over the world fast from sunrise to sunset. This fasting means abstaining completely from food, drink, and sexual intercourse from dawn to sunset (Abdalati, 1996). Fasting is done for spiritual purposes in Islam. The Quran (2:183) declares, "O ye who believe! Fasting is prescribed to you as it was prescribed to those before you, so that ye may learn self-restraint." As Woodward (1985) stated, "Fasting is thought to purge the body of passion and sin and reduce the risk of disease. Once passion has been controlled, it is possible to clear the mind (an element of the spiritual body) of conscious thought. This allows the mystic to establish contact with saints, spirits, sources of magical power and ultimately with Allah." Fasting also teaches patience and unselfishness, for when a person fasts, he or she can identify with the pains and deprivations of others less fortunate (Abdalati, 1996).

In naturopathic medicine, fasting is used as a method of detoxifying the body (see Chapter 21). It is a rapid way to increase the elimination of wastes within the body to facilitate healing. Also, a number of medical conditions have been treated with fasting, ranging from obesity, allergies, and chemical poisoning to irritable bowel syndrome (Murray et al, 1991). Obesity is becoming epidemic in the United States. Furthermore, intermittent fasting, caloric restriction, and undernutrition (but not malnutrition) have been associated with increased life span in both animals and humans (Walford, 1983). As suggested by Rumi, one of the maladies that come with overeating may be a shorter lifespan.

MEDITATION

When you neglect your meditation, you contract with pain. This is God's way of telling you that your inner pain can become visible. Don't ignore it.

—RUMI (1991)

Meditation is one of the most important Sufi tools for drawing nearer to Allah by "remembering" God and thus treating one's inner heart that has become distant, diseased, and hardened. Worshipful meditation is an integral part of Sufism and is also known as "Divine Remembrance," *Dhikr*, or *Zekr* (Chishti, 1991). As noted in the Quran, "Then do ye remember Me, I will remember you" (2:152). The place of worship or the *takiya* is also known as the "house of remembrance." These Sufi meditation practices are above and beyond the traditional prayers.

Such meditation practices involve a prescribed number of recitations of verses from the Quran using prayer beads (i.e., a rosary to keep count), such as "la illaha illa Allah," or "there is no god but Allah (the God)" (Ansha, 1991), or other remembrances, such as "the beautiful names" of Allah. For some *tariqas* (e.g., Tariqa Casnazaniyyah), this recitation is done aloud with accompanying head movements symbolizing a hammer slamming a heart that has become "hardened like a stone." The remoteness from Allah causes this hardness, and the remembrance is the remedy. As noted in the Quran (2:74), "Thenceforth were your hearts hardened: they became like a rock and even worse in hardness." Other tariqas use silent remembrances or employ different movements altogether. Meditation has been suggested to help treat diseases (see Chapter 9). It has been recommended that to

treat diseases the number of recitations end with a zero (e.g., 100, 300) (Chishti, 1991). Again, from the Sufi perspective, worshipful meditation is a means of drawing near to Allah, and with that connection may come transcendent events.

Research has documented the many health and physiological benefits of meditation, including decrease in blood pressure, rate of breathing, heart rate, and oxygen consumption (see Chapter 9). The positive effects of meditation are associated with the production of a physiological "relaxation response" that is opposite to the "fight-or-flight response" (Benson, 1975). Thus the regular worshipful meditative practice of Sufism may also contribute to increased health.

PRAYER

Prayers of Salat (the Arabic term) are performed five times a day by Muslims throughout the world as a means of drawing near to Allah. During these prayers all Muslims face the *Kaaba* in Mecca, which is believed to have been built by the Prophet Abraham. These five prayers are performed at dawn, noon, midafternoon, sunset, and nightfall and can be done anywhere, but community prayer at the mosque on Fridays also serves the function of bringing the community together, as in other religious traditions, with all the health benefits of social support. Hygiene or ablution, known as *wudu*, is a traditional part of Muslim prayers. This practice of hand washing was done routinely many centuries before the discovery of germs and antisepsis, and it is interesting to note that although it was quite an accepted part of religious and magic ceremonies, hygiene was very slow to come to the practice of medicine and was met with much resistance (Hall, 1995). Today the health benefits of good hygiene practices are acknowledged, and they are the standard of care. In addition to the benefits of hygiene, the healing benefits of prayer are now becoming recognized within the disciplines of science and medicine (Dossey, 1996, 2001). "Prayer works. More than 130 controlled laboratory studies show, in general, that prayer or a prayer like state of compassion, empathy, and love can bring about healthful changes in many types of living things, from humans to bacteria. This does not mean prayer always works, any more than drugs and surgery always work, but that, statistically speaking, prayer is effective" (Dossey, 1996).

THE PSYCHOLOGY OF SUFISM

The notion of the heart and the ego or lower self (Arabic, *nafs*) has played a prominent role in Sufi psychology (Ansha, 1991; Chishti, 1991). The spiritual path of Sufism is geared toward inner spiritual development by helping the follower in the purification or extinction (*fana'*) of the ego or lower self (nafs) or more basic appetitive aspects of the body and selfish and mean-spirited desires. A system that helps manage excessive appetitive urges would have positive health benefits for a number of disorders of over-indulgence, such as weight problems and addictions. Disorders of excess are significant causes of morbidity within the West, with obesity one of the most serious threats.

The heart, in Sufism, is related to one's spiritual self. As mentioned earlier, the head movement that accompanies the recitation meditation, or Dhikr practice, symbolizes a hammer slamming a heart that has become a stone so that its true luster can shine through. Muhammad stated, "There is a polish for everything that taketh away rust; and the polish of the Heart is the invocation of Allah" (Lings, 1977). It is within the heart or inner being that spiritual development and battles occur. It is to this internal battleground that the true concept of *jihad* relates.

JIHAD

One of the most misunderstood concepts in Islam is the term *jihad,* usually associated with the notion of "holy war" and terrorism. The definition of jihad in the Quran is to "exert the best efforts," or engage in some type of "struggle" or "resistance," to achieve some goal (Fatoohi, 2002). The Quran discusses two types of jihad, "peaceful jihad" and "armed jihad." Armed jihad was permitted for Muslims as a temporary response against armed aggression. The early Muslim community lived for 14 years under the guidance of the Prophet's revelations before they were given permission from Allah to fight back to defend themselves. The Quran uses a different term, *qital,* when referring to fighting an enemy. It is also forbidden in Islam to take an innocent life, because killing one innocent person is like killing the whole group; conversely, saving one person is like saving the whole community (Quran 5:32).

Peaceful jihad, on the other hand, is the permanent struggle in which every Muslim must continuously engage against evil desires within the lower self. Shaikh Muhammad al-Casnazani refers to this perpetual internal holy war or jihad as "Spiritual sport." This ongoing inner struggle uses facilities such as intuition to allow the individual to overcome lower drives and draw nearer to Allah, with all the spiritual, material, and metaphysical benefits. This struggle often comes down to a choice. Mathematics professor Jeffrey Lang pointed out the following:

> The Qur'an presents human history as a perennial struggle between two opposing choices: to resist or to surrender oneself to God. It is in this conflict that the scripture immerses itself and the reader; it could be said to be the very crux of its calling. This choice must be completely voluntary, for the Qur'an demands, "Let there be no compulsion in religion—the right way is henceforth clearly distinct from error" (2:256). (Lang, 2000, p. 27)

AFFLICTIONS

One of the greatest challenges people currently face in the world is trying to understand and endure personal crises, illness, and afflictions. The Islamic and Sufi perspective holds that whatever happens to an individual occurs only by the will of Allah. However, one might ask, "Why would Allah allow bad things to happen to people?" Sufi Shaikh Gaylani notes that, given the oneness of Allah, afflictions bring people closer to God:

> The people of Allah accustom themselves to afflictions and do not get annoyed like your annoyance.... Afflictions are of various kinds; some affect the body, while some affect the heart. Some of them are suffered in relation to creatures, while others in relation to the Creator. There is no good in someone who has not been subjected to suffering. Afflictions are the hooks of the True One (i.e. Allah). (Al-Casnaszani al-Husseini, 1999, p. 183)

Shaikh Gaylani goes on to point out the oneness of Allah in terms of afflictions and the lessons learned from such adversities:

> Obey and do not disobey. Believe in the oneness of Allah and do not attribute partners to Him. Your reliance on creatures is a form of polytheistic idolatry. Woe unto you! You are mad! Dissatisfaction and protestation do not give you something or take away another. Your anger cannot delay something or bring forward another. Affliction and the removal of affliction are both in the hand of Allah. It is He who has sent down the disease and the remedy. It is He who has created the disease and has created the remedy. He afflicts you with tribulations to make you come to know Him through affliction, to show you His signs and His power in sending down the affliction and in removing it and to show you the removal and the putting down of His plate (of grace). Afflictions show the way to the door of Allah ('Azza wa Jall) and knock on it. They bring the heart and the True One ('Azza wa Jall) together. They promote the status. Do not hate afflictions for you have many benefits in these things that you hate. Set aside asking "why" and "how." If you endure the afflictions with patience, they will purify you of outward and inward sins. The Prophet (Salla Allah ta'ala 'alayhi wa sallam) is reported to have said: "Afflictions will continue to come the believer's way until he comes to walk on the earth carrying no sin." His sins will be erased from his scrolls and the angels who recorded them will forget them. (Al-Casnaszani al-Husseini, 1999, p. 186)

Thus, affliction teaches humility, patience, and thankfulness to Allah. It is our lower self that rebels against Allah during afflictions and distances one from the source of needed help. The psychology of human behavior is keenly noted in the Quran (C:4), which declares that people tend to "boast in prosperity, and curse in adversity." Faith in the oneness of Allah and enduring these struggles is the heart of peaceful jihad and brings one closer to the God.

FAITH

Faith has also been suggested as an important factor in the psychology of healing from a Sufi perspective as in other healing traditions. A contemporary Sufi, M.R. Bawa Muhaiyaddeen (1991), notes the following:

> Illnesses can be treated in many ways, but no matter how many different treatments are used, they may still fail to heal the patient. In order for a treatment to work, first of all, even if the patient does not have faith in God, he must have faith in the doctor and in whatever treatment he suggests. Secondly, the doctor who is performing the treatment must have faith in God; he must have God's qualities, His love, and His patience. The doctor must give all responsibility to God, instead of thinking that he is the one who is responsible for curing the patient.
>
> When these conditions exist, when the patient has faith in the doctor and the doctor has faith in God, then treatment becomes very easy and the illness will be cured, at least to a certain extent. (p. 253)

PAN-ISLAMIC SUFISM AND HEALING TRADITIONS

Although the primary focus of Sufism is on attainment of nearness to Allah, some Sufis have developed a particular focus on healing. Often there is a blend of Sufi philosophy with other healing traditions, as well as incorporation of the use of herbs and food, and other practices (Chishti, 1991).

The Sufi Healing Order, currently under the guidance of Himayat Inayati, offers both training and services in spiritual healing. Some healing services are conducted within a group prayer circle, where divine help is requested for healing. Members also visit ill persons, offering spiritual support. Himayat Inayati incorporates a number of different traditions within his Sufi healing approach.

Sufi philosophy has played a major role in influencing traditional medical practices on the Indonesian island of Java. Woodward (1985) noted the following:

> The Javanese medical system draws on a wide variety of symbols, roles and interactional patterns, none of which may be understood as uniquely medical. Concepts of personhood, cosmology, power and knowledge are melded into a corpus of closely related theories explaining the origins of disease and motivating highly diverse treatment strategies. Medical pluralism is, therefore, an inherent feature of Javanese traditional medicine. There are two primary modes of medical practice. One practiced by Sufi saints (wali) is based on Islamic mystical concepts of miracles and gnosis. The other, practiced by dukun (curers), involves the use of morally suspect forms of magical power.

COMPLEMENTARY AND ALTERNATIVE MEDICINE

Sufism fits well in the current complementary and alternative medical movement. The 1990s were the era of a "silent revolution" in health care for some of the wealthiest, most highly educated mainstream citizens of major industrialized countries of the world, from the United States to Europe. A U.S. survey conducted in 1990 revealed that Americans with chronic non–life-threatening conditions made about 427 million visits to alternative medicine practitioners in the previous year, compared with 388 million visits to all primary care physicians (Eisenberg et al, 1993). By 1997, the number of visits to alternative medicine practitioners had increased to 629 million visits per year, eclipsing the number of visits to all U.S. primary care physicians (386 million per year) (Eisenberg et al, 1998). When these data were examined in terms of the percentage of people using "unconventional medicine," for the 1990 survey about 34% of individuals interviewed had used at least 1 of 16 alternative therapies in the previous year. By 1997 this number had increased to 42%, and it continues to rise. These alternative therapies ranged from relaxation techniques, hypnosis, biofeedback, imagery, herbal medicines, and chiropractic manipulations to such healing practices as acupuncture, homeopathy, and folk remedies (Eisenberg et al, 1993). In 1990, Americans spent about $15 billion on services for alternative medicine practitioners, and by 1997 this figure had increased to more than $21 billion.

This growing use of alternative medical practices by highly educated Americans with chronic non–life-threatening health conditions may not represent irrational behavior when one considers the finding that a combined total of about 225,000 deaths occur each year in the United States from medication errors and adverse effects, hospital mistakes, unnecessary surgeries, and nosocomial infections. This places our "high-tech" medical interventions as the third leading cause of death in the United States, after heart disease and cancer (Starfield, 2000). Medical interventions for emergency situations are critical, but interventions for chronic non–life-threatening conditions can prove lethal.

There is a paradigm shift within mechanistic medicine best described by Dossey's three eras. Larry Dossey (1993) described medicine as moving through three distinct eras. *Era I* was mechanical, material, or physical medicine; this was the Newtonian view of the world in which the human body was viewed as operating like a machine. At present this is our reductionistic, high-tech medicine. *Era II* was the mind-body medicine movement; in the United States, one can place relaxation, meditation, and many Sufi approaches within the alternative medicine movement. *Era III* is "spiritual healing" or "energy healing"; Dossey also called this "nonlocal" or "transpersonal" medicine. The metaphysical aspects of Sufism can be viewed in this context.

ERA III: Energy Medicine or Spiritual Healing (Nonlocal, Transpersonal Medicine or Vitalism)

The silent revolution or paradigm shift of the 1990s incorporated global healing traditions from other cultures that are thousands of years old. These non-Western practices involved nonmechanistic and whole-person approaches to healing. Such global healing traditions included Ayurveda medicine of India with its various yogas (see Chapters 29 and 31), Chinese medicine with acupuncture (Ergil, 1996), and qigong (McGee et al, 1996) (see Chapters 26 and 27). Western religious traditions provided intercessory prayer and distant healing intention research (Dossey, 1993).

Daniel Benor, a practicing holistic psychiatrist, addressed the evidence-based question of spiritual healing as follows:

"Does spiritual healing work? Does research confirm that healing is an effective therapy?" An impressive number of studies with excellent design and execution answer this question with a "Yes." If we take a broad view, out of 191 controlled experiments of healing,... close to two thirds (64.9 percent) of all the experiments demonstrate significant effects. (Benor, 2001, p. 371)

Spiritual healing effects can be demonstrated on animals, plants, single-celled organisms, bacteria, yeasts, and DNA. Similarly, cellular biologist and physiologist James Oschman states the following:

Medical research is demonstrating that devices producing pulsing magnetic fields of particular frequencies can stimulate the healing of a variety of tissues. Therapists from various schools of energy medicine can project, from their hands, fields with similar frequencies and intensities. Research documenting that these different approaches are efficacious is mutually validating. Medical research and hands-on therapies are confirming each other. The common denominator is the pulsating magnetic field, which is called a biomagnetic field when it emanates from the hands of a therapist. (Oschman, 2000, p. xiv) (see also Chapters 10 and 11).

With the silent revolution, people are moving toward whole-person health and global healing traditions (see Chapter 38). One global healing tradition from the Middle East that has received little attention in the West (probably for geographical and political reasons) is the spiritual practice of rapid healing of wounds from deliberately caused bodily damage as demonstrated at a major Sufi school in Iraq. This has been the focus of my research for the past several years.

THE METAPSYCHOLOGY OF SUFISM AND RAPID WOUND HEALING

The extraordinary phenomenon of instantaneous healing of wounds from deliberately caused bodily damage (DCBD) has been reported by the Tariqa Casnazaniyyah

School of Sufism in Baghdad, one of the largest Sufi schools in the Middle East (Hussein et al, 1994a, 1994b, 1994c, 1997). Followers (dervishes) of this Sufi school have been observed to demonstrate instantaneous healing of DCBD. For example, dervishes have inserted a variety of sharp instruments (e.g., spikes, skewers) into the body, hammered daggers into the skull bone and clavicle, and chewed and swallowed glass and sharp razor blades without harm to the body and with complete control over pain, bleeding, and infection, as well as rapid wound healing within 4 to 10 seconds (Figure 33-1). This Sufi school's name, Tariqa Casnazaniyyah, is an Arabic-Kurdish word meaning "the way of the secret that is known to no one" (Hussein et al, 1997). Researchers report that such extraordinary abilities are accessible to anyone and are not restricted to only a few talented individuals who have spent years in special training. These unusual healing phenomena have also been reproduced under controlled laboratory conditions and are not similar to hypnosis (Hall et al, 2001).

Similar DCBD phenomena have been observed in various parts of the world in a variety of religious and nonreligious contexts (Don et al, 2000; Hussein et al, 1997). For example, trance surgeons in Brazil have employed sharp instruments to cut, pierce, or inject

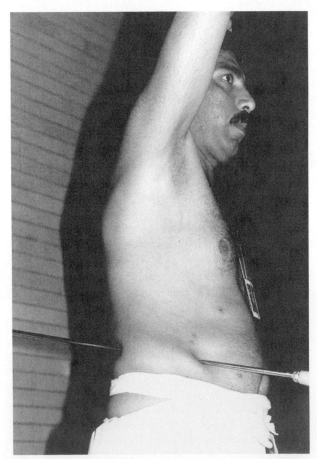

Figure 33-1 A dervish at the major Sufi school in Baghdad demonstrating Sufi wound healing.

substances into a patient's body for therapeutic purposes. Laboratory electroencephalographic (EEG) investigation of trance surgeons has shown that this "state of spirit possession" of the healers was associated with a hyperaroused brain state (waves in the 30- to 50-Hz band) (Don et al, 2000). Unfortunately, not only has little scientific attention been given to the investigation of these claims of rapid healing in the United States, but such claims of extraordinary healing abilities have been met with scorn and have even been challenged by so-called skeptic groups, such as the Committee for the Scientific Investigation of Claims of the Paranormal. These groups offer monetary incentives to discredit such claims in unscientific and dangerous settings (Mulacz, 1998; Posner, 1998). (See Dossey, 1999, and Fatoohi, 1999, for a response.)

Followers of the Tariqa Casnazaniyyah School of Sufism describe the ability to accomplish DCBD healing as an "others-healing phenomenon" within the context of healing energies (Hussein et al, 1994a, 1994b, 1994c). This "higher energy" is alleged to be instantly transferable mediated through a spiritual link from the current shaikh of the Sufi school and through the chain of masters to Muhammad (P) and ultimately to Allah (Hussein et al, 1997). As noted in the Quran, "The Prophet is closer to the Believers than their own selves" (33:6). When I became aware of DCBD phenomena, the first question that naturally arose was, How might Western scientists empirically investigate such unusual claims of healing? From a scientific perspective this would demand a series of systematic observations of the Sufi rapid wound healing phenomenon in both field and laboratory settings. Of course, the first question that needed to be addressed was whether this healing phenomenon was real. This would require a field trip to directly observe, video record, and possible even experience DCBD healing. If these initial observations showed the phenomenon to be genuine, then the question becomes, Can the phenomenon be explained by traditional paradigms, such as hypnosis or the placebo effect? Because I had conducted research in hypnosis and psychoneuroimmunology (Hall, Minnes, Tosi et al, 1992; Hall, Mumma, Longo et al, 1992; Hall et al, 1982, 1989, 1993, 1996) as well as clinical work in hypnosis for over 20 years, I was very interested in comparing this rapid healing with hypnotic phenomena. I will describe my visit to Iraq for field observations and my first direct experience of DCBD healing. It was my impression following that visit that what I had seen and experienced represented a phenomenon that went beyond classical Newtonian mechanics. I argued that explanations for DCBD healing involving psychological factors that influence healing, such as the placebo effect, hypnosis, or altered states of consciousness, have little logical, theoretical, or empirical support (Hall, 2000).

The next question in my series of systematic observations was, Can this unusual healing phenomenon be exported to the United States and observed within a traditional medical setting? If the phenomenon could be brought to the States, what measures should be employed to help us understand underlying processes of DCBD healing, particularly if it represented a new paradigm as defined by Thomas Kuhn (1970) in describing the structure of scientific revolutions? After we found that DCBD healing could be transported to the United States, I then undertook a series of structured observations of this phenomenon with myself as the subject to explore possible underlying mechanism, using both traditional and novel instruments and measures.

These systematic observations laid the foundation for more traditional follow-up laboratory studies that can be conducted with randomized control groups or what Kuhn (1970) might refer to as the puzzle-solving process of "normal science." Kuhn does caution, however, that anomalous observations that do not fit within existing paradigms can result in a crisis and lead to the revolutionary process of a paradigm shift. Because I am a scientist as well as a clinician, my ultimate interest lies in the more important area of the translational application of this research to the healing of clinical conditions. Normal science in general has been criticized for it lack of interest in translating basic science into practical applications (Shapley et al, 1985). For me, translating anomalous findings into practical use is an exciting venture. Below I outline my studies.

In 1998, with an invitation from the shaikh of the Tariqa Casnazaniyyah School of Sufism in Baghdad and support from the Kairos Foundation in Illinois, I traveled alone to Baghdad to meet with the spiritual leader of this group, Shaikh Muhammad al-Casnazani, and witnessed a group demonstration of DCBD healing at their major school (Hall, 2000). At this meeting, which was professionally videotaped, I had the opportunity to examine firsthand the objects that were employed during the DCBD demonstrations, such as knives, razor blades, and glass, and observe them being inserted into various parts of the body. What I witnessed and recorded was consistent with the extraordinary claims made by this group about rapid wound healing and lack of apparent pain.

Although I saw no evidence of a ruse, I imagined that some skeptics might question if I had somehow been deluded, even with video footage. Thus, I had requested permission while at this demonstration to experience DCBD healing by having my cheek pierced (Hall, 2000). After I had witnessed several demonstrations of DCBD healing, an assistant asked if I were ready. I said yes, and he asked me to face the shaikh to ask permission to allow the healing energy for rapid wound healing. The shaikh nodded, indicating that I had his permission. What was most striking was that I did not feel any different or in an altered state, and my cheek was not numb. The assistant then inserted a metal ice pick through the inside of my left cheek to the outside. It felt like a poke, but with no pain (Figure 33-2). I walked around the group circle with

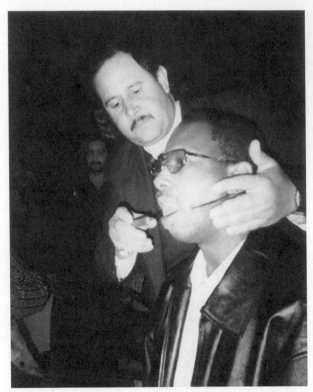

Figure 33-2 The author having his cheek pierced at the major Sufi school in Baghdad.

the ice pick in my cheek, introspecting on how it was not hurting, bleeding, or numb. I could feel the weight of the object and notice the metal taste in my mouth, but I felt no discomfort. Again, consistent with the reports, my cheek healed rapidly in minutes with only a couple of drops of blood. This personal experience was very compelling to me despite the fact that I had much doubt and am not particularly fond of pain. Nonetheless, I still imagined that skeptics would question whether such practices could be demonstrated outside this religious context and exported to the West.

A demonstration of such rapid wound healing was clearly needed within a Western medical setting, given the scientific implications of such healing. If such spiritually based healing approaches are genuine, they hold much promise for addressing some of today's most serious medical issues.

The investigation of such unusual healing phenomena in the West raises many questions. What should be measured within a scientific context? Would standard measures of brain and immune activity be associated with changes in rapid wound healing, or should standard measures, such as EEG activity, be used in less standard ways? Would high-frequency EEG activity need to be examined for hyperaroused brain states? Would new approaches be needed to detect "fields of consciousness," such as the examination of changes in the output of a random event generator?

Case Study

Again with the support of the Kairos Foundation of Wilmette, Illinois, a Sufi practitioner (J.H.) was invited from the Middle East to a local radiology facility in Cleveland, Ohio, on July 1, 1999. He had permission from the shaikh of the Casnazaniyyah Sufi school to perform a demonstration of rapid wound healing after insertion of an unsterilized metal skewer, 0.38 cm thick and approximately 13 cm long, while being videotaped by a film crew in the presence of scientists and health care professionals (Hall et al, 2001). This was apparently the first demonstration by a practitioner from this Sufi school in the United States. The practitioner consented to sign a release of liability for the medical facility and personnel against claims from possible injuries. Emergency medical technicians were present. The major goal of this demonstration was to observe the authenticity of rapid wound healing following a deliberately caused injury within a medical setting.

The demonstration was also conducted with radiological, immunological, and EEG evaluations, as well as a Zener noise diode random event generator (REG), similar to the one employed at Princeton University by Dr. Robert Jahn and colleagues. Based on previous studies in Brazil with healer-mediums engaged in quasisurgical practices, it was hypothesized that DCBD healing would be accompanied by alterations in brain waves and effects on REGs. The alterations in brain waves found with the Brazilian healer-mediums showed statistically significant enhancement of broadband 40-Hz brain rhythms (Don et al, 2000). A statistically significant deviation from random behavior in REGs was found in a test run covertly while the Brazilian healer-mediums were in trance. This methodology was developed by Robert Jahn and associates at the Princeton Engineering Anomalies Research Laboratory (PEAR) (Nelson et al, 1996, 1998). Such energy fields have been considered as theoretically associated with rapid wound healing (Don et al, 2000).

Nineteen-channel EEGs were recorded during baseline resting conditions, while the dervish inserted the skewer through his cheek, and immediately after removal of the instrument.

An REG, plugged into the serial port of a computer, was run in the background without informing the dervish. The distribution of binary digits was tested for possible significant deviations from random behavior. Data were acquired before and after the self-insertion, as well as during the skewer insertion. Before insertion of the skewer and about 1 hour after the piercing, blood was collected from the practitioner and three volunteers for an immunological analysis of the percent change in CD4, CD8, and total T-cell counts.

Results

Radiological images were made while the skewer was inserted. Computed axial tomographic images through the lower mandibular region showed artifact from dental metal. In addition, a horizontally oriented metallic bar elevated the left lateral soft tissues just anterior to the muscles of mastication. There was no associated underlying mass. A single frontal fluoroscopic image showed a presence of EEG leads over the maxilla and mandibular regions. A transverse metal was superimposed extending from the soft tissues on the right through to the left without interval break.

Because of movement and scalp muscle artifacts throughout the experimental self-insertion condition, it was impossible to assess the EEG for the hypothesized 40-Hz brain rhythms. The frequency spectrum of scalp muscle discharge overlaps the 40-Hz EEG frequency band of interest.

The REG output during baseline periods did not differ significantly from random behavior. However, during the self-insertion condition, there was a trend toward significant nonrandomness. The chi-square test result was 3.052, $df = 1$, and P was approximately .07.

Discussion

The behavior of the REG was in the predicted direction of nonrandomness. This has been interpreted by our laboratory and the PEAR laboratory as being associated with states of heightened attention and emotion. Further, the PEAR group has proposed that a "field of consciousness" is associated with such nonrandomness. Unfortunately, the 40-Hz brain wave hypothesis was not testable because of the excessive amount of scalp artifact and thus awaits further exploration. The presence of increased theta rhythms after the insertion condition (and a slight decrease in average alpha power) suggests a mild hypoaroused altered state of consciousness. The Sufi performing this feat was doing so for the first time. With further practice or with testing of more experienced subjects, it may be feasible to obtain EEG data without large amounts of scalp artifact. Because the subject reported no perceived pain during the self-insertion, preliminary relaxation exercises might eliminate all or most of the artifact. This would enable us to test the 40-Hz hypothesis definitively. Clearly, further work is indicated.

The immunologic analysis did not reveal any major difference between the Sufi practitioner and the control subjects. These data suggest that the variation found in the practitioner was not different from that of normal controls.

The radiological film documented that the skewer had actually penetrated both cheeks, which addresses the arguments of skeptic groups that such practices are the result of fakery. After the removal of the skewer, there was a slight trickle of blood, which stopped with application of pressure to the cheek using clean gauze. The physicians and scientists present documented that the wound healed rapidly within a few moments. The practitioner also reported that there was no pain associated with the insertion or removal of the metal skewer. This demonstration was conducted outside the traditional religious context, where chanting, drumming, and head movements are generally part of the ceremony when it is done in the Middle East. Thus, our case study argues against the view that a religious context, with its accompanying state of consciousness, is important to the successful outcome of such a demonstration. This case study also demonstrated that DCBD healing could be done when a large distance separated the dervish from the master (from Baghdad to Cleveland). This would suggest that this is a robust phenomenon independent of the

distance separating the source and the scene where the DCBD phenomenon occurs.

It should also be noted that the skewer stayed in the dervish's cheeks for more than 35 minutes, longer than the few minutes I had observed during my field observations at the major school of Tariqa Casnazaniyyah. Thus, this case study argues against the necessity of a brief piercing for a successful outcome of DCBD rapid healing. Further, the dervish of this demonstration reported that there was no pain associated with this piercing, minimal bleeding, and no postprocedural infection. Finally, about a half-hour after the completion of the demonstration, the dervish, along with seven other people who witnessed the DCBD event, had dinner together.

PERSONAL EXPERIENCE OF RAPID WOUND HEALING

After witnessing rapid wound healing in the Middle East and experiencing it myself there, I was initiated into the Sufi order with the ritualistic handshake, which took about 2 to 3 minutes. After a subsequent visit with the shaikh in the United Kingdom in June 2000, I was given a license to perform DCBD rapid healing.

I first requested permission from the shaikh in Baghdad to perform a cheek piercing on myself in May at the 2001 World Congress on Complementary Therapies in Medicine in Washington, DC. After lecturing on DCBD rapid healing, I informed the audience that I needed to take an earlier flight home because of a family medical emergency in Cleveland. Skipping a break, I went right into the cheek piercing for the first time on my own. My mind was on the family medical crisis back home, but I was instructed to focus on connecting with the shaikh, asking mentally for spiritual energy for rapid wound healing before the piercing. This took about a minute. One physician in the audience was particularly skeptical, so I invited him to stand next to me when I did the piercing. Please note that this was about 4 months before September 11, so I had brought a skewer from my kitchen drawer to be used for the demonstration.

After the 1-minute mental connection with the energy from the shaikh and with much nervousness, I pushed a very dull skewer through my left cheek. Yes, I was quite worried about the medical situation at home. The most difficult aspect of this experience was getting this dull object through my cheek. Eventually it went through with no pain. My skeptical medical colleague was very quiet after that. I pulled it out and there were a couple of drops of blood, which I blotted with a tissue until the bleeding stopped. From there, I had a friend take me directly to the airport.

The second time I demonstrated DCBD healing on myself (making this my third experience with DCBD healing including Baghdad) was at the Fifth World Congress on Qigong in November 2002. Because this was after September 11, 2001, I had to shop for a better piercing instrument. This demonstration was preceded by a video interview by some of the leading scientists in the field of energy healing attending the conference. The video camera was then set on a stand on the side of my left cheek. I again focused on connecting with the energy of the shaikh for rapid wound healing. I did not feel different, but I had faith that the connection was there, despite the distance in space. Again, I found that pushing the metal pick through my cheek was very difficult. After some effort (jihad), both physical and mental, it went through. I also spoke on camera about how I was feeling with the object through my cheek. After the interview, I pulled the pick out and padded a tissue against my cheek to absorb the few drops of blood. The wound closing was also documented on film for the first time. I had cut myself shaving early in the morning flying to California, and the piercing was the next day. The shaving cut was more noticeable than the piercing after the demonstration. I went out for a late dinner after this demonstration.

The next day after the demonstration I had the opportunity to meet and be evaluated by Dr. Konstantin Korotkov, professor of physics at St. Petersburg State Technical University in Russia, using his gas discharge visualization (GDV) technique, which measures human energy fields as did the earlier Kirlian photography (Korotkov, 2002, 2004; Korotkov et al, 2005). Dr. Korotkov first took a baseline measure of my energy field from my fingers and displayed the results on a screen to the audience. He then asked me to invoke the Sufi energy. I again took about a minute and requested energy from the shaikh for this demonstration. It should be noted that this energy reading was not planned by me nor had I obtained prior permission from the shaikh for this energy demonstration. After about 1 minute I said I was ready for the second (after-energy) measure. Dr. Korotkov outwardly expressed surprise at how quickly I had invoked energy. This time when he took the energy reading from my hand the computer malfunctioned, and another one had to be brought in. After the new computer was in place, the GDV reading revealed a major increase in my energy field after the quick 1-minute energy invocation.

My fourth experience with DCBD healing occurred in response to a request by National Geographic Television and Film (Washington, DC) to participate in a program to be aired for the cable network series "Is It Real?" titled "Superhuman Powers," in 2005. This demonstration was performed in collaboration with Gary Schwartz, PhD, at his Human Energy Systems Laboratory, Center for Frontier Medicine in Biofield Science, at the University of Arizona in Tucson (Hall et al, 2004). Again I obtained permission from the shaikh to conduct another DCBD demonstration, and we also explored whether there were any changes in brain activity associated with this process or any changes in my energy field or aura as indicated by the GDV measures. A 19-channel EEG along with GDV recordings were taken before and after I pierced my left cheek with a 5-inch ice pick and while being filmed by National Geographic. This demonstration took about 90 minutes to complete as I connected with the current shaikh and other masters who are part of this Sufi school's chain of shaikhs (i.e., silsila).

During the demonstration my brain did reach a more relaxed state as measured by EEG recordings. There was, however, no anomalous neurological activity, such as seizures, sleep, or hyperaroused brain states. Pre- versus post-piercing changes on GDV measures did show, for the first time ever, a selective decrease in the energy field where the cheek was pierced, revealing a gapping hole in my aura in that area. As with my prior experiences with DCBD healing, there were a few drops of blood after the ice pick was removed, but the wound healed very quickly and was not noticeable after a few minutes. Again, even with these additional scientific measures, traditional paradigms offered little insight to account for the rapid wound healing phenomenon. Such an observation was consistent with the results of the demonstration involving the Sufi practitioner from the Middle East, described earlier in the case report, in which we also failed to find any correlations between DCBD healing and any of the blood tests or imaging studies. The only hints of associations were the GDV energy measures and the trend of the REG output, which also suggested some change in the energy field. Work in this area might take us beyond Newton's classical mechanics to quantum mechanics and quantum physics to account for possible subtle energy constructs. Eric Leskowitz (2005) proposes a multidimensional model of wound healing incorporating energy concepts to help shift our current paradigm of wound healing beyond the physical and psychological dimensions or, as he describes it, from biology to spirit.

How does Sufism explain how rapid wound healing can occur?

Sufism can form a unified theory for mechanistic, mind-body, and spiritual healing. Traditional Islamic theology recognizes that Allah (God) created a world that can apparently operate under mechanistic and Newtonian principles. As noted in the Quran (6:95-99), Allah (God) created order in this world, causing seeds to sprout, the sun to rise and set, and the rain to fall. "Such is the judgment and ordering of (Him) the exalted in Power, the Omniscient" (6:96).

This is consistent with the mechanistic Newtonian view of the world and humans. Thus, there is no rejection of mechanistic views in traditional Islamic philosophy. Sufi philosophy goes further, noting that mechanistic views can also be explained within a vitalistic perspective. From this point of view, Sufism can predict both mechanistic and energy-based DCBD healing phenomena in ways that Newtonian models cannot.

Sufi Shaikh Gaylani explains it as follows:

> The belief of the followers of the Book and the Sunna of the Messenger of Allah (Salla Allah ta'ala 'alayhi wa sallam) is that the sword does not cut because of its nature, but it is rather Allah ('Azza wa Jall) who cuts with it, that the fire does not burn because of its nature, but it is rather

Allah ('Azza wa Jall) who burns with it, that food does not satisfy hunger because of its nature, but it is rather Allah ('Azza wa Jall) who satisfies hunger with it and that water does not quench thirst because of its nature, but it is rather Allah ('Azza wa Jall) who quenches thirst with it. The same applies to things of all kinds; it is Allah ('Azza wa Jall) who uses them to produce their effects and they are only instruments in His hand with which He does whatever He wills. (Al-Casnazani al-Husseini, 1998, p. 42)

Thus, most of the time the world operates by mechanical laws allowed by Allah, but mediation by a Sufi shaikh based on the shaikh's nearness to Allah and through Allah would allow for fire not to burn or a knife not to cut, so that mechanistic laws are suspended. The Quran is clear in several verses that so-called natural laws can be suspended by Allah. For example, 2:117 says, "when He (Allah) decreeth a matter, he saith to it: 'Be,' and it is."

The goal of the Sufi and all spiritual paths is nearness to God. In Sufism, this is done by following the Sufi path and practices and engaging in jihad or struggling against the lower self or nafs. It is the lower self that keeps humans distant from God. Islam and Sufism are about surrendering to the will of God by following this path. Once this nearness to God has been achieved, alterations of mechanistic laws may occur. This nearness to Allah is the explanation for "miracles" performed within religious contexts in ancient times and today.

Rapid wound healing is a very impressive phenomenon to observe and experience, but Islam and Sufism teach that one's heart is the center of one's being and becomes diseased (5:52) and hardened (6:43) from wrong acts (sins). Sufism, however, offers healing for the heart, as noted in the Quran: "O mankind! There hath come to you a direction from your Lord and a healing for the (diseases) in your hearts—and for those who believe a guidance and a Mercy" (10:57). Thus, when the heart has been purified through jihad, the nearness and true healing will occur.

SUMMARY

Sufism is a mystical tradition within Islam and is based on drawing nearer to Allah through the spirituality of Muhammad. Masters of present Sufi schools trace their origins back to Muhammad through a chain of masters. Sufism can be described as a path or way of attain of nearness to Allah with its possible paranormal powers, knowledge, and healing. The psychology of Sufism is geared toward this attainment. The Sufi way involves following orthodox Islamic practices such as daily prayer, fasting, and some dietary prohibitions, as well as frequent worshipful meditation. These practices may have not only spiritual purposes, but also many positive health implications.

Although Sufism generally is focused on spiritual development, some Sufi schools have focused on healing. This healing is a blend of Sufi philosophy and other Islamic healing traditions. Paranormal Sufi healing abilities have been observed and explained on the basis of a spiritual link mediated by the Sufi master back to the Prophet and Allah. Such phenomena from the Sufi way do not appear to result from meditative or altered states of consciousness but may be caused by a higher consciousness.

The implications of Sufism for integrative health is that Western high-tech medicine can be helpful for medical and surgical emergencies but may not be as helpful for chronic non–life-threatening conditions. What is needed today is a blending of "high tech" with "high touch." Sufism is one of the least-studied approaches that offered an integration of eras I, II, and III of medicine.

The Sufi way is the universal path for spiritual traditions, including prayer, fasting, and meditation; avoidance of intoxicants, pork, and sex outside marriage; engagement in jihad (or battle against the lower self); and ultimate attainment of nearness to the God (Allah). Dossey (2001) anticipated the "respiritualization of medicine" when he noted the following:

Modern medicine has become one of the most spiritually malnourished professions in our society. Because we have thoroughly disowned the spiritual component of healing, most healers throughout history would view our profession today as inherently perverse. They would be aghast at how we have squeezed the life juices and the heart out of our calling. Physicians have spiritual needs like anyone else, and we have paid a painful price for ignoring them. It simply does not feel good to practice medicine as if the only thing that matters were the physical; something feels left out and incomplete. (p. 242)

Acknowledgments

Thanks go to Jeanie Hall, PhD, Lillian Hawkins, and Hadele Banna for their comments on earlier drafts of this chapter.

⊖ Chapter References can be found on the Evolve website at http://evolve.elsevier.com/Micozzi/complementary/

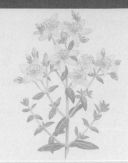

CHAPTER

34

INDIGENOUS KNOWLEDGE SYSTEMS: SOUTHERN AFRICAN HEALING

MARIANA G. HEWSON

This section completes the text, providing a similar presentation of traditional ethnomedical systems, as did Section Five, for Africa and the Americas. The section concludes with a summary of the global dimensions of what in the United States is called alternative complementary medicine but which, according to the World Health Organization (WHO), represents primary care for 80% of the world's people. In an effort to "cover the globe," some of these healing systems are based on historically documented "classical" systems of medicine continuously in practice since antiquity (as with Chinese and Ayurvedic medicine, for example). Others are best described using an essentially ethnographic approach of description and observation of what is currently being practiced in the world around us (as with much of traditional healing in Africa and the Americas). Please refer to the Evolve site at http://evolve.elsevier.com/Micozzi/complementary for an appendix on Native American Medical Plants. ∾

We waited patiently for the healer to call us for the interview. The waiting room was small, containing only six chairs and a dresser.

Prepared with the specified money and gift, we reviewed our questions, how the interpretation would be handled, and how our notes would be taken. Eventually, the traditional healer appeared in full regalia: copious strands of white beads around her neck, wrists, and ankles; decorative strands of animal skins hanging from her waist; her legs clad in animal skins decorated with beads, shells, and beer bottle tops; and an impressive headdress (much like a bishop's miter) made of cowhide. She had several ceremonial tools, highly decorated with intricate beadwork: a fly whisk (made of a cow tail) to signify the healer's status, a long-handled spear for slaughtering animals, and a smoking pipe and drum that she used to contact ancestral spirits. Two younger apprentices in more modest dress stayed close at her side and ministered to her needs. To initiate my interview, I put the required fee (about $20) plus a gift on the floor of the waiting room. One of the apprentices burned a local dried plant, bepo, in an open dish, and the master healer ceremonially smoked her long pipe to invoke the spirits to be present in our conversation. She tipped a little ash onto the money and gifts to bless them, a necessary part of developing our relationship.* ∽

*This interview was one of eight similar interviews with female traditional healers in southern Africa. (Hewson, In preparation.)

This chapter outlines the professional components of traditional African healing based on interviews with traditional healers (Hewson, 1998). The value of studying a phenomenon outside of one's own culture is to identify aspects of one's own culture that are not readily apparent to those who practice within that culture (see Chapter 5).

PROFESSIONALISM AND THE HEALING ARTS

Is traditional African healing a profession? In the Western view the medical profession consists of specialists who diagnose and prescribe in areas that draw on comprehensive knowledge and skills that transcend those available to non-specialists. Education for the professions involves questions about legitimate knowledge, license to practice, arrangements for providing services, entry to education and training, the curriculum offered, standards of achievements, and assessment (Goodlad, 1984). Similarly, Cassidy describes professional considerations of a health care system in Chapter 5 of this volume. Following Cassidy's categories, I discuss (1) the explanatory model of illness that underlies traditional healing in southern Africa, (2) the educational process of healers, (3) the professional accreditation of the practitioners, (4) the professional organization of practitioners who monitor and maintain standards of care, and (5) the social mandate through which the community influences the provision of care. Finally, I highlight unique aspects of traditional healing that can transcend both the traditional and the allopathic system of healing.

EXPLANATORY MODEL UNDERLYING TRADITIONAL HEALING IN SOUTHERN AFRICA

CONCEPTS OF HEALTH, ILLNESS, AND HEALING

Traditional healing in southern Africa existed long before the arrival of modern medicine, and it remains an intact system of caregiving among many African people. This system of healing is shamanic in nature. The term *shaman* refers to medicine men and women, and *shamanism* is a methodology (not a religion) used to describe the practices of healers in the regions of central and north Asia. Shamanism represents "the most widespread and ancient methodological system of healing known to humanity" (Harner, 1990, p. 40). This practice, including assumptions and methods, occurs all over the world, in areas as diverse as Australia, New Zealand, North and South America, Siberia, Central Asia, eastern and northern Europe, and Africa. In this chapter I refer to healing practices found in southern African countries such as Botswana, Lesotho, Swaziland, Mozambique, Zimbabwe, and South Africa. In all these regions, the shaman is seen as "the great specialist of the human soul: he alone 'sees' it, for he knows its 'form' and its destiny" (Eliade, 1964, p. 8). Shamanic practitioners generally make use of "nonordinary reality" or controlled entrancement, to access the information they seek on behalf of their patients.

Africa, in particular southern Africa, is thought to be the cradle of humankind, but little has been written about the traditional healers of southern Africa. Traditional healers in southern Africa are not called "shamans," yet their practices are similar to those described by Eliade (1964) and Harner (1990). At present, their ancient practices coexist in a modern society that subscribes to and practices allopathic medicine. Despite regional differences throughout southern Africa, there appears to be a common system aimed at relieving illness and disease (feelings of being "out of sorts," or ill at ease socially and spiritually).

In the southern African view, illness is thought to be caused by psychological conflicts or disturbed social relationships with persons living or dead. The accompanying disequilibrium is expressed as physical or mental problems (Frank, 1973). Traditional healers believe that psycho-social-spiritual imbalances must be rectified before a patient can recover physically. Traditional healing thus focuses on psychological and spiritual suffering, as well as on physical suffering, and aims to correct the disequilibrium. Traditional healers view healing as the removal of impurities from the body or disequilibrium from the patient's mind, with the hope of reducing the anxieties it has produced. For example, a common concept of healing involves purification by draining the body of harmful substances, which results in wide use of purgatives and emetics. Healing also involves appeasing the patients' spirits (in particular the recently departed members of the family), who might be angry with the patient for some reason. Warding off bad spirits, such as the *tokoloshe* (a mischievous or evil spirit responsible for life's misadventures and accidents), the curses from living people, or the ill will of angry ancestral spirits constitutes a version of preventive medicine. Furthermore, in several southern African groups, such as the Basotho of Lesotho, the state of disequilibrium manifests in the form of being "hot" (not feverish) (Hewson et al, 1985), and treating people who are "hot" involves cooling with appropriate agents such as ash, water plants, or aquatic animals. These views are quite distinct from modern allopathic medical concepts of disease as the malfunctioning of physiological systems.

TRADITIONAL HEALING PROCESSES

Traditional healers hold an esteemed and powerful position in society, especially in traditional African societies, and their role is a combination of physician, counselor, psychotherapist, and priest. Traditional healers prevent and treat illnesses mainly with plant and some animal products in combination with divination. There are two types of traditional healers: those who are mainly herbalists and those who use divination. However, the distinction between the two is becoming increasingly blurred, and most traditional healers appear to practice both types of medicine. The majority of traditional healers are "called" to practice benevolently—their role is to serve their people. Sorcery (evil or malevolent actions for the purpose of harming others, e.g., for revenge) is practiced by some people in southern Africa but is not considered further in this chapter.

Traditional healers appear to work most successfully with illnesses that have a high psychological or emotional content related to envy, frustration, or guilt (Frank, 1973). In allopathic medicine, these might be called *somatic illnesses.*

Currently, healers also appear to concentrate on illnesses for which allopathic medicine has little effective curative power, such as stroke, tuberculosis, cancer, and human immunodeficiency virus infection and acquired immunodeficiency syndrome (HIV/AIDS). Traditional healers claim to be effective in helping to treat pregnancy, malaise, arthritis, and social problems, especially those involving interpersonal disputes. The healers seem to be increasingly able to distinguish between those illnesses that need to be helped by Western medicine (e.g., broken bones, hernias) and those that respond to traditional healing methods. The claims to heal illnesses such as stroke, cancer, and HIV/AIDS appear to relate to the psychosocial and emotional components of the illness rather than the pathological or pathophysiological conditions. For example, traditional healers make no claims to be able to deal directly with bacterial or viral impurities, but rather with the patient's ability to cope with and eliminate them. This view of healing suggests that if one takes care of the psychodynamics of illness, the body will heal. This is in contrast to the modern view that if one takes care of the body, the mind will heal itself (Hewson, 1998).

As part of the diagnostic process, traditional healers "throw the bones." The "bones" consist of a set of 10 to 15 items, such as bones and shells and various collectibles (e.g., dice, coins, bullets, domino pieces). These are usually thrown (like dice) in the belief that clues to the problem can be read in the configuration of the items. The bones are made up of an idiosyncratic collection of items that have attributed meanings, depending on the context and the meaning attributed by particular healers. Each item signifies an important aspect of a person's life (e.g., happiness, children, bad luck, ancestral spirits). The consistencies among these items are in the attributions for the items rather than in the items themselves. For example, a traditional healer from Mozambique had a red die signifying war (the country had experienced a civil war for many years), and a healer from South Africa had a bullet signifying death or misfortune (South Africa was, at that time, engulfed in violence).

Traditional healers use drumming and dance to augment the diagnostic and therapeutic processes. Drumming helps the healer enter nonordinary reality. Sustained dancing has the same effect. In nonordinary reality, healers use their dreams as manifestations of the higher wisdom of the spirits, especially their ancestors. The healers use their own spiritual powers, as well as those of the patient, to discern causes of the patient's spiritual, psychological, or social disequilibrium that cause physical ailments and bad luck. To encourage their own dreams, healers wash with herbal solutions, drink herbal potions, smoke a pipe, or use snuff (all of which appear to have psychotropic effects).

Healers prepare and prescribe therapeutic herbal remedies for their patients. A traditional healer must know the symptoms of a disorder and the conditions of the patient's life before prescribing a treatment. There is a lack of uniformity, however, about the prescribed remedies for particular illnesses. A medicine may be used for multiple problems. The actual prescription depends on the spiritual advice received by the healer through normal dreams and through the dreams of nonordinary reality or entrancement. Each prescription is driven by the particulars of the patient and the details of the situation in which the patient became ill. The lack of a systematic, generalized approach to healing promotes individualistic practices that often seem idiosyncratic to Westerners. This phenomenon is one of the reasons African traditional healing remains so baffling and inscrutable to Western scientists.

Traditional healers seek causes for illness from a variety of areas. The common areas concern relationships with family, friends, and people at work. Healers are especially concerned about disturbed relationships involving jealousy, anger, loss, grief, and resentment. They seek to identify possible causes of illness from the following situations: someone wishes the patient ill; the patient wants something he or she does not or cannot have; the patient has known or unknown enemies; the patient experiences unrequited love or loss of a loved one; the patient has an unfaithful spouse or partner; the patient longs for progeny; and the patient's ancestors (the "recently departed") may be displeased with the patient for some reason, known or unknown. The healer inquires into every aspect of a patient's present and past activities, focusing on behaviors that would be most likely to provoke conflict with others in the community or even internal psychological conflict (e.g., in personal values). This is a process of divination commonly referred to as "seeing." A healer must "see" forward into the future as well as backward into the past. The process is similar to that used by shamans around the world (Harner, 1990). Although southern African healers do make some use of totemic animal spirits, their emphasis is mainly focused on the spiritual forces of the recently departed family members. These ancestors are the source of key information and are powerful forces in the lives of their living family members.

If the divination process does not provide immediate answers, the process may take longer. In this situation the healer may say, "The bones are not talking today," and request subsequent visits. When healers cannot find an answer to the patient's problems, they will refer the patient to another traditional healer or to a Western physician. All healers are concerned with truth and trust in their relationship with a patient. If the healer discerns a lack of either, he or she will ask the patient to leave.

EDUCATIONAL PROCESS

SELECTION: THE CALL TO BE A HEALER

Traditional healers are "called" to become healers and need to be validated by the group's elders, who check whether the call is real or not. First, the future healer experiences an unusual, mysterious illness that does not respond to usual herbal or allopathic treatment. Some examples recounted by my respondents included heart problems, lung problems, abdominal pain, swollen abdomen unrelated to pregnancy, amenorrhea, problems with feet, dizziness, headaches, mental problems (e.g., forgetfulness), pains throughout the body, and "fevers that are not real fevers" (which may relate to the cultural metaphor of being "hot"; see Hewson et al, 1985).

The illness is often followed by dreams with significant, recognizable components. The future healer then asks his or her elders (e.g., parents, aunts, uncles, grandparents) about the dreams. If an elder recognizes the special components of the dream, the elder advises the future healer to consult a traditional healer. At the discretion of the traditional healer, the patient is then both treated and taken as an apprentice for several years. A traditional healer named Emily tells how she was called by her ancestral spirits to be a healer (Hewson, In preparation):

> First I was sick for a whole year, like I didn't know where I was, like becoming mad, my mind wasn't working properly. I felt pains everywhere and I didn't know what to do. I was forgetful. I forgot what I did the day before, like washing dishes, and I felt like sitting alone and no one should come near me. I went to the doctors and they could not see what the problem was with me. Then I had a dream. In my sleep I saw three grand people, old people, sitting next to me. One was holding a bible. My father's mother was holding beads in a dish and some bones—little bones—with two hands. And my mother's father was

holding a bible. They said to me I must wear a white dress. And I dreamed I was in this big hall and on the other side was a church. The people were dancing and preaching. And in the hall the *sangomas* and *nyangas* [widely used terms for traditional healers in southern Africa] were dancing and beating drums. And I said "What kind of a dream is this?"

> Then I told my aunty that I had this kind of funny dream. I described the old people and she said they really were my grand people whom I had never seen before in life. And she called another woman [a healer], and I told her this same dream. Then she took me to the river and prayed and talked to my old people [ancestral spirits] who are called *amanyangas*. And then she prayed there for me and I took the water. She made beads for me and put them round my neck, and then I was alright. I never got sick again.

A second healer, Elizabeth, described her sickness (headaches and fevers that were not really fevers) followed by a dream in which her ancestor came to her and told her to go to the forest to find herbs. This she did and encountered a man, sitting in the light, who instructed her. This dream was interpreted as being a call to be a healer. A third healer described her mysterious sickness and said that she went to consult a healer, who made a mixture of stringy roots mixed with a grated rhizome-like substance in water. A twig was used as a mixer, and this solution created a profusion of bubbles. The future healer was asked by her trainer to drink the bubbles, which induced dreams that "helped me see what I should do to help people." She used the same techniques for inducing the spirits in her apprentices.

To refuse the calling by the ancestors is to invite worse sickness, madness, and possible death. One healer recounted the story of a woman who had denied the call and had become "mad." A man in Cape Town, a renowned drunkard, believed he was being called to be a healer, but the elders of his family disabused him of this idea, saying that his dreams and sickness were the consequence of alcohol.

TRAINING

Training involves an apprenticeship, usually with a well-known master healer. If the master healer lives far away, the apprentices live in the master healer's compound (many small dwellings inhabited by extended family members) for the duration of the training. The art of the healer is thought to be transmitted through the ancestral spirits who speak to healers through dreams. Apprentices are encouraged to have dreams and to learn how to interpret them on behalf of their patients. Dreams can be induced by herbal potions, inhaled smoke, or snuff. As one traditional healer put it, "Through the dreams, your ancestors open your eyes to signs. I trust the dreams every time." Another said that anyone can learn about the practice of traditional healing, but "unless you have contact with the spirits through dreams, you cannot be a healer."

The master healer first demonstrates the use of herbs and animal parts and then teaches the apprentices how to administer them. Then, in a progressive weaning process, the master healer withdraws and expects the apprentices to perform independently. One healer described being taken into the bush by her teacher to find *muti* (medicinal substances, such as herbs, roots, and barks, and animal parts, such as hooves, bones, and horns) that are used for healing. She had to rise at 4:30 AM "because the spirits only come early in the morning." She had to prepare herself to obtain the muti by bringing on the ancestral spirits. This she did by taking an herbal bath, drinking herbal concoctions, beating the drums, and dressing in a special outfit.

The training process is strenuous and challenges the mental and physical strength of the apprentices. One healer said, "I went to the bush for many days with my teacher to seek muti, with only *putu* [cornmeal porridge] and black tea. It was hard to live like that, but it is necessary for nyangas to suffer because this kind of work is *swarig*" (Afrikaans word for "heavy" or "burdensome"). Because this process is so exacting, not every apprentice completes the training.

Apprentices help their master healers with patient consultations, seemingly acting as a team for the duration of the training program. On one occasion I observed an apprentice and master healer in a Lesotho mountain village who entered a trancelike state in which both danced with extremely rapid movements to the accompaniment of drums. In a trancelike state, they called on the ancestors and revealed spiritual insights to the assembled small crowd (Hewson, 1993).

PROFESSIONAL ACCREDITATION OF PRACTITIONERS

TESTS AND STANDARDS

Throughout training, apprentices are tested on their ability to find things, to identify and administer herbs, and to contact the ancestors through dreams to discern people's physical, psychological, or spiritual problems. Some of the objects to be found become part of the divining bones, and others are used as medicines. The items that are needed are often given to the apprentice by patients, friends, or family members in recognition of the demonstrated healing skills and power of the apprentice. The master healer may also help the apprentices find things they need. For example, one healer described how, on occasions, the very item she had been instructed to find would be given to her by someone, apparently in a serendipitous manner (McCallum, 1992). Another described how she went to the beach with her teacher and collected the perfect shells for her set of bones. Other objects must be gleaned from the countryside, found in the bush, or

purchased from stores that specialize in the healers' equipment and accoutrements.

Several levels of tests must be passed by the apprentice healers. Tests of competence may involve oral examinations. For example, one healer described how her master healer asked all the apprentices in her cohort "to stand like a choir" and to answer numerous questions. Then, each apprentice was asked to declare whether he or she was able to cure.

The final test often involves finding a hidden object. For her final test, one healer had to find an unknown object that had been hidden somewhere in the vicinity of a village (McCallum, 1992). The final test also involves "finding" the animal(s) that will be slaughtered as part of the graduation ceremony, such as a chicken, goat, or cow. The apprentice first dreams about the animal(s) and notes the color and the type of spots or other distinguishing characteristics. This dream is viewed as a message from the ancestors, and it must be followed to the last detail. The procurement of these specific animals may involve gifting by the apprentice's family, friends, or satisfied patients. It is an additional social accreditation that represents faith and trust in the apprentice as a healer. The apprentice can also buy the animals from a market, if none is given.

An apprentice graduates when the master healer is satisfied that he or she has passed all the tests (i.e., through dreams, the ancestral spirits have confirmed the apprentice's readiness) and the apprentice has paid the stipulated fees, including procuring the necessary animal(s) for slaughter. The master healer consults his or her own ancestral spirits concerning the sufficiency of each apprentice's knowledge and skills. When all the criteria have been satisfied, the master healer may give each apprentice a gift, such as a set of bones or a braided bracelet. Thus, both the teacher and the apprentice, and indirectly the community, assess the readiness for graduation. Patients also play a part in this judgment through their gifts.

More importantly, the ancestral spirits indicate, through dreams, when a trainee is ready. One healer explained that she knew that she was ready to graduate when she had a dream in which her ancestor (grandfather) "sent me to a *rondavel* [Afrikaans for 'small round dwelling'] that had a half door made of glass. There was a man standing behind the door who asked, 'What do you want here? I don't know what you are doing here any more.'" Then she heard the words coming from behind her, "Go and help people." At this point, she went through the final graduation ceremony, collected all her medicines and divining tools, and traveled back to her home, some 300 miles away.

Graduation often involves a final test of slaughtering an animal with the ceremonial spears. The apprentice drinks the animal's blood and selects various body parts, such as pieces of hoof or bone, to become part of his or her healer's tools (bones) or to be used as muti. For example, the skin of the slaughtered goat may be used as the mat for throwing bones, the animal's stomach may be used as a pouch for carrying other medicine, or a vertebra may become part of the divining tools. The rest of the animal is then consumed by the community to celebrate the occasion.

PROFESSIONAL ORGANIZATION: MONITORING STANDARDS OF CARE

CONTINUING EDUCATION

Traditional healers engage in meetings with other healers. One group described meetings that occurred on weekends, in which they would assemble, fully dressed in their ceremonial costumes (clothing, wigs, necklaces, anklets), to discuss healing matters, to share their latest healing stories, and to compare notes. The group may collectively criticize certain healers for dangerous or unwise practices. The regular meetings also include singing, dancing, drumming, drinking herbal potions, and engaging the ancestral spirits. These meetings are important social events in the lives of traditional healers.

The business of traditional healers includes their formal organization (South African healers are now organized and provide their healers with certificates), their practice in the context of new diseases (e.g., HIV/AIDS), and their relationship with Western medicine. The World Health Organization has recognized traditional healers in Mozambique and elsewhere, and traditional healers are being increasingly recognized and incorporated into the general medical system.

ONGOING RELATIONSHIPS WITH TEACHERS

Traditional healers typically maintain a lifelong relationship with their master healers, who serve as mentors. These relationships appear to be deep and profound. One healer from Maputo in southern Mozambique returned approximately once a year to visit her teacher in northern Mozambique. These visits were casual in nature, and the master healer might teach "depending on his mood. If he is not happy he doesn't teach anything!" This particular healer had trained five of her own apprentices, and she used the same methods as those used by her own teacher. She liked to teach, but reflected that to be a teacher, "You have to be happy all the time," which suggests that the essential relationship between teacher and learner involves enthusiasm and effort.

MUTUAL CARING

Mutual caring among healers becomes necessary under stressful or strained conditions, especially death. According to one healer, when a patient dies, the traditional healer becomes spiritually contaminated and loses his or her healing powers because the relationship with the patient has been broken, and the healer, of necessity, grieves. In this situation the healer removes his or her necklaces, ceremonial clothes, and artifacts and does not practice as a healer. This afflicted healer must be treated by another healer in a purification ceremony that restores the healing powers.

Being a traditional healer does carry dangers. One source of danger is that a healer may cure a patient of an intrusive spirit that has caused him or her to be sick, only to find that this spirit has entered the body of the healer. In such a case, the healer must be treated. Professional jealousies between healers concern access to patients as well as access to countryside where they collect their herbs for medicines. There are tacit agreements concerning the use of particular pieces of land by specific healers, but infringements are common. Healers thus may practice in a team context, which also provides them with a measure of protection in terms of the accuracy of their diagnoses and treatments. In addition, team practice helps protect a healer against the malevolent practices of other healers or sorcerers in this competitive field.

SOCIAL MANDATE: COMMUNITY INFLUENCE ON PROVISION OF CARE

Community control is exerted through remuneration and accreditation systems. Traditional healers are paid according to the type of service they provide. For straightforward dispensing of muti, patients pay over-the-counter fees for the medicines they receive. For diagnosis of physical, psychological, social, or spiritual problems, the patient must first open his or her pockets and pay a flat fee at the beginning of the process. This amount is prorated based on the approximate cost of one head of cattle and appears to be approximately one sixth of the total cost. When cured, the patient must pay an additional fee that appears to be independent of time spent or cost of medicines but is measured in proportion to the patient's satisfaction with the care, the cure, or both. Thus a moderately satisfied patient might provide a modest offering, such as food bought from a store (sugar, flour, or vegetables) or picked from a vegetable garden, whereas a highly satisfied patient might offer a live animal, such as a chicken or a goat. This offering would be ceremonially slaughtered at a later date. In urban areas, money is the usual mode of payment. The amount of money is often a loose translation of the worth of a cow, goat, sheep, chicken, or pumpkin.

For training services, an apprentice needs to pay a relatively large fee, equivalent to at least one head of cattle, and must also provide the animal(s) for the graduation ceremony. Apprentices are helped in paying the required fees by other people (patients, friends, family members), who pay or provide necessary items in proportion to their belief in the healing powers of the apprentice. This linking of the payment, patient satisfaction, and the accreditation process provides a complex system of checks and balances in an otherwise unregulated training system.

The healers refer to their own satisfaction in terms of "happiness." For example, one healer said that "to heal someone is to give life to that person," and when the person is healed, "both the traditional healer and the patient become happy." This happiness is manifest at a celebration in which the food offered is consumed in thanksgiving for the healing and for the continued goodwill of the spiritual beings whose power over the living is great.

UNIQUE ASPECTS OF TRADITIONAL HEALING

Differences between traditional and allopathic professionalism are summarized in Tables 34-1 and 34-2. Despite these differences, interesting phenomena characterize traditional healing and the professional training of the healers that are important to the fundamental, perhaps archetypal, contract between healer and patient.

SPIRITUAL CONTEXT OF HEALING

Spiritual powers are loosely defined within African cosmology as those spiritual powers that derive ultimately from God (within the African worldview) and that are present in decreasing amounts through the various levels of spirits of the ancestors (the forefathers) and the recently departed family members, living people, animals, vegetation (e.g., trees), and the earth itself (Mbiti, 1969).

Traditional healing relates to spiritual powers that are manifest through an integrated conception of body and mind at all levels. For example, in the call to be a healer, the person experiences a mysterious physical illness and has dreams that reveal a connection with ancestral spirits. In the training process the apprentice learns both the physical skills of an herbalist and the spiritual skills of interpreting problems through dreams that involve the ancestral spirits. When traditional healers graduate, the tests involve knowledge and skills in both herbal medicine and spiritual healing.

TRUTH AND TRUST IN THE HEALER-PATIENT RELATIONSHIP

The traditional system of healing in southern Africa is consistent with the worldview of the people indigenous to this region. This worldview constitutes a paradigm that emphasizes some ways of thinking (e.g., the body-mind connection) and deemphasizes others (e.g., the objective, rational scientific approach). To be effective, traditional healing requires that patients who seek healing within this paradigm must subscribe to it. Thus, traditional healers are cautious in checking the adherence of patients to their traditional African way of thinking. In addition, there is the "dark side" to this practice: malevolent sorcery. For reasons similar to those that make benevolent traditional medicine effective, sorcery is powerful and greatly feared. Traditional healers need to discern the

TABLE 34-1

Steps to Becoming a Professional in Traditional Healing and in Western Medicine

Step	Traditional healing	Western medicine
Call to healing	Mysterious illness, significant dreams, interpreted and sanctioned by elders in community	Individual, personal "call" to become a clinician, family suggestion, augmented by academic counseling
Selection of trainees	Based on mysterious illness and recognizable evidence of healing capability and spiritual power	Based on standardized test scores, essay(s), and interviews with medical school personnel
Training	Rigorous, prolonged, relatively expensive; emphasis on subjective witness of healing powers by patients and/or trainers	Rigorous, prolonged, expensive; emphasis on objective measures of competence designed by professional boards
Accreditation	Approval by master healer, community members, and guidance from ancestral spirits	Approval on basis of national test scores in certifying/licensing examinations
Continuing education	Regular and frequent meetings and celebrations with other healers, and regular ongoing communication with trainer	Regular and frequent conferences, with regulated continuing medical education accreditation
Professional relationships	Lifelong relationship with trainer and ongoing relationships with colleagues	Occasional mentors, ongoing relationships with professional colleagues, especially focused on research

TABLE 34-2

Characteristics of the Practice of Traditional Healing and Western Medicine

Step	Traditional healing	Western medicine
Concepts of curing the patient	Take care of the mind and the body will take care of itself.	Take care of the body and the mind will take care of itself.
Diagnosis	Use spiritual powers and psychological techniques involving nonordinary reality to "see" causes of spiritual, psychological, or social disequilibrium.	Use technological and scientific tools to recognize directly or indirectly the pathology or pathophysiology. Use clinical reasoning and evidence-based medicine
Prevention	Very important to ward off negative spirits and harmful circumstances.	Increasing importance of preventive medicine.
Treatment	Resolve disequilibrium and return person to harmonious state.	Treat the biological causes of disease.
Relationship to patient	Subjective, interpersonal involvement, counselor, confessor.	Objective, scientific, rational, clinical relationship.
Relationship to community and individual patients	Paternalistic relationship based on healers' spiritual and social status and reputation.	Paternalistic relationship based on clinicians' accreditation level, social status, and reputation.
Professional satisfaction and rewards for healing	Directly linked with patient satisfaction and monetary payment or in-kind gifts.	Indirectly linked with patient satisfaction; salary negotiated with health care organization.

intentions of their patients, and they are alert to desires for "dirty witch doctoring." If a patient is thought to be untruthful or distrustful, the healer will send the patient away.

PSYCHOSOCIAL MEDICAL MODEL AND INTERPERSONAL COMMUNICATIONS

Based on the central premises concerning the connection between body and mind and between the earthly and spiritual realms, traditional healing is a form of integrated biopsychosocial healing. The role of the healer is to "see" the cause of the problem that afflicts the patient, and this seeing includes spiritual dimensions. Healers pay close attention to the ways in which their patients describe their illnesses and to the contexts within which the illnesses occur. Healers concentrate on looking for signs that indicate the reasons for the disequilibrium that causes sickness. The holistic approach allows traditional healers to integrate body-mind phenomena and to provide healing, despite being extremely limited in terms of modern medical science.

PATIENT CONTRIBUTION TO ACCREDITATION OF PROFESSIONALS

In the training of traditional healers, patients have the opportunity to play a role in certifying the apprentice through the voluntary gifts they make. To the extent that patients believe they are healed by a particular

healer, they gift that healer. These gifts are often in the form of materials needed in the practice, for example, a special necklace or a medicine pouch. These gifts may be worn to signify the healing power of the particular healer.

ESTABLISHMENT OF LIFELONG, MENTORING RELATIONSHIP

Traditional healers in southern Africa appear to engage in lengthy apprenticeships with one master healer. Although the length of training may last from one to many years, the relationship with the master healer does not end at graduation. Instead, these relationships are treasured and maintained for life, which suggests that trainees benefit from the deeper, more sustained relationships, similar to those in traditional apprenticeships. The cross-fertilization of styles and standards of practice takes place at regular meetings of traditional healers. These gatherings can be seen as analogous to grand rounds and national and regional conferences.

APPRENTICESHIP METHODS

The apprenticeships of traditional healers initially involve being shown how to do things (e.g., to recognize herbs, to interpret dreams) through role modeling and coaching. As the apprentice become more competent, the master healer allows the apprentice more independence and takes on a role more akin to that of an evaluator, in which the apprentice is tested for knowledge and skills and for evidence of the power of healing. At the same time the teacher personally rewards the apprentice with small, highly desired gifts that are needed as part of the prescribed collection of accoutrements (e.g., divining bones, various medications). In addition, the apprentice might wear some of the gifts from the master healer as a visible testament to the healer's skills.

This apprenticeship style of teaching is effective in developing professional competence. It makes use of several teaching approaches, such as role modeling (performing so that the learner can see what the teacher does) and coaching (helping the learner by providing assistance as well as feedback). The strategies also include experiential learning throughout the training process, such as collecting and preparing herbs and animals for medicines and helping with all patients seen by the master healer. The apprentices are expected to do much of the work around the master healer's practice. This includes helping the master healer to dress in ceremonial clothes, which often involve an elaborate ensemble of beads, skins, necklaces, anklets, and headdresses, as well as gathering and carrying the items needed for healing processes.

HARDSHIP AS A NECESSARY PART OF PROFESSIONAL TRAINING

The training of traditional healers is strenuous because the practice of medicine is difficult. Healers are expected to lead a lifestyle characterized by a high level of personal and social responsibility, and their training is thus a test of physical and mental endurance. The requirement for this type of physical and mental testing is also present in the cultural initiation rites that take place at puberty for boys and girls in southern African cultures. Indeed, in Xhosa, the word for a healer-in-training is *mkweta,* which is the same word used for young boys and girls who undergo initiation.

SUMMARY

In the practice of traditional medicine in southern Africa and the training of these traditional healers, there are substantial differences between this tradition and Western practice and healers. Although traditional healers lack the science and power of modern medicine, however, they are highly effective in a way that has stood the test of time for 20,000 to 30,000 years. As in modern medicine, the knowledge and skills of traditional healers are based on empirical experiences, and interesting similarities exist in the professional training of the practitioners. These similarities may reduce the negative perceptions of traditional healers and offer possibilities for a synergism between the two traditions, with potential mutual benefits for both types of healers, for the training of these healers, and ultimately for patients.

Ⓔ Chapter References can be found on the Evolve website at http://evolve.elsevier.com/Micozzi/complementary/

CHAPTER 35

NATIVE AMERICAN HEALING

RICHARD W. VOSS

OPENING NOTE

Indian people are understandably wary of the written word. Some may criticize the inclusion of this chapter in this edition. This criticism is understandable, because often the written word objectifies understandings and can be manipulated outside the relationship in which the understanding was shared. This possibility is a concern and a risk in contributing this chapter to the fourth edition of *Fundamentals of Complementary and Alternative Medicine.* However, not to include a chapter on American Indian views about medicine and health care would also be a concern, because it helps perpetuate the invisibility of Indian people amidst the dominant social, political, and religious factions. The untold history of Native American people is a sobering context in which one must view contemporary concerns. The purpose of this chapter is to honor the continuing journey of understanding between medical science practitioners and traditional Indian medicine practitioners to see how these two pathways can help restore health to

people and bring about increased understanding—*wo'wa'bleza*—among peoples. This chapter is not intended to encourage "mixing" of Indian medicine with mainstream allopathic, or "alternative," medicine (as yet another example of so-called "integrative medicine"), but rather to emphasize the importance of respecting the integrity of each of these paths in bringing health and help to people in need.

> It is this loss of faith that has left a void in Indian life—a void that civilization cannot fill. The old life was attuned to nature's rhythm—bound by mystical ties to the sun, moon, stars; to the waving grasses, flowing streams and whispering winds. It is not a question (as so many white writers like to state it) of the white man "bringing the Indian up to his plane of thought and action." It is rather a case where the white man had better grasp some of the Indian's spiritual strength. I protest against calling my people savages. How can the Indian, sharing all the virtues of the white man, be justly called a savage? The white race today is but half civilized and unable to order his life into ways of peace and righteousness. (Standing Bear, 1931)

These words of Luther Standing Bear provide a sobering orientation toward understanding a pan-Indian perspective of medicine and health. Long before Columbus landed in what he thought was Hindustan, the indigenous peoples of the Americas practiced a highly advanced medicine that was effective in combating diseases then common in the Americas (Iron Shell, 1997; Little Soldier, 1997; Looking Horse, 1997; Red Dog, 1997; Standing Bear, 1933). These medicine ways emphasized the "right order of things" and viewed humans not as some higher intellectual being above lower animal and inanimate beings but as a kindred partner in the universe (creation), reliant on the other beings in creation for life itself.

The worldview of the new European visitors to the Americas, from the beginning, prompted misunderstandings and exploitation of the peoples they called *Indios*, actually a corruption of the Spanish, derived from Columbus's perception of the people he encountered in the New World. He described them as *"una gente en Dios,"* which literally means "a people in with God" (Means, 1995).

Tragically, this early perception of the natural peacefulness, harmony, and ease of temperament of these "Indians" prompted Columbus to conclude that "they would make excellent slaves" (Means, 1995). This set the stage for the subsequent historical events that led to the degradation of the indigenous, or natural, people of the Americas who were called *Indians*. The "natural" style of these people was to be perceived as "brutish" and "savage"(words that could have been taken from Thomas Hobbes in his description of seventeenth century European society [see Chapter 7]); their attentiveness to primal experience would be perceived as "primitive"; their understanding of the creation (all of the universe) as infused with life and spirit would be seen as "animistic." In all these assessments, what was "Indian" was evaluated as inferior to the European cultural standards, including advanced technology and "higher" (theistic) religion(s).

The single term *Indian* was imposed on the indigenous peoples of the Americas erroneously, because they were not a homogeneous group but rather distinct "nations" or "peoples" with different languages, beliefs, customs, social and political structures, and historical rivalries. The term *American Indian* is used today to talk about common values and a certain shared identity among many Native American people, and it is also used as the legal title of federally recognized tribes holding jurisdiction on reservation lands in the United States. The indigenous people of Canada and the Six Nations' People (Iroquois) preferred the term *Natives,* which is the official term used by the Canadian government to identify indigenous people. The terms *American Indian, Native American,* and *Indian people* are used interchangeably throughout this chapter, with an awareness of the historical and political complexity associated with these terms (Means, 1995).

HISTORY

To understand American Indian health care and approaches to medicine, one needs to get the history right and take a critical look at the "other" American history that most Americans were never taught, that was never included in their textbooks, and that continues to be glossed over in mainstream American classrooms—the largely invisible history of Native Americans in the United States. Non-Indian people need to learn both sides of American history, to understand the "bad medicine" that has infected relations between Indians and non-Indian people. Recall the interaction between Tosawi, chief of the Comanches, and General Sheridan (who had put the torch to the Shenandoah Valley of Virginia during the Civil War) after Tosawi brought in the first band of Comanches to surrender. Addressing Sheridan, Tosawi spoke his own name and two words in English: "Tosawi, good Indian." Sheridan responded with the now-infamous words: "The only good Indians I ever saw were dead" (Ellis, 1900, cited in Brown, 1970, p. 170).

Beyond the larger cultural-historical context, one also needs to consider the distinctive Indian tribal culture. It is important to know how each tribe dealt with its own survival in the wake of U.S. expansionism, policies of extermination, and level of exposure of each tribe to racial and cultural genocide. It is also important to understand how its tribal leadership related with the U.S. government and to assess the degree of broken trusts and treaties. With this background information, one can then develop an awareness of, and sensitivity to, the issues that have an impact on the consciousness and sense of well-being or disease and distrust of government and other social institutions by many Native American people today. One needs to be informed about the issues of loss of land and culture, repeated broken trusts, and unenforced treaties. One must be sensitive about the forced assimilation policies and programs, and depersonalizing attitudes directed toward Indian people, both formally and informally, by the U.S. government, missionaries, and other social institutions that were embedded in the "progressive American consciousness" and committed to civilizing and incorporating the Indian into this larger consciousness.

Although some Indian people claim to have benefited from their boarding school experience, the greater number of Indian people are beginning to speak out about the cultural trauma of the boarding school systems. Through assimilation programs, what was "natural" and basic to Indian self-identity was suppressed, discouraged, and literally beaten out of Indian people through systematic resocialization. Indian children were separated from their families and their traditional ceremonial practices, which were intimately linked to the extended family and reinforced by social, moral, political, and spiritual life, and introduced to what was perceived as a more civilized (materialistic) view of life, which devastated Indian society (Clark, 1997; M Clifford, 1997; Douville, 1997a; Little Soldier, 1997; Mestheth et al, 1993; White Hat, 1997). For Indian people, all aspects of life were intimately connected to good health and well-being. The interconnections among family, tribe or clan, moral, political, and ceremonial life all contributed to a sense of harmony and balance that was called *wicozani* (good total health) by the Lakotas and *hozhon* (harmony, beauty, happiness, and health) by the Navajos.

Traditional Navajo healing practices revolve around the notion of *hozho*, a term that embodies the concepts of balance, harmony, and spirituality. When people achieve a life of hozho, they walk the "Beauty Way," and their lives are filled with peace, contentment, and positive health—physically, mentally, emotionally, and spiritually. Positive interconnections among family, clan, tribe, nature, all living things, and ceremonial life all contribute to a sense of harmony and balance, which is the achievement of hozho. When a Navajo medicine man performs a healing ceremony, a circle of healing is formed by the interconnection among the sick person, family, relatives, the spirits, and singers who help with ceremonial songs. For traditional Navajo, the world is a dangerous place requiring due caution and respect; there is an emphasis on preventing harm from occurring through prevention-type ceremonies *(hozonji)* to better meet this dangerous world. Navajo healers *(hatalie)* use sand painting to cure the sick person. A very stylized sand painting is drawn using various colors of sand; on its completion, the patient is instructed to sit on the painting while the healing ceremony is performed. Healing takes place as the sick person absorbs the power or spirits that exist in the sand painting (Figure 35-1) (Edwards, 2004).

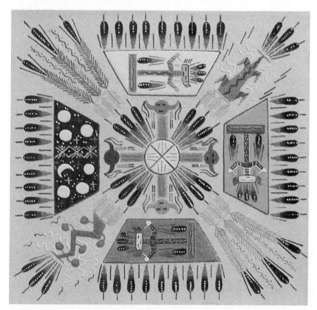

Figure 35-1 Traditional sand painting (Artist: Frank Martin). (Courtesy Penfield Gallery of Indian Arts, Albuquerque, NM, http://www.penfieldgallery.com.)

Case Study

Robert, a full-blood American Indian, has lived most of his life in a large metropolitan area. He was hospitalized in a residential treatment facility for depression, anxiety, weight loss, verbal and social regression, agitated moods, hysterical behaviors, and night terrors. During his hospitalization, these behaviors worsened, and he was noncompliant with the treatment plan, which included group and individual psychotherapy. Additional background included the following: Robert lived with his mother and two half-siblings; his mother was recently divorced from his stepfather; and Robert's father died 6 years earlier.

An urban American Indian social worker from Robert's tribe was called in as a clinical consultant to the hospital staff regarding Robert's deteriorating mental and physical health status. The clinical consultant met first with staff and then with Robert. In their initial meeting, Robert and the American Indian clinical consultant conversed in their native language regarding their parents, siblings, clans, home reservation areas, and cultural activities in which they both participated. They then talked about Robert's current situation, including his hospitalization, his separation from his family, and his fears. Robert believed that his father had been hexed (someone had placed an evil spell on him) and died as a result of evil forces associated with this hex. Robert also believed that these evil forces could be unleashed on him, and that he, too, might die.

The clinical consultant talked with Robert about the spiritual ceremonies that could be arranged for him on his home reservation to restore balance and harmony in his life. Robert knew and understood the significance of these healing ceremonies and was willing to participate with the clinical consultant in arranging the ceremony for him. The clinical consultant, an enrolled member of a recognized American Indian tribe, gave Robert an eagle feather and talked to Robert about the power and protective nature of the eagle feather, the value of his cultural healing traditions, and the importance of his native culture in restoring balance and harmony in his life. A healing ceremony was arranged for Robert on his home reservation, where the Indian medicine people were able to provide information and healing to Robert, effectively allaying much of his anxiety, to the point where he was amenable to participating in the recommended clinical treatment available at the hospital. The combined therapies contributed to a positive treatment outcome.

Native American Church and Peyote

The term *Peyote religion* describes a wide range of spiritual practices primarily of tribes of the American Southwest that have expanded into a kind of pan-Indian movement formally recognized as the Native American Church. Peyote religion incorporates the ritual use of

(Continued)

Native American Church and Peyote—cont'd

peyote, the small spineless peyote cactus *Lophophora williamsii,* into its spiritual and healing ceremonies. The peyote ceremony is led by a recognized practitioner who is referred to as a "roadman" and is sponsored by an individual or family requesting a ceremony, usually for some specific need or healing or to recognize some event, such as a birthday or an important life transition.

The term *peyote* is derived from the Aztec word *péyotl.* The Peyote Way religions have expanded their spheres of influence from an area around the Rio Grande Valley, along the current U.S.-Mexican border, to indigenous groups throughout Central and North America (Anderson, 1996).

The ritual use of peyote has roots in antiquity. A ritually prepared peyote cactus was discovered at an archeological site that spans the U.S.-Mexican border dated to 5700 years before the present. Other archeological evidence, paintings and ritual paraphernalia, indicates that the indigenous people of that region have been using both peyote and psychoactive mescal beans ritually for over 10,500 years (Bruhn et al, 2002).

The Peyote Way is a complex bio-psycho-social-spiritual phenomenon that encompasses much more than the pharmacologically active plant. The contemporary peyote practice found in the United States and Canada, and among *mestizo* peoples in Mexico differs significantly from the older rites that continue to be practiced by the Huichol, Cora, and Tarahumar peoples in Mexico (Steinberg et al, 2004). The forebears of the modern Native American Church were the Lipan Apaches, who brought the practice from the Mexican side of the Rio Grande to their Mescalero Apache relatives around 1870. From the Mescaleros it spread to the Comanches and Kiowas in Oklahoma and Texas. It quickly expanded to most of the eastern tribes forcibly relocated to the Oklahoma Territory. The quick spread from the Mescaleros to most of the Oklahoma tribes has been attributed to the loss of traditional religions because of oppression (Anderson, 1996).

The psychedelic properties of peyote are just one part of the whole spiritual package. "This is not to say that peyote does not facilitate visions but rather that it is only one influence in a total religious setting" (Steinmetz, 1990, p. 99). It is important to note that describing peyote as a "psychedelic," although accurate, is fraught with problems, particularly when the Peyote religion is studied outside its indigenous context. Here, one needs to differentiate the ritual use of peyote by indigenous practitioners, or roadmen, and Native American Church participants from use or abuse of peyote by curiosity seekers and experimenters who are simply seeking a "high" devoid of a ceremonial and cultural context. Peyote has

been described as both a psychedelic and an entheogen. Entheogens are chemical or botanical substances that produce the experience of God within an individual, and it has been argued that such drugs must be included as a necessary part of the study of religion (Roberts, 2002). Entheogens have also been defined as psychoactive sacramental plants or chemical substances taken to induce a primary religious experience. In keeping with this understanding, the complementary use of the peyote ceremony within the context of mental health treatment has been viewed as a form of cultural psychiatry (Calabrese, 1997). Other entheogens include psilocybin mushrooms and dimethyltryptamine-containing *ayahuasca,* which, like peyote, have been used continuously for centuries by indigenous people of the Americas (Tupper, 2002).

Mental health practitioners across several disciplines may view Peyote Religion and the Native American Church with some degree of suspicion, if not with downright skepticism. Mack (1986) discussed the medical dangers of peyote intoxication in the peer-reviewed *North Carolina Journal of Medicine.* Mack refers to the users of peyote as "the more primitive natives of our hemisphere" (p. 138) and gives repeated attention to details of nausea, vomiting, and bodily reactions which occur at doses that he failed to mention were 150 to 400 times higher than the ceremonial amount reported nearly a century earlier (Anderson, 1996). So there is need for reasoned and open discourse on this important resource and potential partner for the mainstream mental health practitioner.

Psychiatric researchers Blum et al (1977) looked at the mildly psychedelic effects of the peyote coupled with Native American Church ritual and exposure to positive images projected by the skillful use of folklore by the roadman. They found that these components facilitated an effective therapeutic catharsis. Albaugh and Anderson (1974) hypothesized that peyote created a peak psychedelic experience similar to that found when lysergic acid diethylamide (LSD) was used as an adjunct to psychotherapy in alcoholics. In a study of a group of lifelong drug- and alcohol-abstaining Navajos, Halpern et al (2005) found no evidence of psychological or cognitive deficits associated with regularly use of peyote in a religious setting. However, the placement of peyote, LSD, and other psychedelics on Schedule I of the federal drug classification has eliminated public funding of research into psychedelic drugs (Strassman, 2001) and has limited scientific inquiry into their effects. The current biomedical opinion on the efficacy of entheogens is that data are inconclusive (Halpern, 2001), but there is limited evidence that further study is warranted. Wright (2002) has suggested that those in the behavioral sciences should once again open their minds to incorporating mind-expanding substances in the psychiatric and psychotherapeutic treatment milieu. As science takes a more benign look at the

Native American Church and Peyote—cont'd

effects of traditional healing practices on brain chemistry, new pathways for treatment may be opened up for study and discussions about traditional indigenous healing methods may be renewed (see Hwu et al, 2000).

Acknowledgments to Robert Prue, enrolled member of the Lakota Sioux, for his contribution.

This case study illustrates a number of important components of the relationship between traditional healing methods and Western medicine practices relevant to this discussion. First, the clinical consultant was able to speak the native language of the patient and could comprehend the cultural significance of the problems Robert was facing, as well as the corresponding cultural resources available to address these problems in a culturally compatible manner. Second, the consultant was able to explain to the non-Indian hospital staff Robert's perceptions of his problems and desire to participate in a traditional healing ceremony. Third, the clinical consultant, as an enrolled member of a recognized tribe, was able to give Robert, also an enrolled member, an eagle feather (illegal for non-Indians to possess), which requires considerable generosity on the part of the giver and is a sign of utmost respect for the person to whom the gift is given. Fourth, it is important to note that regardless of the current residence or length of time Native people have lived off the reservation, identification with Native traditions and cultural practices may play a very important role in their construction of meaning in life events, as well as in their understanding of health and well-being. Finally, the case study illustrates well how Western medicine and traditional Indian medicine may complement each other in promoting good health and wellness among traditional American Indians living both on the reservation and off the reservation. (A version of this case study appeared in *Social Work: A Profession of Many Faces* [Edwards et al, 1998, pp. 477-478].)

For Indian people, life is like a circle: continuous, harmonious, and cyclical, with no distinctions. Medicine was a coming together of all the elements in this circular pattern of life. The circle of healing was formed by the interconnections among the sick person, his or her extended family or relatives, the spirits, the singers who helped with the ceremonial songs, and the medicine practitioner (Figures 35-2 and 35-3).

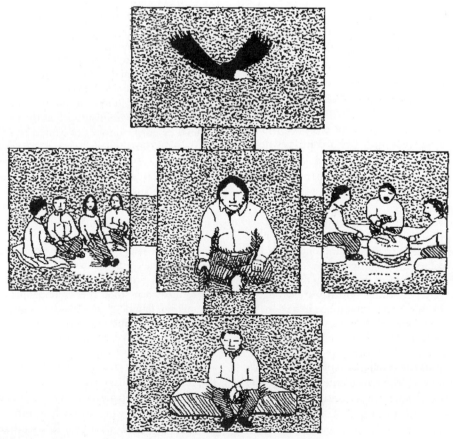
Figure 35-2 Spirits, relatives, singers, and sick person in the shape of two intersecting lines. (Courtesy Sinte Gleska University.)

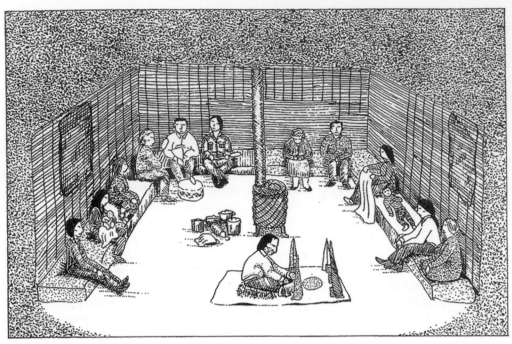

Figure 35-3 All of the elements from Figure 35-2 are depicted in this ceremony of the extended family in the healing process. The drawing shows a quiet gathering of people in a darkened room. (Courtesy Sinte Gleska University.)

Therefore, as ceremonial practices were suppressed and as government policies undermined the integrity of traditional Indian practices, the cultural fabric of Indian peoples was also torn. Official U.S. government assimilation policies forced many traditional Indian medicine practitioners underground for risk of being cited for committing actions prohibited by government regulation or being accused of "devil worship" and held up to public ridicule. Archie Fire Lame Deer and Richard Erdoes note, "Between 1890 and 1940, the Sundance, as well as all other native ceremonies, were forbidden under the Indian Offenses Act." They recall the following:

> One could be jailed for just having an Inipi [a sweat-lodge ceremony] or praying in the Lakota way, as the government and the missionaries tried to stamp out our old beliefs in order to make us into slightly darker, "civilized" Christians. Many historians believe that during those fifty years no Sundances were performed, but they are wrong. The Sundance was held every year . . . but it had to be done in secret, in lonely places where no white man could spy on us. (Lame Deer et al, 1992, p. 230)

Clyde Holler notes that the official ban on the Sundance began on April 10, 1883, with the enforcement of the Rules for Indian Courts; these rules were in effect until 1934, and the ban on piercing was in effect until 1952 or later, depending on interpretation (Holler, 1995; see also Commissioner of Indian Affairs, 1883).

Luther Standing Bear reflected on the profound shift that was occurring as he recalled his experience traveling to the Carlisle Indian School as a boy. He wrote as follows:

> It was only about three years after the Custer battle, and the general opinion was that the Plains people merely infested the earth as nuisances, and our being there simply evidenced misjudgment on the part of Wakan Tanka. Whenever our train stopped at the railway stations, it was met by great numbers of white people who came to gaze upon the little Indian "savages." The shy little ones sat quietly at the car windows looking at the people who swarmed on the platform. Some of the children wrapped themselves in their blankets, covering all but their eyes. At one place we were taken off the train and marched a distance down the street to a restaurant. We walked down the street between two rows of uniformed men whom we called soldiers, though I suppose they were policemen. This must have been done to protect us, for it was surely known that we boys and girls could do no harm. Back of the rows of uniformed men stood the white people craning their necks, talking, laughing, and making a great noise. They yelled and tried to mimic us by giving what they thought were war-whoops. We did not like this. (Standing Bear, 1933)

To this day many older Indian people are reluctant to talk about their traditional ways, and many middle-aged Indian people who were educated in the boarding school system were literally removed from their tribes and forced to assimilate. Resocialized in often abusive environments, many never learned the older traditions and their native languages. Often, students from western tribes were sent east to the Carlisle Indian

School in Carlisle, Pennsylvania, and students from eastern tribes were sent west (e.g., the Nanticokes of Delaware were sent to the Haskell Indian School in Kansas) (Clark, 1997).

Other Indians whose behavior seemed odd or troublesome were sent to the infamous Hiawatha Insane Asylum for Indians, also known as the *Canton Insane Asylum,* which was the only segregated asylum built exclusively for American Indians in the United States, located in Canton, South Dakota (Hoover, 1997; Iron Shield, 1992; Putney, 1984). This institution was opened in 1902 as the second federal institution for the insane (predated by St. Elizabeth's Hospital in Washington, DC, now long closed) to provide psychiatric care exclusively to Indian people by an act of Congress, despite opposition from the Department of the Interior and the Superintendent of St. Elizabeth's Hospital when the bill was first passed by Congress in 1898 (Iron Shield, 1988, 1992). Under the abusive administration of Dr. Harry Hummer, the institution would become the subject of a 150-page report filed by Dr. Samuel Silk in 1929 detailing the abhorrent conditions endured by the patient-residents there.

As a result of Dr. Silk's report, Dr. Hummer was dismissed, and in December 1933, after further study, the Hiawatha Asylum for Indians was closed and its remaining 71 Indian patients were transferred to St. Elizabeth's Hospital. Over the 31 years of operation, the asylum housed 370 Indians. There are 121 Indians buried on the grounds of the former asylum; the causes of these deaths are unknown. The asylum was founded "as a place to alleviate the suffering of mentally ill tribesmen from the Indian reservations; it ended as an institution that itself caused genuine human misery" (Putney, 1984). The asylum was turned into a community hospital in the 1950s and is now the Canton-Inwood Memorial Hospital. The Indian burial ground is now located next to the Hiawatha Golf Course, which sits adjacent to the grounds of the asylum in Canton (Iron Shield, 1991, 1994, 1997). Harold Iron Shield is currently leading a movement to identify relatives of those buried at the Canton (Hiawatha) asylum and is seeking to repatriate their remains to their respective tribes, when possible, and to preserve the cemetery as a National Historic Site.

Medical treatment and health care for American Indians was historically grossly inadequate and often seen as antagonistic to traditional Indian medicine ways. There was no supervision of agency doctors, and "not until 1891 were physicians placed in a classified service and required to pass examinations in addition to having a medical degree" (DeMallie et al, 1991). Charles Alexander Eastman, a Lakota Sioux Indian who served as an agency physician at Pine Ridge from 1890 to 1892, observed the practice of government-sponsored medical care. He wrote as follows:

> The doctors who were in the service in those days had an easy time of it. They scarcely ever went outside of the agency enclosure, and issued their pills and compounds after the most casual inquiry. As late as 1890, when the Government sent me out as a physician to ten thousand

Ogallalla Sioux and Northern Cheyennes at Pine Ridge Agency, I found my predecessor still practicing his profession through a small hole in the wall between his office and the general assembly room of the Indians. One of the first things I did was to close that hole; and I allowed no man to diagnose his own trouble or choose his pills. (DeMallie et al, 1991)

Physicians in the Indian Service had to use their own funds and gifts of money from friends to buy medicines and supplies. Drugs supplied to the Indians were "often obsolete in kind, and either stale or of the poorest quality" (DeMallie et al, 1991). In 1893, Dr. Z.T. Daniel recommended that the procedures for Indian Service doctors be reappraised, modernized, and compiled in serviceable form. He also recommended that an agency physician be sent annually as a representative of the American Medical Association, and he urged that Indian Service doctors be supplied with medical textbooks and medical journals.

In light of the inadequate health care provided to Indian people, it is important to keep in mind the decimation Indian people faced through exposure to Old World diseases. Henry Dobyns (1983) estimated that Native people faced serious contagious diseases that caused significant mortality at approximately 4-year intervals from 1520 to 1900. The pandemics affecting Indian people are often treated by white historians and others as types of "natural disasters," never intended by Europeans (Jaimes, 1992). However, Indian people are cognizant of their history and remember their oral history in which forms of germ warfare were related to have been conducted in military operations against them. One example often cited was the distribution of smallpox-infected blankets by the U.S. Army to Mandan (Indians) at Fort Clark on June 19, 1837, which was thought to be the causative factor in the smallpox pandemic of 1836 to 1840 (Chardon, 1932; Jaimes, 1992).

The shame caused by decades and centuries of efforts to "civilize the heathen Indian" has taken its toll on our American consciousness. One cannot begin to appreciate traditional Indian medicine ways without a profound awareness at a gut level of how much effort went into the eradication of what is now being perceived as "alternative medicine." This is the uneasy starting point of understanding traditional Indian medicine. Within this historical context, one can better perceive the basis for many Indian peoples' objections to the growing "popularity" of their traditional spirituality and healing practices among non-Indians—by the *wasicun.* This Lakota word described the early white hunter's propensity to take the fatty, choice portion of the buffalo, and leave the rest to rot. Buechel (1983) translates it as "one who takes things." This term is still used today to express Indian people's perception of the narrow, materialistic, and destructive worldview of mainstream white culture. Interest among whites in seeking out "Indian medicine men and shamans" and the resultant exploitation of Indian ceremonies (e.g., buying Indian spirituality in weekend or half-day workshops and seminars, paying fees for sweatlodge ceremonies) have prompted some Lakota leaders to issue a "declaration of war" against such exploitation (Mestheth et al, 1993). There are strong feelings about the contemporary curiosity of whites about Indian medicine ways.

WILLIAM PENN'S ACCOUNT OF TENOUGHAN'S SWEATBATH

One of the earliest accounts of a European observing an American Indian healing ceremony is in *William Penn's Own Account of the Lenni Lenape or Delaware Indians* (Meyers, 1970). The account portrays many factors relevant to understanding Indian medicine ways and the quality of interaction of Indian people with Europeans. The portion cited here is Penn's observation of a Lenape man named Tenoughan involved in a healing sweatbath (Figure 35-4).

> I called upon an Indian of Note, whose Name was Tenoughan, the Captain General of the Clan of Indians of those Parts. I found him ill of a Fever, his Head and Limbs much affected with Pain, and at the same time his Wife preparing a Bagnio for him: The Bagnio resembled a large Oven, into which he crept, by a Door on the one side, while she put several red hot Stones in a small Door on the other side thereof, and fastened the Doors as closely from the Air as she could. Now while he was Sweating in this Bagnio, his Wife (for they disdain no Service) was, with an Ax, cutting her Husband a passage into the River, (being the Winter of 83 the great Frost, and the Ice very thick) in order to the Immersing himself, after he should come out of his Bath. In less than half an Hour, he was in so great a Sweat, that when he came out he was as wet, as if he had come out of a River, and the Reak or Steam of his Body so thick, that it was hard to discern any bodies Face that

stood near him. In this condition, stark naked (his Breech-Clout only excepted) he ran into the River, which was about twenty Paces, and duck'd himself twice or thrice therein, and so return'd (passing only through his Bagnio to mitigate the immediate stroak of the Cold) to his own House, perhaps 20 Paces further, and wrapping himself in his woolen Mantle, lay down as his length near a long (but gentle) Fire in the midst of his Wigwam, or House, turning himself several times, till he was dry, and then he rose, and fell to getting us Dinner, seeming to be as easie, and well in Health, as at any other time (Surveyor General Thomas Holme's letter, dated 5th Month [May] 7, 1688, concerning the running of a survey line). (Meyers, 1970)

Penn made this observation when he was on a surveying expedition of the "farthest northern region of his Provence," which was actually near Monocacy, Berks County, Pennsylvania, today about a 45-minute commute from Philadelphia. The river would be the Schuylkill River, now polluted by a century of industrial contaminants and washoff from coal mines and agriculture farther north. This old account provides a powerful illustration of the cultural chasm that separated Penn from Tenoughan's world of medicine and health care. This story conveys the tremendous gap in appreciating what was happening during the observation. Penn was intent on buying land from the Lenape people, so it was on an economic venture that he stumbled on a healing bath taken by Tenoughan, a Lenape leader of some stature.

The story provides a model for understanding the complexity and the obstacles that confront non-Indian people, embedded in Eurocentrism, who do not comprehend Indian medicine ways. Penn was struck by the exotic and the unusual nature of the event he witnessed, as well

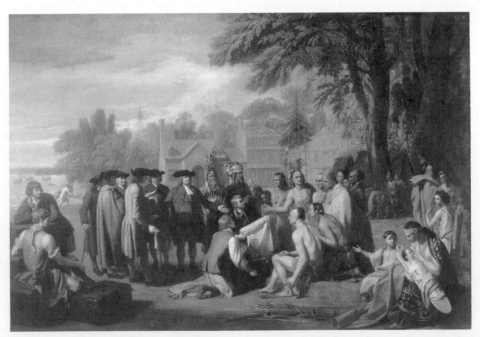

Figure 35-4 Benjamin West's painting of William Penn's treaty with the Indians. (Courtesy Pennsylvania Academy of the Fine Arts, Philadelphia, gift of Mrs. Joseph Harrison, Jr.)

as the apparent efficacy of the sweatbath on Tenoughan, but the observation lacks any description of a real personal encounter between Penn and Tenoughan, although we read that *Tenough* served dinner for his guests after the sweatbath. As old and as minimally detailed as is this account, it provides a number of important insights into American Indian medicine and health care.

First, the sweatbath was located near Tenoughan's home. It was familiar—literally in his backyard. Second, the practice included the assistance of a family member, Tenoughan's wife, who actually prepared the sweatbath for him, carried the red hot stones into the bagnio, and assisted in closing the door securely. Much of Indian medicine is family oriented; it is not something that is done by strangers. Medicine is a family matter; family is intimately involved and plays a significant role in the healing process. Later, Tenoughan's wife assisted in the arduous task of cutting a path through the ice for the "patient" to plunge into the river. Indian medicine often brings the patient into close interaction with the natural world and the elements. After the sweatbath, Tenoughan rests by the fire in his wigwam, and he then serves dinner to his guests. For many Indian people, stone, fire, air, water, food, spirits, and social and familial relationships are seen as medicine.

CULTURE

Sutton and Broken Nose cite a powerful clinical vignette about how cultural differences can create real tension between the expectations of clinical practitioners from the dominant culture and Indian sensibilities and practices. Although they cite the experience of a social worker sent to run an alternative school program on a Montana Indian reservation, the setting could be any health care or service-oriented setting. The vignette is quoted in the following:

> One day I came into work and no one was there. There were no teachers, students, or counselors. At first I thought it was Saturday or some holiday I had forgot about. I checked my calendar and the one the tribe printed to see if it was some special kind of Indian holiday, but it was not. Finally, I went riding around in my car. I saw one of the counselors and asked where everyone was. He said Albert Running Horse had died. I found out later that Albert was one of the oldest men in the tribe and was somehow related to almost everyone at school. When I tried to find out when everyone would be back at work, I couldn't get a definite answer because they weren't sure when some of Albert's relatives would come in from out of state. I was upset because I felt we had been making progress with some particularly difficult cases. I was concerned about the continuity of therapy and the careful schedule we had all worked out. When I expressed my frustration to one of my counselors she just shrugged her shoulders and said we all have to grieve. All I could think of is how am I going to explain this to my superiors. (McGoldrick et al, 1996)

This example illustrates the fundamental difference in worldview between Indian and non-Indian Americans and presents a common clinical dilemma that is likely to occur when mainstream approaches to health care come up against the "natural" approach to healing and human relationships typical among Indian people. Which is the better medicine: following the prescribed treatment plan or attending to the sense of community loss and grief on the death of an esteemed elder? Health care practitioners need to look for ways to affirm and support the values, beliefs, and needs of Indian people. Conversely, these values, beliefs, and needs may well be the same for non-Indian people as well, but be denied in the face of economic expediency. Appreciating the impact of diverse cultures on medical and health care practice is essential and is perhaps the most important thing the health care practitioner needs to address in developing cultural competence with Indian people or with any group not often credited or valued by the larger, dominant culture.

First, the concept of "professional helper/healer" is foreign to traditional Indian peoples and has no precedent in prereservation Lakota society. The idea of paid professionals conflicts with the tradition that helping other people is a social responsibility for everyone, not just for a few. Professional or paid health care practitioners are often viewed with suspicion by traditionalists as governmental agents of forced assimilation. Along with government-sanctioned missionary activity, the legacy of Indian boarding schools, and psychiatric hospitalization, health care professionals were associated with oppressive social structures that were intended to "civilize the Indian." Thus, a Lakota-centric view of health care starts with the awareness of the power of the institutionalized systems (e.g., social, health care, educational systems) to influence and assert social control, which although aimed at "improved health care" or social well-being, may also reflect and enact the larger, more pervasive oppression of racist attitudes, policies, and procedures for "civilizing the Indian."

Although no permanent or paid professional "health care providers" were among the Lakota bands or tribes in prereservation days, various individuals, groups, and societies within Lakota bands provided health care to the people. In effect, every tribal member was expected to follow the "natural law of creation," or the *wo'ope*, the unwritten natural law that guides Lakota life, which emphasizes unselfishness and generosity. The wo'ope embodies the philosophy of *mitakuye oyas'in*, which, according to White Hat "is what keeps us together." It is the knowledge "that we come from one source, and we are all related." However, to make this work, "we must identify the good and evil in us, and practice what is good" (White Hat, 1997). Lakota philosophy does not separate good and evil, sickness and health, or right and wrong as distinct realities, they coexist in each person, in every creation; even in the most sacred thing there is good and evil. The important thing is to understand that there is the negative and the positive within everyone and everything, and to be responsible in one's life to live in a good, moral, healthy way, in balance with all creation.

The natural law is the way nature acts. Understanding Lakota philosophy begins with understanding the natural law or the seven laws of the Creator (Iron Shell, 1997; Looking Horse, 1997; Lunderman, 1997). The natural law or the wo'ope required each person to exercise shared values, which, if acted on in one's life, gave the person as well as the extended family *(tios'paye)* and the tribe *wicozani*, which was understood as total or perfect health, balance and harmony, good social health, and well-being (Iron Shell, 1997); it implies physical and spiritual health (White Hat, 1997).

Another orienting value of helpers and healers among the Lakotas is *nagi'ksapa* or self-wisdom, the awareness of your aura or spirit (Iron Shell, 1997). Albert White Hat, Sr. (1997) translates and explains the nagi'ksapa as "one's spirit, the wise spirit in a person." White Hat notes that "the Lakotas are very much aware of the spirit within [us]—we talk to our spirit—we ask our spirit to be strong and to help us in our decisions" and life. *Iha'kicikta* is the ability to look out for one another. If you move camp, you should be concerned that everyone is going to move together. You want to make sure there is enough water and food for everyone (Iron Shell, 1997). *Wo'onsila* is the ability to have pity on each other (Iron Shell, 1997). White Hat explains the word as "recognizing a specific need of someone or something, and you address that (specific) need." According to White Hat, Lakota philosophy does not encourage people to "stay stuck" or dependent. *Iyus'kiniya* is the ability to go do things with a happy attitude (Iron Shell, 1997). *Wi'ikt ceya* is the measure of wealth by how little one has; it is the capacity to give to others; it is one's capacity for self-sacrifice (Iron Shell, 1997). *Teki'ci'hilapi* is the ability to cherish, esteem, and treasure each other (Iron Shell, 1997). Putting into practice these social values ensured good social functioning.

The primary orientation of traditional Indian medicine was universalistic. Health and welfare resources were made available to everyone through the family and community. Prereservation Lakota society emphasized tribalism over individualism, social harmony over self-interest, and a commitment or loyalty to the people or the larger extended family relations over individual success. Health care functions were accomplished by one's extended family (tios'paye); it was the extended family that provided for the social support and material assistance of all its members. Wealth was distributed through the practice of the giveaway ceremony *(wopila)*, which is still practiced by traditional Lakotas. This practice ensured that no one person's or one family's wealth or resources dominated.

Mental health and physical health were viewed as inseparable from spiritual and moral health. The good balance of the one's life in harmony with the wo'ope, or natural law of creation, brought about wicozani, or good health, which was both individual and communal. Rather than viewing the individual as a mind-body split, which

has influenced much of Western psychiatric thinking, traditional Lakota philosophy viewed the individual person as an unexplainable creation with four constituent dimensions of self. The *nagi* is one's individual soul; Buechel (1983) translates the word as "the soul, spirit; the shadow of anything, as of a man *(wicanagi)* or of a house *(tinagi)*." The *nagi la* is the divine spirit immanent in each human being. The *niya*, or "the vital breath," gives life to the body and is responsible for the circulation of the blood and the breathing process. The fourth element of the person is the *sicun*, or intellect (Goodman, 1992, p. 41). Albert White Hat, Sr., however, describes the sicun as "your (spirit's) presence [that] is felt on something or somebody." Beuchel (1983) translates the word as "that in a man or thing which is spirit or spiritlike and guards him from birth against evil spirits." Often a person appeals to his or her nagi la for assistance. This is a power within each person that can help him or her overcome obstacles. When one goes on the *hanbleceya*, or pipe fast, one leaves the physical world as a nagi.

According to Gene Thin Elk, "We are not humans on a soul journey. We are nagi, 'souls,' who are making a journey through the material world" (Goodman, 1992). The nagi la has been described as the "little spirit," which is the "divine spirit immanent in each being" (Goodman, 1992). Existence in the material world is tenuous for the newborn, according to Lakota philosophy: Edna Little Elk commented, "The most important things for infants and little children are to eat good, sleep good and play good," and doing so persuades the nagi of the child to become more and more attached to its own body (Goodman, 1992). Traditional Lakota philosophy views abuse, rejection, or neglect as affecting the child's nagi, which may detach from the child's body and not come back. In this case, ceremonies are conducted by a medicine man to find the child's nagi and bring it back (Goodman, 1992). Such a condition has been called *soul loss*. Thus, good mental or emotional health is intimately related to good spiritual, moral, and physical health; these cannot be separated out. (See the Evolve site for a discussion of Native American herbs and medicinal plants.)

CONTRIBUTIONS OF INDIAN PEOPLE TO MEDICINE AND HEALTH CARE

Despite the fact that Native American people have ancient oral traditions of healing and helping tribal members in need during reservation times, prereservation times, and the traumatic transition periods in between (Douville, 1997a; Lunderman, 1997; Red Dog, 1997), much of the health care literature reviewed focused on practice issues concerning Native American people and viewed them primarily as a special client or health care risk group in need of a specialized approach to treatment (DuBray, 1985, 1992; Garrett et al, 1994; Good Tracks, 1973; Williams et al,

1996). This literature generally treats "Native Americans" as a generic, homogeneous group and does not examine specific tribal traditions or practices of help and healing.

DuBray calls for a more holistic approach to treatment intervention based on Native American (Lakota) practices. DuBray (1992) discusses the use of the vision quest, the importance of food as a symbol of love and respect, the role of cultural healing ceremonies, and the importance of the collective unconscious in Indian experience of reality. The contributions of Native American practices, philosophies, and traditions of help and healing have also been discussed in anthropological studies (Wallace, 1958), rehabilitation medicine (Braswell et al, 1994; Hodge, 1989), nursing (Reynolds, 1993; Turton, 1995), and psychiatric literature (Garro, 1990; Hammerschlag, 1988, 1992; Lewis, 1982, 1990). There is a growing use of traditional medicine ways in alcohol treatment programs for American Indians, both on and off the reservation (Hall, 1985, 1986; Red Dog, 1997; Thin Elk, 1995a, 1995b, 1995c), as well as in health programs for Indian children and youth (e.g., Healthy Nations Program of the Cheyenne River Sioux tribe) (Red Dog, 1997).

The timing is ripe for health care and medical educators to look carefully at how native practices, traditions, and values can shape theory, practice, and policy at a foundational level. This is particularly important as tribal governments develop strategies and responses to welfare reform with the implementation of the Temporary Assistance to Needy Families (TANF) program, which is being met with great concern by many Native American tribal leaders and health care providers (Goldsmith, 1996).

ORIENTING CONCEPTS TO INDIAN MEDICINE

In a report to the National Institutes of Health, *Alternative Medicine: Expanding Medical Horizons* (1992), the Lakotas (Sioux tribe) were cited for the use of healing ceremonies by specialists who are essentially shamanic in their approach to treatment.(The use of the term *shamanic* for Native American healers is not ethnographically precise because the term was coined for the peoples of Trans-Siberia, notwithstanding the Bering Strait land bridge of the Ice Age.) Although the report cites key ceremonies and practices used by healers and helpers, the report shows a number of important inaccuracies in addition to the use of the term *shaman*, which now has been perpetrated throughout the CAM community. To understand Indian medicine ways, one cannot rely solely on written accounts. Although written ethnographical studies may provide a wealth of descriptive data, it is best to talk to authoritative sources personally.

Although the sweatlodge, Sundance, and vision quest are all used by Lakotas for health, help, and healing, not all were always conducted by "medicine women" or "medicine men." The report tends to project an exclusivity of these ceremonies, when in fact there is considerable variation and scope for these practices, most of which were family oriented (Douville, 1997b).

The sweatlodge or "purification ceremony," for example, is very common and may be conducted by anyone who has "been on the hill" or completed the *hanbleceya*, often called the vision quest (Figure 35-5). Although the

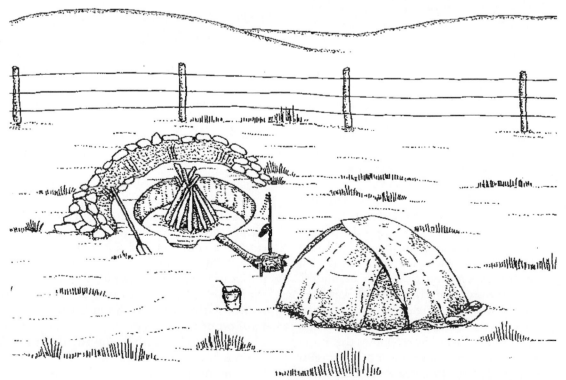

Figure 35-5 Sweatlodge. (Courtesy Sinte Gleska University.)

English name emphasizes the physiological reaction of the sweat, this ceremony of the common man (Lakota *ikce wicasa*), it is really an encounter with one's spiritual self and one's spirit relatives. This is a purification that "gives life" (*inipi'kogapi,* "that which gives life") to the participants and represents a form of rebirth. It is a family-oriented ceremony and is an integral part of all other Lakota ceremonies. Participants enter a small lodge made of willow saplings (for support) and covered with heavy, darkening canvas. Between 7 and 16 or more red hot stones are brought into this little lodge, which can be 10 to 15 feet in diameter. The stones represent the "first creation" and have deep spiritual meaning in this ceremony. Water is poured over the stones by someone who is permitted to conduct this ceremony, and the steam from this generates intense heat. There is deep spiritual significance to this.

Family members usually participate in this ceremony on a regular basis. Often, sweatlodges are located behind people's homes. There is a prohibition that excludes menstruating women from ceremonies out of respect for the ceremony the woman's body is undergoing (i.e., menstruation, which is seen by Lakota people as a purification with its own proper spiritual power). This is often viewed by white culture as discriminatory, but the tradition is not intended to be discriminatory. It is an affirmation of the natural feminine power, which white culture tends to minimize, often viewing menstruation as a handicap or a problem (e.g., premenstrual syndrome).

There are also different types of "medicine" people among the Lakotas. It is difficult to generalize about the diverse functions using the English term "medicine man" or medicine woman." The Lakotas practiced common medicines that included the use of herbal remedies known to families, whose primary medical care was prevention and geared to building up the immune system (Douville, 1997b). The various common medicines included teas, ointments, and smudging (smoke from burning certain herbs, such as prairie sage or "flat cedar"). This first line of medical care was performed by knowledgeable family members or friends. When required, more spiritual consultations were sought from a shaman medicine man or an interpreter for the *wakantanka* (the great mystery in all creation), which represents sacred medicine.

A "ceremony" could be requested by the patient and was usually held at night with family members, close friends, and singers (see Figure 35-3). Usually the patient presented a sacred pipe to the medicine man, who would smoke it if he accepted the request. The ceremony (which was usually described as a *lowanpi* or a spirit ceremony) took place in a darkened room in the home. All furniture was removed, and the windows were covered. Certain ceremonial objects were used (e.g., various-colored flags, tobacco offerings, earth). During the ceremony, the spirits instructed the medicine man or interpreter on what remedies would be provided by *Unci Maka* (Grandmother Earth) to heal the patient. This process was done with the support of the tios'paye, or the extended family, for the wicozani (good health) of the patient.

Along with these practices, family members actively participated in a ceremonial life that revolved around the wo'ope, or natural law of creation, which included the behaviors and attitudes for right living. The wo'ope is embodied in the philosophy of mitakuye oyas'in, which recognizes that all things, persons, and creations (both animate and inanimate, seen and unseen) are related (White Hat, 1997). These laws were not written down; they were learned through observing the creation. These behaviors for right living were reinforced by the ceremonial life of the extended family system, or tios'paye.

Health care was primarily an extended family matter. Medical care was common and free to everyone who needed it, because the herbs or materials for ceremonies used natural elements that could be harvested from nature's bounty. Although medical care was "free," it was not provided without cost, because in Lakota philosophy, when someone gives you something, you are expected to return it at fourfold the value. When treated by healers, the people who received help gave something back. The concept of receiving "something for nothing" is not part of Indian philosophy (White Hat, 1997). The Lakota philosophy encourages self-reliance *and* mutual relations. Something changed when white man's medicine became institutionalized in the United States, emphasizing intervention over prevention, the individual over the tribe or extended family, materialism over spirituality, and the physical body-self over the spirit-body-self.

TRENDS IN CONTEMPORARY INDIAN MEDICINE AND HEALTH CARE

Today, many of the old Indian healing traditions are experiencing a renaissance and are beginning to be viewed with a renewed sense of respect and credibility as an alternative and complement to more invasive or secular Western medical models of treatment (*Alternative medicine,* 1992; Hall, 1985, 1986; Thin Elk, 1995a, 1995b, 1995c). For example, on the Cheyenne River Indian Reservation at Eagle Butte, the tribal council approved alcohol treatment programs and delinquency prevention programs based on traditional methods and approaches to helping people with alcoholism, viewed as a problem with social, emotional, physical, and spiritual dimensions (Red Dog, 1997). These traditional methods include the *inipi,* or purification ceremony (popularly called the sweatlodge); the *hanbleceya,* or pipe fast (vision quest), and the *wi'wang wacipi,* or the gazing-at-the-sun dance (Sundance). The infusion of these ceremonies within the treatment process, collectively, has been called the *Red Road approach* (Thin Elk, 1995a, 1995b, 1995c).

A number of medical facilities on various reservations include medicine men as consultants on a formal and informal basis (M Clifford, 1997; Douville, 1997a; Erickson, 1997; Twiss, 1997), and the use of traditional ceremonies in health care settings is encouraged and respected (Erickson [Rosebud Indian Health Services Hospital], 1997; Richards [Rapid City Regional Hospital], 1997). Although the ceremonial burning of sage (a common medicinal herb burned for purification) had been discouraged in the past, hospital staff report increased acceptance of this practice and now arrange appropriate space for traditional ceremonial practices both within the health care facility and outside on hospital grounds (Erickson, 1997; Richards, 1997). One Lakota friend commented on his recent hospitalization at an allopathic hospital. He was visited by a medicine man, who placed a bundle of sage under his pillow. This made him feel better and showed how simple cooperation can be between allopathic medicine and alternative health care practices.

Rapid City Regional Hospital has initiated a Diversity Committee to discuss cultural sensitivity in both employee-administration and staff-patient relationships and credits this committee for improved retention rates of Indian staff (Montgomery, 1997). The Diversity Committee, which meets monthly, provides an opportunity to identify areas of cultural awareness, tension, and misperception, so that understanding across cultures can take place. Conflicts in cultural views and values are inevitable, but there are growing opportunities for understanding and joint efforts.

Mike Richards, discharge planner and liaison with the tribes at Rapid City Regional Hospital, noted one situation in which a Lakota client was discharged to his extended family. The plan was for the child to live in a tent in the backyard. This plan was challenged by the state social services department, which failed to recognize that it is not uncommon for Lakota children to share close space in the family home or home of a relative. During my visits and stays with Lakota friends, I might see many children from an extended family share a small space in the family dwelling or occupy outbuildings or tents on the family compound or community (tios'paye) during the summer months. Although this practice might be considered inappropriate based on middle-class white standards, it affirms the Lakota value of close kinship bonds and enjoyment of children and illustrates the "bifurcating-merging family structure," a traditional Lakota kinship structure that considered parallel family relationships (e.g., one's aunts and uncles as "mothers" and "fathers"). Close kinship among all family members was reinforced by this family structure, whereby households and family resources were shared generously (Douville, 1997a; Driver, 1969).

The mental health liaison to the tribe advocated the child's return to his extended family, and the plan was eventually approved. This case illustrates how simple cultural misunderstanding can occur when service delivery is not centered on the values, family system organization,

and beliefs of the traditional Indian perspective. Further illustrating this cultural insensitivity at a structural level is the fact that reservation housing financed by U.S. Housing and Urban Development (HUD) grants is assigned on a lottery basis and "invents" communities that are not based on natural, extended family relationships. This social invention (i.e., building housing developments and populating them on the basis of governmental criteria) often conflicts with the natural, familial basis of the tios'paye, or extended family system, of Lakota people (Lunderman, 1997). Such practices undermine the natural sense of community among Indian people and unwittingly create community tensions.

There is active cooperation between medical practitioners and traditional medicine men on Lakota reservations. Referrals are made both ways; medicine men will refer patients to medical doctors when they have exhausted their repertoire of remedies, and medical doctors will refer to medicine men when they have exhausted their treatment repertoire. The relations between traditional and medical health care providers appear cooperative and fluid. Antagonism between these distinct and complementary approaches to health care has subsided somewhat, although suspicions toward Western approaches to medicine remain among some traditional Indian people, which is understandable.

Whereas traditional Western psychiatric thought has emphasized the mechanics of the mind, traditional American Indian philosophy looks at the natural flow of the individual's spirit-body-mind-self in relation to "everything that is." The Lakota term *mitakuye oyas'in* is often heard during ceremonies, reminding and reaffirming the participants of their relationships to ancestral spirits, powers, and energies of creation and to their kinship relatives, or tios'paye, the extended family and community. All these elements are considered essential for wicozani, or good health. The notion of mitakuye oyas'in is consistent with family systems theory that examines the impact of intergenerational family dynamics on the present functioning of family members.

Shamanic traditions and healing practices are very active among traditional American Indians today and seem to be gaining ground after generations of official and unofficial prohibitions and sanctions. There is diversity among traditional Indian tribal practices. The Lakotas have been open and receptive to sharing knowledge and technology with other nations. Lakota medicine people rely on their spirit helpers to "give them permission" to treat people and conduct ceremonies (Holler, 1995; Little Soldier, 1997; Smith, 1987; Twiss, 1997). This permission is very specific; for example, a medicine man may be instructed to use certain herbal medicines for men only, women only, or people in general. The spirits work through the healer. The medicine man is only as effective as the spirits working through him. He is responsible and accountable to the spirits for everything. This is a serious responsibility that these healers accept.

Although many similarities exist in approaches to health and healing practices among American Indian healers (e.g., emphasis on prevention, involvement of family and community in healing ceremonies), important differences must be taken into consideration as well when treating American Indians. The best advice is for the health care practitioner to ask patients about their traditional practices, assuring them that the practitioner may not understand all their cultural traditions but that he or she is interested in learning about these practices and, perhaps most importantly, is willing to work in a collaborative way that incorporates traditional healing practices without dismissing them. Individuals who use traditional methods of help and healing need to sense that their traditions will be respected when they seek medical care in mainstream medical facilities, or they may not accurately inform their physicians about what traditional measures and remedies they are using to restore health, balance, and healing in their lives (Lunderman, 2004).

One of the most important trends in Indian health care today may be the concern about the impact of welfare reform on Indian peoples, along with the widespread tendency of individual states to reduce welfare rolls and move Medicaid services under managed care providers. An article in the *Journal of the American Medical Association* noted that American Indians know a lot about government program reforms. "If some people had had their way, Native American tribes would have been reformed out of existence a century ago. So it's not surprising that members of some 500 federally recognized tribes that remain are wary when talk in their locality turns to 'health care reform'" (Goldsmith, 1996, p. 1786).

At present, the Indian Health Service (IHS), a federally administered Indian health care program that is accredited by the Joint Commission (formerly the Joint Commission on Accreditation of Healthcare Organizations, or JCAHO), is facing severe budget deficits, overall receiving only 50% to 75% of what it needs to operate (Goldsmith, 1996, p. 1787). At the same time, IHS director Michael H. Trujillo, MD, MPH, reported that the service population has increased by more than 2% per year. Although there have been increasing federal appropriations for IHS over the years, the actual amount of "real money" has gone down. For many Indian people, the IHS is the only medical provider in their often-remote areas, serving a population with disproportionately higher incidence rates of diabetes and cervical cancer, for example, than the general American population. In the context of anticipated health care reform, Dr. Gerald Hill, the director of the Center for American Indian and Minority Health in the Institute for Health Services Research at the University of Minnesota, reminds health care planners of the statistic that, in the American Indian population, 31% of the people die before their forty-fifth birthday (Goldsmith, 1996). Indian health care remains at a critical crossroad. *Trends in Indian Health 2000-2001* (IHS, 2004) reports that the age-specific death rate for American Indians and Alaska Natives from 1996 to 1998 was more than double the U.S. white rate in 1997 for the age groups 1 to 4 years and 15 to 54 years. Interestingly, the only age group with a lower death rate than the U.S. white rate was the 85 and older group (p. 70). Recent evidence provides some reason for optimism in that the overall death rate for American Indians and Alaska Natives for individuals under 45 years of age was 28% during 1996 to 1998 (p. 72).

QUESTIONS FOR FURTHER DISCUSSION

In light of the growing interest in and expanding practice of traditional healing methods across American Indian communities, a number of questions deserve further study. First, it is important to note that, in raising these questions, the authors recognize the complex cultural context in which these questions are framed as they straddle the divide between Western diagnostic categories that relate to empirical facts and traditional methods of healing that relate to the subject's belief system and spiritual practices. Thus, what is being questioned here is not traditional spirituality, but the specific medical implications of certain physical activities, often part of the spiritual healing practices. These questions are raised for both Western health care practitioners and traditional healing practitioners to consider as both seek continuing understanding in promoting good health among all people.

Because diabetes is a leading cause of death among American Indian people, 291% greater than the U.S. mortality rate for all races (IHS, p. 7), the question is raised as to the effect of moderate, sustained, or prolonged fasting from food and water on the renal system. Some traditional healing practices, such as the hanbleceya (pipe fast, vision quest) and the wi'wang wacipi (Sundance), involve fasting from food and water from 1 to 4 days, and we still do not know the long-term effect of such practices on renal functioning. Traditional Indian people differentiate physical healing and spiritual healing; sometimes both occur during a ceremony, and at other times a spiritual healing may take place without a physical cure. A powerful example of this is the sobering account reported by Archie Fire Lame Deer (1992, pp. 186-188), in which a man with diabetes died while on a vision quest, having fasted without food or water for 4 days. Lame Deer noted, "Ron's autopsy showed that, besides diabetes, he had been suffering from three other deadly conditions. He had already been in the process of dying when he went to the mountain to leave this world in prayer" (p. 186). In this case, the individual faster was advised to take his insulin during the vision quest, but as Lame Deer later reports, "He had not touched his insulin."

Although this case may represent a rare occurrence, researchable questions can be asked, such as, What are the physiological effects of such prolonged fasts on individuals with early, middle, and advanced stages of diabetes?

Because practices vary among traditional healers in the use of fasting, other questions could focus on the effects on the individual faster of complete or absolute fasts, partial fasts from sundown to sundown, and partial fasts that include some liquid nourishment (e.g., herbal teas, medicines). It would be interesting to know which of these practices offers the best opportunity for physiological healing or cure. Some might argue that such inquiry is not appropriate for, or perhaps even disrespectful to, traditional healing practices. However, the authors also note the long tradition of holding so-called medicine men (and women) accountable to demonstrate their power in public ways before the tios'paye, or extended family or community. For example, the test of a true *heyoka* (medicine man) has been the demonstration of plunging his hand into a boiling hot kettle and pulling out the medicine for the people. This ceremony was (and is) conducted publicly and in full daylight. The witnessing community attests to the power and truth of the heyoka, so there are precedents for such demonstrations of efficacy among traditional healers.

Another aspect of these questions is to challenge any romanticized notion or exploitation of traditional healing, particularly among or by non-Indians, who may attempt to engage in such healing practices without the appropriate guidance or understanding. This is an extremely serious concern among genuine traditional practitioners and healers, and it has been repeatedly raised as an issue by the elders, traditional spiritual leaders, and others.

Ayahuasca: Master Healer of the Forest

The first time I drank ayahuasca I went into complete catharsis. I lost all track of time and I lost all control over my thoughts. Visions began to appear. I was suddenly about 5 years old experiencing very real traumatic childhood memories. Ayahuasca is said to completely shut down your conscious mind and take you directly to whatever issues may lurk in your subconscious mind. Ayahuasca took me straight to the deepest, darkest, most painful corners of my subconscious mind. All the dull, aching childhood memories that have shaped my life and that I have carried with me for so many years came back alive and came to pass.

My experience was extremely painful. I cried and screamed as I relived my past. As time seemed so altered, years and years of my childhood and young adult life passed in those few hours of the ceremony.... I definitely died on some level during my experience. I released so much pain that finally I was empty. I cried out, "I don't want to live! There's nothing left for me! Life is too hard!" With the release of the past I felt empty and lost. Physically, I became uncomfortable.

Drinking ayahuasca is said to be a purging experience. It is almost inevitable for people to either vomit or have diarrhea. I had the latter. However, after I physically purged, my experience became easier. My purge on the physical level mirrored my purge on the spiritual level. I suppose it was my higher self that kicked in right after my purge. Suddenly there was a voice in the back of my head telling me, "You can do this. You have the power now. You can live your life and find your happiness." All of the horror had passed and I was free. A burden had been lifted. At four or five in the morning the day after the ceremony, when the sun was beginning to come up, I finally snapped out of my trance. I was back to reality, feeling quite empty and lost. The next day, and the next few weeks for that matter, would be about processing my experience. I think the ayahuasca brought my life into perspective, helping me release old wounds and gain my power, and leading me closer to my life's purpose.

Writing about my ayahuasca experience is difficult. It is hard to explain how a little bit of tree bark can liberate a person from so much pain. As far as my journey goes, ayahuasca was a positive healing experience, but only the tip of the iceberg.... Shamanism and ayahuasca, I believe, are incredible healing mechanisms. My trip to Peru opened my eyes. There is so much wisdom in the trees and plants of the earth. (Personal communication from an ayahuasca patient and colleague, December 2008)

The preceding account of a personal experience with an ayahuasca ceremony told by a colleague is very similar to an account given by Kira Salak (n.d.), whose experience with an ayahuasca ceremony in Peru was videotaped by a National Geographic Channel film crew and published as a video exclusive in *National Geographic Adventure* magazine.

Field Research with Indigenous People on the Tambopata River, Peru

This author learned about the ayahuasca ceremony from a number of sources, including actual interviews with shamans who were active practitioners, patients who had positive experiences with the healing ceremony, and a patient who went to a "bad shaman" and "got lost" in the healing experience; an unpublished article, "Ayahuasca-Wasi: Proyecto de Investigación Shamánico Transpersonal" (n.d.); and Professor Mustalish, director of the Amazon Center for Environmental Education and Research.

First of all, it was clear that the "master healer" was the vegetation—the forest plants (including woody vines, tree bark, and herbs) that are boiled together to produce the ayahuasca, which is taken by both shaman and patient. The ayahuasca forms the spiritual pathway or the connection ("la conexión mágico-espiritual") between the patient and the shaman that enables the

(Continued)

Ayahuasca: Master Healer of the Forest—cont'd

healing to take place. The ayahuasca is a hallucinogen that often acts as a purgative and may cause vomiting and/or diarrhea; it is viewed as both a medicine and a cleansing agent. The concoction produces vivid hallucinations that reflect the power of the healing.

The ayahuasca ceremony takes place at the shaman's house, which is often located in the middle of the forest. The use of the *cha'pa'ka* (a rattle made from the leaves of certain forest plants tied together at the base, which forms the handle) is significant in this ceremony. According to a shaman, the shaking of the cha'pa'ka awakens the spirit of the leaves, and the sound (the songs) produced by the movement of the leaves makes the shaman and patient dizzy. The shaman then begins to dance with the shaking of the leaves. The sound of the cha'pa'ka also helps keep the patient from getting lost while experiencing the effects of the ayahuasca. It is the sound of the shaking leaves that helps the patient stay connected to the shaman during the ayahuasca ceremony. If one takes the ayahuasca medicine alone (without a shaman present) one can become lost or lose control. A real shaman provides control during the ceremony while the ayahuasca helps the patient to see his or her dreams. When the question was asked, "How does one know a real shaman from a fake shaman?" the answer was that the ayahuasca shows you this, "You see who the shaman really is." Of course, the outcome here can be either reassuring or devastating depending on the findings of the patient.

Clinical Applications

Clinical applications of ayahuasca are currently being studied by Jacques Mabit, director of the Centro de Rehabilitación de Toxicomanos (Rehabilitation and Detoxification Center) at Takiwasi Center, Peru. Mabit combines the traditional use of ayahuasca with psychotherapy techniques and holistic methods (consciousness-expanding techniques such as fasting, hyperventilation, and use of nonaddictive plants), largely in the treatment of coca paste addiction. The center is funded by the French government. Conventional allopathic medicines are not used (except in unusual circumstances).

Physical detoxification is accomplished through the use of medicinal plants. Conventional Peruvian approaches to addiction treatment are based on prison or military models, which have raised human rights concerns among health care workers.

All studies of the clinical use of ayahuasca have European or South American sponsorship, and the results of most are published in Spanish (Mabit, 1995; http://www.unsm.edu.pe/takiwasi).

Healing Ceremony

Although this author did not participate in an ayahuasca ceremony, when he asked one of the shamans interviewed to demonstrate a typical song used in the ceremony, the author was invited back to the shaman's one-room house later that evening. After a friendly conversation, the author was invited to sit on the edge of the bed as the shaman actually performed a healing ceremony on the author. The author was sprinkled with rose water as the shaman began to sing. The song itself sounded more like a bird's whistle. Smoke from a hand-rolled tobacco cigarette was also blown on the author at various times during the ceremony. The cha'pa'ka (leaf rattle) was used and proved to be a very significant part of the ceremony. As noted earlier, the cha'pa'ka is a bunch of leaves tied at the base to form a handle. The "rattle" results from the sound of the shaken leaves. At one point the author recalls the cha'pa'ka being shaken over his entire body and then focused on his head, and as the rattle continued the author had an overwhelming sensation that the entire forest was dancing around him, and the small cha'pa'ka made it feel like all the vegetation in the forest was singing and dancing in a much larger cosmic ceremony. Now this is quite remarkable, because ayahuasca was not used during this ceremony, and yet the effect of the ceremony was still quite magical.

Songs Used in the Ayahuasca Ceremony

Although the circumstances precluded taping of the healing songs being sung during the author's own healing experience with the shaman, the author did find a collection of songs used in the ayahuasca ceremony. The author reviewed Senen Pani Antonio Muñoz's collection of ayahuasca songs recorded on the music CD entitled, *Bewa Icaro, Songs of Preparation* (2005). As in the peyote ceremony of the Native American Church, there are songs used while the ayahuasca is being prepared for the ceremony followed by the actual healing songs (elevation songs), which are used during the central action of the ceremony. Two songs from the Muñoz collection (2005) are included here:

I am the son of old Metsarawa, my name is Senen Pani and my wife is Raipena. Tonight I will take ayahuasca so that I can see the body of each one of you; with flower water I will blow on you.

I will control the fine ray of powerful light straightening it to guide your medicine well. I will sing my song of luminous patterns for every woman, every man. I will call up the power of light to heal my family. As I sing, thus sang the ancients when they still lived on this earth. Ayahuasca made them wise raised them up with its strength, my powers have connected with that same energy and from that position I light up and am guiding each and every one of you to heal your spirit from the space of

Ayahuasca: Master Healer of the Forest—cont'd

this light. With each being, man and woman, I am connecting in the deepest of ways. I am not important in this world but cloaked in my power I have become a king to bring solace to my brothers; on Mother Earth my throne is raised.

I have taken my ayahuasca, with my beautiful song I envelope the men and women, I adorn them with my luminous patterns. Connecting with the spirits of the air I unite with other beings with healing powers. Men and women from different places have admired them. Now that we have prepared both men and women, now that we have cleansed them, now that I am ready with my beautiful words, we begin the icaros we sing for healing.

Ayahuasca song of elevation:

I am cloaked in the power of the air, with my song of luminous patterns, with sufficient strength to enter each one of you. My magical drum is beating to bring relief, with my crown of air with my protection. My crown of air bears the sun at its front to blind the enemy.

My crown of air has the moon at its back for heightened awareness. My crown is covered with stars. I come with my crown of air I come playing my flute, my drum. I come by a serpent bridge. As I pass, water and space thunder. I bring, too, my serpent maraca. It brings happiness, awakening the spirits. On a golden table I carefully place those who are here. Adding strength to my song. I look down from on high, I guide my song like a magnet. We the kings to the Creator god accept that our light is divine. Two serpent princesses sing at my side; from each medicinal plant comes the healing light. I am not alone here; from the heights of the world come many merayas,* men and women, they come rotating. Whilst I remain alive I will conduct the energy, ancient knowledge of the old healers, with my crown of light.

Rising through space I beautify with the wondrous songs I am singing carefully placing women and men on my table of gold, enveloping them in luminous patterns to bring them solace. The serpent's power issues forth from the tip of my tongue. I raise them up with my words, and even higher with my medicinal words have I raised myself to bring them relief. ∞

*Shamans of the highest level.

Healing Rites and Civil Rights

From seemingly every corner psychedelics are making their way back into the news, and science is asking whether psychedelics can have a role in psychiatry (Sessa, 2005). On the legal front, recently in the case of *United States v. O Centro Espírita Benefiente União do Vegetal,*

et al the Supreme Court ruled in favor of the defendant, a New Mexico religious group affiliated with a Brazilian church of the same name (Mauro, 2005). The religious group uses ayahuasca, a psychedelic plant medicine that has its origins in indigenous South American shamanism (Moir, 1998). The active ingredient in ayahuasca (sometimes called *yagè*) is N,N-dimethyltryptamine (DMT), a potent short-acting hallucinogenic agent (McKenna, 2004) that is thought to be the substance released during a near-death experience (Strassman, 2001). In the context of the religious healing ceremony of the União do Vegetal (UDV) ayahuasca is more properly called an entheogen, which is a psychoactive sacramental plant or chemical substance taken to induce a primary religious experience. The UDV is a syncretic religion, blending elements of Christianity and African religions with the indigenous Amazonian shamanistic rites (Weiskopf, 2002).

Indigenous people in South America have used ayahuasca for centuries, and the ritual has become common among the mestizo populations in urban areas of the Amazon, particularly as a curing ritual for drug addiction (Dobkin de Rios, 1970; Moir, 1998). Like peyote in the United States (Calabrese, 1997), ayahuasca use among the indigenous people of the Amazon is a form of cultural psychiatry. Although entheogens are regularly being discovered by academic and popular presses, their use for spiritual and healing purposes, especially by indigenous peoples, has continued unabated. One mixed-lineage Spanish and mestizo Indian Peruvian *ayahuascera* claimed a spiritual lineage extending 17,000 years (C.M.M., personal communication, March 2002).

During three ceremonies I attended facilitated by a Peruvian healer and his protégé, I noted the tendency of many of the Euro-Americans present to "do their own thing" to some extent, whereas the Hispanic and indigenous people present tended to comply with the ritual instructions. Most notable was the recommendations regarding dietary restrictions. The facilitator of these ceremonies insisted that the participants abstain from foods high in salt or fat and particularly recommended that only steamed vegetables and steamed fish be eaten. The lead shaman noted that the physical problems of many of those present could be solved by adopting these dietary recommendations on a permanent basis.

The interaction between the healer and the participants is vital, and important contextual meaning is lost when cultural and linguistic barriers are encountered. Words, music, and phrases are an important part of the ceremony, and ayahuasca shamans manipulate participants' consciousness with their ceremonial songs and sayings (Dobkin de Rios et al, 1975). However, as with the peyote ceremony (Prue, 2008), the effects of the

(Continued)

ayahuasca in the context of the ritual environment produce a heightened sense of empathy. A poignant example came the morning after a ritual. I had accompanied a friend who was in need of a healing, and because this was a serious healing of a physical problem (a tumor) the shaman took special note of the case. During this after-ceremony doctoring session, because I had accompanied the patient I was asked to assist in the preparations. Since I understood very little Spanish, the interpreter joined us. As the shaman and I worked together for a while, the sense of being empathically connected heightened, and at one point, I felt sufficiently connected to him that when the translator ran into words she did not know, I found myself able to tell her the meaning. This echoed an experience we had had in the ceremony the night before. This occurrence came at the end of the ceremony, when people were asked to share their experiences with each other and with the shaman. Many shared experiences of psychedelic ecstasy or deep soul-searching journeys; in my case it was a sense of superempathic connection, not so much with the group, but through the shaman and to the collective indigenous experience. To honor that experience I expressed my gratitude to the shaman in my best attempts at the Lakota language. The translator was baffled, but I understood her to tell him that I was speaking in some indigenous language; his response was that he understood what I had said, and he proceeded to tell her what I had said and then gave the response he wanted for me.

Biological Mechanisms

A recent double-blind brain imaging study suggests that "ayahuasca interacts with neural systems that are central to interoception and emotional processing and point to a modulatory role of serotonergic neurotransmission in these processes" (Riba et al, 2006, p. 93). Other types of psychedelics cause elevated blood levels of oxytocin and vasopressin (Jerome et al, 2003), which have been linked to inhibition of development of tolerance to opiates in studies in rats (Sarnyai et al, 1994). Tolerance to drugs is a necessary part of drug addiction. Oxytocin and vasopressin also have social and emotional dynamics associated with them. Neurobiological research has highlighted their importance to the dynamics of falling in love (Marazziti, 2005) and to commitment-making behaviors in primates, particularly those playing a role in monogamy (Young et al, 1998). Social interactions are also known produce increased levels of oxytocin. In a study of stress adaptation in humans, social interactions alone provided better relief from stress than did the administration of oxytocin alone; however, the combination of the two provided the highest relief in that study group

(Heinrichs et al, 2003). The administration of an oxytocin and vasopressin–producing substance during a culturally meaningful and often highly intimate social interaction is but one element of the set and setting necessary to produce change in entheogenic rituals.

Abuse problems with these types of substances tend to arise after entheogens have "passed from ceremonial to purely hedonic or recreational use" (Masters et al, 1966). The use of some types of entheogens is integral to some indigenous people's spiritual and healing practices. Indigenous healing systems have mechanisms by which one can rise to the status of shaman or facilitator of a healing ritual, but few if any of the Western practitioners have fulfilled these requirements. Take the example of the shaman's apprentice who assisted at two of the ayahuasca ceremonies I attended and facilitated the third alone. After my second meeting with her, I asked if she would be returning the following year. Her reply was "Maybe?" She explained that the last ordeal she had to endure to become an independent ayahuasca practitioner was to live among the indigenous people in the rain forest for 6 months under the tutelage of their shaman. She further indicated that if she had not properly learned the religion at the end of that 6 months she would not be allowed to leave, so closely did the indigenous people of the Amazon want to maintain their control of their intellectual property.

SUMMARY

A pan-Indian perspective of health care and medicine challenges the intervention model and offers a prevention model as the starting place for social health and assistance. A Lakota-centric view of health and wellness prioritizes a universal approach to health care as opposed to the exceptional approach typical of most Western medicine currently in the United States. Traditional Lakota values emphasize the participation of the family in the healing process, including the extended family, as well as the larger kinship of community to bring about *wicozani*, or good health. The help and healing process is not impersonal, but rather is highly personalized and individualized around specific needs. This personal dimension touches on all of reality (creation) as fundamentally relational and ecological, challenging the mechanism of Cartesian dualism. For the Lakotas and other Indian peoples, there is no split or dualism in reality or creation. Health and sickness, good and evil, and mind and body are intrinsic, interrelated, and unified. The roles of medicine practitioners include that of healer, counselor, politician, and priest (Figure 35-6).

Another important contribution of a pan-Indian perspective of health is that it provides a rich topology of spirit. The human creation, like all creations, is a

WHAT IS A MEDICINE MAN?

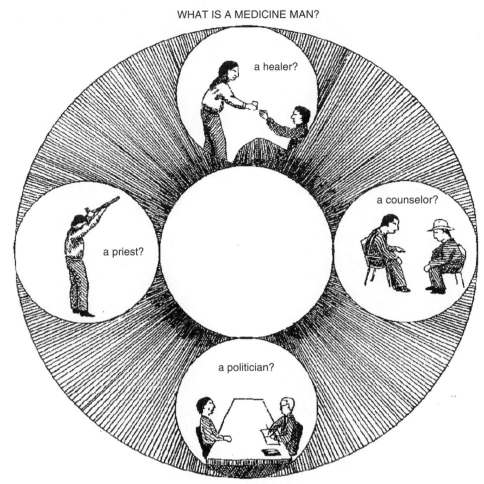

Figure 35-6 Illustration of the multiple roles of the medicine man: healer, priest, counselor, and politician. (Courtesy Sinte Gleska University.)

spirit-being composed of multilayered aspects of spirit. "Spirit" here is not some supernatural reality outside the human being, but rather an intrinsic dimension of everything that is, including the human creation (person). To speak of humans is to speak about spiritual reality. Medical treatment or any form of social or human/mental health service is first and foremost a spiritual endeavor. A pan-Indian view of medicine and health care forces us to look at the human person from a broader, more encompassing perspective. Rather than taking a narrow biomedical approach, a pan-Indian view of health and well-being looks at the human as part of a lively and interacting bio-psycho-social-spiritual creation, in which the human person is viewed as a peer to other beings in a highly personalized universe and is intimately related to all of creation (i.e., the natural world of plants, animals, insects, fish, stone, earth, fire, air, water, wind, and spirit entities).

The human being, or to use the Lakota term, *the ikce wicasa*, is the common man/woman—a peer to all other beings. He or she is not above creation, and as a peer depends on good relations with all the other elements of creation for survival and good health. If anything, the human creation is the most needy of all the created beings and depends on the medicine of other beings (e.g., plant nations and various animal nations) to overcome sickness. The Lakota view of life is based on a radical mutuality, interrelationships, and respect among all the members or peoples of creation. They have no word for "animal"; the birds belong to a nation and have status, as does everything (Smith, 1987; White Hat, 1997).

The most obvious implication of a pan-Indian perspective of health care and medicine is that it compels health care educators and practitioners to begin "indigenizing" our own consciousness, not only about the "missing chapter" in our introductory textbooks, but also about the fundamental influence of Western materialism and Eurocentrism on our thinking.

As we begin to take multicultural perspectives seriously, the Eurocentrism of our epistemologies, pedagogies, and professional practice of medical and health services will come under greater scrutiny, and we may even question some long-held beliefs about how to provide medical and health services. There will be a greater awareness of the role and importance of spirituality, shamanic practices, and common or herbal remedies as a complement to clinical practice. Finally, there will be a reaffirmation of the importance of grassroots community development in health care delivery services, an expanding awareness of the prescribed limitations of our dominant Eurocentric models of help and healing in the United States, and the increasing need, as well as opportunities, to incorporate integrative, alternative, and complementary models of health care into our mainstream health care services (see Chapter 1).

The increasing cooperative relations between medical and health care service personnel and traditional Indian medicine practitioners provide grounds for encouragement that a multicultural approach not only is possible but also is actually taking root in Indian country. It is time for the diverse medical and health care disciplines to learn more about Native American and pan-Indian ways of healing and health. Not only will this cross-cultural collaboration benefit Indian people, but everyone in the larger culture will benefit from wider implementation of a more holistic health care model that recognizes both the physiological and the spiritual causes of disease and sickness, as well as the efficacy of both biological and spiritual remedies.

Hecetu'yelo! (Lakota, "the way it is").

⊖ Refer to the Evolve website at http://evolve.elsevier.com/Micozzi/complementary for an appendix on Native American Medicinal Plants by Daniel E. Moerman.

⊖ Chapter References can be found on the Evolve website at http://evolve.elsevier.com/Micozzi/complementary/

CHAPTER 36

SOUTH AMERICAN SPIRITISM

EMMA BRAGDON

If the spirit is not acknowledged as existing and real, psychiatrists will only pay attention to effect. They will be impeded from divining the root causes and will never cure effectively.... New theories—with solid experimental foundation—point at the spirit, illuminating and unveiling. But, we need courage, not only to acknowledge these theories, but also to examine them.

—JL AZEVEDO, MD (1997)

SPIRITIST HOSPITALS AND HEALING CENTERS IN BRAZIL

There is a form of spiritual healing practiced by Spiritists that touches the lives of 20% of Brazil's people, up to 40 million Brazilians. Although only 3% of the population of 180 million claim formal membership in the 1650+ Spiritist centers in Brazil (Instituto Brasileiro de Geografia e Estatística [IBGE], 2007; Datafolha, 2007), many more come to these ecumenical centers seeking healing. There are also approximately 50 Spiritist psychiatric hospitals in Brazil, founded from the 1930s through the 1970s (Souza et al, 1980), where

spiritual healers collaborate with conventional medical doctors.

According to a 2000 census (IBGE, 2000) membership in these Spiritist centers is growing strongly among the most well educated and wealthy in Brazil. There are also 161 Spiritist centers in 31 countries outside Brazil (United States Spiritist Council, 2004) with 70 of these in the United States. The centers in Brazil, which have been functioning since 1865, are the models for the centers in other countries, the majority of which cater specifically to Brazilians who have emigrated.

All of these healing centers and hospitals drew their original inspiration from books written by Léon Dénizarth-Hippolyte-Rivail (1804-1869), a French academic living in Paris who used the nom de plume Alan Kardec. A few Brazilians (Franco, 2004, 2005; Xavier, 2000a, 2000b) have recently become popular Spiritist authors. The main principle of Spiritism is the premise that life does not end at physical death, but our individual spirits go on for lifetimes, alternating between this life and an afterlife. The goal of these lives is for the spiritual self to increasingly become more aware, wiser, and more loving. According to

551

Spiritism, disincarnate spirits can impact the lives of incarnated human beings, either negatively or positively, depending on the level of evolution of the incarnate and the disincarnate. Essential to Spiritism is the encouragement to relate to, think about, and evoke the more evolved spirits in prayer and to practice charity and fraternity. Jesus Christ is considered an important model for the right way to live, and many perceive Spiritism as both a revitalization of Christianity and a practical path of Christianity. At its core, however, Spiritism welcomes people of all faiths.

We distinguish Spiritist centers from other spiritual healing centers in Brazil that have been more frequently described because of the dramatic healing practices by unique individuals (Bragdon, 2002, 2004, 2008; Don et al, 2000; Fuller, 1974; Greenfield, 1994, 1997) or colorful rituals associated with African traditions that were brought to Brazil beginning in the sixteenth century by the African slaves, or the indigenous Amazonian shamanic tribal traditions. Traditional Spiritist healers embrace a form of healing that is performed in small groups by healers who bring a dedication to *personal transformation* founded on study and discussion of philosophical texts. Kardec (2004) wrote, "You recognize a true Spiritist by their moral transformation and the effort they make to dominate their negative tendencies." Spiritists prefer not to practice their healing work alone. The possibility of becoming ego inflated as a result of one's personal success—or deflated if a patient does not improve—can erode one's ability as a medium, a healer, or be disempowering for a balanced, healthy person.

Spiritist healers are trained at Kardecist spiritist centers and hospitals. In some cases, these healers have already qualified as medical physicians. Spiritist hospitals have integrated the Spiritist healing practices and philosophy into their treatment protocols.

QUANTIFIED SUCCESS

Statistics currently available in Brazil report unusual success in healing at specific Spiritist centers. The statistics are few, however, and may lack objectivity because they come from members at the centers. In April 2004, the president of the Federation for Spiritism of the State of São Paulo (FEESP), Avildo Fioravanti, remarked in an interview that FEESP has a more than 90% success rate in helping addicts and the suicidally depressed recover normal functioning, without dependence on drug therapy. Another center in São Paulo, Grupo Noel, was formally profiled by Cleide Martins Canadas (2001), a social psychologist. She reported that 70% of the community experienced great improvement and a definite cure of their problems. These included all manner of physical and emotional disease, including cancers. Rigorous scientific studies are needed to confirm what has been reported.

Bear in mind that in the United States in 2002 an estimated 22 million people suffered from substance dependence or abuse (U.S. Department of Health and Human Services, 2003). A 1999 report by Fuller et al noted that the highest success rate (in outpatient care) for treatment of alcoholism after only 1 year is 35%. Major depressive disorder affects approximately 10 million American adults in any given year (National Institutes of Health, 2001). The most typical therapeutic interventions are pharmaceuticals, which frequently have detrimental side effects. Ascertaining whether Spiritist therapies can improve the outcomes for depressive patients and addicts could be extremely valuable for patients, their loved ones, their employers, and insurance and health care providers.

At this time no data are available from North American studies examining the efficacy of the healing practices of Spiritist hospitals in randomized controlled double-blind trials. The only such trial of Spiritist therapy completed in Brazil was conducted at an institution for the cognitively disabled and reported by Frederico Leão and Francisco Neto (2007).

Before casting aspersions on Spiritists for rarely employing the holy grail of research, we must recognize that using randomized controlled trials as the standard method of research may not be able to do justice to the subject matter of Spiritist work. Spiritist healers in Brazil work with each individual as a unique entity, in aspects of each person's body, mind, and spirit covering a span of lifetimes. They also work in a cultural environment in which many people accept notions of reincarnation as well as karmic consequences for actions. It is possible that all the variables in Spiritist healing cannot be considered within the typical confines of randomized controlled trials.

Nevertheless, the standards for establishing the statistics quoted earlier could be further studied to validate their correctness. Judging by the numbers of people attending Spiritist centers, the current expansion of their popularity, and the fact that some centers have been developing their protocols for more than 130 years, we must assume that the protocols used have unusual success. The FEESP serves between 7000 and 10,000 people each day. Most of these people are coming to attend classes and/or obtain spiritual healing. Why would they bother to come if they were not receiving something they find valuable?

CENTER ACTIVITIES

My knowledge of Spiritist centers and hospitals in Brazil comes from 30 trips I took to Brazil visiting and participating in Spiritist activities from 2001 through 2008 (Bragdon, 2002, 2004, 2008).

An individual attending a Spiritist center in Brazil has access to a wide variety of free services. Mediums, teachers in study groups and training sessions, physicians serving the poor, and healers see their tasks as charitable work. First, as in many public welfare systems, the individual begins by meeting with a social worker to determine his or her needs and/or the needs of the family. Most Spiritist centers then offer laying on of hands (called "pass," or transfer of energy), blessed water, counseling, and/or consultations. Physicians, who may give nutritional supplements and therapeutic drugs, as well as lawyers, dentists, and financial counselors are all available for free consultations at many Spiritist centers. Some Spiritist centers also offer classes in life skill training, self-awareness, and acceleration of spiritual evolution. In addition, some centers offer classroom and practical training for those who are naturally gifted so that they can harness their talents to serve others as mediums and healers.

Just as individuals find support for financial, legal, physical, emotional, and spiritual needs, the centers also become axes for community and social get-togethers as well as coordination of volunteer service programs. The golden thread weaving its way through all activities is the notion that we, as incarnate spirits in body, are all spiritually evolving through lifetimes in and out of a physical body, and that the most powerful positive step to progress is *charitable work.* Spiritist centers typically emphasize that the treatment they provide is complementary to conventional medical treatment. Thus, patients are strongly encouraged to seek medical treatment if they have a medical issue.

The educational classes are offered to discuss life principles, awakening the mind and the will through the sharing of many points of view, including those derived from modern science. Attending a *basic class* is sometimes a prerequisite for those who seek the services of the center. This class emphasizes the concept that every action has a consequence—what the Eastern philosophies refer to as the natural law of *karma,* or cause and effect. Under the guidance of a teacher, students discuss the most essential life questions: Why are we alive? Is there a God? What happens at death? Does life go on for our loved ones who have passed on? Who models the correct way of living life? The books of Kardec and Chico Xavier are read to stimulate discussion, along with news from contemporary media. Chico Xavier (1910-2002), who wrote more than 400 books, is the most popular author in this lineage of Spiritualism.

Belief that our purpose in life is continued progression and that we are influenced by cause and effect helps the individual to take charge of his or her life. This orientation leads to a positive outlook and mental equanimity. Practicing positive thinking, feeling joy and gratitude for life, grows with the practice of prayer, meditation, and deliberate exercises to attune to the divine aspects of the self. This attunement opens each person to inspiration and guidance. Being positive strengthens the immune system, enhancing physical functioning as well as emotional and spiritual well-being.

Participation in a loving "community learning center" to accelerate spiritual progress keeps attracting more members to these centers. The well-educated people come to learn, to come to terms with pressing life issues, and be

of service to others. The poor also come to introspect, learn, find support to establish an independent lifestyle, and become part of a positive community. The activities are not dependent on blind faith, but founded on everyone's natural desire to progress.

The centers are maintained by private donation. They are not extensions of the government or of any religion. Only a few key administrators and janitorial staff are paid a wage. This keeps operating costs at a minimum. There are no membership dues.

DYNAMICS OF SPIRITIST HEALING

What kind of healing occurs in these centers? The most often-used form, energy transference, or passes, involves a healer who focuses on transmitting a powerful subtle energy to the patient. The healer sometimes receives the help of benevolent disincarnates who "step down" the power, just as a transformer steps down the electrical current of high-voltage power lines, adapting it to the capacities of ordinary houses. First the healer becomes focused, which usually involves shifting to a deeper state of consciousness (alpha or delta brain wave pattern with a lower frequency). The healer then passes his or her hands 3 to 6 inches above the body of the patient. Although this is typically regimented to circumscribed gestures, individual styles are permitted; however, physical touch is avoided. At times, a second healer will stand behind the patient's healer, giving energy to the healer by placing a hand above the healer's head. A variation of this assistance occurs when a group of healers hold hands in a circle with the patient attended by one healer in the center of the circle. Directing their spiritual energy to the patient is thought to break up congestion or strengthen an area of weakness in the patient.

Some mediums perform "psychic surgery" through incisive prayer and positive intention. This can be done at a distance without the patient's being present. Whether the patient is present or not, healing takes place through the uninterrupted transmission of energy from the spiritual source to the spirit of the incarnate healer, and from the healer to the spiritual body, or *perispirit,* of the patient.

Kardec (2004) described the perispirit as "a subtle, ethereal, nearly massless covering . . . a kind of energy body that serves as a blueprint for the human form." This etheric body permeates the physical body in every detail, creating an exact duplicate of every organ and limb. Its main function is to transmit energy to the physical body. Imbalance of energy in the perispirit, or a weakening caused by stress, negative thinking, overly judgmental attitude, lack of forgiveness of self or others, or depression, can link to a particular organ or system in the body, causing a physical manifestation of illness.

Intervention through psychic surgery, passes, and/or prayer focuses a high vibration (associated with pure love) that changes the subtle energetic blueprint in and around the physical body and lays the foundation for the physical body of the patient to become healthy. These same interventions are also practiced as preventative care to stop the development of disease states by maintaining an appropriate flow of energy in the perispirit and, in turn, the body.

The soul ... forms a single unity with the perispirit, and integrates with the entire body, which constitutes a complex human being. ... We can imagine two bodies similar in form, one interpenetrating another, combined during life and separated at death, which destroys one while the other continues to exist. During life, the soul acts through the vehicles of thought and emotion. It is simultaneously internal and external—that is, it radiates outwardly, being able to separate itself from the body, to transport itself considerable distances, and there to manifest its presence.

—A. KARDEC (2004)

From the point of view of Spiritism, mental illness that does not stem from organic brain disorders or specific psychosocial stressors originates through interaction with negatively motivated spirits who attach themselves to a weakened individual for a period of time, negatively influencing that person's willpower, thoughts, and feelings (Kardec, 1986; Moreira-Almeida and Neto, 2005; Moreira-Almeida et al, 2008). These negatively motivated spirits are considered confused, not knowing whether they are dead and still attached to the pleasures of material life (e.g., drinking alcohol), or are perceived as seeking retribution for harm caused in previous lifetimes (e.g., having been murdered by the person to whom they are attached). Spiritists believe that when a patient is often motivated to engage in some negative behavior, such as abusing drugs or alcohol, caused by their own weakness accentuated by the attachment of a spirit, they are *obsessed*. If the obsession progresses to a more severe stage so that the patient has no ability to exercise will over the negative influence, the patient is considered to be *possessed*.

Although most of the therapies (e.g., laying on of hands, prayer, short lectures,) occur with the patient present, disobsession sessions are performed "at a distance" with the patient not present and often unaware that the treatment is being done. These sessions typically happen in a room similar to a boardroom, around a large table, with approximately eight mediums. Lights are turned low, calming classical music is played on a CD player, and a prayer is said to initiate the session, elevating the thoughts of those present and helping them to make contact with the spirit realm more immediately by decreasing other distractions. While mediums sit focusing, eyes closed, the appointed scribe reads from notes about the person having the problem. One or two mediums inevitably begin to sense the exact obsessing thoughts of the patient through mental telepathy—and also to sense the nature of the spirit that might be "obsessing" the patient. Disobsession is then twofold: the patient is relieved of the obsessor, and the obsessor is guided into its next step in evolution

through oral counseling by one of the mediums assigned to the specific task of counseling the spirit.

Another avenue of healing, equally important, is to encourage the patient to make amends for prior negative behaviors and reorient his or her life to more loving action. This path of healing is similar to the protocol in 12-step programs, in which the person seeking healing takes a moral inventory of past behavior and subsequently makes some positive contributions to make amends for prior behaviors that have caused others pain. This may involve changing behaviors and renegotiating relationships. Spiritists believe we must also study books related to Spiritism to deepen our understanding of life and death and the way to accelerate spiritual growth. Without such study, a person does not understand the steps of spiritual evolution and has difficulty staying both focused on and inspired to ethical and charitable action.

OBSERVATIONS IN THE FIELD: SPIRITIST HOSPITALS

In both 2003 and 2004 I spent several days in Palmelo, a town founded by Spiritists in 1929, at that time serving approximately 3000 visitors who come to Palmelo each month for healing of various kinds. I observed several depossession and disobsession sessions in Euripedes Barsanulfo Hospital, a freestanding Spiritist psychiatric hospital in Palmelo, and spent time interviewing several people on staff. In 2005 I was given a tour of Casa André Luís, a Spiritist residence for more than 300 intellectually disabled individuals, in the suburbs of São Paulo. In 2007 I visited disobsession sessions at the Spiritist Psychiatric Hospital of Anápolis and later filmed these sessions and interviewed the physician responsible for this therapy at the hospital (Bragdon, 2008). In 2008 I spent a week in Curitiba getting to know the Spiritist Psychiatric Hospital Bom Retiro and a week in Porto Alegre visiting the Spiritist Psychiatric Hospital of Porto Alegre. I was also able to spend 2 days observing activities at a Spiritist hospital dedicated to helping those dealing with cancer near Florianópolis, where 35 patients are in residence each week for four days at a time.

The Spiritist movement does not have a central regulatory agency that controls Spiritist practices (like the Vatican for Catholicism). Each Spiritist group is free to behave as it prefers, even if this includes doing things that are not supported by (or are even in contradiction to) Spiritist theory. Thus, I was able to witness several practices that are not necessarily based on Spiritist theory or Kardec's works because some Spiritist groups combine their practices and theories with African-Brazilian, New Age, or Eastern traditions. I endeavor to report here only on those practices that dovetail with Spiritist theory.

In each hospital the patients were first treated in the conventional manner. They were initially interviewed by a physician for a medical assessment, including an assessment for psychosocial stressors. The interview included questions related to special dietary needs, allergies, and preferences regarding religious and spiritual practices. Those wanting Spiritist therapies were given the opportunity to have them. Those not wanting these therapies were able to be treated using conventional medical practices. Attending nurses and doctors were a blend of Spiritists and people of other philosophies and religions. The only exception was the facility for treating those with cancer, because it was dedicated to serving Spiritists and therefore only Spiritists requested treatment there. Nurses and physicians at this hospital were all Spiritists. In some cases the doctors conducting conventional medical assessment for entering patients were also accomplished spiritual healers in the treatment room.

In April 2008 at the Spiritist Psychiatric Hospital of Porto Alegre I observed a well-organized facility on the hospital grounds dedicated to community education, Spiritist therapies, and training. Physicians and psychologists associated with the hospital offered evening classes for students and professionals wanting to study the relationships between quantum physics, medicine, and Spiritist therapies. A meeting room was provided once a week for a group of doctors associated with the Brazilian Medical Spiritism Association to facilitate a deeper understanding of Spiritism. Specific rooms were used each day for disobsession work, accomplished by well-trained mediums under the kind and disciplined eye of a supervising medium. Records noting which patients were treated and the outcomes were carefully kept to support present and future research. Teams of volunteers, all trained healers, would enter hospital wards at specific times to offer "energy passes" to the patients, assembled in rows of chairs. The head nurse, not a Spiritist herself, said to me, "Patients are noticeably more calm for 3 days after receiving these treatments."

Visiting the day treatment center for patients with chemical addictions at the Spiritist Psychiatric Hospital of Bom Retiro in Curitiba in April 2008 I noticed a remarkable ambience. The lines of authoritarian hierarchy were less rigid than I expected to see. Undoubtedly the presence of many Spiritist volunteers, there to create a fraternal, loving home atmosphere, facilitated this. I believe it was also a product of the Spiritists' practice of evoking the energy of highly evolved spirits to help staff, patients, and disincarnates in the work of spiritual evolution.

EXPLANATORY VIEWPOINTS

Does this kind of focused, spiritually based attention make a difference in healing mental illness? Arthur Guirdham (1978, 1980), an English psychiatrist, believes so. He is one of a handful of psychiatrists who write that possession may be a contributing factor in mental illness (Grof, 1985; Sanderson, 2008; Weiss, 1994).

I was personally impressed by two interviews I had in Palmelo in 2003 with a patient named Marcel (Bragdon,

2004). Diagnosed with schizophrenia by psychiatrists in São Paulo, Marcel had been brought to Euripedes Barsanulfo Hospital by his concerned parents. At that point Marcel was suffering from delusions and had frequent outbursts of violently aggressive behavior. In the hospital Marcel took psychiatric medication under the supervision of a psychiatrist and, as he was able, began to study Spiritism, participate in disobsession, and be checked regularly by Bartólomo Damo, who is gifted as a medical intuitive. After weeks, Damo saw that Marcel was a natural medium with healing abilities, who needed to learn how to harness his abilities to help others. This gift became increasingly more evident as Marcel was released from obsessing entities. Months later he began training to practice healing while he continued his therapy in the hospital, which still included minimal amounts of psychiatric drugs. His healing necessitated his making amends for prior wrongdoing in this and other lifetimes, as well as deliberately being dedicated to serve others in this lifetime. His parents and the support staff at the hospital were essential to the process. By the time I met him, Marcel was taking a very small amount of antipsychotic medication, still being supervised by a physician and several medium-healers, and was becoming part of the team of healers attending others at the hospital. Inacio Ferreira published descriptions of several similar cases in the 1930s and 1940s (Moreira-Almeida et al, 2008).

In the Spiritist tradition, healing offered to disincarnates can take many forms. In April 2004, I attended a group meeting of healers at FEESP in São Paulo who were helping a spirit who was releasing from the body of a man who had just "died" in Maryland in the United States. His wife informed us by cell phone that the man had died within seconds, unexpectedly, of a critical heart condition, while sitting at his desk. In São Paulo one healer-medium allowed her body to be overcome with the emotions of the spirit of the man who was passing on. She became full of emotion: regret, fear, and anxiety. Another healer-medium verbally counseled the spirit, advising "him" that his physical body had died, and "he" must reach out to the spirits ready to take "him" to the spiritual realm. Five other healer-mediums made a circle around the two who were most actively engaged in the process. The process, including the counseling, took approximately 20 minutes, most of which was taken up with the emotional outburst of the person who engaged the spirit of the man who had died. When it was complete, everyone in the healers' circle was relaxed and in a peaceful state. They believed that the spirit of the man who had "died" was also at peace.

The problem of the nature of man and his destiny after death of the physical body was relegated to religions. Those religions could not find a solution that would agree with science, consequently man is facing a paradox: he knows more about his environment than about himself and his real destination in time and space.

—H.G. ANDRADE (1974)

LIMITATIONS OF FURTHER RESEARCH AND INTEGRATION

Even though practicing a Spiritist way of life brings benefits of peace of mind and increased well-being to participants, for the most part Spiritists protect the privacy of their affiliation with Spiritist centers. This inhibits collection of data on the demographics of participants. It also inhibits further examining the centers and enlisting participants in clinical trials.

It is easy to sympathize with the reason for wanting privacy. For almost a century in Europe, the United States, and Brazil, Spiritism was regarded as a diabolic phenomenon or a major cause of insanity (Moreira-Almeida, Almeida et al, 2005). In 1861, by order of the Catholic Church, Spiritist books were confiscated and publicly burned in Spain. In the early 1890s Brazil's penal code banned all forms of Spiritism. Spiritists were legally prosecuted through the 1920s, and their activities were still considered illegal during the 1930s and 1940s. From the 1940s through 1988, Spiritist activities were regarded with suspicion and disfavor.

All forms of Spiritualism have been denigrated in the United States as well. Although Spiritualists are not publicly persecuted today, we can easily recall the horrific graphic illustrations of Puritan women being burned at the stake or drowned if it were even suspected that they communicated with spirits (and thus defied the hegemony of the church and its priesthood).

With this history in our cultural memory, how many of us can easily apply scientific thinking to explore the rationale of Spiritism? First we must make our way through the dense undergrowth of centuries of cultural conditioning, taboos encrusted with deep emotions, which would have us dismiss anything Spiritist.

Pioneering researchers, willing to risk public ridicule, are opening the way to the reconsideration of what happens at death and the real possibility that the spirit survives death. Ian Stevenson, MD, Carlson Professor of Psychiatry at the University of Virginia, has published several books (1980, 1997) reporting on his very credible research of the subject that spans continents. Recently, many researchers combined efforts to renew the conversation about reincarnation in *Irreducible Mind: Toward a Psychology for the 21st Century* (Kelly et al, 2007). Dean Radin, PhD, laboratory director of the Institute of Noetic Sciences, and Dr. Gary Schwartz, former director of the Yale Psychophysiology Center and currently a professor of psychology, medicine, and psychiatry at the University of Arizona, are finding substantial evidence of life after death and reincarnation (Radin, 1997, 2006; Schwartz et al, 2002). However, the public at large in the United States is still reluctant to make such a conceptual leap.

There are other limitations in integrating Spiritist centers in the United States: the services of these centers in Brazil are free to all, even when professionals are made available for a day at a time. This level of goodwill

donation is rare in the United States. Our real estate and overhead expenses are much higher in the United States than in Brazil. We are a materialistic culture. Most people in the United States find it reasonable and right to charge for any service rendered. The view of Brazilian Spiritists that "what is freely given from God should be freely donated to people" is not embedded in our culture. Spiritual healers, medical intuitives, and mediums typically charge for their services in the United States and Europe.

If we find in future research that Spiritist centers offer a viable path for healing, more effective than our own, there is a challenge in finding adequate teachers for classes, mediums, and healers, as well as sufficient written material for classes in the United States. Of the 70 centers in the United States, 10% conduct all their activities in English. Fifty percent have at least one activity per week in English. There are few Spiritists with developed skills as Spiritist mediums and healers in the United States who are as fluent in English as they are in Portuguese—although young Brazilian Americans are already beginning to teach and will soon fill that gap. Many books are available in English and can be downloaded for free at http://www.usspiritistcouncil.com. Spiritist books and research, until now published only in Portuguese, are becoming available in English. At this time the translations of talks and literature are not consistently of good quality, which can obstruct the learning process, but these obstacles are manageable. The U.S. Spiritist Council is encouraging U.S. Spiritist centers to offer more study groups, training, and events in English.

HISTORY OF SPIRITISM

Belief in discarnate spirits and communication with spirits has been a part of most cultures throughout the world for thousands of years (Krippner et al, 1987). Saints and sages of all religions have demonstrated diverse forms of spiritual healing. Jesus Christ was acknowledged for casting out evil spirits as a form of healing. However, the mid-nineteenth century is considered the birth time of *modern Spiritualism* (Weisberg, 2004), when communicating with spirits was first practiced in "technologically advanced" society.

Separated from the traditions of shamanic culture and the sanctions of a particular church, Spiritualists believed that death is a time when the physical body dies, but the spirit of the individual continues on in another form, in another dimension. The first Spiritualists developed their own ways of communicating with spirits in living rooms and assembly halls, using musical instruments, pens, tables, and chairs to facilitate communication.

Beginning in 1848, two sisters, both adolescents, Maggie and Kate Fox of Hydesville, New York, invited the public to witness their extraordinary communications with the spirits. The women put themselves on display in public auditoriums and submitted themselves to tests by numerous groups of doctors to establish that the rappings, playing of musical instruments, and moving of furniture, including levitation of heavy tables, came from a nonphysical source. Although these occurrences might be ascribed to psychokinesis (mind over matter), in some of their meetings the Foxes divined messages from the departed containing information to which they could not have formerly been privy. Those who found these displays authentic had to engage the belief in life after death, the idea that our spirits never die but go on to new life, a life that may intersect with human life. Despite the antagonism of many physicians and religious men who could not accept these ideas, many more found the evidence compelling. Horace Greeley, the famous editor of the *New York Tribune* (who also was known for his interest in exploring new frontiers, as evidenced by his admonition, "Go west, young man"); Charles Partridge, a publisher; Charles Hammond and R. P. Ambler, both Universalist ministers; Judge John Worth Edmonds, chief justice of the New York State Supreme Court; and Nathaniel Tallmadge, former governor of Wisconsin publicly supported Spiritualism and attended related activities. Interest in séances (group gatherings for the purpose of communicating with the spirits) began to expand throughout the United States as well as in Europe. By the mid-1850s there were several hundred thousand Spiritualists in the United States. By 1890, there was estimated to be up to 11 million in the United States.

Like many of his contemporaries in Paris in the 1850s, Rivail became interested in the phenomena of spirit communication. Rivail was an earnest intellectual, a professor of languages, physics, anatomy, and mathematics, dedicated to improving public education. He approached Spiritualism with the discipline of an academic employing the methodology of a scientist.

Rivail crafted over 1000 questions concerning the reason for human life on earth, the nature of the spiritual realms, and the dynamics of spiritual evolution. He then carefully observed, collected, and collated answers to these questions from 10 different mediums, each unknown to the others. More than 1000 Spiritualist centers contributed answers to questions, given to their mediums by higher spirits. Rivail was thus in a position to make note of the answers that were "universal," that is, repeated by all the mediums questioned. He found that these universal answers created a comprehensive and rational philosophy of life—what he named *Spiritism*. Soon, he published five books under the pen name Alan Kardec: *The Spirits' Book* (1857), which presents the philosophy, based on the existence, manifestations, and teachings of the spirits; *The Mediums' Book* (1861), which explains the practical, experiential aspects of Spiritism; and *The Gospel According to the Spirits* (1864), which illumines the ethical ramifications of Spiritism. *What is Spiritism?* (1859) and *Spiritism in Its Simplest Expression* (1865) were booklets introducing the basics of Spiritism. *Heaven and Hell* (1865) and *Genesis*

(1868) elaborate on the concept that heaven and hell are psychological constructs related to the workings of our own conscience. Together these works formulate the precepts of Spiritism—sometimes known in Brazil as "Kardecist Spiritism" to distinguish it from other forms of Spiritualism that sprang from the indigenous Indians or Africans who were brought to Brazil as slaves.

Why did he call this philosophy *Spiritism,* as separate from *Spiritualism?*

Strictly speaking, Spiritualism is the opposite of Materialism; every one is a Spiritualist who believes that there is in him something more than matter, but it does not follow that he believes in the existence of spirits, or in their communication with the visible world. ... We say, then, that the fundamental principle of the spiritist theory, or Spiritism, is the relation of the material world with spirits, or the beings of the invisible world; and we designate the adherents of the spiritist theory as spiritists.

—A. KARDEC (1857:1996)

Kardec's books advocate a high degree of discipline and perseverance in life—to effect personal transformation ("reforma íntima" in Portuguese) and transcend the selfish desires of more basic motivations. Thus, Spiritists take on a demanding life path. The precepts also advocate communicating with highly evolved spirits for the purposes of healing and the study of deeper truths, rather than communing with spirits who are less evolved for the sake of amusement or curiosity. Spiritists are attending not only to the regulation of their own behavior, thoughts, and will, but doing what they can to assist disincarnate spirits to evolve to higher levels. Knowledge of the spiritual worlds, acquired through study, is regarded as *essential* in this task.

As mentioned earlier, Spiritists believe that spiritual healing and the gifts of mediumship originate with God and are given freely to humankind, and that what is received for free must be given for free. Therefore, all Spiritist healing is without charge or "suggested donation." Furthermore, Spiritists believe that when a spiritual healer or medium charges money for his or her services the healer opens the door to less evolved spirits who downgrade the spiritual work and possibly damage the healer or medium by causing addiction and mental and/or physical disease. Given this belief, it is interesting to note the downfall of Kate and Maggie Fox, both of whom became victims of alcoholism after making a commercial venture of their mediumship.

Why did Kardec's Spiritism develop in Brazil? In the late nineteenth century it was customary for wealthy Brazilian families to send their male offspring to European universities. Because Kardec's books were in fashion in Europe at the time, they came to Brazil tucked under the arms of the university students returning home and then passed on to the parents and the upper classes of Brazilian society. Kardec's philosophy also found an enthusiastic following among homeopathic physicians trained in Europe who were practicing in Brazil. These physicians had already been trained to accept and use some aspects of spiritual healing, because Samuel Hahnemann (1755-1843), the founder of homeopathy, encouraged the use of intuition in diagnosis and a form of laying on of hands for healing (see Chapter 24). Charitable homeopaths in Brazil were the first to organize groups to study and practice Spiritism in Brazil. The upper classes were primed to participate, and the lower classes quickly availed themselves of the charity these Spiritist groups offered—free food, free medical services, free dental care, financial and legal advice, orphanages for children and abandoned elders, and institutional living for the intellectually disabled or those suffering from dementia.

According to a recent census (IBGE, 2007), Brazil is 64% Catholic, 25% Evangelical/Protestant, and 3% Spiritist, and 17% declare that they attend religious services of other religions besides their own. Some 44% of Catholics state that they believe fully in reincarnation. In the general population, 37% declare that they believe in reincarnation. Although it is impossible to quantify exactly, the majority of Brazilians are practicing *syncretistism*, that is, participating in spiritual activities of diverse traditions, including attending ceremonies of their churches. However, deeply embedded in their approach to life is the golden rule of Christian tradition: to practice charity and goodwill. That Spiritism is infused with this same ethic and endorses the continued development of moral values associated with Christianity made Kardec's precepts easy for Brazilians to assimilate.

In fact, Kardec's philosophy is considered both a path of revitalization and a path of practical Christianity—but without rituals, priesthood, or churches, and without fear of hell and damnation. Spiritists believe in a loving God, the supreme intelligent force, with whom all people may have direct communication.

SPIRITUALISM'S PROGENY

Because of disenchantment with the personal shortcomings of Spiritualism's first public personalities, North Americans' fascination with Spiritualism was on the decline by the end of the nineteenth century. Those still intrigued by the afterlife, mysticism, and invisible worlds transferred their loyalty to organizations like the Theosophical Society, which combined study of Eastern mysticism with Western spirituality, and founded Theosophical medicine (see Chapters 6 and 7).

In the twentieth century channeled teachings addressing universal questions continued to be published by some individuals who gained international fame, such as Alice Bailey (1880-1949), who produced more than 23 books; Chico Xavier, the aforementioned Brazilian, who wrote more than 400 books that sold millions of copies (he never received any payment for these books but donated all copyrights to charity institutions) and were distributed internationally in numerous translations; and Helen Schucman, whose *Course in Miracles* was published in 1975. Channeling of personal advice and the practice of *medical intuition* (diagnosing accurately without use of physical examination, technical diagnostics, or even meeting the person face to face) was taken up by individuals such as Edgar Cayce (1877-1945) and, more recently, Carolyn Myss, an energy healer, who first gained her reputation by working with C. Norman Shealy, MD. As of 2004, Dr. Shealy offered a doctoral program in medical intuition at his Holos University Graduate Seminary. The practice of laying on of hands continued in various religious ministries, as well as by notable independent healers such as Harry Edwards (1893-1976) and Olga Worrall (1906-1985) and, more recently, practitioners of reiki, a Japanese form of laying on of hands, and therapeutic touch, among others (see Chapter 16).

In the 1930s, Dr. Joseph Rhine coined the term *parapsychology* as an umbrella for the scientific studies he was conducting to explore psychic phenomena, or "psi." This research at Duke University continues in the United States and abroad. Hernani G. Andrade (1912-2002), director of the Brazilian Research Institute of Psycho-Biophysics, devoted the last 40 years of his life to research and writing on spiritual phenomena and parapsychology. Dr. Sergio Felipe de Oliveira is presently documenting the biophysics of mediumship at the Pineal-Mind Institute of Health in São Paulo. He is associated with both the Brazilian and international branches of the Medical Spiritist Association (AME). The international organization, founded in 1999, hosts a biannual international convention to stimulate research and cross-cultural exchange among scientists, physicians, and psychologists of all faiths who are interested in the relationship between spirituality and health. AME published a special magazine, *Health and Spirituality* (Associação Médico-Espírita, 2003), in English that documents the 2003 convention. Dr. Marlene Nobre, author (Nobre, 2003; Nobre et al, 1994) and president of AME-Brasil and AME-International, finds that Spiritist principles are clearly aligned with quantum physics, pointing to the mind as a key factor in the manifestation of all phenomena. She writes that doctors have a responsibility to teach their patients "that all pathologies originate in the addictions of the mind, and that's why diseases are opportunities for introspection and resolving imbalances" (AME, 2003).

Three physicians have recently been especially prolific in writing about the crossover between spirituality and medicine. Koenig cites evidence in numerous books that a strong spiritual life is an indicator of longer life span and increased well-being (Koenig, 2004; Koenig et al, 2004). Benor (2001, 2004) documents scientific validation for spiritual healing. Dossey (1993) cites evidence for the positive effects of prayer on healing.

Currently, there are almost 4000 members in the National Spiritualist Association of Churches—the most prominent association of Spiritualists in North America.

A truer indicator of the popularity of mediums and healers is the results of a Gallup poll. In 1996, a Gallup poll concluded that 52% of North Americans believe in mediums and ghosts.

At its birth, modern Spiritualism was mainly a commercial phenomenon that amused or aggravated the public in North America but never took root. The process of fascinating and disarming the public who seek the dramatic phenomena produced by charismatic mediums and healers continues in large groups today. These healers, like TV evangelist Bennie Hinn in the United States and John of God in Brazil, may attend a stadiumful of people in a day, displaying phenomena that convince people that spiritual healing is effective. These are the strong personalities who stand at the portals of the field of spiritual healing—they introduce it to others.

Once through the portals, one finds a different field, related less to drama and personal ego and more to steady, humble, personal work. Those who follow *Spiritism* have created a deeply rooted tradition that continues to spread today, quietly engaged with profound personal transformation and anonymous charitable giving. There are millions of Brazilian Spiritists who go about the work of "reforma íntima," channeling, healing, praying, and doing charity work—without commercialization, self-serving promotion, or flamboyant display. Some of them consider Spiritism their religion. Call it what you will, their way of life may, in fact, be the essence of a healing life of the spirit. It is a way of life that allows the individual to become whole, more healthy, more knowledgeable, more giving, and more connected to community and "higher power," and consistently to progress on the path of spiritual evolution.

Your intentions must remain pure. You work to be of service, for love. When you work alone, it is easier to lose your ethical standards, get greedy, or get lost in the glamour.

—ELSIE DUBUGRAS, SPIRITIST
AND EDITOR OF *PLANETA* MAGAZIN (2001)

SUMMARY

In their healing centers and hospitals Spiritists employ highly developed spiritual healing techniques to complement allopathic medicine. These may be more effective than the therapeutic practices such as reiki and therapeutic touch that are more familiar to us in the United States. Although some reports indicate extraordinary successes in healing both mental and physical diseases at the centers that use Spiritist techniques, there is need for more rigorous research.

Spiritism addresses many of our current socioeconomic needs. Because the therapies are given by highly trained volunteers (as part of their spiritual practice), Spiritist therapies provide a partial answer to the skyrocketing costs of our current health care system. They can also nourish those looking for a philosophy of life and spiritual practice distinct from conventional religion. Spiritists answer the need of those natural mediums and healers who wish to harness their gifts. This is particularly significant for those who may be misdiagnosed as having mental illness when, in fact, they are suffering from a "spiritual problem"—namely, mediumistic abilities that need to be channeled positively, to help others. These natural mediums need the direction and spiritual community that Spiritist centers offer.

Several organizations are bringing Brazil's Spiritism to the United States. The International Medical Spiritist Association in Brazil increases dialogue about spirituality and health through annual conferences. The Center for the Study of Religious and Spiritual Problems in São Paulo, founded by Alexander Moreira-Almeida, MD, and Francisco Lotufo Neto, MD, is furthering scientific research and publishing in Portuguese and English. The Foundation for Energy Therapies in the United States offers mobile classrooms in Brazil to introduce Spiritist therapies to students and health professionals outside Brazil and collaborates with Brazilians in research studies in Spiritist hospitals. Although there are independent researchers in the United States who have been looking into spiritual healing in various cultures, there is a need and opportunity to generate a more organized effort that includes the Kardecist Spiritist tradition. Fortunately, many Spiritists are encouraging this initiative by translating more of the seminal books into English and welcoming English-speaking participants into their activities.

Acknowledgments

The author gratefully acknowledges the kind support of J.L. Grobler, MD, as well as the editorial comments on earlier versions of this chapter by Alexander Moreira-Almeida, MD; Vanessa Anseloni, MA; Ily Reis, Esquire; and Joby Thompson.

Research for this article was funded by Laurance Rockefeller, Mr. and Mrs. Edmund Kellogg, the Lloyd Symington Foundation, the Foundation for Energy Therapies, Inc., and the Marion Institute.

Chapter References can be found on the Evolve website at http://evolve.elsevier.com/Micozzi/complementary/

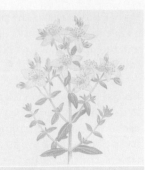

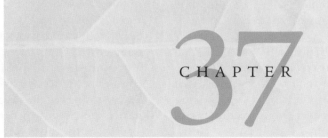

CHAPTER

37

LATIN AMERICAN CURANDERISMO

ROBERT T. TROTTER II

HISTORY

Curanderismo, from the Spanish verb *curar* (to heal), is a broad healing tradition found in Mexican American communities throughout the United States. It has many historical roots in common with traditional healing practices in Puerto Rican and Cuban American communities, as well as traditional practices found throughout Latin America. At the same time, curanderismo has a history and a set of traditional medical practices that are unique to Mexican cultural history and to the Mexican American experience in the United States.

Seven historical roots are embedded in modern curanderismo. Its theoretical beliefs partly trace their origins to Greek humoral medicine, especially the emphasis on balance and the influence of hot and cold properties of food and medicines on the body. Many of the rituals that provide both a framework and a meaningful cultural healing experience in curanderismo date to healing practices contemporary to the beginning of the Christian tradition and even to earlier Judeo-Christian writings. Other healing practices derive from the European Middle Ages, including

the use of traditional medicinal plants and magical healing practices in wide use at that time.

The Moorish conquest of southern Europe is visible in the cultural expression of curanderismo. Some common Mexican American folk illnesses originated in the Near East and then were transmitted throughout the Mediterranean, such as belief in *mal de ojo,* or the evil eye (the magical influence of staring at someone). Homeopathic remedies for common health conditions such as earaches, constipation, anemia, cuts and bruises, and burns were brought from Europe to the New World to be passed down to the present time within curanderismo. There also is significant sharing of beliefs with Aztec and other Native American cultural traditions in Mexico. Some of the folk illnesses treated in pre-Columbian times, such as a fallen fontanelle *(caída de la mollera)* and perhaps the blockage of the intestines *(empacho)* are parts of this tradition. The pharmacopeia of the New World also is important in curanderismo (and added significantly to the plants available for treatment of diseases in Europe from the 1600s to the present). Some healers *(curanderos)* keep track of developments in parapsychology and New Age spirituality, as well as acupuncture and Eastern healing traditions, and have incorporated these global perspectives into their own practices.

Finally, curanderismo is clearly a deeply rooted traditional healing system, but it also actively exists within the modern world. Biomedical beliefs, treatments, and practices are very much a part of curanderismo and are supported by curanderos. On the border between the United States and Mexico, it is not unusual for healers to recommend the use of prescription medications (which can often be purchased in Mexico over the counter) to treat infections and other illnesses. These healers also use information obtained from television and other sources to provide the best advice on preventive efforts such as good nutrition and exercise as well as explanations for biomedical illnesses.

Individual healers vary greatly in their knowledge of the practices that stem from each of these seven historical sources. The overall system of curanderismo is complex and not only maintains its cultural link to the past but evolves toward accommodation with the future as well.

Cultural Context

This chapter is based partly on research that was conducted in the Lower Rio Grande Valley of Texas for more than 15 years. That information is enhanced by data from other regions near the U.S.-Mexican border, and from Mexican American communities in Colorado, Nebraska, Chicago, and Florida. Multiple research environments, both rural and urban, have affected the practice of curanderismo. Alger (1974) described one possible outcome of urbanized curanderismo, in which the folk healing system mimics the modern medical system, but this mimicry does not exist to any significant extent in southern Texas, where both curanderos and their patients have extensive knowledge of the medical system in urban and rural areas. However, unlike those whose attitudes were reported in earlier studies of the area (Madsen, 1961; Rubel, 1966), curanderos and their patients accept the use of modern medicine. These multiple environments of curanderismo practice create a complex healing system with core elements that are common to each place and modifications that respond to local cultural, political, and legal circumstances.

The earliest systematic research on curanderismo was done in the late 1950s, when modern medicine was inaccessible or only recently available to significant segments of the Mexican American population. Since that time, the efficacy of modern medicine has been demonstrated empirically numerous times, so it is an integrated part of the cultural system, although many access barriers still exist to prevent its full use by everyone. These barriers are part of the reason that the holistic health movement and the charismatic healing movements are becoming increasingly popular. Although traditional healers in Mexican American communities believe that modern medicine is

as capable in certain types of healing, their experience shows that their own practices are not recognized in hospitals and clinics and that they can accomplish those same tasks better than modern medicine. Thus, curanderismo and modern medicine often assume complementary roles in the minds of the curanderos and their patients, although not necessarily in the minds of the medical professionals of the area.

The information in this chapter has been checked and updated by periodic visits and, at this time, by virtual contacts (through the Web and E-mail) with practitioners in South Texas and all along the U.S.-Mexico border, with the basic finding that the core elements of curanderismo remain very stable through time. There are curanderos who were practicing in the 1970s and 1980s who are still practicing, and there are new healers emerging in communities that need their services.

Intellectual Tradition

Traditional Mexican American healers perceive health and illness to involve a duality of "natural" and "supernatural" illnesses. This duality forms the theoretical base on which curanderismo is constructed. Views of the natural source of illness essentially conform to a biomedical model of illness that includes lay interpretations of some diseases inspired by Mexican American culture. Biomedical aspects such as the germ theory of disease, the genetic basis of some disorders, the existence of psychological conditions, and dietary causes for medical conditions are accepted. These natural illnesses are treated by physicians with herbal remedies. A parallel supernatural source of illness also is recognized by this healing tradition. These illnesses are not considered amenable to treatment by the medical establishment. They can be repaired only by the supernatural manipulations of curanderos. The curanderos fault the scientific medical system for its failure to recognize the existence of magic or of supernatural causation. One curandero commented that as many as 10% of patients in mental institutions were really *embrujados* (hexed or bewitched), and because physicians could not recognize this condition, it went untreated. This curandero was willing to test his theory scientifically in any way that the mental health professionals set up as a research project. However, the mental health professionals were not willing to allow the tests to be conducted because of their attitudes toward curanderismo. In this case, it appeared to the anthropologists that the curanderos had a stronger belief and trust in science, even when it was directed at the supernatural, than did the physicians and other health professionals.

Supernaturally induced illnesses are most often said to be initiated by either evil spirits (*espíritos malos*) or by *brujos* (individuals practicing antisocial magic). They form a significant part of the curanderos' work. These healers explain that any particular illness experienced by a patient could be caused theoretically by either natural or supernatural processes. For example, they believe that there is a natural form of diabetes and a form that is caused by a supernatural agent, such as a brujo. The same is true for alcoholism, cancer, and other diseases. Identifying the nature of the causal agent for a particular illness is a key problem for the curandero. Some identify more supernatural causes for illnesses, and others take a more biomedically balanced approach. In either case, there is much less dichotomizing of physical and social problems within curanderismo than within the medical care system (Holland, 1963; Kiev, 1968).

Curanderos routinely deal with problems of a social, psychological, and spiritual nature, as well as physical ailments. Many cases overlap into two or more categories. Bad luck in business is a common problem presented to curanderos. Other problems include marital disruptions, alcoholism or alcohol abuse, infidelity, supernatural manifestations, cancer, diabetes, and infertility. One healer distinguishes between the problems presented by women and men. The central focus of the problems brought by women is the husband: the husband drinks too much, does not work, does not give the wife money, or is seeing other women. Men bring problems of a more physical nature, such as stomach pain, headaches, weakness, and bladder dysfunction. Men also bring problems that deal directly with work: they need to find a job, cannot get along with people at work, or are having trouble setting up a business. The wife rarely is the focal point of their problems. The total list of problems presented to curanderos includes almost every situation that can be thought of as an uncomfortable human condition. Curanderismo seems to play an important, culturally appropriate psychotherapeutic role in Mexican American communities (Galvin et al, 1961; Klineman, 1969; Torrey, 1972).

Another element of curanderismo that forms an important intellectual foundation for its practices is the concept that healers work by virtue of "a gift of healing" (el don) (Hudson, 1951; Madsen, 1965; Romano, 1964; Rubel, 1966). This inherent ability allows the healer to practice his or her work, especially in the supernatural area. In the past this was believed to be a gift from God. However, a secular interpretation of the don is competing with the more traditional explanation. Many healers still refer to the don as a gift from God and support this premise with biblical passages (Corinthians 12:7 and James 5:14), but other healers explain the don as an inborn trait that is present in all humans, just like the ability to sing, run, or talk. Almost any person can do these things, but some do them better than others, and a few people can do them extremely well. Curanderos, according to this theory, are the individuals with a better ability to heal than is normal for the population as a whole. Healers refer to this concept as "developed abilities."

Another element common to Hispanic-based folk medicine is the hot-cold syndrome (Currier, 1966; Foster, 1953; Ingham, 1940). The hot-cold belief system is not common in southern Texas (Madsen, 1961), where the only indications of belief in a hot-cold syndrome found among patients were scattered folk beliefs such as that one should not eat citrus during menses, not iron barefoot on a cement floor, and not take a cold shower after prolonged exposure to the sun. None of these beliefs was organized systematically or shared extensively within the Mexican American population. In other areas, there is extensive knowledge and use of this system of classifying foods, treatments, and elements of illnesses to provide the basis for deciding which remedies apply to specific illnesses.

THEORETICAL BASIS

The community-based theoretical structure for curanderismo has three primary areas of concentration, called *levels* (*niveles*) by the healers: the material level (*nivel material*), the spiritual level (*nivel espiritual*), and the mental level (*nivel mental*). More curanderos have the don for working at the material level, which is organized around the use of physical objects to heal or to change the patient's environment. This theoretical area can be subdivided into physical and supernatural manipulations. Physical treatments are those that do not require supernatural intervention to ensure a successful outcome. *Parteras* (midwives), *hueseros* (bone setters), *yerberos* (herbalists), and *sobadores* (people who treat sprains and tense muscles) are healers who work on the nivel material and effect cures without any need for supernatural knowledge or practices. All the *remedios caseros* (home remedies) used in Mexican American communities are part of this healing tradition.

The supernatural aspect of this level is involved in cures for common folk illnesses found in Mexican American communities, such as *susto, empacho, caída de mollera, espanto,* and *mal de ojo*. These illnesses are unique to Hispanic cultural models of health and illness. This area of healing also includes the spells and incantations that are derived from of medieval European witchcraft and earlier forms of magic, such as the cabala, that have been maintained as supernatural healing elements of curanderismo. Supernatural manipulations involve prayers and incantations in conjunction with objects such as candies, ribbons, water, fire, crucifixes, tree branches, herbs, oils, eggs, and live animals. These treatments use a combination of common objects and rituals to cure health problems.

The spiritual level (nivel espiritual) is an area of healing that is parallel to the channeling found in New Age groups and in shamanistic healing rituals around the world (Macklin, 1967, 1974a, 1974b, 1974c; Macklin et al, 1973). Individuals enter an altered state of consciousness and, according to the curanderos, make contact with the spirit world by one or all of the following methods: opening their minds to spirit voices, sending their spirits out of the body to gain knowledge at a distance, and allowing spirits the use of the body to communicate with this world.

The mental level (nivel mental) is the least often encountered of the three levels. One healer described working with the mental level as the ability to transmit, channel, and focus mental vibrations *(vibraciones mentales)* in a way that affects the patient's mental or physical condition directly. Both patients and healers are confident that the curanderos can effect a cure from a distance using this technique.

The three levels are discrete areas of knowledge and behavior, each necessitating the presence of a separate gift for healing. They involve different types of training and different methods of dealing with both the natural and the supernatural world. The material level involves the manipulations of traditional magical forces found in literature on Western witchcraft. Spiritualism involves the manipulation of a complex spirit world that exists parallel to our own and the manipulation of *corrientes espirituales,* spiritual currents that can both heal and provide information or diagnosis from a distance. The mental level necessitates the control and use of the previously mentioned vibraciones mentales. Thus the levels are separate methods of diagnosing and treating human problems that are embedded into a single cultural tradition.

Not all problems can be dealt with successfully using each level. An example of this is serious alcohol abuse (Trotter, 1979a, 1979b; Trotter et al, 1978). Alcohol abuse and alcoholism are treated by curanderos using techniques of both the material and the mental level. The techniques of the spiritual level, however, are considered ineffective in dealing with alcohol-related problems. Therefore, if one has the don for working with the spiritual level alone, he or she is excluded from the process of curing alcohol problems.

One theme that is common to the practices of all three levels is the use of energy to change the patient's health status. On the material level, this energy often is discussed in relation to the major ritual of that level, known as the *barrida* or *limpia* (a "sweeping" or "cleansing"). In this ritual a person is "swept" from head to foot with an object that is thought to be able either to remove bad vibrations *(vibraciones malos)* or to give positive energy *(vibraciones positivos)* to the patient. The type of object used (e.g., egg, lemon, garlic, crucifix, broom) depends on what the patient's problem is and whether it is necessary to remove or to replace energy. On the spiritual level, the energy used for both diagnosis and healing is the previously mentioned corrientes espirituales. The mental level is almost totally oriented around generating and channeling vibraciones mentales. The following sections provide more detail on the actual practices of the curandero's work on each level.

MATERIAL LEVEL (NIVEL MATERIAL)

The material level is the easiest of the three levels to describe; it is the most extensively practiced and the most widely reported. At this level the curandero manipulates physical objects and performs rituals (or *trabajos,* spells). The combination of objects and rituals is widely recognized by Mexican Americans as having curative powers. Practitioners of the material level use common herbs, fruits, nuts, flowers, animals and animal products (chickens, doves, and eggs), and spices. Religious symbols such as the crucifix, pictures of saints, incense, candles, holy water, oils, and sweet fragrances are widely used, as are secular items such as cards, alum, and ribbons. The curandero allows patients to rely extensively on their own resources by prescribing items that either are familiar or have strong cultural significance. Thus a significant characteristic of the objects employed at the material level is that they are common items used for daily activities such as cooking and worship.

Natural Illnesses and Herbal Cures

Curanderos recognize that illnesses can be brought about by natural causes, such as dysfunction of the body, carelessness or the inability of a person to perform proper self-care, and infection. Curanderos practicing at the material level use large amounts of medicinal herbs *(plantas medicinales)* to treat these natural ailments. Some traditional curanderos classify herbs as having the dichotomous properties considered essential for humoral medicine, based on a hot-cold classification system common throughout Latin America (Foster, 1953). They use these dual properties to prescribe an herb or combination of herbs, depending on the characteristics of the illness. If a person's illness supposedly is caused by excessive "heat," an herb with "cold" properties is given. Conversely, if a person's illness is believed to be caused by excessive "coldness and dryness," a combination of herbs having "hot and wet" properties is administered.

Other curanderos recognize herbs for their chemical properties, such as poisons *(yerba del coyote, Karwinskia humboldtiana* Roem. et Sch.), hallucinogens (peyote, *Lophaphora williamsii* Lem.), sedatives *(flor de tila, Talia mexicana* Schl.), stimulants *(yerba del trueno),* and purgatives *(cascara sagrada).* These individuals refer to the beneficial chemical properties of the herbs that allow them to treat natural illnesses.

Curanderos prescribe herbs most frequently as teas, baths, or poultices. The teas act as a sort of formative chemotherapy. *Borraja* (borage, *Borago officinalis* L.), for example, is taken to cut a fever; *flor de tila,* a mild sedative, is taken for insomnia; *yerba de la golondrina (Euphorbia prostrata* Ait.) is used as a douche for vaginal discharges; and *pelos de elote* is used for kidney problems. Herbal baths usually are prescribed to deal with skin diseases; *fresno* (ash tree, *Fraxinus* species) is used to treat scalp problems such as eczema, dandruff, and psoriasis; and *linaza* is prescribed for body sores. For specific sores such as boils, leaves of *malva* (probably a *Malvastrum)* are boiled until soft and then applied to the sores as a poultice. Other herbs are used as decongestants. A handful of *oregano* (*Origanum vulgare* L.) is placed in a humidifier to treat someone with a bad cold.

Some herbal lore is passed on through an oral tradition, and other information is available in Spanish-language books for Mexico that are widely circulated among both curanderos and the public (Arias, n.d.; Wagner, n.d.). These works describe and classify numerous herbs. Herbal remedies are so important to Mexican American folk medicine that their use often is confused with the art of curanderismo itself by the mass culture. Indeed, some curanderos, known as *yerberos* or *yerberas,* specialize in herbs, but their knowledge and skills go beyond the mere connection of one disease to one herbal formula. For curanderos to be genuine, even at the material level, an element of mysticism must be involved in their practice. Herbs are typically used for their spiritual or supernatural properties. Spiritual cleansings (barridas) often are given with *ruda* (*Ruta graveolens* L.), *romero* (rosemary, *Rosmarinus officinalis* L.), and *albacar* (sweet basil, *Ocimum basilicum* L.), among others. Herbs are used as amulets; *verbena* (*Verbena officinalis* L.), worn as an amulet, is used to help open a person's mind to learn and retain knowledge.

Some curanderos have successful practices on the material level without resorting to the use of herbs. Some nonherbal treatments are described in the following section.

Supernaturally Caused Illnesses and Ritual Cures

Supernatural illnesses, which occur when supernatural negative forces damage a person's health, sometimes can be confused with natural illnesses. One healer stated that these supernatural illnesses may manifest as ulcers, tuberculosis, rheumatism, or migraine headaches, but in reality, they are believed to be hexes that have been placed on the person by an enemy. Supernatural influences also disrupt a person's mental health and his or her living environment. Physicians cannot cure a supernatural illness. The curandero usually deals with social disruption, personality complexes, and sometimes serious psychological disturbances. One healer gave the following description of a case that contained several of these elements:

> This patient worked for the street maintenance department of (a small city in south Texas). Every day after work a voice would lead him out into the brush and sometimes keep him there until 2:00 AM. This activity was wearing out the man and his family and he was going crazy. A bad spirit was following this man and would not leave him alone. The man was cured, but it took three people to cure him: myself, a friend, and a master *(maestro)* from Mexico. This man was given three *barridas* each day for seven days, one by each of us. The tools used were eggs, lemons, herbs, garlic, and black chickens. The man was also prescribed herbal baths and some teas to drink. He was also given a charm made from the *haba mijrina* designed to ward off any more negative influences which might be directed at him. This patient regained his sanity.

Also, a number of illnesses are both supernaturally caused and of a supernatural nature and can be treated on the material level. The following account is an example of such an illness and cure:

> My brother-in-law was working at a motel...in Weslaco. When he started working they laid off this other guy who had been working there for several years. This guy didn't like it, and he's been known to be messing around with black magic. I don't know what he did to my brother-in-law, but every other day he'd have to be taken home because he was sick. He started throwing up, had shaky knees, and weak joints. So my mother and I went over to see this lady in Reynosa, and she told my mother just what to do. My sister rubbed her husband with a lemon every night for three days. She also gave him some kind of tea.... On the third day, a big black spot appeared on the lemon, so we threw it away, and he's been fine ever since.

Rituals and the Material Level

Curanderos use several types of rituals for supernatural cures. The barrida is one of the most common rituals. These cleansings are designed to remove the negative forces that are harming the patient, while simultaneously giving the patient the spiritual strength necessary to enhance recovery. Patients are always swept from head to toe, with the curandero making sweeping or brushing motions with an egg, lemon, herb, or whatever object is deemed spiritually appropriate. Special emphasis is given to areas in pain. While sweeping the patient, the curandero recites specific prayers or invocations that appeal to God, saints, or other supernatural beings to restore health to the patient. The curandero may recite these prayers and invocations out loud or silently. Standard prayers include the Lord's Prayer, the Apostles' Creed, and Las Doce Verdades de Mundo (The Twelve Truths of the World). Many of the tools used in barridas are plants that are available in people's yards; others can be purchased at local *yerberías* or *botánicas* (Figure 37-1).

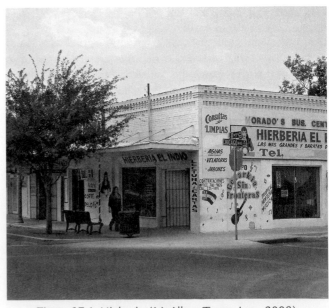

Figure 37-1 Hieberia (McAllen, Texas, June 2008).

The following description of a barrida illustrates how the material objects, the mystical power of these objects, the invocations, the curandero, and the patient come together to form a healing ritual designed for a specific patient and a specific illness. In this case, five eggs, four lemons, some branches of albacar (sweet basil), and oil are used. To begin the healing process, the lemons and eggs are washed with alcohol and water to cleanse them spiritually. Before beginning the ritual, the participants are instructed to take off their rings, watches, and other jewelry; high-frequency spiritual and mental vibrations can produce electrical discharges on the metal, which might disturb the healing process. The sweeping itself is done by interchanging an egg and a lemon successively. Sweeping with the egg is intended to transfer the problem from the patient to the egg by means of conjures *(conjures)* and invocations *(rechasos)*. The lemon is used to eliminate the *trabajo* (magical harm) that has been placed on the patient. The patient is swept once with albacar (sweet basil) that has been rinsed in *agua preparada* (prepared water). This sweeping purifies the patient, giving strength and comfort to his or her spiritual being. The ritual ends by making crosses with *aceite preparado* (specifically prepared oil) on the principal joints of the patients, such as the neck, under the knees, and above the elbow. This oil serves to cut the negative currents and vibrations that surround the patient, which have been placed there by whoever is provoking the harm. The crosses protect against the continued effect of these negative vibrations. Agua preparada is then rubbed on the patient's forehead and occiput *(cerebro)* to tranquilize and to give mental strength. All the objects used in the barrida are then burned to destroy the negative influences or harm transferred from the patient.

Another common ritual is called a *sahumerio,* or "incensing." The sahumerio is a purification rite used primarily for treating businesses, households, farms, and other places of work or habitation. This ritual is performed by treating hot coals with an appropriate incense. The curandero may prepare his or her own incense or may prescribe some commercially prepared incense, such as *el sahumerio maravilloso* (miraculous incense). A pan with the smoking incense is carried throughout the building, with care taken to ensure that all corners, closets, and hidden spaces, such as under the beds, are properly filled with smoke. While incensing, the healer or someone else recites an appropriate prayer. If the sahumerio maravilloso is used, the prayer often is one to Santa Marta, requesting that peace and harmony be restored to the household. After the sahumerio, the healer may sprinkle holy water on the floor of every room in the house and light a white candle that stays lit for 7 days. The sahumerio is an example of the curandero's treating the general social environment, seeking to change the conditions of the persons who live or work there. Incensing of a house removes negative influences such as bad luck *(salaciones),* marital disruptions, illness, or disharmony. For business and farms, incensing helps ensure success and growth and protects against jealous competitors. These rituals are designed to affect everyone in the environment that has been treated.

Another type of ritual, called a *sortilegio* (conjure), uses material objects such as ribbons to tie up the negative influences that harm the curandero's patients. These negative influences are often personal shortcomings, such as excessive drinking, infidelity, rebellious children, unemployment, or any other problem believed to be imposed by antisocial magic (trabajo). One sortilegio that I observed required four ribbons in red, green, white, and black, each approximately 1 yard in length. The color of each ribbon represents a type of magic, which the curanderos can activate to deal with specific problems. Red magic involves domination, green deals with healing, white with general positive forces, and black with negative or debilitating forces.

When working with a specific area of magic, one uses material objects that are the appropriate color naturally or that have been made that color artificially. The color-based division of magic also is carried over into another type of ritual system used on the material level, *velacione,* or burning candles to produce supernatural results. The velaciones and the colored material objects used in the sortilegios tie into the energy theme that runs throughout curanderismo, because the colors and objects are believed to have specific vibratory power or energy that can affect the patient when activated by the incantations used in conjunction with the objects. For example, blue candles are burned for serenity or tranquility; red candles are burned for health, power, or domination; pink candles are burned for goodwill; green candles are burned to remove a harmful or negative influence; and purple candles are burned to repel and attack bad spirits *(espíritus obscuros)* or strong magic. Once the proper color of candle has been chosen to produce the proper mental atmosphere, the candles are arranged in the correct physical formation and activated by the *conjuros y rechasos.* If a patient asks for protection, the candles might be burned in a triangle, which is considered to be the strongest formation, one whose influence cannot be broken easily. If the patient wants to dominate someone—a spouse, a lover, or an adversary—the candles might be burned in circles. Other formations include crosses, rectangles, and squares, depending on the results desired (Buckland, 1970).

Another relatively common use of candles is to diagnose problems by studying the flame or the ridges that appear in the melted wax. A patient may be swept with a candle while the healer recites an invocation asking the spirit of the patient to allow its material being to be investigated for any physical or spiritual problems that may be affecting the person. This ritual also can be performed by burning objects used in a barrida. Lighting the candle or burning the object after the barrida helps the curandero identify the cause and extent of the patient's problems. Similarly, if a petitioner asks for candling, the wax of the candles burned for the velacione may be examined for figures or other messages that point to the source of a patient's problems.

One of the organizing principles of the material level of curanderismo is synchronicity with Christianity in general and the Catholic Church in particular. Special invocations often are directed at saints or spirits to bring about desired results. For example, San Martín de Porres is asked to relieve poverty, San Martín Caballero to ensure success in business, San Judas Tadeo to help in impossible situations, and Santa Marta to bring harmony to a household. Ritual materials used by the Church, such as water, incense, oils, and candles, are extensively used by folk healers. The ways in which these religious objects are used and the theories for their efficacy closely mirror the concepts found within the healing ministry of the Church, which are not incompatible with European witchcraft, from which curanderismo partly derives.

Spiritual Level (Nivel Espiritual)

Curanderos who have the don for working on the spiritual level (nivel espiritual) of curanderismo are less numerous than those who work on the material level. These practitioners also must go through a developmental period *(desarrollo)* that can be somewhat traumatic. Spiritual practices in communities revolve around a belief in spiritual beings who inhabit another plane of existence but who are interested in making contact with the physical world periodically. Healers become a direct link between this plane of existence and that other world. In some cases the curanderos claim to control these spirit beings, and in other cases they merely act as a channel through which messages pass. Some of these practices are carried out by individual healers, whereas other activities occur in conjunction with spiritual centers *(centros espiritistas)* that are staffed by trance mediums and other individuals with occult abilities. These centers often work through two prominent folk saints: El Niño Fidencio from Northern Mexico and Don Pedrito Jaramillo from southern Texas (Macklin, 1974a, 1974b, 1974c). This trend in visiting spiritualist centers appears to be relatively recent, not having been reported during the 1950s and 1960s by those doing research on Mexican American folk medicine (Clark, 1959a, 1959b; Madsen, 1964a, 1964b; Rubel, 1960, 1966).

The practice of spiritualism rests on "soul concept," a belief in the existence of spirit entities derived from once-living humans. The soul is thought to be the immortal component, the life and personality force of humans, an entity that continues to exist after physical death on a plane of reality separate from the physical world. This concept is important not only to curanderismo but also to the religions and mystical beliefs found in all Western cultures.

The soul is alternatively described by curanderos as a force field, ectoplasm, concentrated vibrations, or group of electrical charges that exists separate from the physical body. It is thought to retain the personality, knowledge, and motivations of the individual even after the death of the body. The soul is ascribed the ability to contact and affect persons living in the physical world under proper conditions. Although souls occasionally can be seen as ghosts or apparitions by ordinary humans, they exist more often in the spiritual realm previously mentioned. Some people view this realm as having various divisions that have positive or negative connotations associated with them (e.g., heaven, limbo, purgatory, hell). Other people see the spiritual realm as parallel to the physical world. They state that the spiritual is a more pleasant plane on which to live, but few attempt any suicidal test of this belief. One healer commented that "spirits" *(espíritos)* and "souls" *(almas)* are the same thing. The activities of these spirits closely parallel their former activities in this world. Because the personality, knowledge, and motivation of the spirits are much the same as they were for the living being, there are both good and evil spirits, spirits who heal and spirits who harm, and wise spirits and fools.

These spirits might communicate with or act on the physical plane. Some have left tasks undone in their physical lives that they want to complete; others want to help or cause harm; and many want to communicate messages to friends and relatives, telling them of their happiness or discontent with their new existence. Therefore, curanderos with the ability to work on the spiritual realm become the link between these two worlds. Some curanderos believe that there are multitudes of spirits who want to communicate with the physical world and that these spirits tend to hover around those who have the don to become a medium, waiting for an opportunity to enter their bodies and possess them. This explains the cases of spirit possession in Western cultures. Individuals who become possessed are people with a strong potential to be trance mediums who have not had the opportunity to learn how to control this condition.

The ability to become a medium is thought to be centered in the cerebro, that portion of the brain found at the posterior base of the skull. Those with the gift are said to have a more fully developed cerebro, whereas those who do not are said to have a weak cerebro *(un cerebro débil)*. This weakness has no relationship either to the intelligence or to the moral nature of the individual, only to his or her ability to communicate with the spiritual realm. Weak cerebros represent a danger for anyone who wants to become a medium. Only rare individuals demonstrate mediumistic potential spontaneously and can practice as mediums without further training. Therefore, curanderos often test their patients and friends for this gift of healing, and those with the gift are encouraged to develop their ability.

The development of this ability is called *desarrollo* and is a fairly lengthy process that might last from 2 months to more than 6 months initially, with periodic refresher encounters often available from the maestro (teacher). Desarrollo is a gradual process of increasing an apprentice's contact with the spirit world, giving the apprentice more and more experiences in controlled trances and possessions, as well as the knowledge necessary to develop and protect the apprentice as a spiritualist. The teacher also is responsible for giving the apprentice knowledge at a safe pace. The curandero does not always explain what each sensation means; each person, as he or she develops, becomes more sensitive to the environment. The apprentice must expect to encounter odd sensations, such as bright lights, noises, changes in pressure, and other sensations associated with developing powers. At the end of these desarrollo sessions, the conversation reverts to social chatting for some time before the apprentice leaves. This developmental process continues, with variations, until the apprentice is a fully developed medium.

Fully developed mediums control how, where, and when they work, and several options are available to them. Some mediums work alone and treat only family problems (Box 37-1); others might use their abilities only for their own knowledge and gratification. Some mediums work in groups with other mediums or with other persons whom they believe have complementary spiritual or psychic powers. Some mediums work in elaborate spiritual centers (centros espiritistas) that are formal churches, often dedicated to a particular spirit (e.g., Fidencio, Francisco Rojas, Don Pedrito Jaramillo). The spiritual centers and the activities surrounding them take on the major aspects of a formalized religion.

Sometimes a trance session is open to more than one person at the same time. This group session can be carried out by a lone curandero but more often is seen at spiritual centers. The process of the development of these centers is described elsewhere (Trotter et al, 1975a). Once a temple has been established, it may house from 1 to 20 mediums. The more mediums, the better; otherwise, a medium may have to let his or her body be used by too many different spirits, which exhausts the medium and lays the medium open to supernatural harm. Larger temples might have four or five *videntes* (clairvoyants), as well as the mediums, and might be putting several apprentices through desarrollo at the same time. Many of the accounts about spiritual healing were from individuals who had had experiences with spiritual temples in Mexico. Some temples were located in Espinazo, the home of El Niño Fidencio and a center of pilgrimage for mediums practicing in his name, and others were in urban centers such as Tampico and Mexico City. Large numbers of people make pilgrimages to these healing centers in Mexico to deal with health care problems that they have not resolved in the United States.

One healing center is called *Roca Blanca*, after the spirit that speaks most often in that place. The owner, Lupita, founded it about 30 years ago, after discovering her ability to cure. She was granted permission to practice by a

BOX 37-1

Curanderos

Many curanderos able to work on the spiritual level prefer to work at home, alone. Their practices tend to be less uniform than the practices of mediums working at spiritual centers, because they do not have to conform to the calendric and ritual structure found in more formalized temples. However, there is enough commonality to their actions to provide an accurate description of a lone medium. In the following dialogue a healer is described by a student in his early twenties who was one of her patients; she had been handling problems for him and his family for several years.

R: Can you describe how this curandera works, in as great detail as you can?

S: We drive up into the driveway of a fairly decent-looking place. She walks out and greets us, shakes our hands, asks how we are doing and how we have been. Then we go inside. She's got a small room perhaps 8 by 10 feet. She has an altar with saints and candles and flowers on it. She has a small vase shaped like a crystal ball sitting on a table. Sometimes it has water on it and sometimes turned upside down.

You walk in there and sit down and she's talking with you. She's not in her trance; it's just social talk. Then she sits and puts her hand on that crystal deal. She taps it, closes her eyes, and she starts asking you what kind of problem you have or whatever you want to ask her.

R: Her voice changes?

S: Yes, it does. It's a lot lower. All of a sudden her voice becomes soft, sort of like whispering. Really mild.

R: Does she keep her hands on the glass all of this time?

S: No. Sometimes she grabs a folder with papers in it and starts writing down things on it, using her finger.

R: Can she read what she has written?

S: I'm pretty sure she can.

R: How does she cure people?

S: She does it in a number of ways. Some time ago my mother had pains on both of her heels. She went to the doctor and the doctor didn't find anything wrong. So she went over to this lady again, who said it was something (a *trabajo* or hex) that [a woman across the alley from my house] had put in the yard. When my mother's out hanging up clothes she's barefooted and she stepped on it. And that's what was hurting her. So the curandera gave her a "shot" on her arm like a regular shot. And that cured her.

R: How did she give her the shot?

S: (Simulates the action of giving an injection without a syringe or hypodermic.)

R: Could your mother feel it?

S: She told me she didn't. But it cured her.

The informant went on to tell of several other cures that this curandera had performed for his family. She had prescribed herbs, suggested the use of perfumes to ward off the *envidia* (envy) of their neighbors, and

(Continued)

BOX 37-1

Curanderos—cont'd

recommended that the mother perform a series of *barridas* on her son-in-law to remove a hex against him that was making him ill and keeping him from work. Each of these cures could just as easily have been suggested or performed by a curandero working on the material level of curanderismo, but this curandera did it from a trance state. Therefore, what sets this curandera apart from those working strictly on the material level is not the tools she uses or the rituals she suggests to her clients, but the source of her diagnosis and cure—her contact with a spirit world.

spiritual association. The following report is from a visitor to Lupita's healing center:

> I went to this place simply because I was curious. I was swept with *albacar* and the medium was at my side. While I was being swept, the medium went into trance. The sister who was sweeping me asked the spirit who he wanted to talk to. He said, "with the one you are sweeping." Then, the sister finished sweeping me and directed me to talk with the person who was addressing me. When she (the medium in trance) talked to me, she sounded like a man. He asked me, "Do you know who I am?" I have a cousin who got killed in a place in Tampico. "You must be my cousin," I said. "Yes, exactly, I am your cousin." "Look," he said, "You have come here with your husband." On other occasions I really had been there with my husband, mother and different relatives. "You have come here with your husband because you think he is hexed and that is why he is sick. But that's not true. He has a physical illness that the doctor can cure. Don't believe it's anything bad."
>
> He said, "I'm going to prove who I am by coming to your house. Tell my cousin I'm going to see her." You see, I have a sister who's not nervous at all and who isn't afraid of anything. On Tuesday, as my sister was leaning by the window watching a television show, she felt someone embrace her. She turned and saw no one.

These spiritual centers vary in their size, their owners, and the spirits who are associated with them, but there is considerable consistency in the services they perform. Sometimes mediums prescribe simple herbal remedies for physical problems. These recipes are virtually identical to the ones presented in the previous section on the material level, although occasionally it is said that a spirit will recommend a new use for an herb. The mediums might suggest that the patient perform the already familiar rituals of curanderismo, such as the barrida. The spirits are thought to be able to influence people's lives directly, in addition to imparting knowledge about remedies. The curanderos state that spirits control spiritual currents (corrientes espirituales) and mental vibrations (vibraciones mentales); they can manipulate the patient's health by directing positive or negative forces at them from the spiritual realm.

During spiritual sessions observed at a developing spiritual center in southern Texas, a spirit repeatedly presented himself over the course of several weeks to treat several patients. One of these patients was a man with lower back pain. One week the spirit told him to buy a bandage and bring it to the next session. The man did so, but then the spirit chided him for not following instructions correctly. The bandage was too narrow and not long enough. The man was instructed to buy a new bandage and place it on the window ledge to catch the morning dew, which is thought to have healing properties. He then was to place a glass of water under the head of his bed and a jar of alcohol at the side of the bed. He was to wrap himself in the bandage according to instructions given and lie quietly on his bed for no less than 2 hours, during which time the spirit promised to visit him and complete the cure. The man followed these instructions and stated that he did gain relief from his back pain. The same spirit treated a young college girl who periodically had asthma attacks. The girl's mother, a regular member of the group, brought her to the session. The spirit, in the person of the medium, stood and clasped the girl's head with one hand on her cerebro and the other on her forehead, sending corrientes espirituales through her brain. The spirit then told her to take a sip of agua preparada and sit back down in the circle. The treatment was successful in overcoming this particular attack, and the mother mentioned after the session that these cures relieved her own asthma for several months.

Another patient requested a social and emotional treatment. Her husband recently had begun to practice witchcraft (*brujería*), and she was worried that he or his friends might attack her or members of her family. A considerable amount of tension existed between the couple's families. She felt under continual stress and had gone to a doctor for help. The physician prescribed a mild sedative, which she had taken for 3 weeks without relief. The medium's spirit probed her mind and told her to take three sips of agua preparada to break any spells that had been cast on her. The spirit promised to provide her with protection and help from the spiritual realm to counteract anything that her husband might do. She appeared to be content with the spirit's activities on her behalf and was greatly relieved.

Several aspects of the spiritual level of curanderismo have not been covered in this brief description but were originally described in more detail elsewhere (Trotter et al, 1975a, 1975b, 1975c). These aspects include the actual techniques of testing for el don, the physical and supernatural dangers of trance mediumship, the acquisition of spiritual protectors to overcome those dangers, detailed descriptions of the trance state from the subjective perspective of the developing medium and the objective perspective of an observer, and, finally, the existence and purpose of mediums' associations.

MENTAL LEVEL (NIVEL MENTAL)

Conducting observational, descriptive, and experimental research on the practices of the mental level has proved to be the most difficult task in exploring all the aspects of curanderismo. The mental level has the fewest rituals and the least outward complex behavior associated with it. To date, it has the fewest practitioners, which severely limits the number of people who can be approached for an opportunity to investigate the phenomenon. All the cases the author observed followed a similar pattern. The following is an example:

> After the curandero chatted with the patient and asked [him or her] about the basic problem, he asked the patient to state [his or] her complete name (el nombre completo). The curandero wrote the name on a piece of paper. Sitting behind the desk he used for consultations, he leaned his arms on the desk, bent forward slightly, closed his eyes, and concentrated on the piece of paper. After a few minutes, he opened his eyes, told the patient more about his or her problem, and stated that it was being resolved.
>
> The curandero stated that he had learned to use his mind as a transmitter through desarrollo. He could channel, focus, and direct vibraciones mentales at the patient. These mental vibrations worked in two ways—one physical, one behavioral. If he was working with a physical illness, such as cancer, he channeled the vibrations to the afflicted area, which he already had pinpointed, and used the vibrations to retard the growth of damaged cells and accelerate the growth of normal cells. In a case of desired behavioral changes, he sent the vibrations into the person's mind and manipulated them in a way that modified the person's behavior. The curandero gave an example of one such case in which a husband had begun drinking excessively, was seeing other women, was being a poor father to his children, and was in danger of losing his job. The curandero stated that he dominated the man's thought processes and shifted them so that the husband stopped drinking to excess, and became a model husband and father. (Trotter, 1981a, 1981b, 1981c)

A number of syncretic beliefs drawn from other alternative healing traditions—such as New Age practices, the "psychic sciences," and Eastern philosophy—also have been incorporated into this area of curanderismo. For example, some healers state that they are able to perceive "auras" around people and that they can use these auras to diagnose problems that patients are encountering. They reach the diagnosis on the basis of the color or shape of the patient's aura. Some state that they learned these practices from other healers, whereas others indicate that they learned them from books on parapsychology.

The mental level is practiced most often by individual healers working with individual patients, rather than in groups. It appears to be a new addition to this healing system and does not have, as yet, a codified body of ritual associated with it. It therefore constitutes an area in which additional descriptive work will be necessary to unify healers' behavior.

THEORETICAL UNIFICATION

The three levels of curanderismo unify the theories of disease and illness found in the Mexican American folk medical model. They create a framework for determining the therapeutic approaches of curanderos in southern Texas. The system emphasizes a holistic approach to treatment and relies heavily on the intimate nature of the referral system and the extensive personal knowledge of the patient's social environment that is normally held by the curandero. Christian symbols and theology provide both tools (candles, incense, water) and organizational models (rituals, prayers, animistic concepts) for the material and the spiritual levels, but not to a similar degree for the mental level. An *energy* concept is the central idea that integrates the three levels and defines a systematic interrelationship among them. This energy concept derives from belief in forces, vibration, and currents that center in the mind of those who have the gift for healing and that can be transmitted to cause healing from a distance by affecting the patient's social, physical, spiritual, or psychological environment.

All three levels of healing are still evolving. The variations in the practices of curanderismo can be explained partly by differences in the curanderos' personality, differences in their treatment preferences or abilities, and differences in their emphasis on theoretical or experiential approaches. There also are variations produced by individual interpretations of an underlying body of theory. A study of these variations would be useful, now that the underlying theoretical system has provided a common starting point and common objectives.

SETTINGS FOR THE CURANDERISMO HEALING SYSTEM

Curanderismo is a community-based healing system. It is complex and widespread. At one level, it may be practiced in any area where Mexican Americans know about it. Part of this healing tradition is the information that is spread throughout the Mexican American culture on home treatments for common physical ailments (colds, flu, arthritis, asthma, diabetes) and for common spiritual or "folk illnesses" (susto, mal de ojo, and empacho). This is analogous to the biomedical information that is spread throughout all European cultures, including the Mexican American culture, in which the home is the first line of defense for the diagnosis of illnesses that eventually might necessitate a physician or hospital. On the other hand, some aspects of curanderismo require the use of special locations, preparations, and tools. This is especially true for spiritual practices on the spiritual level and for treatment of supernatural harm on the material level.

The first setting in which this knowledge is used is at home. When people become ill, they use their existing

570 FUNDAMENTALS OF COMPLEMENTARY AND ALTERNATIVE MEDICINE

cultural model of health and illness to come up with solutions. One type of solution is home diagnosis and home treatment. Therefore, both biomedical concepts and folk medical concepts are applied immediately, and home treatments are attempted. In the case of curanderismo, this often results in the use of home remedies *(remedio caseros)* that have been part of the culture for generations, especially herbal cures. When the diagnosis identifies a magical or supernaturally caused illness, the illness results in a home-based ritual. These interventions are done by mothers, grandmothers, cousins, friends, or knowledgeable acquaintances.

Illnesses that appear to be too serious to handle at home, both natural and supernatural, are taken to professional healers who have a locally widespread reputation for being able to treat both biomedical and traditional health problems. Most of these healers work in a silent, but positive, partnership with physicians, although the physicians often are unaware of the link. The curanderos interviewed in various studies of Mexican American folk medicine are consistent in their positive regard for modern medicine. They regularly refer patients to modern health care services in cases in which they see the efficacy of that approach to be equal to or greater than their own. At the same time, they note significant differences in the models of health and illness between their own practices and modern medicine, especially in the areas of treating supernatural illnesses, addressing social (marital, business, interpersonal) problems, and dealing with psychological problems. In these cases the treatments take place either in the patient's home or work environment or in special workrooms established by the curanderos as part of their practices. The cure might call for working directly in the environment that is affected. In other cases the venue of choice is the curandero's area, because the cure depends on careful preparation and protection from outside influences. These work areas contain altars, medicinal plants, tools for supernatural rituals, and other items, and the atmosphere is considered most beneficial for the healing process, particularly in the case of supernatural problems and treatments (Trotter et al, 1981).

RESEARCH AND EVALUATION APPROACHES

The research that is available on curanderismo is broad in interest and historical depth. Unlike specific healing techniques, such as acupuncture, which can be studied in relation to specific illnesses with relative ease, curanderismo is a complex brew of both theoretical approaches to healing and an interrelated set of healing techniques. The techniques range from herbal cures, which must be approached from an ethnopharmacological perspective; to rituals, which can be studied symbolically as projective psychiatric techniques; to methods such as massage, natural birth, nutritional prescriptions, and dietary practices. Some

studies have investigated the scientific efficacy of the practices of curanderismo, whereas others have approached it from a sociopolitical or symbolic viewpoint. Some practices have not been studied at all. Therefore, although the efficacy of some parts of the system is clearly defined, other parts remain to be explored.

Early research on curanderismo can be found in the classic anthropological works on Mexican American folk medicine, published primarily in the 1960s (Clark, 1959a; Currier, 1966; Kiev, 1968; Madsen, 1961, 1964a, 1964b; Romano, 1965; Rubel, 1960, 1964, 1966). These authors produced descriptive baseline data on the prominent folk medical practices of Hispanic communities in the United States. They provide an initial view of curanderismo that is rich in descriptions of Mexican American folk illnesses, such as susto, empacho, mal de ojo, caída de mollera, bilis, and espanto (Nall et al, 1967). These works generally treat traditional healing in Mexican American communities as a body of knowledge that is widely distributed throughout the culture, rather than as a theoretical healing system. Therefore the works consider the consensual data on what is available to a significant segment of the existing Mexican American population but spend less time describing the professional actions of curanderos, because these mass cultural phenomena are generally thought of as having themes or unifying elements rather than a theoretical structure. This viewpoint is well represented in articles about curanderismo and its form and function within Mexican American communities (Clark, 1959b; Edgerton et al, 1970; Foster, 1953; Martinez et al, 1966; Torrey, 1969).

Later research maintains the strengths of this approach but adds folk theoretical concepts. Early epidemiological approaches to folk illnesses give an idea of the geographical spread and variation in beliefs, illnesses, and healing rituals, whereas later studies identify or discuss the common denominators that unify curanderos, including their underlying perception of illness. Traditional anthropological research techniques were used to gather the data for these studies, primarily participant observation and interviewing over prolonged periods. Most of the authors used personal networks to identify individuals who were known locally as healers. Emphasis often was placed on finding individuals who were full-time healers rather than talking to those who treated only family members and neighbors. Therefore a curandero can be defined as an individual who is recognized in his or her community as having the ability to heal, who sees an average of five or more patients a day, and who has knowledge of and uses the theoretical structure described in this chapter. These people can be viewed as both specialists and professionals. Several areas of curanderismo have received a considerable amount of research attention.

HOME REMEDIES

Herbal and chemical treatments for both natural and supernatural illnesses are common in Mexican American communities. More than 800 remedios caseros have been identified on the U.S.-Mexican border alone (Trotter, 1981a, 1981b). Some of the remedies have been tested for biochemical and therapeutic activities (Etkin, 1986; Trotter, 1981a, 1981b, 1981c, 1983a, 1983b, 1983c; Trotter et al, 1986). Overall, the tested remedies are not only biochemically active, but more than 90% have demonstrated therapeutic actions that matched the folk medical model for their uses. At the same time, only a small proportion of the herbs have been tested. This lack of information is being overcome by an ongoing project to study the efficacy of the complete range of herbal cures available in Mexican American communities (Graham, 1994) through the use of combined ethnographic and biomedical methods (Browner et al, 1988; Croom, 1983; Ortiz de Montellano et al, 1985; Trotter, 1985).

The exceptions to the general rule of efficacy are the use of remedies for illnesses such as the common cold, for which the remedies relieve symptoms but do not directly treat the illness. These remedies, some of which were described earlier, include diuretics, treatments for constipation, abortifacients, analgesics, sedatives, stimulants, cough suppressants, antibacterial agents, coagulants and anticoagulants, vitamin and mineral supplements, and plants with antiparasitic actions. Most have proved safe and effective when used in the manner described and recommended by the curanderos. This area and the therapeutic, culturally competent counseling practices of the healers are the most clearly acceptable and useful approaches for articulation with modern medicine.

ADDITIONAL INFORMATION ON EPIDEMIOLOGY OF FOLK ILLNESSES

Of all the complex areas of Mexican American traditional healing, the one that has received the most research attention has been the study of common folk illnesses that are experienced and treated in Mexican American communities. The most frequently reported are susto, an illness caused by a frightening event; mal de ojo, an illness that can be traced to the Near East, which involves a magically powerful glance that takes away some of the vital essence of a susceptible person; empacho, a blockage of the intestines caused by eating the wrong type of food at the wrong time or by being forced to eat unwanted food; and caída de la mollera, a condition of fallen fontanelle in infants. A number of others also are well defined, if not as commonly studied, but these four receive most of the research attention.

The epidemiology and the cognitive models of these illnesses have been well documented (Rubel, 1964; Trotter, 1982a, 1982b, 1985; Weller et al, 1993). These illnesses have been studied both singly and in combination (Baer et al, 1989; Rubel et al, 1964; Weller et al, 1993) in terms of their cognitive structure within and between Hispanic cultural groups, their frequency of treatment, the belief in and mention of them in various communities, and their relationships to medical conditions and to

the treatment of medical conditions (Collado-Ardon et al, 1983; Trotter, 1991; Trotter et al, 1989). In the case of susto, clear evidence indicates that it is linked directly to serious morbidity patterns in Latin American communities and acts as an excellent indicator of the need for biomedical personnel to investigate multiple conditions and problems among patients complaining of its symptoms. Caída de la mollera, on investigation, is a folk medicine label that corresponds to severe dehydration in infants caused by gastrointestinal problems. It is life threatening and, when identified by parents, is an excellent indicator of the need to bring in the child immediately for medical care. Empacho is a severe form of constipation based on its description and is treated with numerous remedies that cause diarrhea. Because it is thought to be a blockage of the intestines, a purgative effect from these remedies signals that treatment has been effective. To date, no studies have linked mal de ojo to any biomedical condition; however, because the symptoms include irritability, lethargy, and crying, some connection may be made in the future.

HEALING AND PSYCHIATRY

Another area of significant endeavor in curanderismo is the identification of parallels and areas of compatibility between the processes and rituals of curanderismo and the use of psychiatry in cross-cultural settings (Kiev, 1968; Klineman, 1969; Torrey, 1969; Trotter, 1979a, 1979b; Velimirovic, 1978). The parallels are clear, especially when healers concentrate on psychological conditions that they recognize from their knowledge of psychology and psychiatry. A number of successful collaborations have been conducted in this area between traditional healers and individuals from modern medical establishments in several states.

UNEXPECTED CONSEQUENCES

It is clear that Mexican American folk medicine contains a very high proportion of useful, insightful, and culturally competent healing strategies that work well in Hispanic communities. As seen previously, these range from proven herbal cures to therapeutic models to culturally important labeling systems that can help physicians identify the cultural labels for certain types of biomedical problems. The complexity of curanderismo ensures that these findings will increase.

At the same time, no health care system exists that does not have side effects and unexpected results. With allopathic medicine, these range from the birth defects of thalidomide to the dreadful side effects of chemotherapy and the limited ability of psychology to deal with chronic mental health conditions such as alcohol and drug abuse. In curanderismo, allopathic conditions do not constitute the bulk of its application, but a few unexpected consequences have been discovered in treating empacho (Baer et al, 1988, 1989; Trotter, 1983b). These occurrences are rare but must be taken into account and understood within the overall cultural context of curanderismo and within the context of the much more pervasive positive benefits that the communities derive from having these alternative health care practices available.

Given the complexity and the diversity of practices within this traditional healing system, there remains a great deal of useful and insightful research that can be conducted beneficially in relation to curanderismo.

Acknowledgments

The initial phase of the research findings reported by the author was supported by a grant from the Regional Medical Program of Texas (RMPT Grant No. 75-108G). Further data collection efforts were supported by the Texas Commission on Alcoholism, Pan American University, and the author himself.

⊖ Chapter References can be found on the Evolve website at http://evolve.elsevier.com/Micozzi/complementary/

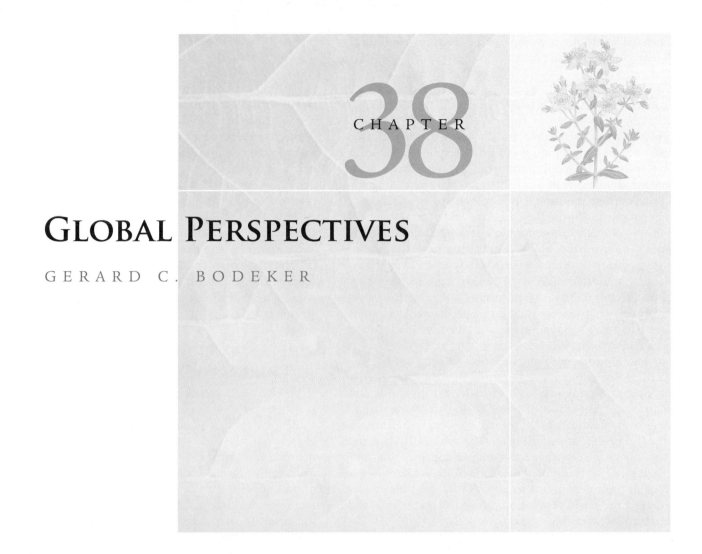

CHAPTER 38

GLOBAL PERSPECTIVES

GERARD C. BODEKER

At the basis of global concern about the ever-increasing cost of health care lies the issue of *sustainability*. Developing countries recognize that their health care systems are based on expensive imported medicines and technologies, and that if they continue to rely on these systems then health care costs will consume national financial resources and stifle national economic growth.

Industrialized countries are struggling with decisions over who pays for health care—state, employer, the public—and how the escalating costs of high-technology medicine can be made manageable. At the same time, in a number of industrialized countries almost half of the population now regularly uses some form of complementary medicine, whereas the figures for Canada and Germany are 70% and 75%, respectively.

Considerable use of traditional (i.e., indigenous) medicine also exists in many developing countries: 40% in China and Colombia, 71% in Chile, and up to 80% in some African countries (Kasilo et al, 2005).

In the developing world, basic questions are now being asked about priorities in health expenditures and national economic development: How can countries address the health needs of their people without continuing to rely on expensive imported pharmaceuticals? How can existing local systems of health care be utilized to provide basic health services to rural and poor communities?

Increased attention is being paid to the potential of locally available medicinal plants and inexpensive herbal medicines in providing effective primary health care. This consideration has in turn raised concerns about the sustainable use of wild sources of medicinal plants, the conservation of biodiversity, appropriate forms of local cultivation and production, the safety and effectiveness of natural medicines, and the regulatory environment that should accompany the incorporation of traditional systems of health into national health care.

In this chapter, recent trends are discussed and illustrated with experiences from countries and communities in Africa, the Americas, and Asia. We consider economic, cultural, environmental, and other factors that have led to the resurgence of interest in traditional systems of health. We conclude with a discussion of policy options for incorporating traditional ecological (see Chapter 4) and medicinal knowledge into national and international environmental, health, and economic policy and planning.

BACKGROUND

The terms *traditional medicine* and *traditional systems of health* refer to the longstanding indigenous systems of health care found in developing countries and among the indigenous populations of industrialized countries. The paradigms of these traditional medical systems view humanity as being linked intimately with the wider dimensions of nature (Bodeker, 2000; Bodeker et al, 2008). Long relegated to marginal status in the health care plans of developing countries, traditional medicine—or, more appropriately, traditional systems of health care, because they provide comprehensive approaches to prevention and treatment that are beyond the scope of medicine alone (see Chapter 5)—has undergone a major renewal in the past decade or more.

The World Health Organization (WHO) has referred to these systems as *holistic,* meaning that their perspective is "that of viewing man in his totality within a wide ecological spectrum, and of emphasizing the view that ill health or disease is brought about by an imbalance, or disequilibrium, of man in his total ecological system and not only by the causative agent and pathogenic evolution" (WHO, 1978). Traditional medicine has been described as "one of the surest means to achieve total health care coverage of the world population, using acceptable, safe, and economically feasible methods."

The treatment strategies utilized by traditional systems of health include the use of herbal medicines; mind-body approaches such as meditation; physical therapies including massage, acupuncture, and exercise programs; and approaches that address both physical and spiritual well-being. These methods incur limited costs, are available locally, and, according to WHO, are utilized as the primary source of health care by 80% of the world's population.

An essential feature of traditional systems of health is that they are based in cosmologies or paradigms that take into account mental, spiritual, physical, and ecological dimensions in the conceptualization and evaluation of health and well-being. Assumptions of causality frequently differ from those of Western medicine, and treatments are designed to reflect those underlying theories of causality. Indeed, classifications of diseases, medicinal plants, and ecosystems in traditional knowledge systems may vary substantially from those of Western taxonomies.

A fundamental concept found in many systems is that of *balance:* the balance between mind and body; between different dimensions of individual bodily functioning and need; between individual and community; between individual, community, and environment; and between individual and the cosmos or universe. Disease is understood to arise from a breakdown in the state of balance in

one or more of these areas. Treatments are designed not only to address the locus of the disease, but to restore a state of systemic balance to the individual and his or her inner and outer environment.

Historically, the paradigms of traditional knowledge systems have been considered "primitive" by modern or Western science. However, recent advances in environmental sciences, immunology, medical botany, and pharmacognosy have led to a new appreciation of the precise descriptive nature and efficacy of many traditional taxonomies, as well as of the efficacy of the treatments employed and the appropriateness of their use in terms of their impact on the environment, the community, and the society. There is an emerging awareness that any meaningful appraisal of a traditional system of health and its contribution to health care must take into account the paradigm or cosmology that underlies diagnosis and treatment.

ORGANIZATIONAL RELATION BETWEEN MODERN AND TRADITIONAL MEDICINE

Under colonial influence, traditional medical systems were frequently outlawed by authorities. In the postcolonial era, the attitudes of Western medical practitioners and health officials have maintained the marginal status of traditional health care providers, despite the role that these practitioners play in providing basic health care to the rural majority in developing countries and within indigenous communities in industrialized countries.

Traditional medicine and modern medicine have interfaced with each other in one of four broad ways:
1. *Monopoly:* Modern medical doctors have the sole right to practice medicine.
2. *Tolerance:* Traditional medical practitioners are not officially recognized, but are free to practice on the condition that they do not claim to be registered medical doctors.
3. *Parallelism:* Practitioners of both modern and traditional systems are officially recognized. They serve their patients through separate but equal systems, such as in India.
4. *Integration:* Modern and traditional medicine are merged in medical education and jointly practiced within a unique health service, such as in China and Vietnam.

FACTORS INFLUENCING POLICY DEVELOPMENT

Despite the historic suppression of traditional medicine by modern medical interests, an increasing number of developing countries are displaying policy interest in traditional approaches to health care, which has led to a resurgence of interest in research, investment, and program development in this field (Bodeker et al, 2002). Several factors underlie this new interest.

ECONOMIC FACTORS

The majority of the rural populations of developing countries cannot afford Western medical health care. In Vietnamese peasant communities, there is a common saying that traditional medicine costs one chicken, modern medicine costs one cow, and modern hospital treatment costs many cows. Rural people may have to travel for a day or more to reach a modern medical clinic or pharmacy. This results in lost wages, which is compounded by the cost of transport and the relatively high cost of the medicines themselves.

Typically, more than 80% of health budgets in developing countries is directed to services that reach approximately 20% of the population. Of this, 30% of the total health budget is spent on the national pharmaceutical bill.

In Asia, traditional systems of health care have been incorporated as formal components of national health care for approximately 20 years. The Indian Medicine Central Council Act of 1970 gave an official place in national health programs to the Ayurvedic and Unani medical systems of India (see Chapter 29). India now has over 200,000 registered traditional medical practitioners, the majority of whom have received their training in government colleges of Ayurvedic or Unani medicine. China has had a policy of integrating traditional medicine into national health care for more than three decades and has an extensive national program in which modern and traditional medicine are combined as formal components of health care provision (see Chapters 26 and 27). In both India and China the traditional health sector provides the majority of health care to the poor and rural communities, which are not considered "profit centers" by the Western biomedical enterprise.

In recent years, other countries have begun to provide increased support for their longstanding traditional medical systems, recognizing that they cannot afford Western medicine. In Thailand, for example, the Ministry of Health promotes the use of 66 traditional medicinal plants in primary health care, based on scientific evidence of the efficacy of these plants, as well as on traditional patterns of utilization. The Fourth Public Health Development Plan of Thailand (1977 to 1981) stated the country's general policy to promote the use of traditional medicinal plants in primary health care. The Seventh Plan (1992 to 1996) promoted the integration of traditional Thai medicine into community health care and prioritized research on medicinal plants. The Thai Ministry of Health also promotes the use of medicinal plants in state-run hospitals and health service centers (Koysooko et al, 1993). A study by the Royal Tropical Institute of the Netherlands found that traditional herbal medicines were used most effectively in primary health care in Thailand when self-administered.

Because most rural people treat themselves before seeking help from either modern or traditional medical practitioners, herbal medicines offer a low-cost intervention in the early treatment of disease and provide a safe alternative in the face of the growing problem of self-medication with inappropriate dosages and harmful combinations of over-the-counter drugs (Le Grand et al, 1990).

In Korea, between 15% and 20% of the national health budget is directed to traditional medical services, and government reports indicate that traditional medicine is favored equally by all levels of society. Health insurance coverage is available for Oriental medical treatments. In Japan, where physicians have been authorized to prescribe and dispense medications, over two thirds of all physicians reportedly prescribe herbal medications (Norbeck et al, 1987).

CULTURAL FACTORS

Cultural factors play a significant role in the continued reliance on traditional medicine. Often villagers seek symptomatic relief with modern medicine and turn to traditional medicine for treatment of what may be perceived as the "true cause of the condition" (Kleinman, 1980). Traditional medical knowledge typically is coded into household cooking practices, home remedies, and health prevention and health maintenance beliefs and routines. The advice of family members or other significant members of a community has a strong influence on health behavior, including the type of treatment that is sought (Nichter, 1978).

Decolonization and increased self-determination for indigenous groups has led some countries to reevaluate and promote their traditional medical systems. At a 1993 Pan American Health Organization conference on indigenous peoples and health, representatives from South America reported increasing activity and interest in traditional medicine in their countries (Zoll, 1993). Several Latin American countries have departments or divisions of traditional medicine within their health ministries.

Mexico has undertaken an extensive program of revitalizing its indigenous medical traditions: over 1000 traditional medicines have been identified as a result of a program of ethnomedical and pharmacognostic research; training centers have been established by the government to pass traditional medical knowledge on to new generations of health care workers; and hospitals of traditional medicine have been established in a number of rural areas. The Mexican constitution is currently being revised to include traditional medicine in the provision of national health care (Argueta, 1993). Nongovernment organizations have played a strong role in revitalizing traditional health in Mexico, organizing national and international meetings on traditional approaches to health care. More than 50 different traditional medicine associations were represented at a 1992 meeting of the Instituto Nacional Indigenista.

Native North American communities have been incorporating traditional forms of treatment into health programs for some years (see Chapter 35). In the United States, Indian Health Service (IHS) alcohol rehabilitation programs include traditional approaches to the treatment of alcoholism. An analysis of 190 IHS contract programs revealed that 50% of these programs offered a traditional sweatlodge at their site or encouraged the use of sweatlodges (Hall, 1986). Treatment outcomes improved when a sweatlodge was available. Often these sweatlodges include the presence of medicine men or healers, and the presence of a traditional healer greatly improved the outcome when used in combination with the sweatlodge. In northern Canada, the Inuit Women's Association developed a program to revitalize traditional birth practices (Flaherty, 1993). Women who had been midwives in their own communities for many years were interviewed and recorded on videotape, and these tapes are being used to train young midwives in the use of traditional methods.

NATIONAL CRISES

In addition to economic and cultural factors, national crises have spurred governments to evaluate their indigenous medical traditions as a means of providing affordable and available health care to their citizens. War and national epidemics are two common crises faced by these nations.

War

During the war in Nicaragua, there was an acute shortage of pharmaceutical supplies. In 1985, out of necessity, the country turned to its herbal traditions as a means of fulfilling the country's medical needs. A department was established within the health ministry to develop "popular and traditional medicine as a strategy in the search for a self-determined response to a difficult economic, military and political situation" (Castellon, 1992).

The department of traditional medicine initiated a program of ethnobotanical research in the midst of war. More than 20,000 people nationwide were interviewed regarding their use of traditional and popular remedies, the methods of preparing these remedies, and the sources of plant ingredients. Previously, nurses and health workers in rural areas frequently manned outposts without medical supplies. They often were surrounded by medicinal herbs of which they knew nothing.

A national toxicology program was begun, based on the extensive survey. Over a period of 6 to 7 years, pharmacognostic studies attempted to determine the chemistry and medicinal properties of commonly used plants. As a result of this effort, inexpensive medicines were produced locally and sustainably in rural areas to treat a wide range of conditions, including respiratory ailments, skin problems, nervous disorders, diarrhea, and diabetes.

Following Vietnam's war of independence from France, an official policy was articulated by President Ho Chi Minh in 1954, asserting the importance of preserving and developing traditional medicine as a basic component of health care throughout the country, because a significant proportion of the population could not afford modern medicine.

A national heritage program in traditional medicine was established to ensure that the medical knowledge of experienced practitioners was gathered, recorded, and passed on to future generations through formal training programs. Simultaneously, a policy was developed to promote the modernization of traditional medicine and to incorporate it into the provision of health services in integration with modern medicine. This policy was expanded and strengthened during the 1960s and 1970s, during the war between the north and the south. Emergency medical strategies were generated, including the development of a traditional medical program for the treatment of burns.

After several decades of pharmacognostic and toxicological research, the Institute of Materia Medica in Hanoi has developed a list of 1863 plants of known safety and efficacy in the treatment of common medical conditions. Traditional medicine now accounts for one third of all medical treatments provided (Institute of Materia Medica, 1990).

Forced migration due to war or persecution of political dissidents can remove people from mainstream medical care and force an increased reliance on medical practices from their cultural traditions, even in the face of unfamiliar biodiversity. In one study of Burmese refugees at the Thai-Burma border, high use of traditional medicine was found despite health officials' views that there was little or no traditional medicine use among these displaced groups (Bodeker, Neumann et al, 2005).

In surveys of outpatients at a refugee-run clinic at the Thai-Burma border, 59 refugee respondents listed 271 traditional remedies used to treat common health conditions. Research on psychosocial health found that separation from ancestral spiritual practices and shrines in the home country may exacerbate and even prolong mental health conditions.

Refugee aid agencies set the global agenda for refugees and ultimately determine the fate of refugees' health and well-being. By not looking at traditional systems of health care, these agencies may be overlooking a valuable sustainable resource, as well as contributing unknowingly to a loss of important cultural knowledge. By contrast, by harnessing this knowledge and its practices, agencies could help facilitate new global strategies for coping and new prospects for development.

Epidemics

Acquired Immunodeficiency Syndrome. In Africa, governments face huge drug bills for the growing acquired immunodeficiency syndrome (AIDS) crisis and are looking to their indigenous medical traditions and medicinal plants for inexpensive and effective methods of at least alleviating the suffering of AIDS victims. The Health

Ministry of Uganda has been active in generating research into the role of traditional medical practitioners in treating people with AIDS. The Uganda AIDS Commission and the Joint Clinical Research Centre in Kampala have worked with traditional healers' associations to evaluate several traditional treatments for opportunistic infections associated with human immunodeficiency virus (HIV) infection and AIDS. An official of the Uganda AIDS Commission commented on research findings, saying that traditional medicine is better suited to the treatment of some AIDS symptoms such as herpes zoster, chronic diarrhea, shingles, and weight loss (Kogozi, 1994).

As the AIDS crisis leads an increasing number of countries to question their priorities in health expenditures, there is an emerging awareness that traditional health practitioners can play an important role in delivering an AIDS prevention message. There is growing recognition that some traditional health practitioners may be able to offer treatment for opportunistic infections. At the same time, there are concerns about unsafe practices and a growth in claims of traditional cures for AIDS. Partnerships between the modern and traditional health sectors are a cornerstone for building a comprehensive strategy to manage the AIDS crisis.

In Uganda, where there is only one doctor for every 20,000 people, there is one traditional health practitioner per 200 to 400 people (Green, 1994). In such settings, partnerships may be the only way that effective health care coverage can be achieved in managing the twin epidemics of AIDS and malaria. Clearly, such partnerships not only make good public health sense but, based on a growing body of pharmacological evidence, may also yield important preventative and treatment modalities.

In light of the widespread availability of traditional health care services and the reliance of the population on these services, it is inevitable that people with AIDS will turn to traditional health care practitioners for treatment. Collaborative AIDS programs have been established in many African countries, including Malawi, Mozambique, Uganda, Senegal, South Africa, Swaziland, Zambia, and Zimbabwe.

As a result of information sharing and educational programs in South Africa, traditional health practitioners have provided correct HIV/AIDS advice as well as demonstrations of condom use. One such program trained 1510 traditional health practitioners, and it was calculated that during the first 10 months of the program, some 845,600 of their clients may have been reached with messages regarding prevention of AIDS and sexually transmitted diseases (STDs). In similar programs in Mozambique, traditional healers learned that AIDS is transmitted by sexual contact, by blood, and by unsterile razor blades used in traditional practice. In a follow-up evaluation, 81% of those trained reported that they had promoted condom use at least with their STD patients (Green, 1997).

One of the challenges in such workshop situations is to move beyond "training" to genuine information sharing. It has been noted that it is difficult to modify the manner in which health professionals teach about AIDS—a style that tends toward the didactic and use of scientific jargon. Removing communication barriers such as these is a necessary first step in ensuring that training is an effective tool in mobilizing traditional health practitioners as partners in AIDS control.

An important example of how this may be done is provided by Brazil, where a face-to-face educational intervention by healers blended traditional healing—with its language, codes, symbols, and images—with scientific medicine and simultaneously addressed social injustices and discrimination. New information about HIV/AIDS transmission was conveyed using language and concepts intimately familiar to traditional health practitioners. A controlled evaluation found significant increases in AIDS awareness, knowledge about risky HIV behavior, information about correct condom use, and acceptance of lower-risk, alternative ritual blood practices among the 126 members of the trainee group compared with 100 untrained controls. There were also significant decreases in prejudicial attitudes related to HIV transmission among the trainee group compared with controls (Nations et al, 1997).

The Ugandan nongovernment organization Traditional and Modern Health Practitioners Together Against AIDS (THETA) was established in 1992 to conduct research on traditional medicines potentially useful in managing HIV-related illness and to promote a mutually respectful collaboration between traditional and modern health workers in the fight against AIDS. THETA has conducted workshops to share knowledge on AIDS prevention and also treatment of opportunistic infections using local herbal remedies.

Traditional healers participating in clinical observational studies of their herbal medicines have subsequently sought training in prevention, education, and counseling as well as in basic clinical diagnostic skills. A 1998 evaluation of THETA sponsored by UNAIDS (Joint United Nations Programme on HIV/AIDS) found that it had reached 125 traditional health practitioners (44 women and 81 men) in five districts of Uganda. Some 50,000 people were found to have benefited from the improved services offered by traditional health practitioners over a period of 2 years (Kabatesi, 1998).

Malaria. The emergence of multidrug-resistant strains of malaria that has accompanied the introduction of each new class of antimalarial drugs may be viewed as one of most significant threats to the health of people in tropical countries. Although there is widespread agreement that a fresh approach to the prevention and treatment of malaria is urgently needed, solutions have tended to focus on the development of new classes of drugs. More recently, there has been an emphasis on promoting combination therapy with existing drugs as a means of preventing resistance.

Historically, however, local communities in tropical regions have used local flora as a means of preventing and treating malaria (Kirby, 1997). It can be argued that these traditional medicines, based on the use of whole plants with multiple ingredients or of complex mixtures of plant materials, constitute combination therapies that may well combat the development of resistance to antimalarial therapy.

RESISTANCE, SYNERGISM, AND TRADITIONAL MEDICINE

Although combination therapy in malaria, cancer, and AIDS is based on the principle of synergistic action among multiple drugs, little significance has as yet been given to the obvious point that all of the major antimalarials have been derived from plants and that combinations existed in the traditional formulations before the process of extraction took place. For example, flavonoids in *Artemisia annua* that are structurally unrelated to the antimalarial drug artemisinin enhance the in vitro antiplasmodial activity of artemisinin (Kirby, 1997).

Elsewhere, synergism has been observed among the alkaloids of the antimalarial plant *Ancistrocladus peltatum*. A total alkaloid extract of this plant had far greater antiparasitic activity than any of the six alkaloids isolated subsequently. In studies of antimalarial plants from Madagascar, the alkaloids bisbenzylisoquinoline, novel pavine, and benzyl tetrahydroisoquinolines all were found to potentiate the antiparasitic activity of chloroquine in vitro and, in some case, in vivo. Preparations of these plants are currently being tested as adjuvants to chloroquine therapy in Madagascar (Kirby, 1997). In Uganda, there are data from clinical case reports and a cohort study that a traditional Ugandan herbal remedy is effective against malaria (Bitawha et al, 1997; Willcox, 1999).

As do people with other conditions, individuals with malaria will often combine conventional drugs and traditional medicines, sometimes simultaneously, as first- or second-line treatments (Agyepong et al, 1994; Bugmann, 2000; Gessler et al, 1995; Jayawardene, 1993; Lipowsky et al, 1992; McCombie, 1996; Pagnoni et al, 1997), with herbalists reporting their view that this combination gives an additional therapeutic effect (Rasaoanaivo et al, 1994). Perceived efficacy is an important reason that people use traditional antimalarial medicines. Affordability is another. However, when patients themselves were asked why they choose traditional medicine over conventional drugs, a study in Burkina Faso found that the cost of medicines was cited by only 50% of respondents. Lack of faith in doctors was the reason that the other 50% resorted to traditional medicine (Abyan et al, 1993). Elsewhere it has been reported that medical staff at Burkina Faso hospitals are less trusted because they are frequently young, do not speak the local languages, and are not courteous or welcoming to patients (Bugmann, 2000).

Several cohort studies have been conducted to evaluate the outcomes of traditional herbal treatments used by herbalists in managing malaria. A few of these have been shown to produce complete parasite clearance by day 7 (Willcox et al, 2004). Makinde et al showed 100% parasite clearance in adults after treatment with a leaf extract of *Morinda lucida*. However, there was not full parasite clearance from infected children. Further preclinical and clinical studies on the antimalarial effects of plants have been reviewed in the book *Traditional Medicinal Plants and Malaria* (Willcox et al, 2004).

WORLD HEALTH ORGANIZATION POLICY

In response to rising demand for traditional medicines globally and the call from health ministries for formal regulation of this sector, WHO developed a Traditional Medicines Strategy (2002 to 2005) that focuses on four areas identified as requiring action if the potential of traditional medicines to play a role in public health is to be maximized. These areas are (1) policy; (2) safety, efficacy, and quality; (3) access; and (4) rational use. Within these areas, WHO identified the following respective challenges for action.

NATIONAL POLICY AND REGULATION

- Lack of official recognition of traditional, complementary, and alternative medicine (TCAM) and TCAM providers
- Lack of regulatory and legal mechanisms
- Lack of integration of TCAM into national health care systems
- Need for equitable distribution of benefits in indigenous knowledge and products
- Inadequate allocation of resources for TCAM development and capacity building

SAFETY, EFFICACY, AND QUALITY

- Inadequate evidence base for TCAM therapies and products
- Lack of international and national standards for ensuring safety, efficacy, and quality control
- Lack of adequate regulation of herbal medicines
- Lack of registration of TCAM providers
- Inadequate support of research
- Lack of research methodology

ACCESS

- Lack of data measuring access levels and affordability
- Lack of official recognition of the role of TCAM providers

- Need to identify safe and effective practices
- Lack of cooperation between TCAM providers and allopathic practitioners
- Unsustainable use of medicinal plant resources

RATIONAL USE

- Lack of training for TCAM providers
- Lack of training for allopathic practitioners in TCAM
- Lack of communication between TCAM and allopathic practitioners and between allopathic practitioners and consumers
- Lack of information for the public on rational use of TCAM

The WHO Centre for Health Development in Kobe, Japan, has brought out the *WHO Global Atlas on Traditional, Complementary and Alternative Medicine* to provide policy makers with a frame of reference on global utilization and policy trends as well as a set of examples from different countries illustrating policy development in this field (Bodeker, Ong et al, 2005).

INTERNATIONAL PRESSURE TO CONSERVE BIODIVERSITY

Traditional health systems intersect with areas of the national economy other than health care: they interface with environmental concerns as well.

Environmental factors such as land degradation through erosion or development have contributed to the loss of natural habitats. Loss of natural habitats can affect the availability of medicinal plants and, hence, local health standards. In countries where this has occurred, herb gatherers must walk increasingly longer distances to find herbs that previously grew nearby. This contributes to increasing the cost and reducing the availability and sustainability of naturally occurring sources of medicines that traditionally provided basic health care to rural communities.

National economic development may be linked to the cultivation and use of traditional medicines. Wild harvesting of medicinal plants can provide an additional source of family income and also saves expenditure on other forms of medicine. However, overharvesting constitutes a serious threat to biodiversity. Overharvesting of medicinal plants occurs in China, where approximately 80% of the raw materials (animal and plant) for traditional medicines come from wild sources. This raises the need for new policies to integrate health, environmental, and economic perspectives. Investments are needed to develop appropriate cultivation and harvesting strategies that will meet the demand for inexpensive and accessible medicines while ensuring the conservation of diverse biologic resources.

Most developing countries lack the information and resources to apply the contemporary methods of studying the inventory of flora and fauna. It has not been possible systematically to track resource depletion of medicinal plants or animal species that are used in traditional formulas. International collaboration in developing the taxonomic capabilities of environmental and forestry departments is one means by which donor agencies can protect diverse medicinal plant species and thus influence the long-term health of local populations in developing countries.

Although the world's medicinal plant resources have been used primarily to address local health needs, there has been interest in traditional medicine on the part of the international pharmaceutical industry as well as the natural products industry in Europe and America. Pharmaceutical interest has declined in the past decade as challenges have arisen regarding intellectual property rights (Bodeker, 2007), and a low yield of positive hits in high-throughput screening programs has caused genetic and marine sources to be of more interest to large pharmaceutical companies.

The other source of interest in traditional medicine is the natural products industry in Europe and the United States. In Europe, where there is a large industry in phytomedicines, extracts of medicinal plants are sold in purified form to treat and prevent a wide variety of conditions.

These trends have led to a situation in which traditional medicine is considered as a source for the production of other medicines, rather than viewed in terms of its intrinsic value. Concern over these developments has been expressed by the traditional medicine community. A prevailing view is that these trends do not contribute to the development of traditional medicine as a health care system for poor or rural communities, the main constituency of traditional medical care. Rather, the international drug development initiative is seen to take medicinal knowledge from these communities to serve the demand for new drugs in industrial countries. The drugs that are being developed are for the treatment of cancer and heart disease, which are the major killers in industrialized societies, rather than for the treatment of malaria and other endemic diseases that decimate the populations of the developing countries from which the knowledge derives.

There has been no attempt, to date, to develop a scientific understanding of the efficacy of medicinal plants in addressing the primary health care needs of the populations in the areas from which the plants derive. Some projects, however, have recognized this imbalance—the New York Botanical Garden's ethnobotany program in Belize, for example—and are addressing the situation through community-based projects to produce natural medicines for local consumption. They also are working to include knowledge of medicinal plants in school curricula as a means of conserving endangered traditional medical knowledge as well as conserving medicinal plants and rain forest areas. The National Institutes of Health is supporting research and policy evaluation on the role of traditional medicine in the provision of cost-effective primary health care in developing countries (http://www.nccam.nih.gov).

A broader economic perspective would recognize that the health status of developing countries is central to the economic health of those countries and thus to the health of the world economy. Traditional medicine and medicinal plants play an important role in meeting the basic health needs of the majority of the world's population.

SUMMARY

Currently, there is wide variability in the consideration given by health planners to traditional health systems. In some countries, traditional medicine is incorporated routinely into health planning. However, this occurs in only a minority of cases, primarily in Asia. In most cases, the revival has come from nongovernment organizations. National and international funding currently is directed to the provision of Western-style health services in developing countries and indigenous communities. Research consistently links reductions in morbidity and mortality rates to economic conditions; educational levels, particularly to years of female education; and large-scale public health measures such as sanitation and safe water supply. Although these factors—rather than the availability of Western medicines—have been found to lead to improved levels of health, health planners continue to operate under the view that Western medicine provides the primary means of improving health in these communities. This belief is not based on a scientific appraisal of the world's natural systems of health. Some traditional treatments are still more effective than modern treatments, as has been noted in this chapter.

Although old and limited views of traditional systems of health continue to exist, there is an emerging intellectual and policy climate that is giving expression to a fresh perspective. Whereas the old view favors the marginalization of traditional systems of health, the new view looks to them to provide complementary therapy and, in some cases, new solutions to major health crises. This new view is consonant with the ancient or traditional concepts of health and human potential that underlie many of the world's traditional systems of health.

Finally, the global move toward a view of optimal health and well-being as the goal of health care has found expression in the wellness movement. According to the U.S. National Wellness Institute (NWI), wellness is "an active process through which people become aware of, and make choices towards, a more successful existence." The NWI identifies six dimensions of wellness: social, occupational, spiritual, physical, emotional, and intellectual. Similarly, Lifestyles of Health and Sustainability (LOHAS) is a framework that focuses on "health and fitness; the environment; personal development; sustainable living; and social justice." Included in this framework is a strong nutritional emphasis and a focus on integrated health care and positive living. The magnitude of this momentum is reflected in part by the growth of the global spa industry into a $255 billion global industry (Cohen et al, 2008; SRI International, 2008).

From the harnessing of local forest herbs to treat everyday common ailments in rural parts of the developing world, to the widespread use of standardized complementary medicines and licensed therapies in Europe and the United States, to the focus on wellness and healthy living through diet, natural products, and mind-body approaches to stress reduction, the complementary and medicine revolution appears to be maturing into an integrated and mainstream trend. Naturally, further clinical evidence is always needed, and a global research endeavor is moving in this direction. The central shift has been that now consumers are active participants in and managers of their own health care.

Chapter References can be found on the Evolve website at http://evolve.elsevier.com/Micozzi/complementary/

Index

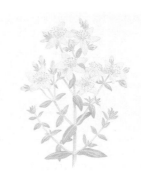

Note: Entries followed by "b" indicate boxes; "f" figures; "t" tables.